COLD SPRING HARBOR SYMPOSIA ON QUANTITATIVE BIOLOGY

VOLUME LIV

COLD SPRING HARBOR SYMPOSIA
ON QUANTITATIVE BIOLOGY

VOLUME LIV

Immunological Recognition

COLD SPRING HARBOR LABORATORY PRESS
1989

COLD SPRING HARBOR SYMPOSIA ON QUANTITATIVE BIOLOGY
VOLUME LIV

© 1989 by The Cold Spring Harbor Laboratory Press
International Standard Book Number 0-87969-057-7 (cloth)
International Standard Book Number 0-87969-058-5 (paper)
International Standard Serial Number 0091-7451
Library of Congress Catalog Card Number 34-8174

COLD SPRING HARBOR SYMPOSIA ON QUANTITATIVE BIOLOGY

Founded in 1933 by
REGINALD G. HARRIS
Director of the Biological Laboratory 1924 to 1936

Previous Symposia Volumes

All Cold Spring Harbor Laboratory publications may be ordered directly from Cold Spring Harbor Laboratory Press, Box 100, Cold Spring Harbor, New York 11724. Phone: 1-800-843-4388. In New York (516)367-8423.

SYMPOSIUM PARTICIPANTS

ABRAHAM, KRISTIN, University of Washington, Howard Hughes Medical Institute, Seattle

ACUTO, ORESTE, Immunologie Moleculaire, Institut Pasteur, Paris, France

AIR, GILLIAN, Dept. of Molecular Biology, University of Alabama, Birmingham

AIREY, JEREMY, Dept. of Pathology and Immunology, Cambridge University, England

ALÉS-MARTÍNEZ, JOSE, University of Rochester Cancer Center, New York

ALLEN, PAUL, Dept. of Pathology, Washington University School of Medicine, St. Louis, Missouri

ALT, FRED, Howard Hughes Medical Institute, Columbia University College of P&S, New York, New York

AMENTO, EDWARD, Genentech, Inc., South San Francisco, California

AMSTUTZ, HANSPETER, Theodor Kocher Institut, University of Berne, Switzerland

ANSARI, AFTAB, Good Samaritan Hospital, Johns Hopkins University School of Medicine, Baltimore, Maryland

ARANEO, BARBARA ANN, Dept. of Pathology, University of Utah, Salt Lake City

ASANO, YOSHIHIRO, Dept. of Immunology, Faculty of Medicine, University of Tokyo, Japan

ASHTON-RICKARDT, P., Dept. of Pathology, University Medical School, Edinburgh, Scotland

AUSTIN, PENELOPE, *Nature*

AYANE, MOHAMED, Max-Planck-Institut fur Immunbiologie, Freiburg-Zahringen, Federal Republic of Germany

BACKSTROM, THOMAS, Dept. of Immunobiology, University of Auckland School of Medicine, New Zealand

BACON, PAUL, National Institutes of Health, Bethesda, Maryland

BALARAM, GHOSH, Dept. of Clinical Immunology, Johns Hopkins University School of Medicine, Baltimore, Maryland

BAND, HAMID, Laboratory of Immunochemistry, Dana Farber Cancer Institute, Boston, Massachusetts

BANIYASH, MICHAL, National Institutes of Health, Bethesda, Maryland

BANSAL, GEETHA, Molecular Vaccines, Inc., Gaithersburg, Maryland

BARBER, BRIAN, Dept. of Immunology, University of Toronto, Canada

BARBOSA, JAMES, Cellular Genetics, Molecular Diagnostics, Inc., West Haven, Connecticut

BARON, JODY LYNN, Dept. of Immunobiology, Yale University School of Medicine, New Haven, Connecticut

BARRY, PATRICK, Dept. of Pediatrics, University of Massachusetts Medical Center, Worcester, Maryland

BENACERRAF, BARUJ, Dana Farber Cancer Institute, Boston, Massachusetts

BENDELAC, ALBERT, Cellular and Molecular Immunology, National Institutes of Health, Bethesda, Maryland

BENJAMIN, RICHARD, Dept. of Cell Biology, Stanford University School of Medicine, California

BERG, LESLIE, Dept. of Microbiology and Immunology, Stanford University School of Medicine, California

BERKOWER, IRA, Center for Biologics, Food and Drug Administration, Bethesda, Maryland

BERZOFSKY, JAY, Dept. of Molecular Immunogenetics and Vaccine Research, NCI, National Institutes of Health, Bethesda, Maryland

BEVAN, MICHAEL, Dept. of Immunology, Scripps Clinic and Research Foundation, La Jolla, California

BHATNAGAR, PRADIP, Smith Kline & French Laboratories, Philadelphia, Pennsylvania

BIKOFF, ELIZABETH, Dept. of Obstetrics and Gynecology, Mount Sinai Medical School, New York, New York

BIX, MARK, Dept. of Biology, Massachusetts Institute of Technology, Cambridge

BJORKMAN, PAMELA, Dept. of Biology, California Institute of Technology, Pasadena

BLANKENHORN, ELIZABETH, Depts. of Microbiology and Immunology, Hahnemann University, Philadelphia, Pennsylvania

BLEICHER, PAUL, Dana Farber Cancer Institute, Boston, Massachusetts

BLUESTONE, JEFFREY, Ben May Institute, University of Chicago, Illinois

BLUMBERG, RICHARD, Dept. of Molecular Immunology, Dana Farber Cancer Institute, Boston, Massachusetts

BODMER, HELEN, Dept. of Clinical Medicine, J. Radcliffe Hospital, University of Oxford, England

BODMER, JULIA, Imperial Cancer Research Fund Laboratories, London, England

BODMER, WALTER, Imperial Cancer Research Fund Laboratories, London, England

BODO, IMRE, St. Luke's/Roosevelt Hospital, New York, New York

BOND, JULIAN, ImmuLogic Pharmaceutical Corporation, Cambridge, Massachusetts

BOON, THIERRY, Ludwig Institute for Cancer Research, Brussels, Belgium

BOREL, YVES, Center for Blood Research, Boston, Massachusetts

BOYLSTON, ARTHUR, Dept. of Pathology, University of Leeds, England

BRACIALE, THOMAS, Dept. of Pathology, Washington University School of Medicine, St. Louis, Missouri

BRAIT, MARYSE, Dept. of Animal Physiology, University of Brussels, Belgium

BRANDWEIN, HARVEY, Pall Corporation, Glen Cove, New York

BRODSKY, FRANCES, Pharmacy, University of California, San Francisco

BRONSON, RICHARD, Dept. of Reproductive Endocrinology, State University of New York, Stony Brook

BROOKS, COLIN, The Medical School, University of Newcastle-Upon-Tyne, England

BROWN, MARION, Cell Surface Biochemistry Laboratory, Imperial Cancer Research Fund Laboratories, London, England

BUDD, RALPH, Genentech, Inc., South San Francisco, California

BUELL, GARY, Pharmacia Genetic Engineering Inc., La Jolla, California

BURDETTE, SUSAN, Depts. of Hematology and Oncology, New England Medical Center, Boston, Massachusetts

BURKE, RAE LYN, Dept. of Virology, Chiron Corporation, Emeryville, California

BURSTEIN, HAROLD, Brigham & Women's Hospital, Harvard Medical School, Boston, Massachusetts

BUTCHER, GEOFFREY, Institute of Animal Physiology, AFRC, Cambridge Research Station, England

CAIN, JUDITH, Tumor Institute, University of Alabama, Birmingham

CAMMISULI, S., Preclinical Research, Sandoz, Basel, Switzerland

CAPON, DANIEL, Dept. of Molecular Biology, Genentech, Inc., South San Francisco, California

CATERINI, JUDY, Center for Biotechnology Research, Connaught Research Institute, Willowdale, Canada

CATON, ANDREW, Wistar Institute, Philadelphia, Pennsylvania

CELIS, ESTEBAN, T Cell Sciences, Inc., Cambridge, Massachusetts

CHAMBERS, CYNTHIA, Depts. of Research, Immunology and Neurology, Mt. Sinai Hospital, University of Toronto, Canada

CHAN, BOSCO, Dept. of Biology, Massachusetts Institute of Technology, Cambridge

CHEN, JOSEPH, Dept. of Veterinary Biologics, APHIS, U.S. Department of Agriculture, Hyattsville, Maryland

CHEN-KIANG, SELINA, Dept. of Immunobiology, Mt. Sinai School of Medicine, New York, New York

CHISHOLM, PATRICIA, Immunology Section, King College, University of London, England

CHISWELL, DAVE, Pollards Wood Laboratories, Amersham International plc, Buckinghamshire, England

CHOI, YONGWON, Howard Hughes Medical Institute, National Jewish Hospital, Denver, Colorado

CLAYTON, LINDA, Dana Farber Cancer Institute, Boston, Massachusetts

COHEN, IRUN, Dept. of Cell Biology, The Weizmann Institute of Science, Rehovot, Israel

COLBERT, ROBERT, Dept. of Pediatrics, University of Rochester Medical Center, New York

COLLINS, MARY, Genetics Institute, Cambridge, Massachusetts

CONNELLY, MARGERY, Dept. of Pathology, State University of New York, Stony Brook

COOPER, MAX, Depts. of Medicine, Pediatrics and Microbiology, University of Alabama, Birmingham

CORTI, ANGELO, Tecnogen, S.P.A., Milan, Italy

COUTINHO, ANTONIO, Dept. of Immunology, Institut Pasteur, Paris, France

CRESSWELL, PETER, Depts. of Microbiology and Immunology, Duke University Medical Center, Durham, North Carolina

CROMWELL, MANDY, Dept. of Pediatrics, University of Massachusetts Medical Center, Worcester

CRUMPTON, MICHAEL, Imperial Cancer Research Fund Laboratories, London, England

DAVID, CHELLA, Dept. of Immunology, Mayo Clinic/Mayo Medical School, Rochester, Minnesota

DAVIES, DAVID, National Institutes of Health, Bethesda, Maryland

DAVIS, MARK, Dept. of Medical Microbiology, Stanford University School of Medicine, California

DAVIS, SIMON, Cellular Immunology Unit, Medical Research Council, Sir William Dunn School of Pathology, Oxford, England

DE LA CRUZ, VIDAL, Dept. of Immunology, Molecular Vaccines, Inc., Gaithersburg, Maryland

DEFRANCO, ANTHONY, Depts. of Microbiology and Immunology, Karl Friedrich Meyer Laboratories, University of California, San Francisco

DELOVITCH, TERRY, Banting & Best Dept. of Medical Research, University of Toronto, Canada

DIU, ANITA, Unite d'Immunogenetique Cellulaire, Institut Pasteur, Paris, France

DORNMAIR, KLAUS, Stauffer Laboratory of Physical Chemistry, Stanford University, California

DUSTIN, LYNN, Renal Division, Brigham and Women's Hospital, Boston, Massachusetts

DUSTIN, MICHAEL, Center for Blood Research, Boston, Massachusetts

DWYER, EDWARD, Dept. of Rheumatic Diseases, Hospital for Joint Diseases, New York, New York

ECKELS, DAVID, Dept. of Immunogenetics Research, Blood Center of S.E. Wisconsin, Milwaukee

EDGEWORTH, JONATHAN, Macrophage Laboratory, Imperial Cancer Research Fund Laboratories, London, England

EISEN, HERMAN, Whitehead Institute, Massachusetts Institute of Technology, Cambridge

ELLIOTT, TIMOTHY, Whitehead Institute, Massachusetts Institute of Technology, Cambridge

ENFIELD, DAVID, Kallestad Diagnostics Inc., Chaska, Minnesota

ERARD, FRANCOIS, Pharmaceutical Research Division, Ciba-Geigy Ltd., Basel, Switzerland

ERTL, HILDEGUND, The Wistar Institute, Philadelphia, Pennsylvania

ETLINGER, HOWARD, Hoffman La Roche, Basel, Switzerland

EZQUERRA, ANGEL, BRB/NIAID, National Institutes of Health, Bethesda, Maryland

FALLISE, JEAN-PIERRE, Dept. of Clinical Research, Bayer Research Center, Wuppertal, Federal Republic of Germany

FERNANDEZ-LUNA, JOSE, Dept. of Pathology, Washington University School of Medicine, St. Louis, Missouri

FIELD, ELIZABETH, Dept. of Internal Medicine, University of Iowa, Iowa City

FIERZ, WALTER, Innere Medizin, Universitatsspital Zurich, Switzerland

FISCHER, HANS, Dept. of Tumor Immunology, The Wallenberg Laboratory, Lund, Sweden

FISCHER LINDAHL, KIRSTEN, Howard Hughes Medical Institute, University of Texas, Dallas

FISH, LEONARD, Dept. of Research Operations, AMGen Inc., Thousand Oaks, California

FLAHERTY, LORRAINE, Wadsworth Center for Laboratory Research, New York State Department of Health, Albany

FLAVELL, RICHARD, Dept. of Immunobiology, Yale University, New Haven, Connecticut

FLYER, DAVID, Depts. of Microbiology and Immunology, Milton B. Hershey Medical Center, Hershey, Pennsylvania

FOERSTER, OTHMAR, Institut fur Experimentelle Pathologie, University of Vienna, Austria

FONG, SHERMAN, Dept. of Pharmacological Sciences, Genentech, Inc., South San Francisco, California

FORMAN, MARK, Depts. of Cellular Physiology and Immunology, Rockefeller University, New York, New York

FOUSER, LYNETTE, Genetics Institute, Cambridge, Massachusetts

FRANCUS, TOVA Dept. of Medicine, Cornell University Medical College, New York, New York

FREED, JOHN, Dept. of Medicine, National Jewish Center for Immunology, Denver, Colorado

FREITAS, ANTONIO, Dept. of Immunology, Institut Pasteur, Paris, France

FURNEAUX, HENRY, Dept. of Neurology, Memorial Sloan Kettering Cancer Center, New York, New York

GALELLI, ANNE Dept. of Immunology, Institute Pasteur, Paris, France

GAO, MEIHUA, Dept. of Laboratory Medicine, Yale University, New Haven, Connecticut

GARRETT, THOMAS, Depts. of Biochemistry and Molecular Biology, Harvard University, Cambridge, Massachusetts

GEFTER, MALCOLM, Dept. of Biology, Massachusetts Institute of Technology, Cambridge

GEHA, RAIF, Children's Hospital, Harvard Medical School, Boston, Massachusetts

GERHARD, WALTER, Wistar Institute, Philadelphia, Pennsylvania

GILBOA, ELI, Dept. of Molecular Biology, Memorial Sloan Kettering Cancer Center, New York, New York

GOLDMAN, JACKI, Dept. of Biology, Massachusetts Institute of Technology, Cambridge

GOLDSBY, RICHARD, Dept. of Veterinary and Animal Sciences, University of Massachusetts, Amherst

GOODMAN, JOEL, Depts. of Microbiology and Immunology, University of California, San Francisco

GOODNOW, CHRISTOPHER, Clinical Immunology Research Centre, University of Sidney, Australia

GOUDSMIT, JAAP, Depts. of Virology and Human Retrovirology, Academic Medical Center, Amsterdam, The Netherlands

GOVERMAN, JOAN, Dept. of Biology, California Institute of Technology, Pasadena

GREENSPAN, NEIL, Institute of Pathology, Case Western Reserve University, Cleveland, Ohio

GREENSTEIN, JULIA, ImmuLogic Pharmaceutical Corporation, Cambridge, Massachusetts

GREGERSEN, PETER, Dept. of Rheumatic Diseases, Hospital for Joint Diseases, New York, New York

GREGORY, SUSAN, University of Chicago, Illinois

GREY, HOWARD, Cytel Corporation, La Jolla, California

GRONBERG, ALVAR, Dept. of Inflammation Research, Pharmacia Leo Therapeutics AB, Uppsala, Sweden

GÜSSOW, DETLEF, LMB, Medical Research Council, Cambridge, England

HALL, BRUCE, Dept. of Nephrology, Stanford University Medical Center, California

HAMMERLING, ULRICH, Dept. of Immunology, Memorial Sloan Kettering Cancer Center, New York, New York,

HANAHAN, DOUGLAS, Dept. of Biochemistry and Biophysics, University of California, San Francisco

HANSBURG, DANIEL, Dept. of Pathology, Fox Chase Cancer Center, Philadelphia, Pennsylvania

HANSON, DOUG, Dept. of Immunology, Pfizer Central Research, Groton, Connecticut

HARDING, CLIFF, Dept. of Pathology, Washington University School of Medicine, St. Louis, Missouri

HATAKEYAMA, MASANORI, Institute for Molecular and Cellular Biology, Osaka University, Japan

HAYDAY, ADRIAN, Dept. of Biology, Yale University, New Haven, Connecticut

HEBER-KATZ, ELLEN, The Wistar Institute, Philadelphia, Pennsylvania

HEDLUND, GUNNAR, Dept. of Immunology, Pharmacia Leo Therapeutics, Malmo, Sweden

HERZENBERG, LEONARD, Dept. of Genetics, Stanford University School of Medicine, California

HERZENBERG, LEONORE, Dept. of Genetics, Stanford University School of Medicine, California

HILBORN, DAVID, Life Sciences Research Laboratories, Eastman Kodak Company, Rochester, New York

HODGKINSON, SUZANNE, Dept. of Neurology, Stanford University Medical Center, California

HOFFMANN, MICHAEL, Dept. of Immunology, Memorial Sloan Kettering Cancer Center, New York, New York

HOLSTI, MATTHEW, Dept. of Biology, Massachusetts Institute of Technology, Cambridge

HONJO, TASUKO, Dept. of Medical Chemistry, Kyoto University, Japan

HOOD, LEROY, Dept. of Biology, California Institute of Technology, Pasadena

HOSMALIN, ANNE, National Cancer Institute, National Institutes of Health, Bethesda, Maryland

HOWARD, FRANK, Dept. of Medical Oncology, Dana Farber Cancer Institute, Boston, Massachusetts

HOWARD, JONATHAN, Institute of Animal Physiology, AFRC, Cambridge Research Station, England

HOZUMI, NOBUMICHI, Depts. of Molecular Immunology and Neurobiology, Mt. Sinai Hospital Research Institute, Toronto, Canada

HSIANG, YUN-HUI, Dept. of Biology, Massachusetts Institute of Technology, Cambridge

HUANG, SHAU-KU, Dept. of Clinical Immunology, Johns Hopkins University, Baltimore, Maryland

HUDSON, PETER, Division of Biotechnology, CSIRO, Victoria, Australia

HÜNIG, THOMAS, Molekulare Biologie Genzentrum, Ludwig Maximillians Universitat, Martinsried, Federal Republic of Germany

ICHIHARA, YOSHIKAZU, Institute for Comprehensive Medical Science, Fujita Gakuen Health University, Japan

INGLIS, JOHN, Cold Spring Harbor Laboratory, New York

ISAACS, JOHN, Dept. of Pathology, Immunology Division, University of Cambridge, England

ISHIDA, ISAO, Center for Cancer Research, Massachusetts Institute of Technology, Cambridge

ITO, KOUICHI, Center for Cancer Research, Massachusetts Institute of Technology, Cambridge

ITOHARA, SHIGEYOSHI, Center for Cancer Research, Massachusetts Institute of Technology, Cambridge

JANEWAY, CHARLES, Dept. of Pathology, Yale University School of Medicine, New Haven, Connecticut

JARDETZKY, TED, Depts. of Biochemistry and Molecular Biology, Harvard University, Cambridge, Massachusetts

JERNE, NIELS, Basel Institute for Immunology, Switzerland

JOLLIFFE, LINDA, Biotech Division, R.W. Johnson Pharmaceutical Research Institute, Raritan, New Jersey

KAGNOFF, MARTIN, University of California, San Diego

KAMIN-LEWIS, ROBERTA, Dept. of Microbiology, University of Maryland, Baltimore

KANAGAWA, OSMAI, Lilly Research Laboratories, La Jolla, California

KANG, JOONSOO, Depts. of Molecular Immunology and Neurobiology, University of Toronto, Canada

KANNO, TOMOHIKO, The First Dept. of Internal Medicine, Tohoku University School of Medicine, Sendai, Japan

KANNO, YUKA, The First Dept. of Internal Medicine, Tohoku University School of Medicine, Sendai, Japan

KAPLAN, DON, Central Research Dept., Dow Chemical Corporation, Midland, Michigan

KAPPES, DIETMAR, Dept. of Biology, Massachusetts Institute of Technology, Cambridge

KAPPLER, JOHN, Immunology and Respiratory Medicine, National Jewish Center, Denver, Colorado

KARR, ROBERT, Dept. of Internal Medicine, University of Iowa VA Medical Hospital, Iowa City

KAWAGUCHI, TAKAAKI, Memorial Sloan Kettering Cancer Center, New York, New York

KEARNEY, JOHN, Dept. of Microbiology, University of Alabama, Birmingham

KERR, WILLIAM, Dept. of Genetics, Stanford University School of Medicine, California

KIM, MOON-GYO, Dept. of Microbiology, State University of New York, Stony Brook

KIMURA, SHOJI, Memorial Sloan Kettering Cancer Center, New York, New York

KINASHI, TATSUO, Dept. of Medical Chemistry, Kyoto University, Japan

KISHI, HIROYUKI, Basel Institute for Immunology, Switzerland

KISHIMOTO, TADAMITSU, Institute for Molecular and Cellular Biology, Osaka University, Japan

KLAUS, GERRY, National Institute for Medical Research, MRC, London, England

KLAUSNER, RICHARD, Cell Biology and Metabolic Branch, National Institutes of Health, Bethesda, Maryland

KNIGHT, KATHERINE, Dept. of Microbiology, Stritch School of Medicine, Loyola University, Mayood, Illinois

KNOWLES, ROBERT, Memorial Sloan Kettering Cancer Center, New York, New York

KOBRIN, BARRY, Dept. of Cell Biology, Albert Einstein College of Medicine, Bronx, New York

KOCH, FRIEDRICH, Immunologie, Universitat Hamburg, Federal Republic of Germany

KOCH, NORBERT, German Cancer Research Center, Heidelberg, Federal Republic of Germany

KOCKS, CHRISTINE, Institut fur Genetik, University of Cologne, Federal Republic of Germany

KONING, FRITS, Dept. of Immunohematology and Blood Bank, University Hospital, Leiden, The Netherlands

KORMAN, ALAN, Whitehead Institute, Cambridge, Massachusetts

KORN, LAURENCE JAY, Protein Design Labs, Inc., Palo Alto, California

KOSZINOWSKI, U., Dept. of Virology, University of Ulm, Federal Republic of Germany

KOURILSKY, PHILLIPE, Dept. of Immunology, Institut Pasteur, Paris, France

KRAFFT-CZEPA, Institute for Immunology & Genetics, German Cancer Research Center, Heidelberg, Federal Republic of Germany

KRAMER, STEVEN, Oncogene Science, Inc., Manhasset, New York

KRUISBEEK, ADA, National Cancer Institute, National Institutes of Health, Bethesda, Maryland

KUBO, RALPH, National Jewish Center for Immunology, Denver, Colorado

KUMAR SADANA, DEVINDER, FAO Fellow from India, Cold Spring Harbor, New York

KYES, SUSAN, Dept. of Biology, Yale University, New Haven, Connecticut

LACY, LIZ, Dept. of Molecular Biology, Memorial Sloan Kettering Cancer Center, New York, New York

LAFAILLE, JUAN, Center for Cancer Research, Massachusetts Institute of Technology, Cambridge

LANZAVECCHIA, ANTONIO, Basel Institute for Immunology, Switzerland

LARSEN, BODIL, Dept. of Immunology, Health Sciences Center, Memorial University of Newfoundland, Canada

LARSSON-SCIARD, EVA-LOTTA, Institut Pasteur, Paris, France

LASSILA, OLLI, Dept. of Medical Microbiology, University of Tarku, Finland

LAWETZKY, ALEXANDRA, Dept. of Molecular Biology, University of Munich, Federal Republic of Germany

LE DOUARIN, NICOLE, Institut D'Embryologie Cellulaire et Moleculaire, CNRS and College of France, Nogent-sur-Marne

LE MOAL, MIKAEL, Immunologie Imm. Phy. Moleculaire, Institut Pasteur, Paris, France

LECLERC, CLAUDE, Biologie des Regulations Immunitaires, Institut Pasteur, Paris, France

LEE, JANET, Memorial Sloan Kettering Cancer Center, New York, New York

LEIDEN, JEFFREY, Howard Hughes Medical Institute, Ann Arbor, Michigan

LERNER, RICHARD, Dept. of Molecular Biology, Research Institute of Scripps Clinic, La Jolla, California

LIAO, NAN-SHIH, Center for Cancer Research, Massachusetts Institute of Technology, Cambridge

LIBERATOR, PAUL, Dept. of Biochemical Parasitology, Merck Sharp & Dohme Research Laboratories, Rahway, New Jersey

LINDSTEN, TULLIA, Howard Hughes Medical Institute, Ann Arbor, Michigan

LOH, DENNIS, Howard Hughes Medical Institute, Washington University School of Medicine, St. Louis, Missouri

LONGLEY, JACK, Dept. of Dermatology, Yale School of Medicine, New Haven, Connecticut

LUNDKVIST, INGER, Dept. of Immunohemotology, University Hospital, Leiden, The Netherlands

MACDONALD, HUGH ROBSON, Ludwig Institute for Cancer Research, Epalinges, Switzerland

MACH, BERNARD, Dept. of Microbiology, University of Geneva Medical School, Switzerland

MADDEN, DEAN, Dept. of Biophysics, Harvard University, Cambridge, Massachusetts

MAIO, MICHELE, Dept. of Immunology, Centro Di Riferimento Oncologico, Aviano, Italy

MAIZELS, NANCY, Dept. of Molecular Biophysics and Biochemistry, Yale University, New Haven, Connecticut

MAK, TAK, Dept. of Medical Biophysics, Ontario Cancer Institute, Toronto, Canada

MALISSEN, MARIE, CNRS, Centre d'Immunologie de Marseille-Luminy, France

MALKOVSKY, MIROSLAV, Dept. of Biomedical Research, Xenova, Berkshire, England

MANSER, TIM, Dept. of Biology, Princeton University, New Jersey

MARCU, KEN, State University of New York, Stony Brook

MARGALIT, HANAH, Dept. of Mathematical Biology, NCI, National Institutes of Health, Bethesda, Maryland

MARRACK, PHILIPPA, Howard Hughes Medical Institute, National Jewish Center, Denver, Colorado

MARSH, DAVID, Good Samaritan Hospital, Johns Hopkins University Medical School, Baltimore, Maryland

MARSHALL, W.H., Dept. of Immunology, Health Sciences Centre, Memorial University of Newfoundland, Canada

MARTINEZ, CARLOS, Dept. Biologia Molecular, Universidad Autonoma, Madrid, Spain

MARYANSKI, JANET, Ludwig Institute for Cancer Research, Epalinges, Switzerland

MATHIS, DIANE, Laboratoire de Genetique Moleculaire, INSERM Institute de Chimie Biologique, Strasbourg, France

MATTHEWS, REGINALD James, Dept. of Pathology, Washington University School of Medicine, St. Louis, Missouri

MATZINGER, POLLY, Basel Institute for Immunology, Switzerland

MCCARTHY, ROBERT, Boehringer Mannheim Corp., Indianapolis, Indiana

MCCLUSKEY, JAMES, Dept. of Pathology and Immunology, Monash Medical School, Melbourne, Australia

MCDEVITT, HUGH, Dept. of Medical Microbiology, Stanford University School of Medicine, California

MCVAY, LAILA, Dept. of Biology, Yale University, New Haven, Connecticut

MELCHERS, FRITZ, Basel Institute for Immunology, Switzerland

MELIEF, KEES, Dept. of Immunology, The Netherlands Cancer Institute, Amsterdam

MEZES, PETER, Dow Chemical Corporation, Midland, Michigan

MICELI, CARRIE, Dept. of Immunology, Stanford University Medical Center, California

MILLER, GERALDINE, Baylor College of Medicine, Houston, Texas

MILLER, J.F.A.P., Walter & Eliza Hall Institute for Medical Research, Royal Melbourne Hospital, Australia

MITCHELL, RICHARD, Dept. of Pathology, Brigham and Women's Hospital, Harvard Medical School, Boston, Massachusetts

MITCHISON, AVRION, Dept. of Biology, University College, London, England

MIZUOCHI, TOSHIAKI, Dept. of Blood Products, National Institutes of Health, Tokyo, Japan

MOMBAERTS, PETER, Dept. of Biology, Massachusetts Institute of Technology, Cambridge

MONOS, DIMITRI, Depts. of Biochemistry and Molecular Biology, Harvard University, Cambridge, Massachusetts

MOULDER, KEVIN, BRB/NIAID, National Institutes of Health, Bethesda, Maryland

MURAOKA, SHIZUKO, Trudeau Institute, Saranac Lake, New York

MURPHY, DONAL, Wadsworth Center for Laboratories and Research, New York State Dept. of Health, Albany

NARDIN, ELIZABETH, Dept. of Medical and Molecular Parasitology, New York University Medical Center, New York

NASSERI, SCHEHERAZADE, Dept. of Biophysics and Biochemistry, FDA/CBER, National Institutes of Health, Bethesda, Maryland

NATHENSON, STANLEY, Depts. of Microbiology and Immunology, Albert Einstein College of Medicine, Bronx, New York

NELL, LAURA, Baylor College of Medicine, Houston, Texas

NEZLIN, ROALD, Dept. of Chemical Immunology, The Weizmann Institute of Science, Rehovot, Israel

NISHIKAWA, SHIN-ICHI, Dept. of Immunopathology, Kumamoto University Medical School, Japan

NOSSAL, GUSTAV, Walter and Eliza Hall Institute for Medical Research, Royal Melbourne Hospital, Australia

NUCHTERN, JED, Dept. of Cell Biology and Metabolism, NICHD, National Institutes of Health, Bethesda, Maryland

NUSSENZWEIG, RUTH, Dept. of Parasitology, New York University Medical Center, New York

NUSSENZWEIG, VICTOR, Dept. of Pathology, New York University Medical Center, New York

O'HARA, BRYAN, Lederle Laboratories, American Cyanamid Company, Pearl River, New York

OBATA, YUICHI, Laboratory of Immunology, Aichi Cancer Center Research Institute, Nagoya, Japan

OCHI, ATSUO, Research Institute, Mount Sinai Hospital, Toronto, Canada

OHNISHI, KAZUO, Dept. of Cellular Immunology, National Institute of Health, Tokyo, Japan

OKUMURA, KO, Dept. of Immunology, Juntendo University School of Medicine, Tokyo, Japan

OLSEN, NANCY, Depts. of Medicine, Rheumatology and Immunology, Vanderbilt University, Nashville, Tennessee

OSBORNE, BARBARA, Dept. of Veterinary and Animal Sciences, University of Massachusetts, Amherst

OSMAN, GAMAL, Dept. of Biology, California Institute of Technology, Pasadena

OSTRAND-ROSENBERG, SUZANNE, Dept. of Biological Sciences, University of Maryland, Catonsville

OTTENHOFF, T.H.M., Dept. of Immunohaematology and Blood Bank, University Hospital, Leiden, The Netherlands

OVARY, ZOLTAN, Dept. of Pathology, New York University Medical Center, New York

PADLAN, EDUARDO, NIDDK, National Institutes of Health, Bethesda, Maryland

PALMER, EDWARD, Division of Basic Sciences, National Jewish Center, Denver, Colorado

PARHAM, PETER, Dept. of Cell Biology, Stanford University School of Medicine, California

PARIKH, VANDANA, Dept. of Microbiology, University of Texas Southwestern Medical Center, Dallas

PARKHOUSE, R.M.E., Dept. of Immunology, National Institute for Medical Research, London, England

PARNES, JANE, Dept. of Immunology, Stanford University Medical Center, California

PAUL, SUDHIR, Depts. of Pathology and Microbiology, University of Nebraska Medical Center, Omaha

PERKINS, DAVID, Dept. of Biology, Massachusetts Institute of Technology, Cambridge

PETERMAN, GARY, Dept. of Immunology, Pfizer Central Research, Groton, Connecticut

PHILLIPS, J., Dept. of Neurology, University of Texas Southwestern Medical Center, Dallas

PHILLIPS, RODERICK, Dept. of Immunology, National Institute for Medical Research, London, England

PIERRES, MICHEL, Centre d'Immunologie, INSERM-CNRS, Marseille, France

PILLAI, SHIV, MGH Cancer Center, Harvard Medical School, Boston, Massachusetts

POLJAK, ROBERTO, Immunologie Structurale, Institut Pasteur, Paris, France

POLLOCK, ROBERTA, Dept. of Biochemistry, Columbia University College of P & S, New York, New York

PURE, ELLEN, Depts. of Cellular Physiology and Immunology, The Rockefeller University, New York, New York

QIN, SHIXIN, Dept. of Pathology, University of Cambridge, England

QUAKYI, ISABELLA, NIAID/LPD, National Institutes of Health, Bethesda, Maryland

QUEEN, CARY, Protein Design Labs, Inc., Palo Alto, California

RADA, CRISTINA, AFRC Institute of Animal Physiology and Genetics Research, Cambridge, England

RADOUX, VICTOR, Dana Farber Cancer Center, Boston, Massachusetts

RAJEWSKY, KLAUS, Institute for Genetics, University of Cologne, Federal Republic of Germany

REINHERZ, ELLIS, Laboratory of Immunobiology, Dana Farber Cancer Institute, Boston, Massachusetts

REYNOLDS, FREDERICK, Oncogene Science, Inc., Manhasset, New York

RIA, FRANCESCO, Dept. of Biology, Massachusetts Institute of Technology, Cambridge

RIJNDERS, TON, Dept. of Cell Culture and Microbiology RDL, Organon International BV, The Netherlands

ROCK, KENNETH, Dept. of Lymphocyte Biology, Dana Farber Cancer Institute, Boston, Massachusetts

RODEWALD, HANS-REIMER, Dana Farber Cancer Institute, Boston, Massachusetts

ROEDERER, MARIO, Dept. of Genetics, Stanford University, California

ROMERO, PEDRO, Dept. of Medical and Molecular Parasitology, New York University School of Medicine, New York

RONCHESE, FRANCA, Istituto di Oncologia, Universita di Padova, Italy

ROOPENIAN, DERRY, The Jackson Laboratory, Bar Harbor, Maine

ROTHBARD, JONATHAN, Dept. of Molecular Immunology, Imperial Cancer Research Fund Laboratories, London, England

SAITO, TAKASHI, Depts. of Molecular Immunology and Neurobiology, Chiba University School of Medicine, Japan

SANCHO, JAIME, Dept. of Molecular Immunology, Dana Farber Cancer Institute, Cambridge, Massachusetts

SANZ, INAKI, Dept. of Medicine, University of Texas Health Science Center, San Antonio

SARVETNICK, NORA, Dept. of Developmental Biology, Genentech, Inc., South San Francisco, California

SASAZUKI, TAKEHITO, Dept. of Genetics, Kyushu University, Fukuoka, Japan

SCHARFF, MATTHEW, Cancer Research Center, Albert Einstein College of Medicine, Bronx, New York

SCHERER, MARK, Dept. of Biology, Massachusetts Institute of Technology, Cambridge

SCHIFFER, MARIANNE, Dept. of Biology, Argonne National Laboratory, Illinois

SCHWAB, RISE, Dept. of Medicine, Cornell University Medical College, New York, New York

SCHWARTZ, RONALD, NIAID, National Institutes of Health, Bethesda, Maryland

SCHWOCHAU, MARTIN, Institut fur Genetik, Heinrich Heine Universitat, Dusseldorf, Federal Republic of Germany

SCOTT, DAVID, Dept. of Immunology, University of Rochester, New York

SCOTT, DIANE, Dept. of Transplantation Biology, Clinical Research Centre, Middlesex, England

SEKALY, RAFICK-PIERRE, Dept. of Molecular Immunology, Clinical Research Institute of Montreal, Canada

SEONG, RHO, Dept. of Immunology, Stanford University Medical Center, California

SERCARZ, ELI, Dept. of Microbiology, University of California, Los Angeles

SHAANAN, BOAZ, Dept. of Molecular Biology, NIDDK, National Institutes of Health, Bethesda, Maryland

SHARPE, MELANIE, Laboratory of Molecular Biology, Medical Research Council, Cambridge, England

SHAW, ALBERT, Dept. of Genetics, Harvard University Medical School, Boston, Massachusetts

SHEAR, HANNAH, Dept. of Medical and Molecular Parasitology, New York University Medical Center, New York

SHIH, CHARLES, Dept. of Pediatrics, Medical College of Wisconsin, Wilwaukee

SHULMAN, MARC, Dept. of Immunology, University of Toronto, Canada

SILVER, JACK, Dept. of Molecular Medicine, North Shore University Hospital, Manhasset, New York

SILVERSTEIN, ARTHUR, Dept. of Opthamology, Johns Hopkins University, Baltimore, Maryland

SIMISTER, NEIL, Dept. of Biomedical Research, Whitehead Institute, Cambridge, Massachusetts

SIMON, THOMAS, Institut fur Genetik, University of Cologne, Federal Republic of Germany

SINGER, ALFRED, Experimental Immunology Branch, NCI, National Institutes of Health, Bethesda, Maryland

SLANETZ, ALFRED, Dept. of Immunobiology, Yale University School of Medicine, New Haven, Connecticut

SMART, JOHN, Dept. of Protein Biochemistry, Hoffmann-La Roche, Inc., Nutley, New Jersey

SMITH, CLAIRE, Dept. of Immunology, Medical Research Council, London, England

SMITH, LAURIE, Depts. of Experimental Oncology and Pathology, Stanford University School of Medicine, California

SOLVASON, H. BRENT, Dept. of Microbiology, University of Alabama, Birmingham

SORGER, PETER, Laboratory of Molecular Biology, Medical Research Council, Cambridge, England

SPENCER, DAVID, Dept. of Biology, Massachusetts Institute of Technology, Cambridge

SPRENT, JONATHAN, Dept. of Immunology, Scripps Clinic and Research Foundation, La Jolla, California

SPRINGER, TIMOTHY, Center for Blood Research, Boston, Massachusetts

STAEHELIN, THEOPHIL, Pharmaceuticals Division, Ciba-Geigy Ltd., Basel, Switzerland

STAHL, PHILIP, Dept. of Cell Biology and Physiology, Washington University School of Medicine, St. Louis, Missouri

STAUNTON, DONALD, Blood Research Center, Harvard Medical School, Boston, Massachusetts

STEINER, LISA, Massachusetts Institute of Technology, Cambridge, Massachusetts

STEINMETZ, MICHAEL, Central Research Units, F. Hoffmann-La Roche and Company, Basel, Switzerland

STEMME, STEN, Viacor, Menlo Park, California

STOCKINGER, HUBERTUS, Boehringer Mannheim GmbH, Penzberg, Federal Republic of Germany

STROMINGER, JACK, Depts. of Biochemistry and Molecular Biology, Harvard University, Cambridge, Massachusetts

SU, BING, Dept. of Immunobiology, Yale University School of Medicine, New Haven, Connecticut

SUNG, SUN-SANG, Oklahoma Medical Research Foundation, Oklahoma City

TAKAGAKI, YOHTAROH, Center for Cancer Research, Massachusetts Institute of Technology, Cambridge

TAKATSU, KIYOSHI, Dept. of Biology, Institute for Medical Immunology, Kumamoto University Medical School, Japan

TAKIGUCHI, MASAFUMI, Institute of Medical Science and Immunology, Tokyo, Japan

TAMMINEN, WENDY, Dept. of Immunology, University of Toronto, Canada

TAN, KUT-NIE, Dept. of Molecular Biology, Dana Farber Cancer Institute, Boston, Massachusetts

TANIGUCHI, TADATSUGA, Institute for Molecular and Cellular Biology, Osaka University, Japan

TEH, HUNG-SIA, Dept. of Microbiology, University of British Columbia, Vancouver, Canada

TEMPLE, GARY, Life Technologies, Inc., Gaithersburg, Maryland

TEPPER, ROBERT, Dept. of Genetics, Harvard Medical School, Boston, Massachusetts

TERHORST, COX, Dept. of Molecular Immunology, Dana Farber Cancer Institute, Boston, Massachusetts

THIELE, H., Dept. of Immunology, University of Hamburg, Federal Republic of Germany

THOMAS, BRIAN, MRC National Institute for Medical Research, London, England

THOMAS, JAMES, Baylor College of Medicine, Houston, Texas

THOMAS, MATTHEW, Dept. of Pathology, Washington University School of Medicine, St. Louis, Missouri

THOMPSON, CRAIG, Howard Hughes Institute, University of Michigan, Ann Arbor

THORNTON, GEORGE, R.W. Johnson Pharmaceutical Research Institute, San Diego, California

TINDALL, RICHARD, Dept. of Neurology, University of Texas Southwestern Medical Center, Dallas

TONEGAWA, SUSUMU, Center for Cancer Research, Massachusetts Institute of Technology, Cambridge

TORBETT, BRUCE, Lilly Research Laboratories, La Jolla, California

TOWNSEND, ALAIN, Nuffield Dept. of Clinical Medicine, University of Oxford, England

TRIPPUTI, PASQUALE, Tecnogen, S.P.A., Milan, Italy

TROWSDALE, JOHN, Human Immunogenetics Laboratory, Imperial Cancer Research Fund Laboratories, London, England

TULIP, WILLIAM, Parkville Laboratory, CSIRO, Parkville, Australia

UHR, JONATHAN, Dept. of Microbiology, University of Texas Southwestern Medical Center, Dallas

ULLRICH, STEPHEN, National Cancer Institute, National Institutes of Health, Bethesda, Maryland

UNANUE, EMIL, Dept. of Pathology, Washington University School of Medicine, St. Louis, Missouri

URBAIN, JACQUES, Dept. of Animal Physiology, University of Brussels, Rhodes, Belgium

VAKIL, MEENAL, Wallace Tumor Institute, University of Alabama, Birmingham

VAN PEL, ALINE, Ludwig Institute for Cancer Research, Brussels, Belgium

VEROMAA, TIMO, Dept. of Medical Microbiology, Turku University, Finland

VIDOVIC, DAMIR, Basel Institute for Immunology, Switzerland

VIGUIER, MIREILLE, Dept. of Chemistry, Stanford University, California

VITETTA, ELLEN, Dept. of Microbiology, University of Texas Southwestern Medical Center, Dallas

VIVES, JORDI, Servei d'Immunologia, Hospital Clinic i Provincial de Barcelona, Spain

VON BOEHMER, HARALD, Basel Institute for Immunology, Switzerland

WADE, NANCY, Dept. of Immunology, Wadsworth Center for Laboratories & Research, Albany, New York

WALDMANN, HERMAN, Dept. of Pathology, Cambridge University, England

WALLNER, BARBARA, Dept. of Molecular Biology, Biogen, Cambridge, Massachusetts

WANECK, GERALD, Surgery Unit, Massachusetts General Hospital, Charlestown

WARD, REBECCA, Research Dept., Genentech, Inc., South San Francisco, California

WARDLAW, ANDY, Center for Blood Research, Boston, Massachusetts

WARNER, CAROL, Dept. of Biology, Northeastern University, Boston, Massachusetts

WARNER, GARVIN, University of Rochester Cancer Center, New York

WATERS, J., St. Mary's Hospital School of Medicine, London, England

WATSON, JAMES, Cold Spring Harbor Laboratory, New York

WATTS, COLIN, Dept. of Biochemistry, University of Dundee, Scotland

WATTS, TANIA, Dept. of Immunology, University of Toronto, Canada

WEIGERT, MARTIN, Fox Chase Cancer Center, Institute for Cancer Research, Philadelphia, Pennsylvania

WEISSMAN, IRVING, Dept. of Pathology, Stanford University Medical Center, California

WILEY, DON, Depts. of Biochemistry and Molecular Biology, Harvard University, Cambridge

WILLIAMS, ALAN, Medical Research Council, Sir William Dunn School of Pathology, University of Oxford, England

WILLIAMS, IFOR, Dept. of Pathology, Washington University School of Medicine, St. Louis, Missouri

WILLIAMS, MEGAN, Dept. of Pathology, Brigham and Women's Hospital, Boston, Massachusetts

WILLIAMSON, ALAN, Merck Sharp & Dohme Research Laboratories, Rahway, New Jersey

WINOTO, ASTAR, Whitehead Institute, Cambridge, Massachusetts

WINTER, GREGORY, Medical Research Council, Laboratory of Molecular Biology, Cambridge, England

WLOKA, JERZY, St. Luke's/Roosevelt Hospital, New York, New York

WRIGHT, STEPHEN, Texas Tech University HSC, Amarillo

WU, GILLIAN, Dept. of Immunology, University of Toronto, Canada

ZALLER, DENNIS, Dept. of Biology, California Institute of Technology, Pasadena

ZERLER, BRAD, Molecular Therapeutics, West Haven, Connecticut

ZIEGLER, STEVEN, Immunex Research and Development Corporation, Seattle, Washington

ZINKERNAGEL, ROLF, Institute of Pathology, University of Zurich, Switzerland

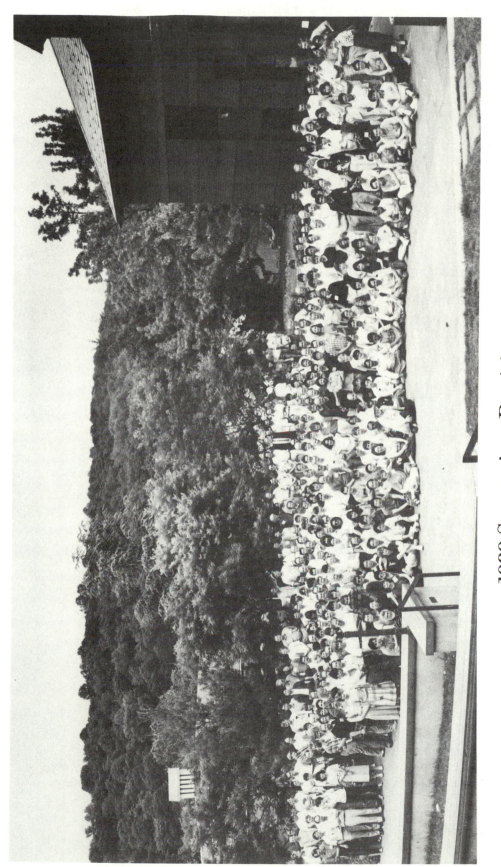

1989 Symposium Participants

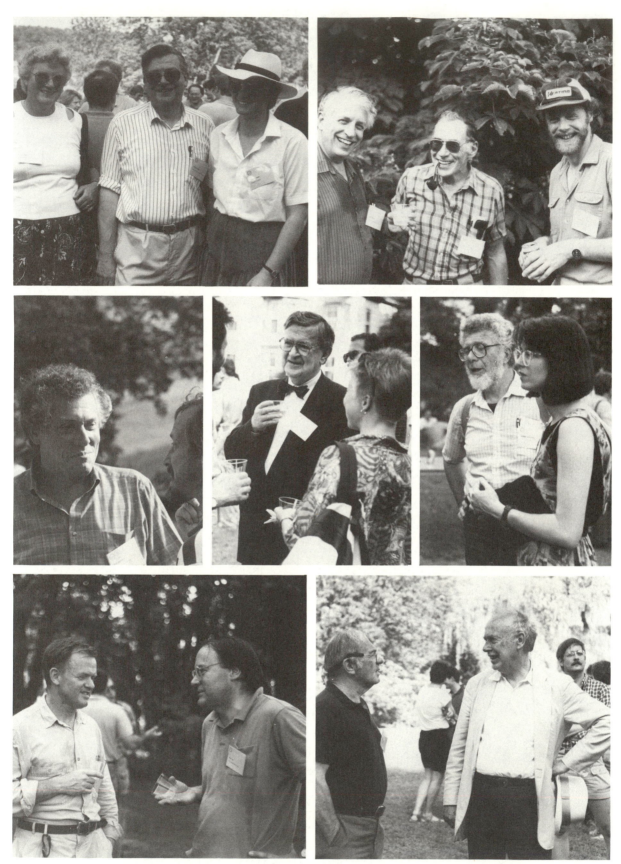

First row: J. Bodmer, W. Bodmer, H. Bodmer; G. Nossal, A. Silverstein, J. Inglis
Second row: F. Melchers, A. DeFranco; N. Jerne; L. Herzenberg, C. Kocks
Third row: A. Williams, B. Hall; J. Strominger, J.D. Watson

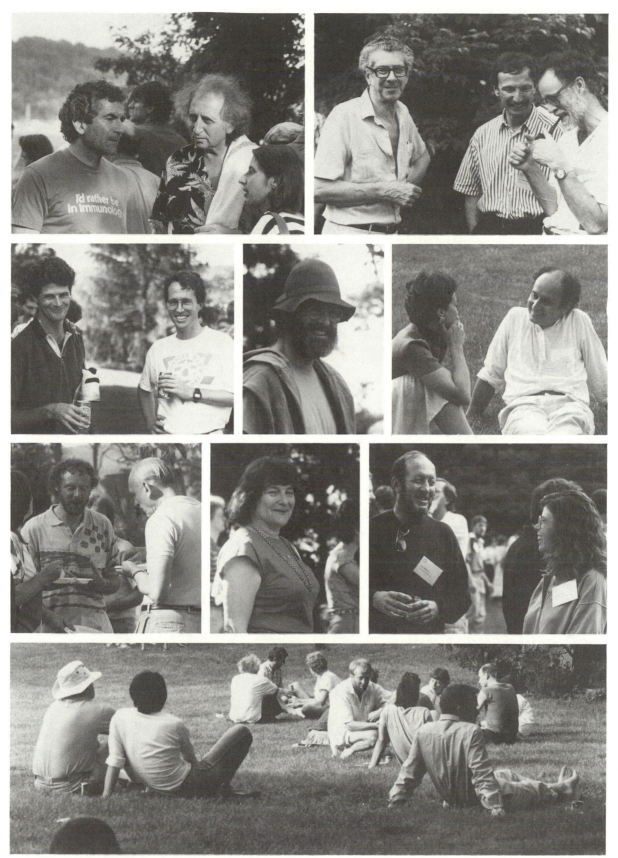

First row: D. Scott, E. Sercarz, N. Sarvetnick; J. Miller, R. Zinkernagel, J. Sprent
Second row: C. Goodnow, S. Grant; C. Janeway; P. Matzinger, J. Howard
Third row: J. Inglis, D. Davies; L. Herzenberg; I. Weissman, R. Wood
Fourth row: Picnic

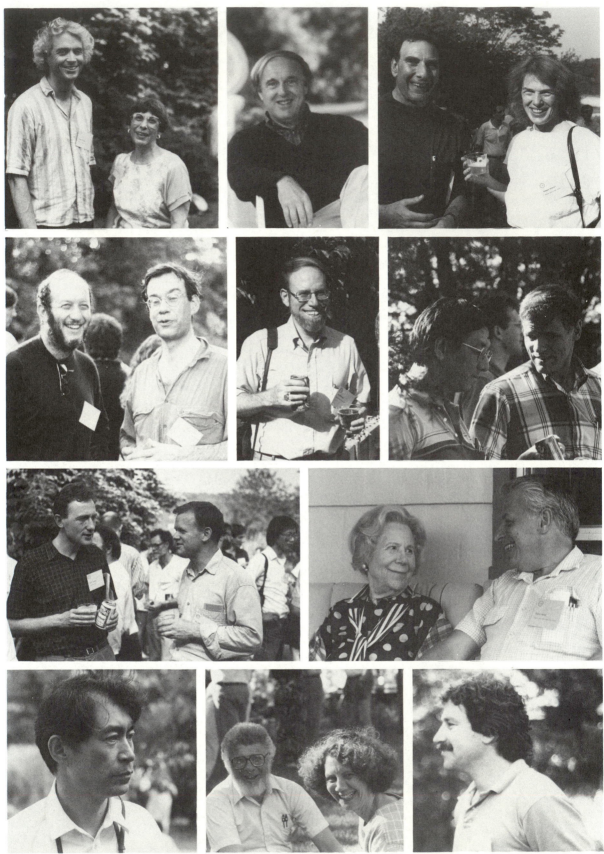

First row: D. Hanahan, M. Cozza; R. Lerner; M. Gefter, P. Marrack
Second row: I. Weissman, C. Terhorst; J. Berzofsky; D. Loh, L. Hood
Third row: A. Townsend, A. Williams; L. Hazen, G. Nossal
Fourth row: T. Honjo; L. Herzenberg, N. Maizels; R. Klausner

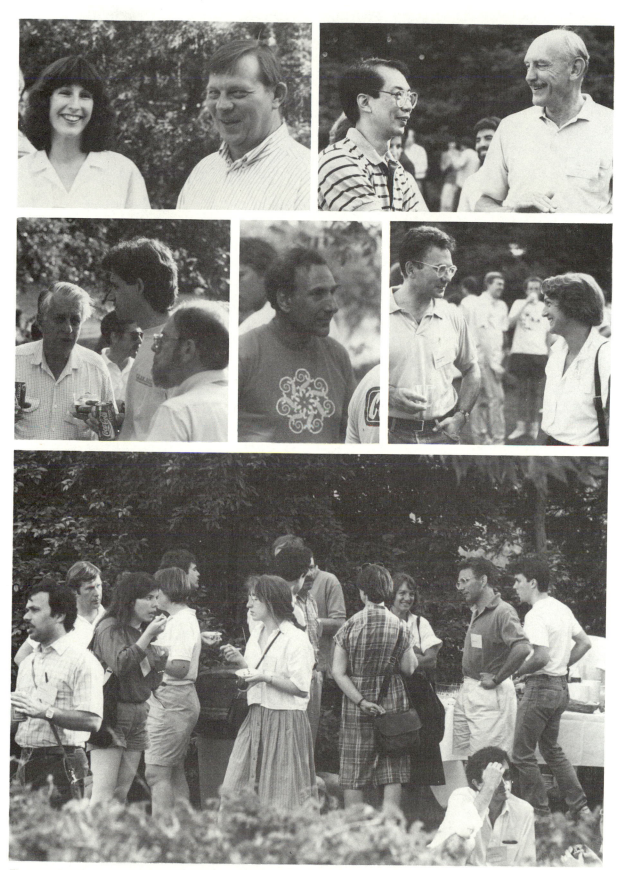

First row: M. Sharp, A. Boylston; S. Fong, D. Davies
Second row: G. Nossal, B. Stillman, J. Berzofsky; M. Gefter; P. Kourilsky, J. Maryanski
Third row: Picnic

Foreword

Our 1967 Symposium on antibodies marked the acceptance of the theories advanced by Jerne and Burnet that antigen, on entering the immune system, selected and expanded clones of lymphocytes with immunoglobulin receptors that best fitted the antigen. Yet, even then, it was apparent that this was not a whole explanation. Induction of antibodies to a hapten seemed to require specific recognition of the carrier molecule, not just the hapten. By 1976, and our next immunological Symposium, the separation of lymphocytes into two classes had been established, and for most antibody responses, interaction between T and B cells with separate specificities was known to be necessary. Clearly, the antibody-like membrane receptors of B cells could bind free antigen. The target for T cells, however, seemed to be cell-bound antigen, but only if effector and target cell were identical for genes at the major histocompatibility loci. Although speculation at the Symposium was intense, the nature of the T cell's receptor, and of its ligand, remained mysterious.

Work in the 1980s clarified these events at a molecular level, greatly aided by the advent of monoclonal antibody technology and the ability to clone T cells and manipulate lymphocyte genes. Antigen receptor molecules from T cells were identified and found to be encoded in a unique set of rearranging gene segments, separate from but evolutionarily related to the immunoglobulin genes. The analysis of other cell-surface molecules revealed diversity among T cells that correlated with differences in function. Crucially, it was observed that the products of MHC loci could bind peptide fragments of antigen and deliver them to the surface of antigen-presenting cells. A structural basis for T-cell antigen recognition became apparent when the solution of the crystal structure of the class I histocompatibility molecule HLA-A2 showed it to have a groove in which both peptide and the variable T-cell receptor might bind. X-ray crystallography also shed light on the interaction between an antibody and its ligand, with the solution of the structure of an immune complex.

By 1989, therefore, the time was clearly ripe for another Cold Spring Harbor Symposium on immunology, the third in the series, this time focusing on the molecular, cellular, and structural aspects of immunological recognition. The themes of the meeting were the interactions among MHC molecules, peptides, and T-cell receptors; the shaping of T-cell and B-cell repertoires by these events; and their consequences for lymphocyte activation and tolerance. Our aim was to bring together the leaders in this now very diverse field, and as principal organizers, we benefited greatly by advice from many sources. In particular, we thank Jay Berzofsky, Malcolm Gefter, Tasuko Honjo, Richard Lerner, Philippa Marrack, Fritz Melchers, Matthew Scharff, Susumu Tonegawa, and Don Wiley for their help.

The final program consisted of 114 speakers, and there were 446 participants. Every available seat in Grace Auditorium was occupied throughout the week, and the aisles overflowed. The meeting opened with splendid presentations from Leroy Hood, Philippa Marrack, Don Wiley, Emil Unanue, and Hugh McDevitt, whose talks highlighted the themes of the coming week. Following 14 sessions of great intensity, Jonathan Howard concluded with an elegant and wide-ranging summary.

Such a meeting requires many sources of financial support; we gratefully acknowledge the help of the National Cancer Institute, the National Institute of Allergy and Infectious Diseases, the National Science Foundation, and the Lucille P. Markey Charitable Trust. Essential funds also came from our Corporate Sponsors: Alafi Capital Company; American Cyanamid Company; Amersham International plc; AMGen Inc.; Applied Biosystems, Inc.; Becton Dickinson and Company; Beecham Pharmaceuticals; Boehringer Mannheim Corporation; Ciba-Geigy Corporation/ Ciba/ Geigy Limited; Diagnostic Products Corporation; E. I. du Pont de Nemours & Company; Eastman Kodak Company; Genentech, Inc.; Genetics Institute; Hoffman-La Roche Inc.; Johnson & Johnson; Life Technologies, Inc.; Eli Lilly and Company; Millipore Corporation; Monsanto Company; Oncogene Science, Inc.; Pall Corporation; Perkin-Elmer Cetus Corporation; Pfizer Inc.; Pharmacia Inc.; Schering-Plough Corporation; Tambrands Inc.; The Upjohn Company; The Wellcome Research Laboratories, Burroughs Wellcome Co.; and Wyeth-Ayerst Research.

Registration and housing for the participants were organized with care and courtesy by the staff of the Meetings Office: Maureen Berejka, Barbara Ward, Karen Otto, Diane Tighe, Michela McBride, and Marge Stellabotte. Jim Hope and his staff provided admirable catering, and once again Herb Parsons and his assistants delivered a flawless audiovisual service, rising to the challenges of double projection (requested by nearly every speaker) and the presentation of a movie. The enormous correspondence required for a Symposium was ably handled by Andrea Stevenson and P.J. Harlow. These books were edited by Dorothy Brown, Patricia Barker, and Ralph Battey, assisted by Joan Ebert, Mary Cozza, and Inez Sialiano, and their production was overseen by Nancy Ford.

James D. Watson
John R. Inglis
November 24, 1989

Contents

Part 1

Part 2

Signals for Lymphocyte Activation, Proliferation, and Adhesion

Tolerance and Self Recognition

Summary

Appendix

COLD SPRING HARBOR SYMPOSIA ON QUANTITATIVE BIOLOGY

VOLUME LIV

Approaching the Asymptote?
Evolution and Revolution in Immunology

C.A. JANEWAY, JR.

Section of Immunology, Howard Hughes Medical Institute at Yale University School of Medicine
New Haven, Connecticut 06510

It is a great privilege to introduce this Cold Spring Harbor Symposium on quantitative biology on the subject of immune recognition. My predecessors in this role, Macfarlane Burnet (1967) and Niels Jerne (1976), had a profound effect on the development of ideas in our field, and many of the participants have made great contributions to our understanding of the subject of this symposium and are clearly more qualified than I to introduce it.

The first Cold Spring Harbor Symposium to consider the immune system was held in 1967 on the subject of antibodies. It marked the acceptance of the clonal selection theory as the central paradigm of immunology (Jerne 1967). That meeting also brought together sufficient data on antibody structure to promote the idea that immunoglobulins are encoded in two distinct types of gene segments, variable segments and constant segments, and that a genetic mechanism must exist to direct the association of these segments in antibody-producing cells. Finally, it was becoming clear at the 1967 symposium that, although antibody molecules might be both the receptor on and the secreted product of single cells, the specificity of immune activation was distinct from the specificity of the antibodies themselves. Thus, the stage was set for the discovery over the succeeding years that lymphocytes were divided into two major populations, the B cells that bear antibody molecules as their surface receptor for antigen and secrete antibody molecules upon activation, and the T cells that mediate all other specific immune responses, including the activation of B cells to produce antibody.

This discovery provided the focus for the second Cold Spring Harbor Symposium on the immune system, held in 1976 under the title of *Origins of Lymphocyte Diversity*. This meeting was dominated by three themes: the function and specificity of T lymphocytes, with special emphasis on the recent discovery that T cells only responded to antigens presented by cells genotypically identical at the major histocompatibility complex (MHC), termed MHC restriction; the structure and genetics of the MHC and its products; and the structure and genetics of immunoglobulin molecules. It is clear that the discovery of T cells as a separate lineage of cells with distinctive recognitive properties had released a flood of experimentation that could explain many of the mysteries of immunology. The most important of these was the role of the MHC in controlling immune responses, and much effort was directed to understanding the MHC molecules and the genes that encode them. Finally, the 1976 symposium saw the first description of immunoglobulin gene rearrangement in antibody-forming cells by Susumu Tonegawa (1976), opening the way to an understanding of the greatest genetic puzzle of the antibody molecule, its possession of variable and constant structural motifs.

APPROACHING THE ASYMPTOTE?

This year's symposium on immunological recognition carries on in the tradition of its precursors. Its dominant theme is well captured in Figure 3 of Madden et al. (this volume), showing the structure of a class I MHC molecule with a peptide fragment bound to its outer face (Bjorkman et al. 1987). This is the structure recognized by T cells, and the high degree of resolution provided by this picture has given a firm structural basis for understanding immunological recognition by T cells. A second set of pictures, again provided by X-ray crystallography (see Amit et al. 1986), allows us to visualize the interaction between an immunological receptor, the antibody molecule, and its protein ligand. The intervening years have also fulfilled Edelman's (1976) prediction in summarizing the 1976 symposium that "we should have satisfactory answers to many of the major questions of immunology." Edelman himself appears to have believed this prediction, and he now graces a different field, neurobiology. His specific predictions for the future of immunology have proven remarkably accurate. Again to quote from his 1976 summary: "I think it likely that we are going to see the T-cell receptor characterized, the major histocompatibility complex understood in terms of its functions, and the origin of diversity reasonably well ensconced within a detailed analysis of particular enzymes and their mechanisms." The proceedings of this third Cold Spring Harbor Symposium on the immune system will bear out this forecast, although the enzymology of rearranging immunological receptor genes is an area that has not quite arrived as of this writing; it could someday form the subject of a different symposium. Edelman has the wisdom to add: "We shall, of course, hear of more surprising discoveries," and indeed we have, and shall continue to do so. Finally, it is perhaps fair to point out that we have yet to obtain the three-dimensional structure we all hope to see at a future symposium, namely, the trimolecular complex of T-cell receptor:antigenic peptide:MHC molecule. Nevertheless, I believe it is safe to state that our understanding of immunological recognition is approaching some sort of asymptote, where future experiments are obvious, technically difficult to perform, and aim to achieve ever higher degrees of precision rather than revolutionary changes in our understanding. Thus, this is a good time to take stock of immunology, to catalog what is known, to ask how we arrived where we are, and to look ahead to where we might go.

Although our understanding of immunological recognition by clonally distributed receptors is approaching an asymptote, I have ended my main title with a question mark, because I believe that immunological recognition extends beyond antigen binding by the clonally distributed receptors encoded in rearranging gene segments detailed in this volume and that there is still much to learn. In this introduction, I shall present the known and indicate what is unknown about immunological recognition. I use the evolutionary development of the immune system to account for some of the apparent complexity of these recognitive processes. Finally, I return to Macfarlane Burnet's (1967) introduction to the first Cold Spring Harbor Symposium on immunology, entitled *The Impact of Ideas on Immunology*. Although it is clear that ideas can provide an impetus for experiment, as was the case for the clonal selection theory of Burnet, I believe that ideas, especially good ideas, can so satisfy our desire to explain what we are studying that they can inhibit our ability to explore and to understand. I agree with Burnet that it is the unfettered empirical exploration of a subject that makes it move forward, whereas ideas are better suited for organizing existing knowledge into understandable pictures and thus to make the available information readily understandable to expert and student alike. Here, I would like to echo Jerne's (1976) introduction, in which he points out the virtue of structural studies for their own sake. Much of what we have learned in the past and shall learn in the future rests on analyses of gene and protein structure. This can lead directly to questions about function, as is beautifully illustrated by the discovery of the γ/δ T-cell receptor (see Janeway 1988) or the finding that CD45 has tyrosine phosphatase activity (Charbonneau et al. 1988).

EVOLUTION IN IMMUNOLOGY

The immune system clearly exists to protect the host from infectious agents; the disastrous impact of these agents on immunodeficient patients allows us to make this statement with some conviction (Janeway et al. 1953). The immune system must recognize the presence of an infectious agent and then respond appropriately to contain and remove this threat to the integrity of the internal milieu. Thus, it is easiest to understand the processes of immune recognition in terms of the microorganisms that the system has evolved to recognize and destroy. I will use defense against infection to explain why the multiple recognitive and effector systems present in contemporary organisms were necessary to the effective functioning of the immune system. In contrast, viewed in isolation, antigen processing, MHC-restricted antigen recognition, and T-cell effector functions have a remarkably ad hoc appearance. It is surely no accident that our understanding of these processes has been due in no small part to the analysis of immunity to influenza viruses, a true target of immune surveillance (Morrison et al. 1986; Townsend et al. 1986).

Infectious agents are highly variable in structure, and their short generation time allows them to alter their structure with great rapidity. This is especially true of their protein structure, which can diversify remarkably even during the course of an infection within an individual. It is perhaps not surprising that Macfarlane Burnet, the originator of the clonal selection theory, was studying antigenic variation in influenza viral proteins at the time he fashioned his hypothesis. He realized the necessity for the immune system to develop mechanisms to generate an essentially open and unlimited repertoire of receptors, since evolutionary selection could not provide the immune system with receptors that would recognize the hemagglutinin molecules of next year's strain of virus. Indeed, we now appreciate that the somatic rearrangement of gene segments, including the addition of nucleotides at gene segment junctions, coupled with somatic mutation in antibody variable region genes, provides the immune system with a general mechanism for the generation of diversity that allows the recognition of virtually any molecule by an antibody. Thus, the problem of the generation of diversity has been solved in a unique way in the immune system. The set of germ-line genes has probably been selected over evolutionary time to provide "useful" receptors directed at common pathogens or structural motifs and to provide a broad set of structural possibilities on which to build variants. These gene segments rearrange to form complete variable domain genes, whose products combine with similar variable chains to form complete heterodimeric receptor sites. Further rapid somatic mutation in active B lymphocytes provides antibody molecules with the precision of fit to antigen embodied in the elegant structures made visible by the crystallographers (see Bentley et al.; Davies et al.; Tulip et al.; all this volume).

With such a powerful and adaptable recognitive system as the antibodies in hand, one might ask why there is a need for a second, and quite distinct, recognitive system, the T-cell receptors. Indeed, at the Cold Spring Harbor Symposium in 1976, it was thought by many participants that the answer to this question had to be that T cells simply used the genetic material encoding antibody molecules in a slightly different way to form their receptors. To again quote Edelman's summary of the earlier meeting, "It appears that the T-cell receptor is an immunoglobulin, at least in the sense that it has V_H regions at its active site. We are thus relieved of the repellent possibility of having to invoke two separate origins of diversity, one for B cells and one for T cells." We now know, thanks to the identification of the molecules themselves and of the genes encoding them, that T-cell receptors derive from a separate and unique set of rearranging gene segments. However, it is also absolutely clear from the structures of immunoglobulin and T-cell receptor genes that these two sets of rearranging genes arose by duplication, that many or all of the enzymes involved in gene rearrangement are used in common by developing T and B lymphocytes, and that the essential principle of variable receptor generation by somatic recombination had only to arise once (see Hunkapiller et al., this volume).

What was the evolutionary pressure that selected for the development of these two different sets of receptors and the two distinct recognition mechanisms they employ? I believe that the answer lies in the habitats occupied by different types of parasitic microorganisms. Antibody molecules are ideally suited to bind to extracellular microorganisms and to mark them for removal by activation of complement and Fc-receptor-bearing phagocytic cells. However, antibody molecules cannot bind to those microorganisms that live within cells, such as the *Mycobacteria* and the viruses. For the immune system to recognize infection within a cell, a mechanism was needed to deliver the antigens to the cell surface. The presence of these nonself molecules on a self cell surface had to be recognized by a cell that could mediate an appropriate response. The first requirement is met by the molecules of the MHC. These molecules appear to have evolved primarily, if not exclusively, to deliver peptide fragments of intracellular microorganisms to the cell surface. The complex of foreign peptide bound to self-MHC molecule is then recognized by the cell-surface receptor of a T lymphocyte. Upon activation, these specific T cells induce a change in the infected cell. In the case of an infected macrophage, the T cell secretes macrophage activating factors, such as γ-interferon, that allow the macrophage to destroy those bacteria proliferating in its vesicles; in the case of a virally infected cell, a different T cell kills the infected cell to rid the body of its source of new virions.

Infectious agents can occupy quite distinct intracellular compartments. For instance, *Mycobacteria* reside within cellular vesicles and synthesize their own proteins in this site. In contrast, the influenza virus utilizes the cell's protein synthetic apparatus to produce virion proteins. Two classes of MHC molecules have evolved to deliver peptides from these different intracellular compartments. Class I MHC molecules deliver peptides synthesized in the cell's cytoplasm to the cell surface; complexes of antigen with class I MHC molecules are recognized by a subset of T cells bearing CD8 whose major functional capability is cell-mediated cytotoxicity. Such cells kill virus-infected cells as a mechanism of inhibiting viral replication and continuing infec-

tion. Class II MHC molecules deliver peptides deriving from cellular vesicles, including the endosomes, to the cell surface. The complex of peptide and class II MHC molecule is recognized by the subset of T cells bearing CD4 whose major functional capabilities are the production of lymphokines, molecules that induce various activities in other cells, such as macrophages and B cells. CD4 T cells activate macrophages to kill the bacteria living in their vesicles; they also activate antigen-specific B cells to produce antibody in response to extracellular bacteria bound by the immunoglobulin receptor of the B cell. These pathways of antigen processing and the responses they stimulate are shown diagrammatically in Figure 1. The studies of the past 13 years have given us a remarkably accurate picture of the role of MHC molecules in antigen presentation, the recognition of MHC/peptide complexes by the T-cell receptor, and the types of effector responses elicited by such recognitive events.

Antigen recognition by T cells is thoroughly described in this volume. If one is to understand this complex process fully, it is useful to keep the biological purpose of these recognitive events clearly in mind. In particular, the role of the molecules encoded in the MHC as peptide delivery vehicles should be emphasized. For the MHC molecules to perform this function effectively, they must have two cardinal features. First, they must be able to bind a substantial fraction of all possible peptides sufficiently well to deliver them to the cell surface and hold them there until they can be recognized by a T-cell receptor. This has proven to be the case, although the mechanism by which MHC molecules can bind such a wide variety of peptide ligands so stably is not clear. The chemistry of this interaction is thoroughly explored in many papers in this volume. Second, MHC molecules must be specialized to interact with the T-cell receptor complex. This appears to be the case; the focusing of T-cell recognition on MHC molecules was foreseen by Jerne (1971) and accounts for the apparent violation of clonal selection theory represented by the T-cell response to nonself MHC molecules, discussed at prior symposia by Simonsen (1967) and by Wilson et al. (1976). Indeed, the focusing of T-cell recognition on MHC molecules leads to the potent graft rejection that gave this complex its name; at this point, knowledge of the true function of MHC molecules may allow a more rational nomenclature to emerge. Finally, one may ask why T cells do not simply recognize the foreign component of the antigen on the cell surface, instead of a complex of antigenic peptide and MHC molecule. The requirement for MHC restriction solves two problems in T-cell recognition. First, it directs T cells to antigen recognition at the cell surface, the site of T-cell function. If T cells recognized antigen alone, soluble forms of antigen could prevent T cells from performing their specific effector functions of killing, macrophage activation, and B-cell activation, all of which require cell/cell contact. Second, this peptide delivery system allows virtually all of the proteins of an infectious agent an equal

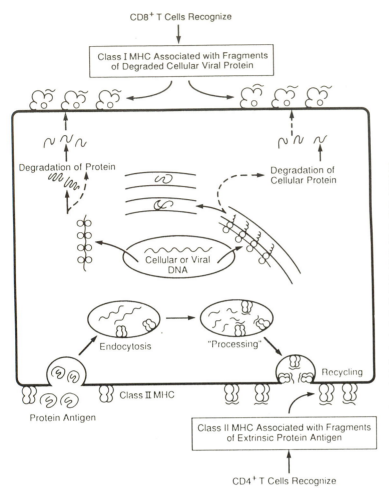

CD8+ T Cells Recognize

Class I MHC Associated with Fragments
of Degraded Cellular Viral Protein

Degradation of Protein

Degradation of
Cellular Protein

Cellular or Viral
DNA

Endocytosis   "Processing"

Recycling

Protein Antigen   Class II MHC

Class II MHC Associated with Fragments
of Extrinsic Protein Antigen

CD4+ T Cells Recognize

Figure 1. The pathways of antigen processing leading to peptides bound to class I and class II MHC molecules, and the T-cell responses elicited, are shown schematically (adapted from Germain 1986). Proteins degraded in cellular vesicles, such as endosomes, bind to class II MHC molecules and are recognized by CD4 T cells at the cell surface. CD4 T cells are involved in inducing activation of other cell types: Macrophages harboring an intracellular infection can be activated to kill the bacteria that are proliferating in macrophage cytoplasmic vesicles by exposure to γ-interferon released by an activated CD4 T cell. Peptides derived from proteins degraded in the cell's cytoplasm, such as viral nuclear proteins, are transported to the cell surface by class I MHC molecules. The mechanism by which such peptides are generated and translocated into the endoplasmic reticulum to associate with class I MHC molecules is not understood at present. Complexes of peptide and class I MHC molecules are recognized by CD8 T cells. The dominant effector function of CD8 T cells is to kill cells bearing the appropriate peptide/class I MHC complex. This allows the elimination of virally infected cells, necessary for clearance of viral infections.

chance of being expressed at the cell surface; in contrast, only those components of bacteria or viruses destined for delivery to the cell surface would be recognizable on infected cells in the absence of this mechanism. Thus, the biological necessity of recognizing which cells are infected with intracellular parasites is likely to explain the many complexities of immunological recognition by T cells, the major topic of this symposium.

Evolutionary selection appears to account for the development of the major pathways of antigen recognition utilized in clonal selection and self/nonself discrimination. The details of many aspects of these processes are clarified in the papers that follow in this volume. We do indeed seem to be approaching an asymptote in our understanding. However, I am convinced that there is a tremendous gap between this asymptote and a full understanding of the induction of an immune response. In the next section, I discuss aspects of immunological recognition that go beyond clonal selection. I argue that these aspects are essential to the immune response, and further, that existing paradigms may have retarded our recognition of their importance.

THE LANDSTEINERIAN FALLACY AND THE IMMUNOLOGIST'S DIRTY LITTLE SECRET

Landsteiner is one of the giants of immunology; his work on the *Specificity of Serological Reactions* (1945) stands with Burnet's (1959) book *The Clonal Selection Theory of Immunity* as one of the few works still read and referred to from the premolecular era of immunology. Landsteiner made many outstanding contributions to the field of immunology, but one of the most important was his finding that simple aniline dyes chemically coupled to pure protein carriers could make excellent antigenic determinants called haptens, thus allowing a chemical characterization of antibody specificity. In making this finding, Landsteiner also led the way to our current understanding of repertoires. It is abundantly clear from this finding that a general mechanism for the generation of diversity must exist that is independent of evolutionary selection of receptor genes specifying the recognition of particular pathogenic microorganisms. The use of simple chemicals as antigenic determinants also made detailed analysis of immune responses easy, since a single, known, and controllable substance was used as antigen. Studies of responses to haptens greatly contributed to the discovery of immune response genes (Kantor et al. 1963), T-cell/B-cell interaction in antibody production (Mitchison 1971), and MHC restriction (Katz et al. 1973; Shearer 1974). Why, then, do I refer in my heading to the "Landsteinerian fallacy?"

The Landsteinerian fallacy is that all foreign macromolecules are equally able to give rise to an immune response, and, therefore, that the immune response shows no special predilection to respond to infectious agents. I believe that this latter conclusion is wrong, which is why I call it a fallacy. It is becoming clear that immunogenicity, the ability to elicit an immune response in the form of clonal expansion of virgin lymphocytes, requires both the presence of a suitable antigenic determinant to signal the lymphocyte through its antigen receptor *and* distinct signals derived from host cells. In the case of T-cell responses, the host cell signal derives from cells we refer to as antigen-presenting cells. In this section, I argue that the ability to deliver the second signal is induced on host antigen-presenting cells by infectious agents as the result of a distinct type of immunological recognition specific for microorganisms, but not resulting from clonally distributed receptors. If this construction is correct, then the interpretation of Landsteiner's famous experiment is incorrect, and we can move beyond clonal selection in our understanding of the specific immune response.

Signals for Lymphocyte Activation: Beyond Clonal Selection

It is now clear that all lymphocyte activation requires two signals, as originally proposed by Bretscher and Cohn (1970). Signal one is conventionally defined as the signal delivered by the interaction of the antigen receptor with its specific ligand. This interaction is the central feature of the clonal selection hypothesis. This symposium is largely devoted to the detailed molecular analysis of this interaction and to the signals transduced by the specific receptor across the lymphocyte membrane upon ligand binding. However, as first appreciated for B cells, simple ligand binding to the receptor does not lead to activation, clonal expansion, and the generation of an immune response; a second signal, most likely in the form of lymphokines, must be delivered by a helper T lymphocyte to generate an effective B-cell response. In the case of T lymphocytes, certain costimulatory factors derived from antigen-presenting cells are required for clonal expansion. The specific interactions and proposed cofactors are shown in Figure 2.

The requirement for two signals for lymphocyte activation has been explained in various ways; Bretscher and Cohn (1970) proposed that this requirement served as a mechanism for avoiding autoimmunity caused by the activation of lymphocytes bearing receptors directed at self-ligands. This is undoubtedly important in the case of B lymphocytes, whose receptors can rapidly

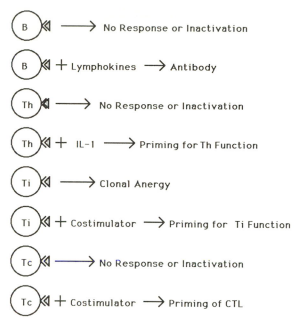

Figure 2. All lymphocyte classes appear to require two signals for their initial activation by antigen leading to clonal expansion. B cells binding ligand via their surface immunoglobulin receptor are inactivated by different mechanisms in the absence of T-cell help. Soluble, monovalent antigens lead to clonal anergy (see Goodnow et al., this volume), the loss of the ability to respond without the loss of the responding cell, whereas multivalent, cell-surface antigens lead to clonal deletion (Nemazee and Burki 1989). The same antigen bound to the receptor in the presence of T-cell help leads to specific antibody production (Metcalf and Klinman 1976). CD4[+] helper T cells (Th) require ligand in the form of a peptide fragment bound to class II MHC molecules. If such ligands are presented by cells expressing surface interleukin-1 (IL-1), priming occurs; in the absence of IL-1, no response ensues, and clonal anergy may be induced. CD4[+] T cells that produce IL-2, γ-interferon, and tumor necrosis factor, which I term inflammatory T cells (Ti), respond to peptide/class II MHC ligands only if they are presented by cells having costimulator activity (see Schwartz et al., this volume). The nature of this costimulator is unknown. In the absence of costimulator activity, encounter of Ti cells with ligand leads to clonal anergy. Finally, CD8[+] cytolytic T cells (Tc) can be activated by peptide/class I MHC ligands only if these are presented by cells, such as dendritic cells, that have high levels of costimulator activity. This costimulator activity can be substituted for by IL-2, either added by the investigator or provided by CD4 T cells in a three-cell interaction (see Fisher et al., this volume). In the absence of costimulator activity or IL-2, no activation of cytolytic T cells is observed; a state of clonal anergy may be induced by this exposure (see Guerder and Matzinger, this volume).

somatically mutate to generate autoreactive clones (see Radic et al.; Behar et al.; both this volume); T-cell dependence normally prevents further stimulation of such autoreactive B cells. T cells appear to have efficient mechanisms for clonal deletion in the thymus (Kappler et al. 1987) and do not somatically mutate, making a two-signal requirement for T-cell activation appear less essential. However, the fact that T cells recognize antigens as peptides bound to MHC molecules, including peptides derived from proteins synthesized within a cell, raises a problem for clonal deletion in the thymus: How can all the peptides of proteins in peripheral tissues be presented to developing T cells in such a way as to cause clonal deletion within the thymus? The answer appears to be that they are not. Rather, recent studies in many systems have made it clear that T-cell tolerance to peripheral antigens may be mediated by an absence of costimulatory factors on tissue cells rather than by clonal deletion of specific T lymphocytes; these studies are well represented in the proceedings of this symposium. Indeed, it appears that in many cases, the encounter of a T cell with its specific ligand in the absence of costimulatory molecules leads to clonal anergy, as detailed by Jenkins et al. (1987). In a later section, I raise the possibility that the second signals arose prior to the development of specific antigen recognition. Under this construction, second signals may be viewed more as positive initiators of immunity than as late adaptations to avoid autoimmunity.

Whichever hypothesis is correct, the requirement for second signals in lymphocyte activation means that self/nonself discrimination is determined not only by the interaction of specific, clonally distributed receptors with their ligand, but also by the presence or absence of costimulators on cells presenting the ligand. The regulation of costimulator expression is as critical as specific antigen recognition for self/nonself discrimination. Thus, I will now turn to a consideration of the costimulators and the regulation of their expression on antigen-presenting cells.

The Immunologist's Dirty Little Secret

In accepting the Landsteinerian fallacy as correct, immunologists have tended to use simple, well-characterized proteins or hapten-protein conjugates as antigens. This has greatly facilitated the analysis of the specific immune response, as illustrated throughout these proceedings. However, in order to obtain readily detectable responses to these antigens, they must be incorporated into a remarkable mixture termed complete Freund's adjuvant, heavily laced with killed *Mycobacterium tuberculosis* organisms or precipitated in alum and mixed with dead *Bordetella pertussis* organisms. I call this the immunologist's dirty little secret. Even the apparently pristine cloned T-cell lines of most T-cell biologists began life as cells exposed to these very messy preparations. Why do we need to use adjuvants? To be quite honest, the answer is not known. However, it seems likely that these substances are required to provide two attributes not found in soluble proteins. The first is effective antigen uptake into macrophages, thus increasing ligand density in the form of peptides derived from the foreign protein bound to class II MHC molecules. The second is the provision of costimulatory activity, induced in macrophages and/or B cells by the bacterial constituent of the adjuvant.

Little is known about the induction of costimulator activity. The apparent requirement for interleukin-1 (IL-1), predominantly a macrophage product, for the priming and clonal expansion of those T cells most

capable of providing helper function to B cells (see Janeway et al. 1988b), and the known potency of bacterial products such as lipopolysaccharide in inducing IL-1 secretion, suggest that one role of adjuvants is to induce IL-1 expression. In vivo studies in chimeric chickens (Lassila et al. 1988) and transgenic mice (van Ewijk et al. 1988; R.A. Flavell, pers. comm.) have provided evidence that both the peptide/MHC ligand for the T-cell receptor and the costimulator must be present on the same cell in order for priming to occur. This in vivo requirement for the coordinate expression of ligand and costimulator on a single antigen-presenting cell means that the regulation of costimulator activity on antigen-presenting cells incorporates a second mechanism of self/nonself discrimination into the immune system (Fig. 3). That the usual means of inducing costimulator activity is exposure of antigen-presenting cells to bacteria would appear to mean that infection is normally required to elicit an immune response and that the experimental immunologist bypasses this requirement by using adjuvant. Finally, this finding implies a means independent of strict clonal selection by which the immune system responds to relevant nonself in the form of infectious agents, but not to innocuous proteins, including self-proteins. This analysis suggests that a critical issue for future study is the analysis of microbial signals that induce second signaling capacity in antigen-presenting cells, and the receptors on antigen-presenting cells that detect these microbial signals.

The one cell that appears to violate this principle by expressing costimulator activity constitutively is the dendritic cell described by Steinman et al. (1989). Such cells would seem to be dangerous components of an

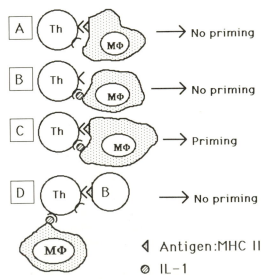

Figure 3. Helper T-cell (Th) priming requires the delivery of ligand in the form of peptide/class II MHC complexes and costimulator in the form of IL-1 on a single cell surface. This requirement has been demonstrated only in complex in vivo experiments (see text), but it is paralleled by the activation requirements of cloned helper T-cell lines (Kaye et al. 1984; Greenbaum et al. 1988; Janeway et al. 1988b).

immune system, since they should present self-antigens in an immunogenic form. However, two aspects of dendritic cell behavior appear to prevent this potential danger from occurring. First, dendritic cells take up and process antigens from surrounding tissues or extracellular fluid extremely inefficiently. Second, dendritic cells are present in the thymus and will thus delete any developing T cell recognizing the self-peptides that a dendritic cell can present. Indeed, dendritic cells are remarkably potent in inducing tolerance in developing thymocytes (Matzinger and Guerder 1989). What protective role have dendritic cells evolved to fulfill in the immune system? I suggest that dendritic cells exist primarily to present viral antigens (Macatonia et al. 1989). Unlike presentation of protein antigens, presentation of viral antigens does not require a specific mechanism of antigen uptake such as phagocytosis. Rather, the virus can infect the antigen-presenting cell, and, if it can replicate in the antigen-presenting cell, that cell will present viral antigens. Thus, I believe that dendritic cells will turn out to have unique mechanisms for allowing viral replication, such as an absence of responsiveness to α,β-interferons. Dendritic cells may have evolved such characteristics in order to stimulate immunity to viruses that could otherwise avoid immune responses because they do not induce costimulator activity. A virus that did not induce costimulator activity and also did not infect dendritic cells might be particularly dangerous. If adjuvants are the immunologist's dirty little secret, and if dendritic cells are "nature's adjuvant," as suggested by Steinman et al. (1989), then perhaps dendritic cells are nature's dirty little secret (at least from the vantage point of a virus that is seduced into replicating in a dendritic cell, only to be attacked and destroyed by the host's immune response elicited by the infected dendritic cell).

The Landsteinerian fallacy, then, is the idea that the immune system has evolved to recognize equally all nonself substances, and that self/nonself discrimination is based solely on clonally distributed receptors encoded in rearranging gene families that can discriminate hapten A from hapten B. I contend that the immune system has evolved specifically to recognize and respond to infectious microorganisms, and that this involves recognition not only of specific antigenic determinants, but also of certain characteristics or patterns common on infectious agents but absent from the host. That one can obtain antibodies and T cells highly specific for nonmicrobial antigens does not disprove this contention. Most or all such specific immune reactants were elicited by making use of the immunologist's dirty little secret, an adjuvant whose essential constituent is a microorganism, or of nature's adjuvant in the case of viral immunity. By ignoring the importance of this microbial component of immunological recognition, I contend that we have collectively ignored a critical feature of self/nonself discrimination, the requirement for a microbially induced second signal. Furthermore, I argue that this form of self/nonself discrimination violates the tenets of clonal selection

theory by proposing that a recognitive function required for immune responsiveness is derived from nonclonally distributed receptors. Indeed, I believe that if we fail to incorporate such ideas into our thinking, we shall fail to understand immune recognition at its most fundamental level, that is, the discrimination of self from nonself, and in the defense of the host against infection. The Landsteinerian fallacy is that all antigens are not only equally recognizable, but also equally immunogenic, that is, equally able to stimulate an immune response. This is clearly not the case. In the next section, I attempt to explain the concept of nonclonal recognition of microbial pathogens and to show how the evolution of microbial recognition preceded a truly revolutionary development in immunity, the use of rearranging, clonally distributed receptors to recognize and destroy foreign microorganisms.

REVOLUTION IN IMMUNOLOGY

Kuhn (1970) describes the progress of a science as occurring by successive revolutions, interspersed with periods of "normal science," the quiet brickmaking that builds up the factual and conceptual edifice he calls a paradigm. Revolutions destroy the old paradigm and point the way to a new one. Talmage (1988), in reviewing the history of immunology's first 100 years, came to a different conclusion: that normal science is what leads to revolutions, and that revolutions can only occur through the continuous efforts of normal science. Biological evolution is characterized in similar terms: The adherents of punctuated equilibrium emphasize the prominence of periods of stasis surrounding bursts of change, and thus resemble Kuhn in their thinking, whereas the neo-Darwinians emphasize the continuity of change required for the major evolutionary modifications in form. A middle way may be found in the homoeotic genes, which control pattern formation (see Hunkapiller et al., this volume); point mutations in such genes can create major changes in body form.

How has the immune system evolved? Have there been revolutions, and if so, what are they? The complexity of effector mechanisms activated by specific antigen receptors is particularly difficult to account for. Did the ability to recognize foreign antigen with clonally distributed receptors encoded in rearranging gene segments arise first, with effector mechanisms then diversifying to meet new needs? Or did the immune system develop nonspecific effector mechanisms, to which specific recognition was then added? For various reasons outlined in this section, I believe that the immune system predates the development of specific immunological recognition mediated by clonally distributed receptors. This primitive immune system is still observable in contemporary vertebrate immune systems where it provides a nonclonal form of host defense. Vertebrates have added antigen recognition by clonally distributed receptors to this earlier immune system; this is the true revolution in immunity, and it is noteworthy that it is shared by all vertebrates but has not been detected in any other phylum. I also propound the hypothesis that nonclonal recognition of nonself patterns plays a major role in immune system function and in host defense. The receptors mediating such recognitive events were the original, nonclonal triggers for immune effector mechanisms. If this idea is correct, it could also revolutionize our thinking about immunity by taking us well beyond clonal selection and the Landsteinerian fallacy to an integrated view of immunological recognition and self/nonself discrimination. In this section, I describe what we know of this area presently and point to the areas that need to be examined to validate or refute this notion.

The Evolution of Effector Mechanisms

There are several different effector mechanisms by which the immune response actually rids the body of infectious agents following specific recognition via antibody or T-cell receptors. As summarized in Table 1, each of these mechanisms exists today in vertebrates in a form that is inducible by means independent of specific antigen recognition. Furthermore, each of these mechanisms is faithfully paralleled by effector mechanisms triggered by receptors encoded in rearranging genes that recognize antigen specifically. A clear example of this principle is seen in the complement system. The alternative pathway of complement activation is a powerful effector mechanism that is selectively triggered by differences in the structure of bacterial as compared to host cell membranes; host cells are further protected by a series of cell surface and soluble proteins that accelerate the breakdown of activated complement components bound to them. The specific arm of this effector system, the classic complement pathway, is initiated by antibody binding to antigen, usually on a cell surface; the proteins of this pathway, with the exception of the components of C1 required to recognize the bound antibody, are encoded by genes that arose by duplication from genes encoding the components of the alternative pathway. It seems almost certain that the alternative pathway of complement activation arose first in evolution, even though it was characterized later and thus named "alternative." Specificity, in the form of complement-fixing antibodies, was later engrafted onto this pathway, presumably to enhance self/nonself discrimination and to promote fixation of complement on surfaces that have developed resistance to alternative pathway activation, such as encapsulated bacteria. Deficiencies of components in one of the two pathways illustrate this nicely. Likewise,

natural killer cells and cytolytic T lymphocytes appear to share most of their lytic machinery. However, natural killer cells can only act on cells infected by certain viruses, whereas the presence of the T-cell receptor allows cytolytic T lymphocytes to detect virtually any virally infected cell by the presence of viral peptide/class I MHC complexes on the infected cell's surface. Thus, it appears that the effector mechanism existed prior to the development of specific antigen receptors and that antigen receptors added to preexisting effector mechanisms enhanced the precision and broadened the scope of recognition that could trigger these effector mechanisms. The clonal distribution of receptors also allowed the development of immunological memory.

The Nonclonal Origins of the Immune System

If effector mechanisms used by lymphocytes in contemporary vertebrate immune systems derived from primitive immune systems lacking the rearranging receptor gene families that allow for clonal selection, how was effector function regulated in primitive organisms? The most likely possibility is that primitive effector cells bear receptors that allow recognition of certain pathogen-associated molecular patterns that are not found in the host. I term these receptors *pattern recognition receptors*. In this section, I argue that pattern recognition receptors are still an important part of vertebrate immune systems. However, because they are not clonally distributed on lymphocytes, they do not confer immunological memory, the hallmark of the specific immune response. Possible examples of pattern recognition receptors would be the uncharacterized receptors that allow natural killer cells to discriminate between target cells, the antigen-presenting cell receptors acted upon by adjuvants to induce second signals, and the many T-cell surface molecules of unknown specificity that can induce T-cell activation upon cross-linking (Table 2). I propose that these pattern recognition systems activated effector functions of primitive immune systems prior to the development of rearranging gene families and continue to play a role in host defense today.

Within the confines of the clonal selection theory of immunity, it is not allowable for these T-cell surface receptors to initiate or mediate an immune response. However, I think we may be on the verge of a new revolution in immunological thinking, in which we will discover that these T-cell surface molecules are in fact the original recognition units of the immune system. They are not clonally distributed. They can, however,

Table 1. Effector Mechanisms in Immunity, Nonspecific and Specific

Nonspecific effector mechanism	Specific effector mechanism
Alternative complement cascade	antibody + classic complement cascade
Phagocytosis	antibody + Fc-receptor-induced phagocytosis
C-reactive protein	specific antibody to phosphocholine
Macrophage sequestration	T-dependent macrophage activation
Natural killer cells	cytolytic T cells

Table 2. T-cell Surface Molecules That Can Cause Activation upon Cross-linking by Antibody

T-cell receptor ($\alpha:\beta$ and $\gamma:\delta$)
Thy-1
CD2
CD23
CD27
CD28
CD43
CD44
CD45
CD54
CD73
Ly6

(For review, see Shaw 1989.)

induce T-cell activation upon cross-linking. It has been proposed that one of these structures, CD43, may recognize bacterial carbohydrate presented on the surface of a specific B cell and allow any T cell to provide help to carbohydrate-specific B cells by triggering the release of lymphokines (Rosen 1989). This nonclonal analysis of CD4 T-cell function and evolution is shown schematically in Figure 4. This explanation has three virtues. First, it provides a postulated function for the many triggering molecules found on T-cell surfaces.

Second, it provides a mechanism to explain the evolution of the immune system, in which specific recognition of antigen by clonally distributed receptors encoded in rearranging gene segments is a late addition to an already elaborate system of pattern recognition by nonclonally distributed receptors encoded in single, nonrearranging genes. Third, it directs one's attention to certain types of ligand for these receptor molecules.

What kinds of ligands or patterns should such nonclonally distributed receptors recognize? I think likely that such receptors will recognize general structural patterns in molecules found in many microorganisms, but not in the multicellular organisms in which this system of defense evolved. Recognition of such structural differences allows the evolutionary selection of those receptors that can efficiently discriminate self from nonself. The pattern recognized should be the product of a complex and critical enzymology in the microorganism. Complex cell wall carbohydrates or lipopolysaccharides are likely ligands. Such structures, unlike the proteins recognized as peptide/MHC complexes by the T-cell receptor, would require multiple mutations and major evolutionary shifts on the part of the microorganism to evade recognition. Presumably, over evolutionary time, the receptors would reach a

〈, ⊏ Non-clonal pattern receptors

丫, Ψ Clonal, rearranging receptors

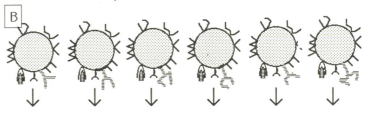

Non-Clonal Response to Pattern

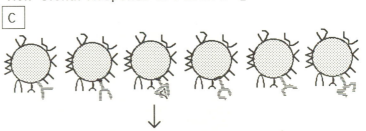

Non-Clonal Response to Pattern

Specific, Clonal Response to Ligand + Co-Stimulator

Figure 4. The development of the immune system. Panel *A* illustrates the proposed nature of lymphocytes in pre-vertebrates. Such cells have several different pattern recognition receptors distributed nonclonally. All such cells can respond to a particular pattern, leading to a protective immune response to a microorganism expressing that pattern. Panels *B* and *C* illustrate the proposed nature of the vertebrate immune system, in which clonally distributed receptors deriving from rearranging receptor genes have been added to cells that retain the pattern recognition receptors of their pre-vertebrate ancestors. In panel *B*, all such cells retain the ability to respond to a particular pattern, leading to protective immunity to microbes expressing that pattern. This type of response does not lead to clonal expansion and, thus, cannot lead to immunological memory. In panel *C*, the response to a specific ligand, recognized by a clonally distributed receptor encoded in rearranging receptor genes, generates specific immunity, clonal expansion, and immunological memory, provided the appropriate costimulatory activity is also present. Both types of response may be important in protective immunity.

standoff with the microorganism at a stage where the possibilities for change in the microorganism have been severely reduced. This form of self/nonself discrimination may be reflected in natural killer cells as well; it has recently been reported that such cells can directly kill many kinds of bacteria (Garcia-Penarrubia et al. 1989). It is of interest in this regard that cloned cytolytic T-cell lines frequently acquire phenotypic properties of natural killer cells, suggesting a close evolutionary relationship of these two cell types. Finally, it may be worth noting that this nonclonal form of immunity is perhaps preferable to clonal selection in smaller organisms that have a limited number of cells available to mount an immune response. In small organisms, a vast potential repertoire distributed clonally in a small number of cells could lead to significant holes or defects in recognitive potential; this difficulty is mitigated if all immunologically competent cells in such an organism can recognize major patterns in pathogens. The disadvantage of such nonclonal responsiveness is that pattern recognition receptors do not discriminate one form of nonself from another and thus are not able to demonstrate clonal selection or its most critical consequence, immunological memory.

B cells also fit this schema. The well-known responses of B cells to polyclonal B-cell activators, such as lipopolysaccharide, presumably represent the action of nonclonally distributed pattern recognition receptors on the B cell. These responses were well characterized in a paper delivered at the 1976 Cold Spring Harbor Symposium by Goran Moller (1976). Moller describes how such responsiveness can be used to elicit specific antibody responses to bacteria, a proposition wholly in keeping with the present analysis.

The immune system appears to have originated as a set of effector cells having multiple distinct receptors that discriminate self from infectious nonself by recognition of patterns found exclusively on microorganisms. In some cases, cells having these characteristics appear to have persisted in contemporary vertebrate immune systems: The action of natural killer cells and macrophage engulfment of certain microorganisms show that infectious nonself can be recognized and destroyed by cells lacking clonally distributed receptors. I argue that most or all cells in the immune system retain this capacity; however, it is usually obscured by the more dramatic responses elicited via the clonally distributed antigen receptors borne by these same cells. This interpretation provides an explanation for the evolution of the complex immune system of vertebrates and for the presence of many molecules of unknown function on lymphocyte surfaces. Experimental verification of this hypothesis is not available.

How Did the Requirement for Signal Two Evolve?

I have proposed above that effector mechanisms to combat infection evolved prior to the evolution of recognitive mechanisms based on rearranging receptors. I have further argued that these effector mechanisms were activated by nonclonally distributed receptors whose specificity developed over evolutionary time to recognize patterns found on the surfaces of large groups of microorganisms. Likewise, I believe that the requirement for a signal delivered from another cell, now called signal two in studies of lymphocyte activation, predates the development of the rearranging receptors that deliver signal one. In modern vertebrates, there are clear examples of cell activation triggered by the action of microorganisms on host cells occurring independently of specific antigen recognition. These are listed in Table 3. Lipopolysaccharide acts on macrophages to induce the production of IL-1, IL-6, and tumor necrosis factor. These molecules in turn act on other cells to induce production of primitive antibody-like molecules such as the phosphocholine-binding, complement-fixing C-reactive protein from hepatocytes. IL-1 and IL-6 are also important costimulators for T-cell activation. Viruses induce the production of interferons α and β, which, in addition to being directly antiviral, also activate natural killer cells. These activated natural killer cells can be documented to play a role in the early elimination of virally infected cells. Recently, a patient with a primary deficiency in natural killer cells has been described who has a profound susceptibility to infections with herpesviruses (Biron et al. 1989). These infections are eventually well controlled in this individual by the production of antibody and cytolytic T cells, but the importance of the natural killer cells in providing the time for these clonally specific responses to develop is clearly emphasized by the intensity of the illness provoked by these viral agents.

The above examples suggest that second signals, that is, lymphocyte-activating signals derived from other host cells, evolved prior to the development of rearranging receptor genes. The substances that trigger second-signal expression, such as lipopolysaccharide, do so very rapidly and do not require recognition by rearranging, clonally distributed receptors. The specificity of these responses for particular bacterial structures suggests that there must be a system for the

Table 3. Responses Directly Stimulated by Microorganisms

Stimulus	Initial cellular response	Induced secondary cellular responses
Lipopolysaccharide	macrophage release of IL-1, IL-6, and TNF	IL-6: acute-phase protein from hepatocytes TNF: alteration of blood flow IL-1, IL-6: T-cell activation
Virus	release of interferons	resistance to viral replication activation of natural killer cells

recognition of these inducers of second signals, again based on pattern recognition rather than on the type of specificity we associate with the immune system. Such receptors must be distributed nonclonally on all antigen-presenting cells. These two characteristics of broad specificity and nonclonal distribution are required to avoid the danger of nonresponsiveness. As in the case of pattern recognition receptors on lymphocytes, these antigen-presenting cell receptors mediate the discrimination of self from infectious nonself.

How Did Immunological Recognition Evolve?

I have outlined my ideas about self/nonself discrimination by primitive, nonclonally distributed pattern recognition receptors on lymphocytes and antigen-presenting cells. I have presented evidence that these receptors are still present on the lymphocytes and antigen-presenting cells we study today, in mouse, rat, chicken, human, and other species. Furthermore, the requirement that lymphocytes receive two signals for activation is probably also present in this primitive response system. However, an immune system based only on pattern recognition has certain severe limitations. First, any new microbial pattern requires the development of a new receptor. Second, the total number of different receptors a single cell can express may be limited. Third, and perhaps most important, such a system does not allow the development of immunological memory. Thus, prior experience with an infectious agent confers no protection against reinfection.

The true revolution in immunity occurred when such cells developed the capacity to make clonally distributed, highly variable receptors by rearrangement of receptor gene segments. For the first time, precise self/nonself discrimination could be applied to all molecules and not just to dominant microbial patterns. Second, any new pattern could be recognized immediately by the host due to the diversity of receptors deriving from genetic processes in somatic cells. Third, through clonal distribution of receptors, immunological memory became a possibility, allowing more rapid and effective clearance of a second infection with any agent. It seems unlikely that all of the seven known rearranging gene families arose at once; rather, I would envision a step-wise evolution of immunological recognition.

First, as outlined above, cells bearing nonclonally distributed, pattern recognition receptors were selected by standard evolutionary mechanisms. Organisms developing the ability to recognize and destroy a pathogenic microbe would survive, whereas those that failed to do so were lost. From this arose the multiplicity of pattern recognition receptors and effector mechanisms that are retained by our lymphocytes. These receptor/ligand systems need to be characterized. Although some T-cell surface molecules with receptor characteristics, such as CD2 (see Dustin et al.; Brown et al.; Reinherz et al.; all this volume), recognize self-ligands and are involved in cell interactions, many may recognize external ligands as well.

Second, some mechanism for using genetic information more efficiently may have developed. A possible example of this is CD45, a molecule having an extracellular domain encoded in several exons that can be spliced differentially to give rise to at least eight distinct extracellular protein domains, connected to an invariant cytoplasmic domain with signal transducing capability in the form of a tyrosine phosphatase. The ligand(s) for CD45 is presently unknown.

The T-cell receptor γ/δ system has some characteristics that suggest that it was the first rearranging receptor system to arise in evolution (Janeway et al. 1988a). It has all the complexity found in the other receptor families but is represented in fewer gene segments. Cells bearing highly restricted forms of this receptor predominate in various epithelia (see Tonegawa et al., this volume), a tissue more prominent in primitive multicellular organisms. There appears to be a type of pattern recognition in this receptor system, with recognition of conserved bacterial proteins like heat shock proteins being a current dominant theme (Holoshitz et al. 1989; Janis et al. 1989; O'Brien et al. 1989). However, these cells share with T cells recognition of MHC molecules and the ability to kill and to secrete cytokines (Matis et al. 1987; Bonneville et al. 1989). Again, determining the ligand specificity of the different γ/δ receptors is a high priority for future studies.

The α/β T-cell receptor probably arose directly from the γ/δ receptors; the intimate chromosomal relationship of the α and δ gene clusters in mouse and man point strongly in this direction. These receptors are predominant in the internal milieu, and they recognize and discriminate a seemingly infinite variety of antigens in the form of peptide/self-MHC products. These systems are described in detail in this volume.

Antibodies may have evolved last, albeit shortly after T-cell receptors, since they are found in all modern vertebrates. There are additional specializations in antibody molecules, such as the ability to be both surface receptors and soluble molecules, bivalency, isotypy, and somatic mutation that all suggest further specialization of these molecules and the genes that encode them. Furthermore, antibody production to most antigens is highly T-cell dependent.

In summary, rearranging, clonally distributed, antigen-specific receptors that discriminate not only self from nonself, but also nonself A from nonself B, appear to have arisen late in evolution. Such receptors provide exquisite specificity to a primitive but nevertheless complex system of effector cells bearing a multitude of distinct pattern recognition receptors that themselves confer a distinct system of self/nonself discrimination on immunologically competent cells. This earlier system persists today and accounts for many attributes of the immune system; one critical attribute is the requirement for induced second signals in T- and B-cell activation. The trigger for these second signals is usually a microbial product, supplied by the immunologist studying the response to a Landsteinerian antigen in the form of the bacterial component of his adjuvant of choice. A critical consequence of this interpretation is that it extends self/nonself discrimination beyond clonal selection. It proposes that the system predominantly discriminates infectious nonself from noninfectious self by means of a system of pattern recognition receptors.

CONCLUSION

The first revolution in immunological thinking came when the advocates of the humoral theory of immunity, that is, immunity mediated by antibodies, vanquished Metchnikov and the cellularists, who believed that phagocytosis was the essential aspect of immunity (see Silverstein 1989). The thinking of the humoralist school so dominated immunology that cells were largely ignored until Burnet's clonal selection theory dramatically placed them back on center stage. However, the clonal selection theory so dominantly focused our collective thinking on clonal mechanisms of self/nonself discrimination that we lost sight of the possibility that other more Metchnikovian, nonclonal forms of self/nonself discrimination were possible and perhaps even important. What clonal selection usually addresses is not self/nonself discrimination but rather discrimination of substance A from substance B (see Nossal and Lederberg 1958), the analysis of which was the dominant theme of Landsteiner's work. In consequence of the dominance of these ideas, innate immunity has usually been treated as a minor curiosity, shunted to the beginning or the end of treatises on immunology, and given short shrift in study sections bound and determined to spare no effort first to solve the antibody problem and later the T-cell receptor and MHC-restricted antigen recognition problems. The approach to the asymptote in our understanding of immunological recognition based on clonal selection and rearranging receptor gene families, so beautifully brought together in this symposium as in its predecessors, lays the groundwork for a new immunology. This immunology will integrate innate and induced immunity by providing explanations for the requirement for induced second signals, for the myriad of T-cell surface molecules with triggering capabilities, and for the dual nature of self/nonself discrimination that includes a role for receptors that recognize patterns of microbial structure. This integrated immunology will require a rediscovery of microbiology by immunologists and a new approach to lymphocyte activation incorporating specific and nonspecific signals.

Beyond this immunology, which can be studied largely at the level of single cells (or cell pairs) and molecules, lies the immunology that was to be in Jerne's introduction to the 1976 Cold Spring Harbor Symposium. Jerne stated at that time: "The common sense of immunology in 1976 retains clonal selection as one of its simpler notions, but cooperative and suppressive clonal interactions have now become the dominant themes. Regulatory feedback is no longer thought to proceed only within clones: it is now clear that different clones speak to one another." This is a far cry from the immunology of the 1989 symposium. Today, we are strict clonalists all, and interclonal communication is viewed as a special case reserved mainly for T-cell/B-cell cooperation leading to specific antibody production. Interclonal regulatory phenomena are not on the agenda of this symposium. Nevertheless, it seems likely that regulation beyond simple antigen clearance does exist, and that, as Jerne predicted in 1976, interclonal communication will provide, once the molecules are defined, a rich area for investigating the sociology of lymphocytes, their population dynamics, the multiple roles of the multitude of lymphokines, and that most vexing of immunological problems, the control of repertoire structure (Jerne 1974). At this symposium, we are grappling with clonal selectionist aspects of repertoire only, with the exception of the fascinating problem of positive selection of self-MHC restriction in the thymus (for discussion, see Marrack et al., this volume). Only when such systems questions are answered can we begin to feel that we understand the immune system, that we are truly approaching the asymptote.

One can foresee at least three new symposium topics just on the basis of what little we know today: the enzymology of gene rearrangement in somatic cells; pattern recognition by lymphocytes and antigen-presenting cells; and the sociology of lymphocytes. It is my hope to attend these future symposia in the pleasant surroundings and lively intellectual atmosphere that the leaders of the Cold Spring Harbor Laboratory have provided to scientists annually for the past 54 years. These symposia (from the Greek "a drinking together") are aptly named: We drink together the knowledge of our collective experience, and distill new ideas in the lecture halls, meeting rooms, and on the lawns and beaches of this magnificent institution.

ACKNOWLEDGMENTS

I thank John Inglis and Jim Watson for asking me to prepare this introduction and for helpful suggestions as to its content and organization. I also thank the introducers and summarizers of previous symposia on the immune system for their thoughts and words, which I have both used and abused. Kim Bottomly, Michael Edidin, and Ron Germain were most helpful with comments on drafts of this manuscript.

REFERENCES

Amit, A.G., R.A. Mariuzza, S.E.V. Phillips, and R.J. Poljak. 1986. Three-dimensional structure of an antigen-antibody complex at 2.8Å resolution. *Science* **233**: 747.

Biron, C.A., K.S. Byron, and J.L. Sullivan. 1989. Severe herpes virus infections in an adolescent without natural killer cells. *N. Engl. J. Med.* **320**: 1731.

Bjorkman, P.J., M.A. Saper, B. Samraoui, W.S. Bennet, J.S. Strominger, and D.C. Wiley. 1987. The foreign antigen binding site and T cell recognition regions of class I histocompatibility antigens. *Nature* **329**: 512.

Bonneville, M., K. Ito, E.G. Krecko, S. Itohara, D.Kappes, I. Ishida, O. Kanagawa, C.A. Janeway, Jr., D.B. Murphy, and S. Tonegawa. 1989. Recognition of a self MHC TL region product by γδ T cell receptors. *Proc. Natl. Acad. Sci.* **86:** 5928.

Bretscher, P. and M. Cohn. 1970. A theory of self-nonself discrimination. *Science* **169:** 1042.

Burnet, F.M. 1959. *The clonal selection theory of immunity.* Vanderbilt University Press, Nashville, Tennessee.

———. 1967. The impact of ideas on immunology. *Cold Spring Harbor Symp. Quant. Biol.* **32:** 1.

Charbonneau, H., N.D. Tonks, K.E. Walsh, and E.H. Fischer. 1988. The leukocyte common antigen (CD45): A putative receptor-linked protein tyrosine phosphatase. *Proc. Natl. Acad. Sci.* **85:** 7182.

Edelman, G.M. 1976. Summary: Understanding selective molecular recognition. *Cold Spring Harbor Symp. Quant. Biol.* **41:** 891.

Garcia-Penarrubia, P., F.T. Koster, R.O. Kelley, T.D. McDowell, and A.D. Bankhurst. 1989. Antibacterial activity of human natural killer cells. *J. Exp. Med.* **169:** 99.

Germain, R.N. 1986. The ins and outs of antigen processing and presentation. *Nature* **322:** 687.

Greenbaum, L., J.B. Horowitz, A. Woods, T. Pasqualini, E.-P. Reich, and K. Bottomly. 1988. Autocrine growth of CD4⁺ T cells: Differential effects of IL-1 on helper and inflammatory T cells. *J. Immunol.* **140:** 1555.

Holoshitz, J., F. Koning, J.E. Coligan, J. De Bruyn, and S. Strober. 1989. Isolation of CD4⁻, CD8⁻ mycobacteria-reactive T lymphocyte clones from rheumatoid arthritis synovial fluid. *Nature* **339:** 226.

Janeway, C.A., L. Apt, and D. Gitlin. 1953. Agammaglobulinemia. *Trans. Assoc. Am. Physicians* **66:** 200.

Janeway, C.A., Jr. 1988. Frontiers of the immune system. *Nature* **333:** 804.

Janeway, C.A., Jr., B. Jones, and A. Hayday. 1988a. Specificity and function of T cells bearing γδ receptors. *Immunol. Today* **9:** 73.

Janeway, C.A., Jr., S. Carding, B. Jones, J. Murray, P. Portoles, R. Rasmussen, J. Rojo, K. Saizawa, J. West, and K. Bottomly. 1988b. CD4⁺ T cells: Specificity and function. *Immunol. Rev.* **101:** 39.

Janis, E.M., S.H.E. Kaufman, R.H. Schwartz, and D.M. Pardoll. 1989. Activation of γδ T cells in the primary immune response to *Mycobacterium tuberculosis. Science* **244:** 713.

Jenkins, M.K., D.M. Pardoll, J. Mizuguchi, H. Quill, and R.H. Schwartz. 1987. T-cell unresponsiveness in vivo and in vitro: Fine specificity of induction and molecular characterization of the unresponsive state. *Immunol. Rev.* **95:** 113.

Jerne, N.K. 1967. Summary: Waiting for the end. *Cold Spring Harbor Symp. Quant. Biol.* **32:** 591.

———. 1971. The somatic generation of immune recognition. *Eur. J. Immunol.* **1:** 1.

———. 1974. Towards a network theory of the immune system. *Ann. Immunol.* **125C:** 373.

———. 1976. The common sense of immunology. *Cold Spring Harbor Symp. Quant. Biol.* **41:** 1.

Kantor, F.S., A. Ojeda, and B. Benacerraf. 1963. Studies on artificial antigens. I. Antigenicity of DNP-poly-lysine and DNP-copolymers of lysine and glutamic acid in guinea pigs. *J. Exp. Med.* **117:** 55.

Kappler, J.W., N. Roehm, and P. Marrack. 1987. T cell tolerance by clonal elimination in the thymus. *Cell* **49:** 273.

Katz, D.H., T. Hamaoka, M.E. Dorf, P.H. Maurer, and B. Benacerraf. 1973. Cell interactions between histoincompatible T and B lymphocytes. IV. Involvement of the immune response (Ir) gene in the control of lymphocyte interactions in responses controlled by the gene. *J. Exp. Med.* **138:** 734.

Kaye, J., S. Gillis, S.B. Mizel, E.M. Shevach, T.R. Malek, C.A. Dinarello, L.B. Lachman, and C.A. Janeway, Jr. 1984. Growth of a cloned helper T cell line induced by a monoclonal antibody specific for the antigen receptor: Interleukin 1 is required for the expression of receptors for interleukin 2. *J. Immunol.* **133:** 1339.

Kuhn, T.S. 1970. *The structure of scientific revolutions,* 2nd edition, revised. The University of Chicago Press, Chicago, Illinois.

Landsteiner, K. 1945. *The specificity of serological reactions.* Harvard University Press, Cambridge, Massachusetts.

Lassila, O., O. Vainio, and P. Matzinger. 1988. Can B cells turn on virgin T cells? *Nature* **334:** 253.

Macatonia, S.E., P.M. Taylor, S.C. Knight, and B.A. Askonas. 1989. Primary stimulation by dendritic cells induces anti-viral proliferative and cytotoxic T cell responses in vitro. *J. Exp. Med.* **169:** 1255.

Matis, L.A., R.Q. Cron, and J.A. Bluestone. 1987. Major histocompatibility complex-linked specificity of γδ receptor-bearing T lymphocytes. *Nature* **330:** 262.

Matzinger, P. and S. Guerder. 1989. Does T cell tolerance require a dedicated antigen-presenting cell? *Nature* **338:** 74.

Metcalf, E.S. and N.R. Klinman. 1976. In vitro tolerance induction of neonatal murine spleen cells. *J. Exp. Med.* **143:** 1327.

Mitchison, N.A. 1971. The carrier effect in the secondary response to hapten protein conjugates. II. Cellular cooperation. *Eur. J. Immunol.* **1:** 18.

Moller, G. 1976. Mechanism of B cell activation and self-nonself discrimination. *Cold Spring Harbor Symp. Quant. Biol.* **41:** 217.

Morrison, L.A., A.E. Lukacher, V.L. Braciale, D.P. Fan, and T.J. Braciale. 1986. Differences in antigen presentation to MHC class I- and class II-restricted influenza virus-specific cytolytic T lymphocyte clones. *J. Exp. Med.* **163:** 903.

Nemazee, D.A. and K. Burki. 1989. Clonal deletion of B lymphocytes in a transgenic mouse bearing anti-MHC class I antibody genes. *Nature* **337:** 562.

Nossal, G.J.V. and J. Lederberg. 1958. Antibody production by single cells. *Nature* **181:** 1419.

O'Brien, R.L., M.P. Happ, A. Dallas, E. Palmer, R. Kubo, and W. Born. 1989. Stimulation of a major subset of lymphocytes expressing T cell receptor γδ by an antigen derived from *Mycobacterium tuberculosis. Cell* **57:** 667.

Rosen, F.S. 1989. T cell:B cell collaboration: The response to polysaccharide antigens. *Semin. Immunol.* **1:** 87.

Shaw, S. 1989. Lymphocyte differentiation: Not all in a name. *Nature* **338:** 539.

Shearer. G.M. 1974. Cell mediated cytotoxicity to trinitrophenyl modified syngeneic lymphocytes. *Eur. J. Immunol.* **4:** 527.

Silverstein, A.M. 1989. *A history of immunology.* Academic Press, San Diego, California.

Simonsen, M. 1967. The clonal selection hypothesis evaluated by grafted cells reacting against their hosts. *Cold Spring Harbor Symp. Quant. Biol.* **32:** 517.

Steinman, R.M., J. Metlay, N. Bhardwaj, P. Freudenthal, E. Langhoff, M. Crowley, L. Lau, M. Witmer-Pack, J.W. Young, E. Pure, N. Romani, and K. Inaba. 1989. Dendritic cells: Nature's adjuvant. In *Immunogenicity* (ed. C.A. Janeway et al.). A.R. Liss, New York. (In press.)

Talmage, D.W. 1988. A century of progress: Beyond molecular immunology. *J. Immunol.* **141:** S5.

Tonegawa, S., N. Hozumi, G. Matthyssens, and R. Schuller. 1976. Somatic changes in the content and context of immunoglobulin genes. *Cold Spring Harbor Symp. Quant. Biol.* **41:** 877.

Townsend, A., J. Rothbard, F. Gotch, G. Bahadur, D. Wraith, and A.J. McMichael. 1986. The epitopes of influenza nucleoprotein recognized by cytotoxic T lymphocytes can be defined with short synthetic peptides. *Cell* **44:** 959.

van Ewijk, W., Y. Ron, J. Monaco, J. Kappler, P. Marrack, M. LeMeur, P. Gerlinger, B. Durand, C. Benoist, and D. Mathis. 1988. Compartmentalization of MHC class II gene expression in transgenic mice. *Cell* **53:** 357.

Wilson, D.B., E. Heber-Katz, J. Sprent, and J.C. Howard. 1976. On the possibility of multiple T-cell receptors. *Cold Spring Harbor Symp. Quant. Biol.* **41:** 559.

Implications of the Diversity of the Immunoglobulin Gene Superfamily

T. HUNKAPILLER, J. GOVERMAN, B.F. KOOP, AND L. HOOD

Division of Biology, California Institute of Technology, Pasadena, California 91125

The vertebrate immune response consists of a complex set of cellular and serologic reactions that provide protection from infectious foreign agents and abnormal or damaged cells. Responses to these insults are mediated by a complex array of immune elements that recognize distinct macromolecular structural patterns (antigens). Characterization of these elements over the past two decades has shown that many share a common evolutionary precursor, a gene element encoding the immunoglobulin homology unit (Cunningham et al. 1973; Strominger et al. 1980; Williams 1984; Hood et al. 1985). Recently, a large number of molecules, with no immunologic function and mostly expressed on a cell surface, have also been shown to share this same ancestral element (Williams 1987; Hunkapiller and Hood 1989). Therefore, the genes encoding these related molecules are defined as belonging to the immunoglobulin gene superfamily. Together, these genes encode an amazingly diverse array of functions from immune recognition to cellular adhesion, reflecting the versatility of the shared immunoglobulin homology unit (Fig. 1).

The immunoglobulin gene superfamily includes many unique genes as well as numerous multigene families. The potential to duplicate, delete, and reorganize informational units at all levels in the hierarchal organization of such a superfamily—nucleotides, exons, genes, and even multigene families—increases the possibilities for rapid evolutionary change of complex phenotypic characters. This potential has profoundly affected views about the driving forces of evolution, emphasizing the possibility of rapid acquisition of novel phenotypic traits. Moreover, the fact that the immunoglobulin homology unit is employed in many different types of systems argues that there is an underlying unity of shared strategies for molecular recognition at the cell surface. Thus, the immunoglobulin gene superfamily is a common thread weaving through the complex patterns of eukaryotic biology and evolution.

In this paper, we first define the homology unit and describe the features that lend particular advantage to its use in such a wide range of biological contexts. We illustrate the diversity and combinatorial advantages of the homology unit through a consideration of the strategies of molecular recognition in the immune system. The ability of the homology unit to accommodate tremendous functional flexibility is discussed primarily in the context of nonimmune receptor molecules. We then discuss the evolution of the immunoglobulin gene superfamily and the implications it has for eukaryotic biology.

Immunoglobulin Homology Unit

Molecules are defined as belonging to the immunoglobulin superfamily by the presence of one or more regions homologous to the basic structural unit of immunoglobulins, the immunoglobulin homology unit (Hill et al. 1966) (Fig. 2). These regions are usually between 70 and 110 residues in length and are characterized by a series of nonparallel β strands that generate a compact sandwich of two β sheets (see Amzel and Poljak 1979). This structure is stabilized by a small series of conserved residues, particularly, two virtually invariant cysteine residues that generate a signature disulfide bond holding the faces of the β sheet sandwich together. The loop sequences connecting the β strands are less significant for the basic homology unit structure and therefore, can accommodate extensive variability.

Three distinct types of immunoglobulin homology units have been identified (Williams 1987; Hunkapiller and Hood 1989). These are compared in Figure 3 and are characterized by type-specific amino acid residues and the presence or absence of particular β strands and loop sequences between the two cysteine residues forming the characteristic disulfide bridge. These homology units include the V and C homology units characteristic of the immune-antigen receptors (discussed later), both defined from crystallographic analysis (Fig. 2). The V unit has an extra β-strand pair and loop sequence relative to C units. The extra loop means the V motif can accommodate even greater variability. We have denoted a third unique homology unit type, H. This motif appears to have a more C-like structure, lacking the same β-strand pair and loop, but it has a slightly more V-like sequence. Also, H homology units are the primary motif of various molecules that seem to predate in evolution the molecules of the immune receptors. Hence, V and C units appear to be the more specialized versions, whereas H units more nearly represent the primordial homology unit motif.

The number and functional diversity of molecules incorporating the immunoglobulin homology unit is proof that it has been a tremendously successful protein motif throughout evolution. Four particular factors have contributed to this success (Hunkapiller and

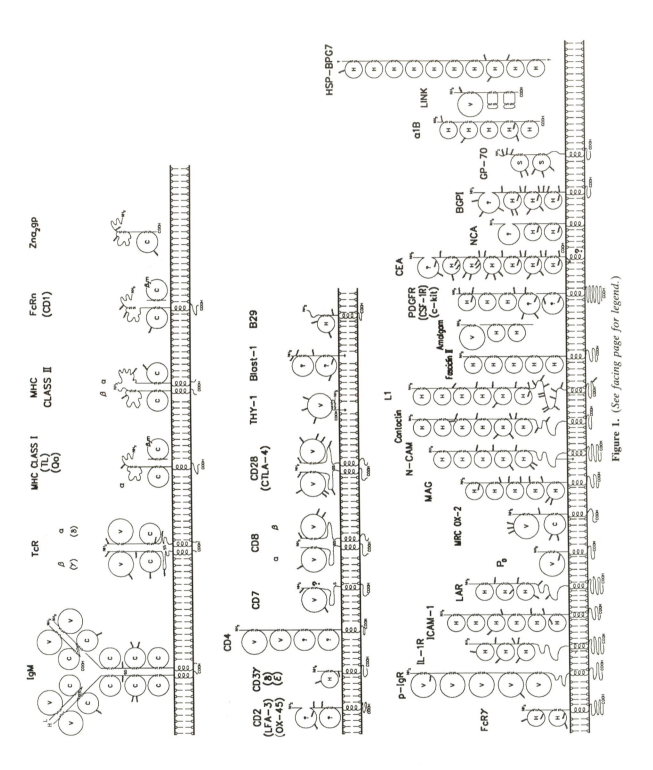

Figure 1. (*See facing page for legend.*)

16

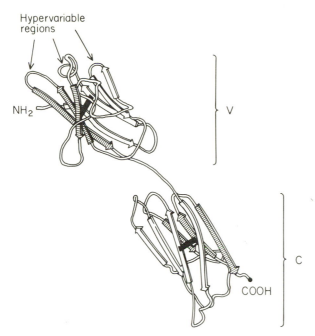

Hypervariable regions

NH₂

V

C

COOH

Figure 2. Tertiary organization of V and C homology units (after Edmundson et al. 1975). This illustrates the tertiary structure of an immunoglobulin light chain. The β strands and their orientations are shown as flat arrows. Opposite faces of the sandwich structure are indicated by either blank or hatched β strands. The disulfide bond is indicated by a solid bar. (Reprinted, with permission, from Hunkapiller and Hood 1989).

Hood 1989). First, apart from the very few conserved residues involved in direct inter- and intrachain interactions, the primary structure of the homology unit can vary dramatically and still generate the same tertiary structure. The loops that connect the β-pleated sheet strands are particularly variable. Thus, because the homology unit is capable of accommodating enormous diversity of primary sequence, it can be the structural foundation for an equally enormous array of highly specific interactions. Second, the tertiary structure of the homology unit is such that homology units tend to interact with one another. This impacts both the development of the homo- and/or heterotypic dimers that are the basis of many receptor structures as well as the protein-protein interactions between different or the same immunoglobulin superfamily members. Combinatorial associations between different protein chains mediated by homology unit interactions increase both the evolutionary and somatic diversification potentials of the gene systems involved. Such interactions should favor the establishment of new functional associations between existing members of the immunoglobulin gene superfamily. The third feature that contributes to the evolutionary advantage of the homology unit is its striking stability. It must be an effective cell-surface display structure for molecular recognition, and, as such, it must be resistant to proteolytic digestion by the enzymes that bathe these external receptors. Thus, the need for a compact, globular structure resistant to proteolysis may have been the initial driving force in the evolution of the homology unit. Finally, most homology units are encoded by discrete exons. The 3' end of each exon ends with the first base of the next codon, whereas each 5' end has the last two bases. These conserved splicing rules ensure correct, in-frame translation of any number of tandemly encoded units regardless of their order. These exons, therefore, serve as a basic unit of evolutionary diversification.

Molecular Recognition in the Immune System

There are four distinct classes of immune receptors, molecules that interact directly with antigen. The immunoglobulin homology unit was first recognized during the study of antibodies, the immunoreceptors of B cells (Hill et al. 1966). Antibodies can be either fixed to the cell surface or expressed humorally; that is, secreted into the blood to carry out their functions at a distance from the cell of origin. T cells, on the other hand, synthesize only a surface-bound antigen receptor. There are also two classes of receptors encoded within the major histocompatibility complex (MHC). Class I MHC molecules are present in varying amounts on virtually all somatic cells. Class II MHC molecules are expressed only on particular antigen-presenting cells (discussed later) such as macrophages and B cells. The multiple roles played by the homology units in these molecules dramatically reflect the versatility of the basic motif.

The basic structure of antibodies is a tetramer composed of identical heterodimers of a light and a heavy chain (Fig. 1) (see Klein 1982). The antibody molecule is divided into variable (V) domains that are responsible for pattern recognition and constant (C) domains that carry out various effector functions. The V domain is constructed of one V homology unit from both the light (V_L) and heavy (V_H) chains. The C region of light chains (C_L) likewise has only a single C homology unit, whereas the C region of heavy chains (C_H) has two to four C homology units, depending on the type of heavy

Figure 1. Schematic diagram of the members of the immunoglobulin gene superfamily (IgGSF). Disulfide bonds are represented by (S–S). Homology units are indicated as loops labeled V, C, or H (see text). Loops of uncertain relationship to homology units are labeled with a question mark. Different-sized loops illustrate the relative differences in length between the conserved disulfide bond of the labeled types. Membrane-spanning peptides are shown as simple helices. Glycophospholipid linkage to the membrane is represented as an arrow. Intracytoplasmic regions are drawn with wavy lines that indicate their relative lengths. Extra- and intracellular orientations are indicated by NH₂ and COOH labels on the protein chains, respectively. Possible asparagine-linked carbohydrates are shown as jagged lines extending from the protein chains. Note that these sites are not necessarily conserved between alleles or across species, but are representative of at least one known example of the labeled protein. Related IgGSF members are illustrated with a single structure, as indicated by the name labels above each structure. For a description of the molecules and their references, see Hunkapiller and Hood (1989).

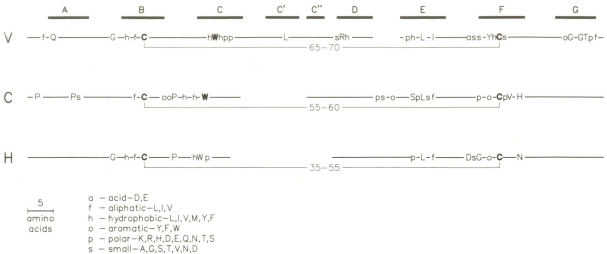

Figure 3. Sequence motifs of each homology unit type. This figure illustrates idealized aligned examples of each homology unit type. Representative amino acid residues of each type are shown in their relative position along the polypeptides. Uppercase letters are single-letter amino acid code. Lowercase letters represent a selection of amino acids with similar functional or physical properties. The key to this code is shown in the lower left. Relative gaps are introduced into each chain to align residues conserved between types. The more nearly invariant cysteine and tryptophan residues are highlighted. The distances between the conserved cysteine residues are shown beneath each chain. The approximate locations of the β strands are illustrated with heavy bars above the sequence representations. Note the two β strands (C' and C'') not found in the C and H domains. It is also clear that β strand D may not be found in the shorter H domain sequences. (Reprinted, with permission, from Hunkapiller and Hood 1989).

chain. As with the V regions, pairs of C-region homology units interact to form discrete structural domains. There are several different C_H genes, each of which defines a different class or isotype of immunoglobulin. Different effector functions and interactions are mediated by different classes of antibodies and facilitate the destruction or elimination of antigen or antigen-associated pathogens.

The T-cell antigen receptor is a simple heterodimer with one V domain involved in antigen recognition and one C domain that interacts with a membrane-bound protein complex, CD3, presumably involved in signal transduction (Fig. 1) (see Davis 1985; Kronenberg et al. 1986). T cells responsible for general antigen recognition use α and β chains (see Hannum et al. 1984; Meuer et al. 1984). A small subset of T cells employs γ and δ chains (Bank et al. 1986; Brenner et al. 1986; Ioannidis et al. 1987). The function of the γ/δ cells is unclear, but some form of interaction with particular antigens appears likely (e.g., Matis et al. 1987). Unlike B cells, T cells do not express different isotypes. Rather, there are subsets of T cells that use common receptor recognition gene elements, but have different functional responses upon activation, presumably due to the expression of other, subset-specific gene products. This is consequent with the lack of direct effector function of the T-cell receptor itself. Cytotoxic T cells (T_C) destroy altered or damaged cells, often as the result of viral infections or neoplastic transformation. Helper T cells (T_H) facilitate the differentiation and activation of B cells and other T cells and, accordingly, play a central role in the regulatory and developmental processes of the immune system.

The primary sequences responsible for antigenic interaction and specificity in immunoglobulins are the four relatively hypervariable loop sequences between the β strands of the V homology unit faces (see Amzel and Poljak 1979). Homologous sequences are presumed to function the same for T-cell receptors (Goverman et al. 1986; Novotný et al. 1986). These hypervariable regions make up the antigen-binding pocket or cleft (Wu and Kabat 1970; Capra and Kehoe 1974) and, consequently, play a critical role in determining the antigen-specific repertoire. The ability of V regions to accommodate diversity is illustrated by the fact that even V gene regions of the same gene family can have less than 20% amino acid similarity.

Molecular recognition in the T and B cell systems is mediated by distinctly different mechanisms. Antibodies recognize the native three-dimensional structure of macromolecules by virtue of their molecular complementarity to the foreign structural pattern. T cells expressing α/β receptors, on the other hand, recognize only peptide fragments of antigens when they are bound by a receptor encoded in the MHC expressed on an antigen-presenting cell (see Schwartz 1984). As a result, T-cell activation requires the formation of a trimolecular complex, the T-cell receptor recognizing portions of both the antigenic peptide and the MHC molecule. Thus, the complex ligand of the T-cell receptor bears no necessary structural similarity to the native antigenic protein. This requirement for direct cell-cell interaction to activate T cells is perhaps the primary operational distinction between T and B cells and is critical to the regulatory role played by T cells in the immune response.

A major aspect of this regulatory role of T cells is establishing and maintaining tolerance to self-antigens. This is accomplished in large part during T-cell development in the thymus as T cells that react strongly to self-molecules are clonally deleted (see Sprent and Webb 1987). A subset of the cells remaining become responsible for regulation of B-cell activation. Communication between B and T cells is established through the role of the B cell as an antigen-presenting cell. That is, B cells bind native antigen with surface-bound immunoglobulin, process the protein, then present denatured fragments via class II MHC molecules to T cells. Thus, T cells are the major arbiters of whether or not B cells proliferate and differentiate to produce quantities of antibodies after they have interacted with their complementary antigen.

There are two unique features shared by both B and T cells. First, through numerous genomic and somatic diversification strategies (discussed later), each set of cells can express an enormous diversity of immune receptors. Second, each individual B and T cell generally expresses only a single clonotype of receptor molecule, a process referred to as allelic exclusion (Luzzati et al. 1973). This clonal expression provides a means whereby each B or T cell can express a unique receptor type with a unique specificity. Therefore, any particular antigen will selectively amplify only the appropriate subset of T or B cells that have complementary receptors. This antigen-specific expansion is referred to as clonal selection. Thus, the primary consequence of allelic exclusion is the ability to regulate finely the immune response to particular antigens in the context of the universe of all possible antigens.

MHC molecules are not classic receptors, in that their association with their ligand peptide does not occur on the cell surface. Rather, the peptides are products of intracytoplasmic enzymatic processing and become associated with MHC molecules before cell-surface expression (see Claverie and Kourilsky 1987). Class I MHC molecules present bound peptide primarily to T_C cells, whereas class II molecules present peptides generally to T_H cells (see Schwartz 1984). The class I molecule is a heterodimer composed of the highly polymorphic class I polypeptide and the invariant, non-MHC-encoded β_2-microglobulin. The class II molecule is a heterodimer composed of two highly polymorphic chains, α and β. All four chains contain one C homology unit (Fig.1) (see Hood et al. 1983). In the case of each pair, the association is mediated by noncovalent interactions of the C homology units. All but β_2-microglobulin also contain other, non-homology unit regions that are responsible for peptide binding and antigen presentation (see Germain and Malissen 1986). Unlike B- and T-cell receptors, each individual expresses only a limited number of different MHC molecules. Therefore, the peptide-binding sites must be very degenerate in order to accommodate the very large number of potential, different peptide fragments. Also, because these genes are not allelically excluded, all the different MHC molecules expressed in an individual are co-expressed on the same cells.

Diversity of the Immune Receptors

The genes encoding antibodies are divided into three unlinked gene families; two encode light chains (λ and κ), and the third encodes heavy chains (Fig. 4) (see Honjo 1983). Likewise, the genes encoding the T-cell receptors are divided into three gene families; two encode the α and β chains, and a third encodes the γ chains (Fig. 4) (Davis 1985; Hayday et al. 1985; Kronenberg et al. 1986). The δ genes are contained within the α-chain locus (Chien et al. 1987). The variable regions of antibodies and T-cell receptors are encoded by two or three gene segments that are separate in the germ line: variable (V) and joining (J) for light, α and γ genes and V, diversity (D), and J for heavy, β and δ genes (Fig. 4). The V, D, and J or V and J elements are brought together through somatic DNA rearrangement events to produce complete, expressible V genes.

A large variety of somatic and evolutionary strategies for diversification are shared by T- and B-cell receptors. The basis of the somatic strategies is the rearrangement process. In mammals, this joining is able to unite virtually any VJ, DJ, or VD gene segments within a family, generating by combinatorial means much greater diversity potential than just the number of germ-line elements would support (Table 1). Also, the joining process itself is imprecise and generates enormous additional molecular diversity at the junctional

Table 1. V Gene Diversity

	α	β	Heavy	κ
V gene segments	100	30	500	200
(subfamilies)	(14)	(17)	(8)	(5)
D gene segments	—	2	15	—
J gene segments	50	6 + 6	4	4
Ds in 3 reading frames	n.a.	++	+	n.a.
N-region sequence	++	++	++	—
Junctional diversity	+++	+++	+++	+
Somatic hypermutation	—	—	+	+
Alternate joining order	—	+?	+?	—
Combinatorial joining	$V \times J$ 100×50	$V \times D \times J$ $(30 \times 3 \times 12)$ $+(30 \times 3 \times 6)$	$V \times D \times J$ $500 \times 15 \times 4$	$V \times J$ 200×4
Total	5000	1620	3×10^4	800
Combinatorial association		$\times$ 8.1×10^6		$\times$ 2.4×10^7

n.a. indicates not applicable.

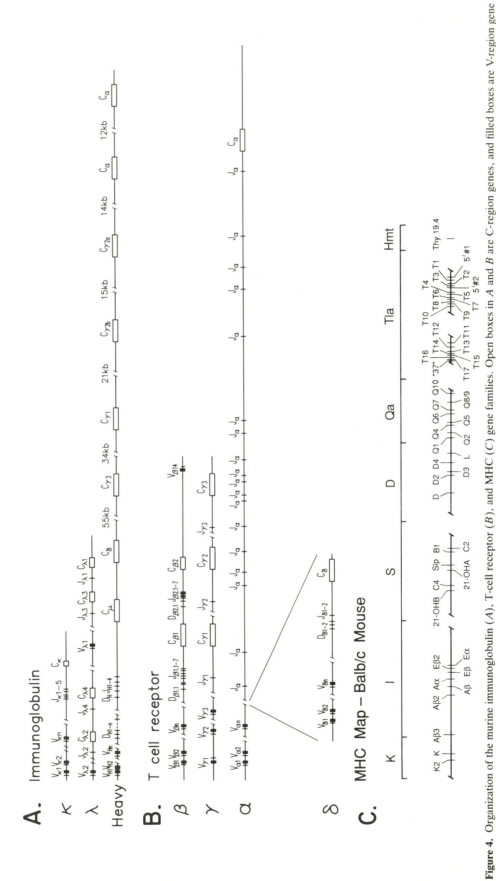

Figure 4. Organization of the murine immunoglobulin (*A*), T-cell receptor (*B*), and MHC (*C*) gene families. Open boxes in *A* and *B* are C-region genes, and filled boxes are V-region gene segments. Vertical lines illustrate D and J gene segments. Numbers between C-region genes in the heavy-chain family are distances in kilobases. Double slashes without numbers indicate unknown distances. Human gene families are organized similarly. The δ gene family is shown as an insert to the α gene family. The MHC map indicates class I regions (e.g., K, I, S, D, Qa, Tla, Hmt), class II regions (A and E), and the complement-associated S-region class III genes. Individual genes are indicated below.

regions through various mechanisms (see Tonegawa 1983; Hunkapiller and Hood 1989). These mechanisms lead to such extreme variability in the junction regions that a window of variability is generated between the V and J elements within which virtually any amino acid may be represented at any position (Elliot et al. 1988; Hunkapiller and Hood 1989). Depending on the gene family, these windows range in size from 3 to 15 residues. This junctional window comprises the third hypervariable loop of the antigen-binding site. Accordingly, variability here has a critical impact on the functional diversity of antibody and T-cell receptor repertoires.

A further mechanism for diversification is a consequence of the fact that essentially any light chain may associate with any heavy chain (or any α with any β). Thus, a final level of molecular diversity is generated through combinatorial association at the polypeptide chain level (Table 1). The fact that the gene families are not linked increases the potential for diversity at the level of populations even further by dissociating the allelism of the families. This provides the possibility, within a population over time, for any V_H allele to combine with any V_L allele.

B cells have an additional mechanism for antigen-specific diversification called somatic hypermutation (Kim et al. 1981; Gearhart and Bogenhagen 1983). This process scatters random single-base substitutions throughout the rearranged V gene, generating variant antibodies with altered affinity for the antigen. Thus, the presence of antigen can selectively expand those B cells producing variant antibodies with an increased affinity for the stimulating antigen. Seen in normal immune responses, this process is called affinity maturation (Gearhart et al. 1981; Clarke et al. 1985; Sablitzky et al. 1985). T cells do not undergo somatic hypermutation. Presumably, this inability to diversify further after leaving the thymus is linked to their role as regulators of the immune response (Barth et al. 1985; Honjo and Habu 1985; Eisen 1986). Clonal deletion of self-reactive T cells occurs during thymic education. If T cells were to mutate randomly their receptors after leaving the thymus, there would be no check on the accidental development of harmful, self-reactive T cells. B cells can take this risk because T cells can still maintain activation control of B cells with receptors for self-antigens.

B cells also employ two other novel strategies for diversifying the immune response potential. However, these do not affect the possible range of antigen specificities, but rather the functional, temporal, and spatial distributions of the possible receptor specificities. Both are related to the lack of any requirement for cell-cell interactions. First, alternative patterns of RNA splicing of heavy-chain transcripts can generate molecules with or without hydrophobic transmembrane regions (Early et al. 1980). Thus, antibodies with the same antigen specificity can be alternatively bound to the cell surface to serve as receptors for the differentiation of B cells or secreted into the blood to serve as end-stage effector molecules. Second, the as-

sembled V_H chain gene can rearrange into juxtaposition with different C_H genes during a process called class switching (Davis et al. 1980). In this manner, the same molecular recognition domain can be expressed with very different kinds of effector or tissue-targeting domains. Thus, the great variability in ligand specificity provided by the V homology unit can be expressed in the context of the functional and structural variability accommodated by the C homology unit.

With the tremendous potential for somatic diversification, the repertoire of unique T- and B-cell receptors generated in one individual is, in theory, limited only by the number of T- and B-progenitor cells that have been generated over the lifetime of that individual. When somatic hypermutation is considered, the potential for variety in antibodies begins to approach the number of actual B cells. This variation is uniquely accommodated by the V homology unit, allowing essentially the somatic tailoring of antigen-receptor repertoires to the current antigenic environment.

Diversity of the MHC genes is based solely on evolutionary mechanisms and the rules of Mendelian genetics. The class I molecules that present antigen in the mouse are encoded by only two or three genes (with a larger number of nonclassic MHC class I genes of unknown function denoted Q, T, and Hmt), and the class II molecules are encoded by two to four α and three to five β genes (Fig. 4) (see Hood et al. 1983; Mengle-Gaw and McDevitt 1985). Those portions of the genes that encode the peptide-binding sites constitute perhaps the most polymorphic non-viral protein-coding sequences known (see Klein and Figueroa 1981). These variations are generated by point mutations as well as recombinational and gene conversion events involving the genes of the non-antigen-binding MHC molecules (see Klein and Figueroa 1986). Thus, although the diversity within populations of expressed collections of MHC molecules can be very large, individuals can only express a relatively small degree of this diversity. The extreme allelism maintained in populations ensures the widest range of variation of peptide-presenting molecules possible for an individual (Hunkapiller and Hood 1989). The class II genes can also generate diversity by combinatorial association of their discrete polypeptide chains. However, the close linkage between the α and β genes tends to reduce this potential within a population.

The diversification strategies of the B- and T-cell receptors, when compared to those of the MHC molecules, reflect basically the different requirements of target and effector cells. B and T cells require clonal expression and specificity in order to respond specifically to antigen. Target cells, on the other hand, must be able to present as wide a range of antigen to the effector cells as possible. Degenerate peptide binding, along with the expression of multiple, highly allelic forms, as with the MHC, accomplishes this.

The mechanisms used for the diversification of these antigen-recognition gene systems operate at the DNA, RNA, and protein levels. This diversity is represented in both the individual and the population as a vast array of different types of molecules employing very different antigen-binding strategies. Most importantly, this ability to respond so specifically to the universe of antigens indicates the tremendous flexibility of the immunoglobulin homology unit in defining both recognition and functional operations.

Features of the Immunoglobulin Gene Superfamily

The immunoglobulin gene superfamily now has more than 40 different identified genes or gene families that fall into a variety of different evolutionary and functional categories (Fig. 1) (Williams 1987; Hunkapiller and Hood 1989). They are expressed by a variety of cell types, including lymphocytes (with an especially large number on T cells), nerve cells, various nervous-system-associated cells, bone-marrow-derived cells, fibroblasts, etc. The superfamily receptors fall into three general categories defined by how they associate with their ligand: homotypic (interaction with an identical subunit), heterotypic (interaction with a nonidentical homology unit), and a ligand without a homology unit. The recognition function of these receptors may be linked to various effector functions such as cellular differentiation or the activation of previously pro-

grammed cellular functions. In other cases, the recognition function serves merely to fix cells in particular positions with respect to other cells through cross-linking of receptor and ligand.

The non-immune receptor members of the immunoglobulin gene superfamily, most of which are involved in molecular recognition at the cell surface, fall into several functionally definable categories (Fig. 5). Morphogenic factors facilitate surface interactions between cells that lead to changes in gene expression and changes in cell movement, shape, and function (e.g., N-CAM, fasciclin II, contactin, MAG, P_0, I-CAM). A second category is represented by kinase growth factor receptors, a specialized group associated with a tyrosine kinase domain (e.g., PDGF receptor, CSF-1 receptor). These molecules play a key role in the proliferation and/or differentiation of specific cell lineages by linking a cascade of intracellular reactions with the recognition of a specific triggering ligand. Third, the specialized differentiation factors include many unrelated molecules responsible for diversity of functions including cellular activation, differentiation, and migration. Many of these molecules facilitate even more complex interactions between other members of the superfamily (e.g., CD3, CD4, CD8). Fourth, the antibody-binding/transport proteins attach to particular C-

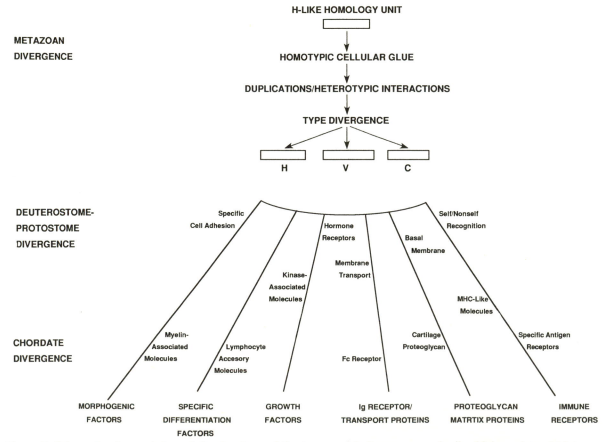

Figure 5. Scheme for the evolution of the functions of the immunoglobulin gene superfamily. Major points of Metazoan divergences are given at the left. Smaller print functions are associated with one of the five major lines of functional categories now evident in the immunoglobulin gene superfamily (see text). The arc is to emphasize that this is not meant to be considered a genealogic tree.

region domains in order to immobilize humoral antibody or ferry specific isotypes across particular membrane/cellular boundaries (e.g., Fc receptors, poly[Ig] receptor). Finally, the proteoglycan-associated proteins stabilize complex connective matrices such as cartilage (e.g., link protein, heparin sulfate proteoglycan [HSP]). They must cross-link other molecules, hence they have multiple binding moieties. The functions of many immunoglobulin superfamily molecules are not known (e.g. CD1, Thy-1, MRC OX2, CEA, Qa, Tla, CD7, CD28, B29). However, most would appear to fall into one of these categories.

Analysis of the non-immune receptor members of the immunoglobulin superfamily reveals that there is a predominance of polyunit structures (Fig.1); that is, most of the molecules are constructed from a series of tandemly repeated homology units. Comparisons at the sequence level indicate that most of these polyunit structures have arisen independently; they are not all the descendants of a primordial polyunit gene (Hunkapiller and Hood 1989). That the same organizational motif arose so many times means both that it must have significant advantages in many different contexts and that it spontaneously appears often enough for selective processes to operate. The general encoding of homology units in discrete exons and the conservation of symmetric splicing rules means that single genetic events can expand, contract, or shuffle any number of exons and still generate an in-frame transcript, mitigating to some degree possible negative selective issues. Therefore, with simple recombinational events, valency for ligand can be multiplied, and novel functional and recognition associations can be generated (Fig. 6).

Essentially all of the polyunit sequences are made up primarily of H units. With the exception of immunoglobulin heavy chains, none of the known homology unit polypeptides have more than a single V or C unit. However, both can be in array with units of a different type (Fig. 1). Also, V and C homology units usually are found in dimeric configurations, generating quaternary domains, whereas there are no known examples of dimeric H-unit proteins. These differences between H proteins and those with V and C units may reflect a greater ability of H units to pack together into a polydomain structure or, alternatively, not pack at all—to exist as open half-domain structures. This latter configuration is consistent with a model of polyunit receptors that interact with their ligands through domain-like interactions of complementary homology units. In support of this idea, essentially all characterized receptor-ligand operations between members of the immunoglobulin superfamily involve at least one, and usually two, H-unit proteins. In either case, it seems that the H unit retains the most flexibility for interaction with different homology units, probably representing the earliest, most basic form of the homology motif.

Two particular examples of the morphogenic members demonstrate the antiquity of the homology unit. Fasciclin II and amalgam are cell adhesion molecules involved in the development of the nervous systems of

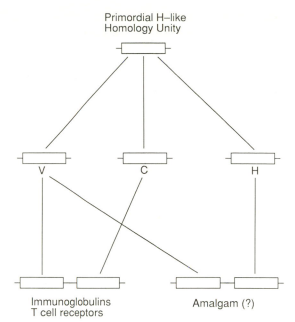

Figure 6. Exon shuffling possibilities between V, H, and C homology units in the immunoglobulin gene superfamily (see Fig. 1 and text).

grasshoppers and *Drosophila*, respectively, in a manner at least analogous to the vertebrate nervous system adhesins, N-CAM and myelin-associated glycoprotein (MAG) (Harrelson and Goodman 1988; Seeger et al. 1988). Both are polydomain sequences with multiple H homology units (Fig. 1), indicating an ancient association of the H motif with morphogenesis. Amalgam may also include a single V motif, illustrating both the early specialization of the V motif and the occurrence of exon shuffling. This means that the homology unit predated the divergence of protostomes and deuterostomes that occurred over 600 million years ago.

Another characteristic of the immunoglobulin superfamily is the association of homology unit regions with other, unrelated functional motifs, presumably through exon shuffling events. Among the best-characterized representatives are the kinase growth factor receptors for PDGF and CSF-1 (Lai et al. 1987). Each has an extracellular array of H homology units for receptor-ligand interaction and an intercellular domain that belongs to the tyrosine kinase superfamily. Also, fibronectin-binding domains are found in various morphogenic members. These examples share a recurring organizational theme, a specific receptor region composed of homology units, and an unrelated reactive moiety. These exon shuffling events broaden the biological contexts in which the homology unit functions.

Evolution of the Immunoglobulin Gene Superfamily

We believe that the immunoglobulin gene superfamily emerged with the radiative evolution of Metazoan organisms when the requirements for increased cell-surface molecular recognition were expanding rapidly, presumably in association with increasing tissue specialization. With this emergence, the gene encoding the primordial homology unit was duplicated many times in many different contexts. This resulted in an explosion of different molecules involved in numerous forms of cell-surface recognition that paralleled the development of Metazoan complexity. Perhaps the most primitive of these functions is evident in modern morphogenic factors.

It is important to emphasize that molecules grouped together by function as in Figure 5 are not necessarily directly linked evolutionarily. In fact, over time, molecules with evolutionary roots in one group can acquire the attributes of another functional system. The development of the V, C, and H homology units seems to have coincided with this radiation of functional groups and the development of Metazoan complexity. The extreme divergence between homology unit sequences belonging to different groups as well as to the same group testifies to the early divergence of the distinct motifs. Indeed, the enormous number of homology unit representatives resulting from this expansion and their current distant relatedness makes the determination of their exact lineage relationships virtually impossible except in the broadest contexts. The genealogical tree for molecules containing homology units is further complicated by the ability of different, unrelated homology unit proteins to interact with each other in novel combinatorial associations (e.g., MHC class I chain and β_2-microglobulin) and the exon shuffling allowed by conserved splicing rules (Fig. 6). For example, it is not likely that V and C units have always been tandemly linked since their divergence from the precursor unit, or they would most likely be more similar to each other than either is to the H unit. MRC OX2, which has a VC structural organization similar to that of T-cell receptor chains, may be a paradigm of the precursor molecule generated by the exon linkage of separate V and C homology units before the evolution of rearrangement (Johnson and Williams 1986). Hence, any detailed evolutionary tree drawn for the members of the immunoglobulin gene superfamily must be considered significantly speculative.

It is important to view the evolution of the immunoglobulin gene superfamily as the result of preadaptive events that generated molecules from precursors that often had no functional relatedness to the descendant molecules. We must be careful, consequently, in developing ad hoc explanations for the evolution of phenotypic systems that involve complex associations between many members of the immunoglobulin superfamily, such as the systems of antigen recognition. It is highly unlikely that the molecules involved in such systems coevolved after their emergence within the context of only one system. They more likely were recruited from many different precursor origins, converging toward an ever more complex association, rather than diverging from simple origins to fill the "needs" of an emerging phenotype. Such coalescence

of immunoglobulin superfamily members was probably facilitated by the tendency of different homology units to interact, establishing the associative possibilities from which complex interactions could arise. Given these caveats, however, we believe that simple generalizations can still be made as to the general flow of the evolution of the immunoglobulin gene superfamily (Fig. 5).

The existence of homology units in invertebrates such as insects is consistent with the idea that the immunoglobulin gene superfamily emerged early in Metazoan evolution. It is likely that the original homology unit exhibited homotypic interactions with homology units on other like cells, perhaps acting as nothing more than a cellular glue (Williams 1982) in a simple, nondifferentiated, multicellular aggregate. The homophyllic character of morphogenic molecules such as the neural cell adhesin, N-CAM, supports the feasibility of this scenario. The duplication of this early homology unit gene enabled the accumulation of a wide variety of novel mutations within the basic structure of the homology unit. This variation generated markers which, with the development of changes in the timing of expression, evolved to become tissue-specific, supporting ever more complex interactions in morphogenesis. Alternatively, of course, it could have been that cellular specialization arose prior to true multicellularity and that it was the communication needs between such cells that drove the emergence of the Metazoa and ultimately the diversity of the homology unit proteins. In either case, this required that early in Metazoan evolution, molecular recognition by homology domains became tied to activation signals that transmitted information from outside to inside the cell. For example, the association of homology units with a tyrosine kinase domain was probably the result of exon shuffling events, linking a specific receptor/ligand interaction to established activation pathways.

The ability of the homology unit to tolerate a wide range of variability no doubt allowed significant allelic variation to arise and generate in effect genotypic or self-markers (and conversely, non-self-markers). A test for non-self could have initially proved useful in favoring the fusion of heterogenetic gametes during sexual reproduction (Burnet 1971; Monroy and Rosati 1979). Members of the immunoglobulin superfamily have been implicated in this process in mammals (Lyon 1984; V. Scofield, pers. comm.). However, the ability to recognize and respond negatively to non-self is also important to any Metazoan organism that competes with its own kind at some time in its life cycle for space or substrate, particularly those that expand through asexual budding. This would require that heterotypic homology unit interactions representing allogeneic interactions become linked to potentially destructive processes. Interestingly, tunicates have a highly polymorphic gene system apparently responsible for both gametic exclusion and histocompatibility (Scofield et al. 1982). Histoincompatibility reactions have been recorded in most multicellular animal phyla (Hildemann et al. 1980), raising the possibility that MHC-like genes were integral to the development of complex Metazoa.

Histocompatibility mechanisms that respond to foreign tissues could presumably also respond to any altered self-markers, for example, arising from the interactions of self-histocompatibility molecules with other macromolecular structures. This suggests that the specific immune response is an outgrowth of these histocompatibility defenses. Early in the evolution of self-defense mechanisms, presumably existing phagocytic operations became linked and targeted to the allogeneic response by the association of the recognition elements with the activation of phagocytic processes, perhaps in a manner analogous to the exon shuffling seen in growth factor receptors. These processes may have represented the first forms of antigen processing. It is possible that MHC-like molecules or at least the precursor to the peptide-binding domain already served as some kind of membrane transport protein that became linked to this process. Facilitated by their membrane cycling, these MHC-like molecules eventually become the receptors for foreign peptide fragments. The ability to present allogeneic antigen on host cells tied to secondary signaling processes allowed an amplification of the antigenic signal. Transport of that signal away from the site of allogeneic contact could recruit by activation even more effector cells. This could explain the present linkage of the MHC and T-cell receptor antigen recognition systems. The acquired ability of MHC molecules to bind and present peptides as "altered self" leads directly to the problem of how the primitive allogeneic recognition system could distinguish MHC complexes with self versus non-self peptides. Although the solution to the problem is not clear, it must involve additional signaling between the antigen-presenting cell and the effector cell. It is also possible that early antigen presentation was restricted to only specific proteins, limiting the problem of tolerance substantially. The example of the highly specific binding and transport of maternal milk antibodies by an Fc receptor that is directly homologous to class I sequences may serve as a paradigm in this regard (Simister and Mostov 1989).

It is probable that the cell-cell interactions involved in morphogenesis arose before the development of immune-type reactions. This branching was no doubt a major event in the evolution of the family, each branch taking advantage of the ability of the homology unit to accommodate variability in a fundamentally different way. Members of the morphogenic differentiation branches became more and more specialized and targeted in their interactions, generating enormous varieties of highly specialized molecules. The immune branch, on the other hand, became more and more dependent on the variation possibilities within one family of genes, allowing that family to have the broadest possibilities for interaction while retaining the highly specific interactions of the individual receptors.

A key event in the evolution of antigen recognition receptors was the acquisition of the ability to rearrange

gene segments. A likely scenario is that a transposon inserted into a primordial V gene separating the initial V and J gene segments (Sakano et al. 1979). Transposon excision with the subsequent joining of the separated elements eventually came under developmental control (e.g., a limited window of time within which the enzymes responsible for rearrangement are active). However, this later process was never precise, generating more nonproductive than productive rearrangements. This had the effect of "excluding" any nonproductively rearranged V gene from generating a functional protein. With only a limited number of V to J possibilities, this would be functionally the equivalent of allelic exclusion because the likelihood of more than one productive rearrangement in one cell would be small. Thus, a single cell could produce only one or a limited number of antigen-specific receptors. With near-clonal expression, the process of clonal selection by foreign macromolecular patterns could now occur, generating selective pressure for ever finer control of allelic expression. The lower the rate of productive rearrangements per number of V-J rearrangement possibilities, the greater the number of such potential pairings allowable while still maintaining near-clonal expression. Therefore, as the control mechanisms for allelic exclusion became more defined, the number of gene segments could be expanded, thereby generating even more receptor diversity potential.

A T-cell-like recognition system probably evolved before that of B cells. It maintained its earlier linkage to non-self cell destruction and thus the recognition of antigen in the context of MHC molecules. Duplications of gene families occurred to generate the various types of T-cell receptors and ultimately the B-cell receptor gene families. Central to this would have been freeing B cells from direct cell-cell interaction requirements and thus the need for MHC binding.

Examination of the antibody genes and diversity in the shark *Heterodontus*, the chicken, and mammals illustrates three different stages in the evolution of rearranging multigene families (Fig. 7). The shark has multiple clusters of tandemly repeated V-D-J-C genes for heavy chains (Kokubu et al. 1987). It is unclear whether V gene segments can only rearrange to their tandemly associated J gene segment, but such possibilities at least seem limited, reducing the combinatorial possibilities. However, junctional variation is still possible. Increase in the effective total number of V-J-C sets possible in one genome is probably limited as well

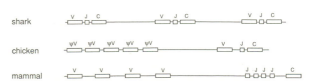

Figure 7. Organization of immunoglobulin light-chain genes in the shark, chicken, and mammal (see Fig. 4 and text).

by the consequent increased likelihood of multiple productive rearrangements, assuming that allelic exclusion
has some stochastic quality. These constraints are consistent with the fact that cartilaginous fish have a more
reduced expressed antibody diversity than other vertebrates (Litman et al. 1982). The chicken, on the
other hand, has a complex antibody repertoire, but has
only a single V and J gene segment for both light and
heavy chains, eliminating all combinatorials. However,
the single V gene can be corrected against 25 or more
closely linked pseudo-V_L gene segments by a process of
random gene conversion, thus generating enormous
diversity (Weill 1986). Certainly, allelic exclusion is
much easier in such a system. Allelic variation may play
an important role in this system as a way to expand the
range of diversity (presumably, the more divergent are
two homologs, the greater the difference in the possible
antigens that can be surveyed by one animal). The most
sophisticated potential for diversity is seen in the mammals. The grouping of V, D, and J gene segments
should allow even tighter control on allelic exclusion,
because each nonproductive rearrangement actually reduces the remaining possible rearrangement target
sites. The number of possible V-J pairings is limited by
the element with the smallest number of copies, usually
D or J. The remaining element(s) can expand without
impact on allelic exclusion. Hence, with this organization there is much less restriction on the expansion of
the number of V gene segments and the consequent
increase in combinatorial and junctional variation
potential. (It is interesting to note that allelic exclusion
of T-cell receptor α chains may not be as complete as
other chains [Malissen et al. 1988]. This may correlate
with the fact that the number of J gene segments far
outnumbers that of any other chain, approaching a
substantial fraction of the size of the V_α gene segment
number. However, experiments with transgenic animals suggest that specific, nonstochastic regulatory
mechanisms also play a role in allelic exclusion [Blüth-
mann et al. 1988].) As diversity and its range increase
in a gene segment family, the importance of allelic
variation is probably reduced.

With the expansion of V gene segments, however, it
becomes more important to link their transcription to
rearrangement. In the case of the mouse V_H family, for
example, the productively rearranged V_H gene is derived from one of over a thousand (including both
chromosomes) V_H gene segments (Livant et al. 1986),
each with its own transcription initiation site. However,
effective transcription is possible only when rearrangement brings a V gene segment into the vicinity of
specific enhancer sequences near the C gene. Thus, the
evolution of rearrangement probably had more to do
with regulation of allelic exclusion and expression than
diversity per se (Hunkapiller and Hood 1989). However, the development of clonal expression is what
freed the constraints on V gene expansion and facilitated the evolution of diverse antigen-specific repertoires.

Implications of the Immunoglobulin Gene Superfamily

The history of the immunoglobulin gene superfamily
reflects both the fundamental diversifying and combinatorial properties of the immunoglobulin homology
unit. New functional possibilities arise by alteration of
the informational units involved (e.g., nucleotides,
exons, genes, and entire multigene families), by shuffling of these elements, and by the linkage of homology
units with other, independent functional processes. The
duplication of a multigene family and the attendant
cis-acting control mechanisms can in a single event
create the genetic basis for a complex new phenotype,
thereby increasing the possibility for very rapid evolutionary change. The evolution of the rearranging gene
families illustrates this principle clearly. On the assumption that the development of rearrangement occurred only once, the proto-immune receptor was probably a homodimer (allowing for allelic forms). Duplication and subsequent divergence of the proto-family led
then to the modern heterodimeric form and, consequently, a whole new diversifying principle. These
duplications promoted the creation of genes whose
products could interact with one another, generating
the combinatorial potentials between the products of
two gene families. Multiple pairs of specifically interacting gene families would coevolve over time.
Changes in the regulation of these pairs would eventually generate the distinctive T- and B-cell receptors
seen today. It seems probable that the development or
addition of antibody effector domains arose after the
regulatory separation of the B- and T-cell lineages.
Thus, the duplication of multigene families can generate new multigene families with entirely distinct functional potential. The duplication of entire or parts of
multigene families, therefore, provides the potential
for extremely rapid evolutionary change and the relatively saltational acquisition of complex new
phenotypes. This is consistent with recent models of
evolution that propose that more punctuated events
may be stronger drivers of large-scale phenotypic
change than the gradualism of simple point mutations
of structural genes (see Gould 1989).

The expansion of the immunoglobulin gene superfamily to carry out a multitude of different major functions in eukaryotic biology is a classic example of evolutionary canalization. This is the process whereby once
an evolutionary branching has been made, a de facto
direction for future evolutionary events has been made
more likely, because the path taken at one juncture
limits the future paths available (i.e., it is hard to go
backwards). The early success of the homology unit
signaled an important early juncture of Metazoan development as regards the possible mechanisms and
motifs employed in cell-cell interactions. Also, the tendency of homology units to interact drives the development of ever more complex associations of proteins
containing homology units. This complexity sub-

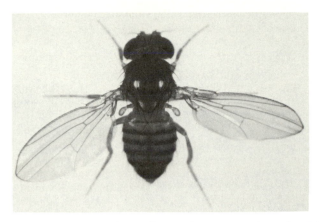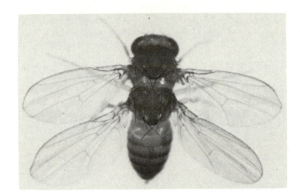

Figure 8. A single homeotic mutation creates a four-winged fly from the wild-type two-winged fly (courtesy of E. Lewis).

sequently generates the building blocks of additional, complex phenotypes. In this regard, the immunoglobulin homology unit motif is repeated in many different variations and contexts, tying together in an evolutionary and sometimes functional sense many areas of eukaryotic biology. Particularly fascinating are the members of the superfamily that are expressed by both the immune and nervous systems (see Parnes and Hunkapiller 1987). This coexpression raises the possibility of shared receptor molecules that facilitate communication between these two complex systems that deal with external stimuli. Indeed, it seems likely that the nervous system plays an important role in regulating the immune response, perhaps mediated by interactions between immunoglobulin superfamily members.

The evolution of control mechanisms is one of the real keys to understanding how the complex phenotypes of eukaryotes have arisen. However, a full understanding of the evolution of regulatory mechanisms is impossible until we understand more of the functional details of current regulatory mechanisms. Hence, the study of developmental biology and evolutionary biology are two sides of the same coin. How is it that a new multigene family can be created and in time its members be expressed in different cell types within different functional contexts? In this regard, it is interesting to consider the evolutionary processes that led to the development of the modern fly from the early annelids. The more specialized descendants of a simple segmental creature had to acquire the developmental programs that led to ever-increasing specialization of their segments (e.g., head, thorax, and abdomen) and their appendages, such as legs and wings. Presumably, these features are encoded by coordinately expressed linked and unlinked genes as well as gene families that must be duplicated and controlled. It seems likely that the required developmental changes were more the result of regulation and timing changes than major modifications to the structural genes. Indeed, a single homeotic mutation can convert a modern two-wing fly to a more ancient four-wing form (Fig. 8), indicating that the

genetic information for generating older phenotypes is still contained intrinsically within contemporary genomes and that it is the context of its expression that determines the final phenotype, not the coding information itself. Such changes in homeotic and multigene systems illustrate that changes in the regulation of complex traits may be more likely to generate selectively tolerable phenotypic changes than direct major alteration of structural genes, thus promoting relatively saltational changes in phenotype.

The immunoglobulin gene superfamily has given us a glimpse into the awesome complexities of modern biology; at the same time, its study offers hope for unraveling some of these complexities. Questions concerning the overall diversity of the immunoglobulin gene superfamily and whether other complex eukaryotic systems employ gene superfamilies of similar complexity await future investigations.

ACKNOWLEDGMENTS

The National Institutes of Health has supported this work. We thank Sue Lewis and all those of the typing staff for help with this paper. B.F.K. is the recipient of a fellowship from the Sloan Foundation.

REFERENCES

Amzel, L.M. and R. J. Poljak. 1979. Three-dimensional structure of immunoglobulins. *Annu. Rev. Biochem.* **48:** 961.

Bank, I., R.A. DePinho, M.B. Brenner, J. Caasimeris, F.W. Alt, and L. Chess. 1986. A functional T3 molecule associated with a novel heterodimer on the surface of immature human thymocytes. *Nature* **322:** 179.

Barth, R.K., B.S. Kim, N.C. Lan, T. Hunkapiller, N. Sobiek, A. Winoto, H. Gershenfeld, C. Okada, D. Hansburg, I. Weissman, and L. Hood. 1985. The murine T-cell receptor employs a limited repertoire of expressed V_β gene segments. *Nature* **316:** 517.

Blüthmann, H., P. Kisielow, Y. Uematsu, M. Malissen, P. Krimpenfort, A. Berns, H. von Boehmer, and M. Steinmetz. 1988. T-cell specific deletion of T-cell receptor transgenes allows functional rearrangement of endogenous alpha and beta genes. *Nature* **334:** 156.

Brenner, M.B., J. McLean, D.P. Dialynas, J.L. Strominger, J.A. Smith, F.L. Owen, J.G. Seidman, S. Ip, F. Rosen, and M.S. Krangel. 1986. Identification of a putative second T-cell receptor. *Nature* **322:** 145.

Burnet, F.M. 1971. "Self-recognition" in colonial marine forms and flowering plants in relation to the evolution of immunity. *Nature* **232:** 230.

Capra, K. and J.M. Kehoe. 1974. Variable region sequences of 5 human immunoglobulin heavy chains of the variable heavy chain. III. Subgroup definitive identification of 4 heavy chain hypervariable regions. *Proc. Natl. Acad. Sci.* **71:** 845.

Chien, Y.-H., M. Iwashima, K.B. Kaplan, J.F. Elliot, and M.M. Davis. 1987. A new T-cell receptor gene located within the α locus and expressed early in T-cell differentiation. *Nature* **327:** 677.

Clarke, S.H., K. Huppi, D. Ruezinsky, L. Standt, W. Gerhard, and W. Weigert. 1985. Inter- and intraclonal diversity in the antibody response to influenza hemagglutinin. *J. Exp. Med.* **161:** 687.

Claverie, J.-M. and P. Kourilsky. 1987. The peptidic self model: A reassessment of the role of the major histocompatibility complex molecules in the restriction of the T-cell response. *Ann. Immunol.* **137:** 425.

Cunningham, B.A., J.J. Hemperly, B.A. Murray, E.A. Prediger, R. Brackenbury, and G.M. Edelman. 1973. Neural cell adhesion molecule structure, immunoglobulin-like domains, cell surface modulation and alternative RNA splicing. *Science* **236:** 799.

Davis, M.M. 1985. Molecular genetics of the T-cell receptor β chain. *Annu. Rev. Immunol.* **3:** 537.

Davis, M.M., S.K. Kim, and L. Hood. 1980. Immunoglobulin class switching developmentally regulated DNA rearrangements during differentiation. *Cell* **22:** 1.

Early, P., J. Rogers, M. Davis, K. Calame, M. Bond, R. Wall, and L. Hood. 1980. Two mRNAs can be produced from a single immunoglobulin μ gene by alternative RNA processing pathways. *Cell* **30:** 313.

Edmundson, A.B., K.R. Ely, E.E. Abola, M. Schiffer, and N. Panagiotopoulos. 1975. Rotational allomerism and divergent evolution of domains in immunoglobulin light chains. *Biochemistry* **14:** 3953.

Eisen, H.N. 1986. Why affinity progression of antibodies during immune responses is probably not accompanied by parallel changes in the immunoglobulin-like antigen-specific receptors on T cells. *BioEssays* **4:** 269.

Elliot, J.F., E.P. Rock, P.A. Patten, M.M. Davis, and Y.-H. Chien. 1988. The adult T-cell receptor δ chain is diverse and distinct from that of fetal thymocytes. *Nature* **331:** 627.

Gearhart, P.M. and D.F. Bogenhagen. 1983. Clusters of point mutations are found exclusively around rearranged antibody variable genes. *Proc. Natl. Acad. Sci.* **80:** 3437.

Gearhart, P.M., N.D. Johnson, R. Douglass, and L. Hood. 1981. IgG antibodies to phosphorylcholine exhibit more diversity than their IgM counterparts. *Nature* **291:** 29.

Germain, R.N. and B. Malissen. 1986. Analysis of the expression and function of class II major histocompatibility complex-encoded molecules by DNA-mediated gene transfer. *Annu. Rev. Immunol.* **4:** 281.

Gould, S.J. 1989. *Wonderful life: The Burgess Shale and the nature of history.* W.W. Norton, New York.

Goverman, J., T. Hunkapiller, and L. Hood. 1986. A speculative view of the multicomponent nature of T-cell antigen recognition. *Cell* **45:** 475.

Hannum, C., J.H. Freed, G. Tarr, J. Kappler, and P. Marrack. 1984. Biochemistry and distribution of the T-cell receptor. *Immunol. Rev.* **81:** 161.

Harrelson, A.L. and C.S. Goodman. 1988. Growth cone guidance in insects: Fasciclin II is a member of the immunoglobulin superfamily. *Science* **242:** 700.

Hayday, A.C., H. Saito, S.D. Gillies, D.M. Kranz, G.

Tanigawa, H.N. Eisen, and S. Tonegawa. 1985. The structure organization and somatic rearrangement of T-cell γ genes. *Cell* **40:** 259.

Hildemann, W.H., C.H. Bigger, J.S. Johnston, and P.L. Jokiel. 1980. Characteristics of immune memory in invertebrates. *Dev. Immunol.* **10:** 9.

Hill, R.L., R. Delaney, R.E. Fellow, and H.E. Lebowitz. 1966. The evolutionary origins of the immunoglobulins. *Proc. Natl. Acad. Sci.* **56:** 1762.

Honjo, T. 1983. Immunoglobulin genes. *Annu. Rev. Immunol.* **1:** 499.

Honjo, T. and S. Habu. 1985. Origin of immune diversity genetic variation and selection. *Annu. Rev. Biochem.* **54:** 803.

Hood, L., M. Kronenberg, and T. Hunkapiller. 1985. T-cell antigen receptors and the immunoglobulin supergene family. *Cell* **40:** 225.

Hood, L., M. Steinmetz, and B. Malissen. 1983. Genes of the major histocompatibility complex of the mouse. *Annu. Rev. Immunol.* **1:** 529.

Hunkapiller, T. and L. Hood. 1989. Diversity of the immunoglobulin gene superfamily. *Adv. Immunol.* **44:** 1.

Ioannides, C.G., K. Itoh, F.E. Fox, R. Pahwa, R.A. Good, and C.D. Platsoucas. 1987. Identification of a second T-cell antigen receptor in human and mouse by an antipeptide γ-chain-specific monoclonal antibody. *Proc. Natl. Acad. Sci.* **82:** 7701.

Johnson, P. and A.F. Williams. 1986. Striking similarities between antigen receptor J pieces and sequence in the second chain of the murine CD8 antigen. *Nature* **323:** 74.

Kim, S., M. Davis, E. Sinn, P. Patten, and L. Hood. 1981. Antibody diversity: Somatic hypermutation of rearranged V_H genes. *Cell* **27:** 573.

Klein, J. 1982. *Immunology: The science of self-nonself discrimination.* Wiley, New York.

Klein, J. and F. Figueroa. 1981. Polymorphism of the mouse H-2 loci. *Immunol. Rev.* **60:** 23.

———. 1986. The evolution of class I MHC genes. *Immunol. Today* **7:** 41.

Kokubu, F., K. Hinds, R. Litman, M.S. Shamblott, and G.W. Litman. 1987. Extensive families of constant region genes in a phylogenetically primitive vertebrate indicate an additional level of immunoglobulin complexity. *Proc. Natl. Acad. Sci.* **84:** 5868.

Kronenberg, M., G. Siu, L. Hood, and N. Shastri. 1986. The molecular genetics of the T-cell antigen receptor and T-cell antigen recognition. *Annu. Rev. Immunol.* **4:** 529.

Lai, C., M.A. Brow, K.-A. Nave, A.B. Noronha, R.H. Quarles, F.E. Bloom, R.J. Milner, and J.G. Sutcliffe. 1987. Two forms of 1B236/myelin-associated glycoprotein, a cell adhesion molecule for post-natal neural development are produced by alternative. *Proc. Natl. Acad. Sci.* **84:** 4337.

Litman, G.W., J. Stolen, H.O. Sarvas, and O. Mäkelä. 1982. The range and fine specificity of the anti-hapten immune response: Phylogenetic studies. *J. Immunogenet.* **9:** 465.

Livant, D., C. Blatt, and L. Hood. 1986. One heavy chain variable region gene segment subfamily in the BALB/c mouse contains 500–1000 or more members. *Cell* **47:** 461.

Luzzati, A.L., I. Lefkovits, and B. Pernis. 1973. Homogeneity of antibodies produced by clones *in vitro*. *Eur. J. Immunol.* **3:** 636.

Lyon, M.F. 1984. Transmission radio distortion in mouse t-haplotypes is due to multiple distorter genes acting on a responder locus. *Cell* **37:** 621.

Malissen, M., J. Trucy, F. Letourneur, N. Rebai, D.E. Dunn, F.W. Fitch, L. Hood, and B. Malissen. 1988. A T-cell clone expresses two T-cell receptor alpha genes but uses one alpha-beta heterodimer for allorecognition and self MHC-restricted antigen recognition. *Cell* **55:** 49.

Matis, L.A., R. Cron, and J.A. Bluestone. 1987. Major histocompatibility complex-linked specificity of γδ receptor-bearing T lymphocytes. *Nature* **330:** 262.

Mengle-Gaw, L. and H.O. McDevitt. 1985. Genetics and expression of Ia antigens. *Annu. Rev. Immunol.* **3**: 367.

Meuer, S.C., O. Acuto, T. Hercend, S.F. Schlossman, and E.L. Reinherz. 1984. The human T-cell receptor. *Annu. Rev. Immunol.* **2**: 23.

Monroy, A. and F. Rosati. 1979. The evolution of the cell-cell recognition system. *Nature* **278**: 165.

Novotný, J., S. Tonegawa, H. Saito, D. Kranz, and H. Eisen. 1986. Secondary, tertiary, and quaternary structure of T-cell specific immunoglobulin-like polypeptide chains. *Proc. Natl. Acad. Sci.* **83**: 742.

Parnes, J.R. and T. Hunkapiller. 1987. L3T4 and the immunoglobulin gene superfamily: New relationships between the immune system and the nervous system. *Immunol. Rev.* **100**: 109.

Sablitzky, F., G. Wildner, and K. Rajewsky. 1985. Somatic mutation and clonal expansion of B cells in an antigen-driven immune response. *EMBO J.* **4**: 345.

Sakano, H., K. Huppi, G. Heinrich, and S. Tonegawa. 1979. Sequences of the somatic recombination sites of immunoglobulin light chain genes. *Nature* **280**: 288.

Schwartz, R.H. 1984. The role of gene products of the major histocompatibility complex in T-cell activation and cellular interactions. In *Fundamental immunology* (ed. W.E. Paul), p. 379. Raven Press, New York.

Scofield, V.L., J.M. Schlumpberger, L.A. West, and I.L. Weissman. 1982. Protochordate allorecognition is controlled by a MHC-like gene system. *Nature* **295**: 499.

Seeger, M.A., L. Haffley, and T.L. Kaufman. 1988. Characterization of amalgam, a member of the immunoglobulin superfamily from *Drosophila*. *Cell* **55**: 589.

Simister, N.E. and K.E. Mostov. 1989. An Fc receptor structurally related to MHC class I antigens. *Nature* **337**: 184.

Sprent, J. and S.R. Webb. 1987. Function and specificity of T cell subsets in the mouse. *Adv. Immunol.* **41**: 39.

Strominger, J.L., H.T. Orr, P. Parham, H.L. Ploegh, D.L. Mann, H. Bilofsky, H.A. Saroff, T.T. Wu, and E.A. Kabat. 1980. An evaluation of the significance of amino-acid sequence homologies in human histocompatibility antigens HLA-A and HLA-B with immunoglobulins and other proteins using relatively short sequences. *Scand. J. Immunol.* **11**: 573.

Tonegawa, S. 1983. Somatic generation of antibody diversity. *Nature* **302**: 575.

Weill, J.C. 1986. Generation of diversity in the avian bursa. *Prog. Immunol.* **6**: 20.

Williams, A.F. 1982. Surface molecules and cell interactions. *J. Theor. Biol.* **98**: 221.

———. 1984. The immunoglobulin superfamily takes shape. *Nature* **308**: 12.

———. 1987. A year in the life of the immunoglobulin superfamily. *Immunol. Today* **8**: 298.

Wu, T.T. and E.A. Kabat. 1970. An analysis of the sequences of the variable regions of Bence-Jones proteins and myeloma light chains and their implications for antibody complementarity. *J. Exp. Med.* **132**: 211.

Diversity, Development, Ligands, and Probable Functions of $\gamma\delta$ T Cells

S. Tonegawa,* A. Berns,† M. Bonneville,* A. Farr,‡ I. Ishida,* K. Ito,* S. Itohara,*
C.A. Janeway, Jr.,§ O. Kanagawa,‖ M. Katsuki,¶ R. Kubo,# J. Lafaille,*
P. Mombaerts,* D. Murphy,** N. Nakanishi,* Y. Takagaki,* L. Van Kaer,* and S. Verbeek†

*Howard Hughes Medical Institute at Center for Cancer Research and Department of Biology, Massachusetts Institute of Technology, Cambridge, Massachusetts 02139; †The Netherlands Cancer Institute, Division of Molecular Genetics and the Department of Biochemistry of the University of Amsterdam, Amsterdam, The Netherlands; ‡University of Washington, Department of Biological Structure SM-70, Seattle, Washington 98195; §Howard Hughes Medical Institute at Yale University Medical School, New Haven, Connecticut 06510; ‖Eli Lilly Research Laboratories, La Jolla, California 92037; ¶Department of DNA Biology, School of Medicine, Tokai University and Central Institute for Experimental Animals, Kanagawa 213, Japan; #National Jewish Center of Immunology and Respiratory Medicine, Denver, Colorado 80206; **The Wadsworth Center, New York State Department of Health, Empire State Plaza, Albany, New York 12201

The most critical step in the vertebrate immune response is the recognition of antigens by lymphocytes. This task is accomplished by two sets of glycoproteins, immunoglobulins (Igs), and T-cell antigen receptors (TCRs). The most extraordinary feature of these proteins is their structural variability, much of which originates from the ability of the encoding gene segments to undergo somatic rearrangement (Tonegawa 1983). All TCRs were initially thought to be composed of a heterodimeric protein composed of α and β subunits. However, the search for the genes encoding these polypeptides led to the identification of a third rearranging gene (Saito et al. 1984; Hayday et al. 1985) that was later shown to code for one of the two subunits of another heterodimeric, TCR$\gamma\delta$ (Bank et al. 1986; Brenner et al. 1986; Weiss et al. 1986).

Despite the striking similarities in the overall structure of their genes and polypeptide chains, TCR$\gamma\delta$ and the T cells that express it are significantly different from their $\alpha\beta$ counterparts. For instance, $\gamma\delta$ T cells are detected in both the thymus (Bank et al. 1986; Lew et al. 1986; Nakanishi et al. 1987) and peripheral lymphoid organs (Brenner et al. 1986; Maeda et al. 1987) in relatively low numbers ($<5\%$ of T cells) but predominate (50–100%) within epithelia such as epidermis (Kuziel et al. 1987; Stingl et al. 1987) and the small intestine (Bonneville et al. 1988; Goodman and Lefrancois 1988). In contrast with most $\alpha\beta$ T cells, the majority of $\gamma\delta$ T cells in the thymus and spleen do not express either CD4 or CD8 (Bank et al. 1986; Brenner et al. 1986; Lew et al. 1986; Maeda et al. 1987; Nakanishi et al. 1987). Neither the specificity of TCR$\gamma\delta$ recognition nor $\gamma\delta$ T-cell function in immune defense is understood. In this paper, we summarize results of our recent studies on the diversity, development, and specificity of $\gamma\delta$ T cells, and we discuss possible functions of these cells.

RESULTS

Anti-mouse TCR$\gamma\delta$ MAbs

To study the nature of the TCR$\gamma\delta$ and the role of $\gamma\delta$ T cells, monoclonal antibodies (MAbs) directed against the native receptor are useful. To generate such antibodies, we immunized Armenian hamsters with the anti-CD3 immunoprecipitate of a lysate of $\gamma\delta$ T hybridoma KN6 (Ito et al. 1989) and prepared three anti-$\gamma\delta$-TCR MAbs (Itohara et al. 1989): MAb 3A10, specific for a C_δ (constant) region determinant, MAb 8D6, specific for (variable) $V_\gamma 4$- and $V_\delta 5$-encoded TCR$\gamma\delta$, and MAb 5C10, specific for a KN6 TCR idiotope.

Appearance of $\alpha\beta$ and $\gamma\delta$ T Cells in the Developing and Mature Thymus

Using appropriate MAbs, we determined the number of thymocytes bearing TCR$\gamma\delta$ (abbreviated hereafter as $\gamma\delta$ thymocytes) or TCR$\alpha\beta$ ($\alpha\beta$ thymocytes) as a function of age (Fig. 1). $\gamma\delta$ Thymocytes were detected at day 14.5 of gestation (E14.5), the earliest time point analyzed. Their number increased until E17.5, remained at this level until birth, dipped, and then gradually increased to the adult level of 1 million cells per thymus. In relative terms, only 0.4–0.6% of total thymocytes at E14.5 are $\gamma\delta$ thymocytes, increasing rapidly to its highest value (5%) at E16.5, then gradually decreasing through embryonic life and the first postnatal week until it reaches a stationary adult level of 0.3–0.5% at about 10 days after birth. $\alpha\beta$ Thymocytes are rare (<100 cells/thymus) at E14.5 but outnumber $\gamma\delta$ thymocytes after E16.5. By E18.5, they are the dominant thymocyte population.

Two-color analysis of thymocytes from E16, E18.5, and adult mice showed that TCR$\alpha\beta$ and TCR$\gamma\delta$

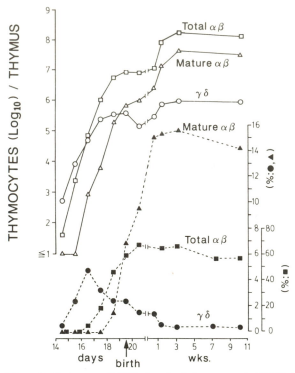

Figure 1. Ontogeny of TCR $\gamma\delta$ and $\alpha\beta$ thymocytes in C57BL/6 mice. Thymocytes of mice at different ages were stained with anti-$\gamma\delta$ (3A10) or anti-$\alpha\beta$ (H57-597) biotin conjugates followed by a streptavidin phycoerythrin conjugate together with an anti-CD3 (2C11) fluorescein isothiocyanate conjugate. The samples were analyzed with FACScan (Becton-Dickinson) using FACScan software.

double-positive cells must be extremely rare or do not exist at all. Thus, a mechanism appears to exist that restricts the surface expression of TCRs to only one of the two types.

$\gamma\delta$ T Cells Compose Minor T-cell Subpopulations in Peripheral Lymphoid Organs

We determined the frequency of $\gamma\delta$ T cells in peripheral lymphoid organs (i.e., spleen, lymph node, and blood) as well as their CD4 CD8 phenotype. The results are summarized in Table 1. In adult mice (7–13 weeks old), the fraction of $\gamma\delta$ T cells among CD3$^+$ T cells is no more than 3% in any of the three sites studied although it is as high as 10% in the spleen of 4-day-old mice. This $\gamma\delta^+$/CD3$^+$ ratio is much lower than that reported for the chicken (Sowder et al. 1988) but is similar to that in humans (1–15%) (Borst et al. 1988; Chen et al. 1989). As suggested in the original report on $\gamma\delta$ T cells (Brenner et al. 1986), the majority of peripheral $\gamma\delta$ T cells do not express CD4 or CD8 (Table 1). However, a significant fraction of $\gamma\delta$ T cells is either CD4$^+$ or CD8$^+$ in all three peripheral lymphoid organs studied, and high CD8 expression can be induced in vitro in peripheral $\gamma\delta$ T cells with the MAb 3A10 (Y. Utsunomiya et al., unpubl.).

Intrathymic Distribution of $\gamma\delta$ T Cells Alters Drastically during the First Postnatal Week

To relate the spatial distribution of $\gamma\delta$ thymocytes to the organization of the thymic environment, we analyzed sections of fetal and adult thymuses using immunohistochemical technique. Adjacent sections of thymus tissue were alternatively labeled with the MAb 3A10 or with the *Ulex europeus* agglutinin (UEA), which we have previously shown to be a reliable marker for medullary thymic epithelial cells in the adult murine thymus (Farr and Anderson 1985). We observed a striking colocalization of $\gamma\delta^+$ thymocytes and UEA$^+$ medullary epithelial cells during late fetal and neonatal periods of development (Fig. 2a,b). In contrast, $\gamma\delta$ thymocytes were scattered throughout cortical and medullary areas of the thymus (Fig. 2c,d) and most concentrated in the subcapsular areas of the thymus in the thymuses of adult mice. Results of ultrastructural immunohistochemistry confirmed the close association between medullary thymic epithelial cells and $\gamma\delta$ thymocytes in the neonatal thymus and also showed that some TCR$\gamma\delta$ molecules were patched to areas of contact with medullary epithelial cells. As shown below, the pattern of TCR$\gamma\delta$ expression in the thymus is limited in diversity and is developmentally ordered. Thus, these histochemical results indicate that changes in receptor repertoire correlate with the changes in the intrathymic distribution of $\gamma\delta$ thymocytes.

$\gamma\delta$ T Cells Are Present in Many Organs Containing Epithelia

Since $\gamma\delta$ T cells are relatively scant in peripheral lymphoid organs (Table 1), we searched for these cells in sections of various organs and tissues. The results are summarized in Table 2. The $\gamma\delta$ T cells were most abundant in the small intestine, moderately abundant in the tongue, stomach, and large intestine, and very scarce in the esophagus. In the tongue and stomach, the vast majority of $\gamma\delta$ T cells were associated with the basal layer of stratified squamous epithelium (Fig. 3a,b). Consistent with previous studies of human and chicken tissues (Bucy et al. 1988; Groh et al. 1989), $\gamma\delta$ T cells were observed in mouse intestines within the columnar epithelium of the villi (Fig. 3c) but not in intestinal crypts nor in the lamina propria.

A substantial number of $\gamma\delta$ T cells was also found to be associated with the columnar luminal epithelium of the uterus (Fig. 3d), the stratified squamous epithelium of the vagina (Fig. 3e), and the transitional epithelium of the bladder. In contrast, no $\gamma\delta$ T cells were found in the liver, pancreas, kidney, or brain.

Unlike the human and chicken epidermis (Bucy et al. 1988; Groh et al. 1989), the mouse epidermis is the site of a major $\gamma\delta$ T-cell subset. About 5×10^6 $\gamma\delta$ T cells are present within epidermis and hair follicles of each mouse (Fig. 3f) (Bergstresser et al. 1983; Tschachler et

Table 1. Frequency and Surface Phenotype of γδ Cells in Periphery

Organ	Age of animals	No. of animals examined	No. of cells bearing[c] (10^{-5}/animal)			γδ Cells among CD3+ (%)	γδ Cells bearing[c] (%)		
			CD3	TCRγδ	TCRαβ		CD4+	CD8+	CD4- CD8-
Spleen	4 days	7[a]	0.74	0.07	0.67	10	5.5	63	32
	7–13 wk	12	300 ± 73	8.2 ± 2.0	279 ± 70	2.8 ± 0.5	10 ± 0.6	15 ± 4.8	75 ± 5.4
Mesenteric lymph node	7–13 wk	12	51 ± 23	1.2 ± 0.5	50 ± 22	2.3 ± 0.3	7.6 ± 2.6	32 ± 14	60 ± 16
Blood	7–13 wk	17[a]	25[b]	0.6	24	2.4	10	18	72

[a] Cells from the indicated number of animals were pooled.
[b] Estimated from the data of Green (1966).
[c] Mean ± S.D.

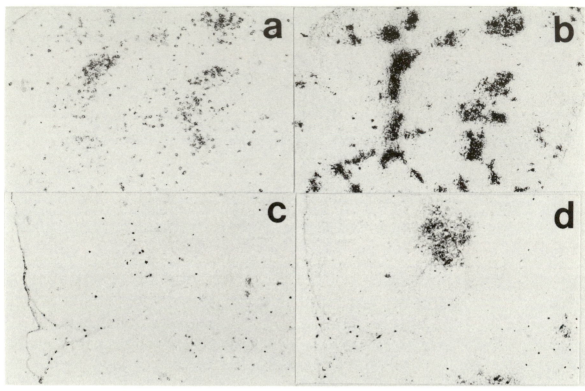

Figure 2. Intrathymic distribution of γδ cells in fetal and adult thymus tissues. Adjacent serial sections of thymus tissue were labeled with anti-γδ MAb 3A10 (*a* and *c*) or with UEA (*b* and *d*). (*a* and *b*) Day 18; (*c* and *d*) adult.

Table 2. Distribution of γδ T Cells in Mice

Organs	Presence of γδ T cells in mice		Contact with epithelial cells	No. of cells per animal	Major V_γ gene segments used	Diversity of TCRγδ
	normal	nude				
Digestive system						
tongue	+		+		6	−
esophagus	+/−		+			
stomach	+		+			
small intestine	+	+	+	1×10^6	7	+
large intestine	+	+	+	1×10^5	7, 4	
liver	−					
pancreas	−					
Reproductive system						
ovary	+/−					
uterus	+	−	+	1×10^5	6	−
vagina	+	−	+	1×10^5	6	−
testis	−					
epididymis	+/−		−			
seminal vesicle					7, 5	
Urinary system						
kidney	−					
bladder	+	−	+			
Others						
skin	+	−	+	5×10^6	5	−
lung					7, 4, 6	
brain	−					
heart	−					
Lymphoid organs						
thymus	+			1×10^6	4, 7	+
spleen	+	−		8×10^5	4, 7, 6	+
lymph node	+	−		1×10^5	4, 7, 6	+
blood	+			6×10^4	4, 7, 6	+

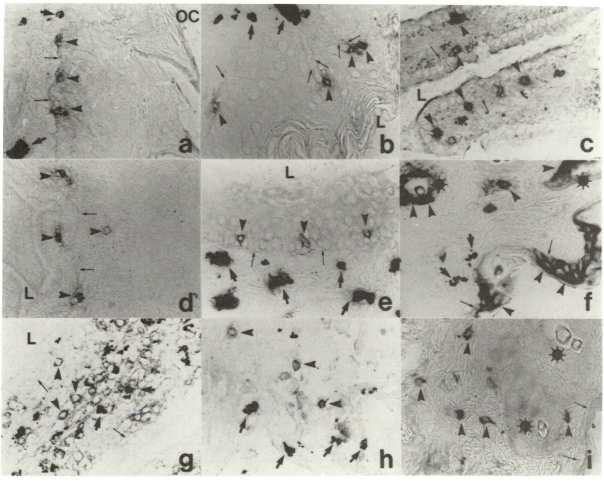

Figure 3. Immunohistostaining of various epithelium-containing organs with anti-γδ and anti-αβ MAbs. Fresh tissues from 8- to 10-week-old BALB/c mice were snap frozen, and 6 μm sections were fixed with cold acetone, stained with a MAb anti-γδ (3A10) (a–f) or anti-αβ (H57-597) (g–i) followed by affinity-purified goat anti-hamster IgG biotin (Caltag Lab., California) and avidin-horseradish peroxidase conjugates. (a) Tongue; (b) stomach; (c and g) small intestine; (d and h) uterus; (e) vagina; and (f and i) skin. Arrowheads indicate some of the stained TCR cells. Endogenous peroxidase activity is indicated by large arrows. Small arrows indicate basal lamina. Asterisks indicate hair follicles. (OC) Oral cavity; (L) lumen. Magnification, 220 ×.

al. 1983). In some areas, these cells tended to form clusters (Fig. 3f).

For comparison, adjacent sections were stained with the MAb against TCRαβ (Fig. 3g,h,i). These T cells were preferentially localized in the lamina propria of the intestines (Fig. 3g), the endometrium and myometrium of the uterus (Fig. 3h), the dermis of the skin (Fig. 3i), and the connective tissue of the vagina. Occasionally, some αβ T cells were observed in association with the epithelia of the intestine, vagina, and uterus. However, the majority of CD3[+] intraepithelial lymphocytes are clearly γδ T cells. In light of these observations, we propose to refer to these T cells as intraepithelial lymphocytes (IEL) as a generic term and to attach the initial of each organ to designate various IEL subpopulations such as i-IEL, s-IEL, r-IEL, and t-IEL for the IELs in the intestine, skin, reproductive organs, and tongue, respectively.

We extended our immunohistological analyses to 8-week-old athymic nude mice. As expected, no αβ or γδ T cells were detectable in most organs analyzed, suggesting a thymus dependency of these T cells. How-

ever, γδ T cells were observed in the small intestines of these nude mice in about half the number present in the strain- and age-matched normal mice (Table 2). These γδ T cells were, as were those of normal mice, IELs.

γδ T Cells of Different Peripheral Sites Use Different V_γ Gene Segments to Encode Their TCR

Previous studies have demonstrated that s-IEL (DEC) and i-IEL use distinct V_γ gene segments, V5 (Asarnow et al. 1988) and V7 (Takagaki et al. 1989a), respectively, to encode the γ subunits of their TCR. To determine whether there was a similar preferential usage of specific V_γ gene segments by γδ T cells present in other sites, DNA extracted from crude lymphocyte preparations from these sites was amplified by the polymerase chain reaction (PCR) technique (Saiki et al. 1988) using a V_γ (V_γ4, V_γ5, V_γ6, or V_γ7)-specific primer in combination with a (joining) J_γ1-specific primer. The PCR products were then analyzed by

Southern blot analysis using a $J_\gamma 1$ oligonucleotide probe. The results are summarized in Table 2. As in adult thymuses (Ito et al. 1989), the $V_\gamma 4/J_\gamma 1$ rearrangements were most abundant in peripheral lymphoid organs (blood, spleen, and lymph nodes) but bands corresponding to $V_\gamma 6/J_\gamma 1$ and $V_\gamma 7/J_\gamma 1$ rearrangements were also detected in these organs. In agreement with previous studies (Asarnow et al. 1988; Takagaki et al. 1989a), strong $V_\gamma 5/J_\gamma 1$ and $V_\gamma 7/J_\gamma 1$ bands were observed in the skin and small intestine, respectively. Apart from these sites, the most conspicuous were the vagina, uterus, and tongue in which $V_\gamma 6/V_\gamma 1$ rearrangement was abundant. Cloning and sequencing of the PCR products indicated that most (12 of 14) $V_\gamma 6/J_\gamma 1$ clones isolated from vaginas and uteruses contained in-frame junctions with an identical nucleotide sequence (S. Itohara et al. in prep.). These results strongly suggest that most $\gamma\delta$ T cells in female reproductive organs use the single V6J1C1 (constant [C]) γ gene to encode the γ subunits of their TCR. Interestingly, $\gamma\delta$ T cells associated with the tongue (t-IEL) also use the same γ gene (S. Itohara et al., in prep.).

$\gamma\delta$ T Cells Associated with Some Epithelial Organs Are Primarily Derived from Fetal Thymocytes and Carry an Entirely Homogeneous TCR$\gamma\delta$

It was previously shown that the use of γ and δ V gene segments is developmentally ordered in thymocytes (Havran and Allison 1988; Ito et al. 1989; Itohara et al. 1989). $\gamma\delta$ Thymocytes from early fetuses (i.e., at around day 15 of the embryonic life) preferentially express TCR encoded by V5J1C1 γ and V1D2J2C δ genes (Havran and Allison 1988; Ito et al. 1989). We found that these TCRs are entirely homogeneous (J.J. Lafaille et al., in prep.) and that they are identical to the TCR$\gamma\delta$ expressed on s-IEL (Asarnow et al. 1988). Thus, s-IEL probably originates from this first wave of fetal $\gamma\delta$ thymocytes. At late fetal and newborn stages, most $\gamma\delta$ thymocytes bear TCR encoded by another pair of γ and δ genes, V6J1C1 γ and V1D2J2C δ (Ito et al. 1989), which are also structurally homogeneous (J.J. Lafaille et al., in prep.). Since the nucleotide sequence of this V6J1C1 γ gene is identical to the sequence of the sole in-frame joined V6J1C1 γ gene present in r-IEL and t-IEL (S. Itohara et al., in prep.), we suspected that these cells are derived from the second wave of fetal $\gamma\delta$ thymocytes. If this were the case, the δ chains of these T-cell populations also should be identical. We therefore cloned and sequenced the PCR products of V1DJ2C δ genes from r-IEL preparations and found indeed that these genes are also homogeneous in their junctional sequences (S. Itohara et al., in prep.) and that the r-IEL δ gene sequence corresponds exactly to the sequence of the δ gene expressed on the surface of the late fetal thymocyte population (J.J. Lafaille et al., in prep.). We conclude from these results that r-IELs are derived from the late fetal wave of thymocytes.

TCR$\gamma\delta$ Expressed in Adult Thymus and Peripheral Lymphoid Organs Are Diverse

Unlike the early and late fetal thymocytes or s-IEL, r-IEL, and t-IEL, adult $\gamma\delta$ thymocytes and $\gamma\delta$ T cells of peripheral lymphoid organs use various combinations of V_γ and V_δ gene segments to encode their TCR. Furthermore, abundant V-(D)-J junctional diversity occurs among the TCR of these adult $\gamma\delta$ T cells (Korman et al. 1988; Lacy et al. 1989; Takagaki et al. 1989b). Taken together, these results indicate that in addition to the difference in the gene segments utilized for surface expression, there is a drastic fetal versus adult shift in the extent of the junctional diversity in the TCR$\gamma\delta$. Since i-IELs preferentially use the $V_\gamma 7$ gene segment (Takagaki et al. 1989a), which is rarely utilized by fetal thymocytes but is used by some adult thymocytes, and since the TCR gene assembled in adult thymocytes and i-IEL show similar extensive deletions and insertions in the junctions (Takagaki et al. 1989a,b), some adult thymocytes may home to intestinal epithelia. The probable developmental relationship between the various $\gamma\delta$ T cell subpopulations is shown in Figure 4.

Developmental Relationship between $\alpha\beta$ and $\gamma\delta$ T-cell Lineages

One interesting issue raised by the discovery of $\gamma\delta$ T cells is their developmental relationship with $\alpha\beta$ T cells. Several observations relevant to this issue can be summarized. First, during thymic ontogeny, rearrangement

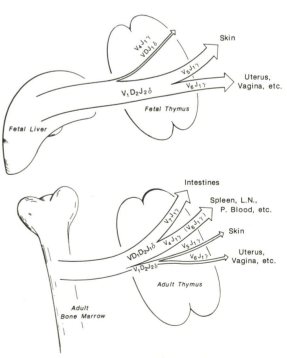

Figure 4. Development of various $\gamma\delta$ T-cell subsets. The arrows indicate the proposed pathways followed by $\gamma\delta$ T lymphocytes expressing the $C_\gamma 1$ region in fetal and adult mice.

and cell-surface expression of at least some γ and δ genes precede that of α and β genes (Raulet et al. 1985; Pardoll et al. 1987; Havran and Allison 1988; Itohara et al. 1989). Second, in peripheral $\alpha\beta$ T cells, some γ genes are almost always rearranged, often in a nonfunctional (i.e., out-of-frame) form (Reilly et al. 1986; Rupp et al. 1986; Heilig and Tonegawa 1987). In contrast, in $\gamma\delta$ thymocytes or peripheral $\gamma\delta$ T cells, β genes are almost always rearranged only incompletely with a diversity (D) gene segment joined to a J gene segment and no V gene segment attached, whereas α genes are never rearranged (Korman et al. 1988; Ito et al. 1989; Takagaki et al. 1989b). Finally, cells bearing both $\alpha\beta$ and $\gamma\delta$ TCRs or "hybrid" TCRs such as $\beta\delta$ or $\alpha\gamma$ heterodimers do not seem to exist (Pardoll et al. 1987; and see above). On the basis of these observations, Pardoll et al. (1987) and Allison and Lanier (1987) proposed that if γ and δ genes rearrange productively (i.e., by in-frame joining), the cell proceeds to surface expression of TCR$\gamma\delta$, which in analogy with the Ig system (Alt et al. 1987) inhibits further rearrangement of any other TCR gene. $\alpha\beta$ T cells are generated only from those cells that failed to rearrange productively both γ and δ genes. We tested this model by constructing and analyzing three different sets of transgenic mice all carrying in their germ line productively rearranged TCR$\gamma\delta$ or TCRγ genes.

Normal Numbers of $\alpha\beta$ T Cells Are Generated in TCR γ and δ Double Transgenic Mice

The first set of transgenic mice (called KN6 transgenic mice) were made by injecting into oocytes a mixture of relatively long γ (40 kb) and δ (43 kb) genomic DNA fragments cloned from the $\gamma\delta$ T-cell hybridoma KN6 (Fig. 5). According to the Pardoll-Allison model, generation of $\alpha\beta$ T cells will be disrupted because all T-cell precursors in these mice should have productively rearranged transgenic γ and δ genes. However, contrary to this prediction neither the absolute number nor the proportion of $\alpha\beta$ T cells is significantly altered in the thymus and spleen of the transgenic mice (Table 3). Furthermore, the thymocytes and splenocytes of these mice exhibit a normal expression pattern of CD4 and CD8 glycoproteins, suggesting that their maturation is normal. The apparently normal generation of $\alpha\beta$ T cells is not due to a failure of the expression of the transgenes in these mice: These mice do contain an elevated level of $\gamma\delta$ T cells, and nearly all of their TCRs are encoded by the transgenes (Table 3).

As in normal mice (see above), $\gamma\delta/\alpha\beta$ double producers are not detectable in these transgenic mice (I. Ishida et al., in prep.). We conclude that there must be a mechanism restricting the expression of TCR to one

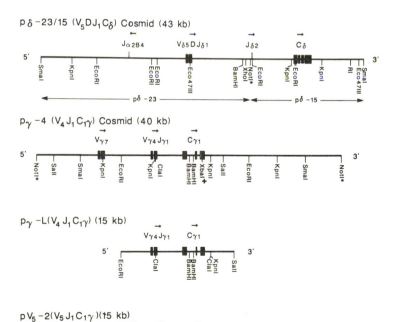

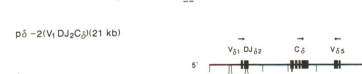

Figure 5. Restriction maps of γ and δ genomic DNA clones used for the construction of transgenic mice. The cosmid clones pδ-23/15 and pγ-4 were cloned from a $\gamma\delta$ T hybridoma KN6 (C57BL/6) and were used to prepare KN6 transgenic mice. Phage λ clone pγ-L was cloned from a T-cell hybridoma 3D10 (C3H, Nakauchi et al. 1984) and was used to prepare the γ-only transgenic mice. The cosmid clones pV5-2 and pδ-2 were cloned from a $\gamma\delta$ T hybridoma KI-129 (C57BL/6) (Ito et al. 1989) and were used to prepare the DEC transgenic mice. (■) Exons or gene segments; ($\rightarrow$) their transcriptional orientation. The *Xba*I ($+$) site was destroyed deliberately in clone pγ-L.

Table 3. Surface Expression of TCRγδ and TCRαβ on Thymocytes and Splenocytes of γδ Transgenic Mice

| Mice | Age (wk) | Total cells | Thymocytes ($\times 10^{-6}$) stained with | | | Total cells | Splenocytes ($\times 10^{-6}$) stained with | | |
			anti-γδ	anti-KN6	anti-αβ		anti-γδ	anti-KN6	anti-αβ
γδ 1313	9	79	1.26 (1.6)	1.02 (1.3)	56.8 (71.9)	153	6.32 (4.1)	6.27 (4.1)	43.0 (28.1)
LM	9	78	0.16 (0.2)	0.00 (0.0)	55.9 (71.7)	167	0.66 (0.4)	0.00 (0.0)	43.6 (26.1)
γδ 1355	8	100	2.66 (2.7)	2.66 (2.7)	72.7 (72.7)	161	4.96 (3.1)	4.83 (3.0)	36.1 (22.4)
LM	8	99	0.10 (0.1)	0.00 (0.0)	74.2 (74.9)	152	0.89 (0.6)	0.00 (0.0)	39.7 (26.1)

Thymocytes and splenocytes were stained with anti-γδ, anti-KN6, or anti-αβ MAb. Proportion (%) of TCRγδ- or TCRαβ-bearing T cells among total thymocytes or splenocytes is also shown in parentheses. LM designates nontransgenic littermates.

of the two types in a given T-cell precursor that is active before either of the two types of TCR is expressed on the cell surface.

A Transcriptional Silencer in the Flanking Region of the γ Gene

We investigated the reason why the γδ transgene products are not expressed on the surface of the αβ T cells in the KN6 transgenic mice by analyzing DNA and RNA of these cells. First, Southern blot analysis of DNA isolated from a T-cell population enriched with TCRαβ⁺ cells as well as from T-cell hybridomas prepared from TCRαβ⁺ cells showed that both the γ and δ transgenes are retained by the αβ T cells. Second, the analysis of the RNA extracted from the αβ T-cell population or from the αβ T hybridomas demonstrated that no transcripts derived from the transgenes accumulate in the αβ T cells. These results suggest that there exists a *cis*-acting DNA element(s) that mediates the repression of γ and δ RNA accumulation in αβ T cells. This putative element(s) must be contained within the 40-kb γ and/or 43-kb δ genomic DNA fragments used for the construction of the transgenic mice.

To test this possibility, we constructed a second set of transgenic mice (called "short γ" transgenic mice) using a γ gene clone containing very limited flanking sequences (Fig. 5, clone pγ-L.). We found that αβ T cells in this set of transgenic mice, in contrast with those in the KN6 transgenic mice, did harbor abundant RNA transcribed from the γ transgene but not from the endogenous γ genes (I. Ishida et al., in prep.). Since these results were obtained with three transgenic founder mice, it is very unlikely that the differential expression of the transgenes and endogenous γ genes is caused by the specific sequence context in which transgenes are integrated. We conclude that the γ gene carries in its flanking regions a *cis*-acting DNA element that down-regulates γ transcription in αβ T cells. This "silencer" element must be in the 5'- or 3'-flanking regions present on the pγ-4 clone but absent on the pγ-L clone.

Silencer Model of αβ and γδ T-cell Lineages

In view of these findings, we propose a model for the differentiation of αβ and γδ T-cell lineages (Fig. 6). γ and δ gene rearrangements occur prior to the completion (i.e., V to DJ joining) of β gene rearrangement and the initiation of α gene rearrangement. In-frame rearrangements of both γ and δ genes are, of course, a prerequisite for the generation of γδ thymocytes. However, we propose on the basis of the normal appearance of αβ T cells in the γδ transgenic mice that the failure to rearrange both γ and δ genes in-frame is not a requirement for the generation of αβ thymocytes. This implies that some αβ thymocytes could be generated from cells that harbor both in-frame rearranged γ and δ genes, and therefore precursors of some αβ T cells may express TCRγδ on their surface. Although this possibility cannot be ruled out, any TCRγδ expression in these cells is likely to be transient because we detected no thymocytes coexpressing both TCRαβ and TCRγδ either in the γδ transgenic mice (I. Ishida et al., in prep.) or normal mice (Itohara et al. 1989).

We propose that the putative machinery acting upon the γ silencer is activated in a fraction of immature thymocytes and that it is from these cells that αβ thymocytes are generated. The activation of the silencer machinery could occur prior to γ and δ gene rearrangements. In this case, αβ and γδ T-cell lineages are completely separate, and no αβ thymocyte precursors will ever express TCRγδ. The activation of the machinery, however, could occur between the completion of γ and δ gene rearrangements and that of α and β gene rearrangements. In this case, precursors of some αβ T cells may express TCRγδ transiently.

One may argue, in support of the Pardoll-Allison model, that the expression of the transgenes in our γδ transgenic mice is abnormally delayed for an unknown reason during the thymocyte differentiation and that this is the reason why rearrangements of the endogenous α and β genes and subsequent generation of αβ T cells are not disrupted in these mice. We argue that this is unlikely for the following two reasons. First, when we examined the cell-surface expression of the transgene-

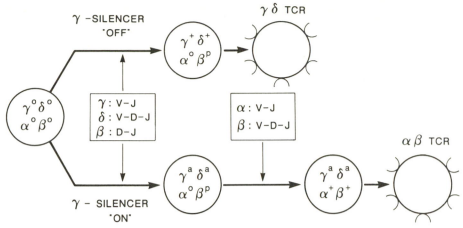

Figure 6. The silencer model of $\alpha\beta$ and $\gamma\delta$ T-cell differentiation. The various states of rearrangement of four TCR genes are indicated by superscripts. (0 and +) The gene is in the germ-line configuration and productively rearranged, respectively; (a and p) gene is in any state (i.e., in germ-line configuration, productively or nonproductively rearranged or deleted); (p) partially rearranged (i.e., D-J joined). The γ gene associated silencer is inactive in the $\gamma\delta$ T-cell lineage (*top*) and is activated in the $\alpha\beta$ T-cell lineage (*bottom*). The activation may occur either before any TCR gene is rearranged or after γ and δ genes are rearranged but before α and β gene rearrangements are completed. See text for more details.

coded TCR$\gamma\delta$ on fetal thymocytes, we found that the transgene-coded TCRs are expressed earlier than TCR$\alpha\beta$ (data not shown). Second, in the $\gamma\delta$1355 transgenic mice, we observed a near complete inhibition of rearrangement of the endogenous γ and δ genes. This inhibition most probably occurred by a mechanism analogous to the one known to form the basis for "allelic exclusion" of Ig and TCR$\alpha\beta$ genes. According to the widely accepted model of allelic exclusion (Alt et al. 1987), Ig or TCR feed back as soon as they are expressed on the cell surface to corresponding genes and inhibit their rearrangement. Thus, if the surface expression of the $\gamma\delta$-transgene-coded TCR$\gamma\delta$ had been abnormally delayed in the $\gamma\delta$ transgenic mice, we would have expected rearrangement of endogenous γ and δ genes and the surface expression of their products. Contrary to this prediction, we detected virtually no rearrangement and no cell-surface expression (Table 3) of the endogenous γ or δ genes in the transgenic mouse $\gamma\delta$1355. We therefore conclude that the transgene expression is not abnormally delayed in this mouse.

A Third Set of Transgenic Mice Support the Silencer Model

One prediction that could be made by the silencer model of T-cell development is that the generation of $\alpha\beta$ T cells would be hampered in a transgenic mouse constructed with γ and δ genes carrying no silencer element. We tested this prediction by constructing the third set of γ/δ double transgenic mice using "short" γ and δ gene clones (Fig. 5, clones pV5-2 and pδ2). As in the KN6 transgenic mice constructed with the "long" γ and δ gene clones, an overwhelming majority of the TCR$\gamma\delta$ in these transgenic mice (called DEC transgenic mice) is encoded by the transgenes (Fig. 7A).

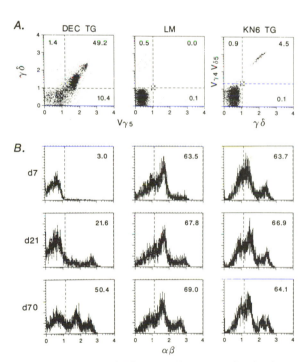

Figure 7. TCR$\gamma\delta$ and TCR$\alpha\beta$ surface expression by thymocytes from DEC transgenic, KN6 transgenic, and nontransgenic mice. (*A*) Thymocytes from 10-week-old DEC transgenic (*left*) and nontransgenic (*middle*) littermate and KN6 transgenic mice (*right*) were analyzed by two-color flow cytometry using anti-V$_\gamma$5 MAb F536, anti-$\gamma\delta$ MAb 3A10, and anti-V$_\gamma$4V$_\delta$5 MAb 8D6. The number in each quadrant is the percentage of cells stained by one or both MAbs. Fluorescence intensity is expressed in $\log_{10}$ units. For comparison, an analysis of age-matched KNG transgenic mice is shown. (*B*) Thymocytes from 7-, 21-, and 70-day-old DEC transgenic (*left*), nontransgenic (*middle*), and KN6 transgenic (*right*) mice were stained with anti-$\alpha\beta$ MAb H57-597. The percentages of positive cells are indicated to the right of each histogram. Fluorescence intensity is expressed in $\log_{10}$ units.

Although the number of TCR$\gamma\delta^+$ thymocytes is 10- to 100-fold higher in the transgenic mice than in the nontransgenic littermates, the total number of thymocytes is greatly reduced because the development of $\alpha\beta$ T cells is severely hampered (Fig. 7B). In older transgenic mice, some $\alpha\beta$ T cells become detectable, most of which coexpress TCR$\gamma\delta$. Southern blot analysis of DNA extracted from the total thymocytes indicated that β gene rearrangement is blocked in these mice (M. Bonneville et al., in prep.).

Recognition of a Self Histocompatibility Complex TL Region Product by TCR$\gamma\delta$

To understand the function of $\gamma\delta$ T cells, it is essential to identify the putative ligand of the TCR. For this purpose, we prepared a number of $\gamma\delta$ T-cell hybridomas from fetal and adult thymocytes and screened them for specificity using a growth-inhibition assay. It was previously shown that cross-linking the TCR$\alpha\beta$, which usually promotes growth of normal T cells, results in growth inhibition of T-cell hybridomas (Ashwell et al. 1987). Assuming a similar effect of TCR$\gamma\delta$ cross-linking by a ligand, we cocultivated the $\gamma\delta$ T-cell hybridomas with a variety of irradiated (6000 rads) test cells, and we measured the effect of these cells on the incorporation of [^{3}H]thymidine into the DNA of the hybridomas. We identified one $\gamma\delta$ T hybridoma, KN6, whose growth was inhibited by syngeneic (C57BL/6) but not allogeneic (BALB/c, CBA/J, and AKR/J) spleen cells (Bonneville et al. 1989). KN6 hybridoma

growth was inhibited efficiently by thymocytes, peritoneal macrophages, splenocytes, cells from the Abelson transformed B6 T-cell line 2052C, and by PCC3 embryonal carcinoma cells. The response to syngeneic spleen cells was observed in three different CD3$^+$ subclones of the KN6 hybridoma (KN6-7, KN6-12, and KN6-10) but not with TCR$^-$ variants of KN6 (KN6-19 and KN6-2), which indicated that growth inhibition was mediated by the TCR. This conclusion was further supported by the finding that the KN6 growth inhibition was blocked in a dose-dependent fashion by the anti-TCR$\gamma\delta$ MAb 3A10 as well as by the anti-KN6 TCR clonotypic MAb 5C10 (Bonneville et al. 1989).

Since the KN6 hybridoma responds to syngeneic but not to allogeneic cells, the gene encoding or controlling the KN6 ligand must be polymorphic. To confirm this and to map the gene, the KN6 hybridoma was screened for reactivity with a panel of spleen cells from various mouse strains (Table 4). Linkage to the major histocompatibility complex (MHC) was demonstrated by results with congenic strains that differ only at H-2. Thus, KN6 cell proliferation was strongly inhibited by cells from H-2^b strains, partially inhibited by cells from H-2^f strains, and not affected by cells from H-2^d, H-2^k, H-2^p, or H-2^s mice. Most importantly, the analysis of recombinant strains showed that the gene controlling the KN6 ligand is located in or distal to the TL region. This conclusion is based on the observation that the hybridoma responds to B6/Boy (K^{b}D^{b}Qa^{b}Tl^b) and A.Tla^b/Boy cells (K^{a}D^{a}Qa^a/TL^b) but not to A/Boy (K^{a}D^{a}Qa^{a}TL^a) or B6.Tla^a/Boy (K^{b}D^{b}Qa^b/TL^a) cells (Table 4).

Table 4. The Ligand Recognized by KN6 is Controlled by MHC Genes Telomeric to the Q Region

Strain[a]	Region[b]				Percentage	
	K	D	Q	TL	phenotype[c]	proliferation[d]
A.BY/SnJ	b	b	b	b	+	−75
C57BL/6J (B6)	b	b	b	b	+	−76 ± 12
C57BL/10SnJ (B10)	b	b	b	b	+	−89 ± 6
A.CA/Sn	f	f	f	f	±?	−37 ± 19
B10.M/Sn	f	f	f	f	±?	−36 ± 29
B10.D2/nSnJ	d	d	d	d	−	+30 ± 17
B10.BR/SgSnJ	k	k	k	k	−	−5 ± 12
P/J	p	p	p	p	−	+31 ± 27
B10.G/Sg	q	q	q	q	−	+8 ± 6
B10.RIII(7INS)/SnJ	r	r	r	r	−	+11 ± 2
B10.S/Sg	s	s	s	s	−	+8 ± 23
A/Boy	a	a	a	a	−	+4 ± 8
B6/Boy	b	b	b	b	+	−85 ± 4
A-Tla^b/Boy	a	a	a	b	+	−66 ± 14
B6-Tla^a/Boy	b	b	b	a		−2 ± 13

^{a} Other + strains include BALB.B/Li, B10.A(2R)SgSnJ, B10.A(R149)-Tla^b/Mrp, B10.A(R410)-Tla^b/Mrp, B10.P(13R)/Sg, B10.SM(70NS)/Sn, and TBR2. Other − strains include AKR/J, A/WySnJ, BALB/c, B6-H-2^k/Boy, B6.K1/Fla, B6.K2/Fla, B10.A/SgSnJ, B10.PL(73NS)/Sn, B10(R297)-Tla^a/Mrp, B10(R310)-Tla^a/Mrp, C3H/HeJ, and MA/MyJ.
^{b} Haplotype origin of region.
^{c} + indicates strong inhibition. ± indicates possible intermediate inhibition. Results variable and not consistent. − indicated no inhibition.
^{d} Data shown are with a single clone, KN6-7. All experiments done at least twice, except with A.BY, which also tested + with the original KN6 line.

Table 5. Percentage of Homology of the cDNAs Encoding the Putative KN6 Ligand with Known Class I Molecules

Region	Gene	Exon					
		I	II	III	IV	V	VI
H-2	H2-K^d	55	71	62	92	43	52
Qa-2, 3	Q10	52	72	60	95	36	49
Tla	T3	48	66	56	92	41	46
	37	52	71	65	95	39	39

TL Gene That May Encode the Class I Molecule Recognized by KN6 TCR$\gamma\delta$

The embryonic carcinoma line PCC3 does not express class I H-2K, D, or L or class II I-A or I-E MHC molecules on their surface (Maher and Dove 1984; Stern et al. 1986), and yet it is specifically recognized by KN6 TCR. To determine the structure of the molecule recognized by KN6 TCR$\gamma\delta$, we made a cDNA library from this cell line and screened the library with a probe composed of the exon 4 region (Weiss et al. 1984), which is conserved among all MHC class I genes known to date. This led to the isolation of 12 cDNA clones that fell into 7 kinds on the basis of their nucleotide sequences. The gene represented by one and only one of these 7 kinds of clones was distinct from all known MHC class I genes and appears to belong to the TL gene family on the basis of the pattern of sequence homology in the various exons (Table 5). Thus, the product of this gene is a good candidate for the TL-mapped ligand recognized by the KN6 TCR$\gamma\delta$.

Fate of Self-reactive $\gamma\delta$ Thymocytes in the KN6 Transgenic Mice

Recent studies suggest that T-cell tolerance is accomplished, at least in part, by intrathymic deletion of self-reactive $\alpha\beta$ T cells (Kappler et al. 1987; Kisielow et al. 1988; MacDonald et al. 1988). We have begun studies to determine whether or not a similar deletion of self-reactive $\gamma\delta$ T cells occurs. Since the KN6 TCR$\gamma\delta$ recognizes syngeneic (TL^b) thymocytes and splenocytes, we analyzed thymocytes and splenic T cells from the KN6 $\gamma\delta$ transgenic mice expressing MHC^b or MHC$^{k/d}$ haplotypes. As shown in Table 6, nearly all $\gamma\delta$ T cells bear TCR encoded by the transgenes regardless of the MHC haplotype of the host (i.e., MHC^b or

MHC$^{k/d}$). Furthermore, the number of $\gamma\delta$ T cells present in either thymus or spleen is not lower in the MHC^b mice than in MHC$^{k/d}$ mice. Thus, there was no obvious deletion of self-reactive $\gamma\delta$ T cells. $\gamma\delta$ Thymocytes isolated from MHC^b hosts but not from MHC$^{k/d}$ hosts propagate rapidly in vitro in the presence of concanavalin A supernatant or recombinant interleukin-2. $\gamma\delta$ Thymocytes derived from MHC$^{k/d}$ transgenic mice require, in addition to the lymphokine, stimulation by TL^b ligand-bearing cells. The average density of TCR$\gamma\delta$ is lower in the MHC^b thymocytes than in MHC$^{k/d}$ thymocytes, suggesting the occurrence of receptor modulation in the former transgenic mice. These results indicate that the $\gamma\delta$ thymocytes recognize and respond to the putative TL^b ligand in vivo in the thymus of the KN6 transgenic mice.

DISCUSSION

Our study sheds considerable light on the characteristics of TCR$\gamma\delta$ and T cells bearing this receptor. Except for some $\gamma\delta$ T cells associated with intestinal epithelia, the majority of $\gamma\delta$ T cells develops in the thymus as $\alpha\beta$ T cells do. However, there are a number of features that distinguish the two types of T cells. First, in mouse, $\gamma\delta$ T cells constitute a relatively minor T-cell subpopulation in peripheral lymphoid organs, and they preferentially home to a variety of epithelial tissues. Second, whereas the TCR$\gamma\delta$ expressed in the peripheral lymphoid organs are diverse, those expressed in some epithelia such as those of the epidermis (DEC or s-IEL) and reproductive organs (r-IEL) are encoded by specific γ and δ genes and exhibit no structural diversity. Third, $\gamma\delta$ thymocyte subsets having the same TCR as those of various peripheral T-cell subsets appear in ontogeny in ordered waves: Thymocytes corresponding to s-IEL and r-IEL appear in early and late

Table 6. Surface Expression of TCR$\gamma\delta$ in KN6 $\gamma\delta$ Transgenic Mice

Mice	H-2	Thymocytes ($\times 10^{-6}$)			Splenocytes ($\times 10^{-6}$)		
		total cells	$\gamma\delta^+$	KN6$^+$	total cells	$\gamma\delta^+$	KN6$^+$
LM	b/k	99	0.1	0	152	0.89	0
$\gamma\delta$	k/d	100	2.66	2.66	161	4.96	4.83
$\gamma\delta$	b/k	44	3.35	3.13	148	4.18	4.02
$\gamma\delta$	b/b	24	1.83	1.79	106	4.16	4.18

Thymus and spleen cell suspensions were stained with anti-δ (3A10) or anticlonotypic KN6 (5C10) MAbs. The H-2 haplotypes of nontransgenic and transgenic mice were determined by using anti-H-2^K MAbs.

embryos, respectively, and thymocytes corresponding to spleen, lymph node, and peripheral blood T cells appear in postnatal animals. Fourth, there is a drastic shift in the diversity of TCRγδ expressed in fetal and postnatal thymuses: Fetal TCRγδ are virtually of two primary structures (those for s-IEL and those for r-IEL), whereas postnatal TCRγδ exhibit both combinatorial and junctional diversity. Fifth, in accordance with the fetal versus postnatal shift in the usage of γ and δ gene segments and the receptor diversity, the intrathymic localization of γδ T cells changes drastically during the first few postnatal days: Fetal and neonatal γδ thymocytes are closely associated with medullary epithelial cells, whereas adult γδ thymocytes are scattered throughout the thymus and are most concentrated in the subcapsular areas. Sixth, although γδ and αβ T cells share common precursor cells, the two cell lineages seem to separate from each other early in differentiation with no coexpression stage. A transcriptional silencer element associated with the γ gene seems to play a critical role in the branching of the two cell lineages. Seventh, at least some γδ T cells recognize a determinant encoded by a self-MHC gene mapped in or distal to the TL region. Preliminary data indicate that this gene encodes a new MHC class I molecule that is not known to present peptides to αβ T cells. Finally, at least some self-reactive γδ T cells, although activated in the thymus, are not deleted in the syngeneic thymus or spleen in contrast with the intrathymic deletion of some self-reactive αβ T cells.

Despite the considerable information that has accumulated during the past few years on TCRγδ and γδ T cells, the biological functions of these cells remain to be determined. Below, we wish to present some thoughts on this issue.

There is considerable evidence indicating that γδ T cells recognize molecules similar to but distinct from the MHC class I molecules that are used to present antigen-derived peptides to αβ T cells (this paper; Bluestone et al. 1988; Bonneville et al. 1989). Although there also are reports that some γδ T cells recognize allogeneic K or D region class I molecules or the I region class II molecules, these specificities may have resulted from cross-reactivity, since strong selective pressure was applied to detect them (Matis et al.

1987; Bluestone et al. 1988). Indeed, the recent finding (Y. Utsunomiya et al., unpubl.) that the subunit structure of CD8 molecules expressed on activated i-IEL and splenic γδ T cells is different from that expressed on αβ T cells supports the hypothesis that γδ and αβ T cells recognize distinct sets of class I (or class-I-like) molecules (Fig. 8).

If γδ T cells generally recognize distinct class I (or class-I-like) molecules, the next question is whether or not these class I molecules present peptides to TCRγδ, as do the MHC class I, K, D, and L molecules to TCRαβ. Although no direct evidence is available at the moment, the structural similarities both between the TCRαβ and TCRγδ and between the class I (or class-I-like) molecules recognized by the two types of TCR suggest that the ligands for TCRγδ generally include antigen-derived peptides (Fig. 8).

Are γδ T cells, then, specific to a variety of antigens as are αβ T cells and is the repertoire of the antigens recognized by TCRγδ more or less identical with that of the antigens recognized by TCRαβ? Here, it would be useful to consider separately the two types of γδ T-cell subsets: one with a high degree of TCR diversity such as i-IEL and splenic γδ T cells and the other with invariant TCR such as s-IEL and r-IEL. In the former case, it is likely that the antigens (hence, the peptides derived from them) recognized by γδ T cells are structurally diverse. However, the antigenic repertoire for γδ T cells may be different from that for αβ T cells. Perhaps the class I molecules recognized by TCRγδ (hereafter, abbreviated as REγδ, antigen-restriction elements for TCRγδ) have evolved to present a special set of antigens to the immune system. The selectivity of REγδ for a particular set of antigens might be explained by postulating a special intracellular pathway of peptide loading for REγδ and/or common structural features of the presented peptides. A hint as to which set of proteins may be presented efficiently by REγδ has come from recent experiments that have shown the recognition of mycobacterial heat-shock-like proteins by some γδ T cells (Holoshitz et al. 1989; Janis et al. 1989; Modlin et al. 1989; O'Brien et al. 1989). It may be that γδ T cells with diverse TCR are primarily directed to a variety of mycobacteria and parasitical protozoa known to produce constitutively structurally

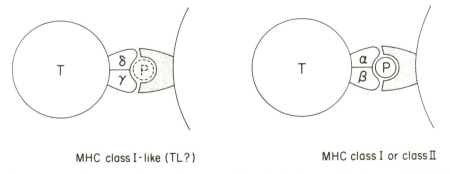

MHC class I-like (TL?)   MHC class I or class II

Figure 8. Comparison of the proposed recognition by a γδ T cell with the established recognition by a αβ T cell.

related but distinct heat-shock-like proteins. The effector function of the γδ T cells is unknown, but one might speculate that these cells play a role in the initiation or regulation of defense reactions by lymphokine secretion or elimination of undesirable cells such as persistent antigen-presenting cells.

In contrast with a γδ T-cell subset capable of recognizing structurally diverse ligands, a γδ T-cell subset with an invariable TCR must recognize an equally invariable ligand. Despite this important difference in the diversity of the ligands, it is likely that the basic composition (i.e., a peptide/RE complex) of the ligand recognized by the invariant TCRγδ is the same as that of the ligands recognized by diverse TCRγδ. Assuming that this is indeed the case, the key issue is again the origin of the peptide. Because it does not make sense for an organism to secure an entire subset of T cells localized in an organ for the protection against just a single foreign antigen, we should consider an alternative role and/or mechanism for the undiversified γδ T cells. Perhaps these γδ T cells recognize a tissue-specific host antigen whose synthesis may be induced in the epithelial cells by a variety of unfavorable stimuli, such as viral infections, toxic chemicals, radiation, heat shock, and malignancy (Janeway et al. 1988). One candidate of such a host antigen is a stress protein whose synthesis may be induced in tissue-specific fashion. Since at least some of these proteins are known to be structurally related to mycobacterial heat-shock-like proteins, it is conceivable that the peptides derived from them could also effectively bind to and be presented by REγδ. Since the postulated antigen is induced only under specific conditions, autoreactivity of these γδ T cells may not have any hazardous consequences but rather play an important regulatory and/or effector role. The peculiar specificity of γδ T cells envisaged in our model is somewhat reminiscent of the specificity of another class of lymphocytes, those called CD5 B cells. These B cells also appear to preferentially recognize common bacterial antigens as well as self-antigens.

ACKNOWLEDGMENTS

We thank Amy DeCloux, Edvins Krecko, Carol Browne, and Sang Hsu for excellent technical assistance and Elly Basel for typing the manuscript. We also thank Werner Haas for useful comments. This work was supported in part by grants from Howard Hughes Medical Institute, National Institutes of Health (NIH), American Cancer Society, and Ajinomoto Co., Ltd. to S.T. as well as the NIH CORE P30-CA-14051. We also thank FUJI Photo Film Co. for the use of the BA100-Bioimage Analyzer.

REFERENCES

Allison, J.P. and L.L. Lanier. 1987. The T-cell antigen receptor gamma gene: Rearrangement and cell lineages. *Immunol. Today* **8:** 293.

Alt, F.W., T. Blackwell, and G.D. Yancopoulos. 1987. Development of the primary antibody repertoire. *Science* **238:** 1079.

Asarnow, D.M., W.A. Kuziel, M. Bonyhadi, R.E. Tigelaar, P.W. Tucker, and J.P. Allison. 1988. Limited diversity of γδ antigen receptor genes of Thy-1⁺ dendritic epidermal cells. *Cell* **55:** 837.

Ashwell, J.D., P.E. Cunningham, P.D. Noguchi, and D. Hernandez. 1987. Cell growth cycle block of T cell hybridomas upon activation with antigen. *J. Exp. Med.* **165:** 173.

Bank, I., R.A. DePinho, M.B. Brenner, J. Cassimeris, F.W. Alt, and L. Chess. 1986. A functional T3 molecule associated with a novel heterodimer on the surface of immature human thymocytes. *Nature* **322:** 179.

Bergstresser, P.R., R.E. Tigelaar, J.H. Dees, and J.W. Streilein. 1983. Thy-1 antigen-bearing dendritic cells populate murine epidermis. *J. Invest. Dermatol.* **81:** 286.

Bluestone, J.A., R.Q. Cron, M. Cotteman, B.A. Houlden, and L.A. Matis. 1988. Structure and specificity of TCR γδ on major histocompatibility complex antigen specific CD3⁺, CD4⁻, CD8⁻ T lymphocytes. *J. Exp. Med.* **168:** 1989.

Bonneville, M., C.A. Janeway, Jr., K. Ito, W. Haser, I. Ishida, N. Nakanishi, and S. Tonegawa. 1988. Intestinal intraepithelial lymphocytes are a distinct set of γδ T cells. *Nature* **336:** 479.

Bonneville, M., K. Ito, E.G. Krecko, S. Itohara, D. Kappes, I. Ishida, O. Kanagawa, C.A. Janeway, Jr., D.B. Murphy, and S. Tonegawa. 1989. Recognition of a self MHC TL region product by γδ T cell receptors. *Proc. Natl. Acad. Sci.* **86:** 5928.

Borst, J., J.J.M. van Dongen, R.L.H. Bolhuis, P. Peters, D.A. Hafler, E. de Vries, and R.J. van de Griend. 1988. Distinct molecular forms of human T cell receptor γ/δ detected on viable T cells by a monoclonal antibody. *J. Exp. Med.* **167:** 1625.

Brenner, M.B., J. McLean, D.P. Dialynas, J.L. Strominger, J.A. Smith, F.L. Owen, J.G. Seidman, S. Ip, F. Rosen, and M.S. Krangel. 1986. Identification of a putative second T-cell receptor. *Nature* **322:** 145.

Bucy, R.P., C.-L.H. Chen, J. Cihak, U. Lösch, and M.D. Cooper. 1988. Avian T cells expressing γδ receptors localize in the splenic sinusoids and the intestinal epithelium. *J. Immunol.* **141:** 2200.

Chen, C.H., J.T. Sowder, J.M. Lahti, J. Cihak, U. Lösch, and M.D. Cooper. 1989. TCR 3: A third T cell receptor in the chicken. *Proc. Natl. Acad. Sci.* **86:** 2351.

Farr, A.G. and S.K. Anderson. 1985. Epithelial heterogeneity of the murine thymus: Fucose-specific lectins bind medullary epithelial cells. *J. Immunol.* **134:** 2971.

Goodman, T. and L. Lefrançois. 1988. Expression of the γδ T-cell receptor on intestinal CD8⁺ intraepithelial lymphocytes. *Nature* **333:** 855.

Green, E.L. 1966. *Biology of the laboratory mouse.* McGraw-Hill, New York.

Groh, V., S. Porcelli, M. Fabbi, L.L. Lanier, L.J. Picker, T. Anderson, R.A. Warnke, A.K. Bhan, J.L. Strominger, and M.B. Brenner. 1989. Human lymphocytes bearing T cell receptor γδ are phenotypically diverse and evenly distributed throughout the lymphoid system. *J. Exp. Med.* **169:** 1277.

Havran, W.L. and J.P. Allison. 1988. Developmentally ordered appearance of thymocytes expressing different T-cell antigen receptors. *Nature* **335:** 443.

Hayday, A.C., H. Saito, S.D. Gillies, D.M. Kranz, G. Tanigawa, H.N. Eisen, and S. Tonegawa. 1985. Structure organisation and somatic rearrangement of T cell "gamma genes." *Cell* **40:** 259.

Heilig, J.S. and S. Tonegawa. 1987. T-cell γ gene is allelically but not isotypically excluded and is not required in known functional T-cell subsets. *Proc. Natl. Acad. Sci.* **84:** 8070.

Holoshitz, J., F. Koning, J.E. Coligan, J. deBruyn, and S. Strober. 1989. Isolation of CD4⁻CD8⁻ mycobacteria-reac-

tive T lymphocyte clones from rheumatoid arthritis synovial fluid. *Nature* **339:** 226.

Ito, K., M. Bonneville, Y. Takagaki, N. Nakanishi, O.
Kanagawa, E. Krecko, and S. Tonegawa. 1989. Different
$\gamma\delta$ T-cell receptors are expressed on thymocytes at differ-
ent stages of development. *Proc. Natl. Acad. Sci.* **86:** 631.

Itohara, S., N. Nakanishi, O. Kanagawa, R. Kubo, and S.
Tonegawa. 1989. Monoclonal antibodies specific to native
murine T cell receptor $\gamma\delta$: Analysis of $\gamma\delta$ T cells in thymic
ontogeny and peripheral lymphoid organs. *Proc. Natl.
Acad. Sci.* **86:** 5094.

Janeway, C.A., Jr., B. Jones, and A. Hayday. 1988. Specificity and function of T cells bearing γ/δ receptors. *Immunol.
Today* **9:** 73.

Janis, E.M., S.H.E. Kaufmann, R.H. Schwartz, and D.M.
Pardoll. 1989. Activation of $\gamma\delta$ T cells in the primary
immune response to mycobacterium tuberculosis. *Science*
244: 713.

Kappler, J.W., N. Roehm, and P. Marrack. 1987. T cell tolerance by clonal elimination in the thymus. *Cell* **49:** 273.

Kisielow, P., H. Blüthmann, U.D. Staerz, M. Steinmetz, and
H. von Boehmer. 1988. Tolerance in T-cell-receptor transgenic mice involves deletion of nonmature $CD4^+8^+$
thymocytes. *Nature* **333:** 742.

Korman, A.J., S.M. Galesic, D. Spencer, A.M. Kruisbeek,
and D. Raulet. 1988. Predominant variable region usage
by γ/δ T cell receptor-bearing cells in the adult thymus. *J.
Exp. Med.* **168:** 1021.

Kuziel, W.A., A. Takashima, M. Bonhadi, P.R. Bergstresser,
J.P. Allison, R.E. Tigelaar, and P.W. Tucker. 1987. Regulation of T-cell receptor γ-chain RNA expression in
murine Thy-1$^+$ dendritic epidermal cells. *Nature* **328:** 263.

Lacy, M.J., L.K. McNeil, M.E. Roth, and D.M. Kranz. 1989.
T-cell receptor δ-chain diversity in peripheral lymphocytes. *Proc. Natl. Acad. Sci.* **86:** 1023.

Lew, A.M., D.M. Pardoll, W.L. Maloy, B.J. Fowlkes, A.
Kruisbeek, S.-F. Cheng, R.N. Germain, J.A. Bluestone,
R.H. Schwartz, and J.E. Coligan. 1986. Characterization
of T cell receptor gamma chain expression in a subset of
murine thymocytes. *Science* **234:** 1401.

MacDonald, H.R., R. Schneider, R.K. Lees, R.C. Howe, H.
Acha-Orbea, H. Festenstein, R.M. Zinkernagel, and H.
Hengartner. 1988. T cell receptor V_β use predicts reactivity
and tolerance to MLs^a-encoded antigens. *Nature* **323:** 40.

Maeda, K., N. Nakanishi, B.L. Rogers, W.G. Haser, K.
Shitara, H. Yoshida, Y. Takagaki, A.A. Augustin, and S.
Tonegawa. 1987. Expression of T$_\gamma$ gene products on the
surface of peripheral T cells and T cell blasts generated by
allogeneic mixed lymphocyte reaction. *Proc. Natl. Acad.
Sci.* **84:** 6536.

Maher, L.J. and W.F. Dove. 1984. Overt expression of H-2
serotypes on EC cells is not necessary for host rejection.
Immunogenetics **19:** 343.

Matis, L.A., R. Cron, and J.A. Bluestone. 1987. Major histocompatibility complex-linked specificity of $\gamma\delta$ receptor-
bearing T lymphocytes. *Nature* **330:** 262.

Modlin, R.L., C. Pirmez, F.M. Hofman, V. Torigian, K.
Uyemura, T.H. Rea, B.R. Bloom, and M.B. Brenner.
1989. Lymphocytes bearing antigen-specific $\gamma\delta$ T-cell receptors accumulate in human infectious disease lesions.
Nature **339:** 544.

Nakanishi, N., K. Maeda, K. Ito, M. Heller, and S. Tonegawa. 1987. T γ protein is expressed on murine fetal
thymocytes as a disulphide-linked heterodimer. *Nature*
325: 720.

Nakauchi, H., I. Ohno, M. Kim, K. Okumura, and T. Tada.
1984. Establishment and functional analysis of a cloned,
antigen-specific suppressor effector T cell line. *J. Immunol.* **132:** 88.

O'Brien, R.L., M.P. Happ, A. Dallas, E. Palmer, R. Kubo,
and W. Born. 1989. Stimulation of a major subset of
lymphocytes expressing T cell receptor $\gamma\delta$ by an antigen
from mycobacterium tuberculosis. *Cell* **57:** 667.

Pardoll, D.M., B.J. Fowlkes, J.A. Bluestone, A. Kruisbeek,
W.L. Maloy, J.E. Coligan, and R.H. Schwartz. 1987. Differential expression of two distinct T-cell receptors during
thymocyte development. *Nature* **326:** 79.

Raulet, D.H., R.D. Garman, H. Saito, and S. Tonegawa.
1985. Developmental regulation of T-cell receptor gene
expression. *Nature* **314:** 103.

Reilly, E.B., D.M. Kranz, S. Tonegawa, and H.N. Eisen.
1986. A functional γ gene formed from known γ-gene
segments is not necessary for antigen-specific responses of
murine cytotoxic T lymphocytes. *Nature* **321:** 878.

Rupp, F., G. Frech, H. Hengartner, R.M. Zinkernagel, and
R. Joho. 1986. No functional gamma-chain transcripts detected in an alloreactive cytotoxic T-cell line. *Nature*
321: 876.

Saiki, R.K., D.H. Gelfand, S. Stoffel, S.J. Scharf, R.
Higuchi, G.T. Horn, K.B. Mullis, and H.A. Erlich. 1988.
Primer-directed enzymatic amplification of DNA with a
thermostable DNA polymerase. *Science* **239:** 487.

Saito, H., D.M. Kranz, Y. Takagaki, A.C. Hayday, H.N.
Eisen, and S. Tonegawa. 1984. Complete primary structure of a heterodimeric T-cell receptor deduced from
cDNA sequences. *Nature* **309:** 757.

Sowder, J.T., C.H. Chen, L.L. Ager, M.M. Chan, and M.D.
Cooper. 1988. A large subpopulation of avian T cells
express a homologue of the mammalian T $\gamma\delta$ receptor. *J.
Exp. Med.* **167:** 315.

Stern, P.L., N. Beresford, S.M. Bell, S. Thompson, R. Jones,
and A. Mellar. 1986. Murine embryonal carcinoma cells
express class I MHC-like antigens. *Immunogenetics*
13: 133.

Stingl, G., K.C. Gunter, E. Tschachler, H. Yamada, R.I.
Lechler, W.M. Yokoyama, G. Steiner, R.N. Germain, and
E.M. Shevach. 1987. ThyI$^+$ dendritic epidermal cells be-
long to the T cell lineage. *Proc. Natl. Acad. Sci.* **84:** 2430.

Takagaki, Y., A. DeCloux, M. Bonneville, and S. Tonegawa.
1989a. $\gamma\delta$ T cell receptors on murine intestinal intraepithelial lymphocytes are highly diverse. *Nature* **339:** 712.

Takagaki, Y., N. Nakanishi, I. Ishida, O. Kanagawa, and S.
Tonegawa. 1989b. T cell receptor γ and δ genes preferentially utilized by adult thymocytes for the surface expression. *J. Immunol.* **142:** 2112.

Tonegawa, S. 1983. Somatic generation of antibody diversity.
Nature **302:** 575.

Tschachler, E., G. Schuler, J. Hutterer, H. Leibl, K. Wolff,
and G. Stingl. 1983. Expression of Thy-1 antigen by
murine epidermal cells. *J. Invest. Dermatol.* **81:** 282.

Weiss, A., M. Newton, and D. Crommie. 1986. Expression of
T3 in association with a molecule distinct from the T-cell
antigen receptor heterodimer. *Proc. Natl. Acad. Sci.*
83: 6998.

Weiss, E.H., L. Golden, K. Fahner, A.L. Mellor, J.J. Devlin,
H. Bullman, H. Tiddens, H. Bud, and R.A. Flavell. 1984.
Organization and evolution of class I gene family in the
major histocompatibility complex of the C57BL/10 mouse.
Nature **310:** 650.

A TCRγδ Cell Recognizing a Novel TL-encoded Gene Product

B.A. HOULDEN,* L.A. MATIS,† R.Q. CRON,* S.M. WIDACKI,* G.D. BROWN,‡
C. PAMPENO,‡ D. MERUELO,‡ AND J.A. BLUESTONE*
*Ben May Institute, University of Chicago, Chicago, Illinois 60637; †Division of Biochemistry and
Biophysics, Food and Drug Administration, Bethesda, Maryland 20892; ‡Department of Pathology and Kaplan
Cancer Center, New York University Medical Center, New York, New York 10016

Two separate lineages of T lymphocytes, bearing different types of CD3-associated antigen receptors have been described: TCRαβ and TCRγδ. The TCRαβ population represents the majority of thymic and peripheral lymphocytes (Hedrick et al. 1985; Kronenberg et al. 1985) and functions by recognizing antigenic peptides in the context of self major histocompatibility complex (MHC) antigens (Marrack and Kappler 1986; Dembic et al. 1986). TCRγδ cells predominate in the epidermis (Koning et al. 1987; Stingl et al. 1987), intestinal epithelium (Goodman and Lefrancois 1988), and during early thymic ontogeny (Bluestone et al. 1987; Pardoll et al. 1987; Havran and Allison 1988) but represent only a small proportion of adult thymic and peripheral T cells (Lew et al. 1986; Cron et al. 1988). It is not known if their role in the immune system is primarily one that operates within the thymus before and after birth to influence TCRαβ development or repertoire and/or if they function in an antigen-recognition capacity in the same way as TCRαβ lymphocytes.

To recognize a diverse array of ligands, TCRγδ cells would require a diverse receptor. Analysis of the germline repertoire has revealed that there are at least seven TCRγ variable (V) regions, which can rearrange to distinct γ constant (C) region exons ($C_\gamma1$, $C_\gamma2$, and $C_\gamma4$) (Hayday et al. 1985; Garman et al. 1986; Iwamoto et al. 1986). There is also diversity within the TCRδ locus, which is composed of at least eight TCRδ V region exons (that may be interchanged with at least some V_α exons) and two diversity (D) elements, often expressed in tandem (Chien et al. 1987; Elliot et al. 1988; Raulet 1989; Takagaki et al. 1989). In addition, variation exists at V-D-joining (J) junctions because of imprecise rearrangement, giving rise to N-region diversity. Overall, this diversity results in multiple permutations of γ and δ rearrangements that could potentially yield distinct individual TCRγδ heterodimers. Our studies and those of other investigators have shown that TCRγδ diversity does appear to be considerable since seven V_γ region genes and multiple V_δ region genes defined in the mouse have been shown to be expressed in normal tissues and/or on cell lines and hybridomas (for review, see Raulet 1989). Thus, TCRγδ cells may recognize multiple but perhaps a somewhat limited number of ligands.

Recent studies of TCRγδ T-cell clones have determined that at least some TCRγδ cells recognize MHC-linked determinants like their TCRαβ cell counterparts (Matis et al. 1987, 1989; Bluestone et al. 1988; Rivas et al. 1989). However, more than one independently derived line recognizes a relatively nonpolymorphic MHC-linked molecule mapping within or to the right of the thymus leukemia (TL) region (Bluestone et al. 1988; Janeway 1988), which may suggest a unique repertoire. This region of the MHC encodes numerous class I molecules that are very homologous to K, D, and L (Fisher et al. 1985) and that are expressed in association with β_2-microglobulin on hematopoietic cells (Vitetta and Capra 1978; Yokoyama et al. 1981).

The TL region encodes three known gene products: Qa-1, maternally transmitted (Mta), and TL antigens (Old et al. 1963; Stanton and Boyse 1976; Rodgers et al. 1986). Qa-1 is a 48-kD cell-surface glycoprotein with four alleles (a–d) (Jenkins and Rich 1983), but the gene encoding the protein remains undefined. Mta is controlled by two genes: the maternally transmitted factor (Mtf) and histocompatibility maternally transmitted factor (Hmt) (Rodgers et al. 1986). Allelic differences are detected by alloreactive cytotoxic thymus lymphocytes (CTLs). Finally, seven specificities define six alleles of the TL antigen (a–f) (Flaherty 1980; Shen et al. 1982). Although not all the genes encoding these specificities have been determined, $T3^b$ and $T13^c$ genes in C57BL/6 and BALB/c respectively encode the TL antigen (Fisher et al. 1985; Pontarotti et al. 1986; Obata et al. 1988). TL expression is restricted to thymocytes, activated peripheral T cells, and leukemia cells. Some mouse strains do not express TL (Tla^b), whereas others express very low levels (Tla^c), but leukemias derived from these strains can have the TL^+ phenotype (for review, see Flaherty 1976). The gene 37 is also located within the TL region, linked to the $T17^c$ gene, and is transcribed in a large variety of cell types, including fibroblasts and brain (Transy et al. 1987), but its protein product has not been identified. Although the above antigens are known to be encoded in the TL region, more than 30 class I genes have been mapped to the Q/TL region (Steinmetz et al. 1982; Winoto et al. 1983; Fisher et al. 1985), which suggests that some of these genes may encode as yet unidentified protein products or alternatively may be pseudogenes.

In this paper, we define a novel MHC molecule recognized by the TCRγδ G8 CTL and confirm that it is TL-encoded. The gene controlling its expression maps to the TL-region near *T15*[b] and restriction-fragment-length polymorphism (RFLP) analyses reveal differences in this region between strains that share the b haplotype. We suggest that the G8 clone may reflect a predominant specificity of TCRγδ cells. This may implicate the TCRγδ subset in the development of TCRαβ cells in the thymus or indicate these cells have a unique repertoire.

METHODS

Mice. BALB/c *nu/nu* mice were purchased from the Frederick Animal Facility (Maryland). A.Tla[b] mice were obtained from R.G. Cook (Baylor College of Medicine, Texas.) B6.K1 and B6.K2 mice were obtained from L. Flaherty (Wadsworth Center for Laboratories and Research, New York). Other mice were purchased from The Jackson Laboratory (Maine).

Monoclonal antibodies and antisera. The monoclonal antibodies (MAbs) used in this study include anti-CD3ε (145-2C11) (Leo et al. 1987a), anti-V$_γ$2 (UC3-10A6) (S.M. Widacki et al., in prep.), anti-CD4 (RL172.4) (Ceredig et al. 1985), anti-CD8 (83-12-5) (Leo et al. 1987b), and anti-TL (HD168) (Obata et al. 1985; Chen et al. 1987). The anti-C$_γ$1/C$_γ$2, anti-C$_γ$4, and anti-V$_γ$1 antisera were provided by J. Coligan (National Institutes of Health, Maryland) and generated by immunizing rabbits with synthetic peptides as described previously (Lew et al. 1986; Cron et al. 1988 and in prep.).

Cell lines and clones. The MHC-specific BALB/c *nu/nu* anti-B10.BR CD3$^+$, CD4$^-$, CD8$^-$ T-cell line was derived as described previously (Matis et al. 1987). The G8 clone was derived from this line by limiting dilution as described previously (Bluestone et al. 1988) and maintained in 100 units of recombinant interleukin-2 (rIL-2)/ml (Cetus Corp., California) in the absence of stimulator cells. L cells and 2M3 cells transfected with the chimeric plasmid KbT3 (construct 3) were obtained from E. Stockert (Memorial Sloan-Kettering Cancer Center, New York) and G. Wanack (Biogen Research Corp., Massachusetts), respectively. This plasmid was derived from the H-2K^b clone pC-H-2Kb (a 10.5-kb *Eco*RI fragment containing the H-2K^b gene from the C57BL/6 mice and its 4.4-kb 5'- and 1.6-kb 3'-flanking regions) (Schulze et al. 1983), and the TL clone P20-TL (an 8.5-kb *Kpn*I fragment containing the T3 TL gene from the C57BL/6 TL$^+$ leukemia ERLD and its 2.9-kb 5'- and 0.4-kb 3'-flanking regions) (Obata et al. 1985). Construct 3 has the 5'-flanking region, and exon 1 (leader sequence) of the H-2^b gene ligated to exons 2–6 and 3'-flanking region of the TL T3 gene (Obata et al. 1988). The MHC mutant R8.15 cell line is a (C57BL/6 × BALB/c)F$_1$ Abelson transformed pre-B cell line that has lost K^b and Qa-2 molecules (Geier et al. 1986)

and has lost H-2^d by chromosomal deletion (S. Geier, pers. comm.). The AKR-derived R1.1 thymoma and β$_2$-microglobulin-negative variant R1.E have been described previously (Parnes and Seidman 1982).

Isolation of CD4$^-$ and CD8$^-$ double-negative cell populations. Double negative (DN) thymocytes were prepared by negative selection using antibodies to CD4 and CD8 and rabbit C' (Cedarlane Laboratories, Canada) as described previously (Fowlkes et al. 1987; Houlden et al. 1988) and were used immediately. DN spleen cells were prepared by negative selection with the same antibodies and C' depletion, using the protocol described previously (Cron et al. 1988). Remaining spleen cells were cultured in vitro for 2 days in the presence of anti-CD3ε MAb and for 5 days further with 100 units/ml rIL-2 (Cron et al. 1988).

Cell-mediated cytolysis assay. Lipopolysaccharide (LPS)-activated spleen cells (2 days old) were radiolabeled with ^{51}NaCrO3 (150 μCi, Amersham International, United Kingdom) for 75 minutes at 37°C. Target cells (10^4) were washed and plated in 96-well U-bottom microtiter plates (Costar, Massachusetts) with effector cells at selected cell ratios. Cells were incubated 4–5 hours at 37°C before the culture supernatant was harvested and counted. The percentage of specific lysis was calculated using the following formula:

$$\% \text{ spec. lysis} = \frac{\text{cpm (experim.-spontaneous)}}{\text{cpm (maximum-spontaneous)}} \times 100$$

Maximum and spontaneous release represent the release of radiolabel in the presence of 0.05 M HCl and in the absence of effector cells, respectively.

Biochemistry. Cells (0.5 × 10^7 to 5 × 10^7) were washed three times with phosphate-buffered saline (PBS) and labeled with Na^{125}I (Amersham, Illinois) by lactoperoxidase-catalyzed iodination as described previously (Lew et al. 1986). Cells were then lysed in 1% digitonin buffer (pH 7.9), centrifuged to remove nuclei, and precleared by overnight incubation at 4°C with rabbit serum and protein-A agarose (BRL) (Houlden et al. 1988). Immunoprecipitation with specific antisera and protein-A agarose and analysis by off-diagonal gel electrophoresis was performed as described previously (Houlden et al. 1988). Briefly, precipitates were electrophoresed under nonreducing conditions in 10% SDS-PAGE tube gels, layered onto 10% SDS-PAGE slab gels, and electrophoresed under reducing conditions in the second dimension. Gels were autoradiographed at −70°C using Kodak XAR-5 film and Lightning-plus intensifying screens.

Southern blot analysis. Genomic DNA (10–20 μg) was digested to completion with the indicated restriction enzymes (BRL), according to the manufacturer's instructions, and electrophoresed in 0.6% submerged agarose gels at 2 volts/cm for 16–24 hours in TBE (50 mM Tris, 50 mM boric acid, and 0.8 mM EDTA). DNA was transferred to nitrocellulose filters (Schleicher and Schuell, Inc., New Hampshire) as described previously (Southern 1975). Filters were baked at 80°C for 2 hours and hybridized (with 50 ng of DNA probe/200 cm² filter) at 42°C in 5× SSC (0.3 M NaCl and 0.3 M sodium citrate), 50% formamide, 10% dextran sulfate, 0.1% SDS, 0.01 M Tris, and 1× Denhardt's (0.02% each of Ficoll, polyvinyl-pyrrolidone, and bovine serum albumin [BSA]). Filters were washed with 2× SSC, 0.1% SDS at room temperature and 0.2× SCC, 0.1% SDS at 65°C, and then exposed to Kodak XAR-5 film at −70°C. Sizes of DNA fragments were calculated relative to bacteriophage λ DNA digested with HindIII.

DNA probes. The 5′-TL.1-flanking probe is an 865-bp fragment from pTLev1 that maps 45 bp 5′ to the TLev1 integration site (Pampeno and Meruelo 1986, 1988). The probe was prepared by subcloning a 5′ pTLev1 BglII/XbaI fragment into plasmid vector pUC19 and excising with HpaII. The T15 region probe is a HindIII/HaeIII 600-bp fragment isolated from the 1.5-kb HindIII fragment 3′ to T15 (Brown et al. 1988). All probes were radiolabeled with [α-³²P]dCTP to a specific activity of 3×10^8 to 9×10^8 cpm/μg using the random hexamer priming method (Boehringer Mannheim, Indiana).

RESULTS

Biochemical and Molecular Analysis of the TCR Diversity Expressed by TCRγδ Cells

To investigate the phenotypic diversity of TCRγδ expression in the periphery, biochemical analysis of C57L DN spleen cells (activated with anti-CD3 and expanded in rIL-2) were undertaken. These studies revealed that at least three discreet types of TCRγδ heterodimers (42–49 kD, 31/46 kD, and 35/36 kD) were immunoprecipitated with anti-CD3 MAb (Fig. 1A). The 31/47- and 35/46-kD heterodimers present in the periphery were reactive with antipeptide serum specific for $C_\gamma 1/C_\gamma 2$ (Fig. 1B). The 42–49-kD heterodimers were immunoprecipitated with antipeptide antisera specific for $C_\gamma 4$-encoded receptor (Fig. 1C). Antisera prepared against V region domains revealed that the majority of $C_\gamma 4$-containing heterodimers utilized $V_\gamma 1$ as did the 31/46-kD heterodimer, which probably contains $V_\gamma 1$-$C_\gamma 2$ (Fig. 1D). These three distinct TCRγδ are also expressed on T-cell hybridomas (Cron et al. 1988). Therefore, the most commonly observed TCRγ rearrangements in DN spleen cells are $V_\gamma 1$-$C_\gamma 4$, $V_\gamma 1$-$C_\gamma 2$, and $V_\gamma 2$-$C_\gamma 1$ (Cron et al. 1989). These findings that TCRγδ cells in spleen use biochemically distinct γ chains and multiple δ chains (Cron et al., 1989) suggest the existence of TCRγδ structural diversity.

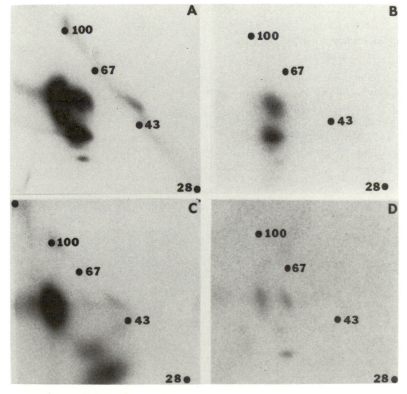

Figure 1. Two-dimensional SDS-PAGE analysis of radioiodinated TCR from C57L DN spleen cells. Immunoprecipitations were performed using anti-CD3 (*A*), anti-$C_\gamma 1$/$C_\gamma 2$ (*B*), anti-$C_\gamma 4$ (*C*), and anti-$V_\gamma 1$ (*D*). Molecular mass standards are indicated in kD.

Analysis of different tissues revealed a predominance of particular receptor classes in the C57BL/10 strain (Fig. 2). C57BL/10 DN spleen cells express distinct TCR compared with C57L, including a nonglycosylated C57BL/10 $V_\gamma2$-$C_\gamma1$ chain, which migrates at 32 kD, masking the 31/46-kD heterodimer (Cron et al. 1988) (Figs. 1A and 2A). Both C57BL/10 DN adult spleen and thymocyte populations express 40–42/43–46-kD $C_\gamma4$- and 32/46-kD $C_\gamma1$-containing heterodimers (Fig. 2A,B). However, the relative proportion of $C_\gamma4$ to $C_\gamma1$ expressed in the thymus is much lower than that seen in the spleen.

Receptor expression has also been shown to be developmentally regulated. Biochemical analysis of TCRγδ heterodimers expressed during fetal ontogeny revealed the presence of a 33/46-kD $C_\gamma1$-containing TCR that was not detected in adult thymocyte or peripheral lymphoid populations (Fig. 2C) and reveal little if any $C_\gamma4$-containing TCR. Studies of N-glycosylation patterns of the unique 33/46-kD heterodimer undertaken using T-cell hybridomas suggest that it contains a rearranged $V_\gamma3$-$C_\gamma1$ gene product (Houlden et al. 1988). This has been confirmed by MAb-staining and mRNA analysis (data not shown). It has been demonstrated previously that this $V_\gamma3$-$C_\gamma1$-containing heterodimer is expressed during a short wave (days 14–16) of fetal thymic ontogeny (Havran and Allison 1988) and on the vast majority of murine dendritic epidermal lymphocytes in the skin (Asarnow et al. 1988). These results in conjunction with others demonstrate that TCRγδ receptor usage is developmentally regulated, which may contribute to repertoire diversity.

Biochemical and Molecular Analysis of TCR Expressed on an MHC-specific TCRγδ CTL

To examine the functional repertoire and antigen-recognition capacity of TCRγδ cells, we generated an MHC-alloreactive TCRγδ cell line from the spleens of BALB/c ($H-2^d$) *nu/nu* mice immunized with B10.BR ($H-2^k$) BSA-enriched spleen cells. A functional $CD3^+$, $CD4^-$, $CD8^-$ CTL line was generated that recognized an MHC-linked gene product, resulting in lymphokine

production and proliferation of the CTL (Matis et al. 1987; Bluestone et al. 1988). This CTL line killed B10.BR stimulator cells ($H-2^k$) but not B10.D2 ($H-2^d$) cells (Fig. 3A). However, the TCRγδ CTL line was broadly cross-reactive on many haplotypes, and it also recognized $H-2^b$ (Fig. 3A), $H-2^f$, $H-2^q$, and $H-2^s$ targets (Bluestone et al. 1988).

To eliminate the possibility that the line was heterogeneous, clones were obtained by limiting dilution and examined for TCR expression and specificity. One of the clones, G8, was selected for further examination. Biochemical analysis revealed that this clone expressed a 35/45-kD TCR that could be immunoprecipitated using anti-CD3 (Fig. 4A) and anti-$V_\gamma2$ (Fig. 4B) MAb, suggesting that the TCR expressed was a $V_\gamma2/C_\gamma1$-containing heterodimer. This was confirmed using molecular analyses, which also revealed that the clone used a member of the $V_\alpha11$ gene family, rearranged to $D_\delta1$, $D_\delta2$, and $J_\delta1$, and contained N-region diversity (Bluestone et al. 1988).

Analysis of the MHC-restricted Specificity of a TCRγδ CTL

The G8 clone was examined for cytolytic activity on a panel of allogeneic targets. It was found to exhibit the same pattern of lysis as the parental line: B10.BR ($H-2^k$) but not B10.D2 ($H-2^d$) stimulator cells were lysed, but lysis was broadly cross-reactive on other haplotypes, including $H-2^b$ (Fig. 3B). This TCRγδ clone and the line it was derived from clearly detects polymorphism based on the degree of cytolysis (high, low, or negative) of LPS blast cells. Whereas 35% of B10.BR stimulator cells were killed by G8 at a 10:1 effector-to-target ratio, the percentage of specific lysis of C57BL/10 blast cells was always higher and often approached 100% (Fig. 3B). Thus, the prototypic strains for the pattern observed in the level of G8 cytolysis are B10.D2 (negative), B10.BR (low), and C57BL/10 (high).

A detailed analysis of the specificity of the clone was performed, using targets derived from various strains and MHC-congenic mice. These and previous studies

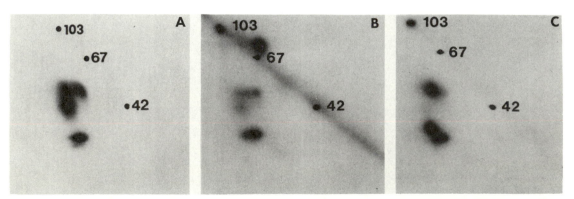

Figure 2. Two-dimensional SDS-PAGE analysis of radioiodinated TCR immunoprecipitated using anti-CD3 from C57BL/10 DN adult spleen (*A*), DN adult thymus (*B*), and day 16 fetal thymus (*C*). Molecular mass standards are indicated in kD.

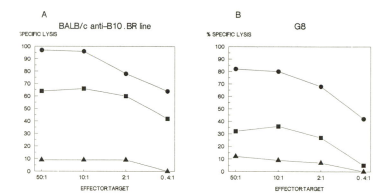

Figure 3. Cytolytic activity of the TCRγδ BALB/c anti-B10.BR line (*A*) and the G8 clone (*B*). LPS blast cells from C57BL/10 (●), B10.BR (■), and B10.D2 (▲) were used as targets in a ^{51}Cr-release cytolytic assay.

localized the target antigen recognized by the TCRγδ CTL to the D end of the MHC or to the right of this region. For example, both C57BL/10 (K^b, I^b, D^b, Qa-2^a, and Tla^b) and B10.HTG (K^d, I^d, D^b, Qa-2^a, and Tla^b) have the high phenotype, whereas BALB/c (K^d, I^d, D^d, Qa-2^a, and Tla^c) was not killed by G8 (Table 1, part I). The antigen recognized by G8 is likely to be a class I molecule, as the H-2^k-expressing tumor line R1.1 was lysed, but the β_2-microglobulin-negative variant R1.E, which does not express class I molecules, was not (data not shown).

Fine Mapping Indicates the Restricting Element Is TL Region Encoded or Regulated

Further analysis using MHC recombinants revealed the specificity was a TL-encoded or -regulated gene. For example, 85% of C57BL/6 and 72% of A.Tla^b LPS blast cells were killed by G8 at an effector:target ratio of 10:1 (high), whereas at this ratio the percentage of specific lysis of A/J was only 45% (low) (Fig. 5A). In the reciprocal experiment, the B6.Tla^a strain expressed the low phenotype, whereas C57BL/6 had the high phenotype in common with C57BL/10 (Fig. 5B). These reciprocal experiments map the high phenotype to the Tla^b region and indicate that the D^b molecule is

not required for the high phenotype since the A.Tla^b strain expresses D^d (like BALB/c) but was killed as was C57BL/6 (Table 1, part I). Additional strains were analyzed, and the emerging pattern was that Tla^b strains were high (C57BL/10, C57BL/6, C3H.SW, and AKR-H-2^b), Tla^a strains were low (B10.BR, C58, A/J, and B10.A[5R]), and Tla^c strains were not lysed by G8 (BALB/c, DBA/2, and B10.D2) (Table 1, parts I and II). There are actually six serologically defined TL haplotypes, and further analysis revealed that Tla^d (B10.M and A.CA) and Tla^e (BDP) strains were also low (Table 1, part II), but Tla^f (C57L, A.By, D1.LP, and 129) strains were high in common with Tla^b strains (Table 1, part II and Fig. 5C).

However, this pattern was not straightforward since not all Tla^b strains had the high phenotype. Several Tla^b strains, including C3H, CBA, and AKR, were killed with the same degree of specific lysis as classic low strains, such as B10.BR (Tla^a) (Fig. 5D, Table 1, part III), as were congenic strains that have a TL region derived from these strains, such as B6.AKR-H-2^k (Fig. 5D). Although these strains are all H-2^k, a direct requirement to have K^k and/or D^k for the low phenotype is ruled out by the A.Tla^b (high) and B6.Tla^a (low) reactivities. In addition, expressing D^b is not sufficient for the high phenotype since B6.K1 and B6.K2 have D^b

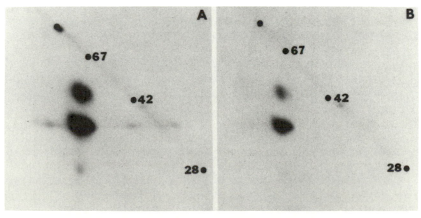

Figure 4. Two-dimensional SDS-PAGE analysis of radioiodinated TCR from the G8 clone. Immunoprecipitations were performed using anti-CD3 (*A*) and anti-V$_\gamma$2 (*B*). Molecular mass standards are indicated in kD.

Table 1. MHC-linked Specific Cytolysis by the TCRγδ G8 CTL

	K	I	D	Qa-2	TL	Qa-1	Lysis[a]
I.							
C57BL/10SnJ	b	b	b	a	b	b	++
B10.HTG/2Cy H-2ᵍ	d	d	b	a	b	b	++
C57BL/6J	b	b	b	a	b	b	++
A.TLAᵇ	k	k	d	a	b	b	++
A/J	k	k	d	a	a	a	+
B6.A-Tlaᵃ/BoyEg	b	b	b	a	a	a	+
BALB/cJ	d	d	d	a	c	b	−
II.							
B10.BR/SgSnJ	k	k	k	b	a	a	+
C58/J	k	k	k	b	a	a	+
B10.A(5R)/SgSnJ	b	b/k	d	a	a	a	+
C3H.SW/SnJ	b	b	b	a	b	b	++
AKR-H-2ᵇ	b	b	b	a	b	b	++
B10.D2/NSgSnJ	d	d	d	a	c	b	−
DBA/2J	d	d	d	a	c	b	−
B10.M	f	f	f	−	d	d	+
A.CA	f	f	f	−	d	?	+
BDP/J	p	p	p	b	e	a	+
C57L/J	b	b	b	a	f	b	++
A.By/SnJ	b	b	b	a	f	b	++
D1.LP/Sn H-2ᵇ	b	b	b	?	f	?	++
129/J	b	b	b	a	f	b	++
III.							
C3H/J	k	k	k	b	b	b	+
CBA/J	k	k	k	b	b	b	+
AKR/J	k	k	k	b	b	b	+
B6.AKR-H-2ᵏ/FlaEg	k	k	k	b	b	b	+
B6.K1	b	b	b	b	b	b	+
B6.K2	b	b	b	a	b	b	+

LPS blast cells from the strains indicated were used as targets in the ⁵¹Cr-release assay.

[a]++, +, or − indicates that the percentage of specific lysis by G8 was equivalent to that observed with C57BL/10, B10.BR, or B10.D2 target cells, respectively.

but express the low phenotype (Table 1, part III). Since identical killing was observed on the Qa-2 congenic B6.K1 and B6.K2 blast cells, G8 does not recognize Qa-2 or any of the determinants coexpressed on this antigen. These results further suggest that the TL regions of Tlaᵇ strain mice are not identical and that G8 recognizes a gene product that is polymorphic or whose level of expression is regulated by a gene that is polymorphic between b strains. Therefore, to distinguish the two groups of Tlaᵇ strains, the group having the low phenotype is hereafter referred to as having the Tlaᵇ' haplotype.

The TCRγδ CTL Does Not Recognize the TL Antigen

The only serologically detected TL antigen in the C57BL/6 strain, encoded by the T3ᵇ gene, is probably not the target antigen recognized by G8. L cells transfected with the T3ᵇ gene express high quantities of the TL antigen (data not shown). However, the transfected line was not lysed by the TCRγδ CTL (Fig. 6) nor was the pre-B cell line 2M3 transfected with the same construct (data not shown). Furthermore, G8 did lyse the R8.15 (C57BL/6 × BALB/c)F1 Abelson transformed

pre-B cell lymphoma (Fig. 6). This cell line does not express TL, as demonstrated by fluorescence-activated cell sorter analysis using the HD168 anti-TL monoclonal antibody (data not shown). In addition, lysis of LPS-activated B cells, which do not express TL, and previous studies indicating that Tlaᵇ and Tlaᵇ' genotypes express common TL specificities (Chen et al. 1987) suggests that the antigen recognized by G8 is probably not encoded by the T3ᵇ gene. Thus, G8 recognizes a novel TL-region-encoded or -regulated molecule.

Southern Blotting and RFLP Analysis

As noted, strains of the Tlaᶠ genotype have the high phenotype. Recent evidence suggests that Tlaᵇ and Tlaᶠ strains share at least some portions of the TL11–15 region, particularly around T14, but that this region is not represented in the Tlaᶜ genome from BALB/c (negative) (Brown et al. 1988; Pampeno and Meruelo 1988). In contrast, restriction maps indicate that T1–T10ᶜ genes in BALB/c are closely related to their counterparts in the C57BL/10 strain (Fisher et al. 1985; Brown et al. 1988). These results suggest that the G8 ligand may be encoded by a gene and/or a regulatory element that localizes to the TL11–15ᵇ region, and its

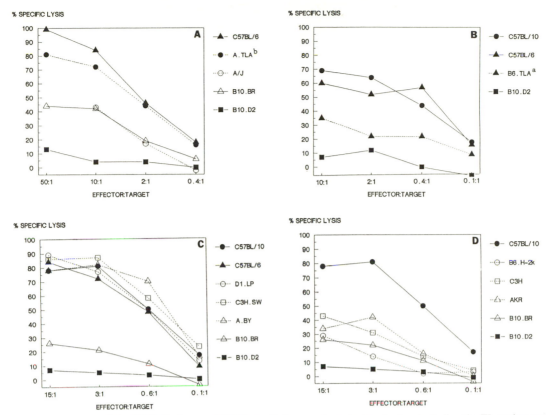

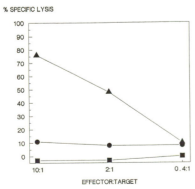

Figure 5. Cytolytic activity of the G8 CTL clone on LPS blast cells from various strains of mice, including the TL-region congenic strains (*A* and *B*), H-2^b (*C*), and H-2^k (*D*) strains.

absence in Tla^c strains may account for their negative phenotype. Therefore, we attempted to identify RFLPs between TL haplotypes that correlate with the high/low/negative phenotypes of G8 cytolysis, using low-copy probes specific for this region.

Previous studies have demonstrated that a retrovirus-like element (TLev1) is located within the TL region of the MHC (Pampeno and Meruelo 1986). The distribution of such sequences among mouse strains has been studied using low-copy probes isolated from the flanking regions of the TLev1 integration sites, including the 5′ TL.1 probe. The patterns of the 5′ TL.1 hybridizing

Figure 6. Cytolytic activity of G8 for R8.15 (▲), L cells (●), and L cells transfected with H-2^b/T3 construct 3 (■) in a ^{51}Cr-release cytolytic assay.

sequences are characteristic for different Tla haplotypes, and *Eco*RI restriction enzyme patterns have shown a conservation of 5′ TL.1 sequence organization within a specific haplotype while also revealing distinctions among different haplotypes (Pampeno and Meruelo 1988). However, fragments produced by digestion with *Bam*HI revealed RFLPs within the classically defined Tla^b haplotype while conserving relationships between haplotypes (Fig. 7). For example, 129/J and C57L (both Tla^f) have a common pattern that is distinct from the pattern of B10.D2 and BALB/c (both Tla^c) strains and different from that obtained with the A/J (Tla^a) (Fig. 7A, lanes 1–5). However, C57BL/6 (Tla^b), C57BL/10 (Tla^b), and C3H (Tla$^{b'}$) do not have an identical pattern. Whereas C57BL/10 and C57BL/6 have 15-, 12-, and 4-kb 5′ TL.1 hybridizing bands (Fig. 7A, lanes 6–7), C3H has 11- and 4-kb hybridizing fragments (Fig. 7A, lane 8). The RFLP revealed by the 5′ TL.1 probe supports the idea that this portion of the TL region of Tla^b and Tla$^{b'}$ strains is divergent.

To determine if Tla^b and Tla$^{b'}$ haplotypes had RFLP patterns that correlated with high/low phenotypes of G8 cytolysis, we analyzed a panel of Tla^b and Tla$^{b'}$ strains. A.Tla^b, C57BL/6. B10.A(2R), and B10.HTG all have the Tla^b haplotype, are highly killed, and have in common 5′ TL.1-hybridizing 15-, 12- and 4-kb fragments (Fig. 7B, lanes 7–10). In contrast, C3H, CBA, AKR, B6.AKR-H-2^b, B6.K1, and B6.K2 are weakly killed and have an 11-kb doublet and 4-kb 5′ TL.1-

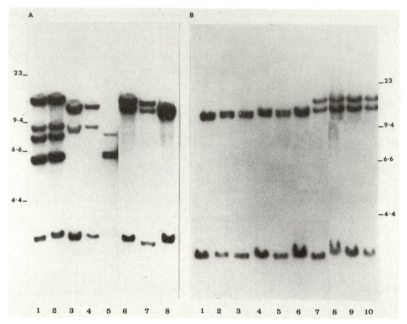

Figure 7. 5' TL.1 probe hybridization to *Bam*HI genomic DNA (10 μg) digests. (*A*) The strains analyzed were 129/J (lane *1*), C57L (lane *2*), B10.D2 (lane *3*), BALB/c (lane *4*), A/J (lane *5*), C57BL/6 (lane *6*), C57BL/10 (lane *7*), and C3H (lane *8*). (*B*) The Tla^b^ strains analyzed were B6.K2 (lane *1*), B6.K1 (lane *2*), B6.AKR-H-2^k^ (lane *3*), AKR (lane *4*), CBA (lane *5*), and C3H (lane *6*), and the Tla^b^ strains analyzed were B10.HTG (lane *7*), B10.A(R) (lane *8*), C57BL/6 (lane *9*), and A.Tla^b^ (lane *10*). Numbers represent the mobility of λ *Hin*dIII fragments in kb.

hybridizing fragments although lacking the 15-kb fragment (Fig. 7B, lanes 1–6). Although the two Tla^f^ strains analyzed have a different pattern than the Tla^b^ strains, the groups share the uppermost 15-kb hybridizing fragment (Fig. 7A, lanes 1–2 and 6–7). Therefore, both b' and f strains share polymorphic bands, which b strains do not possess. Presence of the *Bam*HI 15-kb fragment shows a correlation with the high phenotype of G8 cytolysis, mapping the gene controlling the expression of the antigen to this region.

Further analysis using a 3' T15-region probe on *Hin*dIII-digested DNA revealed a polymorphic fragment that was present in the Tla^b^ strains but absent from the Tla^b'^ strains (Fig. 8). The Tla^b^ strains possess a 1.5-kb T15-hybridizing fragment (Fig. 8, lanes 1–4) that is not present in strains designated as Tla^b'^ (Fig. 8, lanes 5–8). Therefore, the genomic regions of these strains, formerly assumed to be the same, clearly are not identical in this region. This further justifies the use of nomenclature that differentiates these haplotypes.

DISCUSSION

The identification of T cells that express TCRγδ heterodimers has led to an intense interest in determining the specificity and function of this novel T-cell subset. By generating an MHC-specific TCRγδ CTL clone G8, we have demonstrated recognition of relatively nonpolymorphic MHC-linked molecules mapping within the TL region (Bluestone et al. 1988). In this study, we have extended these findings, and we

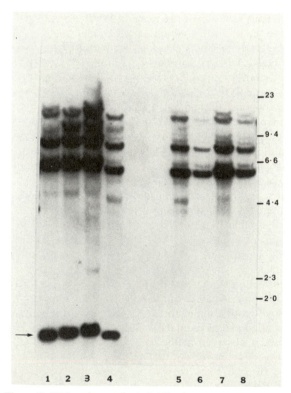

Figure 8. T15-region probe hybridization to *Hin*dIII genomic DNA (10 μg) digests. The Tla^b^ strains (lanes *1–4*) and Tla^b'^ strains (lanes *5–8*) analyzed were A.Tla^b^ (lane *1*), C57BL/6 (lane *2*), B10.A(2R) (lane *3*), B10.HTG (lane *4*), CBA (lane *5*), AKR (lane *6*), C3H (lane *7*), and B6-AKR-H-2^k^ (lane *8*). Numbers represent the mobility of λ *Hin*dIII fragments in kb.

have demonstrated that the ligand recognized by TCRγδ CTL is likely to be a novel TL-encoded class I molecule.

The Q/TL region of MHC determines at least four known class I molecules: Qa-1, Qa-2, Mta, and TL. It is unlikely that any of these are recognized by the TCRγδ G8 CTL. Qa-2 is unlikely to be the ligand because the B6.K1 (Qa-2[b]) and B6.K2 (Qa-2[a]) congenic strains are both killed to the same extent. Furthermore, H-2[f] strains, including B10.M, are recognized by the CTL but have extensive deletions in the Q region from Q1–Q9 that would delete the Qa-2 structural gene (Eastman O'Neill et al. 1986). These strains would also be unable to express the Qa-3, -4, -5, -7, -8, and -9 specificities, which depend on Qa-2 antigen expression (Flaherty et al. 1981, 1982; Sandrin et al. 1983; Sutton et al. 1983), thus eliminating them as potential ligands for G8. Although CTL have been shown to detect Mta and Qa-1 determinants, the polymorphisms in the determinant recognized by the G8 CTL do not correlate with polymorphisms in either of these antigens (Han et al. 1987). For instance, G8 differentiates between the Qa-1[b] strains C57BL/6 (high) and BALB/c (negative). Finally, the TL molecule is unlikely to be the G8 ligand because the CTL recognizes a determinant expressed on both T- and B-activated cells and cell lines, and TL expression has not been demonstrated on B cells; L cells and the pre-B-cell line 2M3 transfected with a T3 gene are not killed by the CTL; and the CTL detects polymorphisms between Tla[b] strains that express the same serologically defined TL specificities.

One unexpected finding was that the TCRγδ CTL detected a polymorphism between classically defined Tla[b] strains of mice. Southern blotting and RFLP analysis supported the conclusion that not all Tla[b] strains are identical throughout the TL region and map the gene of interest to the T15 region. In the C57BL/6 Tla[b] haplotype, T13 is interrupted by a termination codon, and TLev1 is integrated into the coding sequence of T14 (Brown et al. 1988). This integration event would make transcription of a T14-encoded product unlikely, but it is possible that this gene now encodes a fusion protein of H-2 sequences linked to viral sequences recognizable by G8. However, T15 appears to be a complete H-2 gene (Brown et al. 1988) and is thus a possible candidate, although a protein product has not been identified to date. We are currently attempting transfection studies to resolve this issue.

The precise nature of the polymorphism detected by G8 will not be understood until the protein product is identified and its regulation studied. However, the differences observed in the level of plateau-killing seen between strains suggest that perhaps only a subpopulation of LPS blast cells express this determinant in B10.BR strains, whereas all C57BL/10 cells express the determinant recognized by the CTL. Alternative explanations may exist, but all require the interplay of a regulatory element that presumably maps to the TL region. The highly regulated nature of antigens mapping within this region is very characteristic, and it is interesting to speculate on how this regulation may occur for the gene product under study. The integration of retrovirus sequences including TLev1 into the coding sequence of T14 raises the possibility that long-terminal-repeat sequences may regulate genes in this region and thus may account for the differences in expression detected by G8.

Although this report focused on describing the specificity of a TCRγδ CTL clone for a novel MHC class I molecule, it is clear that some TCRγδ cells can also recognize more conventional class I and II molecules. These include C57BL/10 nu/nu anti-B10.BR TCRγδ lines reactive with H-2D[k] (Bluestone et al. 1988), and I-E[k] (Matis et al. 1989). Interestingly, clones and hybridomas derived from the line are very cross-reactive for the products of multiple distinct I-E alleles (Matis et al. 1989). It has also been reported recently that TCRγδ T cells may recognize highly conserved proteins such as heat-shock proteins (O'Brien et al. 1989), and TCRγδ T cells reactive with tetanus toxoid (Kozbor et al. 1989) and immunoglobulin (Wright et al. 1989) have been described previously. Thus, it seems likely that at least a subpopulation of TCRγδ cells are capable of antigen-specific responses, although it remains to be determined if the antigens recognized by this subset are less polymorphic as a general rule when compared with those recognized by TCRαβ.

However, the relatively nonpolymorphic nature of the ligands recognized by TCRγδ cells described to date, coupled with the difficulty associated with generating bulk lines and clones, probably indicate that TCRγδ cells do not express a repertoire as broad as TCRαβ cells. Furthermore, there is an indication that this distinct T-cell subset may be skewed toward recognizing unique cell-surface molecules, such as novel class I antigens encoded in the TL region. TCRγδ cells may therefore occupy a special niche in the immunological system by complementing the repertoire of TCRαβ cells. In fact, the TCRγδ cells that recognize novel self class I molecules may play a role in TCRαβ development during thymic ontogeny or after birth. In addition, the study of the repertoire of TCRγδ cells may be important in discerning the physiological role of non-classical MHC molecules in immune responses.

ACKNOWLEDGMENTS

The authors thank Dr. John Coligan for providing TCR antisera and Drs. E. Stockert and G. Wanack for making TL transfectant cells available. J.A.B. is a Gould Foundation Faculty Scholar with support for the Lucille P. Markey Charitable Trust and both J.A.B. and B.H. are supported by U.S. Public Health Service grant 1-RO1-AI-26847. R.Q.C. is supported by a predoctoral immunology training grant 5-T32AI07090-10.

REFERENCES

Asarnow, D.M., W.A. Kuziel, A. Bonyhadi, R.E. Tigelaar, P.W. Tucker, and J.P. Allison. 1988. Limited diversity of $\gamma\delta$ antigen receptor genes of Thy-1[+] dendritic epidermal cells. *Cell* **55**: 837.

Bluestone, J.A., D. Pardoll, S.O. Sharrow, and B.J. Fowlkes. 1987. Ontogeny, phenotype and functional characterization of murine thymocytes possessing T3-associated T cell receptor structure. *Nature* **326**: 82.

Bluestone, J.A., R.Q. Cron, M. Cotterman, B.A. Houlden, and L.A. Matis. 1988. Structure and specificity of TCR$\gamma\delta$ receptors on major histocompatibility complex antigen specific CD3[+], CD4[−], CD8[−] T lymphocytes. *J. Exp. Med.* **168**: 1988.

Brown, G.D., Y. Choi, G. Egan, and D. Meruelo. 1988. Extension of the *H-2TL*[b] molecular map. Isolation and characterization of *T13*, *T14*, and *T15* from the C57BL/6 mouse. *Immunogenetics* **27**: 239.

Ceredig, R., J.W. Lowenthal, M. Nabholz, and H.R. MacDonald. 1985. Expression of interleukin-2 receptors as a differentiation marker on intrathymic stem cells. *Nature* **314**: 98.

Chen, Y.-T., Y. Obata, E. Stockert, T. Takahashi, and L.J. Old. 1987. Tla-region genes and their products. *Immunol. Res.* **6**: 30.

Chien, Y.-H., M. Iwashima, D.A. Wettstein, K.B. Kaplan, J.F. Elliott, W. Born, and M.M. Davis. 1987. T-cell receptor δ gene rearrangements in early thymocytes. *Nature* **330**: 722.

Cron, R.Q., A. Ezquerra, J.E. Coligan, B.A. Houlden, J.A. Bluestone, and W.L. Maloy. 1989. Identification of distinct TCR$\gamma\delta$ heterodimers using an anti-TCR gamma variable region serum. *J. Immunol.* (in press).

Cron, R.Q., F. Koning, W.L. Maloy, D. Pardoll, J.E. Coligan, and J.A. Bluestone. 1988. A functional subpopulation of peripheral murine T lymphocytes which express a novel T cell receptor structure. *J. Immunol.* **141**: 1074.

Dembic, Z., W. Haas, S. Weiss, J. McCubrey, H. Kiefer, H. von Boehmer, and M. Steinmetz. 1986. Transfer of specificity by murine α and β T-cell receptor genes. *Nature* **320**: 232.

Elliott, J.F., E.P. Rock, P.A. Pattern, M.M. Davis, and Y.-H. Chien. 1988. The adult T-cell receptor δ-chain is diverse and distinct from that of fetal thymocytes. *Nature* **331**: 627.

Eastman O'Neill, A., K. Reid, J.C. Gaberi, M. Karl, and L. Flaherty. 1986. Extensive deletion is the *Q* region of the mouse major histocompatibility complex. *Immunogenetics* **24**: 368.

Fisher, D.A., S.W. Hunt, and L. Hood. 1985. Structure of a gene encoding a murine thymus leukemia antigen, and organization of *Tla* genes in the BALB/c mouse. *J. Exp. Med.* **162**: 528.

Flaherty, L. 1976. The *Tla* region of the mouse: Identification of a new serologically defined locus, Qa-2. *Immunogenetics* **3**: 533.

———. 1980. The Tla region antigens. In *Role of the major histocompatibility complex in immunology* (ed. M.E. Dorf), p. 33. Garland Press, New York.

Flaherty, L., M. Karl, and C.L. Reinisch. 1982. Syngeneic tumor immunizations produce Qa antibodies. Discovery of a new Qa antigen, Qa-6. *Immunogenetics* **16**: 329.

Flaherty, L., E. Rinchik, and K. DiBiase. 1981. New complexities at the *Qa-1* locus. *Immunogenetics* **16**: 339.

Fowlkes, B.J., A.M. Kruisbeek, H. Ton-That, M.A. Weston, J.E. Coligan, R.H. Schwartz, and D.M. Pardoll. 1987. A novel population of T-cell receptor $\alpha\beta$-bearing thymocytes which express a single Vβ gene family. *Nature* **329**: 251.

Garman, R.D., P.J. Doherty, and D.H. Raulet. 1986. Diversity, rearrangement and expression of murine T cell gamma genes. *Cell* **45**: 733.

Geier, S.S., R.A. Zeff, D.M. McGovern, T.V. Rajan, and S.G. Nathenson. 1986. An approach to the study of structure-function relationships of MHC class I molecules: Isolation and serologic characterization of H-2K[b] somatic cell variants. *J. Immunol.* **137**: 1239.

Goodman, L. and L. Lefrancois. 1988. Expression of the γ/δ T-cell receptor on intestinal CD8[+] intraepithelial lymphocytes. *Nature* **333**: 855.

Han, A.C., J.R. Rogers, and R.R. Rich. 1987. Unglycosylated Mta[a] express an Mta[b]-like determinant. *Immunogenetics* **25**: 234.

Havran, W.L. and J.P. Allison. 1988. Developmentally ordered appearance of thymocytes expressing different T cell antigen receptors. *Nature* **335**: 443.

Hayday, A.C., H. Saito, S.D. Gillies, D.M. Kranz, G. Tanigawa, H.N. Eisen, and S. Tonegawa. 1985. Structure, organization and somatic rearrangement of T cell gamma genes. *Cell* **40**: 259.

Hedrick, S., R.N. Germain, M.J. Bevan, M. Dorf, I. Engel, P. Fink, N. Gascoigne, E. Herber-Katz, J. Kapp, Y. Kaufmann, J. Kaye, F. Melchers, C. Pierce, R.H. Schwartz, C. Sorenson, M. Tanaguchi, and M.M. Davis. 1985. Rearrangement and transcription of a T-cell receptor β-chain gene in different T-cell subsets. *Proc. Natl. Acad. Sci.* **82**: 531.

Houlden, B.A., R.Q. Cron, J.E. Coligan, and J.A. Bluestone. 1988. Systematic development of distinct T cell receptor-$\gamma\delta$ T cell subsets during fetal development. *J. Immunol.* **141**: 3753.

Iwanoto, A., F. Rupp, P.S. Ohashi, C.L. Walker, H. Pircher, R. Joho, H. Hengartner, and T.W. Mak. 1986. T cell-specific γ genes in C57BL/10 mice. *J. Exp. Med.* **163**: 1203.

Janeway, C.A. 1988. Frontiers of the immune system. *Nature* **333**: 804.

Jenkins, R.N. and R.R. Rich. 1983. Characterization of determinants encoded by four Qa-1 genotypes and their recognition by cloned cytolytic cytotoxic T lymphocytes. *J. Immunol.* **131**: 2147.

Koning, F., G. Stingl, W.M. Yokoyama, H. Yamada, W.L. Maloy, E. Tschachler, E.M. Shevach, and J.E. Coligan. 1987. Identification of a T3-associated γ/δ T cell receptor on Thy-1[+] dendritic epidermal cell lines. *Science* **236**: 834.

Kozbor, D., G. Trinchieri, D.S. Monos, M. Isobe, G. Russo, J.A. Haney, C. Zmijewski, and C.M. Croce. 1989. Human TCR-γ[+]/δ[+] CD8[+] T lymphocytes recognize tetanus toxoid in an MHC-restricted fashion. *J. Exp. Med.* **169**: 1847.

Kronenberg, M., J. Goverman, R. Haars, M. Malissen, E. Kraig, L. Phillips, T. Delovitch, N. Sucia-Foca, and L. Hood. 1985. Rearrangement and transcription of the β-chain genes of the T-cell antigen receptor in different types of murine lymphocytes. *Nature* **313**: 647.

Leo, O., M. Foo, D.H. Sachs, L.E. Samelson, and J.A. Bluestone. 1987a. Identification of a monoclonal antibody specific for murine T3. *Proc. Natl. Acad. Sci.* **84**: 1374.

Leo, O., M. Foo, D.M. Segal, E. Shevach, and J.A. Bluestone. 1987b. Activation of murine T lymphocytes with monoclonal antibodies: Detection on Lyt-2[+] cells of an activation antigen not associated with the T cell receptor complex. *J. Immunol.* **139**: 1214.

Lew, A.M., D.M. Pardoll, W.L. Maloy, B.J. Fowlkes, A. Kruisbeek, S.-F. Cheng, R.N. Germain, J.A. Bluestone, R.H. Schwartz, and J.E. Coligan. 1986. Characterization of T-cell receptor gamma chain expression in a subset of murine thymocytes. *Science* **234**: 1401.

Marrack, P. and J. Kappler. 1986. The antigen-specific major histocompatibility complex-restricted receptor on T cells. *Adv. Immunol.* **38**: 1.

Matis, L.A., R. Cron, and J.A. Bluestone. 1987. Major histocompatibility complex-linked specificity of $\gamma\delta$ receptor-bearing T lymphocytes. *Nature* **330**: 262.

Matis, L.A., A.M. Fry, R.Q. Cron, M.M. Cotterman, R.F. Dick, and J.A. Bluestone. 1989. Structure and specificity of a class II MHC alloreactive $\gamma\delta$ T cell receptor heterodimer. *Science* **245**: 746.

Obata, Y., T.-T. Chen, E. Stockert, and L.J. Old. 1985. Structural analysis of *TL* genes of the mouse. *Proc. Natl. Acad. Sci.* **82:** 5475.

Obata, Y., E. Stockert, Y.-T. Chen, T. Takahashi, and L.J. Old. 1988. Influence of 5′ flanking sequences on TL and H-2 expression in transfected L cells. *Proc. Natl. Acad. Sci.* **85:** 3541.

O'Brien, R.L., M.P. Happ, A. Dallas, E. Palmer, R. Kubo, and W.K. Born. 1989. Stimulation of a major subset of lymphocytes expressing T cell receptor γδ by an antigen derived from Mycobacterium tuberculosis. *Cell* **57:** 667.

Old, L.H., E.A. Boyse, and E. Stockert. 1963. Antigenic properties of experimental leukemias. I. Serological studies in vitro with spontaneous and radiation induced leukemias. *J. Natl. Cancer Inst.* **31:** 977.

Pampeno, C. and D. Meruelo. 1986. Isolation of a retrovirus-like sequence from the *TL* locus of the C57BL/10 murine major histocompatibility complex. *J. Virol.* **58:** 296.

———. 1988. Genomic organization of the mouse *Tla* locus: Study of an endogenous retroviruslike locus reveals polymorphisms related to different *Tla* haplotypes. *Immunogenetics* **28:** 247.

Pardoll, D., B.J. Fowlkes, J.A. Bluestone, A. Kruisbeek, W.L. Maloy, J.E. Coligan, and R.H. Schwartz. 1987. Differential expression of two distinct T cell receptors during thymocyte development. *Nature* **326:** 79.

Parnes, J.R. and J.G. Seidman. 1982. Structure of wild-type and mutant β_2-microglobulin. *Cell* **29:** 661.

Pontarotti, P.A., H. Mashimo, R.A. Zeff, D.A. Fisher, L. Hood, A. Mellor, R.A. Flavell, and S.G. Nathenson. 1986. Conservation and diversity in the class I genes of the major histocompatibility complex: Sequence analysis of a *Tla^b* gene and comparison with a *Tla^c* gene. *Proc. Natl. Acad. Sci.* **83:** 1782.

Raulet, D.H. 1989. The structure, function and molecular genetics of the γ/δ T cell receptor. *Annu. Rev. Immunol.* **7:** 175.

Rivas, A., M.L. Cleary, and E.G. Engleman. 1989. Evidence for involvement of the γ,δ T cell antigen receptor in cytotoxicity mediated by human alloantigen-specific T cell clones. *J. Immunol.* **142:** 1840.

Rodgers, J.R., R. Smith, M.M. Huston, and R.R. Rich. 1986. Maternally transmitted antigen. *Adv. Immunol.* **38:** 313.

Sandrin, M.S., P.M. Hograth, and I.F.C. McKenzie. 1983. Two "Qa" specificities: Qa-m7 and Qa-m8 defined by monoclonal antibodies. *J. Immunol.* **131:** 546.

Schulze, D.H., L.R. Pease, Y. Obata, S.G. Nathenson, A.A. Reyes, S. Ikuta, and R.B. Wallace. 1983. Identification of the cloned gene for the murine transplantation antigen H-2K^b by hybridization with synthetic oligonucleotides. *Mol. Cell. Biol.* **3:** 750.

Shen, F.-W., M.J. Chorney, and E.A. Boyse. 1982. Further polymorphism of the *Tla* locus defined by monoclonal TL antibodies. *Immunogenetics* **15:** 573.

Southern, E. 1975. Detection of specific sequences among DNA fragments separated by gel electrophoresis. *J. Mol. Biol.* **98:** 503.

Stanton, T.H. and E.A. Boyse. 1976. A new serologically defined locus, *Qa-1*, in the *Tla*-region of the mouse. *Immunogenetics* **3:** 525.

Steinmetz, M., A. Winoto, K. Minard, and L. Hood. 1982. Clustering of genes encoding mouse transplantation antigens. *Cell* **25:** 683.

Stingl, G., F. Koning, H. Yamada, W.M. Yokoyama, E. Tschachler, J.A. Bluestone, G. Steiner, L.E. Samelson, A.M. Lew, J.E. Coligan, and E.M. Shevach. 1987. Thy-1^+ dendritic epidermal cells express T3 antigen and the T-cell receptor γ chain. *Proc. Natl. Acad. Sci.* **84:** 4586.

Sutton, V.R., P.M. Hogarth, and I.F.C. McKenzie. 1983. Description of a new Qa antigenic specificity, "Qa-m9," whose expression is under complex genetic control. *J. Immunol.* **131:** 1363.

Takagaki, Y., N. Nakanishi, I. Ishida, O. Kanagawa, and S. Tonegawa. 1989. T cell receptor-γ and -δ genes preferentially utilized by adult thymocytes for the surface expression. *J. Immunol.* **142:** 2112.

Transy, C., S.R. Nash, R. David-Watine, M. Cochet, S.W. Hunt, L.E. Hood, and P. Kourilsky. 1987. A low polymorphic mouse H-2 class I gene from the *Tla* complex is expressed in a broad variety of cell types. *J. Exp. Med.* **166:** 341.

Vitetta, E.S. and J.D. Capra. 1978. The protein products of the murine 17th chromosome: Genetics and structure. *Adv. Immunol.* **26:** 147.

Winoto, A., M. Steinmetz, and L. Hood. 1983. Genetic mapping in the major histocompatibility complex by restriction enzyme site polymorphisms: Most mouse class I genes map to the *Tla* complex. *Proc. Natl. Acad. Sci.* **80:** 3425.

Wright, A., J.E. Lee, M.P. Link, S.D. Smith, W. Carroll, R. Levy, C. Clayberger, and A.M. Krensky. 1989. Cytotoxic T lymphocytes specific for self tumor immunoglobulin express T cell receptor δ chain. *J. Exp. Med.* **169:** 1557.

Yokoyama, K., E. Stockert, L.J. Old, and S.G. Nathenson. 1981. Structural comparisons of TL antigens derived from normal and leukemia cells of TL^+ and TL^− strains and relationship to genetically linked H-2 major histocompatibility complex products. *Proc. Natl. Acad. Sci.* **78:** 7078.

Phenotypic Analysis of Mice Transgenic for the TCR $C_\gamma 4$ ($V_\gamma 1.1 J_\gamma 4 C_\gamma 4$) Gene

D.A. Ferrick, X. Min, D.A. Gajewski, and T.W. Mak

Ontario Cancer Institute, Departments of Medical Biophysics and Immunology, University of Toronto, Toronto, Canada M4X 1K9

Lymphocyte communication, induced and maintained by antigenic stimuli, is mediated in B cells by immunoglobulin and in T cells by the $\alpha\beta$ T-cell receptor (TCR). It is well established that in B cells free antigen is sufficient for binding to immunoglobulin (Davies and Metzger 1983), whereas in T cells foreign antigenic particles must be associated with the appropriate major histocompatibility antigens (MHC) in order for the TCR$\alpha\beta$ to bind with biological consequence (Ohashi et al. 1985; Dembic et al. 1986; Saito et al. 1987).

Recently, a second TCR, $\gamma\delta$, has been identified (Saito et al. 1984; Brenner et al. 1986; Iwamoto et al. 1986; Chien et al. 1987a,b) and shown to reside in various anatomical locations (Asarnow et al. 1988; Elliott et al. 1988; Goodman and Lefrancois 1988; Havran and Allison 1988; Steiner et al. 1988). As a result of the circumstantial manner in which this second receptor was elucidated, the physiologic role of cells that bear this receptor is still a mystery due to the lack of biological models available to measure their functions. However, rapid progress has been made in the identification of γ and δ genes, their temporal and spatial expression, the cloning of T cells that express $\gamma\delta$ receptors, the development of monoclonal antibodies against $\gamma\delta$ receptors, and the generation of in vivo models that alter the expression of these receptors. This effort has generated an enormous amount of data about the $\gamma\delta$ receptors that are being used to design experimental models to characterize their biological function.

TCR$\gamma\delta$ Diversity and Chromosomal Structure

As shown in Figure 1, there are many fewer variable (V) and joining (J) gene segments available to the γ and δ loci, suggesting a more limited number of receptor-binding conformations for TCR$\gamma\delta$. However, if one takes into account that both (diversity) D_δ segments can exist in tandem or separately and can be read in all three reading frames, plus the extensive amount of N-region diversity observed within rearranged δ-chain genes, then a comparable number of possible unique binding conformations can exist for $\gamma\delta$ as compared with $\alpha\beta$.

A rather unique and intriguing aspect of both receptors is that the δ-chain locus resides in the middle of the α locus, such that, whenever α-chain rearrangement occurs, the intervening δ-gene segments are deleted (Fig. 2). This chromosomal organization and recent experimental evidence, showing the existence of a δ-deleting element (de Villartay et al. 1988; Hockett et al. 1988; P. Ohashi et al. in prep.), have led to the suggestion that lineage determination between $\alpha\beta$ and $\gamma\delta$ may occur before rearrangement. This implies that whatever regulatory mechanism exists for the determination of entry into either the TCR$\alpha\beta$ or TCR$\gamma\delta$ lineages, the site of control most likely exists in the δ locus. In addition, this would imply that there is not a direct precursor relationship between the $\gamma\delta$ and $\alpha\beta$ lineages.

Fetal and Spatial Expression of TCR$\gamma\delta$

Cells that express $\gamma\delta$ receptors are the first immigrants to colonize the thymic rudiment (Havran and Allison 1988) and exist in mice as a major population starting at day 14 of fetal development and declining substantially by day 18 of gestation. Thymocytes that express $\gamma\delta$ are, for the most part, double-negative

	Alpha	Beta		Gamma	Delta
V	100	100		10	6
D	?	≥ 2		?	2 (3)
J	100	13		4	3
C	1	2		2	1
	10^4	10^4		40	40
Recombinations		10^8			10^3
* N-sequences	10^4	10^8		10^4	10^{12}
Total Diversity		10^{20}			10^{19}

* assume 3 a.a. at each junction

Figure 1 Potential diversity of human TCR$\gamma\delta$ and TCR$\alpha\beta$ genes generated from the approximate total number of gene segments available and taking into account N-region diversity. For purposes of calculation, an average of 3 amino acids within each junction (*) was used based on available sequence data.

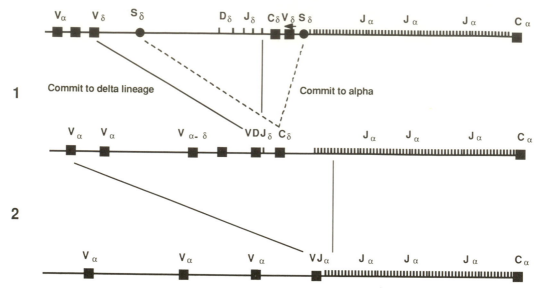

Figure 2 Possible scheme for lineage commitment based on δ-deleting elements (S_δ). The first model (*1*) shows that rearrangement of the δ locus would commit the cell to the γδ lineage. Loss of δ-gene segments because of deletion mediated by S_δ elements would commit the T-cell precursor to the αβ lineage. The second model (*2*) suggests that first δ rearrangement would be attempted (but not necessarily an absolute requirement) followed by further rearrangement of the locus to α.

($CD4^-$ $CD8^-$) (Pardoll et al. 1987; Cron et al. 1988) and in the periphery exist as a minor T-cell population of about 1–5% (Brenner et al. 1987; Cron et al. 1988). However, γδ-bearing cells exist essentially in the absence of αβ are in the skin (Thy-1$^+$ dendritic epidermal cells) (Asarnow et al. 1988; Steiner et al. 1988), the gut (intestinal epithelial $CD8^+$ T cells) (Goodman and Lefrancois 1988), and in athymic mice (Thy-1$^+$ cells) (Yoshikai et al. 1986).

Generation of $C_\gamma 4$ Transgenic Mice

One approach to measure gene effect and function in an in vivo environment is to generate transgenic mice. The over- or inappropriate expression of a TCRγ- or TCRδ-chain gene may produce a phenotype that is related to the normal function of that receptor chain. We recently reported the effect of a (constant) $C_\gamma 4$ ($V_\gamma 1.1J_\gamma 4C_\gamma 4$) transgene on T-cell reactivity in mice (Ferrick et al. 1989). The $C_\gamma 4$ gene was isolated by Iwamoto et al. (1986) and is located within the C_γ locus. This gene shares little similarity with either $C_\gamma 1$ or $C_\gamma 2$ (50%). There is low expression of this gene in the adult thymus (Elliott et al. 1988). However, high levels of TCR $C_\gamma 4$ exist in the spleen beginning at 2–4 weeks and are maintained throughout the life of the mouse, representing approximately half of the splenic γδ cells (J. Bluestone, pers. comm.).

Previously, we demonstrated that $C_\gamma 4$ transgenic mice displayed a significant T-cell-mediated reactivity at a younger age in the periphery as compared with controls (Ferrick et al. 1989). In fact, newborn transgenic splenocytes were capable of generating alloreactive cytotoxic T lymphocytes in primary culture (D.

Ferrick, unpubl.). This difference in T-cell reactivity disappeared with time and was greatest between 2 and 4 weeks after birth (Ferrick et al. 1989).

Phenotype of $C_\gamma 4$ Transgenic Mice during Development

In Table 1, the ratios of the absolute number of transgenic over control thymocytes are shown for various cell-surface phenotypes. It is interesting to note that at the time when the greatest difference exists in peripheral T-cell function between transgenic and control mice (2–4 weeks of age), there is a three- to fourfold increase in the absolute number of thymocytes in the transgenic thymus compared with control (e.g. 2.1×10^8 thymocytes for 4-week-old transgenic mice versus 7.5×10^7 thymocytes for control mice at the same age). However, the absolute number of T cells in the spleen and lymph nodes was not significantly different between control and transgenic mice for all time points tested (data not shown). From Table 1, it is apparent that there was a greater percentage as well as absolute number of γδ T cells at all time points, suggesting that this excess is due to expression of the $C_\gamma 4$ transgene on the surface. In addition, there is an increase in the percentage of CD4 single-positive thymocytes at 2 and 4 weeks of age that correlates with a decrease in the percentage of $CD4^+$ $CD8^+$ double-positive cells at these time points (Table 1). However, what may be most important is that the presence of the $C_\gamma 4$ transgene is not only affecting the number of γδ-bearing cells, but is either directly or indirectly increasing the number of αβ-bearing cells as well, especially between 2 and 4 weeks of age (Table 1). In fact,

Table 1. Thymic Development of T Cells in C$_\gamma$4 Transgenic Mice

Trans/cont	Birth	2 wk	4 wk	6 wk	16 wk
Cells	1.0	1.8	2.8	1.2	0.9
CD3	1.0	1.9	2.7	1.4	0.9
TCR$\alpha\beta$	0.9	1.8	2.7		
TCR$\gamma\delta$	1.7	2.7	3.5		
CD4$^-$8$^-$	1.0	3.8	3.7	2.5	1.5
CD4$^+$8$^+$	0.9	1.6	2.6	1.3	0.8
CD4$^+$8$^-$	1.4	3.1	3.8	1.7	1.1
CD4$^-$8$^+$	1.0	1.8	2.7	0.9	0.9

Thymocytes were isolated and stained with monoclonal antibodies against various surface molecules. The absolute number of positive cells/mouse thymus was calculated and the ratio of transgenic (Trans) over control (Cont) is shown for the ages indicated.

for transgenic mice at 2 and 4 weeks of age, the greatest increase occurs within the subset of thymocytes expressing $\alpha\beta$.

In addition to the phenotypic changes in the T-cell compartment of the transgenic mice, there is also a growth effect as well. In Table 2, preliminary data suggest that the sizes of the transgenic mice and their negative littermates are quite different. From early on, the transgenic mice increase in body weight much sooner than their negative littermates as well as becoming much more alert and active between 1 and 2 weeks after birth. For example, at 6 months of age, a normal male H-2^q × H-2^b mouse will weigh approximately 32.8 ± 1.3 g (average of 4 mice), whereas a transgenic mouse at the same age will weigh approximately 49.2 ± 2.6 g (average of 5 mice).

DISCUSSION

Recently the second described TCR, $\gamma\delta$, has been the subject of intense investigation. The physiologic role of cells that bear this receptor remains an enigma since there are still no good experimental models available to test for their function. In an attempt to alter the expression of one TCRγ gene, we have generated mice transgenic for the V$_\gamma$1.1J$_\gamma$4C$_\gamma$4 TCR chain gene. Our previous results suggested that the T-cell compartment is accelerated during development in these mice (Ferrick et al. 1989).

In this paper, the phenotype of the T cells present and their abundance, as well as some preliminary data on the overall size of these mice as they age, suggest that the transgene is having a drastic effect on the overall development of these mice. The transient in-

crease in the absolute number of thymocytes, peaking between 2 and 4 weeks, along with the increases in both the $\gamma\delta$ and $\alpha\beta$ T-cell subsets (Table 1) correlates with the acute differences in T-cell reactivity measured previously in the periphery at those early time points (Ferrick et al. 1989). The fact that there is no significant increase in the number of T cells in the periphery of transgenic mice between 2 and 4 weeks of age makes it difficult to hypothesize what effect this increase in absolute number has on the observed early appearance of T-cell reactivity. Even harder to envision is why the transgenic mice are larger and appear to develop sooner than their negative littermates. One possibility is that the effect of the transgenic $\gamma\delta$ receptor, when engaged, is to signal the cell to produce growth factors such as interleukins that can have a positive effect on cells other than lymphocytes. This is not so improbable since it is known the $\gamma\delta$-bearing cells can produce biologically active factors such as interleukins and γ-interferon (Nixon-Fulton et al. 1988). We are currently measuring the levels of growth factors in the transgenic mice as well as looking at the relative abundance of hematopoietic precursors to shed some light on these differences.

Given the difficulty of designing biological models for a set of cells that bear a receptor whose physiologic ligand has not been identified has not hindered scientists from developing theories based on the current data. Some of the most widely accepted models are as follows: (1) The $\gamma\delta$ receptor is a primitive first line of defense against highly conserved molecules (e.g., enterotoxins and heat-shock proteins). (2) The $\gamma\delta$ receptor recognizes MHC or MHC-like molecules complexed with antigen (Ia, K, D, Qa, and TL). (3) The $\gamma\delta$ receptor is an adhesion molecule (i.e., homing receptor). (4) Finally, it is an anti-self-receptor involved in the regulation of TCR$\alpha\beta$ development and reactivity. Because of the probable heterogeneity of cells that bear $\gamma\delta$ receptors, some or all of the above may be correct.

In terms of our C$_\gamma$4 transgenic mice, although they do not cast doubt on any of the above potential roles of $\gamma\delta$-bearing cells, they do favor the role of these cells as an anti-self-receptor capable of regulating T-cell development and reactivity. One might speculate, based

Table 2. Weight of C$_\gamma$4 Transgenic Mice during Development

Trans/cont	2 wk	6 wk	12 wk
Whole body[a]	1.52	1.31	1.26
Thymus[b]	1.86	2.33	1.01

[a]Six male littermates (3 control and 3 transgenic) were weighed at various time points and the ratio of transgenic (Trans) over control (Cont) is shown.

[b]The thymus weights were the average of 4–6 mice for each time point and is represented as the ratio of transgenic over control.

on our data and the data of other investigators, that $\gamma\delta$ cells (most likely a subset) could recognize MHC-like molecules (such as Qa or TL) complexed with foreign or self-peptides on activated T cells in both the thymus and periphery. As a result of this binding, the $\gamma\delta$-bearing cell would produce and secrete biological factors to aid in the differentiation and/or activation of the corresponding lymphocyte. This hypothesis is now testable with transgenic mice carrying different chains of γ and δ TCR genes.

ACKNOWLEDGMENTS

The authors thank R. Kubo (anti-TCR$\alpha\beta$) and J. Bluestone (anti-TCR$\gamma\delta$ and anti-CD3) for their generous gifts of antibodies. Also, we thank Irene Ng and Diana Quon for technical assistance. This work was supported by grants from the National Cancer Institute of Canada, the Medical Research Council of Canada (MT-4519 and MT-3017), and a special grant from the University of Toronto. D.A.F. is a recipient of a Cancer Research Institute (New York) fellowship.

REFERENCES

Asarnow, D.M., W.A. Kuziel, M. Bonyhadi, R.E. Tigelaar, P.W. Tucker, and J.P. Allison. 1988. Limited diversity of $\gamma\delta$ antigen receptor genes of thy-1$^+$ dendritic epidermal cells. Cell 55: 837.

Brenner, M.B., J. MacLean, D.P. Dialynas, J.L. Strominger, J.A. Smith, F.L. Owen, J.G. Seidman, D. Ip, F. Rosen, and M.S. Krangel. 1986. Identification of a putative second T-cell receptor. Nature 322: 145.

Chien, Y.-H., M. Iwashima, K.B. Kaplan, J.F. Elliot, and M.M. Davis. 1987a. A new T-cell receptor gene located in the alpha locus and expressed early in T cell differentiation. Nature 327: 677.

Chien, Y.-H., M. Iwashima, D.A. Wittstein, K.B. Kaplan, J.F. Elliot, W. Born, and M.M. Davis. 1987b. T-cell receptor δ gene rearrangements in early thymocytes. Nature. 330: 722.

Cron, R., R. Koning, W.L. Maloy, D. Pardoll, J.E. Coligan, and J.A. Bluestone. 1988. Peripheral murine CD3$^+$, CD4$^-$, CD8$^-$ T lymphocytes express novel T cell receptor $\gamma\delta$ structures. J. Immunol. 141: 1074.

Davies, D.R. and H. Metzger. 1983. Structural basis of antibody function. Annu. Rev. Immunol. 1: 63.

Dembic, Z., W. Haas, S. Weiss, J. McCubrey, H. Kiefer, H. von Boehmer, and M. Steinmetz. 1986. Transfer of specificity by murine α and β T cell receptor genes. Nature 320: 323.

de Villartay, J.P., R.D. Hockett, D. Coran, S.J. Korsmeyer, and D.I. Cohen. 1988. Deletion of the human T-cell receptor δ-gene by a site-specific recombination. Nature 335: 170.

Elliott, J.F., E.P. Rock, P.A. Patten, M.M. Davis, and Y.-H. Chien. 1988. The adult T-cell receptor δ-chain is diverse and distinct from that of fetal thymocytes. Nature 331: 627.

Ferrick, D.A., S.R. Sambhara, W. Ballhausen, A. Iwamoto, H. Pircher, C.L. Walker, W.M. Yokoyama, R.G. Miller, and T.W. Mak. 1989. T cell function and expression are dramatically altered in T cell receptor Vγ1.1Jγ4Cγ4 transgenic mice. Cell 57: 483.

Goodman, T. and L. Lefrancois. 1988. Expression of the γ-δ T-cell receptor on intestinal CD8$^+$ intraepithelial lymphocytes. Nature 333: 855.

Havran, W.L. and J.P. Allison. 1988. Developmentally ordered appearance of thymocytes expressing different T-cell antigen receptors. Nature 335: 443.

Hockett, R.D., J.-P. de Villartay, K. Pollock, D.G. Poplacks, D.I. Cohen, and S.J. Korsmeyer. 1988. Human T-cell antigen receptor (TCR) δ-chain locus and elements responsible for its deletion are within the TCR α-chain locus. Proc. Natl. Acad. Sci. 85: 9694.

Iwamoto, I., P. Ohashi, C. Walker, F. Rupp, H. Yoho, H. Hengartner, and T.W. Mak. 1986. The murine γ chain genes in B10 mice: Sequence and expression of new constant and variable genes. J. Exp. Med. 163: 1203.

Nixon-Fulton, J.L., W.A. Kuziel, B. Santerse, P.R. Bergstresser, P.W. Tucker, and R.E. Tigelaar. 1988. Thy-1$^+$ epidermal cells in nude mice are distinct from their counterparts in thymus-bearing mice. J. Immunol. 141: 1897.

Ohashi, P., T.W. Mak, P. Van den Elsen, Y. Yanagi, Y. Yoshikai, A.F. Calman, C. Terhorst, J.D. Stobo, and A. Weiss. 1985. Reconstitution of an active T3/T cell antigen receptor in human T cells by DNA transfer. Nature 316: 602.

Pardoll, D.M., B.J. Fowlkes, J.A. Bluestone, A. Kruisbeek, W.L. Maloy, J.E. Coligan, and R.H. Schwartz. 1987. Differential expression of two distinct T cell receptors during thymocyte development. Nature 326: 79.

Saito, T., A. Weiss, J. Miller, M.A. Norcross, and R.G. Germain. 1987. Specific antigen-Ia activation of transfected human T cells expressing murine Ti $\alpha\beta$-human T3 receptor complexes. Nature 325: 125.

Saito, H., D.M. Kranz, Y. Takagaki, A. Hayday, H. Eisen, and S. Tonegawa. 1984. A third rearranged and expressed gene in a clone of cytotoxic T lymphocytes. Nature 312: 36.

Steiner, G., F. Koning, A. Elbe, E. Tschachler, W.M. Yokoyama, E.M. Shevach, G. Stingl, and J.E. Coligan. 1988. Characterization of T cell receptors on resident murine dendritic epidermal cells. Eur. J. Immunol. 18: 1323.

Yoshikai, Y., M.D. Reis, and T.W. Mak. 1986. Athymic mice express a high level of functional γ chain, but drastically reduced levels of α and β chain T cell receptor messages. Nature 324: 482.

T-cell Subpopulations Expressing Distinct Forms of the TCR in Normal, Athymic, and Neonatally TCRαβ-suppressed Rats

T. Hünig,* G. Tiefenthaler,* A. Lawetzky,* R. Kubo,† and E. Schlipköter*

*Genzentrum der Ludwig-Maximilians-Universität München, D-8033 Martinsried, Federal Republic of Germany;
†Department of Medicine, National Jewish Center for Immunology and Respiratory Medicine, Denver, Colorado 80262

Two forms of CD3-associated T-cell antigen receptors (TCRs) have been described in humans and mice: The $\alpha\beta$ heterodimer expressed by over 90% of T cells mediates antigen-recognition and alloreactivity by both major histocompatibility complex (MHC) class I- and class II-restricted T cells (for review, see Marrack and Kappler 1987). TCR$\gamma\delta$s, on the other hand, are expressed on a small fraction of T lymphocytes (for review, see Brenner et al. 1988; Raulet 1989). Their preferential location in mouse epidermis (Koning et al. 1987; Kuziel et al. 1987) and in gut epithelium of mice (Goodman and Lefrancois 1988) and chicken (Bucy et al. 1988) and the limited diversity of $\gamma\delta$ receptors expressed by dendritic epidermal T cells (Asarnow et al. 1988) suggest a very specialized and as yet obscure role in host defense.

In the rat, TCR$\alpha\beta$ has been described only recently on cDNA (Morris et al. 1988) and protein (Owhashi and Heber-Katz 1988; Hünig et al. 1989) level. Making use of a monoclonal antibody (MAb) that reacts with all rat TCR$\alpha\beta$, we show here the coexistence of $\alpha\beta$ and $\gamma\delta$ T cells in rat peripheral lymphoid organs and address the question of the contributions of these two subsets to the immune response in vivo and in vitro.

EXPERIMENTAL PROCEDURES

Animals. Young adult Lewis (Zentralinstitut für Versuchstierzucht, Germany) and Wistar (animal facilities of the Max-Planck-Institute für Biochemie, Germany) rats of both sexes were used. Most experiments were carried out with both strains, and no significant differences were observed. BN rats (for stimulation of mixed lymphocyte reaction [MLR]) were also used from the Zentralinstitut für Versuchstierzucht. Aged (>1 year old) LEW/Mol and *rnu/rnu* athymic rats on the same background were obtained from Mollegaards Breeding Centre Ltd.

Antibodies. MAbs W3/25 (anti-CD4, Jefferies et al. 1985), OX-8 (CD8, Brideau et al. 1980), OX-19 (CD5, Mason et al. 1983), OX-22 (CD45R, Spickett et al. 1983), and OX-52 (pan T cell, Robinson et al. 1986) were produced in ascitic forms from cell lines provided by A. Williams. The R73 MAb to a constant determinant of the rat TCR$\alpha\beta$ has been described previously

(Hünig et al. 1989). Antibodies were purified using protein-A-Sepharose (Pharmacia Fince Chemicals). Some were fluoresceine-isothiocynate (FITC, Sigma Chemical Co.)-conjugated or biotinylated according to standard procedures. OX-19-FITC was purchased from Serotec Ltd. Phycoerythrin (PE)-conjugated monoclonal rat anti-mouse-κ antibody was from Becton Dickinson GmbH. The antiserum to human CD3 was prepared by injecting a rabbit seven times (first in complete and then in incomplete Freund's adjuvant) intramuscularly at 2–3-week intervals with CD3 immunopurified from 2×10^9 HPB-MLT cells (Kubo et al. 1987). The rabbit antiserum to peptide 159-187 of the human TCRδ chain (Loh et al. 1987) was a gift from A. Weiss.

Preparation of cells. Suspensions of thymus, spleen, and lymph node cells were prepared as described previously (Hünig et al. 1989). Red blood cells were removed by treatment with 0.83% ammonium chloride in 20 mM Tris (pH 7.2). For enrichment of T cells and natural killer (NK)-cells, cell suspensions were passed over nylon wool. For subset depletion, cell suspensions were treated with a saturating concentration of a relevant MAb and thoroughly washed. A suspension of washed Magnisort-M particles (du Pont, Delaware) (4 μl/10^6 cells) was then added. After 5 minutes, the mixture was centrifuged for 5 minutes at 1500 rpm, gently resuspended, and left for another 5 minutes on ice. Magnetic particles and adhering cells were then removed in a tissue culture flask fastened to a magnetic plate (du Pont). This final step was repeated twice before recovering the unbound cells from the supernatant by centrifugation.

Immunofluorescence and flow cytometry. All antibodies were used at saturating concentrations. For two-color immunofluorescent labeling, 2×10^5 cells in 100 μl of phosphate-buffered saline (PBS)/0.2% bovine serum albumin/0.02% sodium azide were sequentially exposed for 15 minutes on ice (1) to an unconjugated MAb to the first marker, (2) to rat anti-mouse-κ-PE, (3) to 10 μg/ml normal mouse immunoglobulin (Ig), and (4) to FITC-conjugated MAb to the second marker. For three-color analysis, a biotinylated MAb to a third marker was included during step 4, followed by exposure to Duochrome-Streptavidin (Becton Dickinson). Analysis was performed on a FACscan flow cytometer (Becton Dickinson). Light scatter gates were set to include all viable nucleated cells. Where appropriate, an additional fluorescence gate was set to collect single-parameter histograms of defined subpopulations. Then 10,000 events were analyzed using FACscan software and are displayed as dot plots or histograms or as contour plots generated with the LYSYS software (Becton Dickinson).

Cell-surface iodination and radioimmunoprecipitation. Radioiodination, preparation of digitonin lysates, and precipitation and analysis of precipitates were carried out as described previously (Hünig et al. 1989). For precipitation with the antiserum to the human TCRδ chain peptide, 1% SDS was added, and the lysates were heated to 56°C for 30 minutes. A fivefold excess of Nonidet P-40 containing lysis buffer and 5 μl of the antiserum preadsorbed to protein-A-Sepharose was then added. The following steps were as described.

Assay for NK-cell activity. The NK-sensitive mouse YAC-1 lymphoma and the NK-resistant P815 mouse mastocytoma were labeled with $Na_2^{51}CrO_4$ and used as target cells. Varying numbers of effector cells were incubated in triplicates with 10^4 target cells in round-bottom microtiter plates (A/S NUNC) containing 0.2 ml of culture medium (RPMI 1640 plus 5% fetal calf serum)/well. After 4 hours at 37°C, the plates were centrifuged, radioactivity in half the supernatant was determined, and the percentage of specific lysis was calculated as 100 × (cpm experimental, cpm medium/cpm detergent, cpm medium).

Cell culture. For MLR, 10^5 Lewis responder cells were cocultured with 2×10^5 2000-rads-irradiated BN spleen cells in round-bottom microtiter plates (NUNC) containing 0.2 ml of culture medium/well with or without 10 units/ml recombinant interleukin-2 (IL-2) (a gift from Hoechst AG). Relative proliferative activity was determined from days 5 to 6 of culture by [^{3}H]thymidine incorporation as described previously (Hünig et al. 1989). For stimulation with anti-TCR MAb R73 or concanavalin A (Con A), nylon-wool-passed cells were adjusted to 4×10^4 TCRαβ$^+$ cells/flat-bottomed microtiter well with half the usual growth area (Costar). MAb R73 was indirectly cross-linked via rabbit-anti-mouse IgG (Dakopatts) to the tissue-culture plastic. Con A was used at 5 μg/ml, and IL-2 was used at 10 units/ml. [^{3}H]Thymidine incorporation was determined from days 2 to 3 of culture.

In vivo treatment with MAb R73. Litters of newborn Lewis rats were injected twice per week with purified MAb R73 or PBS. The dose of MAb was increased from initially 0.5 mg/wk to 2 mg/wk.

RESULTS

Identification and Functional Analysis of TCRαβ$^+$ and TCR αβ$^-$ Rat T Cells and NK Cells

Three-color flow cytometry was used to define subpopulations of nylon-wool-passed rat spleen cells. In addition to the markers CD4, -5, and -8, the rat pan-T-cell marker OX-52 and TCRαβ were all correlated with one another. The results of these experiments are summarized in Table 1. Among cells expressing the pan-T-cell markers CD5 and/or OX-52, four populations were clearly distinguished. All cells positive for the TCRαβ also expressed CD5 and OX-52 and, as expected, could be divided into the CD4$^+$8$^-$ and CD4$^-$8$^+$ subsets. A small population (4% of all OX-52$^+$ cells) was CD5$^+$ TCRαβ$^-$. More than 90% of these cells expressed CD8.

Finally, a fourth population was identified that was CD5$^-$ but expressed the pan-T-cell marker OX52 although at a roughly fivefold lower density than found on the subsets described above. Most of these OX-52^{low}CD5$^-$TCRαβ$^-$ cells expressed the CD8 antigen and were uniformly negative for CD4. This agrees well with the established phenotype of rat NK cells (Vujanovic et al. 1988), and, as shown in Table 2 the NK-cell activity present in nylon-wool-passed rat spleen cells was indeed highly enriched in that population. Thus, removal of TCRαβ$^+$ cells yielded a roughly 10-fold increase in NK-cell activity, together with an 11-fold enrichment in OX-52^{low}CD5$^-$ cells (from 6.7% to 74%). Additional depletion of the CD5$^+$ TCRαβ$^-$ cells that made up about 24% of this NK-cell-enriched fraction yielded only CD5$^-$ OX-52^{low} cells and a further slight increase in natural cytotoxicity. Not unexpectedly, this population was completely unreactive in the MLR against allogeneic spleen cells. Rather, alloreactivity as detected in MLR was entirely contained within the TCRαβ$^+$ population since depletion of these cells resulted in a complete loss of a proliferative response (Table 2b). In summary, these functional assays detected alloreactivity and NK-cell activity within the TCRαβ$^+$ and the OX-52^{low} CD5$^-$ population, respectively. No function was assigned to the CD5$^+$ TCRαβ$^-$ cells.

Table 1. Cell-surface Phenotype of Rat Spleen Cell Subpopulations Expressing the Pan-T-cell Marker OX-52

Function	TCRαβ	CD4	CD5	CD8	OX-52	OX-52$^+$(%)
Helper/DTH[a]	+	+	+	−	high	66
CTL[a]	+	−	+	+	high	22
Unknown	−	−	+	+(>90%)	high	4
NK-cells[b]	−	−	−	+(>70%)	low	8

[a]Functional assignment from the literature.
[b]This paper and Vujanovic et al. (1988).

Table 2. NK-cell Activity and Alloreactivity of Rat Spleen
Subpopulations

(a) *4-hour ^{51}Cr-release assay*

| | | % specific ^{51}Cr release | |
Effectors	E:T ratio	YAC-1	P815
Nylon-wool-passed (NW)-spleen	100:1	46.3	0.0
	50:1	35.3	0.0
	25:1	18.5	1.8
	12.5:1	13.9	1.2
	6.25:1	12.1	0.0
	3.12:1	0.3	0.0
	1.6:1	0.1	0.2
TCR$\alpha\beta$-depleted	100:1	52.3	12.9
NW spleen	50.1	63.0	11.4
	25:1	53.0	8.5
	12.5:1	49.7	4.6
	6.25:1	37.1	1.3
	3.12:1	27.1	1.2
	1.6:1	15.0	0.6
TCR$\alpha\beta$/CD5-depleted	100:1	69.7	7.0
NW spleen	50:1	73.8	7.4
	25:1	58.8	3.3
	12.5:1	51.0	2.0
	6.25:1	33.1	3.3
	3.12:1	21.4	6.0
	1.6:1	11.7	0.0

(b) *5-day MLR*

Responders	Stimulators	[^{3}H]TdR incorporation[a] (cpm $\times 13^{-3}$)
Lewis NW spleen	—	2269
	Lewis	1641
	BN	56495
TCR$\alpha\beta$-depleted	—	65
NW spleen	Lewis	119
	BN	391
TCR$\alpha\beta$/CD5-depleted	—	134
NW spleen	Lewis	66
	BN	105

[a](TdR) Thymine-2-deoxyriboside.

Identification of Rat TCR$\alpha\beta$ and TCR$\gamma\delta$ by Radioimmunoprecipitation

We have previously described the rat TCR$\alpha\beta$ as a 40–46-kD heterodimeric glycoprotein that, as in all other species investigated, is noncovalently associated with low-molecular-weight polypeptides collectively called CD3 (Hünig et al. 1989). To detect also non-TCR$\alpha\beta$ molecules, immunoprecipitations from digitonin lysates of surface-iodinated cells were performed with an antiserum to human CD3 that cross-reacts with its rat homolog and with an antiserum to a synthetic peptide corresponding to positions 159–187 of the human TCRδ chain (Loh et al. 1987) that had been shown to cross-react with the mouse δ chain (Bonyhadi et al. 1987). The cells used for preparing the lysates were nylon-wool-passed red-cell-depleted spleen cells without further separation (Fig. 1A) or after removal of TCR$\alpha\beta^+$ cells (Fig. 1B).

From a lysate of whole nylon-wool-passed nucleated spleen cells, which contained 80–90% TCR $\alpha\beta^+$ cells,

the anti-CD3 antiserum and MAb R73 to the TCR$\alpha\beta$ precipitated the same spectrum of bands, i.e., the high-molecular-weight TCRα and β chains and the low-molecular-weight CD3 polypeptides. No visible band was obtained with the anti-δ chain antiserum. The lysate prepared from TCR$\alpha\beta$-depleted cells yielded a completely different result when analyzed with the same serological reagents (Fig. 1B). As expected, hardly any TCR$\alpha\beta$ was detected by MAb R73 in this lysate. Still, the anti-CD3 antiserum precipitated the characteristic low-molecular-weight bands together with a major band with a molecular weight of 48K and two faint bands of 40 and 42K. When electrophoresed without reduction, one major band with an apparent molecular weight of 100K was observed (not shown), indicating an at least dimeric molecule. Finally, the anti-human TCRδ-chain antiserum yielded a band of exactly the same molecular weight as the major band found by anti-CD3 coprecipitation. The weaker intensity of the band obtained with the anti-TCRδ-chain antiserum may be due to a weak interspecies cross-reac-

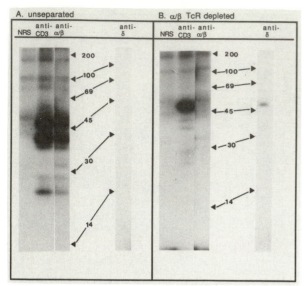

Figure 1. Radioimmunoprecipitation of rat TCR molecules. Digitonin lysates from surface-iodinated unseparated (*A*) or TCRαβ-depleted (*B*) nylon-wool-passed nucleated spleen cells were used for immunoprecipitation with the reagents indicated. Samples were run on 14% slab gels under reducing conditions.

tivity of the antiserum employed or to a consequence of the denaturation required for reactivity of the lysate with this antipeptide antiserum (denaturation also explains the absence of bands corresponding to CD3). These results indicate that at least some, and possibly all, of the CD3-associated molecules precipitated from TCRαβ-depleted cells contained the δ chain and are thus the likely rat homolog of TCRγδ described previously in humans, mice (for review, see Brenner et al. 1988; Raulet 1989), and chickens (Sowder et al. 1988). In further experiments, lysates prepared from CD5⁻ OX-52^low cells were analyzed and found unreactive with any of the anti-TCR reagents employed (not shown). It is thus concluded that a major population of T cells expressing TCRαβ coexists in rat spleen with a minor population containing TCRγδ⁺ cells and a TCR⁻ subset that mediates NK activity. As described above, these three populations can be distinguished and separated on the basis of their different serological phenotypes.

Detection of Functional TCR⁺ Cells in Athymic Rats

T cells normally mature in the thymus. Nevertheless, the existence of functional TCR⁺ positive cells in athymic mice is well documented (for review, see Hünig et al. 1983). Evidence has been provided for an oligoclonal origin of these cells (Hünig 1983; MacDonald and Lees 1984; MacDonald et al. 1987; Maleckar and Sherman 1987), which in old animals can reach near to normal numbers. The availability of a similar mutant in the rat provided the opportunity to extend these studies to another species.

Nylon-wool-passed spleen and lymph node cells from normal and athymic Lewis rats were analyzed by two-color flow cytometry. As shown by the example in Figure 2, both subpopulations of CD5⁺ cells described above, i.e., TCRαβ⁺ and TCRαβ⁻, were found in athymic rats. If the phenotypical characteristics of rat T-cell subpopulations established above for normal rats hold true for T cells found in athymic animals, at least some of these CD5⁺ TCRαβ⁻ express TCRγδ. In some animals, and not always in both lymph node and spleen, we found an enrichment of these presumptive γδ T cells relative to the αβ T-cell population.

As in the athymic mouse model, the origin of T cells in athymic rats remains unclear. The oligoclonality of the nude mouse TCR repertoire mentioned above suggests, however, that very few T cells mature in these animals, which then undergo clonal expansion. A MAb (OX-22) to a CD45R-like form of the leukocyte common antigen that is irreversibly lost from virgin CD4⁺ T cells once they enter proliferation (Powrie and Mason 1989) was therefore used to phenotype cells from normal and athymic rats. As can be seen in Figure 2, the CD45R determinant was indeed absent from most TCRαβ⁺ cells in athymic rats, suggesting that postmaturational expansion may indeed account for the high frequency (> 10% of lymphocytes) of TCR⁺ cells in lymphoid organs of old animals with congenital thymus aplasia. Figure 3 shows that these cells can be triggered via their receptors. Thus, culture of nylon-wool-passed nude rat spleen cells in the presence of immobilized anti-TCR antibody led to a significant proliferative response that, however, was clearly below

Nylon Wool-Passed LN cells

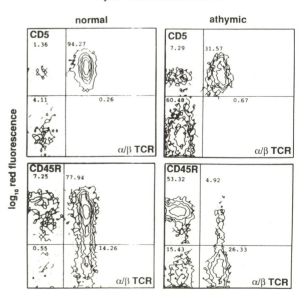

Figure 2. CD45R phenotype of TCRαβ⁺ cells from aged normal and athymic Lewis rats. Nylon-wool-passed lymph node cells were stained by the reagents given and analyzed by flow cytometry. An equal probability contour plot at 20% probability is shown.

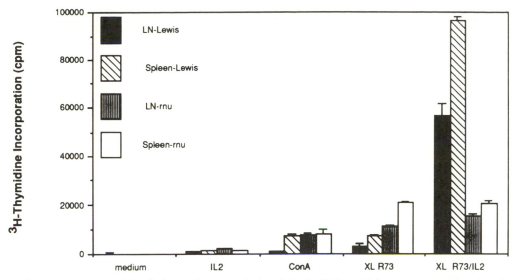

Figure 3. Proliferative response of T cells from athymic rats induced via the TCR$\alpha\beta$. Nylon-wool-passed lymph nodes or spleen cells from an aged normal and an aged athymic Lewis rat were adjusted to the same number of TCR$\alpha\beta^+$ cells and cultured for 3 days with the reagents indicated.

that of cells from a euthymic control animal that had been adjusted to the same number of TCR$\alpha\beta^+$ cells per microculture.

Cellular Composition and Immune Responsiveness of Neonatally TCR$\alpha\beta$-suppressed Rats

It is obvious from the above results that despite the absence of a functional thymus, athymic rats contain TCR$\alpha\beta^-$ and the presumptive TCR$\gamma\delta^+$ T cells. To establish a model system in which the contribution of these T-cell subsets to the immune response in vivo can be studied, we have therefore attempted to suppress the generation of TCR$\alpha\beta^+$ cells by injecting rats with purified R73 MAb from birth.

As shown in Figure 4, the peripheral lymphoid organs of such suppressed animals were virtually devoid of TCR$\alpha\beta^+$ cells. This was not because of modulation of the TCR since (1) the R73$^-$ phenotype persisted after cell culture and (2) there was a concomitant reduction in CD5$^+$ lymphocytes. Interestingly, a small population (3–4%) of lymphocytes in spleen and lymph nodes was consistently observed that expressed TCR$\alpha\beta$ at a roughly fivefold lower level than normal (Fig. 4). At present, we do not know whether such cells, which apparently escape intrathymic deletion or peripheral destruction in the presence of a vast excess of anti-TCR MAb, can also be found in normal animals. As can also be seen in Figure 4, the frequency of CD5$^+$ TCR$\alpha\beta^-$ cells, i.e., the presumptive TCR$\gamma\delta$-expressing T cells, was elevated in suppressed animals above the frequency expected from the reduction in TCR$\alpha\beta^+$ cells. The possibility has to be considered, however, that CD5$^+$ cells without any TCR molecules accumulate in anti-TCR$\alpha\beta$-treated animals that contribute to the CD5$^+$ TCR$\alpha\beta^-$ population.

In the thymus, TCR$\alpha\beta$-suppressed rats lacked mature thymocytes that in control animals expressed a high level (i.e., the same as on peripheral T cells) of TCR$\alpha\beta$. The apparent lack of an effect on immature

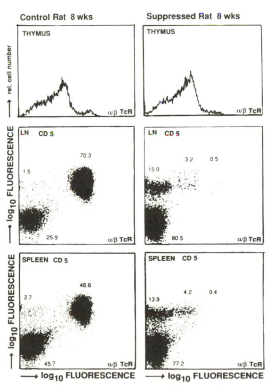

Figure 4. Cell-surface phenotype of lymphoid cells from neonatally TCR$\alpha\beta$-suppressed rats. Rats were injected from birth with either PBS (control, *left* panels) or purified MAb R73 in PBS (*right* panels). At 8 weeks of age, single-cell suspensions of the organs indicated were analyzed by flow cytometry. Here, 10,000 cells are shown in each dot plot.

thymocytes may be because even when a serum concentration of over 200 μg/ml free R73 MAb was reached (data not shown), there was only a partial saturation of available binding sites on these cells, obviously because of a poor penetration of the MAb into the thymus cortex.

The effect of neonatal suppression of TCR$\alpha\beta^+$ cells on immune responsiveness was tested in several functional assays. NK activity of freshly isolated spleen cells was higher in TCR$\alpha\beta$-suppressed rats than in control animals (Table 3a). As calculated from plotted data, this difference was between two- and eightfold in six animals analyzed and thus usually exceeded the increment expected from the absence of TCR$\alpha\beta^+$. In contrast, alloreactivity as measured by MLR was absent from spleen or lymph node cells of the treated animals even when IL-2 was added to facilitate the response (Table 3b). Thus, as in the cell separation experiments described above, no proliferative response to foreign MHC antigens of the presumptive $\gamma\delta$ T cells was detected. This is in line with the acceptance of skin grafts observed in our unpublished experiments (E. Schlipköter and T. Hünig, unpubl.). Finally, the in vivo humoral immune response to the T-dependent antigen keyhole-lympet hemocyanine (KLH), administered in alum with pertussis adjuvant, was studied. In contrast with PBS-injected control animals that produced KLH-specific antibodies with a titer of over 10^{-5} as detected by enzyme-linked immunosorbent assay, suppressed rats produced no detectable antibody to KLH (data not shown), indicating that $\gamma\delta$ T cells cannot functionally replace helper T cells in chronically TCR$\alpha\beta$-suppressed animals.

Table 3. NK Activity and Alloreactivity of Spleen Cells from Neonatally TCR$\alpha\beta$-suppressed Lewis Rats

(a) *4-hour ^{51}Cr release assay: % specific ^{51}Cr release from YAC-1 target cells*

E:T ratio	Control[a]	TCR$\alpha\beta$-suppressed spleen[a]		
		1	2	3
100:1	33.9	63.1	43.1	49.8
30:1	12.6	44.1	23.7	34.9
10:1	11.0	25.5	10.6	19.9
3:1	−1.3	15.9	5.8	7.2

(b) *5-day MLR*

Responders	Stimulators	[^{3}H]TdR incorporation[c] (cpm × 10^{-3})	
		−IL2	+IL-2
Control spleen[b]	—	131	2078
	Lewis	3439	1869
	BN	45873	52669
TCR$\alpha\beta$-suppressed	—	3796	976
spleen[b]	Lewis	3825	1684
	BN	497	3013

[a]Unseparated spleen cells.

[b]T cells were enriched by nylon wool filtration.

[c](TdR) Thymine-2-deoxyriboside.

DISCUSSION

It is shown here that the two types of CD3-associated TCR defined previously in humans and mice, i.e., the major $\alpha\beta$ form expressed by over 90% of T cells that mediates MHC-restricted antigen recognition and the minor $\gamma\delta$ form found on less than 5% of peripheral T cells, can also be identified in the rat and that, in this species, cells mediating natural cytotoxicity are distinct from both populations by cell-surface phenotype. Both types of T cells are present in athymic rats, whereas essentially TCR$\alpha\beta^-$ animals can be obtained by injection of the anti-TCR$\alpha\beta$ MAb R73 from birth. The immunological status of these TCR$\alpha\beta$-suppressed rats indicates that B-cell help and alloreactivity are the domain of T cells expressing TCR$\alpha\beta$. Although we show that, among the small subpopulation of CD5$^+$ TCR$\alpha\beta^-$ cells, CD3 and TCR$\gamma\delta$ are expressed and that the latter has the same apparent molecular weight as the predominantly labeled cell-surface glycoprotein that is associated with CD3 on these cells, it cannot be excluded that T cells with other forms of TCR molecules that remained unidentified are present in that fraction. Thus, the recent discovery of a third form of TCR in chickens (Chen et al. 1989) leaves open the possibility that non-TCR$\alpha\beta$ and non-TCR$\gamma\delta$ exist in other species as well. Without MAbs to rat CD3 and to TCR$\gamma\delta$, this question cannot be resolved. In any event, T cells expressing TCR$\gamma\delta$ are present in the CD5$^+$ TCR$\alpha\beta^-$ fraction isolated and, if subset frequency should be comparable with that found in humans, may account for all CD5$^+$ TCR$\alpha\beta^-$ cells. (We have not observed any CD5$^+$ B cells in rat spleen; data not shown.)

More than 90% of the presumptive $\gamma\delta$ T cells found in spleen (Table 1) as well as in lymph nodes and peripheral blood (not shown) were of the CD4$^-$8$^+$ phenotype. Only a minor subpopulation of "double-negative" and hardly any CD4$^+$8$^-$ cells were detected in that fraction. In mice, $\gamma\delta$ T cells have so far been isolated mostly as CD3$^+$ CD4$^-$8$^-$, i.e., double-negative cells. This procedure was chosen, however, since no MAb to a constant determinant of the mouse TCR$\alpha\beta$ was available for negative selection. The double-negative phenotype may thus not be representative of all mouse $\gamma\delta$ T cells. In fact, TCR$\gamma\delta^+$ intraepithelial lymphocytes isolated from the mouse gut are CD8$^+$ (Goodman and Lefrancois 1988). In humans, up to 70% of $\gamma\delta$ T cells in peripheral blood and spleen are of the "CD8 single-positive" phenotype (Groh et al. 1989).

The specificity of the $\gamma\delta$ T cells is still unresolved. Although individual $\gamma\delta$ T-cell clones with specificity for foreign MHC antigens have been isolated in mice (Matis et al. 1987), a high frequency of alloreactive cells as is characteristic of $\alpha\beta$ T cells has not been reported for freshly isolated $\gamma\delta$ T cells. In our present results, no proliferative response to MHC-disparate cells was detected after in vitro or in vivo removal of $\alpha\beta$ T cells, speaking against alloreactivity as a prominent feature of the $\gamma\delta$ repertoire. No definite conclusions can be drawn, however, before a panel of RT1 haplotypes is screened in MLR and before the possible interference with an MLR of NK cells that were strongly enriched in the responder cell populations presently employed is not excluded.

The demonstration of TCR$\alpha\beta^+$ and TCR$\alpha\beta^-$ T cells in nude rats confirms the existence of a T-cell differentiation pathway in congenitally thymus aplastic animals that has been studied in detail in mice. Although the site where these cells mature remains controversial, we add here another piece of evidence supporting the hypothesis that, in athymic animals, peripheral expansion of mature cells makes a much larger contribution to the T-cell pool observed than in euthymic animals, leading to the oligoclonal T-cell receptor repertoire observed in nude mice (Hünig 1983; MacDonald and Lees 1984; MacDonald et al. 1987; Maleckar and Sherman 1987). Thus, absence of the OX-22 (CD45R) antigen from CD4$^+$ T cells, shown before to indicate a history of proliferation, was characteristic of the minority of TCR$\alpha\beta^+$ cells in aged euthymic rats but was also characteristic of their vast majority in aged athymic rats (and for almost all CD4$^+$ T cells in those animals, not shown). The incompleteness of the TCR repertoire documented for athymic mice provides an explanation for the lack of T-cell responses to "conventional" antigens in animals that contain appreciable numbers ($>10\%$) of TCR$^+$ cells. In addition, we have shown for athymic mice (Lawetzky and Hünig 1988) and show here for athymic rats that TCR$\alpha\beta^+$ cells from these animals may not be fully functional since their responsiveness to stimulation via the TCR is smaller than in normal animals. Whether this reflects a form of "clonal exhaustion" or is due to an aberrant functional phenotype resulting from differentiation outside the normal environment is unclear.

The cellular composition of the immune system in neonatally TCR$\alpha\beta$-suppressed rats is quite different from that found in athymic animals: With the exception of a small population ($<5\%$ of lymphocytes) of cells with an abnormally low level of TCR$\alpha\beta$ that may be functionally inert, these animals are devoid of TCR$\alpha\beta^+$ cells, making them an interesting model system for the contribution of $\alpha\beta$ and $\gamma\delta$ T cells to the immune response. We find here that alloreactivity and T-cell-dependent antibody production are undetectable in such animals. Moreover, unpublished experiments carried out in collaboration with F. Emmrich and colleagues indicate that TCR$\alpha\beta$-suppressed rats are completely resistant to adjuvant-induced arthritis. This is a first example for the usefulness of TCR$\alpha\beta$-suppressed rats in the assessment of the contribution of $\alpha\beta$ T cells to the development of an autoimmune disease.

ACKNOWLEDGMENTS

We thank E. Winnacker for his continued support, A. Williams for antibody-producing cell lines, A. Weiss for the anti-TCRδ-peptide antiserum, and Claudia Heise for large-scale purification of MAb. This work was supported by Genzentrum e.V., by Fonds der Chemischen Industrie e.V., and by grants from the Bundesministerium für Forschung und Technologie and from Deutsche Forschungsgemeinschaft through SFB-217.

REFERENCES

Asarnow, D.M., W.A. Kuziel, M. Bonyhadi, R.E. Tigelaar, P.W. Tucker, and J.P. Allison. 1988. Limited diversity of γ/δ-antigen receptor genes of Thy1 + dendritic epidermal cells. *Cell* **55**: 837.

Bonyhadi, M., A. Weiss, P.W. Tucker, R.E. Tigelaar, and J.P. Allison. 1987. Delta is the Cx gene product in the γ/δ antigen receptor of dendritic epidermal cells. *Nature* **330**: 574.

Brenner, M.B., J.L. Strominger, and M.S. Krangel. 1988. The γ/δ T-cell receptor. *Adv. Immunol.* **43**: 133.

Brideau, R.J., P.B. Carter, W.R. McMaster, D.W. Mason, and A.F. Williams. 1980. Two subsets of T-lymphocytes defined with monoclonal antibodies. *Eur. J. Immunol.* **10**: 609.

Bucy, R.P., C.-L.H. Chen, J. Cihak, U. Lösch, and M.D. Cooper. 1988. Avian T-cells expressing γ/δ receptors localize in the splenic sinusoids and the intestinal epithelium. *J. Immunol.* **141**: 2200.

Chen, E.H., J.T. Sowder, J.M. Lahti, J. Cihak, U. Lösch, and M.D. Cooper. 1989. TCR3: A third T-cell receptor in the chicken. *Proc. Natl. Acad. Sci.* **86**: 2351.

Goodman, T. and L. Lefrancois. 1988. Expression of the γ/δ-T-cell receptor on intestinal CD8 + intraepithelial lymphocytes. *Nature* **33**: 855.

Groh, V., S. Procelli, M. Fabbi, L.L. Lanier, L.J. Picker, T. Anerson, R.A. Walker, A.K. Bhan, J.L. Strominger, and M.B. Brenner. 1989. Human lymphocytes bearing T-cell receptor γ/δ are phenotypically diverse and evenly distributed throughout the lymphoid system. *J. Exp. Med.* **169**: 1277.

Hünig, T. 1983. T-cell function and specificity in athymic mice. *Immunol. Today* **4**: 84.

Hünig, T., H.-J. Wallny, J.K. Hartley, A. Lawetzky, and G. Tiefenthaler. 1989. A monoclonal antibody to a constant determinant of the rat T-cell antigen receptor that induces T-cell activation. Differential reactivity with subsets of immature and mature T lymphocytes. *J. Exp. Med.* **169**: 73.

Jefferies, W.A., J.R. Green, and A.F. Williams. 1985. Authentic T helper CD4 (W3/25) antigen on rat peritoneal macrophages. *J. Exp. Med.* **162**: 117.

Koning, F., G. Stingl, W.M. Yokoyama, H. Yamada, W.L. Maloy, E. Tschaler, E.M. Shevach, and J.E. Coligan. 1987. Identification of a T3-associated γ/δ T cell receptor on Thy1$^+$ dendritic epidermal cell lines. *Science* **236**: 834.

Kubo, R.T., K. Haskins, and S.M. Fu. 1987. Serologic identification of the murine T3 homologue by cross-reactive xenogeneic anti-human T3 antisera. *Mol. Immunol.* **24**: 201.

Kuziel, W.A., A. Takashima, M. Bonyhadi, P.R. Bergstresser, J.P. Allison, R.E. Tigelaar, and P.W. Tucker. 1987. Regulation of T-cell receptor γ-chain RNA expression in murine Thy1 + dendritic epidermal cells. *Nature* **328**: 263.

Lawetzky, A. and T. Hünig. 1988. Analysis of CD3 and antigen receptor expression on T-cell subpopulations of aged athymic mice. *Eur. J. Immunol.* **18**: 409.

Loh, E.Y., L.L. Lanier, C.W. Turck, D.R. Littman, M.M. Davis, Y.-H. Chien, and A. Weiss. 1987. Identification and sequence of a fourth human T-cell antigen receptor chain. *Nature* **330**: 569.

MacDonald, H.R. and R.K. Lees. 1984. Frequency and specificity of precursors of interleukin-2 producing cells in nude mice. *J. Immunol.* **132:** 605.

MacDonald, H.R., R.K. Lees, D. Bron, B. Sordat, and G. Miescher. 1987. T-cell antigen receptor expression in athymic (nu/nu) mice. Evidence for an oligoclonal β chain repertoire. *J. Exp. Med.* **166:** 195.

Maleckar, J.R. and L.A. Sherman. 1987. The composition of the T-cell receptor repertoire in nude mice. *J. Immunol.* **138:** 3873.

Marrack, P. and J. Kappler. 1987. The T-cell receptor. *Science* **238:** 1073.

Mason, D.W., R.P. Arthur, M.J. Dallman, J.R. Green, G.P. Spickett, and M.L. Thomas. 1983. Functions of rat T-lymphocyte subsets isolated by means of monoclonal antibodies. *Immunol. Rev.* **74:** 57.

Matis, L.A., R. Gron, and J.A. Bluestone. 1987. Major histocompatibility complex linked specificity of γ/δ receptor bearing T-lymphocytes. *Nature* **330:** 262.

Morris, M., A.N. Barclay, and A.F. Williams. 1988. Analysis of T cell receptor β chains in rat thymus, and rat Cα and Cβ sequences. *Immunogenetics* **27:** 174.

Owhashi, M. and E. Heber-Katz. 1988. Protection from EAE conferred by a monoclonal antibody directed against a shared idiotype on rat T-cell receptors specific for myelin basic protein. *J. Exp. Med.* **168:** 2153.

Powrie, F. and D. Mason. 1989. The MRC OX22 − CD4 + T-cells that help B-cells in secondary immune responses derive from naive precursors with the MRC OX-22 + CD4 + phenotype. *J. Exp. Med.* **169:** 653.

Raulet, D.H. 1989. The structure, function, and molecular genetics of the γ/δ-T-cell receptor. *Annu. Rev. Immunol.* **7:** 175.

Robinson, A.P., M. Puklavec, and D.W. Mason. 1986. MRC OX-52: A rat T-cell antigen. *Immunology* **57:** 527.

Sowder, J.T., C.-L.H. Chen, L.L. Ager, M.M. Chan, and M.D. Cooper. 1988. A large subpopulation of avian T cells express a homologue of the mammalian Tγ/δ receptor. *J. Exp. Med.* **167:** 315.

Spickett, G.P., M.R. Brandon, D.W. Mason, A.F. Williams, and G.R. Woollett. 1983. MRC OX-22, a mAb that labels a new subset of T lymphocytes and reacts with the high molecular weight form of the leukocyte-common antigen. *J. Exp. Med.* **158:** 795.

Vujanovic, N.L., R.B. Heberman, M.W. Olszowy, D.V. Cramer, R.R. Salup, C.W. Reynolds, and J.C. Hiserodt. 1988. Lymphokine-activated killer cells in rats: Analysis of progenitor and effector cell phenotype and relationship to natural killer cells. *Cancer Res.* **48:** 884.

T-cell Development in Birds

M.D. Cooper, R.P. Bucy, J.F. George, J.M. Lahti,
D. Char, and C.-L.H. Chen

*Division of Developmental and Clinical Immunology, Departments of Medicine, Pediatrics, Microbiology,
and Pathology, and the Comprehensive Cancer Center, University of Alabama at Birmingham, and the
Howard Hughes Medical Institute, Birmingham, Alabama 35294*

The separate developmental pathways of T and B cells were first revealed in comparative studies of birds and mammals. This division of lymphocyte development and function has since been shown to be a fundamental characteristic of the immune system in all vertebrates. Presently, there is considerable phylogenetic information concerning the immunoglobulin (Ig) products of B cells, but relatively little is known about T-cell products other than in humans and mice.

We have embarked on a comparative analysis of T-cell development in birds because of an interest in the evolutionary strategy for this component of the immune system and in search for fresh clues to some of the unresolved issues of the mammalian immune system. These studies began with the production and characterization of mouse monoclonal antibodies (MAbs) that identify a variety of T-cell surface molecules in chickens. These include homologs of the CD3 (Chen et al. 1986), CD4, CD8 (Chan et al. 1988), and T-cell receptor (TCR) molecules (Chen et al. 1988; Cihak et al. 1988; Sowder et al. 1988a). Using this panel of antibody markers, we have traced the development of T-lineage cells in the chicken (Lahti et al. 1988).

Avian T-cell development was found to be remarkably similar to mammalian T-cell development. Because of certain advantages of the avian model for developmental studies and the availability of the first complete panel of antibodies to the different types of TCR, several unanticipated features of the T-cell system were also revealed in these studies. The most striking of these findings are (1) a third type of TCR (Char et al. 1989; Chen et al. 1989) and (2) a third lymphoid lineage that shares some molecules with T cells but is neither thymus- nor bursa-dependent in its development (Bucy et al. 1989b).

Chicken T-cell Antigens

Chick thymocytes express a cell-surface molecule of $M_r = 65,000$ that is recognized by the CT1 MAb (Chen et al. 1984). This molecule is lost as thymocytes become mature T cells. The CD4 and CD8 molecules in the chicken are very similar to their mammalian counterparts in their basic structure, tissue-specific expression, and functional relationships (Chan et al. 1988). The avian CD4 homolog, recognized by the CT4 MAb, is a

polypeptide with $M_r = 64,000$. The CD8 homolog, recognized by the CT8 MAb, is a molecule with $M_r = 63,000$ that is composed of two disulfide-linked chains with $M_r = 34,000$. A majority of the avian thymocytes express both the CD4 and CD8 molecules, whereas mature T cells in the thymic medulla and peripheral lymphoid tissues express either CD4 or CD8. The CD4 subpopulation exhibits helper T-cell characteristics, whereas the $CD8^+$ cells have cytotoxic T-cell capabilities. All of the T cells in the chicken can be identified by the expression of an avian CD3 homolog, which is detected by the CT3 MAb (Chen et al. 1986). This monoclonal antibody immunoprecipitates a complex of three or more polypeptides with M_r values of 20,000, 19,000, and 17,000, as well as the noncovalently associated TCR heterodimers.

It has proven surprisingly easy to produce mouse monoclonal antibodies to the avian TCR, probably because of the phylogenetic distance between mice and birds. The first two TCR heterodimers to be identified in the chicken are recognized by the TCR1 and TCR2 MAbs (Chen et al. 1988; Cihak et al. 1988; Sowder et al. 1988a). TCR1 appears to be the avian counterpart of the mammalian TCR$\gamma\delta$, and TCR2 appears to be the avian counterpart of TCR$\alpha\beta$. The TCR1 and TCR2 molecules are $M_r = 90,000$ molecules consisting of disulfide-linked glycoprotein chains with M_r values of 50,000 and 40,000. Removal of N-linked oligosaccharides reveals core proteins with M_r values of 36,000 and 33,000 for TCR1 and M_r values of 34,000 and 29,000 for TCR2.

Ontogeny of TCR1 and TCR2 Cells

The TCR1 subpopulation of T cells is generated first in the embryonic thymus on the 12th day of embryonic life (E12), approximately 5 days after the first wave of blood-borne precursor cells enters the embryonic thymus (Sowder et al. 1988a). The number of TCR1-positive cells in the thymus rapidly increases over the next few days when they represent the only type of T cells made by the embryo. TCR2 cells begin to appear in the embryonic thymus on the 15th day of incubation, and these quickly become the predominant T-cell subpopulation (Chen et al. 1988). The sequential generation pattern of the avian TCR1 and TCR2 subpopulations appears to recapitulate the developmental patterns of their mammalian counterparts. Moreover, as noted earlier in mammals, the TCR1 cells in the chick thymus rarely express CD4 or CD8, whereas the immature TCR2 thymocytes express both accessory molecules.

The TCR1 and TCR2 subpopulations of T cells are seeded to the periphery in the same order in which they are generated in the thymus. The TCR1 cells begin to appear in the spleen on the 15th day of embryonic life, and the TCR2 splenic cells make their appearance on the 19th day (R.P. Bucy, in prep.).

Special Characteristics of TCR1 Cells

The TCR1 subpopulation is especially accessible for study in the chick model. The TCR1 MAb provided the first specific marker for the entire $\gamma\delta$ population of T cells, which constitutes 20–30% of the peripheral T-cell pool in the chicken (Sowder et al. 1988a).

Relatively high level of TCR1 expression. From the time of their initial appearance in the embryonic thymus, the TCR1 cells express their TCR1/CD3 receptor complex at a relatively high density. In contrast, the TCR2 cells express their receptors in gradually increasing levels as they undergo transition from immature cortical thymocytes to become mature T cells (George and Cooper 1989). Thus, the mean level of TCR1 expression in the E14 thymus (12,000 TCR1/cell) is approximately 20-fold higher than that of TCR2-positive thymocytes three days later (600 TCR2/cell). Even in the periphery, the TCR1 cells have higher mean levels of receptor expression ($\geq 40,000$) than do the TCR2 cells ($\leq 20,000$).

Rapid cortical transit of TCR1 cells. The TCR1 cells thus express their receptors in relatively high levels from the time they begin their development in the outer cortex of the thymus. This subpopulation of cells also appears to divide relatively infrequently as the cells traverse the cortex to enter the medulla or to exit via the corticomedullary vessels to the periphery (R.P. Bucy et al., in prep.). The cortical transit time for the TCR1 cells is approximately 1 day, whereas TCR2 cells require several days for transit from the thymic cortex to the medullary region. At any particular moment in the life of a young chicken, the TCR1 cells can be found scattered, usually as single cells, throughout the cortex and in more focal accumulations in the medulla. The reverse is true for the TCR2 subpopulation of thymic cells, which have a relatively high replication rate, mature relatively slowly, and are more concentrated in the cortex (Bucy et al. 1988).

Selective homing. Distinctive homing patterns are observed for the TCR1 and TCR2 cells in peripheral lymphoid tissues (Bucy et al. 1988). The TCR2 cells, especially the CD4$^+$ subpopulation, are located primarily in the periarteriolar sheaths of the spleen and in the lamina propria of the intestine. In contrast, the TCR1 cells home preferentially to the sinusoidal areas of the splenic red pulp and to the intestinal epithelium; approximately 80% of the intestinal TCR1 cells are in the epithelium and only 20% are in the underlying lamina propria. This homing pattern of TCR1 cells appears to be conserved in both humans (Bucy et al. 1989a) and sheep (W. Heim, pers. comm.). Mice (Koning et al. 1987; Kuziel et al. 1987) and cattle (W. Heim, pers. comm.) differ in that TCR1 cells are also abundant in skin, a site in which few T cells are seen in chickens (Bucy et al. 1988), humans (Bucy et al. 1989a), and sheep (W. Heim, pers. comm.).

CD8 expression by peripheral TCR1 cells. Whereas the TCR1 cells in the thymus and in the blood are largely "double-negative" cells, lacking both CD4 and CD8 (Sowder et al. 1988a), the TCR1 cells in peripheral tissues frequently express CD8 (Chen et al. 1988; Bucy et al. 1988). This is true for approximately two-thirds of the TCR1 cells in both the spleen and intestine. The frequent expression of CD8 is also typical of human $\gamma\delta$ T cells in the spleen (Bucy et al. 1989a) and of murine $\gamma\delta$ T cells in the intestinal epithelium (Goodman and Lefrancois 1988).

Limited expansion of the peripheral TCR1 subpopulation. Development of the TCR1 subpopulation in peripheral lymphoid tissues is very dependent on a prolonged period of thymic seeding. Removal of the thymus during the first week after hatching leads to a more than threefold reduction in the relative proportion of TCR1 cells (Chen et al. 1989; Cihak et al. 1989), the difference being accounted for primarily by expansion of the TCR2 subpopulation in the thymectomized animals. Although the TCR1 cells can be induced to divide by cross-linkage of the TCR1/CD3 receptor complex (Sowder et al. 1988a), it is extremely rare to see follicular expansion of the TCR1 cells. In contrast, follicles of TCR2 cells can easily be found in the spleen and intestinal lymphoid tissues (R.P. Bucy et al., in prep.).

A Third T-cell Sublineage in Birds

Although our studies suggest that T-cell development is remarkably similar in birds and mammals, one very striking difference was observed in our analysis of avian T-cell development. A third subpopulation of T cells is generated following the development of TCR1 and TCR2 cells (Char et al. 1989; Chen et al. 1989). These cells were noted first as a subpopulation of CD3$^+$ cells that were unreactive with either the TCR1 or TCR2 antibodies. These cells, provisionally termed TCR3 cells, increased as a function of age to account for approximately 15% of the circulating pool of T cells by 6 months of age.

To characterize the TCR heterodimer on the CD3$^+$/TCR1$^-$/TCR2$^-$ subpopulation, cells of this phenotype were isolated by negative selection (Ia$^-$, TCR1$^-$, and TCR2$^-$) in immunofluorescence-activated cell sorting (Chen et al. 1989). When these cells were surface-labeled with ^{125}I and the cell-surface TCR/CD3 complex was immunoprecipitated with the CT3 MAb, a heterodimer with $M_r = 88,000$ was identified in association with the CD3 molecules. This heterodimer consisted of disulfide-linked polypeptide chains with M_r values of 48,000 and 40,000. Removal of N-linked oligosaccharides revealed one core protein of novel size, $M_r = 31,000$, and another one similar in size to one of the TCR2 core proteins, namely $M_r = 34,000$. However, following partial proteolysis, electrophoretic analysis of the constituent peptide fragments suggested that both of the TCR3 chains differ from those of the TCR1 and TCR2 heterodimers.

Antigenic analysis also suggests that TCR3 is a novel receptor type. We have produced two monoclonal antibodies that discriminate these receptors from TCR1 and TCR2 (Char et al. 1989 and in prep.). The anti-TCR3 antibodies have been used to demonstrate that the TCR3 cells appear first in the 17-day-old embryonic thymus and are seeded to the peripheral tissues later than the TCR1 and TCR2 cells.

The TCR3 cells most closely resemble the TCR2 subpopulation of cells. In the thymus, they are predominantly CD4$^+$ and CD8$^+$ (Char et al. 1989; Chen et al. 1989), and the relative density of their TCR3/CD3 receptor complexes is low (M.D. Cooper et al., unpubl.). TCR3 cells in the periphery are largely CD4$^+$ (80%), whereas a relatively small subset (20%) of them bear the CD8 accessory molecule. The splenic localization pattern of TCR3 cells also resembles that of the TCR2 cells in that most are located in the periarteriolar sheaths (D. Char et al., in prep.). Interestingly, few TCR3 cells can be found in the intestine.

We have used the TCR1, TCR2, and TCR3 MAbs to examine the lymphoid cells from several avian species in order to determine the extent of conservation of the TCR epitopes (D. Char et al., unpubl.). Varying patterns of cross-reactivity were observed in different Galliformes species, whereas none of the monoclonal antibodies were reactive with lymphoid cells in birds representative of other orders. We conclude that the three types of TCR in the chicken are conserved at least in gallinaceous birds.

Lineage Relationships of TCR1, TCR2, and TCR3 Subpopulations

One method of examining the lineage relationships of these different subpopulations is via the selective suppression of their embryonic development. We have used in ovo injections of the TCR1 and TCR2 antibodies in an attempt to alter T-cell development by cross-linkage of these receptor molecules (Sowder et al. 1988b). Either the TCR1 or the TCR2 antibodies were injected into the circulation on the 11th day of embryonic life, i.e., just prior to the onset of TCR1 expression. Other embryos received the CT3 antibody to cross-link receptor complexes of all three types of TCR. In some experiments, the newly hatched chicks were injected with additional doses of the antibody and then thymectomized to prevent recovery from the sup-

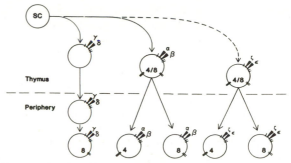

Figure 1. Model of T-cell development in the chicken featuring the sequential intrathymic development of three subpopulations of T cells, each of which expresses a different type of TCR.

pressive effects. The outcome of these experiments supports the model of separate sublineages of T cells outlined in Figure 1.

The suppressive effects of the embryonic TCR2 treatment were especially dramatic (Sowder et al. 1988b; Chen et al. 1989). The TCR2 antibody sharply curtailed growth of this thymocyte subpopulation beginning around the 15th day of incubation when TCR2 cells normally appear. The further development of immature TCR2 thymocytes was aborted by the treatment, and suppression of the TCR2 sublineage was rendered permanent by early thymectomy. The TCR2 antibody treatment had no negative effects on development of the TCR1 and TCR3 subpopulations. Instead, a compensatory increase from 15% to as high as 80% was seen in the proportion of peripheral T cells expressing TCR3 in the TCR2-suppressed birds (Chen et al. 1989; Cihak et al. 1989).

Embryonic treatment with the TCR1 antibody affected the TCR1 subpopulation only (Sowder et al. 1988b; Chen et al. 1989; Cihak et al. 1989). Although this treatment suppressed the expression of the TCR1/CD3 complex, growth of the thymocyte population was not discernibly affected. Seeding of the TCR1 cells to the periphery was inhibited, however, and removal of the thymus after TCR1 antibody treatment resulted in the virtual elimination of the TCR1 sublineage.

Development of T-cell Sublineages in Chick-Quail Chimeras

Chick-quail chimeras were used by Le Douarin (1978) to show that blood-borne stem cells periodically migrate into the thymus in response to chemoattractants produced by thymic epithelial cells. The first wave of precursor cells enters the chick thymus on embryonic days 6.5–8, the second on days 12–14, and the third on days 18–20 (Coltey et al. 1987). The pattern for quail thymus entry is similar but begins slightly earlier (Jotereau et al. 1982). In collaborative studies with Coltey and Le Douarin, we have examined the capacity of the different stem cell waves to give rise to the three sublines of T cells. This analysis was possible because the monoclonal antibody markers of chick T cells do not react with quail T cells. A useful exception to this rule is the CT1 MAb, which identified both chick and quail thymocytes (Chen et al. 1984).

The first important observation made in these studies was that all three sublines of T cells are derived from each precursor cell wave (Coltey et al. 1989; Bucy et al. 1989b). For example, the TCR1, TCR2, and TCR3 subpopulations were generated sequentially in the first wave of thymocyte development, the duration of which was approximately 3 weeks. The corticomedullary migration of thymocytes could be easily traced by the serial examination of chick thymic transplants (E9 donors) into quail embryo recipients (E3). In addition, a sequential seeding of the chick T-cell subpopulations to the peripheral lymphoid tissues of the quail recipients could be demonstrated. Interestingly, migration of chick T cells to the medullary region of the recipient's thymus was also observed. This recirculation pathway of T cells back to the thymus involves all of the mature T-cell phenotypes, but its physiological significance is not obvious.

In this series of experiments, in which the outcome of embryonic spleen, bursa, or intestinal transplants was compared with that of thymic transplants, the development of lymphocytes expressing the three types of TCR was found to occur exclusively within the thymic microenvironment. We were thus unable to confirm the idea that T cells can be generated outside the thymic microenvironment.

A Third Lymphocyte Lineage

While analyzing T-cell development in the chick, we observed an unusual population of CD3[+] cells in peripheral lymphoid tissues (Bucy et al. 1989b). These cells express a cytoplasmic CD3 determinant but have neither CD3 or TCR on their surface. Many of these cells express surface CD8 although none express CD4. For lack of a better name, we call the cytoplasmic CD3[+]/CD8[+]/TCR[−] lymphocyte the TCR0 cells. These cells constitute a numerically significant lymphocyte subpopulation in adult birds and have a restricted anatomical distribution. Approximately 30–40% of the CD3[+] cells in the intestinal epithelium display the TCR0 phenotype, whereas cells with this phenotype comprise 1% or less of the splenic CD3[+] cells.

The first cytoplasmic CD3[+]/surface CD8[+] cells appear in the spleen on embryonic day 8. In comparison, cytoplasmic CD3[+]/surface CD8[−] cells appear in the thymus on embryonic day 9, 2 to 3 days after entry of the precursor stem cells. The origin and fate of the TCR0 cells was examined by constructing interspecies chick-quail chimeras, again taking advantage of the fact that our monoclonal antibodies do not cross-react with homologous molecules on quail T cells. The key issue addressed in these experiments was the lineal relationship between the TCR0 cells and conventional T cells. Splenic transplants from 6- to 8-day-old embryos generated the cytoplasmic CD3[+]/surface CD8[+] cells, the numbers of which increased as a function of age; none

of these cells acquired surface CD3/TCR1, -TCR2, or -TCR3 complexes or surface immunoglobulin. The TCR0 cells of chick splenic origin migrated to the lymphoid tissues of the quail host (spleen, bursa, intestine, and thymus medulla), but they failed to undergo differentiation into T cells or B cells in any of these environments (Bucy et al. 1989b). We conclude that these cells represent an independent lymphocyte lineage. Our current working hypothesis is that the TCR0 cells represent a phylogenetically primitive lineage of cells that is conserved in higher vertebrates and that may serve an important role in body defense. In future experiments, it will be important to determine their relationship with previously described cells with natural killer activity.

CONCLUSIONS

It is interesting that the TCR1 subpopulation of T cells is highly conserved in birds and mammals. This is a relatively large subpopulation in the chicken, comprising 20–30% of the peripheral T-cell pool. Interesting features of the avian TCR1 cells include their (1) rapid maturation and transit through the thymus, (2) relatively high density of TCR1/CD3 expression, (3) relatively limited population expansion in both the thymus and periphery, (4) striking dependence on a prolonged period of thymic seeding, (5) CD8 expression in peripheral lymphoid tissues, and (6) distinctive homing pattern. These clues suggest that the TCR1 thymocyte subpopulation may not undergo the rigorous selection pressures that are so essential in shaping the TCR2 repertoire (Marrack and Kappler 1987). The acquisition of the CD8 accessory molecule by TCR1 cells on homing to the peripheral lymphoid tissues is consistent with the hypothesis of a special role in body defense that is triggered by antigen-presenting cells expressing the major histocompatibility complex class I or class II family of molecules.

The existence of a third type of TCR, which is generated relatively late in avian ontogeny, is an especially intriguing, unprecedented finding. This could be the first indication of a different evolutionary feature of T-cell development in birds, or it could lead to the discovery of a homologous TCR in mammals. The avian TCR3 cells are similar to the TCR2 cells in their developmental pattern of TCR/CD3 acquisition and their utilization of CD4 and CD8 accessory molecules. The TCR2 and TCR3 heterodimers could be related isotypes encoded by different loci, or they may reflect a different mode of TCR repertoire development as is the case of the generation of antibody diversity in birds (Weill and Reynaud et al. 1987). Information on the avian TCR genes is needed to resolve this issue.

The expression of CD3 antigens has been considered a reliable marker for T-lineage cells. However, our avian studies suggest the existence of a thymus- and bursa-independent lineage of lymphocytes that express a CD3-related antigen in the cytoplasm and CD8 on the cell surface. We hypothesize that these cells represent an evolutionarily ancient population of lymphocytes that persist because they serve an important role in body defense. Other investigators have postulated that the CD8 molecule, having both Ig-V and Ig-I sequence homologies could reflect the original antigen-recognition molecule (Davis and Bjorkman 1988). It is interesting to note that ablation of the thymus-dependent system of lymphocytes in *Xenopus* did not eliminate skin allograft rejection by cells capable of a relatively imprecise memory response (Nagata and Cohen 1983). More recently, a population of lymphocytes in humans with similar properties have been shown to express CD3ϵ RNA although they lack TCR/CD3 receptors (Ciccone et al. 1988). It will be interesting to explore the obvious implications of a primitive lymphocyte lineage that may use primordial antigen-receptor molecules for target-cell recognition. It is likely that this trail of exploration will ultimately merge with that of the amorphous natural killer cells.

ACKNOWLEDGMENTS

We gratefully acknowledge the collaboration of Drs. Josef Cihak and Uli Lösch in many of the studies cited here and the help of Ann Brookshire in preparing the manuscript. This work has been supported by grants CA-16673 and CA-13148, awarded by the National Institutes of Health. M.D.C. is a Howard Hughes Medical Institute investigator.

REFERENCES

Bucy, R.P., C.H. Chen, and M.D. Cooper. 1989a. Tissue localization and CD8 accessory molecule expression of T$\gamma\delta$ cells in humans. *J. Immunol.* **142:** 3045.

Bucy, R.P., C.H. Chen, J. Cihak, U. Lösch, and M.D. Cooper. 1988. Avian T cells expressing $\gamma\delta$ receptors localize in the splenic sinusoids and the intestinal epithelium. *J. Immunol.* **141:** 2200.

Bucy, R.P., M. Coltey, C.H. Chen, D. Char, N.M. Le Douarin, and M.D. Cooper. 1989b. Cytoplasmic CD3$^+$ lymphocytes (TCR0) develop as a thymus independent lineage in chick-quail chimeras. *Eur. J. Immunol.* **19:** 1449.

Chan, M.M., C.H. Chen, L.L. Ager, and M.D. Cooper. 1988. Identification of the avian homologues of mammalian CD4 and CD8 antigens. *J. Immunol.* **140:** 2133.

Char, D., C.H. Chen, R.P. Bucy, and M.D. Cooper. 1989. Identification of a third T cell receptor (TCR3) in the chicken with a monoclonal antibody. *Fed. Proc.* **3:** 1507.

Chen, C.H., T.C. Chanh, and M.D. Cooper. 1984. Chicken thymocyte-specific antigen identified by monoclonal antibodies: Ontogeny, tissue distribution and biochemical characterization. *Eur. J. Immunol.* **14:** 385.

Chen, C.H., L.L. Ager, G.L. Gartland, and M.D. Cooper. 1986. Identification of a T3/T cell receptor complex in chickens. *J. Exp. Med.* **164:** 375.

Chen, C.H., J. Cihak, U. Lösch, and M.D. Cooper. 1988. Differential expression of two T cell receptors, TCR1 and TCR2, on chicken lymphocytes. *Eur. J. Immunol.* **18:** 539.

Chen, C.H., J.T. Sowder, J.M. Lahti, J. Cihak, U. Lösch, and

M.D. Cooper. 1989. TCR3: A third T cell receptor in the chicken. *Proc. Natl. Acad. Sci.* **86:** 2351.

Ciccone, E., O. Viale, D. Pende, M. Malnati, R. Biassoni, G. Melioli, A. Moretta, E.O. Long, and L. Moretta. 1988. Specific lysis of allogeneic cells after activation of CD3$^-$ lymphocytes on mixed lymphocyte culture. *J. Exp. Med.* **168:** 2403.

Cihak, J., L. Ziegler-Heitbrock, C.H. Chen, M.D. Cooper, and U. Lösch. 1989. Expression of T cell antigen receptor molecules in the chicken. In *Abstracts of the 7th International Congress of Immunology, Berlin.* (In press.)

Cihak, J., H.W. Ziegler-Heitbrock, I. Schranner, M. Merkenschlajer, and U. Lösch. 1988. Characterization and functional properties of a novel monoclonal antibody which identifies a T cell receptor in chickens. *Eur. J. Immunol.* **18:** 533.

Coltey, M., F.V. Jotereau, and N.M. Le Douarin. 1987. Evidence for a cyclic renewal of lymphocyte precursor cells in the embryonic chick thymus. *Cell Differ.* **22:** 71.

Coltey, M., R.P. Bucy, C.H. Chen, J. Cihak, U. Lösch, D. Char, N.M. Le Douarin, and M.D. Cooper. 1989. Analysis of the first two waves of thymus homing stem cells and their T cell progeny in chick-quail chimeras. *J. Exp. Med.* **170:** 543.

Davis, M.M. and P.J. Bjorkman. 1988. T-cell receptor genes and T-cell recognition. *Nature* **334:** 395.

George, J.F. and M.D. Cooper. 1989. Quantitative analysis of the cell surface expression of $\gamma\delta$ TCR and $\alpha\beta$ TCR in the chicken. *Fed. Proc.* **3:** 1506.

Goodman, T. and L. Lefrancois. 1988. Expression of the γ-δ T-cell receptor on intestinal CD8$^+$ intraepithelial lymphocytes. *Nature* **333:** 855.

Jotereau, F.F. and N.M. Le Douarin. 1982. Demonstration of a cyclic renewal of the lymphocyte precursor cells in the quail thymus during embryonic and perinatal life. *J. Immunol.* **129:** 1869.

Koning, F., G. Stringl, W.M. Yokoyama, H. Yamada, W.L. Maloy, E. Tschachler, E.M. Shevach, and J.E. Coligan. 1987. Identification of a T3-associated gamma delta T cell receptor on Thy-1$^+$ dendritic epidermal cell lines. *Science* **236:** 834.

Kuziel, W.A., A. Takashima, M. Bonyhadi, P.R. Bergstresser, J.P. Allison, R.E. Tigelaar, and P.W. Tucker. 1987. Regulation of T cell receptor gamma-chain RNA expression in murine Thy-1$^+$ dendritic epidermal cells. *Nature* **328:** 263.

Lahti, J.M., C.H. Chen, J.T. Sowder, R.P. Bucy, and M.D. Cooper. 1988. Characterization of the avian T cell receptor. *Immunol. Res.* **7:** 303.

Le Douarin, N.M. 1978. Ontogeny of hematopoietic organs studied in avian embryo interspecific chimeras. *Cold Spring Harbor Conf. Cell Proliferation* **5:** 5.

Marrack, P. and J. Kappler. 1987. The T cell receptor. *Science* **238:** 1073.

Nagata, S. and N. Cohen. 1983. Specific *in vivo* and *in vitro* alloreactivities of adult frogs (*Xenopus laevis*) that were thymectomized during early larval life. *Eur. J. Immunol.* **13:** 541.

Sowder, J.R., C.H. Chen, L.L. Ager, M.M. Chan, and M.D. Cooper. 1988a. A large subpopulation of avian T cells express a homologue of the mammalian T$\gamma\delta$ receptor. *J. Exp. Med.* **167:** 315.

Sowder, J.T., C.H. Chen, J. Cihak, U. Lösch, and M.D. Cooper. 1988b. T cell ontogeny: Suppressive effects of embryonic treatment with monoclonal antibodies to T3, TCR1 or TCR2. *Fed. Proc.* **2:** 874.

Weill, J.C. and C.A. Reynaud. 1987. The chicken B cell compartment. *Science* **238:** 1094.

Developmental Analysis of the Mouse Hematolymphoid System

S. Heimfeld,*† C.J. Guidos,* B. Holzmann,*‡ M.H. Siegelman,* and I.L. Weissman*

*Department of Pathology, Stanford Medical Center, Stanford University, Stanford, California 94305;
†SyStemix, Palo Alto, California 94303; ‡Department of Molecular Biology, Max-Planck Institut für
Biochemie, 8033 Martinsried, West Germany

The development of lymphocytes and blood cells from hematopoietic precursors is one of the most remarkable and mysterious programs in developmental biology. The prime characteristics of this complex vertebrate system that make them accessible for experimental study are the known functional properties of the mature cell types, the identification of phenotypic markers expressed by these cells during several stages of their development, and most importantly, the ability to obtain these cells in suspension, mark them and separate out specific subsets, and place these fractions back in vivo to study their unique developmental and functional capacities. Here, we present studies on four aspects of mouse hematolymphoid development. The first aspect is the purification of mouse hematopoietic stem cells and the identification of a multipotent (nonstem cell) precursor population and several classes of lineage-restricted progenitors. The second is the differentiation sequence of thymic progenitors and the demonstration that loss of mature anti-self (minor lymphocyte-stimulating antigen) Mls-1^a-responding T cells apparently occurs not at the CD4$^+$8$^+$ (double-positive) stage, as proposed from results of transgenic experiments, but instead at a stage somewhere in between the double-positive thymic blast cell and the single-positive thymic mature cell. The third is the identification of the proteins and genes involved in homing to lymph nodes and the demonstration that these genes are unrelated to genes encoding the Peyer's patch (PP) homing receptor or to putative homing receptor genes/molecules previously identified in humans. The fourth is the characterization of novel molecules involved in Peyer's patch homing. Because the mouse system permits both in vitro and in vivo assays for homing, we propose the molecules identified below, if not sufficient, are at least critical for the homing behaviors of both normal and neoplastic lymphocytes.

In several cases, the answers we obtained differ markedly from the conclusions reached by other investigators in studies using in vitro methodologies, molecular techniques, or even transgenic mice. Although in vitro analyses have made many aspects of the understanding of lymphocyte and hematopoietic cell function accessible to reductionist science, developmental systems exist in vivo in microenvironments that have not yet been reproduced in vitro. Therefore, understanding the normal function of immune cells in allograft rejection, in inflammation, in autoimmunity, in tolerance, and in regulation of the immune response, awaits the development of better physiologically relevant technologies. To that point, we have presented elsewhere an in vivo methodology to study experimentally the development and function of the human hematolymphoid system, and we propose that future experiments based on mouse models, such as those presented here, may help elucidate the nature of human hematopoietic precursors, human thymic development, and human lymphocyte homing molecules, using SCID-hu mice (McCune et al. 1988; Namikawa et al. 1988).

Hematopoietic Progenitors

In adult vertebrates, the bone marrow is the primary site of hematopoiesis and contains the precursor cells that ultimately give rise to all the lymphoid and myeloerythroid lineages (Wu et al. 1967; Abramson et al. 1977). The earliest progenitors, termed stem cells, are defined by their capacity for extensive self-renewal and their potential to differentiate into multiple cell types. It is generally believed that these stem cells give rise to more restricted precursor cells, which in turn generate unipotent progenitors through an unknown series of differentiation steps (Till and McCulloch 1980; McCulloch 1983). There is a tremendous heterogeneity of cell types found in normal bone marrow, and the stem cells and progenitor cells are very rare within this tissue. Thus, understanding the mechanisms controlling stem-cell commitment and differentiation into the various mature cell types has proven difficult to study. In this section, we present data on the isolation of different progenitor cell populations, a characterization of their proliferative and developmental potential in vivo, and a discussion of the possible lineage relationships between them.

Using a panel of monoclonal antibodies that label specific antigens found on the surface of bone marrow cells (see Fig. 1), we have described previously several selected subsets that are highly enriched for hematopoietic precursor activity (Muller-Sieburg et al. 1986; Spangrude et al. 1988; S. Heimfeld et al., in prep.). Our experiments have indicated that most, if not all,

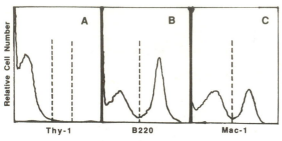

Figure 1. Staining of bone marrow and isolation of Thy-1[low] progenitor cells. Three-color stain of normal mouse bone marrow (BM). Indicated by the dotted lines are the intensities used to designate the 1% of cells that are Thy-1[low] (*A*), B220[+/−] (*B*), and Mac-1[+/−] (*C*). For Thy-1[low] enrichment and purification the methods used were modifications of that described previously (Spangrude et al. 1988). In brief, BM cells were obtained by flushing tibia and femora from mice with Hanks balanced salt solution (HBSS) supplemented with 2% fetal calf serum (FCS) and 10 mM HEPES buffer (pH 7.2). For Thy-1[low], Lineage[−], Sca-1[+/−] purification, the order of reagents was (1) directly fluoresceinated (FL) anti-CD3 plus unmodified anti-CD4, CD8, B220, Mac-1, and Gr-1 (lineage markers); (2) phycoerythrin (PE)-conjugated goat anti-rat plus anti-FL magnetic beads; (3) magnetic separation to deplete CD3[+] (Thy-1[high]) mature T cells; (4) normal rat immunoglobulin (Ig) for 5 min to block any remaining PE anti-rat sites, followed by the addition of FL anti-Thy-1 plus biotinylated (Bio) anti-Sca-1; (5) Texas Red (TX) avidin plus anti-FL beads; (6) magnetic separation to enrich for Thy-1[low] cells. All antibody and/or bead incubations were for 20 min at 4°C followed by a wash through a FCS cushion. After the final wash, cells were resuspended in HBSS containing propidium iodide for live/dead discrimination. For Thy-1[low], B220[+/−], Mac-2[+/−] isolations the above procedure was modified as follows: (1) FL-CD3 plus unmodified Mac-1; (2) TX anti-rat; (4) FL-Thy-1 plus Bio B220; (5) allophycocyanin avidin. Cell analysis and sorting was done on a dual laser FACStar Plus. Reanalysis of sorted fractions indicated ≥90% purity.

progenitor activity falls within the 1% of bone marrow that expresses a tenfold lower level of Thy-1 (Reif and Allen 1964) than that found on mature mouse T cells (Fig. 1A). These cells have been designated as the Thy-1 antigen (Thy[low]) fraction. Using additional markers, the Thy[low] cells have been further subdivided into

five different populations (Table 1). We have isolated very highly purified preparations of these Thy[low] fractions by utilizing a two-step immunomagnetic bead enrichment protocol followed by a six-parameter fluorescence-activated cell sorting (FACS) (see Fig. 1 legend). The resulting populations have been tested in a variety of experimental assay systems to determine their proliferative and differentiative capacities. These data have been summarized in Table 1.

The second column of Table 1 indicates the relative percentages of these different fractions in normal mouse bone marrow. All these Thy[low] populations are very rare, ranging from 1 in 150 for the Thy[low], B220 (B[+]), Mac-1 (M[−]) cells to 1 in 2000 for the Thy[low] lineage (Lin[−]), and stem cell antigen (Sca[+]) cells. It has been proposed that committed progenitor cells are more actively dividing, whereas the earliest precursors remain quiescent (Till 1976; McCulloch 1983). Cell-cycle analyses reveal that two of these fractions, Thy[low], B[+], M[−], and Thy[low], B[−], M[+] have a significantly higher proportion of cells in the S and G_2 phases than whole bone marrow does, suggesting that these populations may represent more committed or restricted stages of differentiation. In contrast, the Thy[low], Lin[−], Sca[+] subset, which we have shown to be the pluripotent stem cells (Spangrude et al. 1988), are not in division cycle.

Spleen colony formation following injection of selected cells into lethally irradiated recipients indicates a capacity for myeloerythroid differentiation (Wu et al. 1967). Furthermore, the time of appearance of the colonies has been correlated with different precursor activity, with those found at day 12 having more stem cell activity than those found on day 8. All the Thy[low] fractions show enrichment for colony-forming unit-spleen (CFU-S) activity (Table 1) with the significant exception of the Thy[low], B[+], M[−] cells. The Thy[low], B[−], M[+] and the Thy[low], Lin[−], Sca[+] cells give rise to more day 8 than day 12 colonies, implying these are more restricted precursors than the Thy[low], B[+], M[+] and the Thy[low], Lin[−], Sca[+] cells.

Table 1. Characteristics of Thy-1[low] Progenitor Cell Subsets

Cell type	BM (%)	Cell cycle[a]	CFU-S[b]	Day 12/day 8	CFU-T[c]	Reconstitution in vivo[d]		
						T-cells	B-cells	M-cells
Bone Marrow	100.0	20.3	+	1	+	+	+	+
Thy[low], B[+], M[−]	0.6	27.5	−	n.d.	−	−	++++	−
Thy[low], B[−], M[+]	0.4	25.3	+++	≤1	−	−	+/−	++++
Thy[low], B[+], M[+]	0.1	12.7	+++	>1	+++	++	+++	+++
Thy[low], L[−], S[−]	0.15	10.2	+++	<1	+/−	−	+/−	+++
Thy[low], L[−], S[+]	0.05	4.5	+++++	≥1	+++++	++++	+++++	+++++

Cell populations were isolated using immunomagnetic beads and FACS as described in Fig. 1 legend. n.d. indicates not determined. (B) B220; (M) Mac-1, (L) cocktail of lineage markers; (S) Sca-1.

[a]Cell cycle, reported as the proportion of the indicated cell population in $S + G_2$.

[b]CFU-S, given as the relative increase or decrease in the number of cells required to obtain a single spleen colony compared to whole bone marrow. The change in the ratio of late-forming day 12 to early day 8 CFU-S is also indicated.

[c]CFU-T were measured by direct intrathymic injection into irradiated congenic hosts. The data are shown as a relative enrichment or depletion for T-cell progenitors.

[d]Reconstitution ability was measured by i.v. injection of 10^3–10^4 sorted cells into lethally irradiated congenic animals along with 10^5 syngeneic bone marrow cells to insure survival. Repopulation was determined by two-color FACS analysis of peripheral blood, staining for donor-type versus individual lineage markers for B, T, and myeloid cells (Spangrude et al. 1988). The data are given as the relative percentage of donor cells found for each of the indicated lineages. See text for further explanations.

Significant enrichment for T-cell progenitors, as measured by direct intrathymic (IT) injection, was found in only two fractions of the bone marrow, the Thy^{low}, B$^+$, M$^+$ and the Thy^{low}, L$^-$, S$^+$ cells (Table 1). Similarly, in the in-vivo-reconstitution experiments, only these two fractions gave rise to detectable numbers of T cells in the peripheral blood. These fractions also repopulated the B and myeloid lineages, indicating these populations are multipotent. In contrast, the Thy^{low}, B$^+$, M$^-$ cells could repopulate only the B-cell compartment whereas the Thy^{low}, B$^-$, M$^+$ and the Thy^{low}, Lin$^-$, Sca$^-$ fractions gave rise only to myeloid cells, implying that these three populations contain only lineage-restricted progenitors. Each of these populations has been tested also for their ability to rescue mice from a lethal dose of irradiation, possibly a better test for true stem-cell activity. Only the Thy^{low}, Lin$^-$, Sca$^+$ cells show that capacity (Spangrude et al. 1988; and data not shown), suggesting that all the other Thy^{low} fractions have only a limited capacity for proliferation and self-renewal.

To summarize, we have identified several classes of pluripotent and restricted progenitor cells in normal mouse bone marrow. These results have been ordered into the lineage scheme shown in Figure 2. All of the precursor populations are characterized by low-level expression of Thy-1. The most primitive stem cells are negative for the cocktail of lineage-differentiation antigens but do have high levels of Sca-1 on their surface. It appears that one of the first steps in stem-cell commitment may result in the coexpression of several lineage markers, giving rise to Thy^{low}, B$^+$, M$^+$ cells. This Thy-1^{low}, B$^+$, M$^+$ subset, as a population, can give rise to at least three lineages (T, B, and myeloid). It should be noted that this does not mean that individual cells in this fraction are multipotent since the low-response frequencies observed make it still formally possible that Thy-1^{low}, B$^+$, M$^+$ are a heterogeneous population of lineage-restricted precursors (S. Heimfeld et al., in prep.). From this point, there is a selective loss of expression of one or more of the lineage markers, and this is correlated with commitment to a single lineage. For example, the Thy^{low}, B$^+$, M$^-$ cells are the earliest stage as yet described for committed pre-B cells, whereas Thy^{low}, B$^-$, M$^+$ and Thy^{low}, Lin$^-$, Sca$^-$ fractions represent very early steps in myeloid/erythroid differentiation. Given this pattern of coexpression of lineage markers, it seems likely that unipotent progenitor cells for other hematopoietic lineages such as T cells, erythroid, mast cells, and megakaryocytes

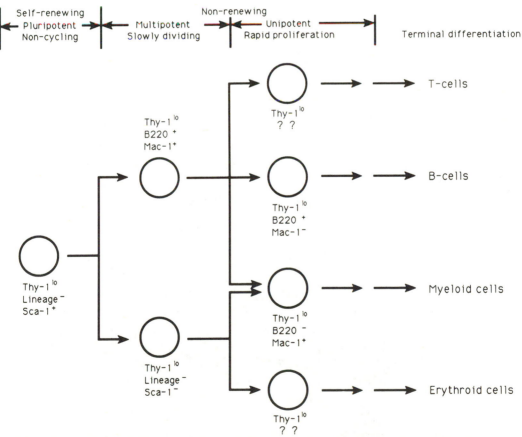

Figure 2. Proposed lineage relationships among the Thy-^{low} progenitor cells. The diagram indicates a progression from the earliest precursor compartment, the Thy-1^{low}, Lineage$^-$; Sca-1$^+$ stem cells (*left*), through the next stage(s) of Thy-1^{low}, B220$^+$, Mac-1$^+$ and/or Thy-1^{low}, Lineage$^-$, Sca-1$^-$ where self-renewal capacity is lost and some restrictions in developmental potential first become apparent, followed by further commitment to a single lineage and then terminal differentiation. See text for further explanations.

are also Thy^{low} and have other as yet uncharacterized differentiation antigens on their surface (Fig. 2).

Having identified all of these different classes of precursor cells, we shall in the future determine whether any of these antigenically defined stages are necessary intermediates in the developmental pathways to mature cell differentiation. We can measure specific responses to defined growth factors and how these change as cells differentiate. We can begin to approach the questions of homeostasis and hopefully learn what controls and governs stem-cell self-renewal, commitment, and differentiation. Finally, we can start applying this knowledge to the study of human cells, using the experimental in vivo system of the SCID-hu mouse (McCune et al. 1988; Namikawa et al. 1988).

Thymus Cell Maturation

Mature T lymphocytes possess clonally diverse heterodimeric T-cell receptors (TCR) specific for cell-surface complexes of foreign peptide antigens and self major histocompatibility complex (MHC) proteins. T cells comprising the mature pool (repertoire) in an individual animal are responsive to foreign antigen self-MHC complexes but are unresponsive or tolerant to self-antigen/self-MHC complexes. Mature T cells with these antigen-recognition properties are produced by positive and negative selective events during intrathymic maturation, both involving interactions between the antigen/MHC recognition complex (CD3/ TCR$\alpha\beta$, CD4, and CD8) on immature T cells and MHC proteins on sessile thymic stromal cells (for re-

view, see Schwartz 1989). Self-MHC-restricted antigen recognition is thought to result from positive selection, whereas self-tolerance can be explained, at least in part, by negative selection (clonal deletion) of autoreactive precursors. The major function of the thymus is to generate a large pool of T-cell precursors bearing distinct TCR clonotypes from which to select those with the appropriate specificities and functions for complete maturation and emigration to the periphery. The majority of thymocytes fail to survive this stringent selection process and die in situ.

Our studies have focused on establishing the developmental pathways by which T lymphocytes mature in order to understand how and at what maturational stage positive and negative events shape the mature T-cell repertoire. We first identified candidate precursor populations based on multiple phenotypic indices of immaturity, and then we assessed the developmental potential of each highly purified subset using the IT technique. To minimize perturbation of the thymic microenvironment and thus examine maturation under physiological conditions, host animals were not irradiated. Donor-derived thymocytes were immunomagnetically enriched and analyzed by three-color flow cytometry for CD3, CD4, and CD8 expression 1–5 days later. The results (Guidos et al. 1989) summarized in Figure 3, showed that the initial stages of T-cell maturation occur in the outer cortex in an apparently linear sequence from the earliest intrathymic progenitors (TCR$^-$/CD4$^-$8$^-$) via CD4$^-$8$^-$ intermediates to the CD4$^+$8$^+$ blast stage. The pathway becomes branched at this point, as demonstrated by the

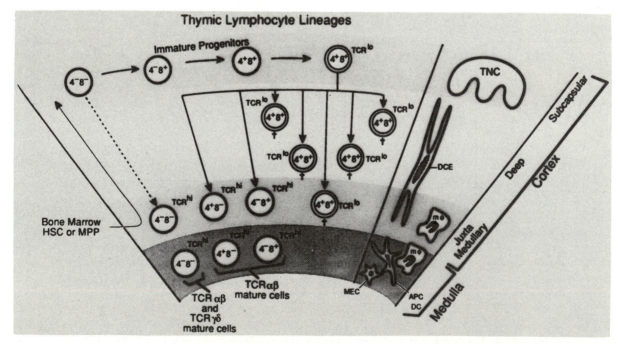

Figure 3. Intrathymic maturation sequence of murine T lymphocytes. Results are summarized from Guidos et al. (1989). Precursors in the subcapsular cortex are blast cells. (DC) Dendritic cell (bone-marrow-derived); (DEC) dendritic epithelial cell; (HSC) hematopoietic stem cell; (MEC) medullary epithelial cell; (MPP) multipotential progenitor cell; (Mf) macrophage; (TNC) thymic nurse cell. Crosses indicate cells destined for intrathymic death.

three types of progeny that develop from purified CD4$^+$8$^+$ blasts 4.5 days after IT injection into unirradiated hosts (Guidos et al. 1989). The majority (65–75%) are small CD4$^+$8$^+$ cells destined for intrathymic death, but 25–35% are CD4$^+$8$^-$ and CD4$^-$8$^+$ cells. The latter two types of progeny express high levels of the CD3/TCR complex (C.J. Guidos et al., in prep.), suggesting that they may be functionally mature. These results define a maturation sequence for both nonmature, small CD4$^+$8$^+$ thymocytes and mature CD4$^+$8$^-$ and CD4$^-$8$^+$ T cells, as well as providing the first direct evidence that TCR$^{-/low}$, CD4$^-$8$^+$, and CD4$^+$8$^+$ blast cells are sequential intermediate stages in the development of both mature subsets.

CD4$^+$8$^+$ thymocytes are reportedly the first maturational stage to express surface TCR$\alpha\beta$ (at low levels) during fetal ontogeny (Roehm et al. 1984), and approximately 50% of adult CD4$^+$8$^+$ thymocytes are TCR^{low} (Havran et al. 1987). Thus, they are potential targets of TCR-mediated selective processes during intrathymic maturation. However, only CD4$^+$8$^+$ blasts (10–15% of total CD4$^+$8$^+$ cells) contain precursors for mature T cells, and their TCR phenotype has not been examined. Because rearrangement and expression of the TCRα locus is thought to be the rate-limiting step for cell-surface expression of TCR$\alpha\beta$ during intrathymic maturation, we looked for TCRα transcripts in small numbers of FACS-purified CD4$^+$8$^+$ thymic blasts. Using the sensitive polymerase chain reaction (PCR), we detected TCRα (variable [V], joining [J], and constant [C]) transcripts in 250 cell equivalents of PCR-amplified material (C.J. Guidos et al., in prep.). Furthermore, a sensitive immunofluorescence staining technique confirmed that the majority of CD4$^+$8$^+$ blasts express very low levels of surface TCR, suggesting that they may be targets of intrathymic repertoire selection.

On the basis of studies of TCR$\alpha\beta$ transgenic mice and lethally irradiated bone marrow chimeras, several groups of investigators have suggested that CD4$^+$8$^+$ thymocytes are the targets of clonal deletion (Fowlkes et al. 1988; MacDonald et al. 1988). However, we have shown that in normal unirradiated mice, the only CD4$^+$8$^+$ thymocytes with precursor activity are the outer cortical blasts (Guidos et al. 1989), and much evidence suggests that the thymic stromal elements responsible for imprinting self-tolerance are bone-marrow-derived cells localized to the medulla and juxtamedullary cortex (for review, see Sprent et al. 1988). In trying to resolve this apparent paradox, we used monoclonal antibodies specific for particular V$_\beta$ regions (e.g., 3, 6, 7, 8.1, and 17a) that have defined recognition specificities (e.g., MHC I-E, Mls-1^a, and Mls-2^a) in an effort to define precisely the targets of clonal deletion in normal unirradiated mice. Clonal deletion of TCR^{low}/CD4$^+$8$^+$ thymocytes in nonpermissive hosts is reportedly evident or not evident, depending on whether the cells were cultured briefly prior to immunofluorescence staining and analysis (Kappler et al. 1987; White et al. 1989). To address this question more definitively, we focused our analysis on the precursor (blast) subset of CD4$^+$8$^+$ thymocytes. Figure 4A shows

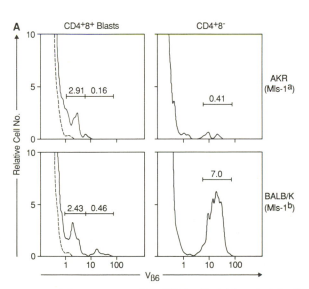
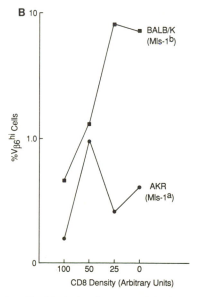

Figure 4. (*A*) Frequency of V$_\beta$6^{low}/CD4$^+$8$^+$ blasts in Mls-1^a and Mls-1^b mice. Freshly isolated young adult thymocytes were stained sequentially with 44-22-1 (anti-V$_\beta$6, solid lines) culture supernatant or R7D4 (isotype-matched control, broken lines), fluorescein isothiocyanate goat anti-rat Ig, 25% normal rat serum, APC-GK1.5 (anti-CD4) and biotin-53-6.7 (anti-CD8) avidin-TR. Fluorescence and scatter signals were computer-gated to display the V$_\beta$6 profile of CD4$^+$8$^+$ blasts and CD4$^+$8$^-$ thymocytes. (*B*) Frequency of V$_\beta$6^{high} cells during CD4$^+$8$^+$ blast to CD4$^+$8$^-$ transition in AKR and BALB.K mice. Cells were stained as for *A*. CD4$^+$ cells expressing an average of twofold or fourfold less CD8 than the peak CD8 fluorescence (100 arbitrary units) were analyzed for the frequency of V$_\beta$6^{high} cells. CD4$^+$8^{low} (25 arbitrary units) cells expressed an average of twofold more CD8 than the highest background level found on CD4$^+$ lymph node T cells.

that the frequency of $V_\beta 6^{low}/CD4^+8^+$ blasts is similar in AKR ($H-2^k$ and $Mls-1^a$) and BALB.K ($H-2^k$ and $Mls-1^b$) mice, whereas, consistent with previous results (MacDonald et al. 1988), the frequency of $V_\beta 6^{high}/CD4^+8^-$ thymocytes is more than tenfold lower in AKR mice. Similarly, there was no phenotypic evidence of clonal deletion in either $CD4^+8^+$ subset (small or blast) for $V_\beta 3$ and $V_\beta 7$ in the appropriate nonpermissive strains (C.J. Guidos et al., in prep.).

Despite the lack of evidence for physical deletion of autoreactive precursors at the $CD4^+8^+$ blast stage, these results did not exclude the possibility that negative signals received by $CD4^+8^+$ blasts result in clonal deletion at a later maturational stage. If this is the case, one would predict that transferring $CD4^+8^+$ blasts from a nonpermissive ($Mls-1^a$) to a permissive ($Mls-1^b$) thymic microenvironment would not rescue development of mature T cells bearing $V_\beta 6^+$ TCR. However, in preliminary experiments, IT injection of AKR $CD4^+8^+$ blasts into unirradiated B10.BR hosts completely rescued production of $V_\beta 6^+$ mature T cells (C.J. Guidos et al., in prep.). Thus, all of our results taken together suggest that the target of clonal deletion in normal unirradiated mice is a post-$CD4^+8^+$ maturational stage.

We have previously observed that $CD4^+8^-$ thymocytes develop from $CD4^+8^+$ blasts via $CD8^{med}$ and $CD8^{low}$ transitional stages (Guidos et al. 1989). The density of surface TCR/CD3 complexes increases concomitantly with the decrease in CD8 density, with the majority of cells not attaining a mature ($CD3^{high}$) phenotype until the latest transitional ($CD8^{low}$) stage (C.J. Guidos et al., in prep.). To define more precisely the maturational stages during which clonal deletion occurs, we determined the frequency of $V_\beta 6^{high}$ cells at each transitional stage in a permissive and nonpermissive strain. Surprisingly, the accumulation of $V_\beta 6^{high}$ cells showed a similar increase in both strains during the early phases of the transition (Fig. 4B). A major difference between the two strains only became evident

during the later ($CD8^{med}$ to $CD8^{low}$) transitional stages. We suggest the following interpretation of these observations. First, clonal deletion of autoreactive precursors occurs late during intrathymic maturation and only after commitment to CD4/8 phenotype (positive selection?). From a teleological perspective, deleting autoreactive cells only from those few (presumably self-MHC-restricted) that have been positively selected for complete maturation would seem to be the most efficient way to achieve a self-MHC-restricted, self-tolerant TCR repertoire. Second, precursors apparently become susceptible to negative signaling very soon after they become TCR^{high}. The fact that $CD4^+8^+$ thymocytes in $TCR\alpha\beta$ transgenic mice become TCR^{high} prematurely (L.J. Berg et al., in prep.) could potentially explain why $CD4^+8^+$ thymocytes appear to be targets of clonal deletion in TCR transgenic but not in normal mice.

In summary, we propose the following speculative but testable view of repertoire selection during intrathymic T-cell maturation in normal unirradiated mice (Fig. 5). Because positive selection is apparently determined by interactions between precursor cells and radioresistant cortical thymic epithelial cells (Sprent et al. 1988), $CD4^+8^+$ blasts represent likely (but not necessarily the only) targets of positive selection by virtue of their TCR^{low} phenotype and outer cortical location. It seems likely that subsequent cell fate (small $CD4^+8^+$ and death versus $CD4^+8^-$ or $CD4^-8^+$ and emigration to the periphery) is determined by the specificity of the expressed TCR (Teh et al. 1988). Positive selection can thus be viewed as TCR-mediated rescue from programmed cell death. Several groups have proposed that the localization (in non-TCR transgenic mice, at least) of positive and negative selection to the cortex and medulla, respectively, reflects differing functional capacities of cortical and medullary stromal cells. However, our results suggest that susceptibility to clonal deletion is an intrinsic property of the precursor cell that is dependent only on TCR density.

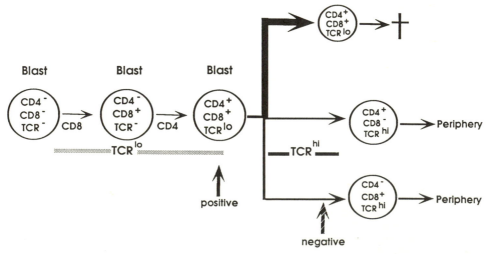

Figure 5. Speculative view of positive and negative selection during intrathymic T-cell maturation.

The current challenge is to devise in vitro systems to study these maturational events using purified thymocyte subsets of defined maturational stages and cloned thymic stromal cells. Such a system would be invaluable for investigating the molecular processes by which TCR-mediated signal transduction results in distinct cellular responses during different phases of intrathymic maturation.

Lymph Node Homing Receptor

Exit of continually recirculating lymphocytes from the vascular compartment is essential not only for delivery of effector cells to a particular inflammatory or otherwise affected site, but also for the proper development and maturation of lymphocytes and lymphoid organs. A fundamental event required for this development and appropriate progression of the immune response resides at the interface between a lymphocyte's mobile circulating phase and the surrounding tissue into which it exits. The specific portal of entry of lymphocytes from bloodstream into peripheral lymphoid organs was identified as specialized postcapillary venules bearing unusually high-walled endothelia (Gowans and Knight 1964; Marchesi and Gowans 1964), subsequently designated high endothelia venules (HEVs) (Stamper and Woodruff 1976). Migration of recirculating lymphocytes from bloodstream to particular sites has been called "homing," and the cell-surface structures mediating recognition and adherence to lymphoid organ HEVs have been called "homing receptors" (Gallatin et al. 1983). Lymphocyte homing appears to be regulated by the expression of complementary adhesion molecules on each of the two participants, the homing receptors on recirculating lymphocytes and the vascular "addresses" on specialized particular organ HEVs (Streeter et al. 1988).

In the mouse, monoclonal antibody MEL-14 (Gallatin et al. 1983), defines the peripheral lymph node homing receptor to be a 90–95-kD glycoprotein, $gp90^{MEL-14}$. The working model of the receptor complex is that of a core protein that is highly glycosylated and apparently conjugated to ubiquitin in isopeptide linkage (Siegelman et al. 1986; St. John et al. 1986). We recently cloned the cDNA encoding the core polypeptide of the mouse lymph node homing receptor, $mLHR_c$, which reveals a highly glycosylated transmembrane protein with an unusual protein mosaic architecture (Siegelman et al. 1989). It consists of four domains, an animal lectin domain, an epidermal-growth-factor (EGF)-like domain, and two precisely identical repeat units, conforming to the homologous repeat structures of complement regulatory protein (CRP) and other proteins.

In the human, a cell-surface molecule, $gp90^{Hermes}$, has also been identified that structurally and functionally had been thought to represent the human counterpart to $gp90^{MEL-14}$ (Jalkanen et al. 1988). However, molecular cloning has recently shown $gp90^{Hermes}$ to be equivalent to CD44, pgp-1, and the ECMIII receptor

(Goldstein et al. 1989; Idzerda et al. 1989; Stamenkovic et al. 1989) and different from the $mLHR_c$. In addition, earlier studies in the rat described molecular species involved in lymph node and PP homing quite disparate from those in mice or humans (Rasmussen et al. 1985; Chin et al. 1986). To help resolve these discrepancies and to address evolutionary issues posed by the unusual $mLHR_c$ composition, we initiated a search for human and rat homologs to $mLHR_c$. In these studies, we describe human (Siegelman and Weissman 1989) and initial rat clones homologous to $mLHR_c$, designated $hLHR_c$ and $rLHR_c$, and we provide primary sequence comparisons. The deduced protein sequences show complete preservation of the unusual protein domain arrangement of $mLHR_c$. The results suggest a structural similarity in the lymphocyte homing system in mice, humans, and rats, and the likelihood of functional homology as well.

The complete nucleotide sequence of apparent full-length cDNA for LHR_c in the mouse (Siegelman et al. 1989) and human (Siegelman and Weissman 1989) has been determined. An initiator ATG codon begins an uninterrupted open reading frame of about 1116 bp for both species. The assignment of the initiator ATG is supported by previous amino acid sequence analysis in the mouse (Siegelman et al. 1986) and by the presence of the flanking sequence falling within those typifying eukaryotic initiator sites in both humans and mice. The TGA stop codon at position 1169 in the mouse is followed by 327 bp of a 3' untranslated region, and the human has 1123 bp of a 3' untranslated region after a TAA stop codon. The deduced mature protein is 334 amino acids in length, with a calculated molecular mass of about 37 kD in mice and humans. Alignment in all three species is precise with identical numbers of amino acids and direct superimposibility of all three varieties of domains without any insertions or deletions required (Fig. 6). As in the mouse, the predicted extracytoplasmic sequence in humans and rats can be segmented into three abutting portions based on homologies with previously described proteins. The amino-terminal 118 amino acids are homologous to the animal lectin family of proteins (Fig. 6A). Positions 120–154 show the conserved cysteine pattern seen in epidermal growth factor (EGF) and other proteins (Fig. 6B), and the succeeding region consists of two 62-amino-acid homologous repeat units sharing the protein motif of CRP (Fig. 6C).

The presence of a lectin domain in $gp90^{MEL-14}$ is entirely consistent with studies that have demonstrated that mannose-6-phosphate and some analogs, but not other carbohydrates, inhibit binding to peripheral lymph node HEV but not to PP (for review, see Stoolman 1989). It is therefore important to note the strong similarity between mouse, rat, and human homing receptors in this domain (Fig. 6A). Human and mouse sequences show 86% identity over this entire region. The rat sequence shows even more marked conservation, having 93% identity with only a single difference in the carboxy-terminal half. In the EGF domain, the

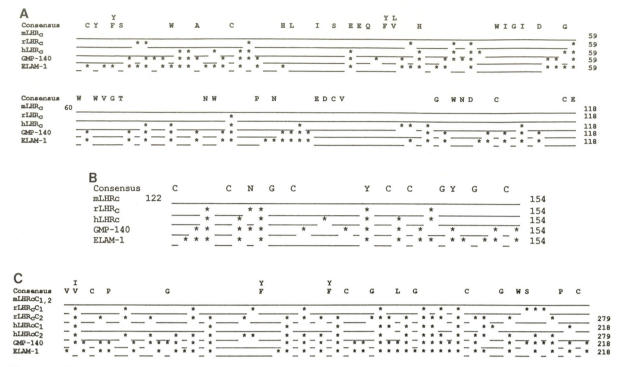

Figure 6. Comparison of recently characterized molecules with tridomain mosaic motif of LHR animal lectin domain (*A*), EGF-like domain (*B*), and CRP domains (*C*). The consensus line represents residues with a frequency of 50% or more in described sequences of each category. Mouse LHR is the index sequence in all three comparisons, differences are indicated by asterisks.

human and mouse sequences share 82% identity, whereas rats and mice are 85% similar.

The last extracytoplasmic domain of $mLHR_c$ consists of a precisely duplicated repeat unit preserving the consensus sequence found in homologous repeat structures of CPR and other proteins. Comparison of the $mLHR_c$ repeat unit with the consensus sequence for this repeat unit of factor H is included in Fig. 6C. The $hLHR_c$ and $rLHR_c$ also contains two repeat units, and yet these are homologous not identical. CRPs generally share the property of binding to C3b and C4b of the complement cascade (for review, see Reid et al. 1986), thereby dampening the cascade at key amplification junctures. It is attractive to consider that the CRP segment in LHRs also has a complement regulatory function that, teleologically, would seem an appropriate role for structures on lymphocytes recruited to and at inflammatory sites.

Both mouse and human cDNAs encode a protein with a hydrophobic leader sequence of 38 amino acids. There is 63% identity and 82% similarity when conserved substitutions are included. This signal sequence has a distinctive composition and is unusually long for a cell-surface protein. The degree of conservation suggests stringent structural constraints for the function of this leader. We have postulated that the unusual nature of the leader may reflect requirements for specific pathways of intracellular traffic for this highly posttranslationally modified receptor molecule, and conservation over this evolutionary distance supports this possibility.

The mature mouse LHR_c begins with a tryptophan by amino acid sequence analysis (Siegelman et al. 1986), and this was confirmed from the cDNA (Siegelman et al. 1989). This is a highly unusual amino-terminal amino acid. An NBRF protein database search revealed only eight sequences in which the initial residue was a tryptophan. Three of these are peptide hormones. Only one of the remaining is a eukaryotic sequence. However, tryptophan also starts the LHRs of the rat and the human, another instance of conservation. The functional significance of this residue is unclear although it should be noted that tryptophan is a destabilizing residue associated with rapid protein turnover according to the N-end rule (Bachmair et al. 1986), and there may be special requirements for rapid turnover and modulation of these molecules.

The mouse sequence possesses ten potential asparagine-linked glycosylation sites, consistent with our protein characterization studies showing extensive glycosylation on endoglycosidase F digestion (Siegelman et al. 1986) and subsequent tunicamycin experiments (M. van de Rijn et al., in prep.). There are eight potential N-linked glycosylation sites in the human and seven in the rat sequence. Both sites in the lectin domain and the single site in the EGF domain align. Therefore, in general, it appears that there is a relative conservation of potential glycosylation sites between mouse, rat, and human. The mature LHRs contain 22 cysteine residues, and their number and position are precisely preserved in all three species.

The putative transmembrane region (296–317) shows complete identity between mouse and human forms with the exception of a single conservative isoleucine/leucine interchange at position 313. The eight residues preceding and initial nine intracytoplasmic residues, following the hydrophobic transmembrane region are also completely conserved, resulting in a 39-amino-acid stretch of virtual identity between mice and humans, the longest region of identity between the molecules. Analysis so far in the rat shows complete identity within the transmembrane region.

The characteristic protein mosaic architecture consisting of an amino-terminal lectin domain, followed by an EGF-like region and a variable number of CRP homology repeats, distinguishes a novel class of cell-surface molecules. The high degree of structural conservation in both rat and human LHRs with a molecule known to confer specific lymphocyte homing activity in another species, the mouse, and the restricted lymphoid expression of the transcript in the human (Siegelman and Weissman 1989) in strict analogy with the mouse strongly suggest a cell-surface molecule, likely mediating similar function in rats and humans, which we provisionally designate rLHR$_c$ and hLHR$_c$. This assembly represents an apparent new family of adhesion molecules structurally unrelated to the immunoglobulin, integrin supergene, or CD44 families. With its unusual tridomain structure and with additional distinct transmembrane and cytoplasmic domains, it represents an ideal single-chain polypeptide with which to study protein structure-function relationships important in cell interactions and development.

PP Homing Receptor

The monoclonal antibody R1-2 was obtained by immunization with TK1 cells, which specifically bind to murine PP-HEV (Holzmann et al. 1989). R1-2 recognizes the α subunit of the $\alpha\beta$ heterodimer, LPAM-1, a member of the integrin family of adhesion molecules (Hynes 1987). When LPAM-1 is isolated by TK1 cells using R1-2, a β subunit can also be immunoprecipitated as long as Ca^{++} is present (Holzmann et al. 1989), suggesting the $\alpha\beta$ heterodimeric association is Ca^{++} dependent. Interestingly, lymphocyte adhesion to PP-HEV requires Ca^{++}, suggesting one of the roles of this ion is to maintain the structural integrity of the PP homing receptor.

When lysates from a panel of lymphoma cell lines were immunoprecipitated with R1-2, two different β chains could be distinguished by their apparent molecular weight (Table 2). Using specific polyvalent antisera, the two subunits were identified as β_1, normally found with the human VLA-4 integrins (Hemler et al. 1987), and a novel β_p integrin chain. Since the α chain appears identical, this suggests that there are two different integrin molecules involved in PP homing. LPAM-1 is distinct from other integrins, whereas LPAM-2 appears to be the murine homolog of the human integrin VLA-4 (Holzmann and Weissman 1989). The association of more than one β subunit with the same integrin α chain is a novel principle for generating structural and functional diversity within the integrin family of cell-adhesion molecules. So far, only receptors consisting of a common β subunit and distinct α chains have been reported (Hynes 1987).

R1-2 antibody was tested for specific inhibition of HEV-binding in vitro. Preincubation of normal lymphocytes with R1-2 strongly inhibited PP-HEV binding while not altering peripheral node adhesion. This inhibition was also seen for all lymphoma lines tested (Table 2). As shown in the last column of Table 2, these cell lines express either or both of the integrin adhesion molecules, LPAM-1 or -2, strongly suggesting that these integrins are specifically involved in the lymphocyte/PP-HEV interactions. To analyze this further, high- and low-LPAM-1-expressing variants were subcloned from TK1. As shown in Table 2, there was a

Table 2. Role of LPAM-1 and LPAM-2 Integrins in Lymphocyte Binding to PP-HEV

Cell type	HEV-binding[b]		Pretreatment with R1-2[c]		Receptor(s)[d] expressed
	PP	PLN	PP	PLN	
TK1 cl14[high] [a]	2.46	0.40	n.t.	n.t.	LPAM-1
TK1 cl14[low]	0.56	0.26	n.t.	n.t.	LPAM-1
MLN	1.0	1.0	0.15	1.07	LPAM-1/LPAM-2
TK1	1.56	0.09	0.06	0.14	LPAM-1
TK23	2.56	1.14	0.99	1.23	LPAM-1/LPAM-2
TK40	2.79	0.07	0.09	0.05	LPAM-1/LPAM-2
TK50	0.87	0.18	0.08	0.17	LPAM-2

[a]FACS-selected variants of the TK1 subclone TK1 cl14 that express high or low levels of LPAM-1.

[b]The in vitro HEV-binding assay has been described in detail previously (Holzmann et al. 1989). Lymphocyte binding to HEV in peripheral lymph nodes (PLN) or Peyer's patch (PP) is presented as relative adherence ratios (RAR). The binding of unlabelled mesenteric lymph node (MLN) lymphocytes defines a RAR of 1.0 (unity).

[c]Cells were incubated with saturating amounts of R1-2 or control antibody and washed to remove unbound antibody. The HEV-binding capacity of antibody-coated cells were determined in the in vitro HEV-binding assay and is presented as RAR.

[d]Lysates of surface-iodinated cells were immunoprecipitated with antibody R1-2. Bound heterodimeric receptors were eluted and dissociated. The β chains associated with α were identified using heteroantisera specific for integrins β_1 or β_p.

direct correlation between the level of LPAM-1 expression and HEV-binding capacity, indicating that the integrin LPAM-1 functions as a lymphocyte cell-surface receptor mediating the organ-specific adhesion to PP-HEV.

ACKNOWLEDGMENTS

This work was supported by U.S. Public Health Services grant AI-09022, National Institutes of Health award OIG-42551 (I.W.), and a grant from the Weingart Foundation. S.H. is a fellow of the Leukemia Society, C.G. is supported by the Medical Research Council of Canada and the Alberta Heritage Foundation for Medical Research, and M.S. is a Bristol-Myers Cancer Research Fellow.

REFERENCES

Abramson, S., R.G. Miller, and R.A. Phillips. 1977. The identification in adult bone marrow of pluripotent and restricted stem cells of the myeloid and lymphoid systems. *J. Exp. Med.* **145:** 1567.

Bachmair, R., D. Finley, and A. Varshavsky. 1986. In vivo half-life of a protein is a function of its amino-terminal residue. *Science* **234:** 179.

Chin, Y.H., R.A. Rasmussen, J.J. Woodruff, and T.G. Easton. 1986. A monoclonal anti-HEBF$_{PP}$ antibody with specificity for lymphocyte surface molecules mediating adhesion to Peyer's patch high endothelium of the rat. *J. Immunol.* **136:** 2556.

Fowlkes, B.J., R.H. Schwartz, and D.M. Pardoll. 1988. Deletion of self-reactive thymocytes occurs at a CD4[+]8[+] precursor stage. *Nature* **334:** 620.

Gallatin, W.M., I.L. Weissman, and E.C. Butcher. 1983. A cell surface molecule involved in organ-specific homing of lymphocytes. *Nature* **304:** 30.

Goldstein, L.A., D.F. Zhou, L.J. Picker, C.N. Minty, R. Bargatze, J.F. Ding, and E.C. Butcher. 1989. A human lymphocyte homing receptor, the hermes antigen, is related to cartilage proteoglycan core and link proteins. *Cell* **56:** 1063.

Gowans, J.L. and E.J. Knight. 1964. The route of recirculation of lymphocytes in the rat. *Philos. Trans. R. Soc. Lond.* B **159:** 257.

Guidos, C.J., B. Adkins, and I.L. Weissman. 1989. Intrathymic maturation of murine T lymphocytes from CD8[+] precursors. *Proc. Natl. Acad. Sci.* (in press).

Havran, W.L., M. Poenie, J. Kimura, R. Tsien, A. Weiss, and J. Allison. 1987. Expression and function of the CD3-antigen receptor on murine CD4[+]8[+] thymocytes. *Nature* **330:** 170.

Hemler, M.E., C. Huang, Y. Takada, L. Schwarz, J.L. Strominger, and M.L. Clabby. 1987. Characterization of the cell surface heterodimer VLA-4 and related peptides. *J. Biol. Chem.* **262:** 11478.

Holzmann, B. and I.L. Weissman. 1989. Peyer's patch-specific lymphocyte homing receptors consist of a VLA-4 like α chain associated with either of two integrin β chains, one of which is novel. *EMBO J.* **8:** 1735.

Holzmann, B., B.W. McIntyre, and I.L. Weissman. 1989. Identification of a murine Peyer's patch-specific lymphocyte homing receptor as an integrin molecule with an α chain homologous to human VLA-4. *Cell* **56:** 37.

Hynes, R.O. 1987. Integrins: A family of cell surface receptors. *Cell* **48:** 549.

Idzerda, R.J., W.G. Carter, C. Nottenburg, E.A. Wayner, W.M. Gallatin, and T. St. John. 1989. Isolation and DNA sequence of a cDNA clone encoding a lymphocyte adhesion receptor for high endothelium. *Proc. Natl. Acad. Sci.* **86:** 4659.

Jalkanen, S., M. Jalkanen, R. Bargatze, M. Tammi, and E.C. Butcher. 1988. Biochemical properties of glycoproteins involved in lymphocyte recognition of high endothelial venules in man. *J. Immunol.* **141:** 1615.

Kappler, J.W., N. Roehm, and P. Marrack. 1987. T cell tolerance by clonal elimination in the thymus. *Cell* **49:** 273.

MacDonald, H.R., H. Kengartner, and T. Pedrazzini. 1988. Intrathymic deletion of self-reactive cells prevented by neonatal anti-CD4 antibody treatment. *Nature* **335:** 174.

Marchesi, V.T. and J.L. Gowans. 1964. The migration of lymphocytes through the endothelium of venules in lymph nodes, an electron microscopic study. *Philos. Trans. R. Soc. Lond.* B **159:** 283.

McCulloch, E.A. 1983. Stem cells in normal and leukemic hemopoiesis. *Blood* **62:** 1.

McCune, J.M., R. Namikawa, H. Kaneshima, L.D. Schultz, M. Lieberman, and I.L. Weissman. 1988. The Scid-hu mouse: Murine model for the analysis of human hematolymphoid differentiation and function. *Science* **241:** 1632.

Muller-Sieburg, C.E., C.A. Whitlock, and I.L. Weissman. 1986. Isolation of two early B lymphocyte progenitors from mouse bone marrow: A committed pre-pre-B cell and a clonogenic Thy-1^{lo} hematopoietic stem cell. *Cell* **44:** 653.

Namikawa, R., H. Kaneshima, M. Lieberman, I.L. Weissman, and J.M. McCune. 1988. Infection of the Scid-hu mouse by HIV-1. *Science* **242:** 1684.

Rasmussen, R.A., Y.H. Chin, J.J. Woodruff, and T.G. Easton. 1985. Lymphocyte recognition of lymph node high endothelium. VII. Cell surface proteins involved in adhesion defined by monoclonal anti-HEBFLN (A.11) antibody. *J. Immunol.* **135:** 19.

Reid, K.B.M., D.R. Bentley, R.D. Campbell, L.P. Chung, R.B. Sim, T. Kristensen, and B.F. Tack. 1986. Complement system proteins which interact with C3b or C4b. *Immunol. Today* **7:** 230.

Reif, A.E. and J.M.V. Allen. 1964. The AKR thymic antigen and its distribution in leukemias and nervous tissues. *J. Exp. Med.* **120:** 413.

Roehm, N., L. Herron, J. Cambier, D. DiGuisto, K. Haskins, J. Kappler, and P. Marrack. 1984. The major histocompatibility complex-restricted antigen receptor on T-cells: Distribution on thymus and peripheral T-cells. *Cell* **38:** 577.

Schwartz, R.H. 1989. Acquisition of immunologic self-tolerance. *Cell* **57:** 1073.

Siegelman, M.H. and I.L. Weissman. 1989. Human cDNA encoding the homologue of the mouse lymph node homing receptor: Evolutionary conservation at tandem cell interaction domains. *Proc. Natl. Acad. Sci.* **86:** 5562.

Siegelman, M.H., M. van de Rijn, and I.L. Weissman. 1989. Mouse lymph node homing receptor cDNA clone encodes a glycoprotein revealing tandem interaction domains. *Science* **243:** 1165.

Siegelman, M., M.W. Bond, W.M. Gallatin, T. St. John, H.T. Smith, V.A. Fried, and I.L. Weissman. 1986. Cell surface molecule associated with lymphocyte homing is a ubiquitinated branched-chain glycoprotein. *Science* **231:** 823.

Spangrude, G.J., S. Heimfeld, and I.L. Weissman. 1988. Purification and characterization of mouse hematopoietic stem cells. *Science* **241:** 58.

Sprent, J., D. Lo, E. Gao, and Y. Ron. 1988. T cell selection in the thymus. *Immunol. Rev.* **101:** 173.

Stamenkovic, I., M. Amiot, J.M. Pesando, and B. Seed. 1989. A lymphocyte molecule implicated in lymph node homing is a member of the cartilage link protein family. *Cell* **56:** 1057.

Stamper, H.B., Jr., and J.J. Woodruff. 1976. Lymphocyte homing into lymph nodes: In vitro demonstration of the selective affinity of recirculating lymphocytes for high-endothelial venules. *J. Exp. Med.* **144:** 828.

St. John, T., W.M. Gallatin, M. Siegelman, H.T. Smith, V.A. Fried, and I.L. Weissman. 1986. Expression cloning of a lymphocyte homing receptor cDNA: Ubiquitin is the reactive species. *Science* **231:** 845.

Stoolman, L.M. 1989. Adhesion molecules controlling lymphocyte migration. *Cell* **56:** 907.

Streeter, P.R., E.L. Berg, B.T. Rouse, R.F. Bargatze, and E.C. Butcher. 1988. A tissue-specific endothelial cell molecule involved in lymphocyte homing. *Nature* **331:** 41.

Teh, H.S., P. Kisielow, B. Scott, H. Kishi, Y. Uematsu, H. Bluthmann, and H. von Boehmer. 1988. Thymic major histocompatibility complex antigens and the T-cell receptor determine the CD4/CD8 phenotype of T cells. *Nature* **335:** 229.

Till, J.E. 1976. Regulation of hematopoietic stem cells. In *Stem cells* (ed. A.B. Cairnie et al.), p. 143. Academic Press, New York.

Till, J.E. and E.A. McCulloch. 1980. Hemopoietic stem cell differentiation. *Biochim. Biophys. Acta* **605:** 431.

White, J., A. Herman, A.M. Pullen, R. Kubo, J.W. Kappler, and P. Marrack. 1989. The Vβ-specific superantigen staphylococcal enterotoxin B: Stimulation of mature T cells and clonal deletion in neonatal mice. *Cell* **56:** 27.

Wu, A.M., J.E. Till, L. Siminovitch, and E.A. McCulloch. 1967. Cytological evidence for a relationship between normal and hematopoietic colony-forming cells and cells of the lymphoid system. *J. Exp. Med.* **127:** 455.

Developmental Regulation of the TCR$\alpha\delta$ Locus

A. Winoto and D. Baltimore

Whitehead Institute for Biomedical Research, Cambridge, Massachusetts 02142; Department of Biology,
Massachusetts Institute of Technology, Cambridge, Massachusetts 02139

The T-cell antigen receptors (TCRs) are heterodimers composed of either $\alpha\beta$ or $\gamma\delta$ chains. The $\alpha\beta$ receptors are expressed mainly in T cells carrying either CD4 (mostly helpers) or CD8 (mostly cytotoxic cells) molecules, whereas the $\gamma\delta$ receptor molecules are expressed mainly in CD4$^-$ CD8$^-$ T cells as well as in some dendritic and epithelial T cells. The TCR$\alpha\beta$ from the cytotoxic T cells recognizes antigen in association with the major histocompatibility (MHC) class I molecules, and the $\alpha\beta$ receptor from the helper T cells recognizes antigen in association with the MHC class II molecules. The ligand(s) for the newly described TCR$\gamma\delta$ are still unknown although some mycobacteria-specific $\gamma\delta$ T cells have been isolated (Kronenberg et al. 1986; Toynoaga and Mak 1987; Davis and Bjorkman 1988; Holoshitz et al. 1989; Janis et al. 1989; O'Brien et al. 1989; Raulet 1989).

During thymus development, the CD4$^+$ CD8$^-$ and CD4$^-$ CD8$^+$ T cells expressing $\alpha\beta$ receptors arise from a class of CD4$^-$ CD8$^-$ T cells distinct from those that express the TCR$\gamma\delta$ (de Villartay et al. 1987, 1988; Berg et al. 1988; Winoto and Baltimore 1989a). The genes encoding the TCRα, -β, -γ, and -δ genes are each formed by joining together several gene segments. The TCRβ, -γ, and -δ genes are rearranged and expressed very early in T-cell ontogeny, by day 14 of the mouse gestation. The TCRα genes are not expressed until day 17 of gestation.

Because the α and δ genes are expressed in different cells, their intermingling in a single $\alpha\delta$ locus requires an intricate regulation of gene expression and gene rearrangement. The genomic organization of the TCR$\alpha\delta$ locus has the δ gene segments located within the α-chain gene segments. At one end of the locus, approximately 200 (variable) V_α and a few V_δ gene segments are interspersed (Satyanarayana et al. 1988). Hundreds of kilobases away is the (constant) C_δ gene segment with associated (diversity) D and (joined) J elements. Just 10 kb after C_δ, the mouse $\alpha\delta$ locus contains approximately 50 J_α gene segments spread across 60 kb of DNA (see Fig. 1). Despite their close physical proximity, the TCRα and -δ genes are expressed in different T-cell lineages and are activated at different stages of T-cell development, suggesting that distinct and strict developmentally controlled transcriptional elements should exist for these two genes. Studying the regulation of these two genes can thus provide insight into how genes are differentially regulated during T-cell development and how the individual properties of the $\alpha\beta$ and $\gamma\delta$ T-cell lineages are established.

Toward this end, we have identified a powerful and T-cell-specific enhancer for the TCRα chain located at the 3' end of the C region (Winoto and Baltimore 1989b). Moreover, the inability of the V_α promoter to be expressed at high level in the absence of an enhancer and the unique organization of the TCRα locus with J_α gene segment spread over 60 kb of DNA suggest that this newly identified enhancer must be able to act over vast chromosomal distances. Several T-cell-specific enhancer-binding proteins have been identified, and we show that both CEM and RS4.2 cell lines can serve as model systems to study the transcriptional activation of this α enhancer during T-cell differentiation (Winoto and Baltimore 1989b).

The α enhancer, however, is functional in both $\alpha\beta$ and $\gamma\delta$ T cells. What provides the cell specificity to the locus are transcriptional silencers that shut off the activity of the α enhancer in $\gamma\delta$ T cells but not in $\alpha\beta$ cells.

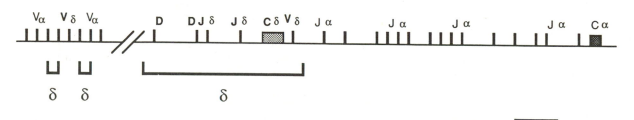

Figure 1. Schematic diagram of the TCR$\alpha\delta$ locus. Several hundred V_α gene segments and a few V_δ gene segments are located at an unknown distance from the D_δ gene segment. The TCRδ locus contains two D, two J, and one C gene segments. A V_δ gene segment is located at the 3' end of the C_δ gene segment. Approximately 50 J_α gene segments and one C_α gene segment are spread across 70 kb of DNA immediately downstream from the C_δ gene segment.

Furthermore, we also found that a V_α promoter in the presence of a heterologous enhancer is $\alpha\beta$-T-cell-specific, being expressed highly only in $\alpha\beta$ T cells. Because expression of TCR gene segments might control their rearrangement, these findings have implications for the regulation of both gene rearrangement and expression at the TCR$\alpha\delta$ locus.

EXPERIMENTAL PROCEDURES

Cell lines. EL4 and YAC-1 are mouse T-cell lines and Jurkat and H-9 are human T-cell lines expressing TCR$\alpha\beta$. The pre-T-cell lines CEM and RS4.2 (derivative of SL12.4 cell line) are of human and mouse origin, respectively, and only express the TCR β-chain transcript. The expression of α-chain mRNA in CEM and RS4.2 cells can be induced by addition of the chemical agent phorbol-12-myristate-13-acetate (PMA). Induction usually is performed for 20 hours at 50 ng/ml PMA. Peer and Molt13 are human T-cell lines expressing TCR$\gamma\delta$. BJAB and EW are human B-cell lines, whereas S194 is a mouse plasmacytoma of B-cell lineage.

Transient transfection and CAT assays. Transfections were done with equimolar amounts of DNA adjusted to the same weight with calf thymus DNA. Transfections were carried out using the diethylaminoethyl (DEAE)-dextran method as described previously (Lenardo et al. 1987) with minor modification in the length of incubation time with DNA for various cell lines: 30 minutes for Molt13 and Peer cells and 20 minutes for the other cell lines. After 48 hours, the cells were harvested, and the heat-treated (7 min at 60°C) cell extracts were assayed for their ability to convert [^{14}C]chloramphenicol to the acetylated form in a 1 hour incubation period (except for cell extracts from Molt13 and Peer where a 2 hr incubation period was used). The resulting samples were analyzed using a thin-layer chromatography (TLC) plate to separate the acetylated form from the unacetylated form of chloramphenicol (Lenardo et al. 1987).

Plasmids. J21 is a plasmid containing the chloramphenicol acetyltransferase (CAT) gene under the c-*fos* minimal promoter (−71–109). DNA fragments assayed for enhancer activity were cloned into polylinker sequences (*Xho*I, *Eco*RV, *Bgl*II, and *Cla*I) and placed 2.5 kb downstream from the c-*fos* promoter. pTCR1700 is a plasmid containing the V_α11.1 promoter (−1700 to +70) expressing the CAT gene. A Moloney long terminal repeat (LTR) enhancer was placed at polylinker sequences in pTCR1700, 2.5 kb away from the start of the CAT gene. The Moloney enhancer was a *Cal*I/*Xba*I fragment containing the 72-bp repeat of the Moloney LTR without the promoter. The *Cla*I site of the Moloney enhancer was converted to *Sal*I, and the *Sal*I/*Xba*I fragment was cloned into a pUC13-based vector. To make the final pTCR1700MoEn construct, the Moloney enhancer was excised using *Sal*I/

*Sma*I enzymes and cloned into *Xho*I/*Eco*RV sites of the pTCR1700 plasmid.

RESULTS

A Powerful TCRα Enhancer Is Located at the 3' End of the C_α Gene Segment

A powerful TCRα enhancer has been identified using a transient transfection assay (Winoto and Baltimore 1989b). Various restriction fragments around the mouse C_α gene were placed in a plasmid vector (J21) containing the CAT gene driven by a minimal heterologous promoter (−71 to +109 of the c-*fos* promoter). The J21 plasmid showed a small background of CAT activity when transfected into various lymphoid cell lines. Insertion of various restriction fragments around the first J-C_α intron and the C_α region into J21 did not give any stimulation of CAT activity in several T-cell lines (EL4, YAC-1, Jurkat, and H9). Fragments containing sequence 3' of the C_α gene, however, gave a large stimulation of CAT activity. This enhancer activity was localized to a 230-bp *Pvu*II/*Bgl*II fragment, 3 kb 3' of the C_α gene segment. It is a powerful enhancer as judged by the five- to tenfold higher activity of this α enhancer compared with that of the TCRβ-chain enhancer (Winoto and Baltimore 1989b). The enhancer placed 2.5 kb away from the promoter is also five- to tenfold more active than the SV40 enhancer placed just upstream of the SV40 early promoter (pSV2CAT). Finally, the activity of the minimal enhancer fragment is T-cell-specific since it is expressed in all the T-cell lines tested (EL4, YAC-1, Jurkat, H-9, Peer, and Molt13) but not in cell lines of the B-cell lineage (BJAB and S194) or the nonlymphoid lineage (Winoto and Baltimore 1989b; A. Winoto, unpubl.).

Several T-cell-specific DNA-binding Proteins Are Crucial for the α-Enhancer Activity

To study the α enhancer in detail, the minimal 0.23-kb *Pvu*II/*Bgl*II-enhancer fragment was sequenced (Fig. 2). No homologies with recognizable AP1-AP4-, Sp1-, Oct-1- (Oct-2), and NF-κB-binding sites or the core polyoma/SV40-enhancer sequences were evident. To identify the DNA-binding proteins responsible for the enhancer activity, footprinting analysis of the enhancer was carried out. Four protected DNA regions in the α enhancer were identified in the heparin fractions of the mouse T-cell nuclear extracts EL4 and RLM11 (NFα1, -2, -3, -4). An additional nuclear factor (NFα5) was readily identified in the nuclear extracts of human T-cell lines Jurkat, Molt13, and CEM (Figs. 2 and 3). Both NFα1 and NFα2 nuclear proteins are not T-cell-specific because they are present in HeLa cell extracts and 40E4 pre-B-cell extracts (Winoto and Baltimore 1989b; A. Winoto, unpubl.). In contrast, NFα3, NFα4, and NFα5 proteins are found only in the nuclear extracts from cells of the T-cell lineage and not in

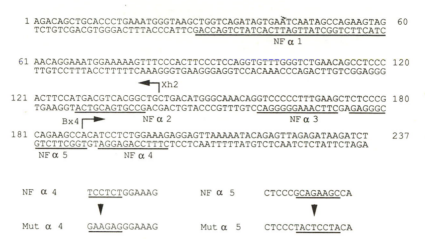

```
  1 AGACAGCTGCACCCTGAAATGGGTAAGCTGGTCAGATAGTGAATCAATAGCCAGAAGTAG  60
    TCTGTCGACGTGGGACTTTACCCATTCGACCAGTCTATCACTTAGTTATCGGTCTTCATC
                                    NFα1

 61 AACAGGAAATGGAAAAAGTTTCCCACTTCCCTCCAGGTGTTTGGGTCTGAACAGCCTCCC 120
    TTGTCCTTTACCTTTTTCAAAGGGTGAAGGGAGGTCCACAAACCCAGACTTGTCGGAGGG
                                          Xh2
121 ACTTCCATGACGTCACGGCTGCTGACATGGGCAAACAGGTCCCCCTTTGAAGCTCTCCCG 180
    TGAAGGTACTGCAGTGCCGACGACTGTACCCGTTTGTCCAGGGGGAAACTTCGAGAGGGC
        Bx4            NFα2                     NFα3
181 CAGAAGCCACATCCTCTGGAAAGAGGAGTTAAAAATACAGAGTTAGAGATAAGATCT 237
    GTCTTCGGTGTAGGAGACCTTTCTCCTCAATTTTTATGTCTCAATCTCTATTCTAGA
    NFα5            NFα4
```

```
NFα4    TCCTCTGGAAAG          NFα5    CTCCCGCAGAAGCCA
            ▼                            ▼
Mutα4   GAAGAGGGAAAG          Mutα5   CTCCCTACTCCTACA
```

Figure 2. DNA sequences of the *Pvu*II/*Bgl*II fragment containing the TCRα enhancer. Sequences protected by nuclear proteins are underlined. At least five proteins (NFα1–5) bind to this region. Correlation between protein-binding sites and enhancer activity was investigated using deletional and mutational analyses. The extents of the two deletion constructs Xh2 and Bx4 are indicated by arrows. Nucleotide changes for mutagenesis of the NFα4 and NFα5 protein binding sites are shown.

the extracts of several non-T cells (see Fig. 3, BJAB, EW, and HeLa).

To correlate the protein-binding sites with enhancer activity, deletion and site-specific mutagenesis analyses were carried out. The enzyme Bal 31 was used to delete progressively the α-chain enhancer from the 5′ and 3′ sides. The resulting fragments were tested for enhancer activity in the J21 plasmid. The relevant deletion points of the mutants are shown in Figure 2, and the resulting CAT activities are listed in Table 1. The Bx4 deletion from the 3′ end, deleting the NFα4-binding site, reduced the enhancer activity to almost background level. Deletion from the 5′ end indicated that the NFα1-binding site contributed only a small amount of

the enhancer activity (data not shown). Further deletion, eliminating both the NFα1- and the NFα2-binding sites (deletion point Xh2), however, has a dramatic effect on the ability of the DNA fragment to mediate enhancer activity. Finally, site-specific mutagenesis was carried out for the protein-binding sites NFα4 and NFα5 as indicated in Figure 2. Mutations at each individual site nearly abolished the α-enhancer activity (Table 1), indicating that both NFα4- and NFα5-binding sites play crucial roles in mediating the powerful T-cell-specific α-enhancer activity.

CEM Cells as a Model for TCRα Development

To obtain a model system for studying transcription activation of TCR genes during T-cell differentiation, we analyzed the ability of several pre-T-cell lines to activate the α enhancer. We chose two pre-T-cell lines, CEM and RS4.2, because both of them lack the TCRα mRNA. Expression of the TCRα chain in these two cell lines can be induced by the addition of PMA, which mimics part of the signal for T-cell activation (Schackelford et al. 1987; Wilkinson and MacLeod 1988). CAT constructs (J21-0.5BgX and J21-0.2BgPv) containing the minimal α-enhancer sequences were transfected into the CEM and RS4.2 cells, and half the cells were treated with PMA for 24 hours. CAT activities were measured 48 hours after transfection. Both constructs gave very little CAT activity without PMA. Treatment with PMA induced the CAT activity severalfold for each construct in both cell lines (Table 1 and data not shown). Similar treatment with PMA did not have any effect on the activity of the α enhancer in B-cell lines (which is undetectable) and in mature T cells (A. Winoto, unpubl.). We conclude that both CEM and RS4.2 cells can serve as models for T-cell activation of the TCRα enhancer during T-cell development.

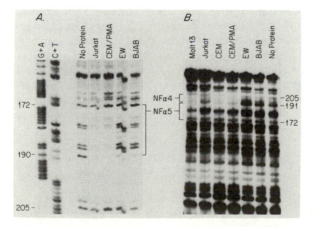

Figure 3. Footprinting analysis of the TCRα enhancer. DNase I footprinting experiments were done using nuclear extracts from the cell lines indicated. The footprints were done on both strands of the *Bgl*II/*Pvu*II enhancer fragment (Fig. 3A,B). Numbers correspond to the numbering of the α enhancer as in Fig. 2.

Table 1. CAT Activities for Various TCRα-chain Enhancer Constructs in
Pre-T-cell Lines CEM and Mature T-cell Lines YAC-1 and Jurkat

Cell lines	Constructs	Chloramphenicol acetylated (%)
YAC-1	J21	0.4
	J21-0.5BgX	31.5
	Bx4	1.3
	Xh2	1.9
Jurkat	J21	1.5
	J21-0.5BgX	90.3
	mutα4	3.2
	mutα5	1.9
CEM	J21	0.3
	J21 (+PMA)	0.3
	J21-0.5BgX	3.1
	J21-0.5BgX (+PMA)	55.6

The J21-0.5BgX construct contains a 0.5-kb *Bgl*II/*Xho*I fragment of the TCRα
enhancer inserted at 2.5 kb downstream from the J21 c-*fos* promoter. The Bx4
and Xh2 deletions are shown in Fig. 2 and described in its legend. mutα4 and
mutα5 are J21-0.5BgX plasmids with changes in the NFα4 and NFα5-binding
sites, respectively, as indicated in Fig. 2.

A Promoter Region from a Vα Gene Segment Is T-cell-specific

To characterize the promoter region of the TCRα
chain, we have isolated genomic clones containing the
Vα11.1 promoter region (Winoto et al. 1986). Vα11.1 is
a variable gene segment used predominantly in the
T-cell response to cytochrome-*c* and MHC class II
molecule I-E. This gene segment has not been found to
be used in γδ T cells although a related Vα11 gene
family, presumably with a different promoter, is used in
some γδ T cells (Bluestone et al. 1988). We placed the
Vα11.1 promoter region in a CAT-based vector and
used it to transfect several T-cell lines. No CAT activity
could be detected in all the cell lines tested, even when
the promoter region was extended to −5000 and CAT
assays were done for a long time (8-hr incubation, A.
Winoto, unpubl.). However, CAT activities from the
Vα11.1 promoter could be detected when a fragment
containing an enhancer element was added to the constructs (see Fig. 4, Moloney LTR enhancer or the
TCRα enhancer). The inability of the Vα promoter to
direct a high level of transcription in the absence of an
enhancer supports the notion that the TCRα enhancer
is required for TCR expression and must be able to act
over a long distance. A Vα gene segment rearranged to
the most distal Jα gene segment would place the promoter at least 69 kb away from the TCRα enhancer.

The Vα11.1 promoter in the presence of the Moloney
enhancer is αβ-T-cell specific. Transient transfection
experiments of the Vα11.1 promoter/CAT construct
with the Moloney enhancer (pTCR1700MoEn) gave
CAT activities only in αβ T cells (Jurkat, EL4, and
YAC-1) but not in several γδ T cells tested (Molt13 and
Peer) nor in cell lines from the B-cell lineage (BJAB
and S194) (Fig. 4). As a control, a plasmid containing
the minimal c-*fos* promoter driving the CAT gene in
the presence of the Moloney enhancer was highly expressed in all cell lines tested (Jurkat, EL4, YAC-1,
Molt13, Peer, BJAB, and S194). We conclude that the
Vα11.1 gene segment promoter contains transcription
elements that confer αβ-T-cell lineage specificity in the
presence of the Moloney enhancer.

γδ-T-cell-specific Silencers in the TCRα Locus

The ability of the TCRα enhancer to activate gene
transcription over large distances poses an interesting
regulatory problem for the TCRδ gene, which is located only 10 kb 5′ of the most 5′ Jα gene segment.
TCRδ gene rearrangement and transcription start very
early during T-cell development, and it is likely it will
have its own transcriptional control elements. Furthermore, if transcription activation explains the targeting
of the gene segment to the recombination machinery

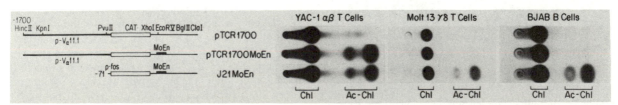

Figure 4. Promoter specificity of the Vα11.1 gene segment. Constructs containing 1.7 kb of the Vα11.1 promoter in the absence
(pTCR1700) or presence (pTCR1700MoEn) of the Moloney LTR enhancer were transfected into different T- and B-cell lines to
assess its transcription specificity. A minimal c-*fos* promoter (−71 to +109) with the CAT gene and Moloney enhancer was used
as a positive control. (Chl) Unacetylated [^14C]chloramphenicol; (Ac-Chl) acetylated [^14C]chloramphenicol.

(Alt et al. 1987; Schlissel and Baltimore 1989), the TCRα enhancer should be inactive in γδ cells.

To determine whether or not γδ T cells are able to activate the α enhancer, we transfected the minimal TCRα enhancer in the J21 plasmid into two γδ-T-cell lines (Peer and Molt13). CAT activity was measured 48 hours later. A dramatic enhancing activity was found for the minimal 0.23-kb α-enhancer fragment (J21-0.2 BgPv), which was comparable to the activity in αβ-T-cell lines (A. Winoto and D. Baltimore, in prep.). Furthermore, DNase I footprinting analysis of the TCRα-enhancer fragment revealed no differences between nuclear extracts of the γδ- or αβ-T-cell origin (Fig. 3). These results suggest that a minimal TCRα enhancer fragment is fully active in γδ T cells.

Remarkably, we found that regions around the minimal 0.23-kb enhancer in the chromosome were able to silence the α enhancer in γδ T cells. This was first indicated when a 7-kb BglII fragment containing the α enhancer in either orientation (J21-C_αBg) was placed in the J21 vector; it showed no enhancing activity in either Peer or Molt13 cell lines. The same constructs gave enormous enhancer activities in all of the αβ-T-cell lines tested (Jurkat, EL4, and YAC-1) with no differences in activities between the J21-C_αBg construct and the J21-0.2BgPv construct containing the minimal α enhancer fragment (A. Winoto and D. Baltimore, in prep.). The presence of negative transcriptional elements in the TCRα locus was confirmed using different combinations of restriction fragments around the C_α locus. Two such elements, one next to the TCRα enhancer (silencer [sil I]) and the other 3' of the C_α region (sil II), were identified and analyzed. Both sil I and sil II were able to turn down the activity of the TCRα enhancer as well as a heterologous enhancer in an orientation- and distance-independent manner (Fig. 5) (A. Winoto and D. Baltimore, in prep.).

DISCUSSION

Using libraries made from the thymus circle DNA, we have shown previously that the αβ and γδ T cells are distinct lineage (Winoto and Baltimore 1989a). Our studies of TCRα gene regulation revealed several transcriptional differences between these two lineages. Two strategies are employed by the TCRα gene to achieve αβ-T-cell lineage-specific expression. First, the V_α11.1 promoter uses positive transcription factors that are presumably αβ-T-cell-specific. Second, the TCRα enhancer is intrinsically T-cell-specific but is further limited to αβ but not to γδ T cells by the action of several silencer elements that work in γδ but not in αβ T cells. The differences in gene expression in αβ versus γδ T cells cannot wholly explain the differences between the cell lineages because TCR genes must be rearranged before they can make functional products. Recent evidence, however, suggests that a key determinant of what rearrangements occur is which germ-line gene segments are being transcribed (Yancopoulos and Alt 1985; Alt et al. 1987; Schlissel and Baltimore 1989). Thus, the transcription control inherent in the promoter/enhancer/silencer system described here could explain both how given gene segments are rearranged and how they are expressed. The functional α silencer in γδ T cells could prevent J_α gene segments from being targets of rearrangement, whereas an as-yet-to-be-located δ enhancer could allow δ gene segments to rearrange in such cells.

How V_α and V_δ gene segments are selected for rearrangement is less clear, especially when they are interspersed along the chromosome. Our studies showing that a V_α promoter is transcriptionally αβ-lineage-specific, however, offers an attractive hypothesis as to how this selective V gene rearrangement can be achieved. As in immunoglobulin genes, the accessibility of a V gene segment to the recombination machinery might be mediated through the existence of a V gene germ-line transcript (Yancopoulos and Alt 1985). Because of the lineage-specific V gene segment promoter, a putative V_α germ-line transcript might only be expressed in αβ but not γδ T cells. This could then result in differential usage of V gene segments in αβ and γδ T-cell subpopulations. Analysis of the transcriptional specificity of more V_α and V_δ promoters, as well as evidence for the existence of V_α/V_δ germ-line transcripts could provide a test for this hypothesis.

In conclusion, studies of the transcriptional regulation of the TCRαβ locus have given insight into how lineage-specific gene expression and gene rearrangement are regulated during T-cell development. Sequences from the TCRα enhancer and promoter provide positive cis-acting elements to mediate specific

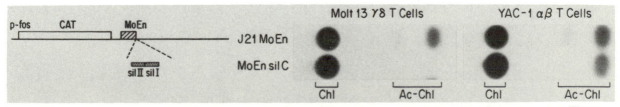

Figure 5. sil I and sil II can decrease the activation of the Moloney enhancer in γδ T cells but not in αβ T cells. A 400-bp fragment containing the sil I sequences and a 350-bp fragment containing the sil II sequences were inserted next to the Moloney enhancer in a CAT construct driven by the −71 c-fos promoter. Both constructs containing Moloney enhancer in the absence (J21-MoEn) or presence (MoEnsilC) of silencer sequences were transfected into Molt13 and YAC-1 T-cell lines using the DEAE-dextran method. CAT activities were assayed 48 hr later. The acetylated (Ac-Chl) and unacetylated (Chl) form of [^{14}C]chloramphenicol were separated on a TLC plate.

transcription activation during the transition from pre-T to the mature $\alpha\beta$ T-cell stage. In addition, lineage-specific *cis*-acting negative elements guarantee that TCRα gene expression will be limited to $\alpha\beta$ but not to $\gamma\delta$ T-cell lineages. The combination of positive and negative transcription elements in the TCR$\alpha\beta$ locus may then lead to selective gene expression and possibly to gene rearrangement in specific T-cell subsets.

ACKNOWLEDGMENTS

We thank Dr. S. Smale for the gift of many of the nuclear extracts used in these experiments, Drs. M. Lenardo and M. Schlissel for the critical reading of this manuscript, and Drs. C. MacLeod and H. Minowada for the gift of some of the cell lines. A.W. was supported by a fellowship from the Jane Coffin Childs Memorial Fund for Medical Research. This work was funded by the National Institutes of Health.

REFERENCES

Alt, F., T. Blackwell, and G. Yancopoulos. 1987. Development of the primary antibody repertoire. *Science* **238:** 1079.

Berg, L.J., B.F. de St. Groth, F. Ivars, C.C. Goodnow, S. Gilfillan, H.J. Garchon, and M.M. Davis. 1988. Expression of T cell receptor α chain genes in transgenic mice. *Mol. Cell. Biol.* **8:** 5459.

Bluestone, J.A., P.Q. Cron, M. Cotterman, B.A. Houlder, and L.A. Matis. 1988. Structure and specificity of T cell receptor γ/δ on major histocompatibility complex antigen specific CD3$^+$, CD4$^-$, CD8$^-$ T lymphocytes. *J. Exp. Med.* **168:** 1899.

Davis, M.M. and P.J. Bjorkman. 1988. T cell antigen receptor genes and T cell recognition. *Nature* **334:** 395.

de Villartay, J.-P., R.D. Hockett, D. Coran, S. Korsmeyer, and D. Cohen. 1988. Deletion of the human T cell receptor δ gene by a site-specific recombination. *Nature* **335:** 170.

de Villartay, J.-P., D. Lewis, R. Hockett, T.A. Waldmann, S.J. Korsmeyer, and D. Cohen. 1987. Deletional rearrangement in the human T-cell receptor α chain locus. *Proc. Natl. Acad. Sci.* **84:** 8608.

Holoshitz, J., F. Koning, J.E. Coligan, J. DeBruyn, and S. Strober. 1989. Isolation of CD4$^-$ CD8$^-$ mycobacteria-reactive T lymphocyte clones from rheumatoid arthritis synovial fluid. *Nature* **339:** 226.

Janis, E.M., S.H.E. Kaufman, R.H. Schwartz, and D.M. Pardoll. 1989. Activation of $\gamma\delta$ T cells in the primary immune response to Mycobacterium tuberculosis. *Science* **244:** 713.

Kronenberg, M., G. Siu, L.E. Hood, and N. Shastri. 1986. The molecular genetics of the T-cell antigen receptor and T-cell antigen recognition. *Annu. Rev. Immunol.* **4:** 529.

Lenardo, M., J.W. Pierce, and D. Baltimore. 1987. Protein binding site in Ig gene enhancer determine transcriptional activity and inducibility. *Science* **236:** 1573.

O'Brien, R.L., M.P. Happ, A. Dalla, E. Palmer, R. Kubo, and W.K. Born. 1989. Stimulation of a major subset of lymphocytes expressing TCR $\gamma\delta$ by an antigen derived from Mycobacteria tuberculosis. *Cell* **57:** 667.

Raulet, D. 1989. The structure, function and molecular genetics of the γ/δ T cell receptor. *Annu. Rev. Immunol.* **7:** 175.

Satyanarayana, K., S. Hata, P. Devlin, M.G. Roncarolo, J.E. de Vries, H. Spits, J. Strominger, and M.S. Krangel. 1988. Genomic organization of the human T-cell antigen-receptor α/δ locus. *Proc. Natl. Acad. Sci.* **85:** 8166.

Schackelford, D.A., A.V. Smith, and I.S. Trowbridge. 1987. Changes in gene expression induced by a phorbol diester: Expression of IL2 receptor, T3 and T cell antigen receptor. *J. Immunol.* **138:** 613.

Schlissel, M. and D. Baltimore. 1989. Activation of immunoglobulin κ gene rearrangement correlates with induction of germline κ gene transcription. *Cell* (in press).

Toyonaga, B. and T.W. Mak. 1987. Genes of the T cell antigen receptor in normal and malignant T cell. *Annu. Rev. Immunol.* **5:** 585.

Wilkinson, M.F. and C.L. MacLeod. 1988. Induction of T-cell receptor α and β mRNA in SL12 cells can occur by transcriptional and post-transcriptional mechanism. *EMBO J.* **7:** 101.

Winoto, A. and D. Baltimore. 1989a. Separate lineage of T cells expressing the $\alpha\beta$ and $\gamma\delta$ receptors. *Nature* **338:** 430.

———. 1989b. A novel, inducible and T-cell specific enhancer located at the 3' end of the T cell receptor α locus. *EMBO J.* **8:** 729.

Winoto, A., J.L. Urban, N.C. Lan, J. Goverman, L. Hood, and D. Hansburg. 1986. Predominant use of a Vα gene segment in mouse T cell receptor specific for cytochrome-c. *Nature* **324:** 679.

Yancopoulos, G. and F. Alt. 1985. Developmentally controlled and tissue-specific expression of rearranged V$_H$ gene segment. *Cell* **40:** 271.

How Important Is the Direct Recognition of Polymorphic MHC Residues by TCR in the Generation of the T-cell Repertoire?

P. Kourilsky, J.-M. Claverie*, A. Prochnicka-Chalufour,*
A.-L. Spetz-Hagberg, and E.-L. Larsson-Sciard
*Unité de Biologie Moléculaire du Gène, U. 277 INSERM, UAC 115 CNRS, *Unité Informatique Scientifique,
Institut Pasteur, 75724 Paris Cédex 15, France*

In line with a long tradition of immunological thinking (e.g., Benacerraf 1978; Winchester et al. 1984), we earlier proposed that peptides derived from somatic self-proteins are presented by class I and/or class II major histocompatibility complex (MHC) molecules on the cell surface (Kourilsky and Claverie 1986). Given the additional notion that MHC molecules select subsets of peptides among all possible ones, the self from the immunological standpoint could be defined as a subset of self-peptides selected (in sequence and shape) by self-MHC molecules. This proposal (the "peptidic self" model, as it was named) had numerous implications, which have been detailed elsewhere (Claverie and Kourilsky 1986; Kourilsky and Claverie 1986; Kourilsky et al. 1987).

To summarize, the following appeared possible:

1. Tolerance to self could be acquired by silencing T cells recognizing self-peptides presented by class I as well as class II MHC molecules (as also proposed by Singer et al. [1986] for self-antigens presented by class II MHC molecules). Correlatively, certain minor histocompatibility antigens might be peptides derived from intracellular as well as extracellular self-proteins displaying polymorphism, whereas certain tumor antigens might be peptides derived from mutant or deregulated (overexpressed) rare host proteins. Finally, certain autoimmune manifestations might be due to disregulation in the expression of internal proteins and/or to mimicry with self-peptides.

2. "MHC restriction" of antigen recognition by T cells might be due to the influence of haplotype-specific (i.e., polymorphic) MHC residues on binding and shaping of peptides not to their direct recognition by the T-cell receptor (TCR). As a direct corollary, alloreactive responses might be directed against the multiple determinants constituted from the nonoverlapping set of self-peptides presented on the surface of cells of different MHC haplotypes (also proposed by Werdelin 1987). Matzinger and Bevan (1977) had suggested that alloreactive reactions might be due to the presentation of a multiplicity of minor histocompatibility antigens. The molecular

nature of the latter was at the time undefined. Along the above view that at least some of the minor histocompatibility antigens are peptides derived from self-proteins, this proposal fits the more molecular postulates of the peptidic self-model.

3. B cells and/or T cells might present "idiopeptides" derived from their own antibody and/or TCR variable (V) parts (see Leserman [1985, 1987] and earlier statements by Benacerraf [1978], Jørgensen et al. [1981], and Janeway [1982]).

The experimental evidence obtained in many different laboratories supports the basic concept. Presentation of self-peptides is now broadly accepted (for review, see Kourilsky and Claverie 1989a). Several implications of the peptidic self-model are also supported by a growing body of experimental data as illustrated by a few selected examples.

Evidence for the silencing of T-cell clones reactive against self-peptides is suggested by the data of Lorenz and Allen (1989a). We do not consider the data involving deletion of T cells expressing certain V_β chains to be necessarily relevant to tolerance to self as discussed later.

To our knowledge, only one minor histocompatibility antigen has been cloned so far, (Fischer Lindahl et al., this volume) but it has been found for example that SV40 T antigen, normally a nuclear protein, causes graft rejection when expressed in fibroblasts from transgenic mice, thus behaving like a minor histocompatibility antigen (Wettstein et al. 1988). The work by Boon and his colleagues (De Plaen et al. 1988; Boon et al., this volume) has highlighted the role of mutant peptides in rejection of tum⁻ tumor cells. Finally, examples of molecular mimicry at the peptide level in autoimmune diseases have been provided (for review, see Oldstone 1987).

Indirect support for the role of self-peptides in alloreactive responses has been gained, particularly from the study of MHC molecules with alterations at the bottom of their binding cleft (for review, see Kourilsky and Claverie 1989a). It may be noted that earlier limiting dilution experiments (Larsson et al. 1985; Beretta et al. 1986) are fully compatible with the fact that alloreactive T cells are made up of highly specific clones. The data are summarized in Figure 1. Polyclonally induced cytotoxic T lymphocyte (CTL) clones, assayed in split clone analysis, distinguish between syngeneic and allogeneic targets (Fig. 1A) and between two different allogeneic targets (Fig. 1B). If such clones are assayed on two syngeneic targets of different cellular origins, about half of the clones lyse both targets, whereas the other half lyse one or the other. If self-peptides are indeed presented, the segregation in reactivities is likely to reflect the array of tissue-specific self-peptides bound to self class I MHC molecules similarly to what was proposed recently by Marrack and Kappler (1988b) for class II determinants. Thus, in this particular case, the 50% of the CTL clones that lyse both targets would recognize MHC-bound self-peptides that are "common," whereas the target-specific CTL clones would be directed against tissue-specific peptides.

Idiopeptides have remained a more elusive matter. The presentation of idiopeptides derived from antibodies opsonized by macrophages appears as a logical and likely possibility, and there is evidence that processed forms of antibodies can be detected by antiidiotypic T cells in several systems. The work of Weiss and Bogen (1989) demonstrates the presentation of a peptide derived from the somatically mutated λ 315 mouse light chain by class II MHC molecules. Also, the work by Bikoff et al. (1988, 1989) on IgG2a alleles strongly suggests presentation of peptides derived from the constant region of processed IgG2a molecules in vivo. A recent interesting observation by Saeki et al. (1989) indicates participation of processed antiidiotypic antibodies in the in vivo rejection of a mouse tumor. To our knowledge, there is no evidence so far for the presentation by T cells of idiopeptides derived from their TCR. Under several circumstances, it was found that nuclear and cytoplasmic proteins yield peptides presented by class I and not class II molecules, whereas proteins secreted or exported to the membrane yield peptides

associated to class II MHC molecules. If this rule was absolute, there would be no obvious way for mature B cells and T cells to expose peptides from their antibody or TCR in association with their class I (or class-I-like, i.e., Qa and Tla in the mouse) MHC molecules. There are, however, several known exceptions to the rule, and this question is not settled. The existence of TCR-derived idiopeptides might be important in T-T networks (T-T interactions so far appear to be mostly MHC unrestricted [for review, see Pereira et al. 1989], but this does not preclude that idiopeptides could be presented by nonpolymorphic molecules). Idiopeptides derived from antibodies could connect the world of B cells to that of T cells. We have noted previously that the connectivity and properties of such idiopeptidic networks would be quite distinct from that of Jerne's network (Kourilsky et al. 1987). The hypothetical role of idiopeptides in repertoire selection is discussed later. The survey of a limited number of antibody sequences has suggested that at least some of the hypervariable regions might be made of sequence motifs that are not or only rarely found in the available sequences of somatic self-proteins (Chalufour et al. 1987).

The peptidic self-model also predicts that it should be possible to find monoclonal antibodies (MAbs) directed against a self-peptide restricted by a given MHC molecule. The question of MHC-restricted antibodies has been debated (Froscher and Klinman 1986; Kievitz et al. 1987), and we are not aware of MAbs that exactly fulfill the above requirements. However, Murphy et al. (1989) described a MAb that recognizes only about 10% of I-A molecules in the medulla but not on the thymic epithelium and only in the presence of I-E. The molecular nature of the 10%-recognized I-A molecules is unknown (one of the investigators' suggestion is that it could be an I-E-derived peptide, but it seems also possible to us that they are loaded with a peptide processed in an I-E-dependent fashion from an abundant serum protein, such as albumin, thus undetectable on thymic epithelial cells and highly represented on the

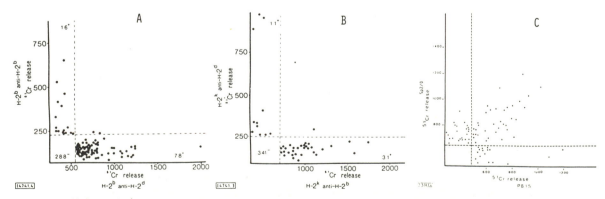

Figure 1. Specificity analysis of polyclonally induced cytotoxic T lymphocyte clones on various allogeneic and syngeneic target cells. Splenic T cells were induced with concanavalin A (Con A) and interleukin-2 (IL-2) under clonal conditions. For each split clone analysis, between 500–700 individual microwells were assayed. Individual clones were assayed for cytolytic activity against different ^{51}Cr-labeled target cells. (Reprinted, with permission, from Larsson et al. 1985.)

immigrant cells from the bone marrow). We (Abastado et al. 1989) have studied a MAb directed against D^d, which similarly recognizes a fraction of about 5–10% of cell-surface D^d molecules. Whether these have a distinctive structure of their own or represent D^d molecules loaded with a given category of self-peptides has not been ascertained at this stage.

Our purpose here is to discuss more thoroughly three points that we think are, for the time being, unsolved and are significant questions in immunological recognition. These questions are the following: Do TCRs recognize polymorphic residues of MHC molecules? What is the meaning of positive selection in the thymus? What is the molecular basis of negative selection in the thymus? For each of these questions, we shall formulate interpretations that fit much of the available data and may provide valuable working hypotheses.

TCR V Segments May Only Contact Nonpolymorphic MHC Residues and Dictate the Geometry of the TCR/Peptide/MHC Complex

By stressing the possible existence of a new class of more or less previously unsuspected molecular elements, namely self-peptides, the peptidic self-model raised the possibility that certain recognition processes might involve self-peptides, rather than MHC molecules, or self-peptides together with MHC molecules. We initially performed an intellectual exercise to see whether TCRs might recognize none of the polymorphic residues of MHC molecules. We concluded that there was no need for TCR to recognize polymorphic residues to explain MHC restriction, alloreactivity, and tolerance to self by negative selection (Claverie and Kourilsky 1986). We failed, however, to explain positive selection in the thymus, which at the time had been established by thymic grafts (Singer et al. 1981, 1982) and has been more recently supported by experiments involving transgenic mice (Kisielow et al. 1988; Loh et al., this volume) and normal mice (Zuniga-Pflucker et al. 1989).

At that time, the human leukemic A antigen (HLA)-A2 structure had not been solved. When it appeared in October 1987 (Bjorkman et al. 1987a,b), it showed only a limited number of residues defined as polymorphic in a position to interact with TCR (only 2–4), whereas many were located in the peptide binding cleft (13) in a position to participate in selecting the peptide and/or in shaping the selected peptide. Accordingly, a few polymorphic residues could still contact the TCR, and their role remained to be appreciated.

To discuss this issue, we shall make use of molecular models. The resolution of the HLA-A2 crystal structure by Bjorkman et al. (1987a,b) has indeed been a major advance in the field. However, as long as additional structural data are not available, molecular models may be helpful. For example, sequence homologies and model-building framed on the HLA-A2 structure have led to the likely conclusion that class II MHC molecules have a roughly similar structure (Brown et

al. 1988), as well as the classical and nonclassical class I molecules in the mouse (see Ajitkumar et al. 1988; Prochnicka-Chalufour et al. 1989).

TCRs have been modeled under the assumption that they are folded like immunoglobulins (Igs) (Novotny et al. 1986). Davis and Bjorkman (1988) and Claverie et al. (1989) have built models of MHC/peptide/TCR complexes. Both groups, as well as Marrack and Kappler (1988a), came to the conclusion that TCR can be positioned in such a way that the most variable sequences (equivalent to CDR3 in antibodies) in both α and β chains face the peptide-binding groove. Amino acid sequences of TCRs recognizing a defined antigenic peptide tend to support this. For example, in the case of the cytochrome c peptide, the recurrence of a given amino acid in the position 100 of the β chain suggests that it fits the peptide (Engel and Hedrick 1988; Hedrick et al. 1988).

Both models are compatible with the additional notion that the CDR1 and CDR2 TCR equivalents are then in a position to interact with MHC. The CDR3 region is generated by the joining process between V and joining (J), or V, diversity (D), and J segments but does not involve amino acids encoded by V genes themselves. Therefore, the segments encoded by V_{α} and V_{β} genes could be involved in interactions with MHC molecules. Accordingly, it has been thought that the use of V genes would correlate with MHC haplotypes with different V genes coding for TCR sequences that would recognize given MHC molecules. This is, in a way, a revival of the "two receptors in one" hypothesis, which states that the TCR carries two specific receptors: one for peptide and another for MHC. The available evidence does not support this view, and we emphasize below a completely different possibility.

The few polymorphic residues (only 2–4) that point up from the HLA-A2 groove are located very close to the peptide-binding site. Accordingly, we propose that these residues, if they make contact with the TCR, are recognized by CDR3. This leaves open the possibility that V gene segments (which include CDR1 and CDR2) do not contact polymorphic MHC residues. On the contrary, we argue that V gene segments, since they work with many different MHC molecules, have evolved in a way to optimize the recognition of nonpolymorphic (conserved) MHC regions. This is also the easiest interpretation of TCR recognition of MHC under alloreactive conditions. This is not to say that certain subsets of V genes may not better fit certain subsets of MHC molecules, sharing one or a few amino acid changes (not necessarily considered polymorphic by the usual standards). However, for us, the (limited) variability in CDR1 and CDR2 regions of V_{α} and V_{β}, instead of being used for haplotype recognition, serves to recognize MHC molecules in different orientations. A given V_{α} or V_{β} chain would in general recognize the same subregion of a given MHC molecule, and this subregion would in general be about the same in most or all MHC molecules. In other terms, V genes would primarily determine the geometry of TCR/MHC interaction largely irrespective of MHC haplotype.

At one extreme, one could imagine the scanning of the MHC peptide-binding site by combinations of V chains, just as in a television screen. One may also visualize one or several preferred points of interactions and rotations around these points. In the former case, the combination of various V_α and V_β genes could probably not be entirely random for geometrical reasons, whereas in the latter case such constraints would be more loose. In recent modeling work, we noted four zones in class I MHC molecules that by calculation appear easily accessible to a large spherical probe (Novotny et al. 1989). These could be preferred anchoring points for V_α and V_β segments.

Positive Selection in the Thymus Does Not Imply That TCRs Recognize Polymorphic Residues

The concept of positive selection in the thymus, primarily based on thymic grafts and bone marrow chimeras, has been supported more recently by experiments involving transgenic mice. The intellectual challenge is to understand how TCRs in the thymus are selected in such a way as to recognize all foreign antigens (which they have never seen) in the context of self-MHC molecules. The idea has gradually emerged that positive selection actually means that the foreign antigens have somehow been seen in the thymus. In other terms, what we interpret as a primary reaction against a foreign antigen encountered in the periphery would in fact be a secondary reaction against an element similar to the foreign antigen found in the thymus. The latter would thus display an internal representation (another "internal image") of the foreign world (Kourilsky and Claverie 1989a,b). Three classes of hypotheses have been put forward as to the molecular origin of these "foreign" or "pseudoforeign" thymic elements.

Three models for positive selection. Since 1986, the idea has spread that the recognition of self-peptides by maturing T cells in the thymus could play a major role in tolerance, the simplest model being that such autoreactive T cells are silenced or deleted (Kourilsky and Claverie 1986; Singer et al. 1986). This has led to the reformulation of an older hypothesis to propose that maturing T cells in the thymus, which strongly recognize self-MHC associated with self peptides, are negatively selected, and that those displaying weak recognition of MHC plus self-peptides grow and serve to build the peripheral T-cell repertoire (Singer et al. 1986, 1987).

It has also been proposed that the thymic epithelium, which apparently plays a major role in positive selection, expresses a special set of peptides. This set of peptides would not be operationally considered as self because the T cells recognizing them would receive an activation signal but not a negative signal delivered by immigrant cells from the bone marrow (macrophages,

dendritic cells, and B cells) (reviewed in Sprent et al. 1988). Accordingly, they would reach the periphery without being negatively selected (Marrack et al. 1988; Marrack and Kappler 1988a).

We proposed still another model in which errors in gene expression would be a major driving force to generate the T-cell repertoire (Kourilsky and Claverie 1989a,b). Such errors would give rise to erroneous self-peptides that, being very rare, would have a low probability to be seen twice by T cells. Thus, a T cell could have received a positive signal from a presented erroneous self-peptide. The probability that this T cell would see the same erroneous self-peptide again would be very low so that it would in general escape a subsequent negative signal. On the contrary, T cells activated by a bona fide self-peptide would in general see it again and be silenced. We initially suggested that the positive signal is delivered by the thymic epithelium and the negative one by immigrant cells from the bone marrow, but this statement may be too restrictive, and the cell types involved in this ping-pong game may not necessarily always be these. Perhaps, activation and deletion (or silencing) can take place on the thymic epithelium alone as well as on immigrant cells from the bone marrow. This is because the determination of whether a thymocyte receives a positive or a negative signal may not depend only upon the antigen presenting cell, but also upon the differentiation stage of the thymocyte. A growing body of evidence indicates that in addition to the TCR, the components of the CD3 complex, the presence of CD2 and perhaps that of CD4 and CD8 (and other differentiation molecules will probably add to this list) determine which intracellular pathways are activated (e.g., breakdown of phosphatidyl inositides, activation of protein kinases, and redistribution of membrane proteins) (R. Klausner et al., pers. comm.).

Errors in gene expression certainly take place in all cell types so that there is no need to postulate a subset of thymic-specific peptides, although it is conceivable that the rate of errors might be increased in the thymic epithelium. We emphasized that an absolute requirement for this model to hold is that T cells can receive a positive signal by recognizing very few or only one of these erroneous self-peptides. This might be true in the thymus and not in the periphery where adhesion and transduction functions may be different.

A list of possible errors in gene expression is shown in Table 1. Translation errors leading to the misincorporation of amino acids are rather frequent ($\sim 2.10^{-4}$) (Kourilsky and Claverie 1989a,b; see also, Buckingham and Grosjean 1986; and earlier work by Loftfield 1963; Loftfield and Vanderjagt 1972; Harley et al. 1981). An interesting possibility, not emphasized earlier, relies on the translational noise derived from the aberrant transcription (followed by translation) of noncoding DNA. It is striking that if noncoding DNA is involved in the generation of the T-cell repertoire its generation and maintenance in higher eukaryotes endowed with an immune system might be under selection pressure. Ac-

Table 1. Genetic Noise, i.e., Errors in the Expression of Genetic Material

Misincorporation of
nucleotides in DNA synthesis (10^{-9})
nucleotides in mRNA synthesis (10^{-6})
amino acids in protein synthesis (10^{-4})

Expression of noncoding DNA
translation of intron sequences
errors in splicing
translational restarts
aberrant transcription starts followed by translation of RNA copied from noncoding DNA

cording to our views, responses to foreign antigens would actually be secondary responses against erroneous self-peptides seen in the thymus. We have previously analyzed the sequences of a number of foreign T epitopes with experimentally demonstrated reactivity. We found that many of them, when compared with somatic cell proteins by an algorithm that deals with the sequences as overlapping sets of tetrapeptides, appear by this criterium to be "far away" from self (Claverie et al. 1988). Keeping in mind the previously underlined uncertainties associated with any analysis of this sort, this observation might suggest that at least some of the presumptive erroneous self-peptides that shaped the responsive T cells involved expression of noncoding DNA rather than single amino acid substitutions in somatic self-proteins.

It should be noted that still other models have been proposed (see references in Marrack and Kappler 1988a). For example, the hypothesis was made that gene conversion would create some mosaicism of MHC molecules in the thymus, which could play a role in generating the T-cell repertoire (Ritzel et al. 1984).

Comparison of the three models. In all three models, which are not mutually excluded, positive selection is interpreted to mean that the peripheral T-cell repertoire has been, at least in part, generated against peptides seen in the thymus, but these peptides are of a different nature. In the first model, they are self-peptides, and the repertoire of responses against foreign antigens derives from cross-reactions with these self-peptides. In the second model, peptides specifically expressed by the thymic epithelium are responsible for the primary response in the thymus. In the third hypothesis, peptides are produced by the overall noise of errors in gene expression. The latter are not specific for the thymic epithelium but could be increased there. Thus, self versus nonself discrimination relies upon three distinct mechanisms: a difference in affinity between various TCRs for self-peptides plus MHC, the tissue-specific expression of a set of peptides, and a difference in the probabilities of a repeated recognition event. In the latter two models, the initial interaction that delivers the positive signal is a bona fide strong recognitive event. We favor the third hypothesis, where the broadest diversity can be generated. In fact, elementary calculations show that the diversity might

be in or close to the desired orders of magnitude to match the world of foreign epitopes presented by the self-MHC molecules (Kourilsky and Claverie 1989b). In addition, it is possible that once a repertoire has reached a certain diversity cross-reactions may become quite significant (one may recall here that alloreactive recognition takes place at a frequency of about 10^{-2}). One may thus wonder whether the so-called immunodominant epitopes in a foreign antigen might be those that match closely erroneous self-peptides that were actually seen in the thymus. It is possible to evoke T-cell responses by immunization with nonimmunodominant peptides, and one may wonder whether such T cells are recruited through relatively weak cross-reactions. Such views suggest that a part of the observed MHC restriction depends on limitation in the T-cell repertoire, at least as far as immunodominant peptides are concerned.

The questionable role of idiopeptides. One intriguing issue is the possible role of idiopeptides in thymic selections. In addition to T cells, the thymus contains relatively large numbers of B cells ($\sim 10^6$ in mice). Under the assumption that these T cells and B cells expose idiopeptides derived from their TCRs and antibodies, should these idiopeptides be classified as self or nonself? We earlier argued that one should make a distinction between the somatic self (including somatic self-proteins) and the immunological self (idiopeptides) because, if idiopeptides play a regulatory role, coincidences between somatic self-peptides and idiopeptides could be a source of disorders (Kourilsky and Claverie 1986; Chalufour et al. 1987; Kourilsky et al. 1987). The question raised here and previously (Kourilsky et al. 1987) is of a different nature, namely that of the tolerization or nontolerization of idiopeptides in the thymus. If tolerized, idiopeptides would play no major role in the regulation of the immune response, except perhaps those derived from somatically mutated antibodies that have not been seen in the thymus. If nontolerized, these idiopeptides might be one source of diversity in the generation of the T-cell repertoire in addition to their regulatory role in the periphery.

Recognition of polymorphic MHC residues. It is remarkable to note that none of the above three models strictly requires that TCRs recognize polymorphic MHC residues as a compulsory feature of positive thymic selection. Exactly as happened in the evolution of our understanding of alloreactivity, the introduction of an intermediate class of elements, namely self- and/or erroneous self-peptides selected by MHC molecules, allows to switch the major requirements for recognition from MHC molecules to these (previously unsuspected) elements. Accordingly, we anticipate that MHC molecules with mutations at the bottom of the peptide-binding cleft (which could hardly be seen directly by the TCR, e.g., K^{bm6}, K^{bm8}, and K^{km2}) will, exactly as they give rise to alloreactive reactions, promote distinctive MHC-dependent positive selection in the thymus (see Loh et al., this volume).

Negative Selection in the Thymus May Be One Component of Tolerance, but All Negative Selection in the Thymus Need Not Be Related to Tolerance

As mentioned above, the notion that self-peptides are presented offers a way by which a number of self-reactive T cells (directed against self-peptides) could be tolerated, for example by deletion, in the thymus (Kourilsky and Claverie 1986; Singer et al. 1986). It should be kept in mind that tolerance has different meanings depending on the experimental system used and that tolerance to grafts, for example, probably involves complex mechanisms that may not only be related to unresponsiveness to self-peptides (Le Douarin et al.; Coutinho et al.; both this volume).

The data that directly address the question of tolerance to self-peptides are just as scarce as those on the presentation of self-peptides themselves. The experiments by Lorenz and Allen (1988, 1989a) using isogenic mice expressing hemoglobin variants do suggest that self-peptides may cause unresponsiveness of T cells in the thymus (Lorenz and Allen 1989b).

We argue here that the experiments that involve the deletion of T cells expressing certain V_α chains in the mouse imply neither that this deletion process is involved in tolerance nor that the specificity of the deletion process with regard to certain V_β chains in certain MHC haplotypes imposes recognition of polymorphic residues of the latter by the former.

Deletion of V_β-bearing cells may improve the specificity of immune responses. The work of many different groups of investigators, but particularly Kappler et al. (1987a,b, 1988) and MacDonald et al. (1988), has shown that T cells bearing certain TCR V_β chains are preferentially eliminated in the thymic cortex by certain class II molecules (I-E) or minor lymphocyte-stimulating antigens (Mls) determinants. For example, $V_\beta 17.a$ (Kappler et al. 1987b), $V_\beta 5.2$ (Okada and Weissman 1989), and $V_\beta 11$ (Bill et al. 1989) are depleted in I-E$^+$ mice contrary to I-E$^-$ animals. Similarly, $V_\beta 6$ (MacDonald et al. 1988), $V_\beta 8.1$ (Kappler et al. 1988), $V_\beta 4$, $V_\beta 7$, and $V_\beta 12$ (see Palmer et al., this volume) are low

in Mls-1^a mice, whereas $V_\beta 3$ (Pullen et al. 1988) is low in Mls-2^a mice. In the elimination of $V_\beta 8.1$, $V_\beta 6$, and $V_\beta 3$, there is some influence of MHC following the hierarchy H-2^k > H-2^d > H-2^b ≈ H-2^q. Interestingly, although Mls reactivities up to now were known to be only directed against class II, we have recently obtained data that point to the fact that class I MHC molecules might present the "Mls determinants." If splenic T cells from an Mls-1^b mouse are stimulated with H-2 mismatched stimulator cells from an Mls-1^a strain, the Mls-associated TCR V_β gene families (in this case, $V_\beta 6$ and $V_\beta 8.1$) are preferentially used by the responding T-cell population, even when T-cell blasts are used as stimulator cells (Table 2). We have also observed that the degree of $V_\beta 6$ and $V_\beta 8.1$ usage among the responder T cells follows the above-mentioned hierarchy of H-2 preference when using class-I-positive T-cell blasts as stimulators (data not shown). Thus, at least in these in vitro assays, we observe more potent effects of Mls determinants with class-I-expressing T cells than with B cells.

The Mls activity has remained elusive. The finding that certain bacterial toxins mimic to a large degree the Mls effects (Janeway et al. 1989) has provided an interesting analogy with one major difference: Bacterial toxins elicit antibody production, whereas no antibodies against Mls have been isolated. This has prompted a number of hypotheses (for review, see Janeway et al. 1989) out of which we briefly describe the two that seem more likely to us, and we add a third one. Kappler and Marrack (1988) suggested that the Mls-1^a product could be a peptide, i.e., the processed product of some (internal?) self-protein. According to Janeway et al. (1989), it could be a protein that helps bridge MHC molecules to the CD3 complex. We would like to emphasize that both models could fuse into a single one, if Janeway's hypothetical ligand was a processed peptide. This is because there is no formal need that the "superpeptide" postulated by Kappler and Marrack lies in the peptide-binding groove. This is in fact somewhat unlikely unless its recognition by TCR occurs in a complex with a completely different geometry so that V_β CDR1 and CDR2 loops would face the groove rather than one of the flanking helixes (see molecular

Table 2. High Frequencies of Mls-associated TCR V_β Gene Usage Are Obtained When Using Allogeneic T Blasts As Stimulators

Responder T Cells[a]	Stimulator cells[c]			
	B blasts		T blasts	
BALB/c (H-2^d, Mls^b)	C3H (H-2^k, Mls^c)	CBA/J (H-2^k, Mls^d)	C3H (H-2^k, Mls^c)	CBA/J (H-2^k, Mls^d)
$V_\beta 6$[b]	9.6%	28.5%	7.2%	41.3%
$V_\beta 8.1$	10.1%	15.7%	9.3%	17.8%

[a] Normal splenic T cells were used at 1×10^6/ml.
[b] Fluorescence-activated cell sorter analysis using MAbs: 44-22-1 (anti-$V_\beta 6$), KJ16 ($V_\beta 8.1$ and 8.2), and F23.2 ($V_\beta 8.2$).
[c] Stimulator cells were either B-cell blasts (stimulated with lipopolysaccharide for 48 hr) or T-cell blasts (stimulated with Con A and IL-2 for 72 hr). Blasts were irradiated 1000 rads and cocultured at 1×10^6/ml as the responder T cells in the presence of IL-2 for 5 days.

models above). A plausible alternative would be that such a putative peptide sticks outside the groove. In the Claverie et al. (1989) model, one sees a kind of cleft on the other side of the α_1 helix of MHC, above which an extra loop of the V_β chain can be positioned (Fig. 2). Perhaps the Mls superpeptide could fit in this hypothetical secondary binding site.

We think, however, that it is not even necessary to postulate the existence of an Mls superpeptide or of any other kind of ligand. We propose instead that the direct binding of the TCR β chain to MHC, perhaps between the above-mentioned extra loop of V_β (named $V_\beta4$ by Claverie et al. 1989) and the edge of one or both of the MHC α helices is enough to trigger selective deletion effects (Fig. 3). This interaction could take place with class I as well as class II MHC molecules, explaining why we find an effect of Mls determinants on T cells (see above). Furthermore, experiments using anti-CD3 antibodies imply that efficient TCR cross-linking can induce apoptosis (Smith et al. 1989). In this context, we propose that the patching of class II MHC molecules on the cell surface induces clustering of those TCRs that have the strongest affinity for MHC molecules. Mls effects could then involve a combination of at least two

types of phenomena. First, Mls alleles could regulate certain posttranscriptional modifications of MHC molecules (e.g., glycosylation pattern) so that extracellular portions of the latter would be made more or less accessible to TCR, as was also suggested previously by Davis and Bjorkman (1988). Second, Mls alleles could influence patching. They could code for or regulate the patching process through some cytoplasmic molecules or molecules embedded in the membrane or through posttranslational modifications of the class II molecules in intra- or extracellular regions that would modify their capacity to aggregate (Fig. 4).

Along this line, we suspect that the transfer of Mls specificity in double bone marrow chimeras (Pullen et al. 1988) might correlate with the transfer of MHC specificities observed in the thymus by Sharrow et al. (1981). Both processes could involve shedded MHC molecules.

Underlying this proposal is the notion that these deletion effects involving certain combinations of V_β chains and MHC molecules do not primarily participate in tolerance but serve the specificity of the immune response. If class II MHC molecules happen to patch during physiological interactions (for example, be-

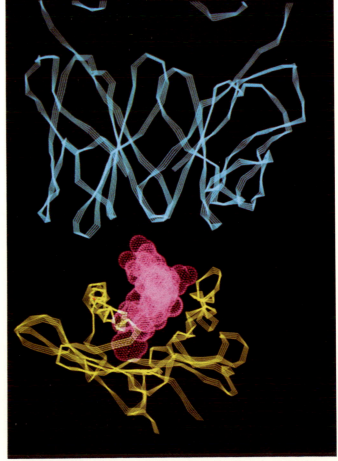

Figure 2. Possible molecular model for the TCR/peptide/HLA-A2 complex. The TCR (top molecule in blue) is modeled after an Ig Fab fold using the HPB-MLT α and β chain sequences followed by the relaxation of stereochemical constraints and energy minimization (Claverie et al. 1989). The constant part is not shown. The antigen is represented as the Van der Waals envelope (red) of a 16-residue peptide (K16F, a HIV-*gag* peptide; Claverie et al. 1988) docked with the binding site (yellow ribbon) of HLA-A2 drawn after the available α-carbon coordinates (Bjorkman et al. 1987a,b). According to the proposed geometry of this complex, the V_α and V_β CDR3 loops (right behind each other above the HLA-A2 cleft) mostly interact with the bound peptide (in a bent extended conformation), whereas the V_α CDR1/CDR2 loops and V_β CDR2/CDR1 loops mostly interact with residues pointing up from the HLA-A2 α_1 and α_2 helices. An additional TCR loop (extreme left) would also be available for interaction with the peptide/HLA-A2 complex in a slightly translated orientation. Details of the various TCR loop contacts with the HLA-A2/peptide complex are presented in Figs. 3 and 4.

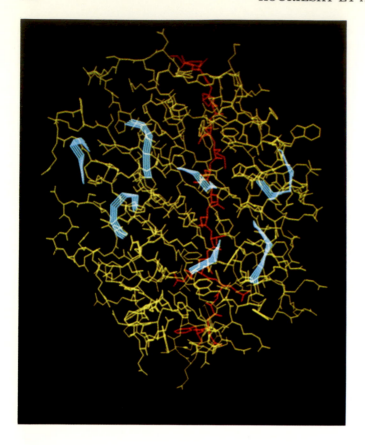

Figure 3. Putative contacts of the TCR variable loops with a HLA-A2/peptide complex. Side chains and backbones of both our HLA-A2 model (yellow) and the docked K16F peptide (red) are shown. Depicted in blue are the parts of the TCR closest to the HLA-A2/peptide complex presented in Fig. 2. This view was obtained by rotating the entire complex, looking down the HLA-A2 site from the TCR point of view, and clipping off the distal parts of the TCR. Fig. 4 identifies the residues involved and shows the dyad symmetry of the loop organization.

tween antigen-presenting cells and helper T cells) this would induce clustering of TCRs that bear overly "sticky" V_β chains and result in a nonantigen-specific activation. Our in vitro results suggest that this could also be the case for the patching of class I MHC molecules. Our view is that the mechanism that circumvents this problem involves nonantigen-specific deletion of the corresponding T cells. The semantic question of whether it is appropriate to refer to Mls as a super antigen becomes a significant one. The present terminology and some of the current models implying that Mls determinants operate as peptides presented by MHC molecules tend to infer that Mls-dependent deletions represent on a large scale what could be observed with specific self-peptides on a smaller scale in the acquisition of central tolerance. Along the above rationale, this view would basically be wrong.

Differences in affinity between different V_β chains and MHC molecules. The deletion of T cells bearing specific V_β chains, be it dependent on known Mls alleles or not, makes it very likely that differences in affinity between various V_β chains and various MHC molecules exist. If we consider one given MHC molecule, several V_β chains must interact differently. Thus, in the simplest interpretation, V_β17.a, V_β5.2, and V_β11 might bind better to I-E than other V_β chains causing their deletion by some unknown mechanism. Reciprocally, a given V_β chain must display different affinities when

interacting with different MHC molecules. For example, in the simplest interpretation, V_β17.a would bind better to I-E than to I-A, explaining I-E-dependent deletion of the corresponding T cells. Do these differences in affinity imply interactions between V_β chains and polymorphic MHC residues? As above, we shall argue that this is unlikely because V_β chains are in fact very promiscuous with regard to MHC molecules. Thus, in I-E⁻ strains, V_β17.a is functional and works with I-A and, more generally, V_α and V_β chains can work (unless they are deleted) in most MHC haplotypes and also with class I as well as class II MHC molecules. This situation therefore is one of rather subtle affinity changes, which could be dependent on several parameters:

1. The overall structure of MHC molecules might be slightly variable. Because of distant amino acid changes, certain atomic positions in conserved regions important for the recognition by V chains might be modified, leading to improved or impaired interaction.

2. Posttranslational modifications could be important. For example, not all class I MHC molecules have the same glycosylation patterns.

3. Local amino acid changes in the interaction region might decrease or increase affinities. Such changes, however, could not be completely random as they should remain compatible with a functional interaction.

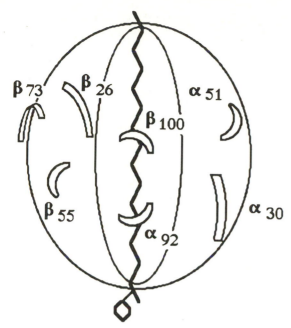

Figure 4 Diagram of the putative contacts of the TCR with a HLA-A2/peptide complex. Identification of the TCR V_α and V_β residues in the best position to interact with an HLA-A2/peptide complex in the geometry corresponding to Figs. 3 and 4. Residue 73, corresponding to the extra-loop found in the V_β chain might be involved in antigen recognition in a different form of the HLA-A2/peptide complex. It is worth noting that this residue is central to a cluster of variable residues in two of three groups of V_β TCR chains (Bougueleret and Claverie 1987).

In summary, the different affinities of V_β chains for MHC molecules, with variations depending rather loosely on MHC class, isotypes, and haplotypes, can be explained (as also suggested by other investigators, cf. Davis and Bjorkman 1988) without invoking interactions of V_β chains with polymorphic MHC residues.

What Do TCRs See?

We have organized the above discussion around the question of recognition or nonrecognition of polymorphic residues in TCR-MHC interactions. This is much more than an academic problem because it draws a line between two broad theories of recognition: one in which the imprint of MHC polymorphism by direct TCR contacts is a compulsory feature of recognition, and one in which MHC polymorphism is primarily reflected by the set of peptides (be it self- or erroneous self-peptides and/or idiopeptides) that are selected and shaped by MHC molecules and where the direct recognition of polymorphic MHC residues becomes an ancillary rather than a constraining feature of the system. On the contrary, the interactions with nonpolymorphic MHC residues might be functionally very important.

In this brief and nonexhaustive survey, we have shown that the second line of thinking is clearly tenable. However, it imposes constraints on the interpre-

tation of a number of observations and experimental data in other areas of molecular immunology.

To summarize, we have proposed that the few polymorphic MHC residues that are in a position to be seen by the TCR are contacted by CDR3 residues. Then, the V_α and V_β segments are not required to contact any polymorphic residues at all (note that the definition of a polymorphic residue in MHC molecules may require some further specification). Accordingly, V chains of TCRs would have been selected to work with most and possibly all MHC molecules in the species. Polymorphic variations in these two sets of coevolving molecules are accommodated in the recognition system provided that they maintain the basic capacity to work with a broad set of partners. Along this view, V chains determine the geometry of the TCR/peptide/MHC complex, and this geometry is more or less independent of isotypic, haplotypic, and, perhaps, class differences in MHC molecules. A variety of V chains could have developed as a means of building complexes with a variety of geometries, increasing the probabilities for the CDR3 regions of recognizing the specific peptide presented by the MHC molecule. In this diverse world of interactions between the various V chains and the subset of polymorphic MHC molecules that are encountered in randomly bred populations, some of these interactions would turn out to be inadequate. The most "sticky" V chains (V_β chains, so far) would need being removed since they would cause nonspecific T-cell activation perhaps when class II molecules (and also class I?) patch on the surface of cells. The spectacular effects of Mls do not, according to us, imply that Mls genes encode real antigens. Rather, Mls could function by influencing patching of MHC molecules and/or their interaction with V_β chains without any involvement of any superpeptide or ligand. The deletion of V_β-bearing T cells would thus be essential for the specificity of immune responses and not for the establishment of tolerance.

This latter point raises a general question on the experimental systems in which so-called positive and negative selection are observed. We feel that it would be appropriate to distinguish clearly between those systems where the response to a well-characterized antigen or peptide is studied and those where large populations sharing an observable phenotypic trait are examined. Thus, the silencing of T cells reacting with self-peptides is very likely to play a role in the establishment of tolerance within the thymus, whereas for us the Mls- or I-E-dependent deletion of T cells may be irrelevant for tolerance. It will become important to make a similar discrimination within phenomena involving positive selection, where large population effects may not be relevant to the activation of T cells with given specificities later found in the periphery. Positive selection in this latter sense, by implying that the thymus displays an internal representation of the foreign world, remains a fascinating possibility. We have proposed that its molecular basis might rely on the noise of errors in the expression of genetic material.

Whether this proposal and others made above are correct or not is indeed open to experimentation. The views developed above show some degree of consistency with the available evidence. This does not imply that they are true but that they need testing.

ACKNOWLEDGMENTS

We are grateful to many colleagues for stimulating discussions and to Drs. Miguel Marcos and Claude Roth for critical reading of the manuscript. We thank Mrs. Viviane Caput for skillful editing of the manuscript.

REFERENCES

Abastado, J.P., S. Darche, H. Jouin, C. Delarbre, G. Gachelin, and P. Kourilsky. 1989. A monoclonal antibody recognizes a subset of the H-2D^d mouse major class I antigens. *Res. Immunol.* **140:** 581.

Ajitkumar, P., S.S. Geier, K.V. Kesari, F. Borriello, M. Nakagawa, J.A. Bluestone, M.A. Saper, D.C. Wiley, and S.G. Nathenson. 1988. Evidence that multiple residues on both the alpha-helices of the class I MHC molecule are simultaneously recognized by the T cell receptor. *Cell* **54:** 47.

Benacerraf, B. 1978. A hypothesis to relate the specificity of T lymphocytes and the activity of I region-specific Ir genes in macrophages and B lymphocytes. *J. Immunol.* **120:** 1809.

Beretta, A., M. Ermonval, and E.-L. Larsson. 1986. Degeneracy of H-2 recognition by cytotoxic T lymphocytes: 10% of the total repertoire is "specific" for a given haplotype and up to 1% is self-H-2 reactive. *Eur. J. Immunol.* **16:** 605.

Bikoff, E.K. and L.A. Eckhardt. 1989. Presentation of IgG2a antigens to class II-restricted T cells by stably transfected B lymphoma cells. *Eur. J. Immunol.* (in press).

Bikoff, E.K., H. Yu, and L.A. Eckhardt. 1988. T cell recognition of endogenous IgG$_{2a}$ expressed in B lymphoma cells. *Eur. J. Immunol.* **18:** 341.

Bill, J., O. Kanagawa, D.L. Woodland, and E. Palmer. 1989. The MHC molecule I-E is necessary but not sufficient for the clonal deletion of V-beta-11 bearing T cells. *J. Exp. Med.* **169:** 1405.

Bjorkman, P.J., M.A. Saper, B. Samraoui, W.S. Bennett, J.L. Strominger, and D.C. Wiley. 1987a. Structure of the human class I histocompatibility antigen, HLA-A2. *Nature* **329:** 506.

————. 1987b. The foreign antigen binding site and T cell recognition regions of class I histocompatibility antigens. *Nature* **329:** 512.

Bougueleret, L. and J.-M. Claverie. 1987. Variability analysis of the human and mouse T-cell receptor beta-chain. *Immunogenetics* **26:** 304.

Brown, J.H., T. Jardetzky, M.A. Saper, B. Samraoui, P.J. Bjorkman, and D.C. Wiley. 1988. A hypothetical model of the foreign antigen binding site of class II histocompatibility molecules. *Nature* **332:** 845.

Buckingham, R.H. and H. Grosjean. 1986. The accuracy of messenger RNA: Transfer RNA recognition. In *Accuracy in molecular biology* (ed. D.J. Galas et al.), p. 83. Chapman and Hall, London.

Chalufour, A., L. Bougueleret, J.-M. Claverie, and P. Kourilsky. 1987. Rare sequence motifs are common constituents of hypervariable antibody regions. *Ann. Inst. Pasteur Immunol.* **138:** 671.

Claverie, J.-M. and P. Kourilsky. 1986. The peptidic self

model: A reassessment of the role of the major histocompatibility complex molecules in the restriction of the T-cell response. *Ann. Inst. Pasteur Immunol.* **137D:** 425.

Claverie, J.-M., A. Prochnicka-Chalufour, and L. Bougueleret. 1989. Immunological implications of a Fab-like structure for the T-cell receptor. *Immunol. Today* **10:** 14.

Claverie, J.-M., P. Kourilsky, P. Langlade-Demoyen, A. Chalufour-Rochnicka, G. Dadaglio, F. Tekaia, F. Plata, and L. Bougueleret. 1988. T-immunogenic peptides are constituted of rare sequence patterns. Use in the identification of T-epitopes in the human immunodeficiency virus *gag* protein. *Eur. J. Immunol.* **28:** 1547.

Davis, M.M. and P. Bjorkman. 1988. T-cell antigen receptor gene and T-cell recognition. *Nature* **334:** 395.

De Plaen, E., C. Lurquin, A. Van Pel, B. Mariame, J.-P. Szikora, T. Wölfel, C. Sibille, P. Chomez, and T. Boon. 1988. Immunogenic (tum$^-$) variants of mouse tumor P815: Cloning of the gene of tum$^-$ antigen P91A and identification of the tum$^-$ mutation. *Proc. Natl. Acad. Sci.* **85:** 2274.

Engel, I. and S.M. Hedrick. 1988. Site-directed mutations in the BDJ junctional region of a T cell receptor beta chain cause changes in antigenic peptide recognition. *Cell* **54:** 473.

Froscher, B.G. and N.R. Klinman. 1986. Immunization with SV40-transformed cells yields mainly MHC-restricted monoclonal antibodies. *J. Exp. Med.* **164:** 196.

Harley, C.B., J.W. Pollard, C.P. Stanners, and S. Goldstein. 1981. Model for messenger RNA translation during amino acid starvation applied to the calculation of protein synthetic error rates. *J. Biol. Chem.* **256:** 10786.

Hedrick, S.M., I. Engel, D.L. McEllogott, P.J. Fink, H.S.U. Meiling, D. Hansburg, and L.A. Matis. 1988. Selection of amino acid in the beta chain of the T cell antigen receptor. *Science* **239:** 1541.

Janeway, C.A., Jr. 1982. The selection of self-MHC recognizing T lymphocytes: A role for idiotypes. *Immunol. Today* **3:** 261.

Janeway, C.A., Jr., Y. Yagi, P.J. Conrad, M.E. Katz, B. Jones, S. Vroegop, and S. Buxzer. 1989. T cell responses to Mls and to bacterial proteins that mimics its behaviour. *Immunol. Rev.* **107:** 61.

Jørgensen, T., B. Bogen, and K. Hannestad. 1981. Recognition of variable (V) domains of myeloma protein 315 by B- and T-lymphocytes. *ICN-UCLA Symp. Mol. Cell. Biol.* **20:** 573.

Kappler, J.W., N. Roehm, and P. Marrack. 1987a. T cell tolerance by clonal elimination in the thymus. *Cell* **49:** 273.

Kappler, J.W., U. Staerz, J. White, and P.C. Marrack. 1988. Self-tolerance eliminates T cells specific for Mls-modified products of the major histocompatibility complex. *Nature* **332:** 35.

Kappler, J.W., T. Wade, J. White, E. Kushnir, M. Blackman, J. Bill, N. Roehm, and P. Marrack. 1987b. A T cell receptor V-beta segment that imparts reactivity to a class II major histocompatibility complex product. *Cell* **49:** 263.

Kievits, F., A. Rocca, A. Opolski, J. Limpens, T. Leuperxs, T. Kloosterman, W.J. Boerenkamp, M. Pla, and P. Ivanyi. 1987. Induction of H-2-specific antibodies by injections of syngeneic Sendai virus-coated cells. *Eur. J. Immunol.* **17:** 27.

Kisielow, P., H.S. Teh, H. Blüthmann, and H. von Boehmer. 1988. Positive selection of antigen-specific T cells in thymus by restricting MHC molecules. *Nature* **335:** 730.

Kourilsky, P. and J.-M. Claverie. 1986. The peptidic self-model: A hypothesis on the molecular nature of the immunological self. *Ann. Inst. Pasteur Immunol.* **137D:** 3.

————. 1989a. MHC-restriction, alloreactivity and thymic education: A common link? *Cell* **56:** 327.

————. 1989b. MHC-antigen interaction: What does the T cell receptor see? *Adv. Immunol.* **45:** 107.

Kourilsky, P., G. Chaouat, C. Rabourdin-Combe, and J.-M. Claverie. 1987. Working principles in the immune system implied by the "peptidic self" model. *Proc. Natl. Acad. Sci.* **84:** 3400.

Larsson, E.-L., A. Beretta, and M. Ermonval. 1985. Clonal specificity of concanavalin A-induced cytotoxic T lymphocytes. *Eur. J. Immunol.* **15:** 400.

Leserman, L. 1985. The introversion of the immune response: A hypothesis for T-B interaction. *Immunol. Today* **6:** 352.

———. 1987. All in the superfamily: Presentation of antigen receptors in the context of the major histocompatibility complex. *Ann. Inst. Pasteur Immunol.* **138:** 53.

Loftfield, R.B. 1963. The frequency of errors in protein biosynthesis. *Biochem. J.* **89:** 82.

Loftfield, R.B. and D. Vanderjagt. 1972. The frequency of errors in protein biosynthesis. *Biochem. J.* **128:** 1353.

Lorenz, R.G. and P.M. Allen. 1988. Direct evidence for functional self protein/Ia complexes *in vivo. Proc. Natl. Acad. Sci.* **85:** 5220.

———. 1989a. Thymic cortical epithelial cells can present self-antigens *in vivo. Nature* **337:** 560.

———. 1989b. Thymic cortical epithelial cells lack full capacity for antigen presentation. *Nature* **340:** 557.

MacDonald, H.R., R. Schneider, R.K. Lees, R.C. Howe, H. Acha-Orbea, H. Festenstein, R.M. Zinkernagel, and H. Hengartner. 1988. T-cell receptor V-beta use predicts reactivity and tolerance to Mls^a-encoded antigens. *Nature* **332:** 40.

Marrack, P. and J. Kappler. 1988a. The T cell repertoire for antigen and MHC. *Immunol. Today* **9:** 308.

———. 1988b. T cells can distinguish between allogeneic major histocompatibility complex products on different cell types. *Nature* **332:** 840.

Marrack, P., D. Lo, R. Brinster, R. Palmiter, L. Burkly, R.H. Flavell, and J. Kappler. 1988. The effect of thymus environment on T cell development and tolerance. *Cell* **53:** 627.

Matzinger, P. and M.J. Bevan. 1977. Why do so many lymphocytes respond to major histocompatibility antigens? *Cell. Immunol.* **29:** 1.

Murphy, D.B., D. Lo, S. Rath, R.L. Brinster, R.A. Flavell, A. Slanetz, and C.A. Janeway. 1989. A novel MHC class II epitope expressed in thymic medulla but not cortex. *Nature* **238:** 765.

Novotny, J., R.E. Bruccoleri, and P. Kourilsky. 1989. On the molecular nature of "restrictive" antigenic elements present on major histocompatibility complex (MHC) proteins. *Res. Immunol.* **140:** 145.

Novotny, J., S. Tonegawa, H. Saito, D.M. Kranz, and H.N. Eisen. 1986. Secondary, tertiary and quaternary structure of T-cell-specific immunoglobulin-like polypeptide chains. *Proc. Natl. Acad. Sci.* **83:** 742.

Okada, C.Y. and I.L. Weissman. 1989. Relative V-beta transcript levels in thymus and peripheral lymphoid tissues from various mouse strains: Inverse correlation of I-E and Mls expression with relative abundance of several V-beta transcripts in peripheral lymphoic tissues. *J. Exp. Med.* **169:** 1703.

Oldstone, M.B.A. 1987. Molecular mimicry and auto-immune disease. *Cell* **50:** 819.

Pereira, P., A. Bandeira, and A. Coutinho. 1989. V-region connectivity in T cell repertoires. *Annu. Rev. Immunol.* **7:** 209.

Prochnicka-Chalufour, A., J.L. Casanova, P. Kourilsky, and J.-M. Claverie. 1989. The extensive structural homology between the H-2K/D/L antigens and the non-polymorphic class I Qa, Tla and "37" molecules suggests they may act as peptide carriers. *Res. Immunol.* **140:** 133.

Pullen, A.M., P. Marrack, and J.W. Kappler. 1988. The T cell repertoire is heavily influenced by tolerance to polymorphic self-antigens. *Nature* **335:** 796.

Ritzel, G., S.A. McCarthy, A. Fotedar, and B. Singh. 1984. Gene conversion may be responsible for the generation of the alloreactive repertoire. *Immunol. Today* **5:** 343.

Saeki, Y., J.-J. Chen, L. Shi, S. Raychaudhuri, and H. Köhler. 1989. Characterization of "regulatory" idiotope-specific T cell clones to a monoclonal anti-idiotypic antibody mimicking a tumor-associated antigen (TAA). *J. Immunol.* **142:** 1046.

Sharrow, S.O., B.J. Mathieson, and A. Singer. 1981. Cell surface appearance of unexpected host MHC determinants on thymocytes from radiation bone marrow chimeras. *J. Immunol.* **126:** 1327.

Singer, A., K.S. Hathcock, and R.J. Hodes. 1981. Self recognition in allogeneic radiation bone marrow chimeras. A radiation-resistant host element dictates the self specificity and immune response gene phenotype of T-helper cells. *J. Exp. Med.* **153:** 1286.

———. 1982. Self recognition in allogeneic thymic chimeras. Self recognition by T helper cells from thymus-engrafted nude mice is restricted to the thymic H-2 haplotype. *J. Exp. Med.* **155:** 339.

Singer, A., T. Mizuochi, T.I. Munitz, and R.E. Gress. 1986. Role of self antigens in the selection of the developing T cell repertoire. In *Progress in immunology: 6th International Congress of Immunology* (ed. B. Cinader and R.G. Miller), vol. 6, p. 60. Academic Press, New York.

Singer, A., T.I. Munitz, H. Golding, A. Rosenberg, and T. Mizuochi. 1987. Recognition requirements for the activation differentiation and function of T-helper cells specific for class I MHC alloantigens. *Immunol. Rev.* **98:** 145.

Smith, C.A., G.T. Williams, R. Kingston, E.J. Jenkinson, and J.T. Owen. 1989. Antibodies to CD3/T-cell receptor complex induce death by apoptosis in immature T cells in thymic cultures. *Nature* **337:** 181.

Sprent, J., D. Lo, E.K. Gao, and Y. Ron. 1988. T cell selection in the thymus. *Immunol. Rev.* **101:** 172.

Weiss, S. and B. Bogen. 1989. B lymphoma cells process and present their endogenous immunoglobulin to MHC-restricted T cells. *Proc. Natl. Acad. Sci.* **86:** 282.

Werdelin, O. 1987. T cells recognize antigen alone and not MHC molecules. *Immunol. Today* **8:** 80.

Wettstein, P.J., L. Jewett, S. Faas, R.L. Brinster, and B.B. Knowles. 1988. SV40 T-antigen is a histocompatibility antigen of SV40-transgenic mice. *Immunogenetics* **27:** 436.

Winchester, G., G.H. Sunshine, N. Nardi, and N.A. Mitchison. 1984. Antigen-presenting cells do not discriminate between self and nonself. *Immunogenetics* **19:** 487.

Zuniga-Pflucker, J.C., D.L. Largs, and A.M. Kruisbeek. 1989. Positive selection of CD4^-CD8^+ T cells in the thymus of normal mice. *Nature* **338:** 76.

T-cell Repertoire and Thymus

P. Marrack,*†‡§** M. Blackman,*† H.-G. Burgert,*† J.M. McCormack,*
J. Cambier,‡¶ T.H. Finkel,† and J. Kappler†‡**
*Howard Hughes Medical Institute at Denver, †Department of Medicine, and ¶Department of Pediatrics, National
Jewish Center, Denver, Colorado 80206; ‡Departments of Microbiology and Immunology, §Biochemistry, Biophysics,
and Genetics, and **Medicine, University of Colorado Health Sciences Center, Denver, Colorado 80206

The α/β T-cell repertoire in any given animal is known to be affected by four factors: the germ line genes available for receptor construction (V_α, J_α, V_β, etc.), positive selection, self-tolerance, and exposure to foreign antigens. In this paper, we discuss two of these phenomena, namely, positive selection and tolerance due to clonal deletion in the thymus.

More than 10 years ago, Bevan (1977) and Zinkernagel et al. (1978) discovered positive selection—thymocytes that mature in a given animal are much more likely to react with a given foreign antigen associated with self-major histocompatibility complex (MHC) than with the same foreign antigen associated with allogeneic MHC. Positive selection, which has since been demonstrated dramatically in transgenic animals (Kisielow et al. 1988a; Sha et al. 1988), is now thought to involve interaction between the receptors on immature thymocytes and MHC molecules on thymus cortical epithelial (TCE) cells. It is very likely that the appropriate thymocyte accessory molecule (CD4 for class-II-restricted cells or CD8 for class-I-restricted cells) is also involved in positive selection (Hung et al. 1988; Zuniga-Pflucker et al. 1989).

Definitive evidence for clonal elimination of self-reactive cells in the thymus has also been produced (Kappler et al. 1987a, 1988; MacDonald et al. 1988b). Elimination appears to involve interaction of α/β receptors on immature thymocytes with MHC molecules (associated with self-antigens) on cells in the thymus (Kisielow et al. 1988b; White et al. 1989). A number of cell types can mediate deletion, including thymus dendritic cells or thymocytes, themselves (Shimonkevitz and Bevan 1988; Matzinger and Guerder 1989). It is possible that any cell bearing the appropriate combination of antigen and self-MHC can cause the elimination of potentially autoreactive immature thymocytes.

The processes of positive selection and clonal deletion appear to be contradictory and self-defeating, since both involve interaction of T-cell receptors and CD4 or CD8 on immature thymocytes with MHC (plus self-antigen) on other cells in the thymus. If both events occur and operate on the same population of thymocytes, how do these cells distinguish between a signal for maturation and a signal for death? Many theories have been put forward to account for this paradox, and they fall into three categories: (1) The receptor on thymocytes changes in some way between the events

inducing selection and deletion (Jerne 1971); (2) selection and deletion are distinguished by the avidity they demand of the thymocyte/MHC interaction (Lo et al. 1986); and (3) selection and deletion involve MHC-presenting cells that bear different versions of self-MHC plus self-peptides (Marrack and Kappler 1987). None of these theories precludes either of the others.

We and other investigators have struggled for a long time to distinguish between these three theories. In this paper, we present data consistent with the first and third of the theories listed above.

MATERIALS AND METHODS

Mice. Mice were purchased from the Jackson Laboratory or bred in the animal care facility at the National Jewish Center. Breeding parents for the 36-2, I-Eα, transgenic animals were kind gifts from Drs. Brinster, Flavell, and Lo. Pregnant females were timed, with the day of plugging termed day zero. To prepare irradiation chimeras, mice were maintained on chlorinated, acidified water and, at the time of irradiation, were protected with gentamicin from acute bacterial infection. As described previously, donors and recipients were given antithymocyte serum 2 days before use (Kappler and Marrack 1978). Animals received 950 rads and 5×10^6 bone marrow cells.

Preparation of TCE cells. TCE cells were prepared as nurse cells, as described previously (Wekerle et al. 1980; Marrack et al. 1989). Treatment with anti-Thy-1 and complement was usually omitted.

Thymus culture. Thymus lobes from day-17 fetal mice were cultured as organs, as described previously (Mandel and Kennedy 1978; Born et al. 1987), with the addition of 20 μg/ml anti-α/β or anti-CD3 antibody.

Analysis of T-cell receptor expression. Peripheral T cells were isolated from lymph nodes after incubation on nylon wool (Julius et al. 1973). Cells from thymuses were analyzed immediately or after 4 hours of incubation. During such incubation, the numbers of receptors on immature thymocytes rise, and analysis of receptors on this population of cells thus becomes easier (Kappler et al. 1988). In some cases, fetal thymuses were cultured as intact organs for several days in the presence or absence of anti-T-cell receptor α/β or anti-CD3 antibody. Such treatment modulates receptor from the surfaces of thymocytes. Therefore, cells from such cultures and controls were incubated for 7–16 hours to allow reexpression of surface receptor prior to analysis.

A collection of biotinylated antireceptor and anti-V_β antibodies was used to stain T cells and thymocytes. Antibodies used included anti-α/β (Kubo et al. 1989), anti-CD3 (Leo et al. 1987), anti-V_β8.1, anti-V_β8.2, and anti-V_β8.3 (Staerz et al. 1985) and anti-V_β17a (Kappler et al. 1987b). Phycoerythrin-conjugated avidin was used to stain cells after incubation with these antibodies, and reactive cells were detected on an EPICS C cytofluorometer.

RESULTS

Factors That Control Positive Selection

Experiments first establishing the existence of positive selection and nearly all experiments studying the phenomenon since have shown that the process involves an interaction between the α/β receptors on developing thymocytes and MHC proteins expressed on thymus stroma (for review, see Sprent and Webb 1987). Consequently, it is of interest to study the structure and function of thymus stromal MHC molecules; this has been done in several ways. Normal T cells do not respond to antigen presented by TCE cells, although we and others have shown that they do present antigen well to T-cell hybridomas (Kyewski et al. 1984; Lorenz and Allen 1989; Marrack et al. 1989). Thymus cortical epithelium is also able to present allogeneic MHC to T-cell hybrids and, in association with MHC, mouse superantigens, such as Mls-1^a, Mls-2^a, and the superantigen engaged by V_β17a$^+$ T cells. Moreover, in some cases, TCE but not spleen cells can be recognized by receptors from syngeneic T cells.

Examples of such presentation are shown in Table 1. Like spleen cells, TCE cells presented exogenously added antigen to antigen-specific, MHC-restricted hybridomas, such as 3DO-8.2 and HTTC. This reactivity was not entirely due to contamination of our TCE preparations with bone marrow-derived cells, because TCE prepared from 36-2 transgenic animals, which express I-E^s on thymus epithelium only, were able to stimulate the T-cell hybrid HTTC in the presence of added cytochrome c.

TCE cells were also able to stimulate allo-specific MHC T-cell hybridomas such as CG4. However, they were not very efficient stimulators of hybridomas, such as QO23, which use V_β17a as part of their α/β receptors and respond to I-E in the presence of a possible superantigen expressed by B cells. TCE cells from BALB/c, I-E^d mice stimulated QO23 poorly. This may have been due to bone-marrow-derived cells contaminating our TCE preparation, because TCE from 36-2 mice did not stimulate QO23 at all. Other V_β17a hybridomas were stimulated by TCE from either BALB/c or 36-2 mice, however (data not shown), suggesting that TCE can, at least sometimes, present the V_β17a ligand (data not shown).

Some T-cell hybridomas, such as 3DO-54.8, were able to respond to syngeneic TCE, but not syngeneic spleen cells, a result that perhaps reflects the phenomenon of positive selection.

Like recognition of antigen/MHC, positive selection seems to pick out receptors based on all of their variable components, V_α, J_α, V_β, and so on. It is therefore quite surprising that, in some cases, the phenomenon of positive selection can be demonstrated even if only one of the variable parts of the receptor is examined—V_β, in all cases studied so far (MacDonald et al. 1988a; Blackman et al. 1989).

For example, as shown in Table 2, CD4$^+$ T cells in SWR animals, which are H-2^q, bear V_β17a quite

Table 1. Recognition of TCE Cells by T Cells

T-cell hybridoma[a]	Specificity	Presenting cell		Class II	Added antigen	Response (IL-2/ml)
CG4	IE^d	BALB/c	sp	IA^d, IE^d	none	2110
QO23	B super/IE	BALB/c	sp	IA^d, IE^d	none	116
3DO-54.8	cOVA/IA^d	BALB/c	sp	IA^d, IE^d	none	<3.2
3DO-8.2	cOVA/IA^d	BALB/c	sp	IA^d, IE^d	cOVA	90
CG4	IE^d	BALB/c	TCE	IA^d, IE^d	none	2490
2Q23	B super/IE	BALB/c	TCE	IA^d, IE^d	none	32
3DO-54.8	cOVA/IA^d	BALB/c	TCE	IA^d, IE^d	none	9.8
QO23	B super/IE	36-2	sp	IA^s	none	<2.2
HTTC	cyt c/IE^s	36-2	sp	IA^s	cyt c	<2.2
QO23	B super/IE	36-2	TCE	IA^s, IE^s	none	<2.2
HTTC	cyt c/IE^s	36-2	TCE	IA^s, IE^s	cyt c	174
QO23	B super/IE	HTT	sp	IA^s, IE^s	none	59
HTTC	cyt c/IE^s	HTT	sp	IA^s, IE^s	cyt c	5040

Abbreviations: (IL-2) Interleukin 2; QO23 is V_β17a$^+$. (sp) Spleen; (B super), a self-superantigen expressed primarily by B cells; (cOVA) chicken ovalbumin peptide 323-339.

[a]Hybridomas were derived and assayed as described previously (Marrack et al. 1989). HTTC, specific for pigeon cytochrome c (cyt c)/IE^s, was the generous gift of Dr. S. Hedrick.

Table 2. Positive Selection Demonstrated by Expression of V_β

Mouse	MHC	$V_\beta 17a$ expression	
		CD4[+]	CD8[+]
SWR	q	18.9 ± 1.0	5.0 ± 0.6
C57BL	b	2.8 ± 0.2	6.3 ± 0.7
(C57BL × SWR)F$_1$	b × q	11.2 ± 0.5	5.2 ± 0.3

Data from Blackman et al. (1989).

frequently. In contrast, CD4[+] T cells in H-2^b, C57BL mice only use $V_\beta 17a$ rarely. F$_1$ animals, expressing both H-2^q and H-2^b, have intermediate levels of $V_\beta 17a$-bearing CD4[+] T cells, indicating that the difference in $V_\beta 17a$ expression between the two MHC haplotypes is not due to deletion of $V_\beta 17a^+$ T cells in the presence of H-2^b, a phenomenon that would be dominant in F$_1$ mice. Experiments with chimeras show that this over-expression of $V_\beta 17a$ in the presence of H-2^q is controlled by the expression of H-2^q by thymus stroma (Blackman et al. 1989). Therefore, this is a manifestation of positive selection demonstrated, in this case, not by a single receptor but by the pool of receptors, including $V_\beta 17a$ and many versions of the other variable receptor components.

Several hypotheses (described above) that have been put forward to account for positive selection have suggested that the process involves recognition by T-cell receptors of MHC-bound peptides, as well as the MHC proteins themselves. We and other workers have published some experiments supporting this idea (Marrack et al. 1989; Murphy et al. 1989). Also, we have noticed that positive selection, at least as measured at the level of V_β expression, involves non-MHC gene products, as well as those of the MHC. Such a result is consistent with the idea that peptides are involved in positive selection.

An illustration of this finding is shown in Table 3. $V_\beta 17a^+$, CD4[+] T cells are present at high levels in SWR mice but are not so frequent in B10.QβBR animals, even though the two strains are identical at MHC.

Again, the phenomenon seems to be due to positive selection, because mice that are F$_1$s of these two strains also contain $V_\beta 17a^+$ T cells at high frequency. Preliminary examination of chimeras between the two strains suggests that this phenomenon is controlled by non-thymus stromal, bone-marrow-derived cells. Although

Table 3. Non-MHC Genes Can Affect Positive Selection

Mouse	$V_\beta 17a$ expression	
	CD4[+]	CD8[+]
SWR[a]	18.9 ± 1.0	5.0 ± 0.6
B10.QβBR[a]	13.2 ± 0.5	3.7 ± 0.2
(B10.QβBR × SWR)F$_1$	17.5 ± 0.5	6.9 ± 0.1
SWR → B10.Q[b]	20.7 ± 0.4	5.5 ± 1.3

All mice in this analysis are H-2^q.
[a]Data from Blackman et al. (1989) and Kappler et al. (1989).
[b]Chimeric animals, created by injection of SWR bone marrow cells into B10.Q, lethally irradiated recipients.

these data are potentially interesting and may introduce a new approach to the study of positive selection, a number of experiments must still be done before we can conclude that this result is really a manifestation of positive selection.

Factors That Control Clonal Deletion

We and other investigators have shown that T-cell tolerance is caused, at least in part, by clonal deletion of potentially self-reactive cells in the thymus. Our recent experiments and those of others have suggested that immature, CD4[+], CD8[+], double-positive cortical thymocytes can be deleted and that both the α/β receptor and CD4 or CD8 are involved (White et al. 1989). Evidence in favor of this stems from the observation that mice expressing a transgenic T-cell receptor and its ligand delete all T cells bearing high levels of the receptor and CD4 or CD8; however, in some cases, T cells bearing the same receptor but lower levels or no CD4 or CD8 are allowed to survive. Such animals also contain no CD4[+], CD8[+] thymocytes (Kisielow et al. 1988b). Also, mice expressing I-E lack $V_\beta 17a^+$, CD8[+], as well as $V_\beta 17a^+$, CD4[+] cells (Kappler et al. 1989). Peripheral T cells bearing CD8 and $V_\beta 17a$ do not, however, often recognize I-E (H.-G. Burgert et al., in prep.), suggesting that the precursors of CD8[+] peripheral T cells must have been deleted by I-E at a time when they bore CD4 as well as CD8.

It has recently been reported that anti-CD3 antibodies cause the death of all developing, receptor-bearing thymocytes in fetal thymus organ cultures (Smith et al. 1989). In the past, we have reported similar experiments, using anti-V_β antibodies, but obtained different results (Born et al. 1987). In our experiments, mature thymocytes bearing the target V_βs did not develop under such conditions, but immature cells bearing the V_βs did. Concerned about this discrepancy, we repeated the organ culture experiments using two hamster monoclonal antibodies, one specific for CD3 and the other specific for T-cell receptor α/β polypeptides. An example of our results is shown in Table 4.

The cells in fetal thymus lobes cultured without antibody continued in an orderly way through their development. Immature cells, bearing variable and low levels of α/β receptor, increased in numbers, and mature thymocytes bearing high levels of receptors subsequently arose, comprising 22% of all thymocytes after 90 hours of incubation. Addition of anti-CD3 caused the disappearance of all receptor-bearing immature and mature cells, as Smith et al. (1989) described. Anti-α/β antibody did not have exactly the same effect, however. Like anti-CD3, it did prevent the appearance of mature, high-density receptor-positive cells, but it only caused the disappearance of about half the immature, low-density receptor-positive cells. We have noticed that a similar percentage of receptor-bearing immature cells are spared deletion due to self- or exogenous antigens in vivo; moreover, our preliminary experiments in vitro suggest that the same cells are

Table 4. Not All Immature α/β Receptor-bearing Thymocytes Can Be Deleted by α/β Ligation

Thymus culture conditions[a]	Cells recovered (% control)/thymus lobe[c]		
	total	immature α/β^+	mature α/β^+
41 hr, no MAb[b]	34.0 (100)	22.5 (100)	0.5 (100)
41 hr, anti-α/β[b]	28.0 (82)	12.5 (56)	0.1 (20)
41 hr, anti-CD3[b]	15.0 (44)	4.8 (21)	0.03 (6)
64 hr, no MAb	34.0 (100)	16.3 (100)	4.5 (100)
64 hr, anti-α/β	18.0 (53)	6.9 (42)	0.02 (0.4)
64 hr, anti-CD3	12.0 (35)	1.6 (10)	0.02 (0.4)
90 hr, no MAb	21.0 (100)	6.1 (100)	4.5 (100)
90 hr, anti-α/β	16.0 (76)	4.4 (72)	0.1 (2)
90 hr, anti-CD3	10.0 (48)	0.4 (7)	0.02 (0.4)

[a]Thymus lobes from 17-day C3H/HeJ fetal mice were cultured for the indicated lengths of time.

[b]Thymuses were cultured with no added antibody (MAb) or with 20 μg/ml anti-α/β or anti-CD3 MAbs.

[c]Results shown are the numbers of cells recovered $\times 10^{-4}$ per thymus lobe. Values in parentheses indicate the percentage of recoveries by comparison with thymuses cultured without antibody.

spared deletion by anti-α/β antibody or by antigen. Therefore, we do not believe that this phenomenon is an artifactual consequence of some peculiarity of the anti-α/β antibody.

In preliminary experiments, we have examined the ability of mature T cells, immature thymocytes, and thymocytes that cannot be deleted by anti-α/β antibody to flux Ca^{++} in response to various stimuli. All cells mobilize Ca^{++} and allow entry of extracellular Ca^{++} in response to anti-CD3 antibody. In contrast, anti-α/β antibody only stimulated a mature Ca^{++} response in mature thymocytes or T cells. The antibody stimulated release of Ca^{++} from intracellular stores only in about half of all immature, receptor-positive thymocytes and caused very little Ca^{++} flux of any description in the immature thymocytes that are resistant to deletion by antigen or anti-α/β.

DISCUSSION

To understand positive selection, our laboratory has focused on two problems: (1) the properties of the cells in the thymus thought to control positive selection, i.e., TCE cells, and (2) the genetics that govern which T cells are selected and which are not.

TCE cells can only be isolated by a very laborious procedure, as thymus nurse cells (Wekerle et al. 1980). Such preparations are, of necessity, contaminated at least with thymocytes, themselves, and also perhaps with bone-marrow-derived cells such as macrophages or dendritic cells. Data from nurse cell experiments must therefore be interpreted cautiously. Some conclusions can be drawn from our experiments, however. Cortical epithelial cells are able to present conventional antigens and at least some superantigens, the latter with efficiences not necessarily the same as those of spleen cells. In some cases, class II molecules on these cells can also be recognized by syngeneic T-cell re-

ceptors, receptors that do not engage class II on syngeneic spleen. At the very least, these data suggest that MHC molecules on thymus cortical epithelium may not always be identical to those found on other cells, perhaps because different self-peptides or self-superantigens are bound to MHC on different cell types to different extents. Because different cells certainly synthesize different spectra of proteins, this is not a particularly surprising idea. Conclusions similar to this have also been drawn from antibody staining experiments (Murphy et al. 1989).

Although subtle and not-so-subtle differences in MHC/peptide complexes expressed by TCE cells and other cell types might account for the paradox of positive selection and self-tolerance, it is not by any means clear from experiments performed so far that this is so. It is particularly unnerving that only about half of the T-cell hybridomas tested so far respond to MHC on syngeneic TCE cells; in addition, it is disappointing that syngeneic responses of this type are always small (Marrack et al. 1989). Perhaps these results in themselves are a clue to the secrets of positive selection and indicate that low avidity interactions are, in fact, part of the process.

Many investigators have pointed out that thymus MHC is implicated in positive selection; this can be measured at the level of individual receptors and even for receptors falling into a large, particular group, such as those bearing the same V_β (MacDonald et al. 1988a; Blackman et al. 1989). A clue to positive selection may be found in the fact that non-MHC genes also seem to control positive selection. SWR and SJL mice all select a higher percentage of $V_\beta 17a^+$ cells than their H-2 identical or similar counterparts on the C57BL background.

Clonal deletion is known to occur in the thymus and operates on double-positive immature and perhaps also single-positive mature thymocytes. Recently, we have shown that in the presence of a superantigen such as Mls-1[a], not all potentially responsive immature thymocytes are eliminated. On the contrary, different superantigens eliminate different percentages of immature cells. The staphylococcal enterotoxin, SEB, for example, eliminates about 50% of all cortical thymocytes, bearing $V_\beta 3$ and $V_\beta 8$s, with which it can interact, whereas Mls-1[a] eliminates about 25% of all $V_\beta 6$-bearing cells. In contrast, all mature cells bearing the appropriate V_β disappear in the presence of a superantigen administered or present at birth (White et al. 1989).

In this paper, we describe similar results using fetal thymus organ culture and an anti-α/β antibody. An anti-CD3 antibody, for comparison, eliminated all receptor-bearing immature thymocytes. These and other results have led us to conclude that immature receptor-bearing cells actually fall into two different subpopulations; one unable to trigger release of intracellular pools of Ca^{++} after engagement of α/β, and another that can release intracellular Ca^{++} stores after a similar event. The two pools of cells appear to differ in the extent to which their α/β polypeptides are coupled to CD3. Perhaps the nondeletable population lacks a component of CD3.

The existence of two populations of immature thymocytes with different receptor/CD3 associations suggests the following possibilities:

1. It seems likely that the two populations are related, e.g., the nondeletable, receptor-positive cells may be the precursors of the deletable, immature thymocytes.
2. The forces of tolerance, which act by receptor engagement of self-MHC plus self-peptides or superantigens, can operate only on the subpopulation of thymocytes that can be killed by receptor engagement.
3. Perhaps some other phenomenon is initiated by engagement of receptor on the nondeletable thymocytes, e.g., positive selection.
4. Given that receptors on the nondeletable population do not transduce signals very effectively, perhaps positive selection is signaled primarily by CD4 or CD8, which will engage the ligand causing selection with the receptor. The receptor, itself, in this case, may serve only to bind the thymocyte to its selecting target and transduce either no signal at all or a signal that does not include changes in Ca^{++} levels.
5. Receptors on the two populations of thymocytes differ in some way in their degree of receptor/CD3 coupling. Perhaps receptors that are relatively "loosely" associated with CD3 can engage MHC molecules more effectively than those that are tightly coupled, such as those on the deletable thymocytes and mature thymocytes and peripheral T cells. Loose coupling may therefore allow binding of receptor to self-MHC in a fashion that is prohibited on a more mature cell. This may account for the ability of the thymus to select cells both positively and negatively for recognition of self.

ACKNOWLEDGMENTS

We thank Ella Kushnir, Rhonda Richards, Terri Wade, and Janice White very much for their excellent technical assistance. This work was supported by grants AI-17134, AI-18785, and AI-22295 from the National Institutes of Health. T.H.F. and H.-G.B. are the recipients of an Arthritis Foundation Postdoctoral Fellowship and a Deutsche Forschungsgemeinschaft Fellowship, respectively.

REFERENCES

Bevan, M. 1977. In a radiation chimera host H-2 antigens determine the immune responsiveness of donor cytotoxic cells. *Nature* **269:** 417.

Blackman, M.A., P. Marrack, and J. Kappler. 1989. Influence of the major histocompatibility complex on positive thymic selection of Vβ17a[+] T cells. *Science* **244:** 214.

Born, W., M. McDuffie, N. Roehm, E. Kushnir, J. White, D. Thorpe, J. Stephano, J. Kappler, and P. Marrack. 1987. Expression and role of the T cell receptor in early thymocyte differentiation in vitro. *J. Immunol.* **138:** 999.

Hung, S.T., P. Kisielow, B. Scott, H. Kishi, Y. Uematsu, H. Bluthmann, and H. von Boehmer. 1988. Thymic major histocompatibility complex antigens and the $\alpha\beta$ T cell receptor determine the CD4/CD8 phenotype of T cells. *Nature* **335:** 229.

Jerne, N. 1971. The somatic generation of antibody diversity. *Eur. J. Immunol.* **1:** 1.

Julius, M., E. Simpson, and L. Herzenberg. 1973. A rapid method for the isolation of functional thymus-derived lymphocytes. *Eur. J. Immunol.* **3:** 645.

Kappler, J. and P. Marrack. 1978. The role of H-2 linked genes in helper T cell function. IV. Importance of T cell genotype and host environment in I region and Ir gene expression. *J. Exp. Med.* **128:** 1510.

Kappler, J.W., E. Kushnir, and P. Marrack. 1989. Analysis of Vβ17a expression in new mouse strains bearing the Vβ[a] haplotype. *J. Exp. Med.* **169:** 1533.

Kappler, J., N. Roehm, and P. Marrack. 1987a. T cell tolerance by clonal elimination in the thymus. *Cell* **49:** 273.

Kappler, J.W., U. Staerz, J. White, and P.C. Marrack. 1988. Self-tolerance eliminates T cells specific for Mls-modified products of the major histocompatibility complex. *Nature* **332:** 35.

Kappler, J., T. Wade, J. White, E. Kushnir, M. Blackman, J. Bill, R. Roehm, and P. Marrack. 1987b. A T cell receptor Vβ segment that imparts reactivity to a class II major histocompatibility complex product. *Cell* **49:** 263.

Kisielow, P., H. Teh, H. Blüthmann, and H. von Boehmer. 1988a. Positive selection of antigen-specific T cells in thymus by restricting MHC molecules. *Nature* **335:** 730.

Kisielow, P., H. Blüthmann, U.D. Staerz, M. Steinmetz, and H. von Boehmer. 1988b. Tolerance in T-cell-receptor transgenic mice involves deletion of nonmature CD4[+]8[+] thymocytes. *Nature* **333:** 742.

Kubo, R.T., W. Born, J. Kappler, P. Marrack, and M. Pigeon. 1989. Characterization of a monoclonal antibody which detects all murine α/β T cell receptors. *J. Immunol.* **142:** 2736.

Kyewski, B., C.G. Fathman, and H.S. Kaplan. 1984. Intrathymic presentation of circulating non-major histocompatibility complex antigens. *Nature* **308:** 196.

Leo, O., M. Foo, D. Sachs, L. Samelson, and J. Bluestone. 1987. Identification of a monoclonal antibody specific for a murine T3 polypeptide. *Proc. Natl. Acad. Sci.* **84:** 1374.

Lo, D., Y. Ron, and J. Sprent. 1986. Induction of MHC-restricted specificity and tolerance in the thymus. *Immunol. Res.* **5:** 221.

Lorenz, R.G. and P. Allen. 1989. Thymic cortical epithelial cells can present self antigens *in vivo*. *Nature* **337**: 560.

MacDonald, H.R., R.K. Lees, R. Schneider, R.M. Zinkernagel, and H. Hengartner. 1988a. Positive selection of CD4[+] thymocytes controlled by MHC class II gene products. *Nature* **336**: 471.

MacDonald, H.R., R. Schneider, R.K. Lees, R.C. Howe, H. Acha-Orbea, H. Festenstein, R.M. Zinkernagel, and H. Hengartner. 1988b. T-cell receptor Vβ use predicts reactivity and tolerance of Mls[a]-encoded antigens. *Nature* **332**: 40.

Mandel, T.H. and M.M. Kennedy. 1978. The differentiation of murine thymocytes in vivo and in vitro. *Immunology* **35**: 317.

Marrack, P. and J. Kappler. 1987. The T cell receptor. *Science* **238**: 1073.

Marrack, P., J. McCormack, and J. Kappler. 1989. Presentation of antigen, foreign major histocompatibility complex proteins and self by thymus cortical epithelium. *Nature* **338**: 503.

Matzinger, P. and S. Guerder. 1989. Does T-cell tolerance require a dedicated antigen presenting cell? *Nature* **338**: 74.

Murphy, D.B., D. Lo, S. Rath, R.L. Brinster, R.A. Flavell, A. Slanetz, and C.A. Janeway. 1989. A novel MHC Class II epitope expressed in thymus medulla but not cortex. *Nature* **338**: 765.

Sha, W., C. Nelson, R. Newberry, D. Kranz, J. Russell, and D. Loh. 1988. Positive and negative selection of an antigen receptor on T cells in transgenic mice. *Nature* **336**: 73.

Shimonkevitz, R.P. and M.J. Bevan. 1988. Split tolerance induced by intrathymic adoptive transfer of thymocyte stem cells. *J. Exp. Med.* **168**: 143.

Smith, C.A., G.T. Williams, R. Kingston, E.J. Jenkinson, and J.J.T. Owen. 1989. Antibodies to the CD3/T-cell receptor complex induce apoptosis (controlled cell death) in immature T-cells in thymic cultures. *Nature* **337**: 181.

Sprent, J. and S. Webb. 1987. Function and specificity of T cell subsets in the mouse. *Adv. Immunol.* **41**: 39.

Staerz, U., H. Rammansee, J. Benedetto, and M. Bevan. 1985. Characterization of a murine monoclonal antibody specific for an allotypic determinant on T cell antigen receptor. *J. Immunol.* **134**: 3994.

Wekerle, H., U.-P. Ketelsen, and M. Ernst. 1980. Thymic nurse cells. Lymphoepithelial cell complexes in murine thymuses: Morphological and serological characterization. *J. Exp. Med.* **151**: 925.

White, J., A. Herman, A.M. Pullen, R. Kubo, J. Kappler, and P. Marrack. 1989. The Vβ-specific superantigen Staphylococcal enterotoxin B: Stimulation of mature T cells and clonal deletion in neonatal mice. *Cell* **56**: 27.

Zinkernagel, R., G. Callahan, A. Althage, S. Cooper, P. Klein, and J. Klein. 1978. On the thymus in the differentiation of H-2 self-recognition by T cells: Evidence for dual recognition? *J. Exp. Med.* **147**: 882.

Zuniga-Pflucker, J.C., S.A. McCarthy, M. Weston, D.L. Longo, A. Singer, and A.M. Kruisbeek. 1989. Role of CD4 in thymocytes: Selection and maturation. *J. Exp. Med.* **169**: 2085.

Control of T-cell Development by the TCRαβ for Antigen

H. von Boehmer,* H. Kishi,* P. Borgulya,* B. Scott,* W. van Ewijk,‡
H.S. Teh,† and P. Kisielow§

*Basel Insitute for Immunology, CH-4058 Basel, Switzerland; †Department of Microbiology, University
of British Columbia, Vancouver, Canada V6T 1W5; ‡Department of Cell Biology II and Immunology,
Erasmus University, Rotterdam, The Netherlands; §Institute of Immunology and Experimental Therapy,
Polish Academy of Sciences, Wroclaw, Poland

Experiments concerned with the selection of the T-cell repertoire have a relatively long history and were conducted even before we knew about the T-cell receptor (TCR) and antigen-presenting major histocompatibility complex (MHC) molecules. Early experiments consistent with clonal deletion (von Boehmer and Sprent 1976; Good et al. 1983) as well as with positive selection (Bevan 1977; von Boehmer et al. 1978; Kappler and Marrack 1978; Zinkernagel et al. 1978) were the subject of much debate because of the indirect nature of these experiments. At the time, it was impossible to reach firm conclusions about mechanisms and extent of selection. Evidence for deletion, for instance, rested on negative experiments failing to reveal suppression in tolerant animals. In addition, it was not clear whether or not deletion could occur at any stage of T-cell development or, as suggested by Lederberg (1959), had to occur early in development. Experiments concerned with positive selection were interpreted as experimental artifacts in X-irradiation chimeras (Doherty et al. 1981; Wagner et al. 1981), an imprecise bending of a T-cell repertoire involving either somatic mutation (Bevan and Hünig 1981) or suppressor cells (Matzinger 1981) or a precise selection implying dual recognition of an MHC molecule and antigen by T cells (von Boehmer et al. 1978; Zinkernagel et al. 1978).

The realization that only one receptor carried the specificity of T cells for antigens and also for presenting MHC molecules (Dembic et al. 1986; Saito et al. 1987), as well as observations that somatic mutation did not contribute significantly to the diversity of TCRs, set a limit for possible interpretations and made it even more of a challenge to address the questions of repertoire selection by more conclusive experimentation. We chose to do this in TCR transgenic mice. This allowed us to follow the selection of MHC-restricted receptors expressed by many T cells in different environments by the use of receptor-specific monoclonal antibodies, rather than assessing selection indirectly by determining T-cell specificity after in vivo priming and restimulation in vitro or after in vitro activation of T cells.

EXPERIMENTAL PROCEDURES

All experimental procedures have been described previously in the papers cited in the Results section.

RESULTS

Expression of TCR Transgenes

The α and β TCR transgenes were obtained from a $CD4^-8^+$ T-cell clone specific for male (HY) antigen in the context of $H-2D^b$ MHC molecules (Krimpenfort et al. 1988; Uematsu et al. 1988; Kisielow et al. 1988b; Blüthmann et al. 1988). Both transgenes are expressed unusually early in T-cell development: In mice carrying the β transgene only the transgenic β chain appears on the surface of $CD4^-8^-$ thymocytes by day 14–15 of gestation. An antibody to these transgenic β chains precipitates a dimer in which the partner chain is encoded by neither α, γ, nor δ TCR chains (von Boehmer et al. 1988; see below). The early expression of the β transgene completely prevents the rearrangement of endogenous V_β gene segments (Uematsu et al. 1988). The surface density of the dimer is relatively low and comparable with that of the $TCR\alpha\beta$ on immature $CD4^+8^+$ thymocytes in normal mice.

The picture is different in $\alpha\beta$ transgenic mice where the transgenic β chain is expressed at high levels on $CD4^-8^-$ thymocytes and is paired with the transgenic α chain (Fig. 1). These pre-T cells in $\alpha\beta$ transgenic mice can be induced to grow by T-cell lectins and interleukin-2. The in vivo progeny of these cells, the $CD4^+8^+$ thymocytes, however, are nonresponsive and express fewer $TCR\alpha\beta$s than their precursors. This implies that during the transition from $CD4^-8^-$ to $CD4^+8^+$ cells the signal transduction is altered and the expression of TCR is reduced probably by some alteration in the expression of CD3 proteins that are associated with the receptor.

The early expression of the $TCR\alpha\beta$ inhibits the rearrangement of endogenous V_β and V_α gene segments to a different extent: On the one hand, in $H-2D^b$ $\alpha\beta$ transgenic female mice, all $CD4^+8^-$ and about half of

CD4⁻8⁻ αβ TRANSGENIC MALE THYMOCYTES

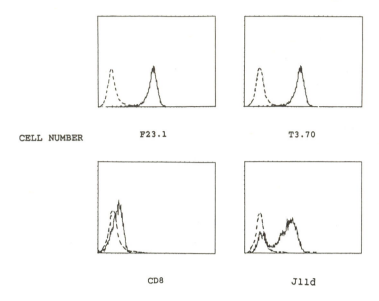

CELL NUMBER   F23.1   T3.70

CD8   J11d

Figure 1. Staining of CD4⁻8⁻ thymocytes by F23.1 (specific for the transgenic β chain), T3.70 (specific for the transgenic α chain), and M1/69 antibodies. The thymocytes were prepared from female TCRαβ transgenic mice.

the CD4⁻8⁺ mature T cells express full-size α RNA transcribed from endogenous TCRα genes in addition to α RNA transcribed from the α transgene. This could be analyzed because the transcripts from the endogenous α locus differ in an 18-bp insertion of the 3′ untranslated regions from the transcripts of the α transgene. By sequential immunoprecipitation, it could be shown that several T-cell clones from αβ transgenic female mice expressed two different receptors, one containing the endogenous and the other the transgenic TCRα chain (Fig. 2). On the other hand, inhibition of rearrangement of endogenous V_β gene segments was much stronger: The vast majority of receptors in the αβ transgenic mice use only the transgenic β chain (Kisielow et al. 1988b; Teh et al. 1988). The early expression of the transgenic β chain with or without α chain in αβ transgenic or β transgenic mice, respectively, affected also the expression of γδ receptors in these mice: The TCR transgenic mice contained no detect-

able γδ cells in their thymus and all CD3-positive cells expressed the transgenic β chain (von Boehmer et al. 1988).

Consequences of TCR Gene Introduction into SCID Mice

Because of the difficulty in analyzing T-cell-repertoire selection in mice expressing different TCRα chains even in a single cell, we introduced productively rearranged TCR genes by breeding into SCID mice (Bosma et al. 1983). By this procedure, we were aiming at mice that express only a single TCR.

In nontransgenic SCID mice the thymus is small, containing 1×10^6 to 2×10^6 lymphoid cells, all of which lack CD4 and CD8 coreceptor molecules. The introduction of productively rearranged α and β transgenes alters this picture drastically in that the thymus of αβ transgenic SCID mice now contains 5×10^7 to $8 \times$

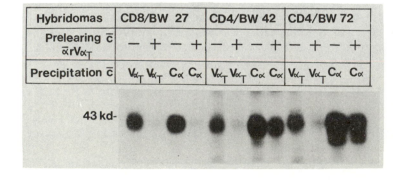

Hybridomas	CD8/BW 27				CD4/BW 42				CD4/BW 72			
Prelearing c̄ / ᾱrVα_T	−	+	−	+	−	+	−	+	−	+	−	+
Precipitation c̄	Vα_T	Vα_T	Cα	Cα	Vα_T	Vα_T	Cα	Cα	Vα_T	Vα_T	Cα	Cα

43 kd-

Figure 2. T-cell receptors on T-cell hybridomas from CD4⁻8⁺ and CD4⁺8⁻ lymph node T cells in αβ transgenic mice. Lymph node T cells from αβ transgenic mice were separated into CD4⁺ or CD8⁺ T cells by sorting and were fused with the BW100 thymoma. CD8/BW27 is derived from a CD8⁺4⁻ T cell. CD4/BW42 and CD8/BW27 are derived from CD4⁺8⁻ T cells. These three hybridomas express transgenic TCRαβ on their surface. Cell-surface proteins of the hybridomas were iodinated. TCR in cell lysates were precleared using rabbit antiserum against recombinant transgenic V_α peptide (V_αT). After or before preclearing, TCRs were precipitated by antirecombinant V_αT or rabbit anti-C_α antibody. Immunoprecipitates were analyzed on 10% SDS-PAGE under reducing conditions.

10^7 lymphoid cells, most of which express CD4 and CD8 coreceptors in addition to the transgenic receptor (Fig. 3). This shows that in SCID mice, the only defect with regard to T-cell development is the defective rearrangement mechanism, which can be corrected by the introduction of productively rearranged TCR genes (Scott et al. 1989).

In normal mice, only about 50% of the CD4$^+$8$^+$ thymocytes express a TCR$\alpha\beta$ on the cell surface (for review, see von Boehmer 1988). This may be due to incomplete α rearrangement in this population. We wished to determine whether β rearrangement was sufficient to allow differentiation of CD4$^-$8$^-$ thymocytes into CD4$^+$8$^+$ progeny. We found that indeed the introduction of the TCRβ transgene into SCID mice allowed the formation of some CD4$^+$8$^+$ thymocytes. The thymuses of various β transgenic SCID mice, however, contained only 2×10^6 to 4×10^6 thymocytes in contrast with $\alpha\beta$ transgenic SCID mice, which contained well over 5×10^7 thymocytes (Fig. 4). This result indicates that α rearrangement is required either for the expansion of CD4$^+$8$^+$ cells or, more likely, for the expression of CD4 and CD8 coreceptors. We think the second possibility is more likely because CD4$^+$8$^+$ thymocytes do not significantly expand and go only through one or two cell divisions. It was noticed by us previously that in TCR transgenic SCID mice, endogenous α genes can

occasionally rearrange productively. Infrequent α rearrangement in β transgenic SCID mice may therefore limit the number of CD4$^+$8$^+$ thymocytes.

Regarding the expression of the TCR transgene in β transgenic SCID mice, we found that all thymocytes expressed the β transgene on the cell surface, again at relatively low density (Fig. 4). This supports our earlier notion that the surface expression of this gene on immature thymocytes does not require any other chain encoded by rearranging genes (von Boehmer et al. 1988): SCID mice are grossly defective in TCR gene rearrangement, and therefore at least a portion of immature SCID thymocytes should lack productive TCR gene rearrangements.

In summary, the introduction of TCR genes into SCID mice has shown that first, the TCRβ chain, encoded by rearranging gene segments, can be expressed on immature thymocytes as a dimer without the participation of any other known TCR chain. Second, only the defective rearrangement mechanism prevents T-cell development in SCID mice. Third, α rearrangement is required to obtain normal numbers of CD4$^+$8$^+$ thymocytes. Fourth, the expression of CD4 and CD8 coreceptors and the expansion of CD4$^+$8$^+$ thymocytes depend on TCR rearrangement but not on the expression of a TCR with a certain specificity on the cell surface since we find near normal numbers of thymocytes in $\alpha\beta$

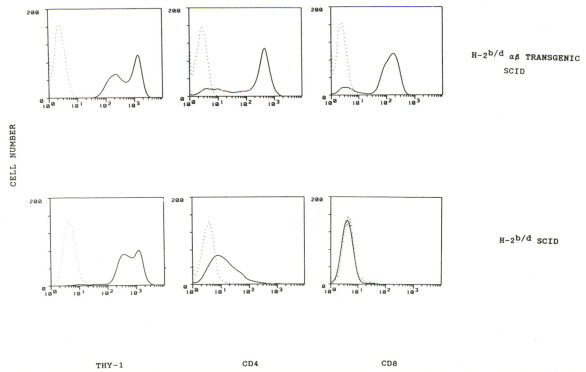

Figure 3. Staining of thymocytes from female TCR$\alpha\beta$ transgenic SCID mice (*top*) and from SCID mice (*bottom*) with CD4 and CD8 antibodies. The thymus of the TCR transgenic mice contained 8×10^7, and the thymus of the SCID mice contained 2×10^6 lymphoid cells. (Reprinted, with permission, from Scott et al. 1989.).

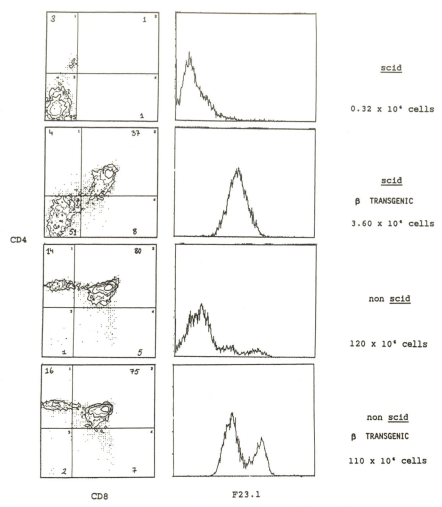

Figure 4. Staining of thymocytes from various offspring of a cross between F_1 (SCID × TCRβ transgenic) hybrids and homozygous SCID mice. The F_1 hybrids expressed the TCRβ transgene. Thymocytes were analyzed by double staining with CD4 and CD8 antibodies (*left*, contour plots) and the F23.1 antibody specific for the transgenic β chain (*right*, histograms).

transgenic SCID mice that express H-2D^d MHC antigens, i.e. antigens not detected by the transgenic TCR (see below).

Development of Mature T Cells Requires an Interaction of the TCR with Thymic MHC Antigen

A significant difference between female αβ transgenic H-2D^d and H-2D$^{b/d}$ SCID mice is not in the number of thymocytes but in the composition of thymocyte subsets: The former contains neither CD4$^+$8$^-$ nor CD4$^-$8$^+$, whereas the latter contains a high proportion of CD4$^-$8$^+$ thymocytes expressing the αβ transgenic receptor (Fig. 5). This observation is well in line with the hypothesis that the development of mature T cells requires a TCR/MHC interaction and that the class of the MHC ligand determines the CD4/CD8 phenotype of the mature T cells (von Boehmer 1986). In other words, binding of the TCRαβ on immature thymocytes to either class I or class II thymic MHC antigens will yield CD4$^-$8$^+$ and CD4$^+$8$^-$ T cells, respectively.

By injecting T-cell-depleted bone marrow cells into various lethally X-irradiated MHC congenic mouse strains, it could be shown that the positive selection of CD4$^-$8$^+$ T cells expressing the transgenic receptor required the presence of the restricting H-2D^b MHC molecule (the transgenic receptor is specific for male antigen in the context of H-2D^b) in the thymus of female mice (Kisielow et al. 1988a). Because all of the hematopoietic reconstitutions were carried out with cells expressing H-2D^b MHC molecules, these experiments indicated that the positive selection required expression of selecting H-2D^b MHC antigens on epithelial cells. By histological examination, the phenotypic changes associated with positive selection are mostly visible in the medulla, which contained a high proportion of CD4$^-$8$^+$-positive cells, whereas the cortex in these αβ transgenic mice appeared normal (W. van Ewijk et al., in prep.). The staining of sections of thymocytes with TCR antibodies did not reveal any clustering of TCRs in lymphocytes in contact with thymus epithelium, i.e., these techniques did not allow

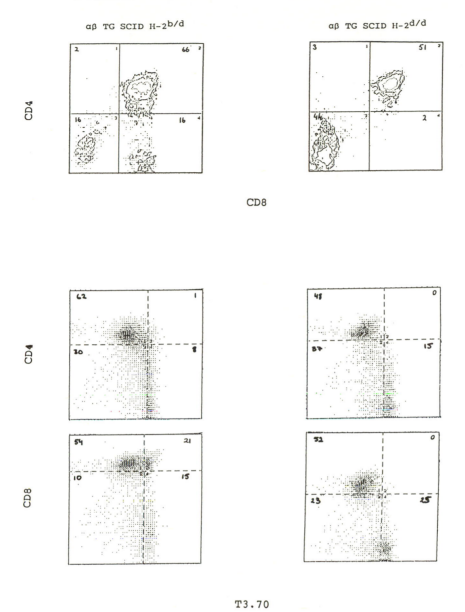

T3.70

Figure 5. Staining of thymocytes from female TCRαβ transgenic SCID mice expressing different H-2 (MHC) antigens. The antibodies used in the double-staining experiments are shown in the Y and X axis of the various plots (Reprinted, with permission, from Scott et al. 1989.)

detection of the binding of the TCR to thymic epithelial cells in female mice.

Binding of the TCR to MHC Plus Peptide Eliminates CD4$^+$8$^+$ Nonfunctional Thymocytes

In male αβ transgenic H-2D^b mice the outer and inner cortex was devoid of CD4$^+$8$^+$immature thymocytes (Kisielow et al. 1988b; W. van Ewijk et al. 1989), and the thymus was small in size. In non-SCID αβ transgenic male mice, the number of peripheral T cells expressing the transgenic receptor and high levels of CD8 was reduced and compensated for by CD4$^-$8$^-$ or CD4$^-$8^{low} cells with normal levels of the transgenic receptor. Curiously, in αβ transgenic non-SCID male

mice, the number of CD4$^+$8$^-$ T cells with the transgenic β but endogenous α chain was also strongly reduced. Because these CD4$^+$8$^-$ T cells are not male-specific (Kisielow et al. 1988b), their reduction in αβ transgenic male mice implied that they were derived from male-specific CD8-positive precursors, which were deleted in male mice. We believe that the precursors must express CD8 because CD4$^-$8$^-$ cells expressing the transgenic TCRαβ are not deleted in male mice. Our conclusion therefore is that the CD4$^+$8$^-$ T cells are derived from CD4$^+$8$^+$ precursors that express transgenic receptors. Thus, in female αβ transgenic mice, endogenous TCRα segments will rearrange in CD4$^+$8$^+$ cells, and certain endogenous α chains will pair better than the transgenic α chain with the transgenic β chain and form new receptors selectable by class II H-2^b MHC antigens. This conclusion is well in line with the observation that all CD4$^+$8$^-$ cells that do not express the transgenic α chain on the cell surface nevertheless contain normal levels of transgenic α RNA. In male mice, CD4$^+$8$^+$ thymocytes can be deleted before the expression of endogenous TCRα chains, and therefore the number of CD4$^+$8$^-$ T cells is reduced. The residual CD4$^+$8$^-$ T cells in these mice must be derived from CD4$^+$8$^+$ precursors that already expressed endogenous α chains even before CD8 molecules appeared on the cell surface.

In contrast with positive selection by MHC antigens in the absence of nominal antigen, which requires MHC antigen expression on thymus epithelial cells, it is sufficient for deletion to occur if MHC molecules and HY antigen are expressed on hematopoietic cells in the thymus. This was concluded from experiments in X-irradiated chimeras where stem cells from αβ transgenic H-2^b male mice were injected in lethally X-irradiated B10.D2 recipients (Fig. 6). In this situation, the thymus epithelium of the recipient expressed inappropriate MHC antigens, and positive selection of T cells with the transgenic TCRαβ did not occur. Nevertheless, the cortex of these mice was depleted of CD4$^+$8$^+$ thymocytes despite the fact that the only tissue expressing H-2D^b MHC antigens and male antigens was of hematopoietic origin.

Have All Peripheral T Cells Undergone Positive Selection by Thymic Epithelial Cells?

It appears that certain T-cell subsets do not have to undergo positive selection by MHC antigens or thymic epithelial cells: In H-2^d αβ transgenic SCID mice, we noted that peripheral lymphoid organs contained CD4$^-$8$^-$ T lymphocytes expressing the transgenic αβ receptor. Actually, the total number of these cells in H-2^d αβ transgenic SCID mice was similar to that detected in the H-2$^{b/d}$ αβ transgenic SCID mice. Thus, peripheral CD4$^-$8$^-$ αβ T cells do not appear to require positive selection by H-2D^b MHC antigens on thymus epithelium.

In chimeras produced by injecting H-2^b αβ transgenic stem cells from male donors into X-irradiated B10.D2 recipients, we detected significant numbers of CD4$^-$8$^+$ T cells expressing the transgenic TCRαβ. These cells expressed relatively low levels of CD8 coreceptors and were unreactive to H-2^b male-stimulated cells. We did not detect significant numbers of such cells in chimeras produced by injecting H-2^b αβ transgenic stem cells from female donors into X-irradiated B10.D2 recipients (Fig. 7). This suggests that the exit of those cells from the thymus either requires the expression of the male antigen on hematopoietic cells or, alternatively, that these cells are more predominant in mice expressing the male antigen at H-2D^b MHC antigens because of the massive deletion of immature CD4$^+$8$^+$ thymocytes in these mice.

CONCLUDING REMARKS

It appears that the experiments in TCR transgenic mice as described here and in independent experiments by Sha et al. (1988a,b) and more recently by Berg et al. (1989) have put an end to the debate whether or not positive selection by thymic MHC antigens plays a crucial role in the selection of the T-cell repertoire. Our

αβ H-2^b ♂ → B10.D2 ♀   αβ H-2^b ♀ → B10.D2 ♀

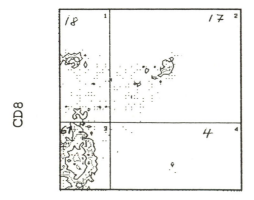 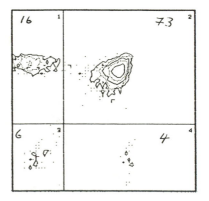

Figure 6. Staining of the thymocytes from lethally X-irradiated B10.D2 mice reconstituted with H-2^b stem cells from male and female TCRαβ transgenic mice. The thymocytes were double-stained by CD4 and CD8 antibodies.

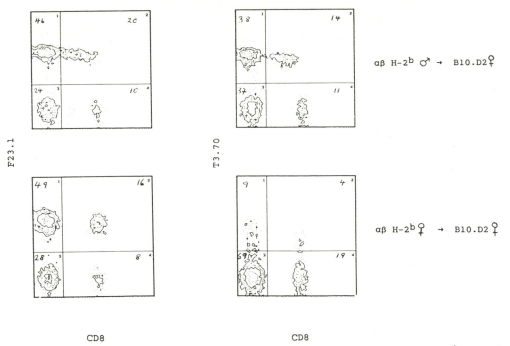

Figure 7. Staining of the lymph node cells from lethally X-irradiated B10.D2 mice reconstituted with H-2^b stem cells from male and female TCR$\alpha\beta$ transgenic mice. The lymph node cells were double-stained with F23.1 and CD8, as well as with T3.70 and CD8 antibodies (F23.1, is specific for the transgenic β chain, T3.70 is specific for the transgenic α chain).

experiments indicate that this interaction is, in fact, essential for the generation of mature T cells, at least for those that express normal levels of CD4 and CD8 coreceptors. In addition, they indicate that the interaction of TCRs with thymic MHC antigens ensures that mature T cells express a "fitting" combination of TCR and CD4/CD8 coreceptors, i.e., class I MHC antigen restricted receptors and CD8 or class II MHC-antigen-restricted receptors and CD4. This constellation ensures that on every peripheral T cell the TCR can be brought into proximity with either CD4 or CD8 accessory molecules by binding to the same MHC ligand. This proximity appears to be required for optimal T-cell activation (Emmerich et al. 1986; Dembic et al. 1987; Gabert et al. 1987).

The experiments on tolerance in TCR transgenic mice were the first to demonstrate that tolerance can be achieved by the deletion of immature CD4$^+$8$^+$ thymocytes, which serve as precursors for the more mature single-positive CD4$^+$8$^-$ and CD4$^-$8$^+$ T cells. As postulated by Lederberg (1959), these cells are not yet ready to respond to antigens by proliferation and differentiation into effector cells, but at this stage contact with antigens is suicidal. More recent experiments by other investigators also indicate that the deletion of autospecific T cells affects CD4$^+$8$^+$ T-cell precursors, even though the extent of deletion of cells with this phenotype may vary according to the nature of antigen and/or the avidity of the T cells for self-antigen (Kisielow et al. 1988b; Berg et al. 1989).

Whereas positive selection requires the expression of selecting MHC antigens on thymic epithelial cells

(Kisielow et al. 1988a), it is sufficient for negative selection if self-antigens are presented by hematopoietic cells. The ligands involved in positive selection are still ill-defined, and the molecular mechanisms of both selection steps are not yet understood.

The experiments in TCR transgenic SCID mice indicate that the TCR$\alpha\beta$ does not only control positive and negative selection through binding to intrathymic ligands, but also controls early developmental steps that require TCR rearrangement but not the binding of TCRs to their ligands: TCRβ rearrangement and expression control rearrangement of other TCRβ gene segments, and this control most likely involves the expression of the TCRβ chain with a so far unknown protein chain on immature T cells. In addition, both β and α TCR rearrangement control the expression of CD4 and CD8 coreceptors, as well as the expansion of immature T-cell precursors. Finally, contrary to expectations by many investigators, it appears that the complete assembly of the TCR$\alpha\beta$ on the cell surface does not shut off the recombinase responsible for TCR rearrangement. The molecular details of all these control mechanisms are unknown and will no doubt be the subject of investigations during the following years.

REFERENCES

Berg, L.J., A.M. Prillem, B. Fazekas de St. Groth, D. Mathis, C. Benoit, and M.M. Davis. 1989. Antigen/MHC specific T cells are preferentially exported from the thymus in the presence of their MHC ligand. *Cell* **58:** 1035.

Bevan, M.J. 1977. In a radiation chimera, host H-2 antigens

determine immune responsiveness of donor cytotoxic cells. *Nature* **269:** 417.

Bevan, M.J. and R.T. Hünig. 1981. T cell respond preferentially to antigen that are similar to self H-2. *Proc. Natl. Acad. Sci.* **78:** 1843.

Blüthmann, H., P. Kisielow, Y. Uematsu, M. Malissen, P. Krimpenfort, A. Berns, H. von Boehmer, and M. Steinmetz. 1988. T cell specific deletion of T cell receptor transgenes allows functional rearrangement of endogenous α and β genes. *Nature* **334:** 156.

Bosma, G.C., P.R. Custer, and M.J. Bosma. 1983. A severe combined immunodeficiency mutation in the mouse. *Nature* **301:** 527.

Dembic, Z., W. Haas, R. Zamoyska, J. Parnes, M. Steinmetz, and H. von Boehmer. 1987. Transfection of the CD8 gene enhances T-cell recognition. *Nature* **326:** 510.

Dembic, Z., W. Haas, S. Weiss, J. McCubrey, H. Kiefer, H. von Boehmer, and M. Steinmetz. 1986. Transfer of specificity by murine α and β T cell receptor genes. *Nature* **320:** 232.

Doherty, P.C., R. Korngold, D.H. Schwartz, and J.R. Bemink. 1981. Development and loss of virus-specific thymic competence in bone marrow radiation chimeras and normal mice. *Immunol. Rev.* **53:** 37.

Emmerich, F., V. Strittmatter, and K. Eichmann. 1986. Synergism in the activation of human CD8 T cells by crosslinking the T cell receptor complex with the CD8 differentiation antigen. *Proc. Natl. Acad. Sci.* **83:** 8298.

Gabert, J., C. Langlet, R. Zamoyska, J.R. Parnes, A. Schmitt-Verhulst, and M. Malissen. 1987. Reconstitution of MHC class I specificity by T-cell receptor and by Lyt-2 gene transfer. *Cell* **50:** 545.

Good, M.F., K.W. Pyke, and G.J.V. Nossal. 1983. Functional clonal deletion of cytotoxic T-lymphocyte precursors in chimeric thymus produced in vitro from embryonic anlagen. *Proc. Natl. Acad. Sci.* **80:** 3045.

Kappler, J.W. and P.C. Marrack. 1978. The role of H-2 linked genes in helper function. IV. Importance of T cell genotype and host environment in I-region and Ir gene expression. *J. Exp. Med.* **148:** 1510.

Kisielow, P., H.S. Teh, H. Blüthmann, and H. von Boehmer. 1988a. Positive selection of antigen-specific T cells in thymus by restricting MHC molecules. *Nature* **335:** 730.

Kisielow, P., H. Blüthmann, U.D. Staerz, M. Steinmetz, and H. von Boehmer. 1988b. Tolerance in T cell receptor transgenic mice involves deletion of nonmature CD4⁺8⁻ thymocytes. *Nature* **333:** 742.

Krimpenfort, P., R. De Jong, Y. Uematsu, Z. Dembic, S. Ryser, H. von Boehmer, M. Steinmetz, and A. Berns. 1988. Transcription of T cell receptor β chain genes is controlled by a downstream regulatory element. *EMBO J.* **7:** 745.

Lederberg, J. 1959. Genes and antibodies: Do antigens bear instructions for antibody specificity or do they select cell lines that arise by mutation? *Science* **129:** 1649.

Matzinger, P. 1981. A one receptor view of T-cell behavior. *Nature* **292:** 497.

Saito, T., A. Weiss, J. Miller, M.A. Norcross, and R.N. Germain. 1987. Specific antigen-Ia activation of transfected human T cells expressing murine Ti ab-human T3 receptor complexes. *Nature* **325:** 125.

Scott, B., H. Blüthmann, H.S. Teh, and H. von Boehmer. 1989. The generation of mature T cells requires an interaction of the αβ T-cell receptor with major histocompatibility antigens. *Nature* **338:** 591.

Sha, W.C., C.A. Nelson, R.D. Newberry, D.M. Kranz, J.H. Russell, and D.Y. Loh. 1988a. Selective expression of an antigen receptor on CD8-bearing T lymphocytes in transgenic mice. *Nature* **335:** 271.

————. 1988b. Positive and negative selection of an antigen receptor on T cells in transgenic mice. *Nature* **336:** 73.

Teh, H.S., P. Kisielow, B. Scott, H. Kishi, Y. Uematsu, H. Blüthmann, and H. von Boehmer. 1988. Thymic major histocompatibility complex antigens and the αβ T cell receptor determine the CD4/CD8 phenotype of T cells. *Nature* **335:** 229.

Uematsu, Y., S. Ryser, Z. Dembic, P. Borgulya, P. Krimpenfort, A. Berns, H. von Boehmer, and M. Steinmetz. 1988. In transgenic mice the introduced functional T cell receptor β gene prevents expression of endogenous β genes. *Cell* **52:** 831.

von Boehmer, H. 1986. The selection of the α,β heterodimeric T cell receptor for antigen. *Immunol. Today* **7:** 333.

————. 1988. The developmental biology of T lymphocytes. *Annu. Rev. Immunol.* **6:** 309.

von Boehmer, H. and J. Sprent. 1976. T cell function in bone marrow chimeras: Absence of host reactive T cells and cooperation of helper T cells across allogenic barriers. *Transpl. Rev.* **29:** 3.

von Boehmer, H., W. Haas, and N.K. Jerne. 1978. Major histocompatibility complex linked immune-responsiveness is acquired by lymphocytes of low-responder mice differing in thymus of high-responder mice. *Proc. Natl. Acad. Sci.* **75:** 2439.

von Boehmer, H., M. Bonneville, M. Ishida, S. Ryser, G. Lincoln, R.T. Smith, H. Kishi, B. Scott, P. Kisielow, and S. Tonegawa. 1988. The early suppression of a T cell receptor β transgene suppresses rearrangement of the V_{γ4} gene segment. *Proc. Natl. Acad. Sci.* **85:** 9729.

Wagner, H., C. Hardt, H. Stockinger, K. Pfizenmail, R. Bartlett, and M. Rollinghoff. 1981. Impact of the thymus on the generation of immunocompetence and diversity of antigen-specific-MAC-restricted cytotoxic T-lyphocyte precursors. *Immunol. Rev.* **58:** 95.

Zinkernagel, R.M., G.N. Callahan, A. Althage, S. Cooper, P.A. Klein, and J. Klein. 1978. On the thymus in the differentiation of "H-2 self-recognition" by T cells: Evidence for dual recognition? *J. Exp. Med.* **147:** 882.

TCR Recognition and Selection In Vivo

M.M. Davis,*† L.J. Berg,† A.Y. Lin,*† B. Fazekas de St. Groth,†
B. Devaux,*† C.G. Sagerstrom,† P.J. Bjorkman,†‡ and J.F. Elliott†§

*Howard Hughes Medical Institute and †The Department of Microbiology and Immunology,
Stanford University School of Medicine, Stanford, California 94305-5428; ‡Biology Division,
The California Institute of Technology, Pasadena, California 95205; §The DNAX Research Institute of
Molecular and Cellular Biology, Palo Alto, California 95304

Much has been accomplished in identifying the molecules and genes responsible for T-cell recognition. We are now familiar with two distinct heterodimers, $\alpha\beta$ and $\gamma\delta$, and we know that the former (at least) confers on a T cell the ability to recognize antigens complexed with specific molecules of the major histocompatibility complex (MHC) (Dembic et al. 1986; Saito and Germain 1987). Because of the recent solution of an MHC class I structure (Bjorkman et al. 1987a,b), its apparent generalization to class II molecules (Brown et al. 1988), as well as the similarity of T-cell receptor (TCR) primary sequences to immunoglobulins (Igs), we can guess a great deal about how they might interact (Chothia et al. 1988, Claverie et al. 1989; Davis and Bjorkman 1988; see also Bjorkman and Davis, this volume). These remain speculations, however, until we can derive real biochemical and structural data from the event itself (e.g., TCR-antigen-MHC interaction). This is required in order to move the current state of affairs beyond the inferences that we are limited to by the indirect nature of current assay methods. Toward such a biochemical resolution of this issue, we have for some years been attempting to express TCR heterodimers in a soluble form, first as immunologic chimerics, with limited success (Gascoigne et al. 1987), and more recently as lipid-linked molecules that can be cleaved off the surface of expressing cells (A. Lin et al.; B. Devaux et al.; both in prep.).

In contrast with the situation in the periphery, where the ligand for TCRs antigen-major histocompatibility complex (Ag-MHC) seems clear, what happens in the thymus with regard to T-cell repertoire selection is not so well understood. In investigating this area, we have made transgenic mice carrying TCRs of defined specificity (Berg et al. 1988, 1989a,b; Ivars et al. 1988; B. Fazekas de St. Groth et al., in prep.). In addition, MHC transgenics provided through a collaboration with C. Benoist and D. Mathis (van Ewjik et al. 1988) have provided an invaluable tool in characterizing some of the TCR/MHC interactions that must occur in the thymus. This has provided useful insights into both positive and negative selection, as discussed below. Although we do not yet know the precise molecules that may be involved, ultimately the combination of soluble TCRs and TCR transgenic mice should provide a solid basis for exploring these phenomena. One

scenario would be that since a particular MHC molecule is all that is required for T-cell export from the thymus (in the absence of nominal antigen) then a TCR/MHC interaction alone (or with a neutral peptide in the structure) may be possible. This should be detectable with a soluble receptor, and the relative affinity of such an event could serve as predictor of the fate of a given TCR in the thymus.

Soluble TCR Heterodimers

Because TCR heterodimers are assembled with the CD3 polypeptides to form complexes of at least seven polypeptides before appearing in the surface (Minami et al. 1987), they may be one of the more difficult types of molecules to produce in a soluble form. On the other hand, the very immunoglobulin-like character of its variable (V), diversity (D), joining (J), and constant (C) region elements, makes it very likely that it can bind to Ag-MHC by itself and that structurally it could exist and bind to its ligand in solution much like an antibody. Thus, the challenge has been to find conditions in which TCR chains can be expressed and form heterodimers free of CD3 molecules, either secreted from cells in culture or in a membrane-associated form that could be easily cleaved from the surface. Initial attempts in our laboratory took the form of TCR(V)-Ig(C) hybrids expressed in myeloma cell lines (Gascoigne et al. 1987). Interestingly, only V_α(TCR) C_H(Ig) chimeras could be assembled or secreted as apparently normal immunological molecules (being expressed with light chains). Neither V_β (Gascoigne et al. 1987), V_γ, nor V_δ (R. Wallich et al.; I.A. MacNeil et al.; both unpubl.) gene segments could be expressed in that same context, suggesting that there is some structural barrier to proper folding. Another category of TCR-Ig chimeras, namely those of Karjalainen and co-workers (Traunecker et al. 1989) have also failed to produce proper heterodimers (with one exception; B. Malissen, pers. comm.). Recent reports of Ig(V) TCR(C) chimeras being expressed and having demonstrable antigen-binding activity (Z. Eshhar; Y. Kurosawa et al.; both pers. comm.) indicate that the reciprocal type of chimera works well. A number of groups have also tried to express soluble TCRs by truncation, that is, by placing a stop codon at the

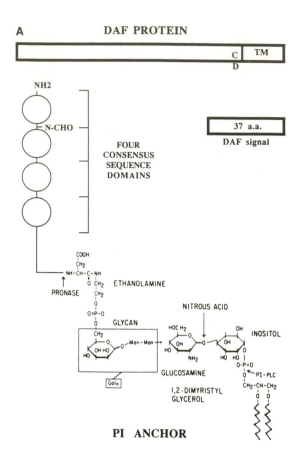

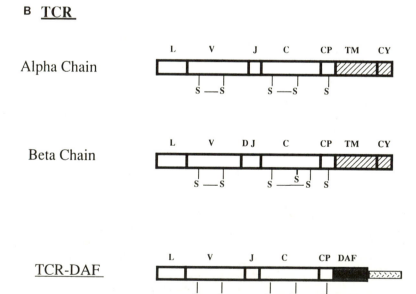

Figure 1. Schematic structure of PtdIns (PI)-anchored protein. (*A*) Structure of membrane-bound DAF. During the maturation of DAF, the last 17 amino acids (TM), containing a highly hydrophobic domain, are proteolytically cleaved. The PtdIns moiety is then attached to the cystein (C). The last 37 amino acids at the carboxyl terminus of DAF that functions as a PtdIns-anchoring signal are highlighted (□). PtdIns is linked to the carboxyl terminus of DAF through glucosamine, glycan, and ethanolamine residues. PtdIns-PLC cleaves at the phosphodiester bond of the PtdIns moiety as indicated. (*B*) Structure of PtdIns-anchored TCR. The domain structure and disulfide bond of TCRs are indicated. In the PtdIns-anchored TCR the transmembrane and cytoplasmic domains are replaced with the PtdIns-anchoring signal. PtdIns-anchored expressed on the cell surface with the PtdIns moiety attached to the carboxyl terminus of the 20 amino acid residues remaining of the PtdIns-anchor signal.

beginning of the transmembrane sequence (O. Acuto and E. Reinherz; K. Arai et al., both pers. comm.). In these cases, it appears that polypeptides are expressed, but there is no heterodimer formation. This is not an infrequent occurrence in truncation experiments, perhaps because of incorrect juxtaposition of the two chains and/or loss of important cell-trafficking signals (in the transmembrane sequence). Recently, through colleagues at Genentech, we became aware of the increasingly large list of surface proteins known to be lipid-linked (for review, see Ferguson and Williams 1988). All such proteins can be cleaved with a specific enzyme, phosphatidylinositol-specific-phospholipase C (PtdIns-PLC), to produce soluble forms. Caras et al. (1987) had shown that the carboxy-terminal 37 amino acids of decay accelerating factor (DAF) could serve as the signal sequence for the lipid-linked expression of a herpes simplex virus membrane protein. Thus, expression of TCR polypeptides as PtdIns-linked molecules might allow them to associate in the plane of a membrane to maximize heterodimer formation and to be cleaved off the surface of expressing cells to produce a soluble form. From a suggestion of P. Travers, we also included experiments with the carboxyl terminus of human placental alkaline phosphatase (HPAP) (Kam et al. 1985) because that PtdIns-linked molecule is normally expressed as a homodimer (DAF is a monomer). Thus, an HPAP "stem" structure may be more compatible with proper heterodimer formation.

Figure 1A shows the native form of DAF with the glycan-PtdIns tail. The enzyme PtdIns-PLC cleaves as indicated. Figure 1B shows schematics of the TCR-DAF fusions with the TCR/HPAP chimeras being done in the same fashion. The characteristics of expression of this type is that a proform of the molecule is translated and that in the endoplasmic reticulum a portion of the carboxyl terminus is cleaved off (17 amino acids in the case of DAF and 23 amino acids in the case of HPAP; Micanovic et al. 1988) and an ethanolamine-carbohydrate-phosphatidylinositol linkage (Fig. 1A, from Ferguson and Williams 1988) is added to the new carboxyl terminus of the protein, which then makes its way to the cell surface.

With respect to TCR expression in both COS cells (for transient transfections) and Chinese hamster ovary (CHO) cells (for long-term transfectants), we found that in most cases single chains of the TCR could be expressed with either the HPAP or the DAF signal sequence with high efficiency (using an expression vector derived from pcDL-SRα296, Takebe et al. 1988) and cleaved off the surface of expressing cells with PtdIns-PLC (in early experiments, a gift from M. Low). Expression could be demonstrated by either the immunoprecipitation of surface-iodinated cells or fluorescence-tagging and analysis by microscopy or a fluorescence-activated cell sorter (FACS). Immunoprecipitation indicates the presence of both dimers and monomers in most cases (A. Lin et al.; B. Devaux et al.; both in prep.). Analysis of CHO cells transfected with both α and β chains from the 2B4 hybridoma modified with

either the DAF or HPAP signal sequences was particularly revealing. As shown in Figure 2, stable transfectants could be isolated that coexpressed both α and β chain determinants (A. Lin et al., in prep.). To demonstrate that heterodimers between α and β were being formed that juxtapose V_α and V_β determinants, we made use of the fact that preincubation of 2B4 TCR-bearing cells with the saturating amounts of anti-Va2B4 (A2B4-2 from Samelson et al. 1983) antibody abolished staining with the anti-V_β3 antibody (KJ25 from Pullen et al. 1988). This cross-blocking phenomenon is shown in Figure 3, showing β^- Jurkat cells (a gift from A. Weiss) transfected with normal 2B4 α and β chain genes as a control. In Figure 3A, the cells were stained with KJ25 (a hamster antibody) and visualized with fluorescinated anti-hamster antiserum. The presence of both negative and positive populations seen in Figure 3 is due to the nonclonal nature of this cell line. In Figure 3B, this same cell line has been pretreated with anti-2B4 (V_α) antibody both prior to and during the KJ25 staining, effectively blocking all anti-V_β reactivity. This same effect can be seen with CHO cells transfected with either α DAF and β DAF chimeras or α HPAP and β HPAP constructs (Fig. 3C, D), indicating that approximately 90% of the 2B4 β-chain polypeptides are being expressed as heterodimers with the complementary α chain (A. Lin et al., in prep.). Mass culture, cleavage with PtdIns-PLC, and isolation on antibody columns also indicates that most of the TCR

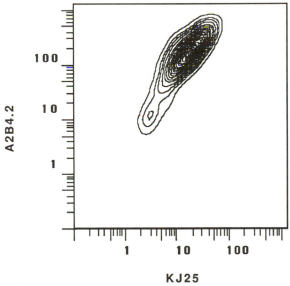

Figure 2. Coexpression of PtdIns-anchored TCR α and β chains on the cell surface. CHO cells were transfected with a plasmid containing the sequences encoding TCR α and β chains with PtdIns-anchor signal sequences (A. Lin et al., in prep.). The stable transfectants were analyzed for surface expression of α and β chains, with FACS, by sequentially staining antibodies KJ25 (anti-V_β3) and biotinylated A2B4.2 (anti-V_α11) with fluorescein-isothyocyanate (FITC)-conjugated goat anti-mouse immunoglobulin and streptavidin as second antibodies, respectively. The data is plotted as log fluorescent intensity in arbitrary units.

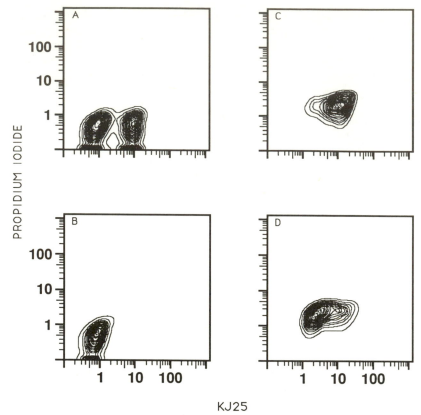

KJ25

Figure 3. Blocking of KJ25 by A2B4.2 on the staining of cell-surface PtdIns-anchored TCR. β^- Jurkat with surface expression of functional 2B4 TCR$\alpha\beta$ (*A* and *B*) and CHO transfectants (*C* and *D*) (as described in Fig. 2) were stained with antibody KJ25, with (*B* and *D*) or without (*A* and *B*) pretreatment with A2B4.2. Following binding of FITC-conjugated goat anti-mouse immunoglobulin, cells were analyzed on the FACS. The data are plotted as log fluorescent intensity in arbitrary scale. CHO has higher fluorescent background than Jurkat as indicated in the propidium iodide staining (A. Lin et al., in prep.)

protein expressed in this fashion is in the form of heterodimers (data not shown). Currently, we are able to purify hundreds of micrograms of soluble receptor. Perhaps the most crucial test is whether TCR expressed in this way can bind to antigen/MHC complexes. Preliminary experiments suggest that it can, but signals are very low and the amount of fluctuation is high.

Selection of the T-cell Repertoire In Vivo

How the T-cell repertoire is shaped in the thymus has long been an interesting but controversial area of immunology. In particular, the concept of "positive selection" or rather the selective export to the periphery of T cells that are best able to interact with self-MHC molecules has been the subject of much controversy. Whereas many laboratories have seen this type of selection in irradiated recipient strains (Bevan 1977; Fink and Bevan 1978; Kappler and Marrack 1978; Sprent 1978; von Boehmer et al. 1978; Zinkernagel et al. 1978; Singer et al. 1981), others have not (Matzinger and Mirkwood 1978; Stockinger et al. 1980; Ishii et al. 1981). Governman et al. (1986) dismissed evidence of positive selection as being the result not of thymic selection but of preferential T-cell expansion in the

periphery. In addition, the nature of the experiments performed was constrained by the facts that mice were heavily manipulated (e.g., irradiated); no single TCR could be followed but only reactivity to particular antigens that must involve many TCRs and probably many epitopes as well; the signal being followed is relatively low because of the small number of cells with a given reactivity at any one time; and because the number of cells being followed is a small fraction of the total, the opportunity to study the biochemistry and physiology of this phenomenon is nil.

The applicability of the transgenic mouse technology (Hogan et al. 1986) to these problems is very clear in that with the proper expression of a given TCR$\alpha\beta$ a large fraction of the T cells in a given individual would be of uniform specificity and subject to the same influences. In this case, different MHC molecules, antigens, and other forces could all be used to modulate expression. The power of this approach can be seen in Figure 4. In this experiment, α- and β-chain genomic constructs for 2B4, a helper T-cell hybridoma that recognizes a fragment of cytochrome c complexed to the I-E^K molecule (Hedrick et al. 1982; Samelson et al. 1983), have been introduced into the mouse germ-line and back-crossed extensively to B10 mice to remove minor lymphocyte-stimulating antigen (Mls-2^A/3^A) ef-

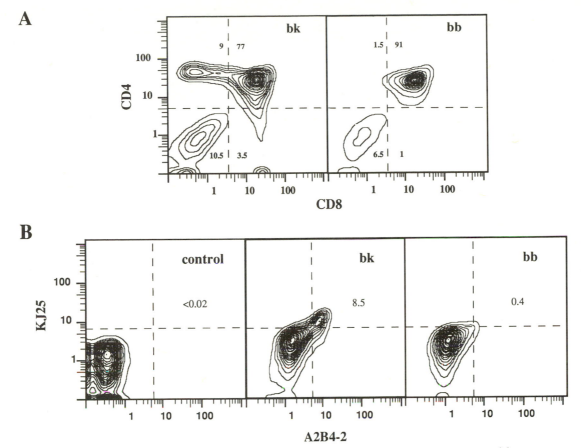

Figure 4. Staining of thymocytes from H-2^{kxb} versus H-2^b $\alpha\beta$ transgenic mice. (*A*) Thymocytes from an H-2^{kxb} (*left*) and an H-2^b (*right*) $\alpha\beta$ transgenic mouse were stained with directly conjugated anti-CD4-phycoerythrin (PE) and the anti-CD8-FITC. The numbers on each profile indicate the percentage of total thymocytes with each phenotype. (*B*) Thymocytes from an H-2^{kxb} nontransgenic control (*left*), an H-2^{kxb} $\alpha\beta$ transgenic (*center*), and an H-2^b $\alpha\beta$ transgenic (*right*) were stained with KJ25 (anti-V$_\beta$3) followed by anti-hamster Texas Red plus directly conjugated A2B4-2-FITC. The number on each profile indicates the percentage of cells staining brightly with both α and β chain antibodies. (Reprinted, with permission, from Berg et al. 1989b.)

fects (Berg et al. 1988, 1989b; Ivars et al. 1988). In this case, the IgH enhancer (Banerji et al. 1983; Gillies et al. 1983) has been used in place of the native α and β enhancers to achieve a high level of expression (Berg et al. 1988; Ivars et al. 1988). Figure 4A shows the very different CD4/CD8 thymic staining patterns of $\alpha\beta$ transgenics having the appropriate MHC (H-2^k) versus those lacking I-E expression altogether (H-2^b). Thymic expression on a (H-2$^k \times$ H-2^k)F$_1$ bK background is relatively normal, whereas the H-2^b BB pattern is distinctly abnormal, with an obviously arrested development at the double-positive stage (CD4$^-$8$^-$) of thymocyte differentiation, as indicated by the greatly reduced numbers of single positive (CD4$^+$ or CD8$^+$) thymocytes. This failure of $\alpha\beta$ transgene-bearing cells to mature in the wrong MHC environment is also seen in Figure 4B, in this case staining with antibodies directed at both chains of the TCR transgenes. Here we see that H-2^K individuals have a large fraction of $\alpha\beta$-2B4 dull cells (in the double-positive compartment) and also significant numbers of $\alpha\beta$ bright cells as well (corresponding to the single-positive compartment). These transgene-TCR dull cells are just as visible in the H-2^b transgenic thymus, but the bright $\alpha\beta$-staining cells are

not. Peripheral expression follows the same pattern, with H-2^K mice having many more $\alpha\beta$ staining cells and a much higher fraction of cytochrome *c* reactive cells than H-2^b littermates, as measured in limiting dilution interleukin-2 (IL-2) assays of antigen-naive mice (Berg et al. 1989b). Also of interest is the heavy bias toward CD4 expression seen in $\alpha\beta$ mice, which have H-2^k, although the 2B4 hybridoma lacks CD4 (or CD8) expression. This suggests that the original T cell expressing the 2B4 antigen receptor was in fact CD4$^+$ and that expression of this molecule was lost sometime after fusion with BW5147. In fact, very few T-cell fusions have persistent CD4 or CD8 expression. Together with the data of von Boehmer and colleagues (Kisielow et al. 1988b) and Loh and colleagues (Sha et al. 1988a,b) with class I MHC-specific transgenics preferentially expressing CD8, this data also indicates that the MHC class preference of a TCR predetermines CD4 or CD8 expression. In addition, to characterize this phenomenon further, we wish also to address the following questions: Is the I-E molecule responsible for this effect? Is thymic expression of I-E necessary and sufficient? What cells in the thymus are most important for positive selection?

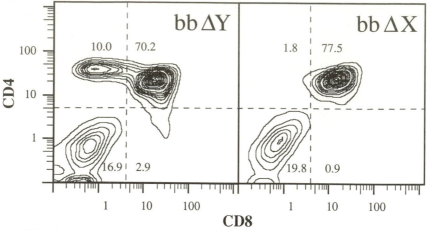

Figure 5. CD4 versus CD8 staining of thymocytes from ΔX and ΔY αβ transgenic mice. Thymocytes for αβ transgenic mice of two MHC types (H-2^b + ΔY and H-2^b + ΔX) were stained with anti-CD4 and anti-CD8. The percentage of thymocytes in each subset is indicated on each profile. Cells were stained with directly conjugated anti-CD4-PE and anti-CD8-FITC. (Reprinted, with permission, from Berg et al. 1989b.)

This we were able to do with the help of C. Benoist and D. Mathis, who kindly provided us with lines of transgenic mice for expressing different versions of E$_\alpha^k$, the gene defective in H-2^b mice and several other I-E$^-$ strains (Mathis et al. 1983; Le Meur et al. 1985; van Ewijk et al. 1988). We will focus here on the ΔY mice, which on a H-2^b background express I-E in the cortical epithelium of the thymus with approximately 1% of normal expression in the medulla (and none elsewhere) and the ΔX mice, which express I-E only in the medullary region of the thymus (van Ewijk et al. 1988). Crossing our 2B4 αβ mice with these E$_\alpha^k$ transgenics produced very clear effects as shown in Figure 5. The first panel shows the CD4/CD8 pattern of thymocytes staining in the thymocytes of ΔY BB mice, whereas the second shows the analogous data for ΔX BB mice. It is thus clear that I-E expression in the cortical epithelium is sufficient to rescue almost entirely the positive selection in these mice (Fig. 4A), whereas medullary expression has no discernible effect (Berg et al. 1989b). Therefore, the basic tenets of positive selection are upheld in that the original restricting element is the important molecule in mediating this effect (for complementary data in a class I MHC-dependent system, see Kisielow et al. 1988a). In addition, these results also offer very strong support that the experiments of Sprent and his colleagues showing the importance of thymic epithelial cells in this phenomenon (Lo and Sprent 1986; Singer 1988; Sprent et al. 1988) are vindicated.

Negative Selection

The other major selective criterion being applied in the thymus involves the removal of self-reactive T cells. Ample evidence for this phenomenon involving the death of such cells has been obtained making use of the Mls-mediated self-reactivity model (Kappler et al.

1987, 1988; MacDonald et al. 1988; Pullen et al. 1988; Pircher et al. 1989; White et al. 1989). These data are consistent with one another and indicate that Mls-reactive cells are absent from the mature single-positive population (CD4$^+$ or CD8$^+$) and the numbers in the double-positive CD4$^+$8$^+$ compartments are not obviously reduced. The limitations of these studies is inherent in the phenomenology of the Mls loci and the related *Staphylococcus* enterotoxin effects, which seem specific only for the germ-line-encoded residues of specific V$_\beta$ molecules and apparently do not involve processed antigens (Janeway et al. 1989). Recent studies (Dellabona et al., this volume) further indicate that *Staphylococcus* enterotoxin B is not affected by mutations in I-A$_\alpha$, which disrupt lysozyme peptide binding, but instead is only disrupted by mutations that point outward (from the putative α helix, that is, away from the peptide-binding groove). Thus, Mls and *Staphylococcus* enterotoxin reactivities are interesting phenomena, but their relevance to the problem of self-tolerance is questionable.

The ability of the Mls deletion data to be generalized has come under further scrutiny with the advent of recent experiments examining the deletion of self-reactive cells in animals transgenic for self-reactive TCRs. In both examples, the HY + D^b system (Kisielow et al. 1988b) and the anti-L^d model (Sha et al. 1988b) T cells bearing both α and β TCR transgenes are specifically deleted from animals that express those targets, but in each case the thymic double-positive compartment is severely affected (as well as the mature single-positive cells). Thus, the timing of negative selection appears to be very early in or even before the CD4$^+$8$^+$ compartment in those systems. In the 2B4 system, we have encountered our own experiences with negative selection based on Mls reactivity, which helps to resolve some of these issues (Berg et al. 1989a). In particular, there was a quantitative removal of cells expressing a high level of the 2B4 β chain because of the combination of its $V_\beta 3$ component and the Mls-$2^A/3^A$ genotype (C3H/HeJ) of one of the parental strains (as defined by Abe et al. 1988; Fry and Matis 1988; Pullen et al. 1988, 1989). We found deletion of mature 2B4 β-positive cells to be evident in the thymuses of both 2B4 TCR$\alpha\beta$ mice, as well as 2B4 β mice. What was interesting, however, was the very different phenotype exhibited by these two types of mice, both of which were undergoing massive and efficient negative selection. The thymic CD4/CD8 profile is shown in Figure 6, indicating that the β mice had a very similar arrest in the double-positive stage as seen in the H-2^b $\alpha\beta$ 2B4 transgenics in Figure 4 or in normal mice undergoing Mls-mediated deletion (Kappler et al. 1987, 1988). In contrast, the $\alpha\beta$ mice that deleted $V_\beta 3$ had a greatly reduced percentage of double-positive cells (2% of the total) and overall less than 1/10 of the normal number of thymocytes, exactly as reported previously by Kisielow et al. (1988b) for HY + D^b and as seen in the high-expressing mice of Sha et al. (1988b). Figure 6 shows a histogram of the absolute numbers of CD4$^+$8$^+$ cells in these mice, making even clearer the conclusion that the presence of TCR$\alpha\beta$ transgenes greatly augments the affects of negative selection, perhaps by speeding up the kinetics of T-cell differentiation and selection in the thymus (Berg et al. 1989a). This, in fact, is predictable from the observations that the TCRα chain is the last TCR to be rearranged and expressed during thymic development, and thus the presence of a rearranged α chain is bound to have an effect on maturation of at least some T cells.

In fact, data (B. Fazekas de St. Groth et al., in prep.) indicate that TCRα transgenics express TCR$\alpha\beta$ fully 2 days before normal (day 15 versus day 17) in fetal mice and at inappropriately high levels. This effect may be due to the absence of normal controlling elements in experiments to date, especially the silencer regions 3' of C_α, recently described by Winoto and Baltimore (this volume). Another important point is that this study of negative selection shows the essential equivalence of Mls-mediated deletion versus antigen plus MHC (Kisielow et al. 1988b) and alloreactive (Sha et al. 1988b) deletion in $\alpha\beta$ transgenic mice. This indicates that Mls-mediated deletion is, in fact, a valid model for the developmental aspects of self-tolerance.

A third conclusion from this study is that death by negative selection in $\alpha\beta$ transgenics is not the same as death by absence of positive selection in any of the three $\alpha\beta$ transgenic systems discussed above. This is indicated in Figure 7, which compares 2B4 $\alpha\beta$ expression on H-2^b and H-2^k background transgenics versus negative selection of these same transgenes because of Mls-$2^A/3^A$-mediated deletion. Thus, although both positive and negative selection are first evident at the same time normally (i.e., toward the end of the double-positive stage of differentiation) and seem to occur in the same location in the thymus (i.e., the cortex), the effect of negative selection on $\alpha\beta$ mice is phenotypically much more severe. One explanation for this might be that self-reactive $\alpha\beta$ transgenic cells arise and are dispatched more quickly; the mechanism of death by negative selection in this instance might be kinetically

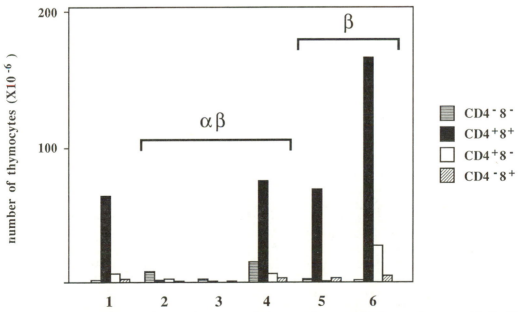

Figure 6. The effects of negative selection on thymocytes of $\alpha\beta$ versus β transgenic mice are shown graphically (Berg et al. 1989a). The total number of thymocytes of each subset (CD4$^-$8$^-$, CD4$^+$8$^+$, CD4$^+$8$^-$, CD4$^-$8$^+$) are indicated for (1) a nontransgenic control, (2) an anti-[D^b + HY] $\alpha\beta$ transgenic (Kisielow et al. 1988a), (3) an anti-[H-2^k + Mls-2^a and/or -3^a] $\alpha\beta$ transgenic, (4) a non-$V_\beta 3$ deleting $\alpha\beta$ transgenic, (5) an anti-[H-2^k + Mls-2^a and/or -3^a] β transgenic, and (6) a non-$V_\beta 3$-deleting β transgenic. Note the severe reduction in CD4$^+$8$^+$ cells in the $\alpha\beta$ transgenics compared with the twofold reduction (back to normal levels) in the β transgenic.

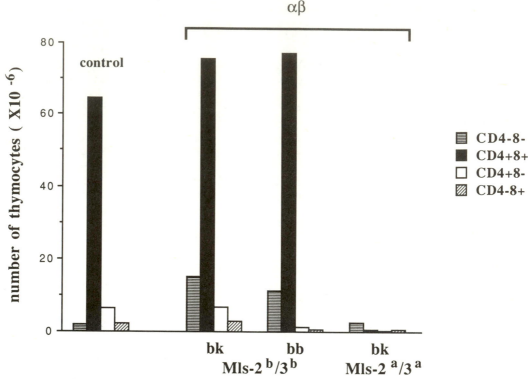

Figure 7. The effects of positive selection versus negative selection on thymocytes of $\alpha\beta$ transgenic mice. The total number of thymocytes of each subset (CD4$^-$8$^-$, CD4$^+$8$^+$, and CD4$^-$8$^+$) are indicated for four mice: one nontransgenic control and three $\alpha\beta$ transgenics. From *left* to *right*, the $\alpha\beta$ transgenics are an H-2^{kxb}, Mls-2^b and -3^b (undergoing positive selection), an H-2^b, Mls-2^b and -3^b (no significant positive selection), and an H-2^{kxb}, Mls-2^a and/or -3^a (undergoing negative selection). Note the radically different phenotype resulting from the absence of positive selection compared with negative selection.

much faster, mediated either by another cell type ($\gamma\delta$ killers?) or by some "active" principal. Thus, $\alpha\beta$ transgenics appear to be illustrating some significant mechanistic differences between positive and negative selection in the thymus.

CONCLUDING REMARKS

Much as issues involving the generation of antibody diversity began to be resolved in the late 1970s, the field of T-cell recognition and selection is beginning to coalesce around the specific molecules and the genes responsible for them. Unlike the antibody "problem," however, knowledge of TCR or MHC genes alone has not been sufficient to explain much of the phenomena important to the T-cell field. Instead, these issues have been starting points in a progressive narrowing of options toward what we hope will be a resolution of some of them in the near future. The successful expression of soluble TCRs will help to bridge the gap between our essentially circumstantial knowledge of T-cell antigen/ MHC interactions to date and a more complete biochemical and ultimately structural appreciation for what is going on. More distant is the expectation that mice transgenic for specific TCRs will not only confirm and extend classical experiments on positive and negative selection but will be the ideal departure point for mechanistic studies of these phenomena.

ACKNOWLEDGMENTS

We wish to thank Dr. J. Bangs for advice concerning PtdIns-linked proteins, Angela Nervi for excellent technical assistance, and Brenda Robertson for preparation of the manuscript. We also thank National Institutes of Health for grant support. M.M.D. is a scholar of the Pew Foundation, L.J.B. is a fellow of the Leukemia Society of Anemia, and A.L. was previously a fellow of the Cancer Research Institute and is now supported by the Howard Hughes Medical Institute. B.F.de S.G. was supported by an Irvington House postdoctoral fellowship and is now supported by a fellowship from the Medical Research Council of Australia. P.J.B. was supported by an American Cancer Society postdoctoral fellowship, and J.F.E. is a centennial fellow of the Medical Research Council of Canada.

REFERENCES

Abe, R., M.S. Vacchio, B. Fox, and R. Hodes. 1988. Preferential expression of the T-cell receptor V$_\beta$3 gene by Mls^c reactive T cells. *Nature* **335:** 827.

Banerji, J., L. Olson, and W. Schaffner. 1983. A lymphocyte-specific cellular enhancer is located downstream of the joining region in immunoglobulin heavy chain genes. *Cell* **33:** 729.

Berg, L.J., B. Fazekas de St. Groth, A.M. Pullen, and M.M. Davis. 1989a. Phenotypic differences between $\alpha\beta$ and β T cell receptor transgenic mice undergoing negative selection. *Nature* **340:** 559.

Berg, L.J., A.M. Pullen, B. Fazekas de St. Groth, D. Mathis, C. Benoist, and M.M. Davis. 1989b. Antigen/MHC specific T cells are preferentially exported from the thymus in the presence of their MHC ligand. *Cell* **58:** 1035.

Berg, L.J., B. Fazekas de St. Groth, F. Ivars, C.C. Goodnow, S. Gilfillan, H.-J. Garchon, and M.M. Davis. 1988. Expression of T-cell receptor alpha-chain genes in transgenic mice. *Mol. Cell. Biol.* **8:** 5459.

Bevan, M. 1977. In a radiation chimera, host H-2 antigens determine immune responsiveness of donor cytotoxic T cells. *Nature* **269:** 417.

Bjorkman, P.J., M.A. Saper, B. Samraoui, W.S. Bennett, J.L. Strominger, and D.C. Wiley. 1987a. Structure of the human class I histocompatibility antigen, HLA-A2. *Nature* **329:** 506.

—————. 1987b. The foreign antigen binding site and T cell recognition regions of class I histocompatibility antigens. *Nature* **329:** 512.

Brown, J.H., T. Jardetzky, M.A. Saper, B. Samraoui, P.J. Bjorkman, and D.C. Wiley. 1988. A hypothetical model of the foreign antigen binding site of Class II histocompatibility molecules. *Nature* **332:** 845.

Caras, I.W., G.N. Weddell, M.A. Davitz, V. Nussenzweig, and D.W. Martin, Jr. 1987. Signal for attachment of a phospholipid membrane anchor in decay accelerating factor. *Science* **238:** 1280.

Chothia, C., D.R. Boswell, and A.M. Lesk. 1988. The outline structure of T-cell $\alpha\beta$ receptor. *EMBO J.* **7:** 3745.

Claverie, J.M., A. Prochnicka-Chalufour, and L. Bougueleret. 1989. Implications of a Fab-like structure for the T-cell receptor. *Immunol. Today* **10:** 10.

Davis, M.M. and P.J. Bjorkman. 1988. T cell antigen receptor genes and T cell recognition. *Nature* **334:** 395.

Dembic, Z., W. Haas, S. Weiss, J. McCubrey, H. Kiefer, H. von Boehmer, and H. Steinmetz. 1986. Transfer of specificity by murine alpha and beta T cell receptor genes. *Nature* **320:** 232.

Ferguson, M.A.J. and A. Williams. 1988. Cell-surface anchoring of proteins via glycosylphosphatidylinositol structures. *Annu. Rev. Biochem.* **57:** 285.

Fink, P.J. and M.J. Bevan. 1978. H-2 antigens at the thymus determine lymphocyte specificity. *J. Exp. Med.* **148:** 766.

Fry, A.M. and L.A. Matis. 1988. Self-tolerance alters T-cell receptor expression in an antigen-specific MHC restricted immune system. *Nature* **335:** 830.

Gascoigne, N.R.M., C. Goodnow, K. Dudzik, V.T. Oi, and M.M. Davis. 1987. Secretion of a chimeric T-cell receptor-immunoglobulin protein. *Proc. Natl. Acad. Sci.* **84:** 2936.

Gillies, S.D., S.L. Morrison, V.T. Oi, and S. Tonegawa. 1983. A tissue-specific transcription enhancer element is located in the major intron of a rearranged immunoglobulin heavy chain gene. *Cell* **33:** 717.

Governman, J., T. Hunkapiller, and L. Hood. 1986. A speculative view of the multicomponent nature of T cell antigen recognition. *Cell* **45:** 475.

Hedrick, S.M., L.A. Matis, T.T. Hecht, L.E. Samelson, D.L. Longo, E. Heber-Katz, and R.H. Schwartz. 1982. The fine specificity of antigen and Ia determinant recognition by T cell hybridoma clones specific for cytochrome *c*. *Cell* **30:** 141.

Hogan, B., F. Costantini, and E. Lacy. 1986. *Manipulating the mouse embryo: A laboratory manual.* Cold Spring Harbor Laboratory, Cold Spring Harbor, New York.

Ishii, N., C.N. Baxevanis, Z.A. Nagy, and J. Klein. 1981. Responder T cell depleted of alloreactive cells react to antigen presented on allogenic macrophages from nonresponder strains. *J. Exp. Med.* **154:** 978.

Ivars, F., L.J. Berg, B. Fazekas de St. Groth, C.C. Goodnow, H.-J. Garchon, S. Gilfillan, and M.M. Davis. 1988. The expression of T cell receptor α chain genes in transgenic

mice. In *The T cell receptor* (ed. M.M. Davis and J. Kappler), p. 187. A.R. Liss, New York.

Janeway, C.A., Jr., J. Yagi, P.J. Conrad, M.E. Katz, B. Jones, S. Vroegop, and S. Buxser. 1989. T-cell responses to Mls and to bacterial proteins that mimic its behavior. *Immunol. Rev.* **107:** 60.

Kam, W., E. Clauser, Y.S. Kim, Y.W. Kan, and W.J. Rutter. 1985. Cloning, sequencing, and chromosomal localization of human term placental alkaline phosphatase cDNA. *Proc. Natl. Acad. Sci.* **82:** 8715.

Kappler, J.W. and P. Marrack. 1978. The role of H-2 linked genes in helper T cell function. *J. Exp. Med.* **148:** 1510.

Kappler, J.W., N. Roehm, and P. Marrack. 1987. T cell tolerance by clonal elimination in the thymus. *Cell* **49:** 263.

Kappler, J.W., U. Staerz, J. White, and P.C. Marrack. 1988. Self-tolerance eliminates T cells specific for Mls-modified products of the major histocompatibility complex. *Nature* **332:** 35.

Kisielow, P., H.S. Teh, H. Bluthmann, and H. von Boehmer. 1988a. Positive selection of antigen-specific T cells in thymus by restricting MHC molecules. *Nature* **335:** 730.

Kisielow, P., H. Bluthmann, U.D. Staerz, M. Steinmetz, and H. von Boehmer. 1988b. Tolerance in T cell receptor transgenic mice involves deletion of nonmature CD4$^+$8$^+$ thymocytes. *Nature* **333:** 742.

Le Meur, M., P. Gerlinger, C. Benoist, and D. Mathis. 1985. Correcting an immune response deficiency by creating E$_\alpha$ gene transgenic mice. *Nature* **316:** 38.

Lo, D. and J. Sprent. 1986. Identity of cells that imprint H-2 restricted T cell specificity in the thymus. *Nature* **319:** 672.

MacDonald, H.R., R. Schneider, R.K. Lees, R.C. Howe, H. Acha-Orbea, H. Festenstein, R.M. Zinkernagel, and H. Hengartner. 1988. T cell receptor V$_\beta$ use predicts reactivity and tolerance to Mls^a-encoded antigens. *Nature* **332:** 40.

Mathis, D., C. Benoist, V. Williams, M. Kanter, and H. McDevitt. 1983. Several mechanisms can account for defective E$_\alpha$ expression in different mouse haplotypes. *Proc. Natl. Acad. Sci.* **80:** 273.

Matzinger, P. and G. Mirkwood. 1978. In a fully H-2 incompatible chimera, T cells of donor origin can respond to minor histocompatibility antigens in association with either donor or host H-2 type. *J. Exp. Med.* **148:** 84.

Micanovic, R., C.A. Bailey, L. Brink, L. Gerber, Y.-C.E. Pan, J.D. Hulmes, and S. Udenfriend. 1988. Aspartic acid-48 of nascent placental alkaline phosphatase condenses with a phosphatidylinositol glycan to become the carboxyl terminus of the mature enzyme. *Proc. Natl. Acad. Sci.* **85:** 1398.

Minami, Y., A.M. Weissmann, L.E. Samelson, and R.D. Klausner. 1987. Building a multichain receptor: Synthesis, degradation, and assembly of the T-cell antigen receptor. *Proc. Natl. Acad. Sci.* **84:** 2688.

Pircher, H., T.W. Mak, R. Lang, W. Balhausen, E. Ruedi, H. Hengartner, R. Zinkernagel, and K. Burki. 1989. T cell tolerance to Mls^a encoded antigens in T cell receptor V$_\beta$8.1 chain transgenic mice. *EMBO J.* **8:** 719.

Pullen, A.M., P. Marrack, and J.W. Kappler. 1988. The T cell repertoire is heavily influenced by tolerance to polymorphic self-antigens. *Nature* **335:** 796.

—————. 1989. Evidence that Mls-2 antigens which deplete V$_\beta$3$^+$ T cells are controlled by multiple genes. *J. Immunol.* **142:** 3033.

Saito, T. and R.N. Germain. 1987. Predictable acquisition of a new MHC recognition specificity following expression of a transfected T-cell receptor beta-chain gene. *Nature* **329:** 256.

Samelson, L.E., R.N. Germain, and R.H. Schwartz. 1983. Monoclonal antibodies against the antigen receptor on a cloned T-cell hybrid. *Proc. Natl. Acad. Sci.* **80:** 6972.

Sha, W.C., C.A. Nelson, R.D. Newberry, D.M. Kranz, J.H. Russell, and D.Y. Loh. 1988a. Selective expression of an antigen receptor on CD8-bearing T lymphocytes in transgenic mice. *Nature* **335:** 271.

————. 1988b. Positive and negative selection of an antigen receptor on T cells in transgenic mice. *Nature* **336:** 73.

Singer, A. 1988. Experimentation and thymic selection. *J. Immunol.* **140:** 2481.

Singer, A., K.S. Hathcock, and R.J. Hodes. 1981. Self recognition in allogenic radiation bone marrow chimeras. *J. Exp. Med.* **153:** 1286.

Sprent, J. 1978. Restricted helper function of F_1 parent bone marrow chimeras controlled by K-end of H-2 complex. *J. Exp. Med.* **147:** 1838.

Sprent, J., D. Lo, E.-K. Gao, and Y. Ron. 1988. T cell selection in the thymus. *Immunol. Rev.* **101:** 173.

Stockinger, H., K. Pfizenmaier, C. Hardt, H. Rodt, M. Rollinghoff, and H. Wagner. 1980. H-2 restriction as a consequence of intentional priming: T cells of fully allogenic chimeric mice as well as of normal mice respond to foreign alloantigens in the context of H-2 determinants not encountered on thymic epithelial cells. *Proc. Natl. Acad. Sci.* **77:** 7390.

Takebe, Y., M. Seiki, J. Fujisawa, P. Hoy, K. Yokota, K. Arai, M. Yoshida, and N. Arai. 1988. SRα promoter: An efficient and versatile mammalian cDNA expression system composed of the simian virus 40 early promoter and the R-U5 segment of human T-cell leukemia virus type 1 long terminal repeat. *Mol. Cell. Biol.* **8:** 466.

Traunecker, A., B. Dolder, F. Oliveri, and K. Karjalainen. 1989. Solubilizing the T-cell receptor—Problems in solution. *Immunol. Today* **10:** 29.

van Ewijk, W., R. Ron, J. Monaco, J. Kappler, P. Marrack, M. Le Meur, P. Gerlinger, B. Durand, C. Benoist, and D. Mathis. 1988. Compartmentalization of MHC class II gene expression in transgenic mice. *Cell* **53:** 357.

von Boehmer, H., W. Haas, and N.K. Jerne. 1978. Major histocompatibility complex-linked immune response is acquired by lymphocytes of low responder mice differentiating in thymus of high responder mice. *Proc. Natl. Acad. Sci.* **75:** 2439.

White, J., A. Herman, A.M. Pullen, R. Kubo, J.W. Kappler, and P. Marrack. 1989. The V_β-specific superantigen staphylococcal enterotoxin B: Stimulation of mature T cells and clonal deletion in neonatal mice. *Cell* **56:** 27.

Zinkernagel, R.M., G.N. Callahan, A. Althage, S. Cooper, P.A. Klein, and J. Klein. 1978. On the thymus in the differentiation of "H-2 self recognition" by T cells: Evidence for dual recognition? *J. Exp. Med.* **147:** 882.

Positive and Negative Selection of the T-cell Antigen Receptor Repertoire in Nontransgenic Mice

H.R. MacDonald,* D. Speiser,† R. Lees,* R. Schneider,†
R.M. Zinkernagel,† and H. Hengartner†
*Ludwig Institute for Cancer Research, Lausanne Branch, 1066 Epalinges, Switzerland; †Institute of Pathology
University Hospital, 8091 Zurich, Switzerland

The T-cell receptor (TCR) repertoire of mature T lymphocytes is shaped by selective events occurring within the thymus (for review, see Möller 1988). Thus, developing T cells that react strongly with self components are deleted and/or inactivated (negative selection), and only those cells with low affinity for self major histocompatibility complex (MHC) components are retained (positive selection). Until recently, these selective processes could only be inferred from functional studies; however, with the recent development of TCR transgenic mice and monoclonal antibodies (MAbs) directed against variable (V) domains of the TCR β chain (V_β), it has become possible to visualize directly and hence follow the fate of T cells with self-reactivity (Kappler et al. 1987, 1988; Kisielow et al. 1988b; MacDonald et al. 1988c; Sha et al. 1988).

In this paper, we will summarize recent findings from our laboratories related to positive and negative selection of the TCR repertoire. The model system employed takes advantage of the fact that most T cells using the $V_\beta 6$ domain react with antigens encoded by the minor lymphocyte-stimulating (Mls-1[a]) and/or I-E genetic loci, thereby allowing a more direct analysis of positive and negative selection events occurring within the thymus (MacDonald et al. 1988b,c).

METHODS

Monoclonal antibodies. Rat anti-TCR MAbs used were directed against $V_\beta 6$ (44-22-1; Payne et al. 1988) or $V_\beta 8$ (KJ16; Haskins et al. 1984).

Mice. MHC congenic mice on a C57BL/10 background were obtained from Harlan Olac, Ltd. (United Kingdom). Mls-1[a] congenic BALB.D2.Mls[a] mice were produced from breeding pairs provided by H. Festenstein (Festenstein and Berumen 1974). Radiation bone marrow chimeras were produced as described previously (Zinkernagel et al. 1978).

Flow microfluorometry. Single- and two-color immunofluorescence was performed as described previously (MacDonald et al. 1988c). Data are in general presented as percentages of positive cells after subtraction of background staining with the fluorescent conjugate alone. Standard deviations are indicated where $\geqslant 3$ individual mice were analyzed.

RESULTS

Clonal Deletion of Autoreactive Cells

The negative correlation of TCR $V_\beta 6$ expression with Mls-1[a] genotype has been documented previously (MacDonald et al. 1988c; Kanagawa et al. 1989). As is the case for deletion of other TCR V_β domains (Table 1), deletion of $V_\beta 6^+$ cells is most efficient in Mls-1[a] mice that express the MHC class II gene product I-E although certain I-A gene products (such as A[b] and A[k]) lead to partial deletion (Table 2).

The requirement for MHC class II molecules for clonal deletion implies that class-II-bearing cells are involved. In the thymus, MHC class II molecules are expressed by epithelial cells (located in both the cortex

Table 1. TCR V_β Domains Imparting Preferential Recognition (and Clonal Deletion) to Self-antigens

TCR domain	Specificity	Reference
$V_\beta 17a$	? + I-E	Kappler et al. (1987)
$V_\beta 8.1$	Mls-1[a] + class II MHC	Kappler et al. (1988)
$V_\beta 6$	Mls-1[a] + class II MHC	MacDonald et al. (1988c) Kanagawa et al. (1989)
$V_\beta 3$	Mls-2[a]/3[a] + class II MHC	Pullen et al. (1988) Fry and Matis (1988)
$V_\beta 11$	? + I-E	Tomonari et al. (1988) Bill et al. (1989)

Table 2. Contribution of MHC Class II Alleles to Clonal Deletion of $V_\beta 6^+$ Cells in Mls-1^a Mice

Class II expression		Mature thymocytes (%)	
I-A	I-E	$V_\beta 6$	$V_\beta 8.2$
b	–	2.1	14.3
d	–	5.1	12.0
f	–	4.8	14.1
k	–	2.3	14.7
q	–	6.2	12.2
s	–	4.9	11.5
d	d	0.6	15.5
k	k	0.5	17.3
s	k	0.9	17.1

Mature (cortisone-resistant) thymocytes were obtained from F$_1$ crosses between BIO congenic strains (Mls-1^b) and DBA/1 (Mls-1^a; A^{q}E$^-$). Data adapted from MacDonald et al. (1989).

and medulla) as well as by hematopoietic-derived cells such as macrophages and dendritic cells (located preferentially in the medulla). To distinguish which of these cell types was required for clonal deletion, we prepared allogeneic radiation bone marrow chimeras in which I-E expression and/or Mls-1^a expression were localized to either the radioresistant (epithelial) or radiosensitive (macrophage/dendritic) compartments. As shown in Table 3, I-E expression on hematopoietic-derived cells was both necessary and sufficient for deletion of $V_\beta 6^+$ mature T cells. It is interesting to note, however, that expression of Mls-1^a by either radioresistant or radiosensitive cells was sufficient for clonal deletion, implying that transfer and/or reprocessing of Mls-1^a antigens can occur in vivo. A more complete discussion of this phenomenon can be found elsewhere (Pullen et al. 1988; Speiser et al. 1989).

In accordance with the apparent role of hematopoietic-derived cells in clonal deletion, elimination of $V_\beta 6^+$ cells could only be observed in the thymic medulla of Mls-1^a mice (Hengartner et al. 1988), whereas no statistically significant reduction was detected in the cortex. This finding was also consistent with the failure to observe significant deletion of $V_\beta 6^+$ cells in the

CD4$^+$8$^+$ thymocyte subset, which is considered to be located primarily (if not exclusively) in the cortex.

Several lines of evidence suggested that CD4$^+$8$^+$ thymocytes might be the target population for clonal deletion. First, both CD4$^+$8$^-$ and CD4$^-$8$^+$ mature T cells were deleted in Mls-1^a mice, despite the fact that only CD4$^+$8$^-$ cells could be shown to react to Mls-1^a in vitro (MacDonald et al. 1988c). Second, in vivo treatment with MAbs directed against CD4 "rescued" CD4$^-$8$^+$ $V_\beta 6^+$ cells that would normally be deleted in Mls-1^a mice (MacDonald et al. 1988a; see also Fowlkes et al. 1988). Both of these observations would be consistent with a model in which CD4$^+$8$^+$ cells are intermediates in the development of CD4$^+$8$^-$ or CD4$^-$8$^+$ mature T cells (Fig. 1A). If clonal deletion were to occur at the CD4$^+$8$^+$ stage, then $V_\beta 6^+$ CD4$^-$8$^+$ cells could be deleted (or alternatively rescued) by the functional contribution (or lack thereof) of the CD4 molecule to self-recognition on $V_\beta 6^+$ CD4$^+$8$^+$ precursor cells (Fig. 1B).

More recent experiments (Table 4) (Schneider et al. 1989) indicate that $V_\beta 6^+$ cells with a CD4$^+$8$^-$ phenotype are in fact transiently present in the early postnatal thymus of Mls-1^a mice. These cells are peculiar in the sense that they express reduced levels of TCR. Furthermore, as shown in Table 5, these cells die selectively when placed in overnight tissue culture, suggesting that their reduced TCR density in vivo may be the consequence of receptor down-regulation upon encounter with self-antigen. The existence of such cells can be accommodated in several ways in the aforementioned model of T-cell development (Fig. 1), most simply by postulating that the CD4$^+$8$^+$ → CD4$^+$8$^-$ transition can occur as a result of CD4/TCR engagement of MHC class II/Mls-1^a ligand, irrespective of committing the cell to ultimate clonal deletion (Fig. 1C).

Positive Selection

In the course of investigating clonal deletion of $V_\beta 6^+$ T cells in Mls-1^a mice, we also observed that the levels

Table 3. Dependence of Mls-1^a-specific Clonal Deletion on I-E$^+$ Hematopoietic Cells in Allogeneic Radiation Bone Marrow Chimeras

Donor (Mls-1^a, I-E)		Recipient (Mls-1^a, I-E)		Percentage lymph node cells (means ± S.E.M.)	
				$V_\beta 6$	$V_\beta 8$
BALB/c	(−+)	BALB/c	(−+)	4.3 ± 0.5	7.7 ± 0.5
BIO.G	(−−)	BIO.G	(−−)	2.4 ± 0.1	5.3 ± 0.6
DBA/1	(+−)	DBA/1	(+−)	2.5 ± 0.1	5.0 ± 0.0
DBA/2	(++)	DBA/2	(++)	0.8 ± 0.4	8.1 ± 0.9
BALB/c	(−+)	DBA/2	(++)	0.8 ± 0.4	10.4 ± 0.4
DBA/2	(++)	BALB/c	(−+)	0.4 ± 0.1	7.4 ± 0.3
BIO.G	(−−)	DBA/1	(+−)	2.5 ± 0.0	8.3 ± 1.3
DBA/1	(+−)	BIO.G	(−−)	3.2 ± 0.4	10.4 ± 0.3
BIO.G	(−−)	DBA/2	(++)	2.8 ± 0.4	8.7 ± 0.7
DBA/2	(++)	BIO.G	(−−)	0.8 ± 0.1	11.2 ± 0.6

Lymph node cells (8–12 weeks after bone marrow reconstitution) were stained with V_β-specific reagents. Some of these data have appeared previously (MacDonald et al. 1989).

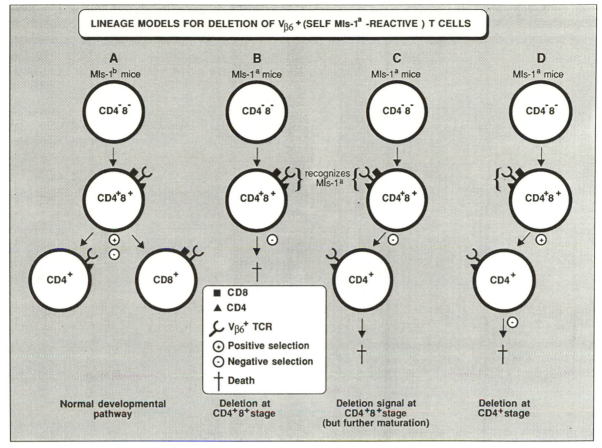

Figure 1. Lineage models for deletion of $V_\beta 6^+$ (self-Mls-1^a-reactive) T cells.

of $V_\beta 6$ expression in the CD4$^+$8$^-$ subset in nondeleting (Mls-1^b) strains were controlled by MHC class II genes and especially I-E (MacDonald et al. 1988b). Thus, BIO.BR (E^k) mice have approximately twofold more $V_\beta 6^+$ CD4$^+$ T cells than congenic BIO.G(E$^-$) mice, and this difference is dominant in F$_1$ animals. More recent experiments in F$_1 \rightarrow$ parent chimeras indicate that this positive selection phenomenon can be entirely accounted for by radioresistant (presumably epithelial) components of the thymus (Table 6). Similar conclusions have been reached in TCR transgenic mice (Kisielow et al. 1988a) and in another V_β correlation model (Blackman et al. 1989).

DISCUSSION

The correlations described here between levels of $V_\beta 6^+$ T cells and Mls-1^a and/or I-E expression provide simple and convincing evidence that both positive and negative selection mechanisms operate to shape the TCR repertoire in the thymus of normal, unmanipulated animals. Furthermore, the chimera data suggest that largely nonoverlapping subsets of nonlymphoid cells in the thymus may be primarily responsible for positive (epithelial cell) and negative (hematopoietic cell) selection events. These conclusions are in good agreement with the bulk of functional thymic selection

Table 4. Presence of CD4$^+$V$_\beta$6$^+$ Cells in Neonatal Mls-1^a Thymus

Strain	Age	V$_\beta$6$^+$ (%)		V$_\beta$8$^+$ (%)	
		CD4$^+$	CD8$^+$	CD4$^+$	CD8$^+$
BALB/c	4 days	9.7	6.7	12.0	13.0
BALB/c	adult	10.3	11.7	22.1	n.d.
BALB.Mls^a	4 days	4.4	0.3	14.8	13.9
BALB.Mls^a	adult	0.4	0.2	21.3	n.d.

Neonatal (4 days) or adult thymus was depleted of CD8$^+$ or CD4$^+$ cells and stained with V_β-specific reagents. Data are expressed as percentage of positive cells in the corresponding (CD4$^+$ or CD8$^+$) subset. n.d. indicates not done.

Table 5. Selective Death In Vitro of Phenotypically Mature (CD4$^+$) V$_\beta$6$^+$ Thymocytes from Neonatal Mls-1^a Mice

Culture	Percentage viable cells	
	V$_\beta$6	V$_\beta$8
4°C	4.0 ± 0.7	12.6 ± 0.8
37°C	1.3 ± 0.4	11.5 ± 0.8

CD8$^-$ thymocytes from 4-day BALB.Mls^a mice were incubated at 4°C or 37°C for 24 hours (1 × 10^6 to 2 × 10^6 cells/ml in normal culture medium) and then stained with V$_\beta$-specific MAbs. Results are expressed as a proportion of the total viable CD3$^+$ cells after subtraction of background staining. Data are mean ± s.d. of four independent experiments.

Table 7. Potential Differences in TCR Expression in TCR Transgenic Versus Normal (V$_\beta$) Model Systems

Parameter	Normal (V$_\beta$)	TCR transgenic
Onset of expression	late	early
Level of expression	low	high
α-Chain diversity	high	low or none

Schematic data are summarized for $\alpha\beta$ transgenic TCR (Kisielow et al. 1988b; Sha et al. 1988; Davis et al., this volume) or for V$_\beta$ correlations in normal mice (Kappler et al. 1987, 1988; MacDonald et al. 1988c; Pullen et al. 1988; Bill et al. 1989).

deletion in vivo in neonatal mice may provide new information regarding the signals and/or mechanisms involved in this terminal selective event.

data obtained previously in radiation bone marrow chimeras (for review, see Sprent et al. 1988); however, they appear to be at odds with some of the more recent data on negative selection in TCR transgenic mice (Kisielow et al. 1988b; Sha et al. 1988; Davis et al.; Zinkernagel et al.; both this volume). At least three important differences in TCR expression exist between the model system presented here and transgenic mouse models (Table 7). In addition, since none of the self-antigens examined so far has been characterized in molecular terms, it is not possible to exclude differences in their ontogeny of expression and/or tissue distribution (e.g., cortex versus medulla) as an explanation for the different patterns of clonal deletion seen under various experimental conditions. Molecular definition of minor self-antigens would therefore seem to be an important goal in our ultimate understanding of the clonal deletion process.

Aside from considerations of positive and negative selection per se, models such as those described in this paper have provided new insights into lineage interrelationships within the thymus. Thus, deletion and rescue of CD4$^-$8$^+$ T cells, in a situation where CD4/TCR recognition of MHC-class-II-associated self-antigens is apparently required for clonal deletion, implies strongly that CD4$^+$8$^+$ precursors are a crucial developmental intermediate in the generation of both CD4$^+$8$^-$ and CD4$^-$8$^+$ mature T-cell subsets. Furthermore, the identification of a novel population of CD4$^+$8$^-$ thymocytes that are apparently in the process of undergoing clonal

REFERENCES

Bill, J., O. Kanagawa, D.L. Woodland, and E. Palmer. 1989. The MHC molecule I-E is necessary but not sufficient for the clonal deletion of V$_{\beta11}$-bearing T cells. *J. Exp. Med.* **169:** 1405.

Blackman, M.A., P. Marrack, and J. Kappler. 1989. Influence of the major histocompatibility complex on positive thymic selection of V$_{\beta17a}$$^+$ T cells. *Science* **244:** 214.

Festenstein, H. and L. Berumen. 1974. Balb.D2.Mls^a—A new congenic mouse strain. *Transplantation* **37:** 322.

Fowlkes, B.J., R.H. Schwartz, and D.M. Pardoll. 1988. Deletion of self reactive thymocytes occurs at a CD4$^+$8$^+$ precursor stage. *Nature* **334:** 620.

Fry, A.M. and L.A. Matis. 1988. Self-tolerance alters T-cell receptor expression in an antigen-specific MHC restricted immune response. *Nature* **335:** 830.

Haskins, K., C. Hannum, J. White, N. Roehm, R. Kubo, J. Kappler, and P. Marrack. 1984. The major histocompatibility complex-restricted antigen receptor on T cells. VI. An antibody to a receptor allotype. *J. Exp. Med.* **160:** 452.

Hengartner, H., B. Odermatt, R. Schneider, M. Schreyer, G. Walle, H.R. MacDonald, and R.M. Zinkernagel. 1988. Deletion of self-reactive T cells prior to entering the thymus medulla. *Nature* **336:** 388.

Kanagawa, O., E. Palmer, and J. Bill. 1989. The T cell receptor V$_{\beta6}$ domain imparts reactivity to the Mls-1^a antigen. *Cell Immunol.* **119:** 412.

Kappler, J.W., N. Roehm, and P. Marrack. 1987. T cell tolerance by clonal elimination in the thymus. *Cell* **49:** 273.

Kappler, J.W., U. Staerz, J. White, and P. Marrack. 1988. Self tolerance eliminates T cells specific for Mls-modified products of the major histocompatibility complex. *Nature* **332:** 35.

Kisielow, P., H.S. Teh, H. Blüthmann, and H. von Boehmer. 1988a. Positive selection of antigen-specific T cells in thymus by restricting MHC molecules. *Nature* **335:** 730.

Kisielow, P., H. Blüthmann, U.D. Staerz, M. Steinmetz, and H. von Boehmer. 1988b. Tolerance in T cell receptor transgenic mice involves deletion of nonmature CD4$^+$8$^+$ thymocytes. *Nature* **333:** 742.

MacDonald, H.R., H. Hengartner, and T. Pedrazzini. 1988a. Intrathymic deletion of self reactive cells prevented by neonatal anti-CD4 antibody treatment. *Nature* **335:** 174.

MacDonald, H.R., R.K. Lees, R. Schneider, R.M. Zinkernagel, and H. Hengartner. 1988b. Positive selection of CD4$^+$ thymocytes controlled by MHC class II gene products. *Nature* **336:** 471.

MacDonald, H.R., R. Schneider, R.K. Lees, R.C. Howe, H. Acha-Orbea, H. Festenstein, R.M. Zinkernagel, and H. Hengartner. 1988c. T cell receptor V$_\beta$ use predicts reactivity and tolerance to Mls^a-encoded antigens. *Nature* **332:** 40.

Table 6. Positive Selection of V$_\beta$6$^+$ CD4$^+$ Cells in Radiation Bone Marrow Chimeras

Chimera	Percentage of V$_\beta$6$^+$ (in CD4$^+$ subset)	
	thymus	lymph node
B10.G → B10.G	3.8 ± 0.4	3.7 ± 0.4
B10.BR → B10.BR	6.5 ± 0.5	7.3 ± 0.8
F$_1$ → B10.G	3.8 ± 0.4	4.9 ± 0.7
F$_1$ → B10.BR	7.4 ± 0.2	7.3 ± 0.6

V$_\beta$6$^+$ CD4$^+$ cells were assessed by two-color immunofluorescence (MacDonald et al. 1988c). Data are mean ± s.d. of four to five individual mice. Chimerism ranged from 83–99% as assessed by allele-specific anti-class I MHC antibodies.

MacDonald, H.R., A.L. Glasebrook, R. Schneider, R.K. Lees, H. Pircher, T. Pedrazzini, O Kanagawa, J.-F. Nicolas, R.C. Howe, R.M. Zinkernagel, and H. Hengartner. 1989. T-cell reactivity and tolerance to Mls^a-encoded antigens. *Immunol. Rev.* **107:** 89.

Möller, G., ed. 1988. The T cell repertoire. *Immunol. Rev.* **101.**

Payne, J., B.T. Huber, N.A. Cannon, R. Schneider, M.W. Schilham, H. Acha-Orbea, H.R. MacDonald, and H. Hengartner. 1988. Two monoclonal rat antibodies with specificity for the V$_{\beta6}$ region of the murine T cell receptor. *Proc. Natl. Acad. Sci.* **85:** 7685.

Pullen, A.M., P. Marrack, and J.W. Kappler. 1988. The T-cell repertoire is heavily influenced by tolerance to polymorphic self antigens. *Nature* **335:** 796.

Schneider, R., R.K. Lees, T. Pedrazzini, R.M. Zinkernagel, H. Hengartner, and H.R. MacDonald. 1989. Postnatal disappearance of self-reactive (V$_{\beta6}{}^+$) cells from the thymus of Mls^a mice. Implications for T cell development and autoimmunity. *J. Exp. Med.* **169:** 2149.

Sha, W.C., C.A. Nelson, R.D. Newberry, D.M. Kranz, J.H. Russell, and D.Y. Loh. 1988. Positive and negative selection of an antigen receptor on T cells in transgenic mice. *Nature* **336:** 73.

Speiser, D.E., R. Schneider, H. Hengartner, H.R. MacDonald, and R.M. Zinkernagel. 1989. Clonal deletion of self reactive T-cells in irradiation bone marrow chimeras and neonatally tolerant mice: Evidence for intercellular transfer of Mls^a. *J. Exp. Med.* **170:** 595.

Sprent, J., D. Lo, E.-K. Gao, and Y. Ron. 1988. T cell selection in the thymus. *Immunol. Rev.* **101:** 173.

Tomonari, K. and E. Lovering. 1988. T-cell receptor-specific monoclonal antibodies against a V$_{\beta11}$-positive mouse T-cell clone. *Immunogenetics* **28:** 445.

Zinkernagel, R.M., G.N. Callahan, A. Althage, S. Cooper, P.A. Klein, and J. Klein. 1978. On the thymus in the differentiation of "H-2 self recognition" by T cells: Evidence for dual recognition? *J. Exp. Med.* **147:** 882.

A Third Set of Genes Regulates Thymic Selection

E. Palmer,*† D.L. Woodland,* M.P. Happ,* J. Bill,* and O. Kanagawa‡

*Division of Basic Sciences, Department of Pediatrics, National Jewish Center for Immunology and Respiratory Medicine, Denver, Colorado 80206; †Department of Microbiology and Immunology, University of Colorado Health Sciences Center, Denver, Colorado 80262; ‡Lilly Research Laboratories, La Jolla, California 92037

The selection of a T-cell repertoire that is both self-major-histocompatibility-complex (MHC)-restricted and self-tolerant involves a number of genetic and biological processes, many of which occur in the thymus. The generation of a germ-line unselected repertoire depends on the rearrangement of a finite number of α- and β-chain gene segments (variable [V_β], diversity [D_β], joining [J_β], V_α, and J_α), as well as the random addition of nucleotides at the VD_β, DJ_β, and VJ_α joints (for review, see Wilson et al. 1988). These rearrangements begin about day 13 of fetal life and are completed by the day of birth (for review, see Fowlkes and Pardoll 1989). There is some polymorphism at the α- and β-chain loci between inbred strains.

Many experiments from many laboratories have described generic T-cell reactivities conferred by particular V_β domains. Several V_β gene segments encode reactivity for the class II MHC protein I-E (Kappler et al. 1987a,b; Tomonari and Lovering 1988; Bill et al. 1989) or gene products encoded by minor lymphocyte-stimulating (Mls) loci (Abe et al. 1988; Kappler et al. 1988; MacDonald et al. 1988; Pullen et al. 1988; Happ et al. 1989; Kanagawa et al. 1989), and T cells with these specificities are deleted from strains that express the appropriate ligands. The fraction of T cells expressing any particular V_β domain is large enough to study experimentally, and investigations of this kind have contributed to our understanding of tolerance. The generation of a self-tolerant repertoire has been shown to involve MHC-bearing cells in the thymus, which are derived from bone marrow precursors. Self-reactive T cells are literally removed from the repertoire by clonal deletion although atypical (nonthymic) expression of MHC gene products results in clonal anergy rather than clonal deletion (Lo et al. 1988). The deletion of self-reactive T cells is thought to occur at the $CD4^+8^+$ (double-positive) stage of thymocyte development in that cells bearing self-reactive TCRs are depleted from both the $CD4^+$ and $CD8^+$ peripheral T-cell subsets (Kappler et al. 1987a, 1988; MacDonald et al. 1988; Pullen et al. 1988; Tomonari and Lovering 1988; Bill et al. 1989; Kanagawa et al. 1989).

Perhaps the most intriguing aspect of T-cell development is the positive selection of self-MHC-restricted T cells into the peripheral repertoire. T lymphocytes recognize antigenic fragments that are physically bound to class I or class II glycoproteins, but this antigen recognition is particularly sensitive to the polymorphic variation that exists between the allelic forms of H-2 proteins (Zinkernagel and Doherty 1975). T cells with the ability to recognize antigen bound to self-MHC molecules are selected in the thymus (Bevan and Fink 1978; Zinkernagel et al. 1978), in the absence of an obvious source of antigen. However, this process requires the expression of the appropriate MHC gene product in the thymic cortex (Lo and Sprent 1986; J. Bill and E. Palmer, unpubl.). Concomitant with the positive selection of T cells is their differentiation from $CD4^+8^+$ (double-positive) into $CD4^+$ or $CD8^+$ (single-positive) thymocytes. Cells that recognize antigens bound to class I gene products coexpress the CD8 accessory molecule, whereas class-II-restricted T cells coexpress the CD4 accessory molecule. All of these features of positive selection have been clearly demonstrated in studies of T-cell receptor (TCR) transgenic mice (Kisielow et al. 1988a; Sha et al. 1988; Berg et al. 1989b).

Alleles of the α and β chains may act as immune response (IR) genes if the response to a particular antigen is absolutely dependent on the presence of a particular allelic form of a TCR gene segment. On the other hand, MHC haplotypes may function as IR genes by several mechanisms. The most obvious is that a particular peptide may not be able to bind any of the MHC molecules expressed in a given strain. Another route by which MHC genes can act as IR loci is the deletion of self-reactive T cells; if the T cells responding to a particular antigen have been deleted as a consequence of self-MHC tolerance, an IR defect should be apparent. Finally, MHC genes can encode IR phenotypes by their failure to select positively T cells capable of recognizing a particular antigen/MHC complex. A third class of genetic loci with the potential to encode IR phenotypes may be encoded by genes other than TCR (α and β chains) structural genes or MHC genes. These gene products might influence the clonal deletion as well as the positive selection of T cells. Moreover, the identification of non-TCR, non-MHC loci with IR properties might implicate a role for this class of gene products in normal thymic selection (positive and negative).

The study of IR genetics has been enhanced by the development of anti-TCR monoclonal antibodies (MAbs). Using these reagents, one can study the development and selection of thymocytes directly in the absence of immunization and expansion of responding

T cells. We have developed monoclonal antibody reagents specific for $V_\beta 5$- and $V_\beta 11$-encoded TCRs, and the experiments presented here describe some of the genetic elements controlling the generation of $V_\beta 5$- and $V_\beta 11$-bearing T cells. Studies with recombinant inbred mice reveal the role of TCR, MHC, and background loci in determining the degree to which these cells comprise the peripheral repertoire.

METHODS

Mice. All mice were purchased from Jackson Laboratories (Maine) or bred in the facilities of National Jewish Center (Colorado).

T-cell hybrids. The T-cell hybrids used in this study have been described previously (Bill et al. 1988). They were generated from mitogen (concanavalin-A)-stimulated peripheral T cells from B10, B10.Q, and B10.BR mice that were fused to BW5147 and maintained in culture as described previously (Kappler et al. 1981). Selected for use in this study were 24 hybrids that expressed mRNA for $V_\beta 5$. Sequencing the β-chain cDNA from the T-cell hybridoma 2HB51 showed that this hybrid expresses an in-frame $V_\beta 5.1$ mRNA transcript. 2HB51.8 is a subclone of 2HB51 selected for high levels of $V_\beta 5$ RNA.

Monoclonal antibody production. SWR mice, which carry a deletion at the V_β locus that includes both functional $V_\beta 5$ genes, were immunized three times intraperitoneally with 10^7 2HB51.8 cells ($V_\beta 5.1$ mRNA$^+$) at 2-week intervals. Three days following an intravenous boost of 10^7 cells, the mice were sacrificed, and spleen cells were fused to P3X63.Ag 8.653/3 using standard procedures (Kanagawa 1988). B-cell hybrids were selected in HAT medium, and culture supernatants were screened for the presence of antibodies capable of stimulating the immunogenic hybrid (2HB51.8) to secrete interleukin-2 (IL-2). Microtiter plates (96 well) were coated with goat anti-mouse immunoglobulin (Ig) (100 μg/ml), washed, and then incubated with B-cell hybridoma culture supernatants to immobilize any antibodies. 2HB51.8 cells (10^5) were added and cultured overnight. The assay depends on the ability of immobilized anti-TCR antibodies to stimulate TCR-bearing hybridomas to secrete IL-2 (detected by the ability of antibody-stimulated 2HB51.8 culture supernatants to support the growth of the IL-2-dependent T cell line, CTLL). Both MR9-4- and MR9-8-producing B-cell hybridomas were subcloned twice by limiting dilution before use. For all studies except the initial characterization of $V_\beta 5.1$ and $V_\beta 5.2$ specificity, which were done with culture supernatants, antibodies were purified over a protein-G-Sepharose column (Pharmacia, New Jersey), according to the manufacturer's directions, and were biotinylated prior to use. Without biotinylation MR9-8 appears to stain a few $V_\beta 5.2^+$ T cells weakly; however, when biotinylated this reactivity is undetectable and the monoclonal antibody is specific for $V_\beta 5.1^+$ T cells. Most likely, biotinylation of MR9-8 changes the binding site of the monoclonal antibody so that its affinity for $V_\beta 5.2$ is markedly reduced.

Flow cytometry. T-cell hybrids, nylon wool-nonadherent peripheral lymph node cells, and thymocytes were examined by indirect immunofluorescent staining to determine surface expression of TCRs composed of $V_\beta 5.1$ and $V_\beta 5.2$. T hybridoma cells (10^5) were stained with biotinylated primary antibody, washed, and stained with phycoerythrin (PE)-conjugated streptavidin (Tago, California). Nylon wool-purified lymph node cells (10^6) were first stained with biotinylated antibodies, washed, and subsequently stained with PE-conjugated streptavidin together with fluorescein-isothiocyanate-conjugated anti-CD4 (GK1.5) (Dialynas et al. 1983) or anti-CD8 (53.6) (Ledbetter and Herzenberg 1979). To compare strains, the percentage of total T cells expressing $V_\beta 5.1$ or $V_\beta 5.2$ was calculated based on a normalized CD4/CD8 ratio of 2:1. Thymocytes were cultured (Kappler et al. 1989) prior to staining to increase the density of TCR on the immature cortical cells. The total percentage of TCR-dull and TCR-bright thymocytes was determined by staining with biotinylated H57-597, which recognizes all $\alpha\beta$ receptors, followed by staining with PE streptavidin (Kubo et al. 1989). Samples were analyzed either on a Coulter Epics C or an EPICS 751 flow cytometer (Coulter Electronics, Florida). The software for the EPICS 751 was purchased from Cytomation, Inc. (Colorado).

RESULTS

Production of MAbs Recognizing $V_\beta 5$-encoded TCRs

SWR mice were immunized with a T-cell hybrid (2HB51.8) that expresses an in-frame mRNA for $V_\beta 5.1$. Since SWR mice carry a deletion encompassing both the $V_\beta 5.1$ and $V_\beta 5.2$ genes, they should respond to recognize a $V_\beta 5$-encoded protein but should be tolerant to many other proteins present on the surface of T-cell hybrids. Immune spleen cells were fused to the myeloma P3X63.AG8.653/3, and culture supernatants from the resultant HAT-resistant B-cell hybrids screened for the presence of antibodies capable of stimulating the immunizing T-cell hybrid (2HB51.8) to produce IL-2. In this way, MAbs MR9-4 and MR9-8 were identified. To determine the specificities of these antibodies, we stained 24 T-cell hybrids that express $V_\beta 5$ mRNA. Of 24, 22 hybrids were stained with MR9-4 while 14 hybrids stained with both MR9-4 and MR9-8. The two hybrids that did not stain with either antibody may express a nonfunctional (out-of-frame) $V_\beta 5$ transcript or lack surface expression of TCR. The hybrids that did stain with these MAbs coexpress a variety of TCR V_α transcripts including Vα2, 3, 4, 5, 8, and 10 (data not shown), implying that these antibodies are specific for $V_\beta 5$-encoded β chains paired with any α chain. DNA sequencing of the junctional regions of

$V_\beta 5$ cDNAs from 13 of these hybrids (data not shown) demonstrated that the MR9-4 MAb stains hybrids expressing either the $V_\beta 5.1$ or $V_\beta 5.2$ gene segments, whereas the MR9-8 MAb stains only $V_\beta 5.1$-expressing hybrids. Although $J_\beta 2.5$ and $J_\beta 2.6$ appear frequently, antibody staining does not appear to require particular D_β or J_β regions. Thus, the fraction of $V_\beta 5.1$-bearing T cells can be determined directly by staining with the MR9-8 MAb, and the fraction of $V_\beta 5.2$-bearing T cells can be determined by subtracting the fraction of cells stained with MR9-8 ($V_\beta 5.1$ only) from that stained with MR9-4 ($V_\beta 5.1$ and $V_\beta 5.2$). The identification and characterization of the anti-$V_\beta 11$ MAb, RR3-15, has been described previously (Bill et al. 1989).

$V_\beta 5^+$ T Cells Are Deleted from Mouse Strains Expressing I-E Molecules

Using $V_\beta 5$-specific MAbs, we stained peripheral lymph node T cells from a panel of B10 MHC congenic mice to understand better the influence of the H-2 haplotype on the number of T cells expressing $V_\beta 5$-encoded TCRs (Fig. 1A). In those strains that do not express an I-E molecule, $V_\beta 5.1^+$ and $V_\beta 5.2^+$ lymphocytes each comprise a significant fraction of the total number of T cells, whereas in I-E$^+$ strains both $V_\beta 5.1$- and $V_\beta 5.2$-expressing cells are rare. Particularly informative are the MHC recombinant pairs, B10.A(4R) versus B10.A(2R) and B10.S(7R) versus B10.HTT. In both pairs, the genetic background and the MHC haplotypes are identical except that the B10.A(2R) and B10.HTT express I-E^k and I-E^s, respectively, whereas B10.A(4R) and B10.S(7R) are I-E$^-$. The expression of an I-E molecule correlates with a dramatic decrease in the fraction of T cells that bear $V_\beta 5$-encoded receptors. Studies of F_1 mice bred from I-E$^-$ and I-E$^+$ parents, e.g., ([B10.A[4R] × B10.A[2R])F_1, (B10 × B10.BR)F_1, and (B6 × DBA/2)F_1 show that the low level of $V_\beta 5^+$ T cells is a dominant trait, suggesting that $V_\beta 5^+$ T cells are clonally deleted from I-E-expressing strains (Fig. 1A). The elimination of $V_\beta 5$-bearing cells is not complete since the fraction of positive cells is clearly above the background seen in C57L ($0.03 \pm 0.01\%$), a strain that carries a germ-line deletion of both the $V_\beta 5.1$ and $V_\beta 5.2$ structural genes.

CD4$^+$ T Cells Rarely Express $V_\beta 5^+$ Receptors

Figure 1B shows the fraction of $V_\beta 5.1$- and $V_\beta 5.2$-bearing T cells in both the CD4$^+$ and CD8$^+$ subsets. There are few $V_\beta 5^+$ cells in either the CD4 or the CD8 subsets of B10.BR mice that express an I-E molecule. This is consistent with the deletion of self-reactive T cells occurring at the CD4$^+$/CD8$^+$ (double-positive) stage of thymocyte development. Surprisingly, in I-E$^-$ strains, there are relatively few $V_\beta 5^+$/CD4$^+$ cells despite appreciable numbers of V$\beta 5^+$/CD8$^+$ cells. This is seen with both $V_\beta 5.1$- and $V_\beta 5.2$-bearing T cells and is

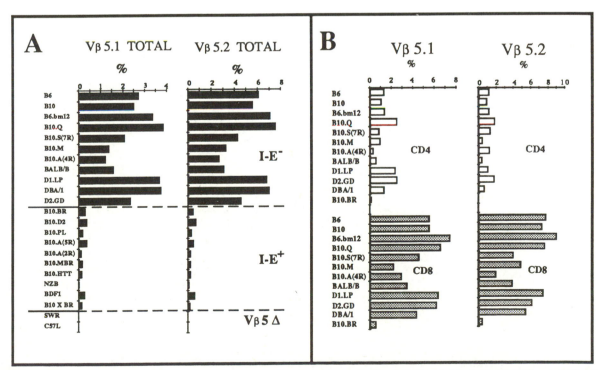

Figure 1. (A) The frequency of $V_\beta 5.1$- and $V_\beta 5.2$-bearing T cells was determined as described in Methods. $V_\beta 5.1^+$ and -5.2^+ cells each comprise 3–8% of peripheral T cells in I-E$^-$ strains, whereas they are very rare ($<0.5\%$) among peripheral T cells in I-E$^+$ strains. The SWR and C57L strains do not carry the $V_\beta 5.1$ and -5.2 structural genes and thus do not express any $V_\beta 5^+$ T cells. (B) The frequency of $V_\beta 5.1$- and $V_\beta 5.2$-bearing T cells in the CD4$^+$ and CD8$^+$ subsets was determined as described in Methods. The majority of $V_\beta 5^+$ T cells are CD8$^+$ in I-E$^-$ strains.

apparent with four I-E⁻ MHC haplotypes (H-2^{b,s,f,q}) as well as with the B10.A(4R) and D2.GD strains, which express I-A^k or I-A^d in the absence of an I-E molecule, respectively. Thus, in six I-E⁻ haplotypes examined, the majority of V$_\beta$5.1- and V$_\beta$5.2-bearing T cells are CD8$^+$.

Sequence Similarities between V$_\beta$ Domains Conferring the Same Reactivity

A large fraction of V$_\beta$ domains confer I-E reactivity to their corresponding T cells. The data in Figure 1A show that V$_\beta$5.1- and V$_\beta$5.2-bearing cells are deleted from I-E-expressing strains, whereas previous work has

shown that V$_\beta$17a- and V$_\beta$11-bearing cells behave in a similar manner (Kappler et al. 1987a; Tomonari and Lovering 1988; Bill et al. 1989). From studies of mitogen-stimulated T-cell hybridomas generated from B10 MHC congenic strains (Bill et al. 1988) and from studies of V$_\beta$ gene expression in mitogen-stimulated T cells (M.S. Vacchio and R. Hodes, pers. comm.), it seems likely that the frequency of V$_\beta$12-bearing T cells is low in I-E$^+$ strains. Thus, V$_\beta$12$^+$ T cells may also be deleted from the repertoire of I-E-bearing mice. We compared the amino acid sequences of the V$_\beta$5.1, -5.2, -11, -12, and -17a domains (Fig. 2A) to determine whether these V$_\beta$ regions share a common sequence motif that might explain their I-E reactivity. These five

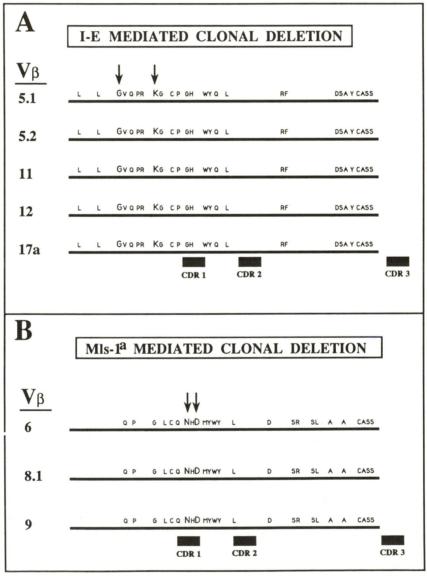

Figure 2. (A) Amino acid sequence comparisons of five V$_\beta$ domains that confer I-E reactivity. These five domains share amino acid identity at 25 positions (excluding the leader). Two residues, Gly-13 and Lys-15 (↓) are shared by these five domains and are not found in any other V$_\beta$ sequence. These residues may contribute to the recognition of I-E. (B) Amino acid sequence comparisons of three V$_\beta$ domains that confer Mls-1^a reactivity. These five domains share amino acid identity at 25 positions (excluding the leader). Two residues, Asn-28 and Asp-30, (↓) are shared by these three domains and are not found in any other V$_\beta$ sequence. These residues may contribute to Mls-1^a recognition.

V_β sequences share sequence identity at 25 of 94 (27%) amino acid residues. However, 23 of the 25 shared amino acids appear frequently in other (I-E unreactive) V_β sequences. What appears to be present in these five sequences but absent from other V_β sequences is a glycine at position 3 and a lysine at position 15. Given the conservation of these two residues, they may play an important role in conferring I-E reactivity. Interestingly, these two residues fall outside the complementarity-determining regions (CDRs) determined by analysis of amino acid variability (Patten et al. 1984; Becker et al. 1986; Chothia et al. 1988).

We have also carried out a sequence comparison between the three V_β domains ($V_\beta6$ [MacDonald et al. 1988; Kanagawa et al. 1989]; $V_\beta8.1$ [Kappler et al. 1988], and $V_\beta9$ [Happ et al. 1989]) that confer reactivity to Mls-1[a]-encoded gene products (Fig. 2B). Although, these three V_β sequences share sequence identity at 25 of 94 (27%) amino acid residues, only the asparagine at position 28 and the aspartic acid at position 30 are unique to these three V domains that confer Mls-1[a] reactivity. These two residues fall within CDR1 (Chothia et al. 1988).

Expression of I-E Is Necessary but Insufficient for the Clonal Deletion of $V_\beta5^+$ T Cells

We noticed that the extent of deletion varied between strains of different genetic backgrounds expressing the same H-2 haplotype. For example, there are more $V_\beta5.2$-bearing cells in DBA/2 than in B10.D2 mice (Table 1). To explore the genetic basis of these non-MHC differences, we determined the frequency of $V_\beta5$-bearing peripheral T cells in 16 B6 × DBA/2 (B × D) recombinant inbred (RI) strains that carry the H-2[d] haplotype (Table 1). Of 16, 11 (approximately 3/4) of these H-2[d] RI strains have a low frequency of CD8[+] $V_\beta5.2^+$ cells (0.7–1.3%) similar to that seen in B10.D2 and (B6 × DBA/2)F$_1$ mice. Another two strains (B × D12 and B × D32) express CD8[+] $V_\beta5.2$-bearing cells at a frequency similar to that seen in DBA/2 mice (2.0–2.9%), whereas three strains (B × D18, B × D31, and B × D28) have more CD8[+] $V_\beta5.2^+$ cells than either the DBA/2 or the B10.D2 parental strains. The marked variation in the frequency of $V_\beta5.2^+$ T cells is not explained by the quantitative expression of the I-E gene product. Table 1 also displays the relative expression of I-E on lymph node cells measured by fluorescence intensity, and all the H-2[d] strains examined express a similar amount of surface I-E[d]. For example, the expression of $V_\beta5.2$-bearing cells differs markedly when comparing the B × D16 and B × D18 strains; however, they express a similar quantity of surface I-E[d]. Thus, the frequency of CD8[+] $V_\beta5.2^+$ cells is not likely to be related to the absolute level of I-E expression.

High Levels of $V_\beta5.2^+$ T Cells in Some I-E[d]-bearing RI Strains Are Due to Poor Clonal Deletion

The high level of $V_\beta5.2$-bearing T cells in some of the H-2[d] B × D RI strains could be explained by poor clonal deletion or by an enhanced level of positive selection. To clarify this issue, we bred the B × D28 strain (expressing I-E[d] and a high level of CD8[+] $V_\beta5.2^+$ cells) with DBA/2 or B10.D2 parents and measured the frequency of $V_\beta5.2^+$ cells in the resulting F$_1$ animals

Table 1. Frequency of CD8[+] $V_\beta5.2^+$ T Cells among I-E[d]-bearing B6 × DBA/2 Recombinant Inbred Strains

Strain	H-2	Relative I-E expression (14-4-4 staining)	$V_\beta5.2^+$/CD8[+] T cells (% ± S.E.)
C57BL/6	b	0	7.5 ± 0.5
DBA/2	d	1.0 ± 0.5	2.5 ± 0.1
B10.D2	d	1.1 ± 0.3	0.7 ± 0.2
BDF$_1$	b/d	0.9 ± 0.2	0.7 ± 0.1
B × D1	d	0.9 ± 0.1	0.3 ± 0.1
B × D5	d	1.0 ± 0.1	0.8 ± 0.1
B × D6	d	1.1 ± 0.2	0.4 ± 0.1
B × D9	d	1.0 ± 0.1	0.6 ± 0.4
B × D12	d	0.8 ± 0.2	2.9 ± 0.6[a]
B × D16	d	1.1 ± 0.1	0.6 ± 0.05
B × D18	d	1.1 ± 0.1	6.8 ± 0.2[b]
B × D21	d	1.0 ± 0.1	0.8 ± 0.2
B × D22	d	0.9 ± 0.3	0.5 ± 0.3
B × D24	d	1.0 ± 0.2	1.1 ± 0.1
B × D25	d	1.0 ± 0.2	1.5 ± 0.2
B × D27	d	1.1 ± 0.1	1.2 ± 0.2
B × D28	d	1.3 ± 0.3	5.3 ± 1.6[b]
B × D30	d	1.3 ± 0.1	0.4 ± 0.1
B × D31	d	0.9 ± 0.1	4.5 ± 0.3[b]
B × D32	d	0.9 ± 0.1	2.2 ± 0.2[a]

[a]Moderate deletion of $V_\beta5.2^+$ cells.

[b]Poor deletion of $V_\beta5.2^+$ cells.

Table 2. Frequency of CD8$^+$ V$_\beta$5.2$^+$ T Cells in Parental and F$_1$ Mice

Strain	H-2	Relative I-E expression (14-4-4 staining)	V$_\beta$5.2$^+$/CD8$^+$ T cells (% ± S.E.)
DBA/2	d	1.0 ± 0.5	2.5 ± 0.1
B10.D2	d	1.1 ± 0.3	0.7 ± 0.2
BDF$_1$	d/b	0.9 ± 0.2	0.7 ± 0.1
B × D28	d	1.3 ± 0.3	5.3 ± 0.1
(DBA/2 × B × D28)F$_1$	d	0.9 ± 0.1	1.9 ± 0.2
(B10.D2 × B × D28)F$_1$	d	0.8 ± 0.1	0.8 ± 0.1

(Table 2). The level of V$_\beta$5.2 cells in (B × D28 × DBA/2)F$_1$ animals is similar to that seen in the DBA/2 parent, whereas the level of V$_\beta$5.2$^+$ cells in (B × D28 × B10.D2)F$_1$ animals is similar to that seen in the B10.D2 parent. In both cases, the B10.D2 and the DBA/2 genetic backgrounds are dominant to the B × D28 genetic background in determining the frequency of V$_\beta$5.2$^+$ T cells. Expression of a gene(s) from the DBA/2 or B10.D2 genome most likely generates a product that acts in *trans* to mediate the clonal deletion of V$_\beta$5.2$^+$ lymphocytes. That a low level of V$_\beta$5.2 expression is dominant in F$_1$ mice is consistent with the idea that a non-MHC gene product plays a major role in deleting V$_\beta$5.2$^+$ cells from the repertoire. This gene product(s) is (are) likely not produced by B × D28 mice.

T-cell Hybridoma 5Q12 Recognizes a Determinant Present on B10.D2 but Absent from DBA/2 Splenocytes

In screening a number of hybridomas for their reactivity to various MHC gene products, we identified a hy-bridoma (5Q12) that recognizes I-E molecules, including I-E^d. The specificity of this hybrid is demonstrated by the fact that an anti-I-E^d antibody (14.4.4) blocks antigen recognition, whereas an anti-I-A^d antibody (MK-D6) does not (data not shown). Surprisingly, the 5Q12 hybridoma is not stimulated by DBA/2 spleno-cytes even though B10.D2, (B6 × DBA/2)F$_1$, BALB/c, and NZB splenocytes are capable of stimulation (Table 3 and data not shown). Examination of the 16 B × D RI strains that carry H-2^d for their capacity to stimulate the 5Q12 hybridoma revealed that spleno-cytes from 9 of the 16 I-E^d-bearing strains are stimula-tory. Table 3 also shows the relative expression of I-E in these strains; the ability to stimulate the hybridoma is clearly unrelated to the degree of I-E expression. That approximately 50% of the I-E^d-bearing RI strains can stimulate the 5Q12 hybridoma is consistent with the idea that a single genetic locus determines this phenotype. Comparing the strain distribution pattern for this phenotype with the list of strain distribution patterns for loci mapped in this set of RI mice identifies a perfect concordance with the Mtv-9 locus on chromo-some 12 (data not shown).

Table 3. Stimulation of the T-cell Hybridoma 5Q12 by Splenocytes Derived from I-E^d-bearing Recombinant Inbred Strains

Strain	H-2	Relative I-E expression (14-4-4 staining)	5Q12 reactivity[a] (IL-2 units/ml)
DBA/2	d	1.0 ± 0.5	<10 (−)
B10.D2	d	1.1 ± 0.3	150 (+)
BDF$_1$	b/d	0.9 ± 0.2	90 (+)
B × D1	d	0.9 ± 0.1	80 (+)
B × D5	d	1.0 ± 0.1	120 (+)
B × D6	d	1.1 ± 0.2	100 (+)
B × D9	d	1.0 ± 0.1	110 (+)
B × D12	d	0.8 ± 0.2	<10 (−)
B × D16	d	1.1 ± 0.1	30 (+)
B × D18	d	1.1 ± 0.1	<10 (−)
B × D21	d	1.0 ± 0.1	40 (+)
B × D22	d	0.9 ± 0.3	70 (+)
B × D24	d	1.0 ± 0.2	310 (+)
B × D25	d	1.0 ± 0.2	<10 (−)
B × D27	d	1.1 ± 0.1	<10 (−)
B × D28	d	1.3 ± 0.3	<10 (−)
B × D30	d	1.3 ± 0.1	390 (+)
B × D31	d	0.9 ± 0.1	<10 (−)
B × D32	d	0.9 ± 0.1	<10 (−)

[a](+) Stimulates 5Q12 hybridoma; (−) does not stimulate 5Q12 hybridoma.

The Locus Encoding the Determinant Recognized by 5Q12 May Be Related to the Deletion of $V_\beta 5.2$-bearing T Cells

The data in Table 4 compare a strain's ability to delete $V_\beta 5.2^+$ cells from the repertoire with its ability to stimulate 5Q12. Two interesting correlations can be drawn from this comparison. First, every strain whose splenocytes can stimulate the 5Q12 hybridoma has efficiently deleted $V_\beta 5.2^+$ T cells from the periphery. In addition, every strain that does not efficiently delete $V_\beta 5.2$-bearing cells is incapable of stimulating the 5Q12 hybridoma. Two strains fit neither of these correlations. B × D25 and B × D27 efficiently delete $V_\beta 5.2^+$ cells despite being unable to stimulate the 5Q12 cell line. The behavior of these two strains is addressed in the Discussion section.

Frequency of $CD8^+ V_\beta 11^+$ T Cells Is Regulated by Non-MHC Genes

We also examined the frequency of $CD8^+ V_\beta 11^+$ T cells in the H-2^d B × D RI strains (Fig. 3). $V_\beta 11$-bearing cells comprise from 1.5–4% of the $CD8^+$ in these various H-2^d strains. Two strains (B × D6 and B × D16) carry a frequency of $CD8^+ V_\beta 11^+$ cells similar to that seen in the B10.D2 strain (1.5%). The other 14 H-2^d B × D RI strains express more $V_\beta 11$-bearing cells in the $CD8^+$ compartment. The lower panel of Figure 3 demonstrates that the frequency of $CD8^+ V_\beta 11^+$ T cells is unrelated to the quantitative expression of surface I-E as measured on the surface of lymph node B cells.

High Frequency of $V_\beta 11^+ CD8^+$ Lymphocytes in the B × D28 Strain Is Most Likely Due to Aggressive Positive Selection

The high level of $V_\beta 11$-bearing T cells in some of the H-2^d B × D RI strains could be explained by poor clonal deletion or by an enhanced level of positive selection. To distinguish between these two alternatives, we generated (B × D28 × B10.D2)F$_1$ animals and measured the frequency of $CD8^+ V_\beta 11^+$ cells in these F$_1$ mice (Fig. 4). The level of $V_\beta 11^+$ cells in (B × D28 × B10.D2)F$_1$ animals is high, similar to that seen in the B × D28 parent. Thus, the B × D28 genetic background is dominant to the B10.D2 genetic background in determining the frequency of $V_\beta 11^+$ T cells. That a high level of $V_\beta 11$ expression in the $CD8^+$ subset is dominant in these F$_1$ mice is consistent with the idea that non-MHC gene products play a major role in the positive selection of $V_\beta 11^+$ cells into the repertoire. These gene products are not likely produced by B10.D2 mice.

DISCUSSION

Previously, we determined that 12% of B10 and 9% of B10.Q T-cell hybridomas expressed $V_\beta 5$ mRNA, whereas less than 1% of B10.BR-derived hybridomas expressed RNA from the $V_\beta 5$ family (Bill et al. 1988). These hybrids were used to generate and characterize $V_\beta 5$-specific MAbs. Our results show that T cells bearing $V_\beta 5.1$- or $V_\beta 5.2$-encoded TCRs are deleted from mouse strains (including B10.BR) that express an I-E molecule. Clonal deletion from I-E-bearing mice has

Table 4. Comparison of B6 × DBA/2 Recombinant Inbred Strains for Their Ability to Delete $V_\beta 5.2^+$ Cells and to Stimulate the 5Q12 Hybridoma

Strain	H-2	Relative I-E expression (14-4-4 staining)	$V_\beta 5.2^+$/CD8$^+$ T cells (% ± S.E.)	5Q12 reactivity[c] (IL-2 units/ml)	
DBA/2	d	1.0 ± 0.5	2.5 ± 0.1	<10	(−)
B10D2	d	1.1 ± 0.3	0.7 ± 0.2	150	(+)
BDF$_1$	b/d	0.9 ± 0.2	0.7 ± 0.1	90	(+)
B × D1	d	0.9 ± 0.1	0.3 ± 0.1	80	(+)
B × D5	d	1.0 ± 0.1	0.8 ± 0.1	120	(+)
B × D6	d	1.1 ± 0.2	0.4 ± 0.1	100	(+)
B × D9	d	1.0 ± 0.1	0.6 ± 0.4	110	(+)
B × D12	d	0.8 ± 0.2	2.9 ± 0.6[a]	<10	(−)
B × D16	d	1.1 ± 0.1	0.6 ± 0.05	30	(+)
B × D18	d	1.1 ± 0.1	6.8 ± 0.2[b]	<10	(−)
B × D21	d	1.0 ± 0.1	0.8 ± 0.2	40	(+)
B × D22	d	0.9 ± 0.3	0.5 ± 0.3	70	(+)
B × D24	d	1.0 ± 0.2	1.1 ± 0.1	310	(+)
B × D25	d	1.0 ± 0.2	1.5 ± 0.2	<10	(−)
B × D27	d	1.1 ± 0.1	1.2 ± 0.2	<10	(−)
B × D28	d	1.3 ± 0.3	5.3 ± 1.6[b]	<10	(−)
B × D30	d	1.3 ± 0.1	0.4 ± 0.1	390	(+)
B × D31	d	0.9 ± 0.1	4.5 ± 0.3[b]	<10	(−)
B × D32	d	0.9 ± 0.1	2.2 ± 0.2[a]	<10	(−)

[a]Moderate deletion of $V_\beta 5.2^+$ cells.
[b]Poor deletion of $V_\beta 5.2^+$ cells.
[c](+) Stimulates 5Q12 hybridoma; (−) does not stimulate 5Q12 hybridoma.

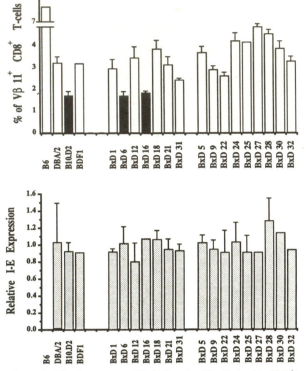

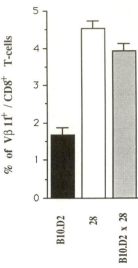

Figure 4. The frequency of $V_\beta 11$-bearing T cells in the CD8$^+$ subset was determined in B10.D2, B × D28, and (B10.D2 × B × D28)F$_1$ mice. The high level of CD8$^+$ V$_\beta 11^+$ T cells seen in B × D28 mice is dominant in (B10.D2 × B × D28)F$_1$ mice. This type of F$_1$ genetics implies that positive selection (not tolerance) is the mechanism determining the level of CD8$^+$ V$_\beta 11^+$ lymphocytes in B × D28 mice.

Figure 3. The frequency of $V_\beta 11$-bearing T cells in the CD8$^+$ subset was determined among parental and H-2^d-bearing B6 × DBA/2 recombinant inbred (B × D RI) strains. Only two RI strains, B × D6 and B × D16, have low V$_\beta 11$ levels similar to the B10.D2 strain. The lower panel displays the relative levels of I-E expression as measured on lymph node B cells. The frequency of CD8$^+$ V$_\beta 11^+$ T cells is unrelated to the quantitative expression of surface I-E.

also been shown to be a property of V$_\beta$17a- and V$_\beta$11-bearing T cells. Amino acid sequence comparisons of the five V$_\beta$ domains engendering I-E reactivity reveal two residues (glycine at position 3 and lysine at position 15) that are shared by these five V$_\beta$ domains but are absent from all other V$_\beta$ domains. Interestingly, these two residues fall outside the CDRs determined by analysis of amino acid variability (Chothia et al. 1988). In contrast, the amino acid residues (asparagine at position 28 and aspartic acid at position 30) shared by the V regions conferring Mls-1^a reactivity fall within CDR1. This implies that amino acids outside the CDRs play an important role in the recognition of I-E by V$_\beta$5.1, -5.2-, -11, -12, or 17a-bearing T cells, and that the analysis of amino acid variability (Chothia et al. 1988) may not have identified all residues important for antigen recognition. Recent investigation (M. Vacchio and R. Hodes, pers. comm.) indicates that the V$_\beta$16 domain may confer reactivity to I-E, as well. Since this domain does not contain the Gly-3/Lys-15 motif, it must use other amino acid residues for the recognition of I-E.

A large fraction of V$_\beta$ domains confers generic reactivity to I-E molecules. Of 20 functional V$_\beta$ gene segments, at least 5 encode receptors with I-E reactivity (V$_\beta$5.1, V$_\beta$5.2 [this paper]; V$_\beta$11 [Tomonari and Lover-

ing 1988; Bill et al. 1989]; V$_\beta$12 [Bill et al. 1988; M. Vacchio and R. Hodes, pers. comm.]; and V$_\beta$17a [Kappler et al. 1987a,b]). Thus, I-E-bearing mice delete approximately 20–25% of their repertoire of T-cells. Presumably, these V$_\beta$ genes have been maintained in the V gene pool because they are advantageous to I-E$^-$ mice.

The effects of I-E on the immune response seem complex. I-E-bearing mice have an additional MHC molecule to select positively (I-E-restricted) T cells and to present (I-E-binding) peptides. The I-E gene product augments the response to several experimental antigens (hen eggwhite lysozyme, cytochrome c, sperm whale myoglobin, influenza hemagglutinin) (for review, see Buus et al. 1987) and presumably to naturally occurring pathogens. On the other hand, the deletion of a large fraction of I-E-reactive T cells may generate holes in the T-cell repertoire through which pathogens can infect hosts. The increased susceptibility of I-E-bearing mice to infections with *Nemtospiroides dubius* and *Trichinella spirali* (Doherty et al. 1985) could result from I-E-mediated deletion of protective T cells. Finally, the expression of I-E may lead to a decreased susceptibility to certain autoimmune diseases. For example, the transgenic expression of I-E in NOD mice prevents the development of insulin-dependent diabetes normally seen in this strain (Nishimoto et al. 1987). V$_\beta$5.1, -5.2, -11, or -12-bearing T cells may play a role in the pathogenesis of this disease.

It is striking that V$_\beta$5$^+$ T cells are not equally distributed among the CD4$^+$ and CD8$^+$ subsets in I-E$^-$ mice. V$_\beta$5.1 and V$_\beta$5.2-bearing T cells each comprise 5–8% of the CD8$^+$ lymphocytes in I-E$^-$ mice. Since each of these gene segments accounts for 5% of the V$_\beta$ gene pool, this represents the expected frequency of the corresponding T cells. On the basis of previous results (Marusic-Galesic et al. 1988), where in vivo administration of an anti-class I MAb abrogated the selection of CD8$^+$ T cells, our data suggest that class I, H-2^K and/or D proteins positively select V$_\beta$5-bearing cells during thymic ontogeny, resulting in their development into mature CD8$^+$ T cells. The class II protein I-E is a potent tolerogen of V$_\beta$5-bearing thymocytes, whereas in the absence of I-E these cells are positively selected by class I gene products. V$_\beta$5-bearing T cells may be cross-reactive for I-E and class I MHC proteins; however, the interaction of V$_\beta$5-bearing immature thymocytes with I-E leads to their deletion from the repertoire, whereas the interaction with the class I molecules (K or D) leads to their positive selection into the repertoire of I-E$^-$ strains.

V$_\beta$5.1 and V$_\beta$5.2-bearing T cells each comprise only 1–2% of the CD4$^+$ lymphocytes in I-E$^-$ strains. This is significantly less than the 5% expected if all of the 20 V$_\beta$ gene segments present in the germ line were equally expressed among peripheral T cells. The class II gene product I-A may be relatively inefficient in the positive selection of V$_\beta$5$^+$ thymocytes, given the paucity of CD4$^+$, V$_\beta$5$^+$ T cells in the periphery of I-E$^-$ mice. Although the low level of V$_\beta$5$^+$ T cells in the CD4$^+$ subset could reflect the I-A-mediated deletion of V$_\beta$5$^+$ T cells, one feature of the data argues against this explanation. In the instances of tolerance by clonal deletion described so far, deletion appears to occur at the double-positive (CD8$^+$/CD4$^+$) stage of thymic development as evidenced by the fact that both the CD4$^+$ and the CD8$^+$ subsets are depleted. This has been observed for I-E-mediated tolerance of V$_\beta$17a (Kappler et al. 1987a,b) and V$_\beta$11 (Tomonari and Lovering 1988; Bill et al. 1989); for Mls-mediated tolerance of V$_\beta$8.1 (Kappler et al. 1988), V$_\beta$6 (MacDonald et al. 1988; Kanagawa et al. 1989), and V$_\beta$3 (Pullen et al. 1988); for the Staphylococcal-enterotoxin-mediated tolerance of V$_\beta$8.2 (Kappler et al. 1989), and the H-Y-, L^d-, or Mls-mediated tolerance seen in TCR-transgenic mice (Kisielow et al. 1988b; Sha et al. 1988; Berg et al. 1989a). In the case of V$_\beta$5-bearing lymphocytes in I-E$^-$ mice, only the CD4$^+$ levels of V$_\beta$5$^+$ cells are less than that expected. Thus, if the low levels of CD4$^+$/V$_\beta$5$^+$ T cells are due to tolerance, it must represent an atypical form of deletion that does not occur at the double-positive stage of thymocyte development. For this reason, we favor the idea that I-A is a weak positive selector of V$_\beta$5-bearing thymocytes.

Studies with recombinant inbred mice clearly show that I-E in and of itself is not sufficient to delete V$_\beta$5.2$^+$ cells from the repertoire. Non-MHC genes are required for this clonal deletion, and the number of B × D RI strains that fail to delete V$_\beta$5.2$^+$ cells implies that only a small number of these genes is involved in this form of tolerance. Approximately three-fourths of the B × D RI strains (11 of 16) that carry H-2^d express a low frequency (0.7–1.5%) of CD8$^+$ V$_\beta$5.2$^+$ cells. This is consistent with the idea that one of two unlinked loci,

in addition to I-E^d, are needed to mediate the full deletion of V$_\beta$5.2-bearing cells. It seems likely that the B6 alleles of these two loci control the phenotype of full deletion because the deletion in the DBA/2 strain is less complete. One-quarter of H-2^d RI strains would be expected to carry the DBA/2 alleles of both of these non-MHC loci and approximately one-fourth of the H-2^d RI strains (5 of 16) do not display the phenotype of full clonal deletion. The other point to be emphasized is that either of these two genetic loci, alone, can mediate the elimination of V$_\beta$5.2$^+$ cells to the full extent. These conclusions are consistent with the observation that three-fourths of the strains display the B10.D2 or the BDF1 phenotype, whereas one-fourth of the strains do not.

The five strains that are weak deletors of V$_\beta$5.2$^+$ lymphocytes can be divided into two groups. One group, composed of B × D12 and B × D32 are similar to DBA/2 mice regarding their elimination of V$_\beta$5.2$^+$ cells (moderate deletion), whereas a second group composed of the B × D18, B × D28, and B × D31 strains deletes even fewer V$_\beta$5.2-bearing cells (poor deletion). The segregation of V$_\beta$5.2 phenotypes among this group of strains supports the idea that the DBA/2 allele of a third genetic locus also contributes to the moderate deletion of V$_\beta$5.2$^+$ cells. Thus, RI strains that carry one or both of two B6 genes fully delete V$_\beta$5.2-bearing T cells from the repertoire. This phenotype is representative of B × D1, -6, -16, -21, -5, -9, -22, -24, -25, -27, and -30. RI strains that have do not carry either of these B6 genes as a consequence of chromosomal segregation but do carry the DBA/2 allele of a third unlinked gene delete V$_\beta$5.2$^+$ cells to a moderate degree, similar to that seen in the DBA/2 parent. The phenotype of moderate deletion is a characteristic of the B × D12 and B × D32 strains. Finally, strains that carry neither of the B6 genes nor the DBA/2 gene poorly delete V$_\beta$5.2$^+$ cells from the periphery. This phenotype is apparent in the B × D18, -28, and -31 strains.

By what mechanism do these genes contribute to the deletion of I-E reactive V$_\beta$5.2-bearing cells? The data in Tables 3 and 4 support the idea that one of the tolerogenic B6 genes encodes a product that is expressed on the surface of splenocytes. We identified a T-cell hybridoma 5Q12 that is I-E reactive and recognizes I-E^d on the surface of B10.D2 and BDF$_1$ splenocytes but not on the surface of DBA/2 splenocytes. Of 16 I-E^d-bearing RI strains, 9 can stimulate the 5Q12, implying that the stimulation is controlled by a single genetic locus. The strain distribution pattern of this phenotype matches that of the Mtv-9 locus on chromosome 12, implying that the expression of this antigenic moiety is controlled by a gene linked to the Mtv-9 marker on chromosome 12.

Recently, a subset of I-A^b molecules has been defined using the MAb Y-Ae (Murphy et al. 1989). This subset of I-A^b molecules is present on peripheral B cells and on thymic medullary cells but is absent from the thymic cortex. Furthermore, this subset accounts for approximately 10% of the I-A^b molecules present on the surface of B cells. One mechanism by which 10% of the I-A molecules can be distinguished is if their binding sites are occupied by a major peptide. By analogy, the B6 gene that encodes the antigenic moiety recognized by the 5Q12 hybridoma may produce a peptide that occupies a large fraction of the I-E on the surface of splenic cells. The DBA/2 allele of this gene may be either nonfunctional or produces a polymorphic form of the peptide.

If this B6 gene does produce a major I-E-binding peptide, it is likely to play a prominent role in the deletion of $V_\beta 5.2^+$ T cells. All H-2^d B × D RI strains that express the cell-surface component recognized by the 5Q12 hybrid, fully delete their CD8$^+$ $V_\beta 5.2^+$ lymphocytes (Table 4). All RI strains that are moderate or poor deletors of $V_\beta 5.2$-bearing cells fail to stimulate the 5Q12 cell line (Table 4). There are two strains, B × D25 and B × D27, that are exceptions to these correlations. Although these strains are "strong" deletors of $V_\beta 5.2^+$ cells, their splenocytes are incapable of stimulating 5Q12. We have proposed the existence of two B6 genes, either of which can mediate the full deletion of $V_\beta 5.2^+$ cells (see above). One of these B6 genes is likely defined by the cell-surface antigen recognized by the 5Q12 hybridoma, whereas the second B6 gene has yet to be characterized. B × D25 and -27 do not carry the 5Q12 gene but do express the second B6 gene as evidenced by the paucity of $V_\beta 5.2^+$ cells.

The data clearly show that the expression of the class II molecule I-E is necessary but insufficient for the deletion of T cells expressing $V_\beta 5.2$-encoded receptors. The most likely explanation for the requirement of additional gene products for this clonal deletion is that the self-ligand for the majority of $V_\beta 5.2$-bearing lymphocytes is a peptide/I-E complex. What is striking is that a small number of genes (two loci in the B6 strain and one locus in the DBA/2 strain) presumably encode a small number of peptides that comprise the self-antigen for a relatively large fraction of the T-cell repertoire. Given the requirement for non-MHC gene products, the I-E- and the Mls-mediated deletions of T lymphocytes can be viewed in the same light. Both types of T-cell recognition (and clonal deletion) require the expression of MHC and non-MHC gene products. The Mls gene products could be considered more promiscuous in that I-A and I-E can present these determinants (Kappler et al. 1988; MacDonald et al. 1988; Happ et al. 1989; Kanagawa et al. 1989). The non-MHC gene products, described here, seem to be presented by I-E only.

When the H-2^d B × D RI strains were examined for their expression of CD8$^+$ $V_\beta 11^+$ cells, we found that similar to the expression of $V_\beta 5.2^+$ cells, the DBA/2 strain contained more $V_\beta 11^+$ cells compared with the B10.D2 strain. However, the strain distribution pattern of the $V_\beta 11$ phenotype does not match the strain distribution pattern of the $V_\beta 5.2$ phenotype. Either a different set of non-MHC genes and/or a different mechanism is controlling the generation of $V_\beta 11$-bearing cells in H-2^d RI mice. That only 2 of 16 (1 of 8) RI strains

have a low level of CD8$^+$ $V_\beta 11^+$ T cells (comparable to the B10.D2 strain) is consistent with the idea that three B6 genes other than the MHC are required to express a low level of CD8$^+$ $V_\beta 11^+$ T cells. We considered the possibility that the B6 genome expresses three non-MHC loci required for the deletion of $V_\beta 11^+$ cells. To confirm this, we bred F$_1$ mice from B10.D2 (low $V_\beta 11$ levels) and B × D28 (high $V_\beta 11$ levels) parents. Surprisingly, the high frequency of CD8$^+$ $V_\beta 11^+$ lymphocytes is dominant in these F$_1$ animals (Fig. 4). This is unlike the frequency of $V_\beta 5.2^+$ cells in the same F$_1$ animals (Table 2) where the low frequency of CD8$^+$ $V_\beta 5.2^+$ lymphocytes is dominant. It is difficult to reconcile tolerance with this type of F$_1$ genetics as the mechanism underlying the low frequency of CD8$^+$ $V_\beta 11$-bearing cells seen in B10.D2 mice. This may be particularly relevant considering the number of non-MHC loci involved in determining the frequency of $V_\beta 11^+$ cells.

Given the dominance of the high frequency of $V_\beta 11$ cells seen in (B10.D2 × B × D28)F$_1$ mice, a more likely explanation of the difference between the B10.D2 and B × D28 parental strains lies in the positive selection of $V_\beta 11^+$ T cells. The deletion of I-E reactive, $V_\beta 11^+$ cells may occur equally well in both strains; however, the B × D28 strain might carry out a more aggressive positive selection of the residual $V_\beta 11^+$ thymocytes. Since this difference is confined to the CD8$^+$ subset, the non-MHC genes segregating in the B × D RI lines may encode gene products that act in concert with the class I molecules, K^d and D^d. The reason that CD8$^+$ $V_\beta 11^+$ T cells are low in B10.D2 mice may be that this strain lacks the polymorphic non-MHC gene products that positively select CD8$^+$ $V_\beta 11$-bearing cells into the repertoire. These data support the notion that the ligands recognized by thymocytes during positive selection are peptide/MHC complexes. That non-MHC genes play a role in the positive selection of T cells was first suggested by Blanden and Ashman (1985) and more recently by Kappler et al. (1988) and Murphy et al. (1989). If one can accept as fact that an MHC/peptide complex is the antigenic moiety recognized by a peripheral T cell (Babbitt et al. 1985; Buus et al. 1986), then it seems reasonable that an MHC/peptide complex was recognized at an earlier time by the developing thymocyte for its positive selection into the repertoire.

ACKNOWLEDGMENTS

We thank Ms. Judy Franconi for preparation of the manuscript and Mr. Bill Townend for assistance with flow cytometry support. This work was supported by National Institutes of Health grants AI-22259, AR-37070, AI-22295 (E.P.), and AI-00863 (J.B.). E.P. is a recipient of a Faculty Research Award from the American Cancer Society.

REFERENCES

Abe, R., M.S. Vacchio, B. Fox, and R.J. Hodes. 1988. Preferential expression of T-cell receptor Vβ3 gene by Mls^c reactive T cells. *Nature* **335:** 827.

Babbitt, G., P. Allen, G. Matsueda, E. Haber, and E. Unanue. 1985. Binding of immunogenic peptides to Ia histocompatibility molecules. *Nature* **317:** 359.

Becker, D., P. Patten, Y.-H. Chien, T. Yakota, Z. Eshhar, M.
Giedlin, N.R.J. Gascoigne, C. Goodenow, R. Wolf, K.-I.
Arai, and M.M. Davis. 1986. Variability and repertoire
size of T-cell receptor Vα gene segments. *Nature* **317:** 430.

Berg, L., B. Fazekas de St. Groth, A. Pullen, and M. Davis.
1989a. Phenotypic differences between αβ versus β T-cell
receptor transgenic mice undergoing negative selection.
Nature **340:** 559.

Berg, L.J., A. Pullen, B. Fazekas de St. Groth, C. Benoist, D.
Mathis, and M. Davis. 1989b. Antigen/MHC specific T-
cells are preferentially exported from the thymus in the
presence of their MHC ligand. *Cell* **58:** 1035.

Bevan, M. and P. Fink. 1978. The influence of thymus H-2
antigens on the specificity of maturing killer and helper
cells. *Immunol. Rev.* **42:** 3.

Bill, J., V.B. Appel, and E. Palmer. 1988. An analysis of
T-cell receptor variable region gene expression in major
histocompatibility complex disparate mice. *Proc. Natl.
Acad. Sci.* **85:** 9184.

Bill, J., O. Kanagawa, D.L. Woodland, and E. Palmer. 1989.
The MHC molecule I-E is necessary but not sufficient for
the clonal deletion of $V_{\beta 11}$ bearing T-cells. *J. Exp. Med.*
169: 1405.

Blanden, R.V. and R.B. Ashman. 1985. Selection of pre-T
cells in the thymus by unique combinations of major and
minor histocompatibility antigens. *Mol. Immunol.*
22(7): 827.

Buus, S., A. Sette, S. Colon, D. Jenis, and H. Grey. 1986.
Isolation and characterization of antigen-Ia complexes involved in T cell recognition. *Cell* **47:** 1071.

Buus, S., A. Sette, S. Colon, C. Miles, and H. Grey. 1987.
The relation between major histocompatibility complex
(MHC) restriction and the capacity of Ia to bind immuno-
genic peptides. *Science* **235:** 1353.

Chothia, C., D.R. Boswell, and A.M. Lesk. 1988. The outline
structure of the T-cell αβ receptor. *EMBO J.* **12:** 3745.

Dialynas, D.P., D.B. Wilde, P. Marrack, M. Pierres, K.A.
Wall, W. Havran, G. Otten, M.R. Loken, M. Pierres, J.
Kappler, and F. Fitch. 1983. Characterization of the
murine antigenic determinant, designated L3T41a, recog-
nized by monoclonal antibody GK1.5: Expression of
L3T4a by functional T cell clones appears to correlate
primarily with class II MHC antigen-reactivity. *Immunol.
Rev.* **74:** 30.

Doherty, D.A., L. Gagliardo, C.J. Krco, C.S. David, and
D.L. Wassom. 1985. H-2 genes influence the kinetics of
lymphocyte responsiveness in trichinell spiralis- infected
mice. In *Genetic control of host resistance to infection and
malignancy*, p. 459. A.R. Liss, New York.

Fowlkes, B.J. and D.M. Pardoll. 1989. Molecular and cellular
events of T cell development. *Adv. Immunol.* **44:** 207.

Happ, M.P., D.L. Woodland, and E. Palmer. 1989. A third T
cell receptor VBβ gene encodes reactivity to Mls-1ᵃ gene
products. *Proc. Natl. Acad. Sci.* (in press).

Kanagawa, O. 1988. Antibody mediated activation of T cell
clones as a method for screening hybridomas producing Ab
to the T cell receptor. *J. Immunol. Methods* **110:** 169.

Kanagawa, O., E. Palmer, and J. Bill. 1989. The T cell
receptor Vβ6 domain imparts reactivity to the Mls-1ᵃ antigen. *Cell. Immunol.* **119:** 412.

Kappler, J.W., N. Roehm, and P. Marrack. 1987a. T cell
tolerance by clonal elimination in the thymus. *Cell* **49:** 273.

Kappler, J.W., B. Skidmore, J. White, and P. Marrack. 1981.
Antigen-inducible, H-2 restricted interleukin-2 producing
T cell hybridomas: Lack of independent antigen and H-2
recognition. *J. Exp. Med.* **153:** 1198.

Kappler, J.W., U. Staerz, J. White, and P.C. Marrack. 1988.
Self-tolerance eliminates T cells specific for Mls-modified

products of major histocompatibility complex. *Nature*
332: 35.

Kappler, J.W., T. Wade, J. White, E. Kushnir, M. Blackman,
J. Bill, R. Roehm, and P. Marrack. 1987b. A T-cell receptor Vβ segment that imparts reactivity to a class II
major histocompatibility complex product. *Cell* **49:** 263.

Kappler, J., B. Kotzin, L. Herron, E.W. Gelfand, R.D. Bigler, A. Boylston, S. Carrel, D.N. Posnett, Y. Choi, and
P.C. Marrack. 1989. Vβ-specific stimulation of human T
cells by staphylococcal toxins. *Science* **244:** 811.

Kisielow, P., H.S. Teh, H. Blüthman, and H. von Boehmer.
1988a. Positive selection of antigen-specific T cells in
thymus by restricting MHC molecules. *Nature* **335:** 730.

Kisielow, P., H. Blüthmann, U.D. Staerz, M. Steinmetz, and
H. von Boehmer. 1988b. Tolerance in T-cell-receptor
transgenic mice involves deletion of nonmature CD4⁺8⁺
thymocytes. *Nature* **333:** 742.

Kubo, R.T., W. Born, J.W. Kappler, P. Marrack, and M.
Pigeon. 1989. Characterization of a monoclonal antibody
which detects all murine αβ T cell receptors. *J. Immunol.*
142: 2736.

Ledbetter, J. and L. Herzenberg. 1979. Xenogeneic monoclonal antibodies to mouse differentiation antigens. *Immunol. Rev.* **47:** 63.

Lo, D. and J. Sprent. 1986. Identity of cells that imprint H-2
restricted T-cell specificity in the thymus. *Nature* **319:** 672.

Lo, D., L.C. Burkly, G. Widers, C. Cowing, R.A. Flavell,
R.D. Palmiter, and R.L. Brinster. 1988. Diabetes and
tolerance in transgenic mice expressing class II MHC molecules in pancreatic beta cells. *Cell* **53:** 159.

MacDonald, H.R., R. Schneider, R.K. Lees, R.C. Howe, H.
Acha-Orbea, H. Festenstein, R.M. Zinkernagel, and H.
Hengartner. 1988. T-cell receptor Vβ use predicts reactivity
and tolerance to Mlsᵃ-encoded antigens. *Nature* **332:** 40.

Marusic-Galesic, S., D.A. Stephany, D.L. Longo, and A.M.
Kruisbeek. 1988. Development of CD4⁻CD8⁺ cytotoxic T
cells requires interactions with class I MHC determinants.
Nature **333:** 180.

Murphy, D.B., D. Lo, S. Rath, R.L. Brinster, R.A. Flavell,
A. Slanetz, and C.A. Janeway, Jr. 1989. A novel MHC
class II epitope expressed in thymic medulla but not cortex. *Nature* **337:** 765.

Nishimoto, H., H. Kikutani, K. Yamamura, and T.
Kishimoto. 1987. Prevention of autoimmune insulitis by
expression of I-E molecules in NOD mice. *Nature*
328: 432.

Patten, P., T. Yokota, J. Rothbard, Y. Chien, K. Arai, and M.
Davis. 1984. Structure, expression and divergence of T-cell
receptor β-chain variable regions. *Nature* **312:** 40.

Pullen, A.M., P. Marrack, and J.W. Kappler. 1988. T-cell
repertoire is heavily influenced by tolerance to polymorphic self-antigens. *Nature* **335:** 796.

Sha, W.C., C.A. Nelson, R.D. Newberry, D.M. Kranz, J.H.
Russell, and D.Y. Loh. 1988. Positive and negative selec-
tion of an antigen receptor on T cells in transgenic mice.
Nature **336:** 73.

Tomonari, K. and E. Lovering. 1988. T-cell receptor-specific
monoclonal antibodies against a Vβ11-positive mouse T
cell clone. *Immunogenetics* **28:** 445.

Wilson, R.K., E. Lai, P. Concannon, R.K. Barth, and L.E.
Hood. 1988. Structure, organization and polymorphism of
murine and human T-cell receptor α and β chain gene
families. *Immunol. Rev.* **101:** 149.

Zinkernagel, R. and P. Doherty. 1975. H-2 compatibility requirement for T-cell-mediated lysis of target T-cells infected with lymphocyte choriomeningitis virus: different cytotoxic T-cell specificity are associated with structure from
H-2K or H-2D. *J. Exp. Med.* **141:** 1427.

Zinkernagel, R.M., G.H. Callahan, J. Klein, and G. Dennert.
1978. Cytotoxic T cells learn specificity for self H-2 during
differentiation in the thymus. *Nature* **271:** 251.

Positive and Negative Selection of T Lymphocytes

D.Y. Loh,* W.C. Sha,* C.A. Nelson,* R.D. Newberry,* D.M. Kranz,‡ and J.H. Russell†

*Departments of Medicine, Genetics, Microbiology, and Immunology, and †Pharmacology, Howard Hughes Medical Institute, Washington University School of Medicine, St. Louis, Missouri 63110; ‡Department of Biochemistry, University of Illinois, Urbana, Illinois, 61801

Precursors of functional T lymphocytes originate in the bone marrow and migrate to the thymus to undergo the necessary developmental events that result in functional T cells. Once within the thymus, genes encoding the antigen-specific T-cell receptor (TCR) undergo somatic DNA rearrangements in a highly regulated manner. The resulting cell-surface TCR allows the differentiating thymocytes to interact with the products of the polymorphic major histocompatibility complex (MHC) displayed in the thymus, allowing "thymic education" to take place. The end result of this process is the presence in the periphery of a TCR repertoire that is skewed toward recognition of antigens in the context of self-MHC molecules (MHC restriction), as well as elimination of T cells that react "too strongly" with self-MHC (self-tolerance). In addition, surface expression of the CD4 or CD8 molecule divides peripheral T cells into mutually exclusive subsets correlating strictly with the nature of the restricting MHC molecules. Lastly, it has been estimated that only a few percent of the dividing thymocytes actually emigrate into the periphery, the majority of them dying as a result of thymic selection. To study these intrathymic developmental events at the cellular and molecular levels, we have made transgenic mice bearing a TCR molecule of known antigenic specificity whose fate can be followed by using an anticlonotypic monoclonal antibody (MAb).

RESULTS AND DISCUSSION

Generation of the 2C TCR Transgenic Mice

One major advantage of the transgenic mouse approach is that it allows the investigators to monitor the effects of the presence of the transgene product throughout development. To follow the fate of developing T cells, we chose to microinject into 1-cell mouse embryos TCR genes whose cell-surface expression can be followed serologically. Cytotoxic T-cell clone 2C originated from a BALB.B (H-2^b) mouse, and it has a specificity for the L^d class I MHC antigen. The 2C TCR can be followed by MAb F23.1, which recognizes the β chain of 2C TCR as well as 1B2, an anticlonotypic antibody that recognizes an epitope dependent on both chains of 2C. We cloned the genes encoding the 2C TCR and constructed cosmid vectors for microinjection purposes (Fig. 1). The use of cosmids containing large amounts of flanking sequences was necessitated because of prior failures in our hands

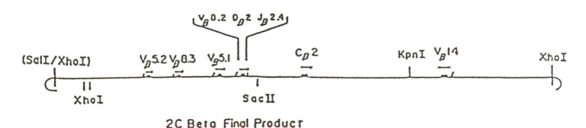

Figure 1. 2C α- and β-chain construction of functionally rearranged genes.

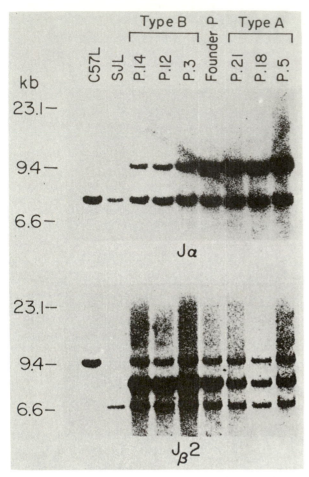

Figure 2. Southern blot analysis of type A and type B offspring of founder P.

in expressing the transgenes using shorter segments. Transgenic mice were produced using fertilized F_2 eggs obtained from mating (C57L × SJL)F_1 mice (Sha et al. 1988a). Southern blot analysis showed that there were two types of transgenic mice (Fig. 2).

Clonal Deletion Model of Self-tolerance

Since the clone 2C has specificity for the L^d molecule, the transgenic mice were mated to BALB/c to generate transgenic mice bearing H-2^d. The fate of self-reactive T cells bearing the 2C TCR can be followed throughout development. The results of experiments using 1B2 and F23.1 antibodies are shown in Figure 3. It is clear from these data that the cells bearing the intact 2C TCR (1B2$^+$) on functional cytotoxic cells (CD8$^+$) are absent in the periphery of H-2$^{b/d}$ animals. This deletion is in fact specific to clonotype-bearing T cells since there are F23.1$^+$ cells still present in the H-2$^{b/d}$ mice. Since there are virtually no CD8$^+$1B2$^+$ in the periphery in the nontolerant (H-2$^{b/d}$) environment, we conclude that self-tolerance against self-MHC antigens known to be present in the thymus is mediated by actual deletion of the self-reactive T-cell clones. The extent of this deletion is functionally complete since cytotoxic activity against L^d cannot be recovered from an H-2$^{b/d}$ mouse (Sha et al. 1988b). To see at what stage of thymocyte development this deletional event was taking place, we performed flow cytometry of the thymocytes. As shown in Figure 4, there are no 1B2$^+$ cells that bear either the CD4 or the CD8 molecule. This would imply that deletion is taking place either before or soon after thymocytes become double-positive (CD4$^+$CD8$^+$). Similar results

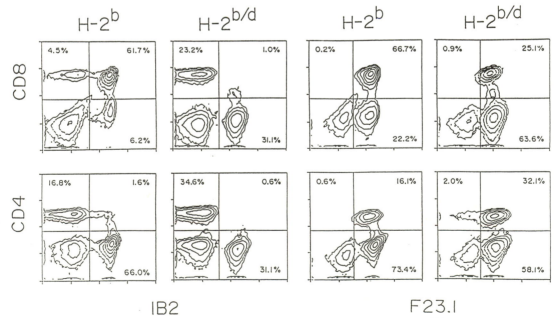

Figure 3. Selective depletion of 1B2$^+$CD8$^+$ spleen cells in type B H-2$^{b/d}$ mice.

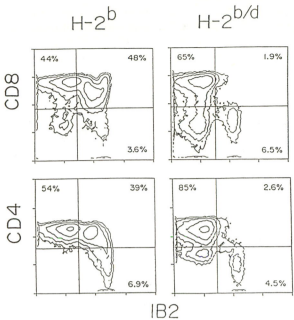

Figure 4. 2C TCR-bearing thymocytes are found among the CD4⁻CD8⁻ subsets in the H-2$^{b/d}$ mice.

have been obtained independently by von Boehmer and colleagues (Kisielow et al. 1988). Our findings are consistent with data obtained by other investigators using anti-(variable) V_β reagents to determine naturally occurring correlations of certain TCR deletions because of self-reactivity (Kappler et al. 1987a,b; MacDonald et al. 1988). Taken together, developing T cells undergo a fate in which they are deleted (programmed cell death?) upon interacting with the MHC molecule to which they are self-reactive. Little is known at this

time about how the TCR/MHC interactions lead to cell death.

Positive Selection Model for MHC Restriction

Since the original embryos that were microinjected were F$_2$ mice, there were three H-2 haplotypes possible (b/b, b/s, and s/s). When transgenic mice of the H-2^s haplotype were analyzed, we found very little expression of 1B2$^+$ cells in the periphery in both CD4$^+$ and CD8$^+$ subsets (Fig. 5). One explanation for this observation is that 2C is reactive against target cells of H-2^s origin. Two pieces of evidence were against this possibility. First, 2C did not react against H-2^s targets in vitro. Secondly, when transgenic H-2$^{b/s}$ mice were analyzed, 1B2$^+$CD8$^+$ cells were found in the periphery. Since clonal deletion or negative selection is dominant in a heterozygote, this too is inconsistent with H-2^s being negatively selecting for the 2C TCR-bearing cells.

We propose here an alternative model to explain the lack of 1B2$^+$ cells in the periphery of H-2^s mice. One way to explain the data is to postulate that the presence of H-2^b is necessary to allow the emergence of peripheral 1B2$^+$CD8$^+$ cells. Thus, in the case of T cells bearing the 2C TCR, the developing T cells must interact with an MHC antigen encoded uniquely in the H-2^b mice (2C originated from a BALB.B mouse, an H-2^b animal). We call this process positive selection and postulate it to be a mandatory step in normal T-cell development. In fact, we hypothesize that the phenomenon of MHC restriction results as a direct consequence of positive selection working on all developing thymocytes, as originally suggested by Zinkernagel et al. (Fink and Bevan 1978; Zinkernagel et al.

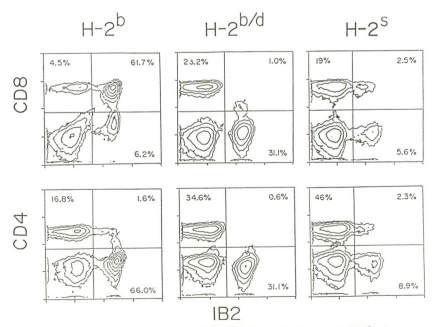

Figure 5. Relative absence of 1B2$^+$CD8$^+$ spleen cells in type A, H-2^s mice.

1978). Further analysis of the data available in positively selecting mice (H-2^b) shows that the 1B2$^+$ T cells show skewing toward CD8$^+$ cells in the periphery. These data are consistent with the notion that the positive selection probably is mediated by not only the heterodimeric TCR but occurs in conjunction with the participation of the CD8 molecule.

Taken together, it is the interaction of the TCR (with CD8) and the MHC antigens that determine the ultimate fate of the developing thymocyte. Under some circumstances where the TCR is self-reactive, the interaction leads to clonal elimination. Conversely, if no interaction occurs as postulated in the H-2^s mice, T cells fail to emerge in the periphery. Only if the TCR "productively" interacts with the self-restricting MHC molecule does a functional T cell emerge in the periphery.

Genetic and Molecular Dissection of the Positive Selecting Element

Having established that an element in the H-2^b haplotype was responsible for the positive selection on the developing 2C-TCR-bearing thymocytes, we sought to identify the locus responsible using mice with intra-H-2 recombination. We postulated that this element was most likely to be a class I or class-I-like MHC locus. Transgene-bearing mice were backcrossed to the following strains of mice (with their H-2 haplotypes, corresponding to K, I-A, I-E, and D loci, indicated in the parentheses): B10.S(26R) (sssb), B10.TBR18 (sssb), B10.AM (kkkb), HTG (dddb), B10.MBR (bkkq), and B10.AKM (kkkq). Analysis of the 1B2$^+$CD8$^+$ cells in the periphery revealed that only B10.MBR but not B10.S(26R) or B10.TBR18 allowed the emigration of these cells. In addition, there was no evidence of negative selection in any of the mice analyzed. These results imply that the element in the H-2^b haplotype responsible for positive selection maps to the K^b but not the D^b or any other class-I-like molecules that map distal to the D^b locus. Thus, we conclude that the 2C clone, which was originally isolated by immunizing a BALB.B (H-2^b) mouse with BALB/c (H-2^d) cells, was positively selected by the K^b molecule prior to immunization. To generalize, this would mean that allospecific T cells are the result of cross-reactive clones that were positively selected by self-restricting MHC elements in the thymus as originally suggested by Bevan and Hünig (1981).

Although the exact nature of the K^b molecule that participates in the positive selection is not known, possibilities include the following: K^b with a polymorphic peptide (i.e., originating from K^b or D^b) in the peptide-binding groove, K^b with a nonpolymorphic peptide of nonthymic origin (i.e., albumin peptide), K^b with thymus-specific peptide, or naked K^b. To dissect in detail the nature of the K^b molecule involved, we have started to use the existence of the bm mutant mice. bm mutant mice are congenic strains of C57BL/6 mice but differ only at the structure of the K^b molecule. Most of the amino acid sequence differences have been determined and the orientation of the amino acid side chains assigned based on the Bjorkman-Strominger-Wiley structure of the human leukemic A antigen molecule (Bjorkman et al. 1987a,b). We initially sought to find the effects of the bm1 mutation, which is comprised of amino acid changes at positions 153, 155, and 156 on the α_2 helix. We postulated that if a direct interaction between the 2C TCR and K^b molecule is necessary for positive selection to take place, changes on the α helix may abrogate positive selection. Preliminary data confirm that indeed bm1 mice behave very differently from the control H-2^b animals. Although preliminary, these findings are consistent with the interpretation that direct interaction between the TCR and MHC is a necessary step for the normal development of MHC-restricted T cells. Further work using all of the available bm mutant mice should shed light on the nature of this important interaction that determines the fate of a developing T lymphocyte.

SUMMARY AND PROSPECTS

The data presented here suggest that it is the nature of the interaction between the TCR (with CD8) and MHC that determines the fate of a developing T lymphocyte. This interaction is very specific in that a few amino acid changes on the MHC molecule can alter the T-cell differentiation pathway. The result of this encounter is profound since it determines if T cells die as a result of negative selection or through neglect (as in H-2^s mice in our case) or emerge as MHC-restricted, self-tolerant T cells. Clearly, much work needs to be done to understand the nature of the ligand as well as the nature of the signals received by the T cells.

ACKNOWLEDGMENTS

This work was supported by funding from the Howard Hughes Medical Institute and National Institutes of Health.

REFERENCES

Bevan, M.J. and T. Hünig. 1981. T cells respond preferentially to antigens that are similar to self H-2. *Proc. Natl. Acad. Sci.* **78:** 1843.

Bjorkman, P., M. Saper, B. Samraoui, W. Bennett, J.L. Strominger, and D.C. Wiley. 1987a. Structure of the human class I histocompatibility antigen, HLA-A2. *Nature* **329:** 506.

———. 1987b. The foreign antigen binding site and T cell recognition regions of class I histocompatibility antigens. *Nature* **329:** 513.

Fink, P. and M.J. Bevan. 1978. H-2 antigens of the thymus determine lymphocyte specificity. *J. Exp. Med.* **148:** 766.

Kisielow, P., H. Blüthmann, U. Staerz, M. Steinmetz, and H. von Boehmer. 1988. Tolerance in T-cell-receptor transgenic mice involves deletion of nonmature CD4$^+$8$^+$ thymocytes. *Nature* **333:** 742.

Kappler, J.W., N. Roehm, and P. Marrack. 1987a. T cell tolerance by clonal elimination in the thymus. *Cell* **49**: 273.

Kappler, J.W., T. Wade, J. White, E. Kushnir, M. Blackman, J. Bill, N. Roehm, and P. Marrack. 1987b. A T cell receptor Vβ segment that imparts reactivity to a class II major histocompatibility complex product. *Cell* **49**: 263.

MacDonald, H.R., R. Schneider, R. Lees, R. Howe, H. Acha-Orbea, H. Festenstein, R. Zinkernagel, and H. Hengartner. 1988. T-cell receptor Vβ use predicts reactivity and tolerance to Mls[a]-encoded antigens. *Nature* **332**: 40.

Sha, W.C., C. Nelson, R. Newberry, D. Kranz, J. Russell, and D. Y. Loh. 1988a. Selective expression of an antigen receptor on CD8-bearing T lymphocytes in transgenic mice. *Nature* **335**: 271.

———. 1988b. Positive and negative selection of an antigen receptor on T cells in transgenic mice. *Nature* **336**: 73.

Zinkernagel, R., G. Callahan, A. Althage, S. Cooper, P. Klein, and J. Klein. 1978. On the thymus in the differentiation of H-2 self-recognition by T cells: Evidence for dual recognition? *J. Exp. Med.* **147**: 882.

Both TCR/MHC and Accessory Molecule/MHC Interactions Are Required for Positive and Negative Selection of Mature T Cells in the Thymus

J.C. Zuniga-Pflücker, L.A. Jones, D.L. Longo, and A.M. Kruisbeek

Biological Response Modifiers Program, National Cancer Institute, National Institutes of Health, Bethesda, Maryland 20892

The development of the T-cell repertoire has been analyzed under conditions where expression of particular MHC-encoded gene products is blocked by in vivo anti-major histocompatibility complex (MHC) monoclonal antibody (MAb) treatments. A particular aim of these investigations was to examine the issue of thymic selection with experimental systems entirely different from hematopoietic and thymic chimeras and to reevaluate in normal mice whether positive selection in the context of thymic MHC indeed forms the basis for the phenomenon of MHC restriction. This approach (Kruisbeek et al. 1983, 1985) demonstrated that $CD4^+CD8^-$ T cells require interactions with class II MHC for their development to occur, whereas the majority of $CD4^-CD8^+$ T cells require interactions with class I MHC (Marusic-Galesic et al. 1988). The main question raised in subsequent studies has been whether such findings are a reflection of blocked TCR/MHC ligand interactions, blocked accessory molecule/MHC ligand interactions, or both. From a variety of experiments, again using the approach of blocking pertinent cell-surface molecules during development, we concluded that both TCR/MHC (Zúñiga-Pflücker et al. 1989a) and (for $CD4^+CD8^-$ T cells) CD4/MHC interactions (Zúñiga-Pflücker et al. 1989b) are crucial for development of T cells to occur. Together with the demonstration that in $TCR\alpha\beta$ transgenic mice (Kisielow et al. 1988; Sha et al. 1988) positive selection in the context of thymic MHC occurs, it now appears that a definite role for TCR/MHC interactions in T-cell differentiation has been established. In the present experiments, we address whether CD8 molecules need to encounter their ligand for the development of CD8 cells to occur. Indeed, it appears that interactions involving CD8 are an absolute necessity for the development of mature $CD4^-CD8^+$ T cells. Together with our previous data, which established a requirement for CD4 interactions in the generation of mature $CD4^+CD8^-$ T cells (Zúñiga-Pflücker et al. 1989b), it is therefore clear that although TCR/MHC interactions are required for positive selection of T cells, such interactions are, in the absence of accessory molecule/MHC interactions, not sufficient: The accessory molecules CD4 and CD8 participate in the selection process as well. The various ways in which these accessory molecules might function in both positive and negative selection are discussed in the context of our current knowledge of repertoire selection.

EXPERIMENTAL PROCEDURES

Mice. Our timed pregnant C57BL/6, C3H, and BALB/c mice were obtained from The Jackson Laboratory. Day 0 was the first day of vaginal plug observation.

Fetal thymus organ culture. Intact fetal thymus lobes were cultured as described recently (Zúñiga-Pflücker et al. 1989b).

Antibodies and treatments. Antibodies for in vivo treatments were purified from ascites as described previously (Zúñiga-Pflücker et al. 1989b) and were GK1.5 (anti-CD4) (Dialynas et al. 1983) and 2.43 (anti-CD8) (Sarmiento et al. 1980). Controls were as described previously (Zúñiga-Pflücker et al. 1989a,b), i.e., nonbinding monoclonal antibodies. In vivo treatments were started either in pregnant mice at day 17 of gestation, i.e., at the time that $TCR\alpha\beta$-bearing $CD4^+CD8^+$ cells are first detectable (Husmann et al. 1988) and/or within 24 hours after birth. Antibodies were administered daily interperitoneally, and doses were either 0.5 mg of MAb to pregnant mice or 0.2 mg to neonatal mice. Mice were sacrificed at 2 weeks of age, and flow cytometry analysis was performed. The MAbs used for in vivo injections were also utilized as staining reagents, as were 2C11 (anti-CD3) (Leo et al. 1987), 53-5.8 (anti-CD8β chain, previously known as Lyt-3) (Ledbetter et al. 1980), 53-7.3 (anti-CD5, previously known as Ly-1) (Ledbetter and Herzenberg 1979), F23.1 (anti-V_β8.1, -2 and -3) (Staertz et al. 1985), RR4 (anti-V_β6) (Kanagawa et al. 1989), and RR3 (anti-V_β11) (Bill et al. 1989). All staining was performed with directly conjugated reagents, using either fluorescein-isothyocyanate or biotin; sample handling was as described previously (Zúñiga-Pflücker et al. 1989a,b). In some experiments, enrichment of mature thymocytes was achieved by one injection of 2.5 mg of hydrocortisone (HC) acetate 48 hours prior to sacrifice.

Flow cytometry analysis. Samples were analyzed on a fluorescence-activated cell sorter 440 (Becton-Dickinson & Co., California) interfaced to a PDP 11/24 computer, and data were collected on 50,000 cells. Data are shown as contour diagrams, with a three-decade log scale of green fluorescence on the x-axis and a three-decade log scale of red fluorescence on the y-axis.

RESULTS

To test the possible contributions of interactions between CD8 and its ligand (presumably, class I MHC antigens) (Swain 1983) to the development of mature T cells, pregnant mice were treated from day 17 of pregnancy with anti-CD8 MAb, and treatment was continued in the neonatal mice until the age of 2 weeks. Analysis of the thymus at that time reveals that expression of most CD8 molecules is completely blocked (Fig. 1, right) but that many CD8$^+$ cells are still present, as visualized by the staining for the CD8β chain (previously known as Lyt-3) (Fig. 1, left). The antibody used for the in vivo treatment is specific for the CD8α chain (Lyt-2) and does not block staining for the CD8β chain either in vitro or in vivo (data not shown), albeit that CD8β chain staining is down-modulated in treated mice (Fig. 1, left). Nevertheless, it appears that CD4$^-$CD8$^+$ cells are no longer detectable in the anti-CD8-treated mice, whereas the CD4$^+$CD8$^+$ cells are still present.

Enrichment of single-positive mature thymocytes can be achieved by in vivo HC treatment and should allow a more sensitive determination of the presence of CD4$^-$CD8$^+$ cells. Additionally, staining for CD5 versus CD4 and CD3 versus CD4 was performed, since such an analysis would not be obscured by blocking effects of the injected anti-CD8 MAb. As shown in Figure 2 (left), only two populations of bright CD3$^+$ T cells are present in HC-treated mice whose thymus glands contain only CD4$^+$CD8$^-$ and CD4$^-$CD8$^+$ cells (data not shown): CD4$^+$ and CD4$^-$ cells. Reciprocal staining demonstrated that the CD4$^-$ cells represent the CD8$^+$ population (data not shown). Strikingly, this subset of bright CD3$^+$CD4$^-$CD8$^+$ cells is completely absent in the anti-CD8-treated mice (Fig. 2, left). Further evidence that CD4$^-$CD8$^+$ cells were unable to develop under these conditions stems from an analysis of CD5 expression versus CD4 expression: Whereas the thymus glands of control mice contain both CD4$^+$

and CD4$^-$ cells (the latter corresponding to CD8$^+$ cells) (Fowlkes et al. 1985) in the CD5$^+$ subsets, there were no CD4$^-$CD5$^+$ cells in the anti-CD8-treated group (Fig. 2, right). Thus, it is clear that generation of CD4$^-$CD8$^+$ cells is abrogated in anti-CD8-treated mice. Specificity of this effect is demonstrated by the fact that generation of the other major population of mature T cells, i.e., the CD3$^+$CD4$^+$CD8$^-$ cells, is unaffected by the anti-CD8 treatment (Fig. 2, left). This is in marked contrast with the studies of Smith (1987) who found that in vivo treatment with anti-CD8 blocked development of the CD4$^+$CD8$^-$ subset as well. However, mixed allogenic tetraparental chimeras were used in those studies (Smith 1987), so that graft-versus-graft reactions, rather than blocking of development, may have caused this subset's elimination. In that context, it should be noted that our data *are* compatible with studies in which anti-CD8-treatment of *syngeneic* bone marrow chimeras was used (Fowlkes et al. 1988) to follow the fate of mature T-cell development.

Two additional observations support the explanation that the observed abrogation of development of CD4$^-$CD8$^+$ cells is not simply due to direct removal of CD4$^-$CD8$^+$ cells by the injected anti-CD8 MAb: (1) Double-positive cells are still present in the anti-CD8-treated mice, as evidenced by the staining for CD8β chain (see Fig. 1), and (2) when treatment with intact anti-CD8 MAb was compared with treatment with F(ab)$_2$ MAb (data not shown), identical effects were obtained. Yet, such F(ab)$_2$ MAbs are unable to acutely deplete CD8$^+$ cells in a 3-day treatment protocol that does effectively deplete CD8$^+$ cells when intact anti-CD8 MAbs are used (data not shown; see Zúñiga-Pflücker et al. [1989b] for similar findings with anti-CD4 MAb). Together, these findings demonstrate that the failure to generate CD4$^-$CD8$^+$ cells in anti-CD8-treated mice is not a reflection of direct removal of these cells but a consequence of blocked interactions between CD8 and its ligands. Furthermore, although it is clear that CD4 and CD8 molecules can function as signal transducers not only in mature T cells (Rudd et al. 1988; Veillette et al. 1988), but also in immature thymocytes (McCarthy et al. 1989; Veillette et al. 1989), it is unlikely that our findings on blocked de-

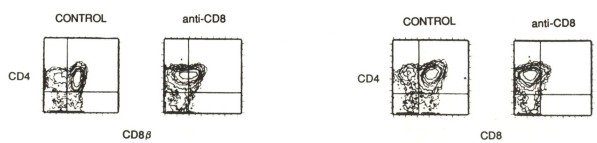

Figure 1. Two-parameter flow cytometry analysis of cell-surface expression of CD4 versus CD8α (Lyt-2) (*right*) or CD4 versus CD8-β (Lyt-3) (*left*) on thymocytes from control and anti-CD8-treated groups. Timed pregnant BALB/c mice and their offspring were treated with 2.43 MAb (anti-Lyt-2.2). Intraperitoneal injections of 0.5 mg were given daily from day 16 of pregnancy and continued at 0.2 mg per day for 12 days after birth. Thymocytes were analyzed on day 13 after birth.

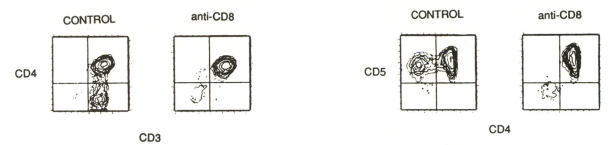

Figure 2. Two-parameter flow cytometry analysis of cell-surface expression of CD4 versus CD3 (*left*) or CD5 versus CD4 (*right*) on thymocytes from HC-treated control and anti-CD8-treated mice. Timed pregnant BALB/c mice and their offspring were treated with 2.43 MAb (anti-Lyt-2.2). Intraperitoneal injections of 0.5 mg were given daily from day 16 of pregnancy and continued at 0.2 mg per day for 12 days after birth. Thymocytes were analyzed on day 13 after birth. Control and anti-CD8-treated mice were injected intraperitoneally with 0.2 mg of HC 2 days prior to analysis.

velopment are due to perturbations caused by antibody-mediated signaling: nonsignaling Fab fragments of anti-CD4 (Zúñiga-Pflücker et al. 1989b) had identical effects as did intact monoclonal antibodies, i.e., blocked generation of CD4$^+$CD8$^-$ T cells equally well. It therefore appears that positive selection of mature T cells is not only a consequence of TCR/MHC interactions, but that CD4/ligand interactions (Zúñiga-Pflücker et al. 1989b) and CD8/ligand interactions (this study) are crucial to the development of mature T cells as well. This may reflect either a direct requirement (i.e., signaling through CD4- or CD8-ligand interactions is necessary) or an indirect one (i.e., TCR/MHC interactions are ineffective in the absence of CD4/ligand or CD8/ligand interactions). The earlier reports of blocked generation of single-positive CD4 and CD8 cells in anti-class-II-treated (Kruisbeek et al. 1985) and anti-class-I-treated (Marusic-Galesic et al. 1988) mice, respectively, may therefore occur not only because of a blockade of crucial TCR/MHC interactions, but also because of interference with accessory molecule/MHC interactions.

It is not clear at which stage of development interactions essential to positive selection occur. Previous studies have demonstrated that interactions involving CD4 participate in the process of negative selection of T cells with a class-II-restricted TCR (Fowlkes et al. 1988; MacDonald et al. 1988): Deletion of CD8 cells with a V$_\beta$17 or a V$_\beta$6 TCR can be prevented by treatment with anti-CD4 MAb. These studies also provided the first evidence that CD4$^+$CD8$^+$ thymocytes are precursors of mature single-positive T cells and that negative selection occurs at the double-positive stage of T-cell development. The observed requirement for CD8 and CD4 interactions in positive selection may reflect blocking at either the double- or the single-positive stage. This issue cannot be resolved on the basis of the present experiments since arguments in favor of each possibility can be presented. A case for effects at the single-positive stage could be made on the basis of the analysis of the T-cell repertoire in HC- and anti-CD8-treated mice: The data shown in Figures 3A

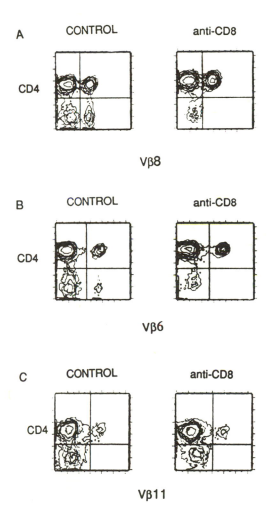

Figure 3. Two parameter flow cytometry analysis of cell-surface expression of CD4 versus V$_\beta$8 (*A*), CD4 versus V$_\beta$6 (*B*), or CD4 versus V$_\beta$11 (*C*) on thymocytes from HC-treated control and anti-CD8-treated groups. Timed pregnant BALB/c mice and their offspring were treated with 2.43 MAb (anti-Lyt-2.2). Intraperitoneal injections of 0.5 mg were given daily from day 16 of pregnancy and continued at 0.2 mg per day for 12 days after birth. Thymocytes were analyzed on day 13 after birth. Control and anti-CD8-treated mice were injected intraperitoneally with 0.2 mg of HC 2 days prior to analysis.

and B reveal that normal numbers of $V_\beta 6$- and $V_\beta 8$-expressing cells are generated in the CD4$^+$CD8$^-$ subset. One might have predicted a skewing of the repertoire if interactions involving CD8 participated in the signaling process leading to the differentiation of single-positive cells out of the double-positive subset. Thus, binding of anti-CD8 MAb to the double-positive subset did not interfere with the overall ability of double-positive thymocytes to participate in positive selection of single-positive CD4 T cells. Furthermore, generation of TCR-bearing double-positive thymocytes is not affected by anti-CD4, anti-CD8, anti-class II, or anti-class I treatment (collective unpublished data from our previous work). On the other hand, one could argue that the very fact that anti-CD4 and anti-CD8 MAbs can be found on the double-positive cells indicates that interference with essential interactions at this stage need to be considered. In any case, the question of where anti-CD4 and anti-CD8 MAb exert their blocking effect in positive selection has been difficult to determine with certainty.

In the course of our investigations, an interesting dichotomy in the effect of anti-CD8 and anti-CD4 on negative selection was observed. In the BALB/c mice used in the present study, I-E molecules are potent tolerogens for T cells expressing $V_\beta 11$ (Bill et al. 1989). Confirmation of this finding is illustrated in Figure 3C and Figure 4, i.e., even in the thymus glands of HC-treated mice, only minute numbers of mature $V_\beta 11^+$ cells can be detected. As was reported previously for $V_\beta 17a$ (Fowlkes et al. 1988) and $V_\beta 6$ (MacDonald et al. 1988), deletion of $V_\beta 11$ in the CD4$^-$CD8$^+$ subset can be prevented by anti-CD4 MAb treatment (Fig. 4), demonstrating that in this experimental system participation of CD4 molecules in negative selection of class-II-restricted T cells occurs at the double-positive stage of T-cell development, as well. In marked contrast, treatment with anti-CD8 MAb had no effect on the generation of $V_\beta 11$-bearing cells (Fig. 3C) under circumstances where positive selection of CD4$^-$CD8$^+$ T

cells was completely prevented (Fig. 3A,B) thus demonstrating effective blocking of all CD8 molecules. Taken together, these experiments suggest that deletion of T cells with a class-II-restricted receptor involves participation of CD4 but not CD8 molecules.

DISCUSSION

The findings described here help to resolve various issues regarding the role of accessory molecules in negative and positive selection. With respect to negative selection, the following picture emerges: In two models of autoreactivity involving self-antigens encoded by class II (I-E) or minor lymphocyte-stimulating (Mls)-self antigens presented by class II, deletion of T cells expressing particular V_β segments is prevented by CD4 blockade (Fowlkes et al. 1988; MacDonald et al. 1988). A similar situation is presented here: I-E-mediated elimination of $V_\beta 11$ cells can be prevented by anti-CD4 MAb. Strikingly, anti-CD8 MAbs do not have a similar effect on $V_\beta 11$ expression. It appears therefore that CD4 and CD8 molecules do not simply function as "avidity enhancers" at the double-positive thymocyte stage since in such a scenario blockade of either CD4 or CD8 might prevent deletion. Instead, the data suggest that, where receptors with class-II-restriction specificity are concerned, only CD4 molecules participate in generating the set of signals causing deletion. Whether the reverse is true for receptors with a class-I-restriction specificity, i.e., blockade of CD8 would rescue the cells from deletion whereas CD4 blocking would have no effect, is currently being analyzed. From studies with TCR transgenic mice expressing a class-I-restricted TCR, it would appear that CD8 plays a similar role in deletion of class-I-restricted T cells as CD4 does for class-II-restricted T cells: The deletion spares cells with a CD8^{low} phenotype, whereas cells with high levels of CD8 are deleted (Teh et al. 1989). These data correspond well with models in which selective interactions between the TCR and accessory molecules are essential for signal transduction to occur, so that class-II-restricted receptors interact with CD4, and class-I-restricted receptors interact with CD8 (Janeway 1988, 1989).

Theories on the role of accessory molecule-mediated and TCR-mediated interactions in positive selection need to take into account the following features of T-cell repertoire development:

1. The T-cell repertoire is nonrandomly expressed in the two main subsets of T cells, i.e., most class-II-restricted T cells are CD4$^+$CD8$^-$ and most class-I-restricted T cells are CD4$^-$CD8$^+$ (Dialynas et al. 1983; Swain 1983).
2. Blocking of CD4 prevents generation of CD4$^+$CD8$^-$ cells, and blocking of CD8 prevents generation of CD4$^-$CD8$^+$ T cells; we presume for the sake of this discussion that antibodies blocking CD4 or CD8 do not prevent TCR/MHC interactions for steric reasons.

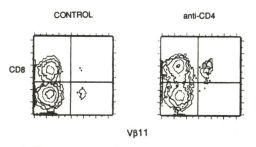

CONTROL   anti-CD4

CD8

$V_\beta 11$

Figure 4. Two-parameter flow cytometry analysis of cell-surface expression of CD8 versus $V_\beta 11$ on thymocytes from HC-treated control and anti-CD4-treated groups. Timed pregnant BALB/c mice and their offspring were treated with GK1.5 MAb (anti-L3T4). Intraperitoneal injections of 0.5 mg were given daily from day 16 of pregnancy and continued at 0.2 mg per day for 12 days after birth. Thymocytes were analyzed on day 13 after birth. Control and anti-CD8-treated mice were injected intraperitoneally with 0.2 mg of HC two days prior to analysis.

3. In TCR transgenic mice with a class-I-restricted receptor, preferential differentiation of CD4$^-$CD8$^+$ cells with the complete transgenic receptor occurs, provided the appropriate MHC antigens are available (Sha et al. 1988; Teh et al. 1988; Scott et al. 1989); similar findings are observed in TCR transgenic mice with a class-II-restricted receptor in that expression of the restricting class II elements leads to preferential differentiation of CD4$^+$CD8$^-$ cells with both transgenic TCR chains (Berg et al. 1989). Thus, the MHC specificity of the TCR determines the CD4 versus CD8 phenotype of mature T cells.

With these findings in mind, and considering previous views on positive selection as a reflection of "rescue from programmed cell death" (von Boehmer 1986), i.e., selective differentiation rather than selective expansion, at least two mechanisms for positive selection and repertoire diversification into CD4$^+$CD8$^-$ and CD4$^-$CD8$^+$ cells can be proposed (see below).

Random Loss of CD4 or CD8 at the Double-positive Stage

Expression of CD4 or CD8 is down-regulated in a random fashion, and only expression of two proper combinations of cell-surface molecules allows for or induces subsequent differentiation: a class-II-restricted TCR with CD4, or a class-I-restricted TCR with CD8. Cells with "nonpermissive" combinations (i.e., CD8 and a class-II-restricted TCR, or CD4 and a class-I-restricted TCR) will not differentiate. TCR/MHC interactions have an "instructional" role in this setting: If TCRs cannot interact with the appropriate restricting MHC elements, interactions between the nonpolymorphic accessory molecules and their ligands are not sufficient, and differentiation does not occur. Yet, the accessory molecules actively participate in generating the set of differentiation-promoting signals when the "permissive" combination occurs because blocking their expression prevents differentiation. This may occur either because CD4/CD8-signaling is required in and of itself or because effective TCR/MHC signaling is dependent on interactions involving CD4/CD8. Obviously, all findings cited above are compatible with the "random loss" hypothesis.

Nonrandom Loss of CD4 or CD8 at the Double-positive Stage

Double-positive cells with a class-I-restricted receptor down-regulate their CD4, and those with a class-II-restricted receptor down-regulate their CD8. Initiation of this process would result from TCR-ligand interactions, and selective differentiation would then be induced only in those cells in which both the TCR and the accessory molecules bind the appropriate ligand. Also, this hypothesis is compatible with both the TCR$\alpha\beta$ transgenic mice studies and with our CD4/CD8/class-I/class-II-blocking studies: prevention of any one of these interactions, through absence of the appropriate MHC molecules or blocking of CD4 and CD8, results in arrested development. The idea that TCR/MHC interactions play an "instructional" role is compatible with this hypothesis as well: In transgenic mice with a class-I-restricted TCR, all T cells with both transgenic receptor chains are of the CD4$^-$CD8$^+$ phenotype, and CD4$^+$CD8$^-$ T cells with both transgenic receptor chains preferentially develop in transgenic mice with a class-II-restricted receptor.

Whichever one of these theories is correct, it appears that the blocking studies with anti-CD8/CD4 have served the purpose of formally proving the earlier suggestions made (von Boehmer 1986; Janeway 1988, 1989) that TCR/MHC interactions alone, in the absence of accessory molecule/MHC interactions, are not sufficient for differentiation to occur. Furthermore, the point is made that interactions involving accessory molecules are crucial participants not only in negative selection (Fowlkes et al. 1988; MacDonald et al. 1988), but also in positive selection.

We lean toward the idea that CD4 and CD8 molecules participate as signaling molecules, rather than as passive enhancers of the avidity of intrathymic interactions between developing T cells and MHC-expressing selecting elements for several reasons: (1) In mature T cells, CD4 and CD8 molecules contribute directly to T-cell activation (Janeway 1988, 1989); (2) models proposing only an avidity role would be unable to explain the bias of the T-cell repertoire, i.e., the preferential expression of CD4 on class-II-restricted T cells and of CD8 on class-I-restricted T cells; (3) anti-class II blockage prevents differentiation of CD4$^+$ class-II-restricted T cells but not of CD8$^+$ class-II-restricted T cells (Mizuochi et al. 1988); (4) the specificity of a given TCR alone determines the outcome of repertoire selection in TCR transgenic mice; (5) in the presence of TCR/MHC but absence of CD4/CD8-MHC interactions (Zúñiga-Pflücker et al. 1989, in prep., and this paper), differentiation-promoting signals are blocked. Among our challenges for the future are to distinguish between the nature of the differentiation-promoting signals (those caused by both TCR and accessory molecule interactions) and those causing clonal deletion.

ACKNOWLEDGMENTS

We thank our colleagues Drs. Ronald N. Germain, Alfred Singer, Jonathan D. Ashwell, and Louis A. Matis for many stimulating discussions throughout these studies and Fran N. Haussman and David A. Stephany of the National Institute of Allergies and Infectious Diseases Flow Cytometry Laboratory for their continued and expert support of our flow cytometry analysis. Furthermore, we thank Drs. Osami Kanagawa and Ed Palmer for generously providing the anti-V$_\beta$11 and anti-V$_\beta$6 MAbs before publication.

REFERENCES

Berg, L.J., A.M. Pullen, B. Fazekas de St. Groth, D. Mathis, C. Benoist, and M.M. Davis. 1989. Antigen/MHC specific T cells are preferentially exported from the thymus in the presence of their MHC ligand. *Cell* **58:** 1035.

Bill, J., O. Kanagawa, D.L. Woodland, and E. Palmer. 1989. The MHC molecule I-E is necessary but not sufficient for the clonal deletion of V_β11-bearing T cells. *J. Exp. Med.* **169:** 1405.

Dialynas, D.P., Z.S. Quan, K.A. Wall, A. Pierres, J. Quintans, M.R. Loken, M. Pierres, and F.W. Fitch. 1983. Characterization of the murine T cell surface molecule, designated L3T4, identified by the monoclonal antibody GK1.5: Similarities of L3T4 to the human Leu-3/T4 molecule. *J. Immunol.* **131:** 2445.

Fowlkes, B.J., R.H. Schwartz, and D.P. Pardoll. 1988. Deletion of self-reactive thymocytes occurs at a CD4$^+$CD8$^+$ precursor stage. *Nature* **334:** 620.

Fowlkes, B.J., L. Edison, B.J. Mathieson, and T.M. Chused. 1985. Early T lymphocytes. Differentiation *in vivo* of adult intrathymic precursors cells. *J. Exp. Med.* **162:** 802.

Husmann, L., R.P. Shimonkevitz, I.N. Crispe, and M.J. Bevan. 1988. Thymocyte subpopulation during early fetal development in the BALB/c mouse. *J. Immunol.* **141:** 736.

Janeway, C.A. 1988. T-cell development. Accessories or coreceptors? *Nature* **355:** 208.

———. 1989. The role of CD4 in T cell activation: Accessory molecule or co-receptor? *Immunol. Today* **10:** 234.

Kanagawa, O., E. Palmer, and J. Bill. 1989. A T cell receptor Vβ domain that imparts reactivity to the Mls^a antigen. *Cell. Immunol.* (in press).

Kisielow, P., H.S. Teh, H. Bluthmann, and H. von Boehmer. 1988. Positive selection of antigen-specific T cells in thymus by restricting MHC molecules. *Nature* **355:** 730.

Kruisbeek, A.M., B.J. Fowlkes, S.A. Bridges, J.J. Mond, and D.L. Longo. 1985. Lack of development of the L3T4$^+$ subset in anti-Ia-treated neonatal mice correlates with absence of thymic Ia bearing APC function. *J. Exp. Med.* **161:** 1029.

Kruisbeek, A.M., M.J. Fultz, S.O. Sharrow, A. Singer, and J.J. Mond. 1983. Early development of the T cell repertoire. *In vivo* treatment of neonatal mice with anti-Ia antibodies interferes with differentiation of I-restricted but not K/D-restricted T cells. *J. Exp. Med.* **157:** 1932.

Ledbetter, J.A. and L.A. Herzenberg. 1979. Xenogenic monoclonal antibodies to mouse lymphoid differentiation antigens. *Immunol. Rev.* **47:** 63.

Ledbetter, J.A, R.V. Rouse, H.S. Micklem, and L.A Herzenberg. 1980. T cell subsets defined by expression of Lyt-1,2,3 and Thy-1 antigens. Two-parameter immunofluorescence and cytotoxicity analysis with monoclonal antibodies modifies current views. *J. Exp. Med.* **152:** 280.

Leo, O., M. Foo, D.H. Sachs, L.E. Samelson, and J.A. Bluestone. 1987. Identification of a monoclonal antibody specific for a murine T3 polypeptide. *Proc. Natl. Acad. Sci.* **84:** 1374.

MacDonald, H.R., H. Hengartner, and T. Pedrazzini. 1988. Intrathymic deletion of self-reactive cells prevented by neonatal anti-CD4 antibody treatment. *Nature* **335:** 174.

Marusic-Galesic, S., D.A. Stephany, D.L. Longo, and A.M. Kruisbeek. 1988. Development of CD4$^-$CD8$^+$ cytotoxic T cells requires interactions with class I MHC determinants. *Nature* **333:** 180.

McCarthy, S.A., A.M. Kruisbeek, I.K. Uppenkamp, S.O. Sharrow, and A. Singer. 1988. Engagement of the CD4 molecule influences cell surface expression of the T-cell receptor on thymocytes. *Nature* **336:** 76.

Mizuochi, T., L. Tentori, S.O. Sharrow, A.M. Kruisbeek, and A. Singer. 1988. Differentiation of Ia-reactive CD8$^+$ murine T cells does not require Ia engagement. Implications for the role of CD4 and CD8 accessory molecules in T cell differentiation. *J. Exp. Med.* **168:** 437.

Rudd, C.E., J.M. Trevillyan, J.D. Dasgupta, L.L. Wong, and S.F. Schlossman. 1988. The CD4 receptor is complexed in detergent lysates to a protein tyrosine kinase pp58 from human T lymphocytes. *Proc. Natl. Acad. Sci.* **85:** 5190.

Sarmiento, M., A.L. Glasebrook, and F.W. Fitch. 1980. IgG or IgM monclonal antibodies reactive with different determinants on the molecular complex bearing Lyt 2 antigen block T cell-mediated cytolysis in the absence of complement. *J. Immunol.* **125:** 2665.

Scott, B., H. Blüthmann, H.S. Teh, and H. von Boehmer. 1989. The generation of mature T cells requires interaction of the $\alpha\beta$ TCR with major histocompatibility antigens. *Nature* **338:** 591.

Sha, W., C. Nelson, R. Newberry, D. Kranz, J. Russell, and D. Loh. 1988. Positive and negative selection of an antigen receptor on T cells in transgenic mice. *Nature* **336:** 73.

Smith, L. 1987. CD4$^+$ murine T cells develop from CD8$^+$ precursors in vivo. *Nature* **326:** 798.

Staertz, U.D., H.G. Rammensee, J.D. Benedetto, and M.J. Bevan. 1985. Characterization of a murine monoclonal antibody specific for an allotype determinant on the T cell antigen receptor. *J. Immunol.* **134:** 3994.

Swain, S. 1983. T cell subsets and the recognition MHC class. *Immunol. Rev.* **74:** 129.

Teh, H.S., H. Kishi, B. Scott, and H. von Boehmer. 1989. Deletion of autospecific T cells in TCR transgenic mice spares cells with normal TCR levels and low levels of CD8 molecules. *J. Exp. Med.* **169:** 795.

Teh, H.S., P. Kisielow, B. Scott, K. Hiroyuki, Y. Uematsu, H. Blüthmann, and H. von Boehmer. 1988. Thymic major histocompatibility complex antigens and the $\alpha\beta$ T-cell receptor determine the CD4/CD8 phenotype of T cells. *Nature* **355:** 229.

Veillette, A., M.A. Bookman, E.M. Horak, and J.B. Bolen. 1988. The CD4 and CD8 T-cell surface antigens are associated with the internal membrane tyrosine protein kinase p56^{lck}. *Cell* **55:** 301.

Veillette, A., J.C. Zúñiga-Pflucker, J.B. Bolen, and A.M. Kruisbeek. 1989. Engagement of CD4 and CD8 expressed on immature thymocytes induces activation of intracellular tyrosine phosphorylation pathways. *J. Exp. Med.* (in press).

von Boehmer, H. 1986. The selection of the $\alpha\beta$ heterodimeric T-cell receptor for antigen. *Immunol. Today* **7:** 333.

Zúñiga-Pflücker, J.C., D.L. Longo, and A.M. Kruisbeek. 1989a. Positive selection of CD4$^-$CD8$^+$ T cells in the thymus of normal mice. *Nature* **338:** 76.

Zúñiga-Pflücker, J.C., S.A. McCarthy, M. Weston, D.L. Longo, A. Singer, and A.M. Kruisbeek. 1989b. Role of CD4 in thymocyte selection and maturation. *J. Exp. Med.* **169:** 2085.

Selection of Lymphocyte Repertoires: The Limits of Clonal versus Network Organization

A. Coutinho, A. Bandeira, P. Pereira, D. Portnoi, D. Holmberg,
C. Martinez, and A.A. Freitas
Uniteé d'Immunobiologie, Institut Pasteur, Paris, France

Over the last 5 years, our laboratory has been engaged in characterizing the immune system of normal, unmanipulated mice. This deviation from the main focus of immunological research commands justification and has required the development of suitable approaches and techniques. A number of our previous concerns and results had paved the way in this direction by demonstrating the importance of immune activities and cellular dynamics in normal animals. Thus, the development of mitogen-driven limiting dilution assays (LDA) (Andersson et al. 1977) had allowed for quantitation of the absolute frequencies of clonal reactivities in the B-cell compartment of unprimed mice and provided evidence for ongoing repertoire selection prior to antigenic challenges (Eichmann et al. 1977; Bernabé et al. 1981b). Furthermore, antibody treatments of normal animals, under conditions that were likely to occur in normal physiology, suggested that immune activities were recursive and that immune components determined, at least in part, their own production (Forni et al. 1980; Ivars et al. 1982). These conclusions brought us close to the notion of autonomy and autopoietic behaviors (Coutinho et al. 1984) and were soon extended to the interactions between T-cell and antibody repertoires (Martinez-A. et al. 1984, 1985, 1987), which again showed circular and apparently autonomous selective influences (Marcos et al. 1988).

Lymphocytes, however, are produced as resting noncycling cells devoid of effector functions. To perform any role at all, even in the context of autonomous activities and repertoire selection, lymphocytes require productive interactions with ligands, activation, and blast transformation, followed by high-rate antibody secretion, and helper or suppressor activities, with more or less extensive multiplication. Therefore, necessarily the notion of autonomous activities is intimately related to the presence and repertoires of *activated* lymphocytes. Methods were then derived to identify and quantitate *effector* B, helper, and suppressive T cells with unknown specificity (Gronowicz et al. 1976; Pobor et al. 1984; Pereira et al. 1985). The quantitation of truly autonomous immune activities would, however, require the analysis of animals secluded from all external antigenic influences. The study of antigen-free mice, established that some 10% of all splenic B and T cells are activated in the internal environment into mitosis and effector functions, such as immunoglobulin

M (IgM) (but no IgG or IgA) secretion, helper (but no inflammatory) and suppressor (but no cytolytic) activities (Pereira et al. 1985, 1986a). We could then start delineating these two compartments in the normal immune system, namely, that composed of activated lymphocytes and serum IgM antibodies versus that of resting lymphocytes.

This notion of functional autonomy, absent from current considerations in immunology, is nevertheless implicit in the network theory (Jerne 1974; Coutinho 1980). The question of variable (V) region connectivity was therefore addressed in a quantitative manner. Unselected collections of hybridoma antibodies derived from naturally activated cells of the newborn mouse were studied for mutual reactivities and revealed a high degree of connectivity: Nearly 25% of all reactions tested in a large matrix were positive (Holmberg et al. 1984). In contrast, collections of hybridoma IgM antibodies derived after polyclonal stimulation of resting lymphocytes in the adult, showed at least one order of magnitude lower levels of V region connectivity (Holmberg et al. 1986). These results lead some of us to associate a network structure and organization with functional autonomy and the compartment of activated cells, whereas we consider the majority of lymphocytes in the immune system as a collection of resting, disconnected clones, integrating no network at all (Coutinho 1989). We had then to consider the rules determining the establishment and maintenance of those two compartments, that is, the structure of their repertoires and how they are selected, as well as the relationships of either with self and nonself and with each other.

Clonal repertoire selection can only occur by activation and expansion of the selected clones (recruitment into the activated compartment) or by differential survival and persistence in a population that is being renewed. Repertoire selection must then also consider lymphocyte turnovers and population dynamics. Novel approaches to quantitate B-cell life-spans and clonal persistence in normal animals were developed (Freitas and Coutinho 1981; Freitas et al. 1982) and provided evidence for high-turnover rates in the mature, immunocompetent cell compartment and among immunoglobulin-secreting cells as well (Freitas et al. 1986b; Lévy et al. 1987). Furthermore, they indicated that the dynamics in the activated lymphocyte population in normal animals was distinct from that expected in conventional immune responses because those cells seemed to undergo very little clonal expansion upon activation (Freitas et al. 1986a). More recently, kinetic studies of natural serum antibodies provided confirmation of these suggestions by showing oscillatory or chaotic dynamics that are sharply different from immune response amplifications (Lundkvist et al. 1989).

We have now used alternative methods to the global assessment of B-cell repertoires by studying the representation of homology families at the V_H locus in the different lymphocyte populations (Freitas et al. 1989a), as well as techniques that allow us to analyze selectively repertoires of B or T cells among activated versus resting lymphocytes (Pereira et al. 1985). Furthermore, provided with the evidence for positive selection of autoreactive cells in the large lymphocyte compartment (Portnoi et al. 1986), we have addressed questions of self-tolerance and ontogenic development of repertoires.

MATERIALS AND METHODS

The methods referred to in this paper have been extensively described previously. For complete information, the reader should consult Freitas and Coutinho (1981), Holmberg et al. (1984), Pobor et al. (1984), Pereira et al. (1985, 1986b), Portnoi et al. (1986), Bandeira et al. (1987), Rocha and Bandeira (1988), Andrade et al. (1989), and Freitas et al. (1989a).

RESULTS

B-cell Production and Population Dynamics

The bone marrow of an adult mouse produces every day some 50×10^6 to 60×10^6 μ-chain-expressing pre-B cells of which roughly half productively rearrange light-chain genes, exit mitotic cycle, and express surface IgM receptors as small lymphocytes (Opstelten and Osmond 1983). As tested by mitogen reactivity, these cells seem as immunocompetent as peripheral B lymphocytes in what concerns proliferative capacity, the ability to switch to the expression of other immunoglobulin isotypes, as well as the competence to differentiate terminally and secrete antibody at a high rate (Benner et al. 1981). Many of these cells, however, do not express surface IgD, the role of which remains a matter of debate. Although several growth factors for precursor B cells have been identified recently (Palacios et al. 1984; Namen et al. 1988), the regulation of the rates of production of B cells in bone marrow remains unclear except for the notion of its existence. Thus, production rates are strikingly similar in a variety of experimental conditions and seem little dependent on T cells, on peripheral B-cell depletion, and on protocols of intense immunization (Fulop and Osmond 1983; Fulop et al. 1983; Osmond 1986). The study of some mutations isolated in the mouse, provided examples of deficient bone marrow B-cell production and could constitute useful tools to investigate those issues.

Thus, whereas the SCID mutant (Bosma et al. 1983) is already reasonably well understood, the basis for low B-cell production in the "moth-eaten" mouse and in the animals carrying simultaneously the *Xid* and the *nude* mutations (Wortis et al. 1982) is much less clear. It is interesting that, in both cases, alterations in the development of the so-called CD5 B cells have been described previously (Herzenberg et al. 1986), suggesting speculations on the role that such cells produced early in development or the antibodies they secrete could have in the regulation of B-cell production.

The majority of newly formed B cells is exported to the periphery (Brahim and Osmond 1970), implying that comparable rates of decay must apply to preexisting peripheral B cells since their total number remains constant. Direct measurements of peripheral B-cell-decay in quasi-physiological conditions confirm this expectation (Fig. 1) (Freitas and Coutinho 1981). The majority of these cells only persist for some hours or a few days. Some of them, however, do persist for longer periods of time, and we have actually found examples of B cells (or their progeny) remaining in the periphery

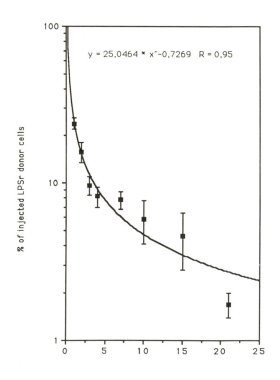

$$y = 25{,}0464 * x^{-0{,}7269} \quad R = 0{,}95$$

DAYS AFTER CELL TRANSFER

Figure 1. Persistence of donor LPS-reactive splenic B cells in the spleen of LPS nonresponder hosts. Spleen cells from LPS responder B6 mice were transferred into LPS nonresponder B10.Cr mice. The number of LPS-reactive B cells in the transferred cell population and those remaining in the recipient's spleen at the indicated times after transfer were determined by LDA. Each point represents the mean and S.E. of the data obtained in 16 different experiments, using pools of 2–3 mice per time point in each experiment. Results were derived from Freitas et al. (1986a,b) and Thomas-Vaslin and Freitas (1989).

for over 3 months. We have previously made conclusions about the existence of two major B-cell populations with life expectancies of about 4 and 10 days, respectively (Freitas et al. 1986b), but the accumulation of data (Fig. 1) shows a continuous distribution of survival times compatible with a large heterogeneity. These conclusions on the short life spans of most B cells have raised some controversy, and a critical assessment of the various methods employed has been published previously (Freitas et al. 1986c). Results obtained in other experimental systems indicate instead that only a minority of B cells show high-turnover rates. It is perhaps not very relevant, however, to discuss whether 40% or 80% of all peripheral B cells are short-lived because the phenomenon remains essentially the same. Nevertheless, it is interesting to note that the high-turnover rates described here are actually necessary to accommodate the rates of bone marrow B-cell production. Given that newly formed B cells in bone marrow

are immunocompetent, it is quite irrelevant where they actually decay.

Of particular interest to us, was the question of recruitment of newly formed B cells into the activated compartment and the persistence of the selected specificities. We have therefore carried out experiments (1) estimating the rates of recruitment and (2) comparing the persistence of resting, nonrecruited cells with that of positively selected cells that are recovered in the activated compartment after transfer of small cells. The results are shown in Figure 2. Assuming that the conclusions of transfer in these experiments do not significantly alter the normal physiology, and, considering that the large majority of transferred small B cells are recently derived from bone marrow, we can conclude that about 5% of newly formed cells are recruited daily into the activated compartment. This means that 1×10^6 to 2×10^6 cells integrate every day a pool of about 10^7 large cells, providing therefore a mean renewal rate of 10–20%/day in the compartment. In other words, recruitment is accompanied by increased life expectancy as compared with nonactivated cells (see Fig. 2). Since our methods measure clonal persistence independently of cell division, the results above could reflect instead amplification of the selected clones. As discussed above, however, cell production in this compartment is low and most probably does not represent more than one or maximally two rounds of division per incoming cell (Freitas et al. 1986a).

At any time point in an adult mouse, only 5–10% of all activated B cells in the spleen are secreting immunoglobulin at a high rate and contributing to the majority of serum IgM. Control of terminal differentiation in vivo remains completely obscure, but as seen below there are indications for V-region-specific regulation at this level. This constitutes one of the several reasons to consider repertoire selection in the context of population dynamics.

Analysis of B-cell Repertoires by V_H Gene Family Representation

A severe limitation in studies of lymphocyte repertoires is the relatively small fraction of the whole that can be analyzed by studying antigenic reactivities. Since the frequencies of clones reacting with a given antigen range from 10^{-5} to 10^{-2}, over 99% of the repertoire is ignored in this type of analysis. The near complete description of the murine V_H locus, leading to the identification of homology families in a relatively low number (Brodeur and Riblet 1984), provided the possibility of studying the globality of repertoires. Clearly, these methods perhaps miss the most interesting aspects of the problem since they do not provide information on reactivities. However, they are the only alternative today to derive general conclusions on major selective steps of repertoire generation. We have been using in situ hybridization of single-cell suspensions (Freitas et al. 1989a) and colony-forming unit-B blot assays (Andrade et al. 1989) to quantitate the

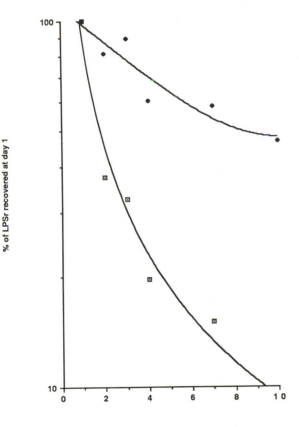

Days after cell transfer

Figure 2. Persistence of LPS-reactive small and large B cells in the spleen of LPS nonresponder hosts. The same as Fig. 1 but studying the fate of purified small spleen cells from B6 mice in the small and large cell fractions of the hosts. Donor small cells were purified by 1g velocity sedimentation, and the recipient's spleen cells were separated into large and small fractions on discontinuous density Percoll gradients (Freitas et al. 1986a). The number of LPS-reactive B cells in the transferred cell populations and in the large (◆) and small (□) spleen cell fractions in the host's spleen were determined by LDA.

representation of 10 of the 11 known V_H gene families. For purposes of description, we will distinguish here several sections in the B-cell repertoire of adult individuals: *emergent* in bone marrow; *available* in peripheral resting cells, *actual* in activated blasts, and *secretory* in plasma cells.

As shown in Figure 3, the emergent V_H family repertoire in adults shows a clear overrepresentation of the 7183 family. This is the case both in relation to the numbers of genes in the germ line and in comparison with peripheral repertoires (Freitas et al. 1989a). It has been established previously that a similar overrepresentation of diversity (D) proximal genes is characteristic

of most B lymphocytes in the developing immune system (Yancopoulos et al. 1984; Perlmutter et al. 1985). The present results, however, would suggest that D proximal preference correlates with the process of differentiation from uncommitted cells, regardless of ontogenic stages. The V_H repertoires of splenic resting B cells, the major site of emigration for newly formed cells, differ from those of bone marrow B cells by a decreased representation of 7183 genes. If total numbers of cells rather than distributions are considered, as shown in Figure 3, it becomes apparent that all families except 7183 increase from bone marrow to spleen. This observation establishes the ongoing selection of B-cell

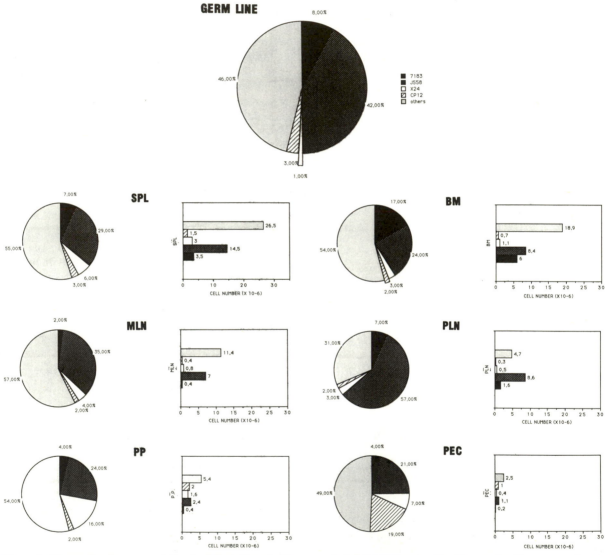

Figure 3. V_H gene family representation in different lymphoid organs of adult BALB/c mice. Ten V_H gene families were analyzed, but the data shown concern only the four most representative, as indicated. The pie plots show the relative representation of each V_H gene family in the different organs of BALB/c mice, as determined by in situ hybridization of single-cell suspensions with V_H-family-specific ^{35}S-labeled cDNA probes (Freitas et al. 1989a). Germ-line distributions are based on current estimates of gene numbers in each family (Blankenstein and Krawinkel 1987). The bar graphs show total numbers of B cells expressing the corresponding V_H families calculated from the relative representation and estimates of B-cell numbers in each organ. (BM) bone marrow; (SPL) spleen; (MLN) mesenteric lymph node; (PLN) peripheral lymph node; (PP) Payer's patch; (PEC) peritoneal resident cells. For BM, cell numbers represent the daily production of B cells based on the estimates of Opstelten and Osmond (1983) and the relative V_H family representation in the population cells (Freitas et al. 1990).

repertoires from the emergent to the available pool. The basis for such a process must involve V-region-specific differential persistence and/or expansion of peripheral lymphocytes. Evidence in this direction was provided by the finding of a very marked increase in J558 family representation among B cells selected for longer life spans (Freitas et al. 1990).

The analysis of V_H gene expression in other anatomical sites, has provided evidence for the local expansion or accumulation of selected specificities. Thus, as shown in Figure 3, whereas mesenteric lymph nodes differ little from those of the spleen, peripheral nodes contain an expanded J558-expressing population, Payer's patches lymphocytes very frequently express X24 genes, and peritoneal resident cells show a marked bias for the expression of V_H11 genes (Andrade et al. 1989). These are likely to be related to particular antibody reactivities described previously in such organs and depend, at least in part, on the continuous challenge by environmental antigens. Thus, similar analysis carried out in germ-free mice reveal no local bias in V_H expression, in relation to spleen and bone marrow (A.A. Freitas et al., in prep.).

The study of the splenic-activated B-cell compartment and of natural plasma cells in normal individuals did not reveal major differences with the available repertoire (Freitas et al. 1989a) except for a particular V_H family (L. Andrade et al., in prep.). To investigate possible selective steps for the entry into the actual repertoire, we had to resume therefore to other kinds of studies, namely those of antibody reactivities.

Analysis of B-cell Repertoires by Clonal Reactivities

Activated lymphocytes can readily be separated from resting cells by their larger size or lower density. Both small and large B cells respond well to lipopolysaccharide (LPS), with comparable cloning efficiencies in vitro. It is possible therefore to compare their repertoires in LDAs, which do not bias the results by depending on factors (e.g., helper-cell activities and antigen concentration) that are extrinsic to the B-cell repertoire itself. So far, such comparisons lead to a major conclusion, namely that the reactivity repertoires of naturally activated B cells are in some instances skewed for autoreactivities (Portnoi et al. 1986; Huetz

et al. 1988; Pena-Rossi et al. 1989). These, in turn, are depleted from the resting lymphocyte compartment. The data show therefore that autoreactivities detected in these assays are not merely the result of low-affinity interactions devoid of functional significance. If this were the case, such reactivities should be found in both compartments of cells. In our minds, the only possible interpretation of the results is that autoreactivity is functionally meaningful for those clones in the normal immune system, so that it leads to their activation and transit from the resting to the activated compartment: We set up the thresholds for the in vitro detection of positive reactions, but the mouse sets up the thresholds for activation as we isolate the cells. In contrast with autoreactivities, it has not been possible so far to show significant differences in the two repertoires for reactivities toward external antigens. A variety of specificities have been analyzed in both cases: heterologous proteins and bacterial polysaccharides, on the one hand, and isologous serum proteins, surface antigens on erythrocytes and nucleated cells, as well as intracellular proteins and DNA on the other. The initial observations had suggested that all reactivities to molecular profiles available in the individual were positively selected into the activated cell pool. More recently, however, we have found at least two examples of self components where we can find neither depletion of reactivities from the small cell compartment nor their increased representation among large lymphocytes. These are antibodies to single-stranded (ss)DNA and rheumatoid factors (RF) with IgG2a specificity (Table 1) (Huetz et al. 1989; Pena-Rossi et al. 1989; M. Weksler et al., in prep.). It is possible that, in these cases, the multimeric nature of the target antigens lowers the threshold of positivity in the assays to the extent that they no longer correspond to those necessary for activation in vivo. It follows that the most frequent anti-ssDNA antibodies are devoid of particular significance. The situation with RF may be different since, in contrast with anti-ssDNA antibodies that are found equally distributed in the resting, the activated, and in the secretory compartments, RF reactivities seem to be selectively depleted from the nonsecretory, large B-cell pool only (Pena-Rossi et al. 1989; P. Pereira; M. Weksler et al., both in prep.). It could then be considered that specific cells are rapidly induced to terminal differentiation with little or no division so that their time

Table 1. Positive Selection of Autoreactive B Cells in Normal Mice

Autoreactivities analyzed	B cells studied[a]		
	resting	activated	secreting
BrMRBC	no	+++	++
Class II	no	++	n.d.
Thyroglobulin	+	++	++
Transferrin	+	++	++
Cytoskeleton proteins	n.d.	n.d.	+++
DNA	++	++	++
Rheumatoid factors	++	+	++

[a] n.d. indicates not determined.

of transit in the large cell compartment is short. This could be due to dual binding of the ligand to both immunoglobulin and Fc receptors of the corresponding cell, and it would explain why RF produced in normal individuals even in secondary, T-cell-dependent responses, are always encoded by unmutated, germ-line V regions (Schlomchik et al. 1987).

A fraction of all activated cells secrete antibodies at a high rate, and these can be tested for reactivities either in single-cell assays or at the level of serum antibodies. Both have been carried out by several groups (e.g., Ishigatsubo et al. 1988; Guilbert et al. 1982) with the same general conclusion, namely, the marked reactivity of secreted antibodies with structural self-components. We have instead analyzed the genetic control of the production of some natural autoantibodies. This type of experiment can indeed provide direct indications of the coincidence or discrepancy between our analysis and the functional reality of the animal since it is possible to analyze transgenic mice and ask questions on how the repertoire of activated cells of such animals compares with those of normal cells (A. Grandien et al., in prep.). Furthermore, the nature of the genetics controls detected given indications on the mechanisms participating in the activation of cells in the internal environment. A typical example was provided by the genetic control of the natural production of RF, where genes linked to the IgH locus as well as to class II I-E genes are determinant (Pereira and Coutinho 1989), suggesting that the activation of such autoreactivities involves specific T/B cell interactions and repertoire selection. Further characterization of T-cell-receptor gene haplotypes will help in these studies.

Analysis of the Activated T-cell Repertoire

These studies have faced a major difficulty, namely, our inability to clone or even to grow in vitro with minimal plating efficiencies activated T cells isolated from normal animals. Interestingly, when freshly isolated, these cells express no receptor for interleukin-2 (IL-2) and rapidly accumulate in G_1, even if exposed to conditions that result in proliferation of in vitro small-cell-derived T cells (Bandeira et al. 1987). This is surprising, since a good fraction of those cells seem to be cycling in vivo, as assessed by their elimination with antimitotic drugs (Rocha et al. 1983) and by their DNA content (Pereira et al. 1985). Furthermore, as shown below, they perform in effector cell assays with an efficiency comparable with in-vitro-derived T cell clones. It is interesting to note in the context of the known functional heterogeneity of CD4 cells (Mosmann and Coffman 1987) that naturally activated T cells seem to belong in the helper T-cell (T_H2) category. Thus, in addition to the lack of expression of IL-2 receptors (Bandeira et al. 1987; Rocha et al. 1989), the majority if not all of these cells fail to secrete IL-2 upon activation by concanavalin A (Con A). As shown in Figure 4, there is around one order of magnitude difference in the frequency of IL-2-producing cells among

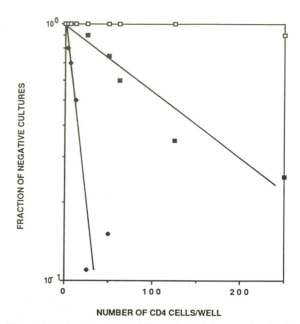

Figure 4. Naturally activated CD4 T cells fail to produce IL-2. Small (◆) and large (■) CD4$^+$ T cells from BALB/c spleen were purified after nylon wool columns and treated with anti-CD8 and anti-I-A antibodies with complement, followed by Percoll gradients (Bandeira et al. 1987). They were stimulated under limiting dilution conditions with Con A (■, ◆) in the presence of syngeneic nude peritoneal cells, and IL-2 production was assayed as described previously (Rocha and Bandeira 1988). (□) Cell cultures without lectin.

large and small CD4 T cells, respectively. The low numbers of IL-2 producers among in-vivo-activated CD4 cells could be real or represent contamination by small lymphocytes in the large cell population. Furthermore, these cells are excellent helpers for B cells, inducing them to proliferation and high-rate antibody secretion, just like cloned helper cells (see Fig. 7). Similarly, naturally activated CD8 T cells belong in what could be designated as the Tc2 functional subset: In addition to similar independence on IL-2, they display no cytolytic activities but are efficient suppressors of B-cell blasts. As few as 10^3 large CD8 T cells isolated from a normal mouse suppress up to 50% of the plaque-forming cell (PFC) response developed by 20 × 10^3 LPS-activated blasts (see Fig. 5); the same cells even at 100-fold-higher effector/target ratios fail to induce significant ^{51}Cr release from the same target B-cell blast population in 4 hour assays (Pereira et al. 1985).

In these conditions, the only possibility we have had so far to assay repertoires of large T cells is limited to effector assays in mass cultures that are therefore only "semiquantitative." The prototype experiment compares the ability of two populations of CD8 T cells to suppress PFC responses by B-cell blasts that are syngeneic or allogeneic to the effector cells: These either are directly isolated from the mouse as large lymphocytes or are activated populations derived by in vitro stimulation of purified small CD8 T cells with Con A or anti-CD3 antibodies. This protocol allows for

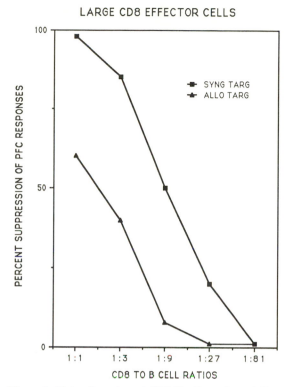

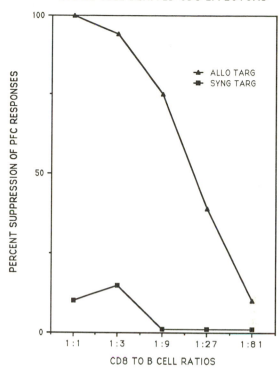

Figure 5. Naturally activated CD8 T cells preferentially react with syngeneic target B cells. Small CD8$^+$ T cells from BALB/c mouse spleen (for purification procedures, see Bandeira et al. 1987) were incubated overnight with Con A and expanded for 4 days with saturating amounts of IL-2 before assay (small-cell-derived CD8 effectors, *right*). Large CD8 T cells were purified ex vivo from normal BALB/c mice (Bandeira et al. 1987) and directly assayed (*left*). Both cell populations were irradiated (1000 rads) and cocultured with syngeneic or allogeneic (C57BL/6) responder B cells in the presence of LPS (25 μg/ml) at the indicated effector/target B-cell ratios in triplicates. All cultures were assayed for the numbers of immunoglobulin-secreting cells on day 4 (see Pereira et al. 1985).

comparing effector reactivities in parallel cultures of essentially the whole set of specificities in either compartment. Results of one such experiment are shown in Figure 5. As can be seen, naturally activated CD8 cells preferentially suppress syngeneic B cells as compared with allogeneic targets, this preference varying in quantitative terms from two- to tenfold in different experiments. Most important, if compared with these in-vivo-activated large cells, small-cell-derived effector CD8 cells consistently show a tenfold enrichment in the suppression of allotargets although being quite completely depleted of reactivity on syngeneic B blasts. The comparison of both effector populations on both targets provides an estimate of selection from one compartment to the other: In the experiment shown in Figure 5, the selection factor is at least 50-fold. Similar experiments are somewhat more complicated in the case of CD4 helper cell activities. Thus, although CD8 effectors directly interact with their targets (B cell blasts), naturally activated effector CD4 cells fail to activate syngeneic small B cells at reasonable effector/target ratios. The population contains helper effector cells, as readily revealed by bridging them to target B lymphocytes with a lectin (see Fig. 7), but most probably their avidity is too low for productive interaction. If syngeneic target B cells, however, are exposed to

anti-μ F(ab)$_2$ fragments, they become suitable interactive targets for in-vivo-activated CD4 helper cells, as in the experiment shown in Figure 6. On the other hand, populations of effector helper cells, derived by in vitro polyclonal activation of purified, small lymphocytes, directly activate allogeneic targets but are completely devoid of reactivities to syngeneic B cells (Fig. 7).

Taken together, these data lead us to the tentative conclusion that in vivo naturally activated CD4 and CD8 cells are selected for reactivities with, respectively, syngeneic B cells that have bound appropriate ligands or with B-cell blasts. Although their specificities remain to be determined with precision (e.g., major histocompatibility complex [MHC] and B-cell peptides), these results allow us to conclude that normal animals display repertoires and interactive conditions that are necessary and sufficient for the ongoing activation and regulation of B-cell activities by T cells. It should be pointed out that in view of the poor growth of such (autoreactive) T cells in vitro, individuals containing proportionally higher fractions of in-vivo-activated T cells will necessarily show as poor responders for T-cell proliferation in vitro. This is actually a consistent finding in autoimmune diseases and in some forms of immunodepression following polyclonal stimulations in vivo.

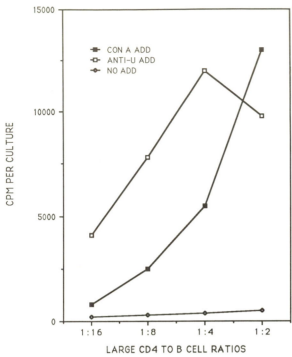

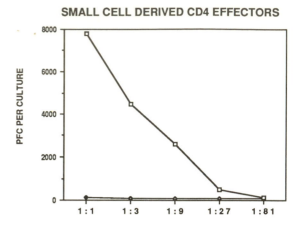

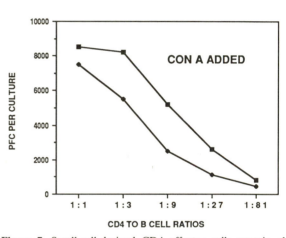

Figure 6. Reactivity of naturally activated CD4 T cells with syngeneic B cells. Irradiated large CD4$^+$ T cells from BALB/c spleen were cocultured with 4×10^4 small syngeneic B cells (purified by anti-Thy-1 and complement treatment, followed by Percoll gradients) either alone, with 5 μg/ml Con A, or with 10 μg/ml F(ab)$_2$ fragments of affinity-purified rabbit anti-mouse μ-chain-specific antibodies, as indicated previously (Pereira et al. 1985, 1986b). Cultures were pulsed with 1 μCi of [^{3}H]thymidine for 3 hr, and the results are expressed as the mean cpm in triplicate cultures. Background values of small B cells alone, with Con A, or anti-μ F(ab)$_2$, were less than 1000 cpm/culture.

Recursive Selection of T/B-cell Repertoires in Normal Animals

If such productive T/B-cell interactions do occur in normal animals, and if they are V-region-directed, it should be expected that T and B cells recursively select their repertoires. Furthermore, since such productive interactions lead to activation of the participating lymphocytes, it should also be expected that selected repertoires were to be found predominantly or exclusively in the activated (but not in the resting) lymphocyte compartment of normal individuals. Experiments analyzing the representation of a given helper T-cell clonotype in normal BALB/c mice have shown that its expression was positively selected in the first few weeks of life by interactions that required a normal B-cell/antibody compartment (Martinez-A. et al. 1988). Indeed, such a T-cell clonotype had its expression controlled both by MHC- and by IgH-linked genes (Martinez-A. et al. 1986). More interestingly, helper CD4 cells expressing the selected clonotype could only be found in the activated compartment of normal animals (Coutinho et al. 1987) and were selectively depleted

Figure 7. Small-cell-derived CD4 effector cells contain alloreactive (but not autoreactive) helper cells. Small CD4$^+$ splenic T cells from BALB/c mice were stimulated with Con A and syngeneic, irradiated peritoneal cells. Afterwards (5 days), activated cells were irradiated (1000 rads) and cocultured with anti-Thy-1 and complement-treated C57BL/6 (□,■) or BALB/c (◇, ◆) spleen cells at the indicated T/B-cell ratios in the absence (*upper*) or in the presence (*lower*) of Con A in triplicates. Numbers of immunoglobulin-secreting cells were measured on day 4 of culture.

from the resting lymphocyte pool. The converse has also been found, namely the strict T-cell dependence of the accumulation in the large cell compartment of autoreactive B cells in normal animals: Nude mice contain undetectable frequencies of clonable, splenic B cells that secrete antibodies directed to autologous erythrocytes, whereas euthymic mice contain high frequencies of such cells in the large cell pool. Moreover, transfer of syngeneic, large CD4 cells to nude recipients leads to the selection of such autoreactivities in the activated B-cell compartment in a matter of weeks (Huetz et al. 1988).

As expected from the biology of activated lymphocyte interactions, such processes of T/B-cell repertoire selection are recursive (Marcos et al. 1988). This was shown by first "educating" B-cell repertoires in nude animals with transfers of normal T cells and thereafter demonstrating the ability of such B cells to select recursively the appropriate T-cell repertoire in B-cell-deficient mice. Such recursive characteristics are obviously very important in the maintenance of the molecular identity of the individual and perhaps in recording its history. Moreover, they suggest the importance of early ontogenic steps, when the learning of self is taking place and maternal influences are predominant (Bernabé et al. 1981a; Martinez-A. et al. 1987), for the whole life time of the individual. All that will happen later is placed in the context of the recursive operation selecting repertoires of activated, autoreactive cells.

The Immune System Starts as a Germ-line-encoded, High-connectivity V Region Network, the Expression of Which Is Developmentally Controlled

Even 10 years after the proposition of the network theory, it was still a matter of debate whether idiotypic interactions did occur in functionally relevant manners within the normal immune system. In our minds, this was essentially due to the fact that no appropriate quantitation of such reactivities had been carried out, and the "network" had been exclusively "used" in the context of the regulation of immune responses to external antigens. It appeared to us that the theory should instead be applied to the globality of the system's operation before introduction of external antigen, namely, to the selection of repertoires and normal immune dynamics. This view implied, of course, the notion of autonomy in immune activities and further elaborations on the question of self-reactivities. Nevertheless, it was also clear that some of the central postulates embodied a number of falsifiable predictions, and we set out to quantitate the frequency of V region interactions (connectivity) to assess the degree of autonomy in the putative network operation and to characterize its dynamics.

Table 2 shows the results from the only three experiments that, to our knowledge, have been carried out to quantitate antibody connectivity in the normal immune system. All three have been independently performed but followed a similar strategy, namely, the isolation of hybridomas from normal, neonatal individuals (because of the difficulty in obtaining significant numbers of hybrids from unmanipulated adult mice), the purification of the corresponding IgM antibodies, and their test for mutual reactivities in vitro. As shown, the three experiments give remarkably similar results: Roughly

25% of all possible interactions among such antibodies are scored as positive by the methods employed. There is no question therefore that the neonatal immune system is a highly connected network of antibody V regions. Unfortunately, the same experiment has not been carried out with adult animals.

Structural studies with some neonatal connected antibodies has revealed their germ-line sequences with a very marked paucity of N-sequence diversity, as if it were important to preserve full germ-line reactivity (L. Carlsson et al., in prep.). Moreover, connected antibodies in the newborn are most often encoded by D-proximal V_H genes (Holmberg 1987), which are the first to be expressed in development for reasons of "accessibility" (Yancopoulos et al. 1984; Perlmutter et al. 1985). In other words, for the developing immune system, there is no possibility other than starting as a highly connected V region network.

Autonomous Immune Activities in Normal Animals: Central and Peripheral Immune System

Together with the demonstrations of a V region network and of the normalcy of autoreactivities, a major acquisition over the last 5 years is, for us, the establishment of the existence of autonomous immune activities. Normal animals, even if secluded from all environmental antigenic contacts, maintain in their spleen a level of mature lymphocyte activities that is actually comparable to conventionally fed mice colonized by all sorts of bacteria and viruses (Pereira et al. 1986a). Autonomy is obviously the consequence of productive V region interactions with other V regions and with somatic autologous antigens, as well. In other words, an immune network of only V regions makes little biological sense, and therefore the final elucidation of network structure and dynamics is likely to include the solution for self-tolerance.

The first thing to note, in the context of autonomous immune activities is that they concern only a part of the lymphocytes in the normal individual. Thus, some 80–90% of all lymphocytes keep resting, implying that, functionally at least, they are disconnected from any network. If a network organization applies to normal immune systems, it only concerns a minority of its components (the compartment of activated cells), the large majority of them showing no autonomy in functional behavior and being structurally disconnected from both "self" and other V regions (Holmberg et al. 1986). In keeping with this proposition, antigen-free mice are severely depleted of allonomous immune ac-

Table 2. V Region Connectivity in Collections of Natural Newborn Antibodies

Possibilities tested	612[a]	756[b]	2704[c]
Positive reactions	173	172	594
Connectivity	0.28	0.23	0.22

[a] Holmberg et al. (1984).
[b] Kearney et al. (1987).
[c] M. Zöller (unpubl.).

Table 3. Partial T-cell-independence of B-cell Activities in Germ-free BALB/c Mice.

Number of cells per spleen ($\times 10^6$)				
	CD3$^+$	CD4$^+$	CD8$^+$	Ig$^+$
Euthymic	28.6	18.7	9.9	29.4
Nude	—	—	—	12.9

Number of activated cells per spleen ($\times 10^5$)				
	CD3$^+$	CD4$^+$	CD8$^+$	Ig$^+$
Euthymic	65	21	8	77
Nude	—	—	—	25

tivities that are stimulated by environmental antigens: Mucosal associated lymphocytes and lymph nodes are absent or markedly underdeveloped, and they produce no IgG or IgA antibodies. Furthermore, repertoire selection processes that are indeed autonomous and relate to T/B-cell interactions in the context of connectivity should contribute to the internal immune activity. We have reported previously that such B-cell activities are extensively suppressed in normal animals upon treatment with anti-CD4 antibodies (Freitas et al. 1989b), and we discussed above other evidence for the T-cell-dependence of B-cell repertoire selection. However, as also suggested by other investigators (Kearney and Vakil 1986; Kearney et al. 1989), there are mechanisms of B-cell selection and autonomous activity that apparently proceed in the absence of T cells (Coutinho et al. 1980). Table 3 shows the levels of B-cell activities in normal and nude germ-free BALB/c mice, indicating that roughly one-third of the autonomous activation of B cells is indeed T-cell-independent.

These results and considerations lead some of us to separate, for simple operational purposes, the central from the peripheral immune system: The latter follows the rules of clonal selection (clonal organization, deletion of autoreactive cells, antigen-dependent regulation and allonomous activities of mature lymphocytes) and provides for immune responses to external antigens, whereas the former conforms to a network organization (V region connectivity and autoreactivity to somatic self) and dynamics and provides for the molecular identity of the individual by self-assertion (Coutinho 1989). It is all the more interesting that recent observations on the dynamics of immune activities in the central and peripheral compartments demonstrate sharp differences between the two: As it could be expected, the activities in the central immune system show typical equilibrium dynamics (Lundkvist et al. 1989) resistant to the induction of large clonal amplifications (Portnoi et al. 1988). The significance of these observations in the context of self-tolerance are yet to be fully investigated.

ACKNOWLEDGMENTS

We thank all our colleagues for stimulating discussions and generous collaboration. More particularly, we thank Dr. M. Zöller for allowing us to refer to her as yet unpublished work and Dr. C. Heusser for providing us with germ-free mice. We also thank J. Badella for excellent secretarial assistance. This work was supported by grants from Association Française contre les Myopathies, Association pour la Recherche sur le Cancer, Direction des Recherches Etudes et Techniques du Ministere de la Defense, the European Economic Community, and the Krupp Foundation.

REFERENCES

Andersson, J., A. Coutinho, L. Lernhardt, and F. Melchers. 1977. Clonal growth and maturation to immunoglobulin secretion *in vitro* of every growth inducible lymphocyte. *Cell* **10**: 27.

Andrade, L., A.A. Freitas, F. Huetz, P. Poncet, and A. Coutinho. 1989. Immunoglobulin V$_H$ gene expression in Ly-1 and conventional B lymphocytes. *Eur. J. Immunol.* **19**: 1117.

Bandeira, A., E.-L. Larsson, L. Forni, P. Pereira, and A. Coutinho. 1987. *In vivo* activated splenic T cells are refractory to interleukin 2 growth *in vitro*. *Eur. J. Immunol.* **17**: 901.

Benner, R., A.-M. Rijnbeek, M.H. Schreier, and A. Coutinho. 1981. Frequency analysis of immunoglobulin V-gene expression and functional reactivities in bone marrow B cells. *J. Immunol.* **126**: 887.

Bernabé, R.R., A. Coutinho, P.-A. Cazenave, and L. Forni. 1981a. Suppression of a "recurrent" idiotype results in profound alterations of the whole B-cell compartment. *Proc. Natl. Acad. Sci.* **78**: 6416.

Bernabé, R.R., A. Coutinho, C. Martinez-A., and P.-A. Cazenave. 1981b. Immune networks. Frequencies of antibody- and idiotype-producing B cell clones in various steady states. *J. Exp. Med.* **154**: 552.

Blankenstein, T. and U. Krawinkel. 1987. Immunoglobulin V$_H$ region genes of the mouse are organized in overlapping clusters. *Eur. J. Immunol.* **17**: 1351.

Bosma, G.C., R.P. Custer, and M.J. Bosma. 1983. A severe combined immunodeficiency mutation in the mouse. *Nature* **301**: 527.

Brahim, F. and D.G. Osmond. 1970. Migration of bone marrow lymphocytes demonstrated by selective bone marrow labelling with ^{3}H-thymidine. *Anat. Rec.* **168**: 139.

Brodeur, P.H. and R. Riblet. 1984. The immunoglobulin heavy chain variable region (Igh-V) in the mouse. I. One hundred IgH V genes comprise seven families of homologous genes. *Eur. J. Immunol.* **14**: 922.

Coutinho, A. 1980. The self-nonself discrimination and the nature and acquisition of the antibody repertoire. *Ann. Immunol. (Inst. Pasteur)* **132C**: 131.

———. 1989. Beyond clonal selection and network. *Immunol. Rev.* **110**: 63.

Coutinho, A., L. Forni, and R.R. Bernabé. 1980. The polyclonal expression of immunoglobulin variable region determinants of the membrane of B cells and their precursors. *Springer Semin. Immunopathol.* **3**: 171.

Coutinho, A., L. Forni, D., Holmberg, F. Ivars, and N. Vaz. 1984. From an antigen-centered, clonal perspective of immune responses to an organism-centered, network perspective of autonomous activity in a self-referential immune system. *Immunol. Rev.* **79:** 151.

Coutinho, A., C. Marquez, P.M.F. Araujo, P. Pereira, M.L. Toribio, M.A.R. Marcos, and C. Martinez-A. 1987. A functional idiotype network of T helper cells and antibodies limited to the compartment of "naturally" activated lymphocytes in normal mice. *Eur. J. Immunol.* **17:** 821.

Eichmann, K., A. Coutinho, and F. Melchers. 1977. Absolute frequencies of lipopolysaccharide-reactive B cells producing A5A idiotype in unprimed, streptococcal A carbohydrate-primed, anti-A5A idiotype-sensitized and anti-A5A idiotype-suppressed A/J mice. *J. Exp. Med.* **146:** 1436.

Forni, L., A. Coutinho, G. Kohler, and N.K. Jerne. 1980. IgM antibodies induce the production of antibodies of the same specificity. *Proc. Natl. Acad. Sci.* **77:** 1125.

Freitas, A.A. and A. Coutinho. 1981. Very rapid decay of mature B lymphocytes in the spleen. *J. Exp. Med.* **154:** 994.

Freitas, A.A., M.-P. Lembezat, and A. Coutinho. 1989a. Expression of antibody V-regions is genetically and developmentally controlled and modulated by the B lymphocyte environment. *Int. Immunol.* **1:** 342.

Freitas, A.A., B. Rocha, and A. Coutinho. 1986a. Lymphocyte population kinetics in the mouse. *Immunol. Rev.* **91:** 5.

————. 1986b. Two major classes of mitogen-reactive B lymphocytes defined by life-span. *J. Immunol.* **136:** 466.

————. 1986c. Life span of B lymphocytes: The experimental basis for conflicting results. *J. Immunol.* **136:** 470.

Freitas, A.A., L. Andrade, M.P. Lembezar, and A. Coutinho. 1990. Selection of V_H gene repertoires: Differentiating B cells of adult bone marrow mimic fetal development. *Int. Immunol.* (in press).

Freitas, A.A., B. Rocha, L. Forni, and A. Coutinho. 1982. Population dynamics of B lymphocytes and their precursors: Demonstration of high turnover in the central and peripheral lymphoid organs. *J. Immunol.* **128:** 54.

Freitas, A.A., P. Pereira, F. Huetz, V. Thomas-Vaslin, C. Pena Rossi, L. Andrade, A. Sundblad, L. Forni, and A. Coutinho. 1989b. B cell activities in normal unmanipulated mice. In *B cells and B cell products. Contributions to microbiology and immunology* (ed. P. Del Guercio), vol. 11, p. 1. S. Karger A.G., Basel.

Fulop, G.M. and D.G. Osmond. 1983. Regulation of bone marrow, lymphocyte production III. Increased production of B and non-B lymphocytes after administering systemic antigens. *Cell. Immunol.* **75:** 80.

Fulop, G.M., Y. Gordon, and D.G. Osmond. 1983. Regulation of bone marrow lymphocyte production. I. Turnover of small lymphocytes in mice depleted of B lymphocytes by treatment with anti-IgM antibodies. *J. Immunol.* **130:** 644.

Gronowicz, E., A. Coutinho, and F. Melchers. 1976. A plaque assay for all cells secreting Ig of a given type or class. *Eur. J. Immunol.* **6:** 588.

Guilbert, B., G. Dighiero, and S. Avrameas. 1982. Naturally occurring antibodies against nine common antigens in human sera. I. Detection, isolation and characterization. *J. Immunol.* **128:** 2779.

Herzenberg, L.A., A.M. Stall, P.A. Lalor, C. Sidman, W.A. Moore, and L.A. Herzenberg. 1986. The Ly-1 B cell lineage. *Immunol. Rev.* **93:** 81.

Holmberg, D. 1987. High connectivity, natural antibodies preferentially use 7183 and QUPC 52 VH families. *Eur. J. Immunol.* **17:** 399.

Holmberg, D., S. Forsgren, F. Ivars, and A. Coutinho. 1984. Reactions amongst IgM antibodies derived from normal, neonatal mice. *Eur. J. Immunol.* **14:** 435.

Holmberg, D., G. Wennerström, L. Andrade, and A. Coutinho. 1986. The high idiotypic connectivity of "natural" newborn antibodies is not found in adult, mitogen-reactive B cell repertoires. *Eur. J. Immunol.* **16:** 82.

Huetz, F., P. Poncet, A. Coutinho, and D. Portnoi. 1989. Ontogenic development of auto-antibody repertoires in spleen and peritoneal cavity of normal mice: Examples of T cell-dependent and independent reactivities. *Eur. J. Immunol.* (in press).

Huetz, F., E.-L. Sciard-Larsson, P. Pereira, D. Portnoi, and A. Coutinho. 1988. T cell dependence of "natural" autoreactive B cell activation in the spleen of normal mice. *Eur. J. Immunol.* **18:** 1615.

Ishigatsubo, Y., A.D. Steinberg, and D.M. Klinman. 1988. Autoantibody production is associated with polyclonal B cell activation in autoimmune mice. *Eur. J. Immunol.* **18:** 1089.

Ivars, F., D. Holmberg, L. Forni, P.-A. Cazenave, and A. Coutinho. 1982. Antigen-dependent IgM-induced antibody responses: Requirement for "recurrent" idiotypes. *Eur. J. Immunol.* **12:** 146.

Jerne, N.K. 1974. Towards a network theory of the immune system. *Ann. Immunol. (Inst. Pasteur)* **125C:** 373.

Kearney, J.F. and M. Vakil. 1986. Idiotype directed interactions during ontogeny play major role in the establishment of the adult B cell repertoire. *Immunol. Rev.* **94:** 39.

Kearney, J.F., M. Vakil, and N. Nicholson. 1987. Nonrandom VH genes expression and idiotype anti-idiotype expression in early BN cells. In *Evolution and vertebrate immunity: The antigen receptor and MHC gene families* (ed. G. Kelsoe and D. Schulze), p. 175. Texas University Press, Austin.

Kearney, J.F., N. Solvason, A. Ploem, and M. Vakil. 1989. Idiotypes and B cell development. *Prog. Allergy* (in press).

Lévy, M., P. Vieira, A. Coutinho, and A.A. Freitas. 1987. The majority of "natural" immunoglobulin-secreting cells are short-lived and the progeny of cycling lymphocytes. *Eur. J. Immunol.* **17:** 849.

Lundkvist, I., A. Coutinho, F. Varela, and D. Holmberg. 1989. Evidence for a functional network amongst natural antibodies in normal mice. *Proc. Natl. Acad. Sci.* **86:** 5074.

Marcos, M.A.R., A. de la Hera, P. Pereira, C. Marquez, M.L. Toribio, A. Coutinho, and C. Martinez-A. 1988. B-cell participation in the recursive selection of T-cell repertoires. *Eur. J. Immunol.* **18:** 1015.

Martinez-A., C., R.R. Bernabé, A. de la Hera, P. Pereira, P.-A. Cazenave, and A. Coutinho. 1985. Establishment of idiotypic helper T-cell repertoires early in life. *Nature* **317:** 721.

Martinez-A., C., P. Pereira, A. de la Hera, A. Bandeira, C. Marquez, and A. Coutinho. 1986. The basis for major histocompatibility complex and immunoglobulin gene control of helper T cell idiotypes. *Eur. J. Immunol.* **16:** 417.

Martinez-A., C., P. Pereira, R.R. Bernabé, A. Bandeira, E.-L. Larsson, P.-A. Cazenave, and A. Coutinho. 1984. Internal complementarities in the immune system: Regulation of the expression of helper T-cell idiotypes. *Proc. Natl. Acad. Sci.* **81:** 4520.

Martinez-A., C., M.A.R. Marcos, P. Pereira, C. Marquez, M.L. Toribio, A. de la Hera, P.-A. Cazenave, and A. Coutinho. 1987. Turning (Ig-gene) low-responders into high responders by antibody manipulation of the developing immune system. *Proc. Natl. Acad. Sci.* **84:** 3812.

Martinez-A., C., M.L. Toribio, P. Pereira, M.A.R. Marcos, A. Bandeira, A. de la Hera, C. Marquez, P.-A. Cazenave, and A. Coutinho. 1988. The participation of B cells and antibodies in the selection and maintenance of T cell repertoires. *Immunol. Rev.* **101:** 191.

Mosmann, T.R. and R.L. Coffman. 1987. Two types of mouse helper T cell clones. *Immunol. Today* **8:** 223.

Namen, A.-E., A.E. Schmierer, C.J. March, R.W. Ourell, L.S. Park, D.L. Urdal, and D.Y. Mochizuki. 1988. B cell precursor growth-promoting activity. *J. Exp. Med.* **167:** 988.

Opstelten, D. and D.G. Osmond. 1983. Pre-B cells in mouse bone-marrow: Immunofluorescence stathmokinetic studies of the proliferation of cytoplasmic μ-chain bearing cells in normal mice. *J. Immunol.* **131:** 2635.

Osmond, D.G. 1986. Population dynamics of bone marrow B lymphocytes. *Immunol. Rev.* **93:** 103.

Palacios, R., G. Henson, M. Steinmetz, and J.P. McKearn. 1984. Interleukin-3 supports growth of mouse pre-B cell clones *in vitro*. *Nature* **309:** 126.

Pena-Rossi, C., P. Pereira, D. Portnoi, and A. Coutinho. 1989. MHC-linked and T cell-dependent selection of antibody repertoires. Quantitation of I-E-related specificities in normal mice. *Eur. J. Immunol.* (in press).

Pereira, P. and A. Coutinho. 1989. I-E linked control of spontaneous rheumatoid factor production in normal mice. *J. Exp. Med.* (in press).

Pereira, P., E.-L. Larsson, L. Forni, A. Bandeira, and A. Coutinho. 1985. Natural effector T lymphocytes in normal mice. *Proc. Natl. Acad. Sci.* **82:** 7691.

Pereira, P., L. Forni, E.-L. Larsson, M.D. Cooper, C. Heusser, and A. Coutinho. 1986a. Autonomous activation of B and T cells in antigen-free mice. *Eur. J. Immunol.* **16:** 685.

Pereira, P., S. Forsgren, D. Portnoi, A. Bandeira, C. Martinez-A., and A. Coutinho. 1986b. The role of immunoglobulin receptors in "cognate" T-B cell collaboration. *Eur. J. Immunol.* **16:** 355.

Perlmutter, R.M., J.F. Kearney, S.P. Chang, and L.E. Hood. 1985. Developmentally controlled expression of immunoglobulin V_H genes. *Science* **227:** 1597.

Pobor, G., A. Bandeira, S. Pettersson, and A. Coutinho. 1984. A quantitative assay detecting small numbers of effector helper T cells, regardless of clonal specificity. *Scand, J. Immunol.* **20:** 189.

Portnoi, D., I. Lundkvist, and A. Coutinho. 1988. Inverse correlation between the utilization of an idiotype in specific immune responses and its representation in pre-immune "natural" antibodies. *Eur. J. Immunol.* **18:** 571.

Portnoi, D., A. Freitas, A. Bandeira, D. Holmberg, and A. Coutinho. 1986. Immunocompetent autoreactive B lymphocytes are activated cycling cells in normal mice. *J. Exp. Med.* **164:** 25.

Rocha, B. and A. Bandeira. 1988. Limiting dilution analysis of Interleukin 2-producing mature T cells. *Scand. J. Immunol.* **27:** 47.

Rocha, B., A.A. Freitas, and A. Coutinho. 1983. Population dynamics of T lymphocytes. Renewal rate and expansion in the peripheral lymphoid organs. *J. Immunol.* **131:** 2158.

Rocha, B., M.-P. Lembezat, A. Freitas, and A. Bandeira. 1989. IL receptor expression and IL-2 production in exponentially growing T cells: Major differences between *in vivo* and *in vitro* proliferating T lymphocytes. *Eur. J. Immunol.* **19:** 1137.

Schlomchik, M., D. Nemazee, J. Van Snick, and M. Weigert. 1987. Variable region sequences of murine IgM and IgG monoclonal antibodies (Rheumatoid factors). *J. Exp. Med.* **165:** 970.

Thomas-Vaslin, V. and A.A. Freitas. 1989. Lymphocyte population kinetics during the development of the immune system. B cell persistence and high span can be determined by the host environment. *Int. Immunol.* **1:** 237.

Wortis, H.H., L. Burklu, D. Hughes, S. Roschelle, and G. Waneck. 1982. Lack of mature B cells in nude mice with x-linked immune deficiency. *J. Exp. Med.* **155:** 903.

Yancopoulos, G.D., S.V. Desiderio, M. Paskind, J.F. Kearney, D. Baltimore, and F. Alt. 1984. Preferential utilization of the most J_H proximal V_H gene segments in pre-B cell lines. *Nature* **311:** 727.

Control of Cell Growth and Differentiation during Early B-cell Development by Stromal Cell Molecules

S.-I. Nishikawa,* S.-I. Hayashi,* M. Ogawa,* T. Kunisada,* S. Nishikawa,*
T. Sudo,† H. Nakauchi,‡ and T. Suda§

*Department of Immunopathology, Kumamoto University Medical School, 860 Kumamoto, Japan; †Biomaterial
Research Institute Co., Ltd., 244 Yokohama, Japan; ‡Laboratory of Molecular Regulation of Aging,
Frontier Research Program, The Institute of Physical and Chemical Research (RIKEN), 305 Tsukuba,
Japan; §Division of Hematology, Department of Medicine, Jichi Medical School,
329-04, Tochigi-ken, Japan

A large number of B lymphocytes are produced daily in the bone marrow of the postnatal mouse by repeating the differentiation from multipotent stem cells into mature B cells (Abramson et al. 1977; Osmond 1986). The most important event to be accomplished in this process is the expression of complete IgM molecules on the cell surface, which functions as the specific receptor to antigens. Because variable regions of immunoglobulin (Ig) are encoded by DNA segments that exist separately in the germ-line gene, each of the segments has to be assembled together to form a complete variable region gene during early B-lineage differentiation. With the advent of a method to produce an immortalized B-cell line by Abelson murine leukemia virus (Ab-MLV: Rosenberg and Baltimore 1976), sequential events during early B-cell development have been characterized extensively (for review, see Alt et al. 1986). The most striking features of this process that emerged from these studies of Ab-MLV-transformed cell lines are the following: (1) The process of Ig gene assembly is an error prone process, thus producing nonfunctional B cells that fail to form productive Ig genes, and (2) Ig gene assembly proceeds in an ordered fashion, starting from H-chain variable (V) gene segments, diversity (D) to joined (J) and subsequently V to DJ joining, followed by L-chain V to J joining. These features indicate, unlike time-scheduled differentiation of cells in other tissues, that the early B-lineage differentiation is a stepwise process where each differentiation step is absolutely dependent on the result of a preceding Ig gene rearrangement.

Despite the clear picture of early B-cell development concerning structural alteration of an Ig gene, nothing essential has been understood regarding how B-cell proliferation during this error prone differentiation process is controlled in adult bone marrow. In the previous study, we have demonstrated that the signals required for the entire process of B-cell development can be divided into two parts, namely, interleukin-7 (IL-7) and other molecule(s) expressed in a stromal cell line PA6, which is defective for the expression of IL-7 (Sudo et al. 1989). Using recombinant IL-7 and PA6 as

separate signals for pre-B cells, we investigate here the process of early B-cell development regarding the growth requirements. On the basis of the results described here, we will propose a model for the control of B-cell growth during intramarrow differentiation.

MATERIALS AND METHODS

Mice. Inbred BDF_1 mice and BALB/c mice were purchased from the Shizuoka Experimental Animal Center (Shizuoka, Japan). CB17 SCID/SCID mice were obtained from S. Habu at Tokai University Medical School. The original stock of SCID mice was introduced from M.J. Bosma (Bosma et al. 1983).

Interleukin-7. cDNA clones encoding the IL-7 gene obtained from a stromal cell line ST2 (Ogawa et al. 1988) and the preparation of recombinant IL-7 were described previously (Sudo et al. 1989).

Bone marrow cell culture. RPMI 1640 containing 5% fetal calf serum (FCS) was used throughout this study. Characteristics and maintenance of stromal cell line PA6 and the bone marrow culture on the PA6 layer were performed as described previously (Kodama et al. 1984; Nishikawa et al. 1988).

Cell-sorting of bone marrow. After lysis of red blood cells by an ammonium chloride potassium buffer, single-cell suspensions of bone marrow were prepared in phosphate-buffered saline supplemented with 3% FCS and 0.1% sodium azide. Cells were stained with fluorescein isothiocyanate- or biotin-conjugated monoclonal antibodies followed by avidin phycoerythrin. Stained cells were sorted on a fluorescence-activated cell sorter (FACStar, Becton Dickinson, California). Antibodies used in this study are rat monoclonal antibodies RA3-6B2 (anti-B220) and 331.12 (anti-mouse IgM).

Colony assay for the cells reactive to IL-7. Methylcellulose culture was used for enumerating the precursor cells that proliferate in response to IL-7 alone.

Cells were incubated in 1 ml of culture medium containing alpha medium (Gibco Laboratories, New York), 1.2% methylcellulose (1500 centipoises, Aldrich Chemical Co., Wisconsin), 30% FCS, 1% deionized bovine serum albumin (Sigma Chemical Co., Missouri), 0.1 mM 2-mercaptoethanol (Sigma), and 10 units of IL-7. On day 7 of the culture, aggregate consisting of more than 40 cells was scored as a colony.

Limiting dilution assay. The frequency of precursor cells whose growth requires both IL-7 and PA6 was analyzed by limiting dilution assay. Prior to the assay (4 days), 2.5×10^5 of PA6 were inoculated into a 96-well cluster dish (2600 cells/well). At the day of assay, varying number of cells (100–1000/well) were inoculated in the well with PA6 monolayer and cultured for 9 days in the presence of 20 units/ml IL-7. Of the individual wells, 96 were initiated for each cell dilution. Half of the medium was exchanged every 3 days. Since this culture condition supports both B lymphopoiesis and myelopoiesis, presence of B cells was determined by light scatter analysis on EPICS PROFIL (Coulter, Florida). After incubation, the cells in each well were individually suspended in 200 μl of medium, and 50 μl was counted and analyzed by EPICS PROFIL. For the analysis, a gate for small lymphocytes was set so as to include a majority of splenic small lymphocytes. When more than 250 cells appeared in this gate, the well was judged as B-progenitor positive.

RESULTS

Characterization of B-precursor Cells Maintained on the PA6 Monolayer

Previously, we have shown that the ability of a stromal cell line to produce IL-7 correlates well with the capability of stromal cells to support B lymphopoiesis (Sudo et al. 1989). Thus, when bone marrow cells are cultured on the PA6 layer that does not produce IL-7, mature lymphoid cells are hardly detectable in the culture although sustained hematopoiesis is able to be maintained (Kodama et al. 1984; Nishikawa et al. 1988). In this section, we investigate the presence of two types of clonogenic B-cell precursors: The first type requires both IL-7 and PA6 for its growth, which is enumerated by the limiting dilution assay in the culture containing both PA6 and IL-7 (B progenitor II: B-pro-II). The second type proliferates in response to IL-7 alone, which is enumerated by a colony-forming cell

assay in semi-solid medium containing methylcellulose and IL-7 (CFU-IL7).

Bone marrow cells were cultured on the PA6 layer, and the cells were harvested 2 weeks later for measuring the frequency of both B-pro-II and CFU-IL7. As shown in Table 1, B-pro-II was present in this culture, whereas no CFU-IL7 was detected. This result suggests that B-pro-II but not CFU-IL7 is generated directly from the B progenitors maintained on the PA6 layer (B-pro-I).

B-pro-II Is the Immediate Precursor for CFU-IL7 and Differentiates into CFU-IL7 Only When It Undergoes Productive Rearrangement in the H-chain Variable Gene

In this section, we investigate whether B-pro-II is the immediate precursor of CFU-IL7 or whether CFU-IL7 belongs to the different cell lineage from B-pro-I to B-pro-II pathway. First, to obtain B-pro-I, bone marrow cells were cultured on the PA6 layer. Then B-pro-II was induced by adding IL-7 to the same culture. Before and 2 weeks after the induction of B-pro-II, the cells were harvested and assayed for CFU-IL7. As shown in Table 2, a significant amount of CFU-IL7 was generated after the addition of IL-7, suggesting that CFU-IL7 is differentiated from B-pro-II.

Lee et al. (1989) have shown that more than 80% of the cells proliferating in response to IL-7 alone are cytoplasmic μ-chain positive. This suggests strongly that CFU-IL7 is pre-B cells that have succeeded to form a productive H-chain gene. This possibility was tested by taking advantage of the fact that the frequency of productive Ig gene rearrangement is extremely low in SCID mice (Schuler et al. 1986; Hendrickson et al. 1988; Malynn et al. 1988; Okazaki et al. 1988). The same experiment as described above was carried out using the bone marrow cells from SCID mice (Table 2). Even in the culture of the SCID mouse, proliferation of B220$^+$ cells was observed after addition of IL-7 (data not shown), suggesting that differentiation from B-pro-I to B-pro-II proceeds in SCID mice. On the other hand, no CFU-IL7 was detected in the culture of the SCID mouse after B-pro-II was induced by adding IL-7. This indicates that a defect of SCID mice to produce productive Ig gene rearrangement results in the arrest of differentiation from B-pro-II into CFU-IL7.

Table 1. Absence of CFU-IL7 in the Bone Marrow Cells Precultured on the PA6 Layer

	Growth signal for assay	
Cell source	PA6 + IL-7	IL-7
Fresh bone marrow	96[a]	97
Bone marrow cells precultured on the PA6 layer for 2 wk	122	0

[a]Number of cells/10^5 cells.

Table 2. Frequency of CFU-IL7 in the Bone Marrow Cell Culture of Normal or SCID Mice

Culture		Source of bone marrow	
1	2	BALB/c	SCID
PA6	—	0[a]	0
PA6	PA6 + IL-7	21	0

[a] Number of cells/10^5 cells.

CFU-IL7 Is B220⁺sIgM⁻, and It Loses the Reactivity to IL-7 upon Maturation into the sIgM⁺ Cell

In this final section, we investigate the surface phenotype of CFU-IL7. Bone marrow cells were sorted into B220⁻, B220⁺ (surface IgM expressing) sIgM⁻, and B220⁺sIgM⁺ populations, and the frequency of CFU-IL7 in each cell population was measured. As shown in Table 3, CFU-IL7 was enriched in B220⁺ sIgM⁻ population. This result suggests that upon maturation of CFU-IL7 into sIgM⁺ cells, it loses the ability to proliferate in response to IL-7.

DISCUSSION

Using an IL-7-defective stromal cell line, PA6, and recombinant IL-7 as separate growth signals, we succeeded to elucidate the sequential change of the growth requirement during B-cell differentiation. In Figure 1, we depicted our model for B-cell development in the postnatal bone marrow of a mouse. Although we know that the entire process from multipotent stem cells into sIgM⁺ mature B cells is observed in our experimental system (H. Nakauchi et al., in prep.), it is not clear whether B-pro-I is identical with the multipotent stem cell or whether it is already committed to B lineage. At present, these stages represent the cells proliferating on the PA6 layer in the absence of IL-7. Further dissection of this process obviously requires the identification of more stromal cell molecules. The second stage, B-pro-II requires both PA6 and IL-7 for its proliferation. Our recent analysis on the clonal growth of B-pro-II demonstrated that the doubling time of the proliferation at this stage is as rapid as 12–15 hours (S.-I. Nishikawa et al., unpubl.). Through such extensive proliferation, B-pro-II continues H-chain gene rearrangement, and only those cells that succeeded to form the complete H-chain variable gene are selected to differentiate into the third stage, CFU-IL7. CFU-IL7 is B220⁺/sIgM⁻ pre-B

Table 3. Surface Phenotype of CFU-IL7

Surface antigen	CFU-IL7/10⁵
B220⁻	5
B220⁺, sIgM⁻	415
B220⁺, sIgM⁺	30

cells, and during this stage it undergoes L-chain rearrangement. Once CFU-IL7 succeeds to form a productive L-chain V gene and expresses complete IgM on its surface, it eventually looses reactivity to IL-7.

We believe that the figure described above is the first comprehensive model for the control of cell proliferation during intramarrow B-cell development. It should be noted that this figure could not have been obtained without two tools, recombinant IL-7 and the IL-7-defective stromal cell line PA6. It is striking that we could detect all four possible types of B cells with these two different growth signals in combination. Therefore, along with identification of additional stromal cell molecules, we will be able to dissect further the differentiation stages, in particular the commitment process from pluripotent stem cells into B lineage. Another striking feature that emerged from the present study is that the shift from one stage that needs a particular growth requirement to another stage seems to be dependent on the result of Ig gene rearrangement during B-lineage differentiation. As shown clearly in this study, differentiation from B-pro-II to CFU-IL7 hardly occurs in SCID mice that have a extremely low frequency of productive Ig gene rearrangement. Moreover, CFU-IL7 loses its reactivity to IL-7 after productive rearrangement in a light-chain gene. Considering that the process of Ig gene rearrangement per se is an error prone stochastic process that generates both functional and nonfunctional B cells, this fashion for controlling the growth of B-lineage cells would be the best solution for selecting only functional cells worth differentiating into a subsequent step. Thus, in the future,

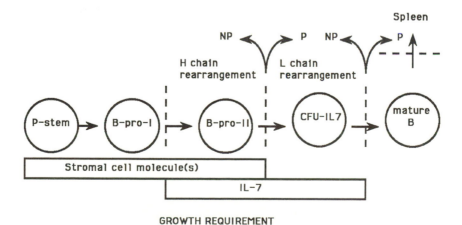

GROWTH REQUIREMENT

P : Productive rearrangement
NP: Nonproductive rearrangement

Figure 1. A model for the control of cell proliferation during intramarrow B-cell development.

it would be important to investigate the mechanisms underlying this close linkage between the status of Ig gene configuration and the growth requirement of the cells. In fact, a recent study clearly showed that transfection of a functionally rearranged μ heavy-chain gene into cIgM$^-$ pre-B cells triggers various cellular events in the subsequent differentiation step (Reth et al. 1987). Moreover, several pre-B-cell-specific molecules that have the potential to associate with the μ heavy chain have been identified and are expected to play a role in regulating the growth of pre-B cells (Sakaguchi and Melchers 1986; Kudo et al. 1987; Pillai and Baltimore 1987). Although it is still premature, we believe that all these findings will be integrated into one scenario in the near future, and that our model proposed here should be tested critically in various experimental systems.

ACKNOWLEDGMENTS

We thank Dr. Max D. Cooper for helpful discussion. This work is partly supported by grants from the Institute of Physical and Chemical Research (RIKEN), Cell Science Research Foundation, and a grant-in-aid for Scientific Research from the Ministry of Education.

REFERENCES

Abramson, S., R.C. Miller, and R.A. Phillips. 1977. The identification in adult bone marrow of pluripotent and restricted stem cell of the myeloid and lymphoid systems. *J. Exp. Med.* **145:** 1567.

Alt, F.W., T.K. Blackwell, R.A. DePinho, M.G. Reth, and G.D. Yancopoulos. 1986. Regulation of genome rearrangement events during lymphocyte differentiation. *Immunol. Rev.* **89:** 5.

Bosma, G.C., R.P. Custer, and M.J. Bosma. 1983. A severe combined immunodeficiency in the mouse. *Nature* **301:** 527.

Hendrickson, E.A., D.G. Schats, and D.T. Weaver. 1988. The *scid* gene encodes a transacting factor that mediates the rejoining event in Ig gene rearrangement. *Genes Dev.* **2:** 817.

Kodama, H., H. Sudo, H. Koyama, S. Kasai, and S. Yamamoto. 1984. *In vitro* hemopoiesis within a microen-vironment created by MC3T3-G2/PA6. *J. Cell. Physiol.* **118:** 233.

Kudo, A., N. Sakaguchi, and F. Melchers. 1987. Organization of the murine Ig related λ 5 gene transcribed selectively in pre-B lymphocytes. *EMBO J.* **6:** 103.

Lee, G., A.E. Namen, S. Gillis, L.R. Ellingsworth, and P.W. Kincade. 1989. Normal B cell precursors responsive to recombinant murine IL-7 and inhibition of IL-7 activity by transforming growth factor-β. *J. Immunol.* **142:** 3875.

Malynn, B.A., T.K. Blackwell, G.M. Fullop, G.A. Rathbun, A.J.W. Furley, P. Ferrier, L.B. Phillips, G.D. Yancopoulos, and F.W. Alt. 1988. The *scid* defect affects the final step of the immunoglobulin VDJ recombinase mechanism. *Cell* **54:** 453.

Nishikawa, S.I., M. Ogawa, S. Nishikawa, T. Kunisada, and H. Kodama. 1988. B lymphopoiesis on stromal cell clone: Stromal cell clones acting on different stages of B cell differentiation. *Eur. J. Immunol.* **18:** 1767.

Ogawa, M., S. Nishikawa, K. Ikuta, F. Yamamura, M. Naito, K. Takahashi, and S.I. Nishikawa. 1988. B cell ontogeny in murine embryo studied by a culture system with a monolayer of a stromal cell clone, ST2: B cell progenitor develops first in the embryonal body rather than in the yolk sac. *EMBO J.* **7:** 1337.

Okazaki, K., S.I. Nishikawa, and H. Sakano. 1988. Aberrant immunoglobulin gene rearrangement in scid mouse bone marrow cells. *J. Immunol.* **141:** 1348.

Osmond, D.G. 1986. Population dynamics of bone marrow B lymphocytes. *Immunol. Rev.* **93:** 103.

Pillai, S. and D. Baltimore. 1987. Formation of disulphide-linked μ 2ω 2 in pre-B cells by the 18K ω-immunoglobulin light chain. *Nature* **329:** 172.

Reth, M., E. Petrac, P. Wiese, L. Lobel, and F.W. Alt. 1987. Activation of Vk gene rearrangement in pre-B cells follows the expression of membrane-bound immunoglobulin heavy chains. *EMBO J.* **6:** 3299.

Rosenberg, N. and D. Baltimore. 1976. A quantitative assay for transformation of bone marrow cells by A-MuLV. *J. Exp. Med.* **143:** 1453.

Sakaguchi, N. and F. Melchers. 1986. λ 5, a new light-chain-related locus selectively expressed in pre-B lymphocytes. *Nature* **324:** 579.

Schuler, W., I.J. Weiler, A. Schuler, R.A. Phillips, N. Rosenberg, T.W. Mak, J.F. Kearney, R.P. Perry, and M.J. Bosma. 1986. Rearrangement of antigen receptor genes is defective in mice with severe combined immunodeficiency. *Cell* **46:** 963.

Sudo, T., M. Ito, Y. Ogawa, M. Iizuka, H. Kodama, T. Kunisada, S.-I. Hayashi, M. Ogawa, K. Sakai, S. Nishikawa, and S.-I. Nishikawa. 1989. Interleukin 7 production and function in stromal cell-dependent B cell development. *J. Exp. Med.* **170:** 333.

Molecular Mechanism for Immunoglobulin Double-isotype Expression

A. Shimizu,* T. Kinashi,† M.C. Nussenzweig,‡ T.-R. Mizuta,†
P. Leder,‡ and T. Honjo*†

*Center for Molecular Biology and Genetics, Kyoto University; †Department of Medical Chemistry,
Kyoto University Faculty of Medicine, Yoshida, Sakyo-ku, Kyoto 606; Japan; ‡Howard Hughes Medical
Institute, Department of Genetics, Harvard Medical School, Boston, Massachusetts 02115

Progeny of a single B lymphocyte can switch the expressed immunoglobulin (Ig) isotype from IgM to IgG or other classes during the course of differentiation without changing the antigen specificity determined by the variable (V) region sequence. Molecular biological analyses of this phenomenon, known as Ig-class switching, have revealed that class switching is accompanied by DNA rearrangement that takes place between S regions located 5′ to each (constant) C_H gene except for the C_δ gene (for review, see Honjo 1983; Shimizu and Honjo 1984). This recombination, named S-S recombination, brings the completed $V_H DJ_H$ exon to the proximity of the C_H gene to be expressed by deletion of other C_H genes located in between on the same chromosome.

Although the studies on myelomas, hybridomas, and normal spleen cells (Cory et al. 1980; Hurwitz et al. 1980; Yaoita and Honjo 1980; Radbuch and Sablitzky 1983) have provided accumulating evidence for the deletion model, the model has faced difficulty in explaining the observation that a single B lymphocyte carries multiple isotypes on its surface (double or triple bearers) (Pernis et al. 1976). Several groups of investigators, including ourselves, suggested the involvement of RNA processing in double-isotype expression by analyzing sorted murine B cells or a murine B-cell line carrying two isotypes and finding no DNA rearrangement in their C_H genes but in the J_H locus instead (Yaoita et al. 1982; Perlmutter and Gilbert 1984; Chen et al. 1986). These findings led to the proposal that the double-isotype expression could be an intermediate stage to class switching (Yaoita et al. 1982; Shimizu and Honjo 1984).

Interleukin-4 (IL-4), previously known as IgG1-induction factor (Lee et al. 1986; Noma et al. 1986), induces switching to IgG1 and IgE and simultaneously up-regulates germ-line transcripts (sterile transcripts) from the $C_\gamma1$ and C_ε genes prior to switching (Lutzker et al. 1988; Rothman et al. 1988). As the existence of such sterile transcripts from a C_H gene seemed to correlate well with switching to that particular C_H isotype, the sterile transcripts were thought to be an indication of the chromatin structure opening of the C_H genes, which makes the putative switch recombinase system accessible (Stavnezer-Nordgren and Sirlin 1986; Yancopoulos et al. 1986; Lutzker et al. 1988; Rothman et al. 1988). The accessibility model (Stavnezer-Nordgren and Sirlin 1986; Yancopoulos et al. 1986; Lutzker et al. 1988; Rothman et al. 1988) thus did not consider that the sterile transcript, which could not encode a meaningful protein, is involved in any physiological function by itself. However, there remains the possibility that the sterile transcript could be a substrate of the trans-splicing reaction for the multiple isotype expression (T. Honjo et al., unpubl.).

In this paper, we first describe human neoplasmic B cells, which express more than one isotype of Ig without deletion of C_H genes, and then we report that the transgenic $V_H DJ_H$ exon can be expressed in conjunction with the endogenous mouse $C_\gamma1$ gene as trans-mRNA in a human Ig transgenic mouse (TG.SA) in which a majority of B lymphocytes express the human μ chain from a nonallelic rearranged human μ transgene and do not completely rearrange the endogenous Ig heavy-chain locus by allelic exclusion. Such trans-mRNA could be produced by either switch recombination between the transgene and endogenous γ_1 gene or by trans-splicing between the transgene and endogenous sterile γ_1-gene transcripts. The results imply that the trans-splicing mechanism could be involved in Ig multiple isotype expression in normal B lymphocytes that do not have the deleted C_H genes.

EXPERIMENTAL PROCEDURES

Transgenic mice. Two transgenic mice lines carrying rearranged human $V_H DJ_H$-C_μ genes that allow expression of either the membrane-bound μ chain (TG.SA) alone or the secretory μ chain (TG.ST) alone were described previously (Nussenzweig et al. 1987, 1988) and were maintained by crossing with FVB/N mice (Taconic Farms). Single-cell suspensions were prepared by passing spleen cells through stainless steel mesh. After adjusting the concentrations of ~3 × 10^5/ml, transgenic spleen cells were cultured in RPMI 1640 medium containing 50 μM 2-mercaptoethanol, 10% fetal calf serum (FCS), 30 μg/ml lipopolysaccharide (LPS) (Sigma), and ~100 units/ml recombinant mouse IL-4 in 7% CO_2 at 37°C.

Surface Ig expression. Mononuclear cells were prepared from peripheral blood of chronic lymphatic leukemic patients or from lymphoid tissues of a lymphoma patient. These cells were stained with fluorescein-isothiocyanate (FITC)-labeled antibodies against human κ, λ, μ, δ, γ, or α chains or human Ig (Dako Patts). Stained cells were counted under a fluorescence microscope. To analyze transgenic spleen cells, cells were washed twice with Hanks balanced salt solution containing 0.01% sodium azide and 1% bovine serum albumin and were preincubated with a mouse monoclonal antibody 2.4G2 (Unkeless 1979) to block the binding through the Fc receptors. Then cells were stained with FITC- or phycoerythrin (PE)-labeled goat polyclonal antibodies against the human or mouse μ or γ chains (Southern Biotechnology Associates, Inc.). Cross-reactivities of these antibodies were excluded by control experiments staining normal mouse spleen cells and a cell line that expresses human IgM on its surface. Stained cells were analyzed by flow-cytometry on a cytofluorograf IIS (Ortho Diagnostic System, Inc.).

Polymerase chain reaction and characterization of amplified DNA. Total cellular RNAs were extracted by homogenizing cells in guanidium isothiocyanate and ultracentrifuging the homogenate through a CsCl cushion (Chirgwin et al. 1979). mRNAs were converted to cDNA from oligo(dT)$_{12-18}$ primers using a cDNA synthesis kit (Boehringer-Mannheim). These RNA/cDNA complexes corresponding to approximately 5 ng of cDNAs were amplified by 25 cycles of polymerase chain reaction (PCR) in a 50-μl reaction mixture (Kim and Smithies 1988) with 1.25 units of *Thermus aquaticus* (*Taq*) DNA polymerase (Perkin-Elmer Cetus) and then by another 25 cycles after the addition of the same amount of the enzyme using an automated DNA Thermal Cycler (Perkin-Elmer Cetus). Primers for the PCR and DNA sequencing were synthesized by an automated DNA synthesizer (models 380A and 381A, Applied Biosystems). Primers used for the PCR were as follows: transgenic V_H primer, 24-mer from 356 bases upstream to the end of the J_H6 in the V_H sequence, sense strand; human C_μ primer, 31-mer from positions 31 to 1 of the C_H1 exon, antisense strand; and mouse $C_\gamma1$ primer, 21-mer from positions 41 to 21 of the C_H1 exon, antisense strand. Amplified DNA fragments were analyzed on 2% low-melt agarose (LGT, FMC Bio Products) gel electrophoresis, were recovered from the gel by heating to 65°C, extracted with a

mixture of water-saturated phenol:chloroform:iso-amyl alcohol (24:24:1), and precipitated with ethanol. The recovered fragment was subcloned into the *Sma*I site of Bluescript KS + vector (Stratagene), and nucleotide sequences were determined by the dideoxy-chain-termination method (Sanger et al. 1977) using alkali-denatured plasmid DNA. The kit for DNA sequencing using 7-deazacytosine, restriction nucleases, and T4 DNA ligase was purchased from Takara (Kyoto, Japan).

RESULTS

Human Neoplastic B Cells That Express Multiple Isotypes without Deletion of C_H Genes

To analyze the molecular mechanism for multiple-isotype expression in B cells, we studied the Ig H-chain gene organization in human neoplastic cells expressing multiple isotypes (three chronic leukemias and one lymphoma). These cells were characterized by flow cytometry and fluorescence microscopic observation after staining with FITC-labeled monocloned or affinity-purified antibodies specific for each class or type of human Ig. As shown in Table 1, major populations of all four specimens expressed more than one isotype because the sum of the fractions expressing each heavy-chain isotype significantly exceeded the fraction expressing human Ig or total light-chain (κ or λ).

The majority of these cells was shown to be of monoclonal origin by Southern blot hybridization analyses using human J_H probe since each DNA had only one or two rearranged J_H bands. Neither S_μ-region rearrangement nor C_H gene deletion was detected by Southern blot analyses using probes for the C_μ, C_γ, C_ε, and C_α genes. Transcripts from the two separate C_H genes were detected in two neoplastic cells by Northern blot hybridization. These data summarized in Table 2 strongly indicate that human neoplastic B cells can express more than one isotype without the C_H gene deletion.

Double Bearers in Cultured Spleen Cells of the Transgenic Mouse TG.SA

To test whether *trans*-splicing can occur, we took advantage of a human Ig transgenic mouse (TG.SA), in

Table 1. Profile of Surface Ig of Human Neoplastic B Cells

Neoplastic specimen	Phenotype	Ig$^+$ (%)	μ^+ (%)	δ^+ (%)	γ^+ (%)	α^+ (%)	κ^+ (%)	λ^+ (%)
145/85	$\mu\delta\alpha$, λ	89	84	58	3	43	4	81
268/85	$\mu\delta\gamma$, λ	n.d.[a]	20	34	83	3	4	95
302/78	$\mu\delta\gamma$, κ	87	83	25	75	<1	78	2
L161	$\delta\alpha$, κ	92	<1	85	<1	60	95	<1

Neoplasmic specimens are from chronic lymphatic leukemia patients except for 145/84, which is from a malignant lymphoma patient. Mononuclear cells from these patients were stained with FITC-labeled antibodies, and positive cells were counted under a fluorescence microscope. Similar results were obtained by flow-cytometric analyses (Kinashi et al. 1987).

[a] n.d. indicates not determined.

Table 2. Summary of Ig Gene Organization and Expression of Human Neoplastic B Cells

Neoplastic specimen	Phenotype	Configuration of J_H[a]	Rearrangement at S_μ[b]	Deletion[b]			Transcript
				C_γ	C_ε	C_α	
145/85	$\mu\delta\alpha$, λ	r/r	-/-	-/-	-/-	-/-	μ, α
268/85	$\mu\delta\gamma$, λ	r/r	-/-	-/-	-/-	-/-	μ, γ
302/78	$\mu\delta\gamma$, κ	r/g	-/-	-/-	-/-	-/-	n.d.[c]
L161	$\delta\alpha$, κ	r/r	-/-	-/-	-/-	-/-	n.d.[c]

DNA rearrangements and mRNA expression in human neoplastic B cells were analyzed by Southern and Northern blot hybridization, respectively, using human J_H, C_μ, C_γ, C_ε, and C_α probes as described previously (Yaoita and Honjo 1980; Kinashi et al. 1987). Data were taken from Kinashi et al. (1987).

[a] Rearranged (r) or germ-line (g) status of each allele.
[b] – indicates not detected.
[c] n.d. indicates not determined because of scarce supply of the cells.

which a vast majority of splenic B lymphocytes express the transgenic human μ chain on their surface and in which the endogenous Ig heavy-chain locus is almost completely excluded (Fig. 1) (Nussenzweig et al. 1987). This observation was confirmed by color flow-cytometry as shown in Figure 2 (first row, left). However, note that a significant number of cells (1.5%) apparently express both human and mouse μ chains on their surface. Few, if any, fresh cells from the TG.SA spleen expressed both the transgene (μ) and the endogenous mouse γ chain simultaneously (Fig. 2, first row, right).

We examined whether spleen cells from the transgenic mouse TG.SA could express both murine γ and human μ chains simultaneously. Since IL-4 is known to enhance the isotype switching to IgG1 or IgE of LPS- or antigen-stimulated B cells (Noma et al. 1986; Snapper et al. 1988), we cultured the transgenic spleen cells with murine recombinant IL-4 (~ 100 units/ml) and LPS (30 μg/ml). On day 4 of the culture, when the

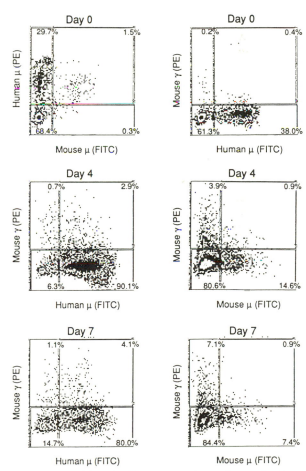

Figure 2. Double color-flow-cytometric analyses of spleen cells cultured with LPS and IL-4 from transgenic mouse strain TG.SA. Horizontal and vertical axes represent relative fluorescence of green (FITC) and orange (PE), respectively, in log scale. Spleen cells were stained with directly labeled antibodies against the human μ, mouse μ, and mouse γ chains. Only live cells ($\sim 10^4$ cells in first and second row and $\sim 5 \times 10^3$ cells in third row) were analyzed. Background levels are indicated by lines. Percentage of cells in each region is shown at the corner.

Figure 1. Schematic representation of a splenic B lymphocyte in transgenic mouse TG.SA. A rearranged human $V_H DJ_H$-C_μ gene, lacking the poly(A) addition site for secretory form of the μ chain, was inserted outside the Ig heavy-chain locus. By the expression of this transgene, the majority of B lymphocytes express human IgM on their surface, and the rearrangements of their endogenous Ig heavy-chain loci were excluded at the DJ or germ-line stage as shown.

Table 3. Double-bearing B Cells in Transgenic Spleen Cells Cultured with IL-4 and LPS

Days in culture	Human IgM$^+$/mouse IgG$^+$ (%)	Mouse IgM$^+$/mouse IgG$^+$ (%)
0	0.4	0.2
4	2.9	0.9
7	4.1	0.9

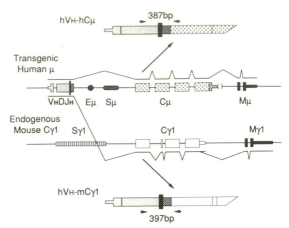

Figure 3. Strategy for detection of the *trans*-mRNA by PCR. Schematic representations of the transgene, endogenous C$_\gamma$1 gene, a part of transgenic μ chain mRNA and a part of expected *trans*-mRNA are shown. Exons are indicated as boxes with different shadings to distinguish functional regions. Enhancer and switch regions are also shown by circles and ellipses, respectively. Parentheses in the transgene indicates the deletion of the poly(A) addition site for the secretory μ chain. Expected sizes of PCR-amplified fragments with transgenic V$_H$ primer and human C$_\gamma$ primer and with the transgenic V$_H$ primer and mouse C$_\mu$1 primer are shown at above and under the mRNA structures, respectively.

proportion of the double bearers from normal mouse spleen cells reached the peak, we could detect a significant number of double bearers of the human μ and mouse γ chains (Fig. 2, second row, left, 2.9% of live cells) among the spleen cells from the TG.SA mouse. A majority of these cells were not triple bearers of human μ, mouse μ, and mouse γ because only 0.9% (Fig. 2, second row, right) of the cells were positive for the mouse μ and γ chains.

Even in a longer culture (7 days) to the stage that most of the double bearers of the normal mice switch to γ single bearers, the population positive for both human μ and mouse γ chains expanded in the spleen cells from TG.SA (4.1%), whereas that for both mouse μ and γ chains did not (0.9%) (Fig. 2, third row). The proportions of the double bearers are also summarized in Table 3. Similar results were obtained with ten times higher concentration of IL-4 (~ 1000 units/ml) (data not shown).

trans-mRNA Consisting of Transgenic Human V$_H$DJ$_H$ and Endogenous Mouse C$_\gamma$ Exons Detected by PCR

Since the endogenous VDJ recombination is largely excluded, the flow-cytometric analyses described above suggest that the mouse γ chain expressed together with the transgenic μ chain might have the V-region sequence derived from the transgenic V$_H$DJ$_H$ exon (Fig. 3). To test this possibility, we extracted RNA from the cultured spleen cells of transgenic mice TG.SA and also from those of TG.ST, which express only a secretory form of human μ chain and do not exclude the endogenous Ig locus. Control RNA was obtained from a human IgM$^+$ cell line (SA210) derived from TG.SA. After converting the mRNAs into cDNAs by reverse transcriptase, we amplified the postulated cDNA sequence that should have been derived from the transgenic human V$_H$DJ$_H$-endogenous mouse C$_\gamma$1 mRNA (*trans*-mRNA) by PCR (Saiki et al. 1985; Kim and Smithies 1988). Two pairs of primers were chosen so that the cDNA of the human transgene mRNA and *trans*-mRNA could be distinguished by the length as well as the sequence (Fig. 3).

As shown in Figure 4, the 397-bp fragment expected from the *trans*-mRNA was amplified only from TG.SA mRNA, whereas the 387-bp fragment from the transgenic μ gene was amplified from all the three mRNAs. Because PCR is so sensitive that it could pick up the sequence of only one or a few molecules (Kim and Smithies 1988), we were very careful to avoid contami-

nation of samples with each other or cloned DNAs, and we had never constructed artificial *trans*-mRNA or cDNA.

Nucleotide Sequence of the *trans*-mRNA Amplified by PCR

To confirm the expected structure of the *trans*-mRNA and to exclude artifacts, the amplified 397-bp fragment was isolated by gel electrophoresis and sub-

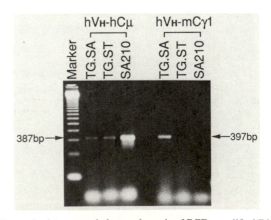

Figure 4. Agarose gel electrophoresis of PCR-amplified DNA fragments. Amplified fragments (20 μl from 50 μl reaction) of mRNA/cDNA from cultured spleen cells of TG.SA, TG.ST, and SA210 cells were applied. Primer pairs used were human V$_H$/human C$_\mu$ (*left*) and human V$_H$/mouse C$_\gamma$1 (*right*). A ladder of multiples of 123-bp fragments was used as a size marker (lane *marker*). Sizes of detected fragments are shown at both sides.

cloned into a plasmid vector for sequencing. Nucleotide sequences of three randomly chosen clones, pTMMG1-4, -5, and -12 (clones 4, 5, and 12), were determined and compared with the transgene and mouse C_γ sequences. All the three subclones had identical sequences except for their orientation in the vector. The clones had the sequence identical to the transgenic $V_H D J_H$ sequence that was linked to the mouse $C_\gamma 1$ sequence at the precise exon-intron junction as shown in Figure 5. The corresponding sequences of the transgenic and the amplified $V_H D J_H$ sequences are identical even at the junctions of the V_H, D, and J_H segments (N regions). All these data unequivocally indicate that the *trans*-mRNA was derived from the human transgene and endogenous $C_\gamma 1$ gene (Fig. 5b).

DISCUSSION

trans-Splicing or S-S Recombination in Transgenic B Cells

We have shown that a significant number of TG.SA spleen cells express both transgenic human μ and endogenous mouse γ chains when cultured with LPS and IL-4 by flow-cytometric analyses. Amplification by PCR and cloning of the amplified fragment have unequivocally demonstrated expression of the *trans*-mRNA containing the transgenic $V_H D J_H$ and endogenous $C_\gamma 1$ sequences. Our data clearly indicate that the transgenic $V_H D J_H$ gene can be expressed with the endogenous $C_\gamma 1$ gene in a primary B lymphocyte. Synthesis of this *trans*-mRNA could be due either to S-S recombination between the transgene and the endogenous $C_\gamma 1$ gene or to *trans*-splicing between the transgene transcript and the sterile transcript from the endogenous $C_\gamma 1$ gene. These two possibilities are not necessarily exclusive to each other, and *trans*-splicing prior to recombination is also possible just as with endogenous genes.

Each TG.SA animal maintained as heterozygous with FVB/N carries two copies of the transgene. The exact location at which two copies of the transgene were integrated is not known although we know that the transgene is not located in the region encompassing the J_H and C_H genes (M.C. Nussenzweig et al., unpubl.).

The combination of exons expressed by *trans*-mRNA does not seem random because we could not detect a *trans*-mRNA with the human V_H and the mouse μ sequences by PCR (data not shown). This could be due to the requirement of specific sequences in the sterile transcript for *trans*-splicing or some specificity of DNA recombination. The fact that we could not detect *trans*-mRNA in the other transgenic mouse (TG.ST), which expresses only the secretory human μ chain and rearranges the endogenous Ig locus (Nussenzweig et al. 1988), could be due to the possible high efficiency of switch recombination between mouse endogenous genes and/or *trans*-splicing between their transcripts, excluding involvement of the transgene.

Durdik et al. (1989) recently reported the expression of the V-region sequence of the transgene in conjunction with the endogenous C_γ gene in the serum Ig and hybridoma lines derived from hyperimmunized transgenic animals. They favor a DNA rearrangement model partly because of multiple copies of the transgenes. More recently, *trans*-rearrangements between the human T-cell receptor γ and δ gene loci were found (Tycko et al. 1989).

Ig Multiple Isotype Expression without C_H Gene Deletion

There are accumulating examples for Ig multiple isotype expression not accompanied by deletions of the C_H genes. In this study, we analyzed four human neoplastic B cells that express multiple isotypes. Two of them were shown to express two isotype-specific

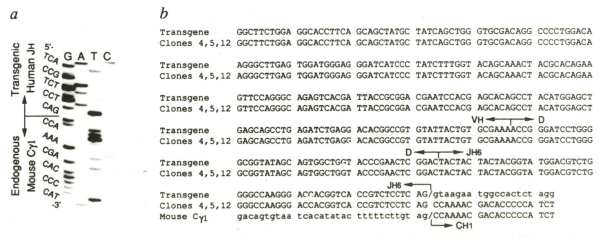

Figure 5. Nucleotide sequence analysis of the amplified fragment of the *trans*-mRNA. (*a*) Autoradiogram of sequence reading at the J/C exon junction. Reading of antisense strand of the exon junction of clone 4 is shown with the sequence converted to the sense strand at left side. The junction is indicated by a horizontal line and arrows. (*b*) Nucleotide sequence of amplified fragment from the *trans*-mRNA. DNA sequence of clones 4, 5, and 12 (without the primer sequences used for PCR) is shown with those of the transgene and mouse $C_\gamma 1$ gene. Junctions of the segments and exon-intron are shown by arrows and vertical lines.

mRNAs. All four cells were shown to be of monoclonal origin and have no deletion of the C_H genes. These results strongly suggest that regulations at the RNA level may be involved in the multiple isotype expression. The mechanism could be either alternative splicing of a long continuous primary transcript or *trans*-splicing between rearranged $V_H DJ_H(-C_\mu-C_\delta)$ gene primary transcripts and sterile germ-line transcripts of the second C_H gene. Careful cytoplasmic staining with isotype-specific antibodies should be able to test a formal possibility that a very small number of cells had already switched, and the second or third isotype was cytophillically associated with most of the unrearranged, unswitched cells.

trans-Splicing Mechanism May Explain Ig Double-isotype Expression in Normal B Cells

In view of the existence of *trans*-mRNA of the transgene and the endogenous $C_\gamma 1$ gene, we would like to propose that *trans*-splicing, which is known to occur in several organisms such as trypanosome, nematode, and tobacco chloroplast (Murphy et al. 1986; Sutton and Boothroyd 1986; Van der Ploeg 1986; Kause and Hirsh 1987; Koller et al. 1987), but not yet in mammals, could be a possible mechanism for multiple isotype expression by a single B lymphocyte that has no deletion of the C_H genes (Yaoita et al. 1982; Perlmutter and Gilbert 1984; Chen et al. 1986; Kinashi et al. 1987; T.-R. Mizuta et al., unpubl.). This *trans*-splicing model is consistent with the existence of the sterile transcripts from specific C_H genes (Stavnezer-Nordgren and Sirlin 1986; Yancopoulos et al. 1986; Lutzker et al. 1988; Rothman et al. 1988; T. Honjo et al., unpubl.) and with significant expression of the *trans*-combination of V_H and C_H allotypic markers on B-cell surface and secretory Ig molecules in F_1 rabbits (Landucci-Tosi and Tosi 1973; Pernis et al. 1973; Knight et al. 1974).

trans-splicing and alternative splicing of a long transcript may not be exclusive with each other. However, the long transcript model is short of explaining the precommitted isotype switching in pre-B-cell lines (Stavnezer-Nordgren and Sirlin 1986; Yancopoulos et al. 1986; Lutzker et al. 1988). We may be able to assess the direct evidence for *trans*-splicing by characterizing mRNA, pre-mRNA, and DNA rearrangements of double bearers from transgenic mice (TG.SA) and F_1 rabbits.

ACKNOWLEDGMENTS

We are grateful to Ms. Juanita Campos-Torres for her excellent assistance in flow-cytometry and Mr. Peter Gentile, Ms. Junko Kuno, and Ms. Masayo Wakino for their technical assistance including the synthesis of oligonucleotides. We are also grateful to Drs. Tore Godal and Noel R. Ling for human neoplastic B cells, and Dr. Kevin Holmes for monoclonal antibody 2.4G2. We also would like to thank Ms. Kazuko Hirano for the preparation of this manuscript. A.S. was supported in part by a fellowship from the Yoshida Scientific Foundation. This work was supported in part by grants from E.I. Du Pont de Nemours & Co. and the Ministry of Education, Science, and Culture of Japan.

REFERENCES

Chen, Y.-W., C.J. Word, V. Dev, J.W. Uhr, E.S. Vitetta, and P.W. Tucker. 1986. Double isotype production by a neoplastic B cell line. II. Allelically excluded production of μ and γ_1 chains without C_H gene rearrangement. *J. Exp. Med.* **164**: 562.

Chirgwin, J.M., A.E. Przybyla, R.J. MacDonald, and W.J. Rutter. 1979. Isolation of biologically active ribonucleic acid from sources enriched in ribonuclease. *Biochemistry* **18**: 5294.

Cory, S., J. Jackson, and J.M. Adams. 1980. Deletions in the constant region locus can account for switches in immunoglobulin heavy chain expression. *Nature* **285**: 450.

Durdik, J., R.M. Gerstein, S. Rath, P.F. Robbins, A. Nisonoff, and E. Selsing. 1989. Isotype switching by a microinjected μ immunoglobulin heavy chain gene in transgenic mice. *Proc. Natl. Acad. Sci.* **86**: 2346.

Honjo, T. 1983. Immunoglobulin genes. *Annu. Rev. Immunol.* **1**: 499.

Hurwitz, J., C. Coleclough, and J.J. Cebra. 1980. C_H gene rearrangements in IgM-bearing B cells and in the normal splenic DNA component of hybridomas making different isotypes of antibody. *Cell* **22**: 349.

Kause, M. and D. Hirsh. 1987. A *trans*-spliced leader sequence of actin mRNA in *C. elegans*. *Cell* **49**: 753.

Kim, H.-S. and O. Smithies. 1988. Recombinant fragment assay for gene targetting based on the polymerase chain reaction. *Nucleic Acids Res.* **16**: 8887.

Kinashi, T., T. Godal, Y. Noma, N.R. Ling, Y. Yaoita, and T. Honjo. 1987. Human neoplastic B cells express more than two isotypes of immunoglobulins without deletion of heavy-chain constant-region genes. *Genes Dev.* **1**: 465.

Knight, K.L., T.R. Malck, and W.C. Henly. 1974. Recombinant rabbit secretory immunoglobulin molecules: Alpha chains with maternal (paternal) variable-region allotypes and paternal (maternal) constant-region allotypes. *Proc. Natl. Acad. Sci.* **71**: 1169.

Koller, B., H. Fromm, E. Galun, and M. Edelman. 1987. Evidence for in vivo *trans* splicing of pre-mRNAs in tobacco chloroplasts. *Cell* **48**: 111.

Landucci-Tosi, S. and R.M. Tosi. 1973. Recombinant IgG molecules in rabbits doubly heterozygous for group *a* and group *e* allotypic specificities. *Immunochem.* **10**: 65.

Lee, F., T. Yokota, T. Otsuka, P. Meyerson, D. Villaret, R. Coffman, T. Mosmann, D. Rennick, N. Roehm, C. Smith, A. Zlotnik, and K.-I. Arai. 1986. Isolation and characterization of a mouse interleukin cDNA clone that express B-cell stimulatory factor 1 activities and T-cell- and mast-cell-stimulating activities. *Proc. Natl. Acad. Sci.* **83**: 2061.

Lutzker, S., P. Rothman, R. Pollock, R. Coffman, and F.W. Alt. 1988. Mitogen- and IL-4-regulated expression of germ-line Ig γ_2b transcripts: Evidence for directed heavy chain class switching. *Cell* **53**: 177.

Murphy, W.J., K.P. Watkins, and N. Agabian. 1986. Identification of a novel Y branch structure as intermediate in trypanosome mRNA processing: Evidence for *trans* splicing. *Cell* **47**: 517.

Noma, Y., P. Sideras, T. Naito, S. Bergstedt-Lindquist, C. Azuma, E. Severinson, T. Tanabe, T. Kinashi, F. Matsuda, Y. Yaoita, and T. Honjo. 1986. Cloning of cDNA encoding the murine IgG$_1$ induction factor by a novel strategy using SP6 promoter. *Nature* **319**: 640.

Nussenzweig, M.C., A.C. Shaw, E. Sinn, J. Campos-Torres, and P. Leder. 1988. Allelic exclusion in transgenic mice carrying mutant human IgM genes. *J. Exp. Med.* **167**: 1969.

Nussenzweig, M.C., A.C. Shaw, E. Sinn, D.B. Danner, K.L. Holmes, H.C. Morse, and P. Leder. 1987. Allelic exclusion in transgenic mice that express the membrane form of immunoglobulin μ. *Science* **236:** 816.

Perlmutter, A. and W. Gilbert. 1984. Antibodies of secondary response can be expressed without switch recombination in normal mouse B cells. *Proc. Natl. Acad. Sci.* **81:** 7189.

Pernis, B., L. Forni, and A.L. Luzzati. 1976. Synthesis of multiple immunoglobulin classes by single lymphocytes. *Cold Spring Harbor Symp. Quant. Biol.* **41:** 175.

Pernis, B., L. Forni, S. Dubiski, A.S. Kelus, W.J. Mandy, and C.W. Todd. 1973. Heavy chain variable and constant region allotypes in single rabbit plasma cells. *Immunochem.* **10:** 281.

Radbuch, A. and F. Sablitzky. 1983. Deletion of C_μ genes in mouse B lymphocytes upon stimulation with LPS. *EMBO J.* **2:** 1929.

Rothman, P., S. Lutzker, W. Cook, R. Coffman, and F.W. Alt. 1988. Mitogen plus interleukin 4 induction of C_ε transcripts in B lymphoid cells. *J. Exp. Med.* **168:** 2385.

Saiki, R.K., S. Scharf, F. Faloona, K.B. Mullis, G.T. Horn, H.A. Erlich, and N. Arnheim. 1985. Enzymatic amplification of β-globin genomic sequences and restriction site analysis for diagnosis of sickle cell anemia. *Science* **230:** 1350.

Sanger, F., S. Nicklen, and A.R. Coulson. 1977. DNA sequencing with chain-terminating inhibitors. *Proc. Natl. Acad. Sci.* **74:** 5463.

Shimizu, A. and T. Honjo. 1984. Immunoglobulin class switching. *Cell* **36:** 801.

Snapper, C.M., F.D. Finkelman, and W.E. Paul. 1988. Differential regulation of IgG_1 and IgE synthesis by interleukin 4. *J. Exp. Med.* **167:** 183.

Stavnezer-Nordgren, J. and S. Sirlin. 1986. Specificity of immunoglobulin heavy chain switch correlates with activity of germline heavy chain genes prior to switching. *EMBO J.* **5:** 95.

Sutton, E.R. and J.C. Boothroyd. 1986. Evidence for *trans* splicing in trypanosomes. *Cell* **47:** 527.

Tycko, B., J.D. Palmer, and J. Sklar. 1989. T cell receptor gene trans-rearrangement: Chimeric γ-δ genes in normal lymphoid tissues. *Science* **245:** 1242.

Unkeless, J.C. 1979. Characterization of a monoclonal antibody directed against mouse macrophage and lymphocyte Fc receptors. *J. Exp. Med.* **150:** 580.

Van der Ploeg, L.H.T. 1986. Discontinuous transcription and splicing in trypanosomes. *Cell* **47:** 479.

Yancopoulos, G.D., R.A. De Pinho, K.A. Zimmerman, S.G. Lutzker, N. Rosenberg, and F.W. Alt. 1986. Secondary genomic rearrangement events in pre-B cells: $V_H DJ_H$ replacement by a LINE-1 sequence and directed class switching. *EMBO J.* **5:** 3259.

Yaoita, Y. and T. Honjo. 1980. Deletion of immunoglobulin heavy chain genes from expressed allelic chromosome. *Nature* **286:** 850.

Yaoita, Y., Y. Kumagai, K. Okumura, and T. Honjo. 1982. Expression of lymphocyte surface IgE does not require switch recombination. *Nature* **297:** 697.

Cellular Stages and Molecular Steps of Murine B-cell Development

F. MELCHERS, A. STRASSER,* S.R. BAUER, A. KUDO,
P. THALMANN, AND A. ROLINK
Basel Institute for Immunology, Basel, Switzerland

During embryonic development of the mouse, B lymphocytes are generated in several waves at different sites in the body (Owen et al. 1974; Melchers et al. 1975; Melchers 1977a,b; Alt et al. 1981; Maki et al. 1982; Reynolds and Morris 1983; Paige et al. 1984). One of these sites is the fetal liver where, at day 13 of gestation, progenitor cells begin to rearrange gene segments of the immunoglobulin (Ig) loci to become precursor (pre-) B cells and later antigen- and mitogen-sensitive B cells. Early stages of progenitor proliferation and inductions to Ig gene rearrangements have been found to be dependent on cells of the environment of B-cell-generating organs, called stromal cells (Kincade et al. 1981; Whitlock et al. 1985; Dorshkind et al. 1986; Gisler et al. 1987; Witte et al. 1987; Kinashi et al. 1988; Pietrangeli et al. 1988; Palacios et al. 1989). Some of the effects of stromal cells appear to be mediated by soluble cytokines, in particular by interleukin (IL)-3 or -7 (Palacios et al. 1984, 1987; Palacios and Steinmetz 1985; Gisler et al. 1988; Namen et al. 1988a,b). Pre-B cells express a series of characteristic genes and surface markers, among them the genes V_{pre-B} (Kudo and Melchers 1987; Bauer et al. 1988), λ5 (Sakaguchi and Melchers 1986), and mb-1 (Sakaguchi et al. 1988), as well as the surface glycoprotein PB76 detected by the monoclonal antibody (MAb) G-5-2 (Strasser 1988). Pre-B cells in fetal liver can therefore be monitored by in situ hybridization analyses of the expressed genes on the mRNA level (Berger 1986) with these pre-B-cell-specific genes and can be enriched by fluorescence-activated cell sorting (FACS) with the MAb G-5-2.

Different tissue culture systems, using serum-substituted, defined media (Iscove and Melchers 1978), have been developed that either allow the development of each B progenitor and precursor in a stromal cell environment or that allow the development of successfully rearranged, i.e., surface-Ig (sIg)-positive pre-B and B cells, to clones of IgM-secreting, plaque-forming cells (PFC) with near 100% plating efficiency (Melchers 1977a,b). These systems allow us to follow the kinetics of progenitor and pre-B-cell development in vivo in fetal liver, as well as in vitro in the time equivalent to in vivo gestation to the states of sIg$^+$ and of mitogen-reactive B cells and to clones of IgM PFC.

MATERIALS AND METHODS

Animals. Adult female C57BL/6, male DBA/2 mice, and 3–6-week-old Lewis rats were obtained from the Institute for Biologisch-Medizinische Forschung AG (Switzerland). (C57BL/6 × DBA/2)F$_1$ (BDF$_1$) embryos from timed pregnant C57BL/6 females were provided by breeding facilities at the Basel Institute for Immunology. The day of appearance of a vaginal plug was counted as day 0 of gestation. Birth occurred at day 19.

Interleukins. Recombinant human IL-1 was obtained from Dr. Lomedico (F. Hoffmann-La Roche, New Jersey) and used at a concentration of 10 units/ml. Recombinant murine IL-2, IL-3, IL-4, and IL-5 were obtained as described previously (Karasuyama and Melchers 1988) and used at a concentration of 5%, i.e., at approximately 5–50 units/ml. Recombinant human IL-6 produced by a cell line transfected with the human IL-6 gene (provided by W. Fiers, Biogent, Belgium) was used at a dilution of 5% (i.e., at 5–50 units/ml). IL-7 (Namen et al. 1988a,b) (a gift from S. Gillis and C. Henney, Immunex, Washington) was used at concentrations between 100 and 1000 units/ml.

Tissue culture. Fetal liver cells were prepared as described previously (Melchers et al. 1975; Melchers 1977a). Total fetal liver cells and G-5-2$^+$ fetal liver cells isolated by cell sorting (see below) were cultured in serum-substituted Iscove's modified Dulbecco's medium (IMDM) (Iscove and Melchers 1978) in the presence or absence of stromal cells and in the presence or absence of IL-1 through IL-7 (Namen et al. 1988a,b; Karasuyama and Melchers 1988), as indicated in the results. Cultures were set up in 0.2 ml in 96-well flat-bottom plastic culture plates (Costar, Massachusetts). Primary fetal liver stromal cell layers were established from 13-day-old BDF$_1$ embryos by overnight culture at a density of 5×10^6 to 1×10^7 cells/ml in IMDM containing 5% fetal calf serum. Nonadherent cells thereafter were removed by extensive washing with serum-free medium. This stromal layer was subjected to 3000 rads of gamma-irradiation before coculturing with MAb G-5-2$^+$ fetal liver cells. Limiting dilution experi-

*Present address: The Walter and Eliza Hall Institute, Melbourne, Australia.

ments were performed in 96-well culture plates in serum-substituted medium in the presence of 3×10^6 rat thymocytes/ml and 50 μg/ml lipopolysaccharide (LPS), (S form of *Salmonella abortus equii*, a gift from Drs. G. Galanos and O. Lüderitz, Max-Planck-Institut für Immunbiologie, West Germany) as described previously (Melchers et al. 1975; Melchers 1977a). Cells were counted under the microscope using a Bürker hemocytometer.

Plaque assay. The total number of IgM-secreting PFCs in a population of cells was determined by the protein-A sheep red-blood-cells plaque assay using a rabbit anti-mouse IgM (MOPC 104E μ/λ) antiserum.

Immunofluorescence analysis and cell sorting. Immunofluorescence staining and analysis as well as cell sorting were done as described previously (Strasser 1988) using biotinylated (Calbiochem, California) MAbs and fluorescein-isothiocyanate-conjugated streptavidin (Amersham, United Kingdom) as secondary reagents.

RESULTS

Development of Pre-B Cells In Vivo in Fetal Liver

The MAb G-5-2 was used to enumerate the number of pre-B cells expressing the glycoprotein PB76 at different days of gestation in fetal liver. The data in Figure 1 show that the number of MAb G-5-2$^+$ cells doubles every day between day 13 and 16 of gestation and then increases by only approximately twofold in the next 3 days of gestation until birth. Thereafter, the number of MAb G-5-2$^+$ cells decreases rapidly to reach 5% of the level measured at birth within a week after birth (data not shown). However, the number of pre-B cells that can develop to clones of IgM PFC in the foreign environment of rat thymus cells under the stimulatory influence of the B-cell mitogen LPS is much lower than the number of MAb G-5-2$^+$ cells at early times of gestation, i.e., between day 13 and 15 of gestation (Fig. 1). This number then increases 100-fold between day 15 and 16 and reaches numbers comparable with those of MAb G-5-2$^+$ cells between days 18 and 19.

When fetal liver cells at days 16 to 19 of gestation were labeled by the MAb G-5-2 and enriched by FACS, the positively sorted populations of cells were also enriched for other markers of pre-B cells. Thus, cells expressing mRNA for μ-heavy (μH) chains and for the pre-B-cell-specific gene λ5 were enriched over 100-fold, and the frequencies of cells developing to clones of IgM PFC in rat filler cells and LPS were increased approximately 1000-fold in these populations.

The MAb G-5-2$^+$ FACS-enriched cell population of fetal liver of days 13 and 14 of gestation were similarly enriched for λ5-expressing cells, but they did not contain similarly high numbers of μH-chain-mRNA-

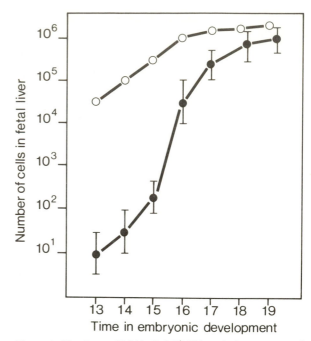

Figure 1. Numbers of MAb G-5-2$^+$ (○) and of precursors of LPS-reactive cells capable of development to IgM PFC in a foreign environment of rat thymus filler cells and LPS (●) in one fetal liver of (C57BL/6 × DBA/2)F$_1$ embryos, as detected by FACS (○) and by limiting dilutions (●). Assays for the development of clones of IgM PFC were done at the equivalent time of day 5 after birth.

expressing cells and precursors of cells capable of development to IgM PFC (Table 1).

All these experiments suggest that pre-B cells at early times of gestation in fetal liver may not be able to express Ig genes and develop into clones of IgM PFC, if they are taken out of their environment in fetal liver and plated under limiting dilutions in the foreign environment of rat filler cells and LPS. Around day 16 of gestation a rapid change occurs so that pre-B cells now are capable of expressing μH-chain mRNA and are more able to develop to IgM PFC in the foreign environment.

Reconstitution of the Ability of Early Fetal Liver Cells to Develop In Vitro to sIg$^+$, Mitogen-reactive B Cells

When unseparated fetal liver cells of day 13 or 14 of gestation were kept in culture until the time equivalent to birth, under conditions that might allow in vivo contacts of cells to continue in vitro (i.e., in concentrations that do not limit the number of fetal liver cells in the foreign environment), the frequencies of cells capable of developing to IgM PFC increased approximately 1000-fold from 1 in 3×10^6 at day 13 to 1 in 3×10^3 at the time equivalent to day 19 (birth).

Adherent stromal cells of B-cell-generating organs, such as bone marrow or fetal liver, have been found to cooperate in the development of mature B cells from progenitors. We therefore attempted to restore the

Table 1. Development of G-5-2$^+$, λ5 mRNA$^+$, and μH mRNA$^+$ Cells in Fetal Liver

Time of embryonic development (days of gestation)	Total cells (% of total cells)					MAb G-5-2$^+$ cells (% of total cells)		
	surface markers			RNA expression of genes		marker	RNA expression of genes	
	B220	BP-1	G-5-2	μ	λ5	G-5-2	μ	λ5
13	1.0	1.0	**1.0**			10–20	**1**	**10**
14	1.3	1.5	**1.0**	1.5	**1**	20–30	**6**	**20–30**
15	1.9	2.0	**1.5**					
16	3.5	3.2	**3.3**	3	**2.5**	50–60	**50**	**50**
17	5.3	4.4	**4.6**					
18	6.0	5.8	**5.7**	5	**5**	>85	**>85**	**>85**

Detection of mRNA by in situ hybridization of single cells (Berger 1986).

capacity of MAb G-5-2$^+$ fetal liver pre-B cells of day 13 and 14 of gestation (see Fig. 1) to develop to sIg$^+$, mitogen-reactive B cells by coculturing them with irradiated adherent fetal liver stromal cells. After various days of coculture, the nonadherent cells were replaced under conditions of limiting dilutions in the foreign environment of rat filler cells and LPS. The results in Figure 2 show that a rapid, approximately 100-fold increase in the frequencies of precursors capable of development to IgM PFC occurred within 24 hours around the time equivalent to day 16 of gestation. This indicates that irradiated adherent stromal cells can provide the environment necessary for B cells to develop

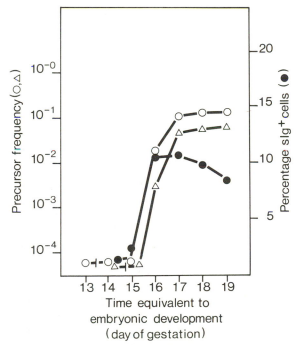

Figure 2. Frequencies of precursors in MAb G-5-2$^+$ fetal liver cells of day 13 (○) and 14 (△) of gestation, capable of development into LPS-reactive B cells, and IgM PFC in rat thymus filler cells and LPS, and the appearance of sIg$^+$ cells (●) in cultures of MAb G52-sorted precursors. Cells were cultured for various days with irradiated fetal liver stromal cells and were either replated under limiting dilution conditions in rat thymus cells and LPS (○,△) or assayed for sIg expression by FACS (●). Assays for the development of clones of IgM PFC were done at the equivalent time of day 5 after birth.

to a mitogen-sensitive stage where they are then independent of stromal cells.

Previous studies (Melchers et al. 1975; Melchers 1977a,b) have shown that reactivity to LPS is gained between days 18 and 19 of gestation in fetal liver. Thus, our results suggest that a stromal-cell-dependent phase of B-cell development between days 13 and 16 is succeeded by a stromal-cell-independent phase between days 16 and 19 to reach the stage of sIg$^+$, mitogen-reactive cells.

Development of sIg$^+$ Pre-B Cells

Cultures of MAb G-5-2$^+$ pre-B cells on irradiated adherent stromal cells were also monitored for the development of sIg$^+$ cells. The results in Figure 2 show that sIg$^+$ cells appear in the nonadherent fractions of these cultures within 24 hours around the time equivalent to day 16 of gestation, i.e., at the time when these cells become independent of stromal cells but 2 to 3 days before they become mitogen-reactive. In different experiments, the level of sIg$^+$ cells in the nonadherent cell fraction varied between 4% and 10%. In the absence of stromal cells, MAb G-5-2$^+$ cells did not develop to sIg$^+$ cells in culture. The development of mitogen-reactive and of sIg$^+$ B cells in cultures of MAb G-5-2$^+$ pre-B cells and of irradiated adherent stromal cells, as well as in the absence of stromal cells, could not be influenced by the addition of IL-1, -2, -3, -4, -5, -6, or -7, alone or in combinations.

DISCUSSION

Several studies have shown that B-cell development from progenitors and precursors to mature B cells depends on interaction with the environment of B-cell-generating organs (Kincade et al. 1981; Whitlock et al. 1985; Dorshkind et al. 1986; Gisler et al. 1987; Witte et al. 1987; Kinashi et al. 1988; Pietrangeli et al. 1988; Palacios et al. 1989). Tissue culture conditions have been established that allow this stromal-cell-dependent B-cell development in vitro. We show that this development in the environment of fetal liver stromal cells takes precursors to a stage where they become sIg$^+$ and at the same time independent of interactions with stromal cells so that they are capable of developing to IgM PFC in a foreign environment of rat filler cells.

The enrichment of precursors for mitogen-reactive cells and the concomitant enrichment of $\lambda5$-expressing and, later, μH-chain-expressing cells by FACS with the aid of MAb G-5-2 suggests that MAb G-5-2$^+$ cells are $\lambda5$ and, later, μH-chain-expressing cells that become sIg$^+$ and mitogen-reactive. Since we have not yet purified early MAb G-5-2$^+$ precursors to homogeneity, and since we have not yet developed an assay that can probe a single cell by in situ staining for MAb G-5-2 binding as well as $\lambda5$ and μH-chain expression, it remains a possibility that different markers might be expressed in (partially) distinct subpopulations. If they are, however, the same, and if the increase of MAb G-5-2$^+$ cells in fetal liver between day 13 and 16 of gestation (Fig. 1) is generated by cell division rather than by recruitment from outside of fetal liver or by differentiation of MAb G-5-2$^+$ precursors inside fetal liver, then the following picture of B-cell generation emerges.

MAb G-5-2$^+$, $\lambda5$-expressing progenitors and precursors divide four times in fetal liver between day 13 and 16 of gestation to become sIg$^+$. Between day 14 and 15 μH-chain gene segments are rearranged, and H-chains are expressed, and around day 16 Ig appears on the surface. The four divisions and the Ig gene rearrangements require interactions with stromal cells. Once pre-B cells are sIg$^+$, they become stromal-cell-independent and mature without much proliferation between day 16 and 19 to mitogen-reactive mature B cells, which can be stimulated to IgM PFC.

The synchrony of B-cell development in fetal liver between days 13 and 19 is striking and suggests that this development occurs in one wave. Since the synchrony is kept for nearly 1 week of embryonic development, tight controls must operate. The wave, like other waves of lymphocyte development (Le Douarin 1978; Melchers 1979; Reynolds and Morris 1983; Pink et al. 1987) might be initiated by progenitors, which populate the fetal liver within a time window of 24 hours around day 13 of gestation when stromal cells of fetal liver are competent to induce four pre-B-cell divisions concomitant with Ig rearrangements. Thereafter, progenitors might continue to exist, but they might not find a competent organ. As an alternative, progenitors might be generated only once around day 13 of gestation, whereas the fetal level might remain a competent organ for a longer time.

Throughout life, the generation of B cells is continuous in bone marrow. It has been estimated that 3×10^7 to 5×10^7 cells are newly generated per day in the adult mouse (Park and Osmond 1987; Thomas-Vaslin and Freitas 1989). If generation of B cells in bone marrow occurs in the same steps with the same number of critical divisions, as we observe in fetal liver, then a pool of approximately 2×10^6 progenitor cells must exist that have not yet rearranged any Ig gene segments. This pool must divide once daily to generate 2×10^6 progenitor cells to be drawn into the stromal-cell-dependent four divisions that induce the Ig gene rearrangements to generate 3×10^7 to 5×10^7 cells

from which the mature B-cell pool of the periphery is replenished.

To generate sIg$^+$ B cells, Ig gene segments have to be rearranged to form functional H- and L-chain genes. These rearrangement processes are known to lead not only to productive, but also to nonproductive forms of rearranged IgH and/or L-chain genes because of incomplete, out-of-frame, or pseudogene rearrangements. Our findings that between 5% and 10% of all MAb G-5-2$^+$ cells develop to sIg$^+$ cells suggest that such nonproductive rearrangements could happen in 90% and more of all precursors. This number is at least within the range of frequencies of productive versus nonproductive rearrangements expected from a stochastic process of rearrangements in which possible corrections of nonproductive to productive rearrangements are not the rule.

Speculations on the Molecular Controls of B-cell Development

Ig gene rearrangements are ordered in time. First, D_H (diversity) segments are rearranged to J_H (joining) segments, then V_H (variable) to $D_H J_H$, followed by V_L to J_L. If rearrangements are controlled by cell divisions, every cell division of a MAb G-5-2$^+$ precursor could carry one of these rearrangements since only four divisions appear to occur.

The rearrangements occur in the stromal-cell-dependent phase of B-cell development. It is therefore tempting to speculate that cell-cell contacts between progenitors or precursors on the one side and stromal cells on the other control Ig rearrangements and the four cell divisions. Soluble cytokine production, especially the production of IL-3 and IL-7, might be induced in stromal cells by these contacts. However, they can only be helping these responses of progenitors since our experiments do not detect any effects of exogenously added ILs on pre-B developments. Cell contacts between progenitors and stromal cells should therefore be mandatory in the signaling to progenitors to proliferate and rearrange Ig gene segments.

We have searched for genes and their products that might be involved in these contacts and in controlling these critical steps of B-cell development. So far, we have found three structures that are good candidates for such contact and control functions. V_{pre-B} and $\lambda5$ are expressed selectively in pre-B but not in B cells (Kudo and Melchers 1987; Sakaguchi and Melchers 1986), whereas *mb-1* is selectively expressed in pre-B and B but not in plasma cells (Sakaguchi et al. 1988). All of them appear to be expressed on the surface of pre-B cells. V_{pre-B} protein might be associated in a noncovalent, Ig-domain-like fashion with $\lambda5$ protein forming a light-chain-like structure with large protrusions of the amino-terminal portion of $\lambda5$ and the carboxy-terminal portion of V_{pre-B} at the site of the third complementarity-determining region (CDR) of a variable region. Both V_{pre-B} and $\lambda5$ proteins have been found associated with μH chains on the surface of pre-B cell lines and tumors (Pillai and Baltimore 1988; S.R. Bauer and F. Melchers, in prep.), suggesting that the dimeric 7-8S IgM found previously on the surface of normal pre-B cells might in fact be μH chains in association with V_{pre-B} and $\lambda 5$ (Melchers 1977c).

mb-1 codes for a 34-kD glycoprotein that appears to be associated with sIg on B cells (Hombach et al. 1988; Sakaguchi et al. 1988). It might have CD3-like properties in anchoring IgM in the surface membrane and in signaling B cells via sIg to reactions controlling proliferation and maturation of B cells. Since *mb-1* is also expressed in pre-B cells, it is a good candidate for similar function in pre-B cells, i.e., to anchor μH chains with V_{pre-B} and $\lambda 5$ proteins in the surface membrane of pre-B cells and to control signaling for proliferation and Ig gene rearrangements.

How could the B lineage of cells control four critical divisions in a precise fashion, so that every division carries one of the four Ig gene rearrangements? We offer here our working hypothesis, which we hope to test in future experiments. This hypothesis predicts that V_{pre-B} and $\lambda 5$ are already expressed on the surface of progenitor cells before Ig gene rearrangement begins and that the two proteins associate with each other to form a light-chain-like structure. V_{pre-B} and $\lambda 5$, by themselves, are expected not to be membrane-bound proteins. To be anchored in the surface membrane, they should be associated with a membrane-bound protein, and that may be an H-chain-like molecule that we call X (Fig. 3). $V_{pre-B}/\lambda 5$ may recognize a structure on stromal cells (Fig. 3, determinant S1). This recognition

may be mediated by X and by the carboxy-terminal, non-Ig-like part of V_{pre-B} and the amino-terminal, non-Ig-like part of the $\lambda 5$, which could be expected to form two long protrusions at the site where the third CDR is located in a V region. As a consequence of this progenitor/stromal-cell interaction, stromal cells could be induced to produce IL-7, whereas progenitors could be induced to the first Ig gene rearrangement, i.e., of D_H segments to J_H segments. After one division, $D_H J_H C_\mu$ can be expressed, which might already suffice to replace X in interactions with $V_{pre-B}/\lambda 5$. $V_{pre-B}/\lambda 5$ in association with $D_H J_H C_\mu$ now may recognize a different stromal cell structure (Fig. 3, determinant S2) that induces another critical division and the rearrangement of V_H to $D_H J_H$. We could also speculate that $D_H J_H C_\mu$ protein associates only with $\lambda 5$ protein but not with V_{pre-B}, if the association between V_{pre-B} and $\lambda 5$ alone is not strong enough. This in turn could lead to the expression of a complete μH chain and the replacement of X and possibly $D_H J_H C_\mu$ in association with $V_{pre-B}/\lambda 5$. $V_{pre-B}/\lambda 5$ in association with the μH chain could recognize a third stromal structure (Fig. 3, determinant S3), and this could induce one more critical division and the rearrangement of L-chain gene segments. The expressed L chains then are expected to replace $V_{pre-B}/\lambda 5$ in association with μH chains. Thereby, contact to stromal cells should be abolished, and cell divisions and further rearrangements should no longer be induced.

Our model predicts that $V_{pre-B}/\lambda 5$, perhaps in association with X, controls H-chain gene-segment rearrangements, that $V_{pre-B}/\lambda 5$ in association with μH

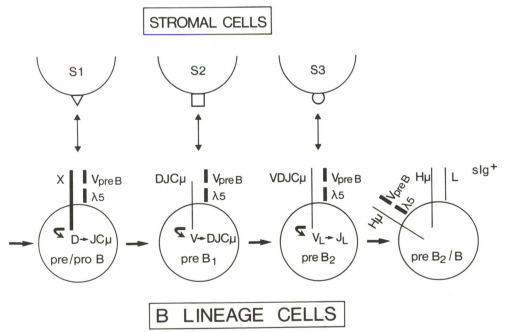

Figure 3. A speculation on possible molecular steps involved in the stromal-cell-dependent steps of critical pre-B-cell divisions and Ig gene rearrangements in the development of sIg$^+$ pre-B cells. S1, S2, and S3 are three possible stromal cell determinants recognized by progenitor, respectively precursor B cells. X, V_{pre-B}, and $\lambda 5$ are the surface-expressed products of the corresponding B-lineage-specific genes that influence the rearrangements and expression of Ig genes, i.e., D_H to J_H and V_H to $D_H J_H$ of the H-chain locus and V_L to J_L of the light-chain loci. For further details see text.

chains controls L-chain gene-segment rearrangements, and that both molecular structures function in recognizing specific and different molecules on the surface of stromal cells. It predicts that inhibition of these interactions should inhibit the rearrangements and that antibodies to $V_{pre-B}/\lambda5$ (and maybe to X and μH chains) might mimic the actions of stromal cells on progenitors and precursors of the B lineage. Since our model predicts a role of $V_H D_H J_H C_\mu$ H-chain protein and maybe $D_H J_H C_\mu$ protein in the recognition of stromal cell determinants, followed by induction of the next Ig gene rearrangement in line, it also predicts that $D_H J_H C_\mu$ could and that $V_H D_H J_H C_\mu$ should definitely be selected for productive rearrangements, i.e., expressed protein. As a consequence, nonproductive $V_H D_H J_H$ rearrangements on *both* chromosomes should never lead to L-chain rearrangements, i.e., cells with two nonproductive H-chain chromosomes and rearranged L-chain chromosomes should not exist in normal B-cell development. The model should also be testable in appropriate transgenic mice where the functions of the normal V_{pre-B}, $\lambda5$, X, and μH chains are altered by mutations.

SUMMARY

Development of B cells in fetal liver occurs in one synchronous wave and involves probably no more than four critical divisions. This leads us to suggest that the main pool of proliferating progenitors that replenish the peripheral B-cell pool are pregenitors before Ig gene rearrangement, that the four Ig gene rearrangements (D_H to J_H, V_H to $D_H J_H$, V_K to J_K, and V_λ to J_λ) might occur in four critical divisions, and that a stromal-cell-dependent phase of pre-B development in which all rearrangements are made is succeeded by a stromal-cell-independent phase of sIg^+ pre-B-cell maturation to mature mitogen-reactive B cells. We speculate on the molecular nature of the tightly controlled steps of Ig rearrangements during pre-B-cell development that might involve the pre-B-cell specific genes V_{pre-B} and $\lambda5$ and the B-lineage-specific gene *mb-1* in interactions with stromal cells.

ACKNOWLEDGMENTS

We thank Anita Imm, Annick Peter, and Diana Thorpe for competent technical assistance. The Basel Institute for Immunology was founded and is supported by F. Hoffmann-La Roche AG, Basel, Switzerland.

REFERENCES

Alt, F., N.E. Rosenberg, S. Lewis, E. Thomas, and D. Baltimore. 1981. Organization and reorganization of immunoglobulin genes in A-MuLV-transformed cells: Rearrangement of heavy but not light chain genes. *Cell* 27: 381.

Bauer, S.R., A. Kudo, and F. Melchers. 1988. Structure and pre-B lymphocyte restricted expression of the $V_{pre\,B}$ gene in humans and conservation of its structure in other mammalian species. *EMBO J.* 7: 11.

Berger, C.N. 1986. *In situ* hybridization of immunoglobulin-specific RNA in single cells of the B lymphocyte lineage with radiolabeled DNA probes. *EMBO J.* 5: 85.

Dorshkind, K., A. Johnson, L. Collins, G.M. Keller, and R.A. Phillips. 1986. Generation of purified stromal cell cultures that support lymphoid and myeloid precursors. *J. Immunol. Methods* 89: 37.

Gisler, R.H., A. Söderberg, and M. Kamber. 1987. Functional maturation of murine B lymphocyte precursors. II. Analysis of cells required from the bone marrow microenvironment. *J. Immunol.* 138: 2433.

Gisler, R.H., C. Schlienger, A. Söderberg, F. Ledermann, and J.D. Lambris. 1988. Functional maturation of murine B lymphocyte precursors. III. Soluble factors involved in the regulation of growth and differentiation. *Mol. Immunol.* 25: 1113.

Hombach, J., L. Leclercq, A. Radbruch, K. Rajewsky, and M. Reth. 1988. A novel 34 kd protein co-isolated with the IgM molecule in surface IgM-expressing cells. *EMBO J.* 7: 3451.

Iscove, N.N. and F. Melchers. 1978. Complete replacement of serum by albumin, transferrin and soybean lipids in cultures of lipopolysaccharide-reactive B lymphocytes. *J. Exp. Med.* 147: 923.

Karasuyama, H. and F. Melchers. 1988. Establishment of mouse cell lines which constitutively secrete large quantities of interleukin 2, 3, 4 or 5 using modified cDNA expression vectors. *Eur. J. Immunol.* 18: 97.

Kinashi, T., K. Inaba, T. Tsubata, K. Tashiro, R. Palacios, and T. Honjo. 1988. Differentiation of an interleukin 3-dependent precursor B cell clone into immunoglobulin-producing cells *in vitro*. *Proc. Natl. Acad. Sci.* 85: 4473.

Kincade, P.W., G. Lee, C.J. Paige, and M.P. Street. 1981. Cellular interactions affecting the maturation of murine B lymphocyte precursors *in vitro*. *J. Immunol.* 127: 255.

Kudo, A. and F. Melchers. 1987. A second gene, $V_{pre\,B}$ in the λ_5 locus of the mouse, which appears to be selectively expressed in pre-B lymphocyte. *EMBO J.* 6: 2267.

Le Douarin, N.M. 1978. Ontogeny of hematopoietic organs studied in avian embryo interspecific chimeras. *Cold Spring Harbor Conf. Cell Proliferation* 5: 5.

Maki, R., J. Kearney, C. Paige, and S. Tonegawa. 1982. Immunoglobulin gene rearrangements in immature B cells. *Science* 209: 1366.

Melchers, F. 1977a. B lymphocyte development in fetal liver. I. Development of reactivities to B cell mitogens "in vivo" and "in vitro." *Eur. J. Immunol.* 7: 476.

———. 1977b. B lymphocyte development in fetal liver. II. Frequencies of precursor B cells during gestation. *Eur. J. Immunol.* 7: 482.

———. 1977c. Immunoglobulin synthesis and mitogen reactivity: Markers for B-lymphocyte differentiation. In *Development of host defences* (ed. M.D. Cooper and D.H. Dayton), p. 11. Raven Press, New York.

———. 1979. Three waves of B lymphocyte development during embryonic development in the mouse. *INSERM Symp.* 10: 281.

Melchers, F., H. von Boehmer, and R.A. Phillips. 1975. B lymphocyte subpopulations in the mouse. Organ distribution and ontogeny of immunoglobulin-synthesizing and of mitogen-sensitive cells. *Transplant Rev.* 25: 26.

Namen, A.E., A.E. Schmierer, C.J. March, R.W. Overell, L.S. Park, D.L. Urdal, and D.Y. Mochizuki. 1988a. B cell precursor growth-promoting activity. Purification and characterization of a growth factor active on lymphocyte precursors. *J. Exp. Med.* 167: 988.

Namen, A.E., S. Lupton, K. Hjenild, J. Wijnall, D.Y. Mochizuki, A. Schmierer, B. Mosley, C.J. March, D. Urdal, S. Gillis, D. Cosman, and R.G. Goodwin. 1988b. Stimulation of B-cell progenitors by cloned murine interleukin-7. *Nature* 333: 571.

Owen, J.J.T., M.D. Cooper, and M.C. Raff. 1974. *In vitro* generation of B lymphocytes in mouse fetal liver, a mammalian "bursa equivalent." *Nature* 249: 361.

Paige, C.J., R.H. Gisler, J.P. McKearn, and M.N. Iscove. 1984. Differentiation of murine B cell precursors in agar culture. Frequency, surface marker analysis and requirements for growth of clonable pre-B cells. *Eur. J. Immunol.* **14:** 979.

Palacios, R. and M. Steinmetz. 1985. IL-3 dependent bone marrow clones that express B-220 surface antigen, contain Ig$^+$ genes in germline configuration and generate B lymphocytes *in vivo*. *Cell* **41:** 727.

Palacios, R., H. Karasuyama, and A. Rolink. 1987. Ly1$^+$ Pro-B lymphocyte clones. Phenotype, growth requirements and differentiation *in vitro* and *in vivo*. *EMBO J.* **6:** 3687.

Palacios, R., S. Stuber, and A. Rolink. 1989. The epigenetic influences of bone marrow and fetal liver stroma liver cells on the developmental potential of Ly1$^+$ pro-B lymphocyte clones. *Eur. J. Immunol.* **19:** 347.

Palacios, R., G. Henson, M. Steinmetz, and J.P. McKearn. 1984. Interleukin-3 supports growth of mouse pre-B cell clones *in vitro*. *Nature* **309:** 126.

Park, Y.H. and A.G. Osmond. 1987. Phenotype and proliferation of early precursor cells in mouse bone marrow. *J. Exp. Med.* **165:** 444.

Pietrangeli, L.E., S.-I. Hayashi, and P.W. Kincade. 1988. Stromal cell lines which support lymphocyte growth: Characterization, sensitivity to radiation and responsiveness to growth factors. *Eur. J. Immunol.* **18:** 863.

Pillai, S. and D. Baltimore. 1988. The Omega and Iota surrogate immunoglobulin light chains. *Curr. Top. Microbiol. Immunol.* **137:** 136.

Pink, J.R.L., O. Lassila, and O. Vainio. 1987. B-lymphocytes and their self-renewal. In *Avian immunology* (ed. A. Toivanen and P. Toivanen), vol. 1, p. 65. CRC Press, Boca Raton, Florida.

Reynolds, J.D. and B. Morris. 1983. The evolution and involution of Peyer's patches in fetal and postnatal sheep. *Eur. J. Immunol.* **13:** 627.

Sakaguchi, N. and F. Melchers. 1986. λ_5, a new light chain-related locus selectively expressed in pre-B lymphocytes. *Nature* **324:** 579.

Sakaguchi, N., S.-I. Kashiwamura, M. Kimoto, P. Thalmann, and F. Melchers. 1988. B lymphocyte-lineage-restricted expression of m6.1, a gene with CD3-like structural properties. *EMBO J.* **7:** 3457.

Strasser, A. 1988. PB:76: A novel surface glycoprotein preferentially expressed on mouse pre-B cells and plasma cells detected by the monoclonal antibody G-5-2. *Eur. J. Immunol.* **18:** 1803.

Thomas-Vaslin, V. and A.A. Freitas. 1989. Lymphocyte population kinetics during the development of the immune system. B cell persistence and life-span can be determined by the host environment. *Int. Immunol.* **1:** 237.

Whitlock, C., K. Denis, D. Robertson, and O.N. Witte. 1985. *In vitro* analysis of murine B cell development. *Annu. Rev. Immunol.* **3:** 213.

Witte, P.L., M. Robertson, A. Henley, M.G. Low, D.L. Stiers, S. Perkins, R.A. Fleischman, and P.W. Kincade. 1987. Relationships between B-lineage lymphocytes and stromal cells in long term bone marrow cultures. *Eur. J. Immunol.* **17:** 1473.

Control of VDJ Recombinase Activity

P. Ferrier,* B. Krippl,† A.J. Furley,* T.K. Blackwell,* H. Suh,*
M. Mendelsohn,* A. Winoto,‡ W.D. Cook,*§ L. Hood,‡
F. Costantini,† and F.W. Alt*

*Howard Hughes Medical Institute and the Departments of Biochemistry and Microbiology;
†Department of Human Genetics and Development, College of Physicians and Surgeons of Columbia
University, New York, New York, 10032; ‡Department of Biology, California Institute of Technology,
Pasadena, California 91125.

B-cell antigen receptors are composed of heterodimers of heavy (H) and light (L) immunoglobulin (Ig) chains, whereas T-cell antigen receptors (TCRs) are heterodimers of α and β or γ and δ TCR chains. The amino-terminal portion of immunoglobulin and TCR chains has a variable amino acid sequence (V region), whereas the remainder of each chain has a constant amino acid sequence (C region); IgH, IgL, and the various TCR chains comprise separate families encoded at distinct loci by homologous genes. The V region genes of immunoglobulin and TCR chains are assembled somatically from two (V and [joining] J) or three (V, [diversity] D, and J) germ-line gene segments depending on the immunoglobulin or TCR family (for review, see Tonegawa 1983; Davis and Bjorkman 1988). Following assembly, transcription of immunoglobulin or TCR genes initiates from a promoter upstream of the V region gene and terminates downstream from the associated C gene. High-level expression of rearranged IgH or IgL chain genes depends on the activity of lymphocyte-specific transcriptional enhancers located in the intervening sequences between assembled V and C region genes (for review, see Sen and Baltimore 1989). Similar enhancer elements appear to direct expression of TCRβ and α genes (Krimpenfort et al. 1988; McDougall et al. 1988; Winoto and Baltimore 1989).

Antigen receptor gene segments are flanked by conserved signal sequences that target a site-specific recombination activity referred to as VDJ recombinase; various lines of evidence suggest that immunoglobulin and TCR genes are assembled by the same VDJ recombinase (e.g., Yancopoulos et al. 1986). Assembly of IgH chain and probably TCRβ V region genes generally is an ordered process that involves initial D to J joining and the subsequent appendage of a V segment to the preexisting DJ complex (Alt et al. 1984; Okazaki et al. 1987). V region gene assembly is tissue-specifically regulated; immunoglobulin genes are assembled completely only in differentiating B-lineage cells (in fetal liver or adult marrow), TCR genes only in differentiating T-lineage cells (in thymus), and neither immunoglobulin nor TCR genes are assembled in non-

lymphoid cells (Kincade 1987; von Boehmer 1988). Within a given lineage, V region gene assembly also is stage-specifically regulated (for review, see Alt et al. 1987); for example, IgH chain genes are generally assembled and expressed before IgL chain genes. Ordered and stage-specific rearrangements are probably intrinsic to regulation of allelically excluded antigen receptor gene expression, a process that involves functional assembly of a given antigen receptor locus on only a single allele. With respect to allelic exclusion of IgH and TCRβ loci, regulation appears to occur at the V to DJ joining step (Alt et al. 1984; Uematsu et al. 1988). In this context, it is notable that IgH D to J_H joining sometimes occurs in T cells (Foster et al. 1980; Kemp et al. 1980; Kurosawa et al. 1981); however, V_H to DJ_H joining usually occurs only in B cells. Clearly, the V to DJ joining event is a critical control point during lymphocyte differentiation.

VDJ recombinase activity appears to be constitutive in precursor lymphocytes and not present in nonlymphoid cells (Blackwell et al. 1986; Lieber et al. 1987; Desiderio and Wolff 1988; Schatz and Baltimore 1988), accounting, at least in part, for lymphoid-specificity of V gene assembly. However, if there is a single VDJ recombinase, then other mechanisms must operate to control and direct its lymphoid stage-, tissue-, and allele-specific activities. Studies of Abelson-murine-leukemia-virus (Ab-MLV)-transformed pre-B-cell lines that actively assemble immunoglobulin V region genes in culture indicated germ-line V gene segments are often transcribed during or prior to their assembly (for review, see Alt et al. 1987). These findings, coupled with results of recombination substrate/gene transfer experiments (see below), suggested that regulation of the various recombination events is effected by modulating accessibility of the substrate gene segments to the common recombinase. According to this accessibility model, cis-acting regulatory sequences should target particular V region gene segments to VDJ recombinase activity.

Candidate regulatory sequences for controlling recombination include elements involved in transcriptional control of antigen-receptor gene expression (Blackwell et al. 1986; Yancopoulos et al. 1986). The IgH-chain transcriptional enhancer element (E_μ) has certain properties consistent with such a control ele-

§Present address: Ludwig Institute for Cancer Research, Melbourne Tumor Biology Branch, Melbourne, Victoria 3050, Australia.

ment including its location in the intron downstream from the J_H segments and its activation very early in B-cell ontogeny (Lenon and Perry 1986; Sen and Baltimore 1989). In this paper, we summarize results of transgenic recombination substrate studies aimed at testing whether transcriptional enhancers can serve as recombination enhancers. These studies also suggest the existence of other potential controlling elements in the VDJ recombination process.

MATERIALS AND METHODS

Probes. DNA fragments used as probes were isolated and prepared as described previously (Alt et al. 1981). The $V_\beta 14$-specific probe used in Southern and Northern blot analyses has been described previously (Ferrier et al. 1989). For RNA protection assay, the $V_\beta 14$-specific probe consisted in a 410-bp *Hae*III/*Sac*I insert composed of a 360-bp *Hae*III/*Acc*I fragment from the 3' portion of the $V_\beta 14$ gene and polylinker sequences subcloned into M13-mp19.

Production and analysis of transgenic mice. Microinjection of purified inserts into fertilized (C57BL/6 × CBA/J)F$_2$ eggs and isolation of tail DNA were as described previously (Costantini and Lacy 1981).

Production of Ab-MLV-transformed cells. Ab-MLV transformation of newborn fetal liver (with Moloney helper) or adult thymus (with radiation leukemia virus helper) from transgenic mice was performed as described previously (Rosenberg and Baltimore 1976; Cook 1985).

Analysis of transgene rearrangements. DNA preparation, restriction enzyme digests, agarose gel electrophoresis, DNA blotting procedures, ^{32}P-labeling of DNA fragments by nick translation, and hybridization procedures were performed as described previously (Alt et al. 1981). Densitometric analyses were performed with a Joyce Loebl Chromoscan 3.

Analysis of transgene expression. Preparation of total RNA, Northern blotting, and S1 nuclease protection methods were as described previously (Yancopoulos and Alt 1985).

RESULTS AND DISCUSSION

Transgenic Recombination Substrates: Experimental Strategy

We have designed transgenic recombination substrates to circumvent potential limitations of experimental systems that involve introduction of recom-

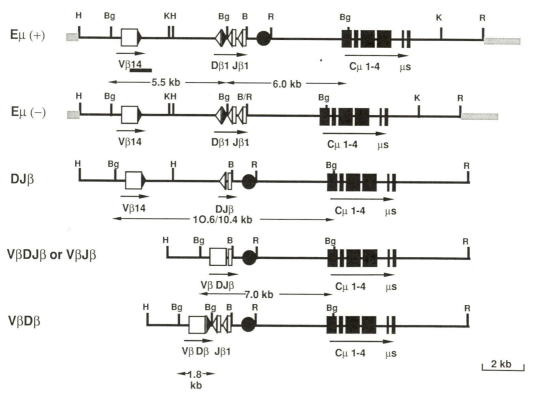

Figure 1. Inserts of recombinant E$_\mu$$^+$ and E$_\mu$$^-$ constructs and partial restriction maps of potential DJ, VDJ, and VD rearrangements predicted from the structure of the E$_\mu$$^+$ construct. The TCRβ V, D, and J variable segments are indicated by open boxes, flanking recognition heptamers and nonamers by closed (23-bp spacer) or open (12-bp or 13-bp spacer) triangles, the E$_\mu$ element by a closed circle, the C$_\mu$ exons by closed boxes, and cosmid sequences by stippled boxes. (→) Directions of transcription of coding elements. The location of the V$_\beta$14 probe used in the blotting analyses is indicated by a closed bar. Restriction endonuclease sites are as follows: (H) *Hind*III; (Bg) *Bgl*II; (K) *Kpn*I; (B) *Bam*HI; (E) *Eco*RI.

bination substrates into cell lines. In particular, we anticipated that gene segments and control elements in the transgenic constructs would undergo activation events associated with normal development; thus, no selection would need to be employed for expression within or around the construct. Two recombination substrates were prepared from genomic fragments of the murine TCRβ and IgH loci (see Fig. 1). Each construct contained a TCRβ V region gene minilocus composed of the germ-line $V_\beta 14$ (Malissen et al. 1986), $D_\beta 1.1$ (Siu et al. 1984), and $J_\beta 1.1$ and $J_\beta 1.2$ (Gascoigne et al. 1984) segments linked to exons that encode the IgH C_μ constant region by a 1.1-kb segment of DNA in which the E_μ element was present (E_μ^+) or absent (E_μ^-). The E_μ-containing segment was in a similar position and orientation relative to the J_β segments as it normally occupies with respect to the immunoglobulin J_H cluster. The signal sequences that flank V region gene segments consist of a palindromic heptamer and an AT-rich nonamer separated by a spacer of 12 or 23 bp; joining occurs only between segments flanked by signal sequences with different spacer lengths (Early et al. 1980; Sakano et al. 1980). On the basis of the spacer lengths of the signal sequences flanking the V_β (23 bp), D_β (5'12 bp, and 3'23 bp), and J_β (13 bp) segments, various rearrangements could occur in accordance with the 12/23 restriction including D_β to J_β, V_β to J_β, or DJ_β, and V_β to D_β joinings (Fig. 1). We oriented the V, D, and J segments within a given construct so that joinings would delete intervening sequences.

We designed the recombination substrates so that all types of site-specific rearrangement events could be assayed by Southern blotting techniques. The assay was based on the presence of three strategic BglII-restriction-endonuclease sites in the constructs: one upstream of the V_β gene, one between the D_β and J_β segments, and one within the C_μ gene. Thus, within a given tissue, germ-line versus rearranged forms of the construct can be distinguished by probing BglII-digested genomic DNA with a $V_\beta 14$-specific probe (Fig. 1). For example, an unrearranged copy of the E_μ^+ construct contains a 5.5-kb BglII fragment that will hybridize to a $V_\beta 14$-specific probe. D_β to J_β joining will remove the intervening BglII site and create new V_β-hybridizing fragments of approximately 10.4 kb or 10.6 kb depending on the J_β fragment used. V_β to DJ_β or direct V_β to J_β joinings will reduce the size of the detected fragment to 7.0 kb by removing V_β/D_β intervening sequences. Finally, joining of V_β to a D_β that had not previously joined to a J_β segment ($V_\beta D_\beta$ joining) will generate a 1.8-kb V_β-hybridizing BglII fragment.

E_μ^+ and E_μ^- Transgenic Lines

The E_μ^+ or E_μ^- inserts were microinjected into fertilized (C57BL/6J × CBA/J)F$_2$ mouse eggs. Southern blot analyses of tail DNA from 14 founder animals showed that each contained multiple, intact copies of the appropriate construct organized in a head-to-tail configuration (not shown). Ten transgenic lines were

established by crossing founders containing the E_μ^+ construct (founders 379, 382, 390, and 392) or the E_μ^- construct (founders 1003, 1006, 1010, 1013, 1016, and 1018) with normal (C57BL/6J × CBA/J)F$_1$ mice. Each line contained mostly intact copies of the construct integrated at a single site; the number of complete construct copies ranged from 2 to 30 (not shown). DNA rearrangement and RNA expression analyses performed on several lines showed no differences between males and females or newborn and adult mice.

Tissue-specific and Ordered Rearrangements within the E_μ^+ Construct

Potential rearrangements of TCR V segments in the transgenic constructs were assayed using genomic DNA from different lymphoid (lymph nodes, spleen, thymus, and bone marrow) and nonlymphoid (skin, liver, kidney, and brain) tissues of the transgenic mice (Fig. 2). With DNA from normal (Fig. 2, lane 1) and transgenic tissues, the $V_\beta 14$ probe hybridized to a 3.7-kb germ-line BglII fragment that contains the endogenous $V_\beta 14$ gene; in all transgenic tissues, the probe also hybridized to the 5.5-kb BglII fragment that contains the unrearranged V and D gene segments of the transgenes. No additional V_β-hybridizing fragments were detected in any tissues of six transgenic lines that contained the E_μ^- construct (Fig. 2A, lines 1010 and 1016; representative data is shown). In contrast, in the four transgenic lines carrying the E_μ^+ transgene, we readily detected two additional V_β-hybridizing fragments that had the correct size to represent substrate DJ_β and $V_\beta DJ_\beta$ joining in DNA from all analyzed lymphoid tissues but not in DNA from nonlymphoid tissues (Fig. 2B, lines 392 and 379). Together, these results demonstrate that the E_μ-containing DNA segment provides dominant activities that, in cis, target associated TCRβ gene segments for rearrangement in lymphoid tissues (see below).

Ordered Rearrangement of Construct V, D, and J Segments

Substantial levels of DJ_β rearrangements within the E_μ-containing construct were apparent in all lymphoid tissues, whereas $V_\beta DJ_\beta$ rearrangements, although present in all lymphoid tissues, were much more prominent in the thymus (Fig. 2B). In contrast, V_β-hybridizing fragments of the size predicted for $V_\beta D_\beta$ joining were not detectable or were only barely detectable in any of these tissues and occurred maximally at less than 5% the level of DJ_β joining (Fig. 2B, lanes 7 and 15). This result indicates that in the constructs direct V_β to D_β joining occurs far less frequently than D_β to J_β or V_β to $(D)J_\beta$ recombinations (see below). We confirmed the structure of the various rearrangements observed by DNA blotting techniques by molecularly cloning and characterizing construct rearrangements from thymus DNA of line 392. Notably, four of six sequenced VDJ joinings contained nucleotides clearly

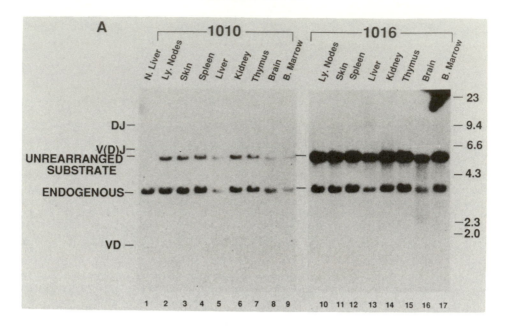

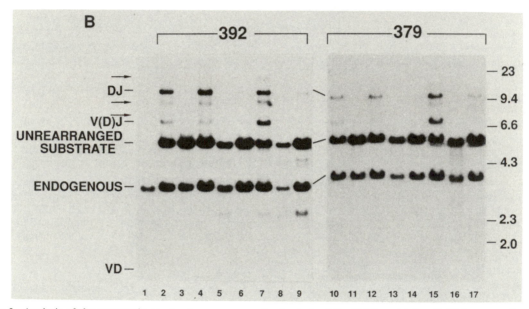

Figure 2. Analysis of the transgenic construct rearrangements. Analysis of the $V_\beta 14$-containing *Bgl*II fragments in transgenic lines containing the E_μ^- (*A*) and E_μ^+ constructs (*B*). DNA (10 μg) from lymphoid ([lanes 2 and 10] lymph nodes; [lanes 4 and 12] spleen; [lanes 7 and 15] thymus; [lanes 9 and 17] bone marrow) and nonlymphoid ([lanes 3 and 11] skin; [lanes 5 and 13] liver; [lanes 6 and 14] kidney; [lanes 8 and 16] brain) tissues of 4-week-old transgenic females was digested with *Bgl*II and analyzed by Southern blot analysis for hybridization to the $V_\beta 14$ probe. DNA from normal (C57BL/6J × CBA/J)F$_2$ liver served as the endogenous germ-line control (lane *1*). Positions of *Bgl*II fragments containing the endogenous $V_\beta 14$ gene and predicted substrate DJ, VDJ, and VD normal rearrangements are indicated in the left margin. Fragment sizes of *Hin*dIII-digested bacteriophage λ DNA are indicated in kb in the right margin.

contributed by the $D_\beta 1.1$ segment, and the others had G residues that could derive from the D segment, confirming that most or all of these joints involved an intermediate DJ_β-joining event. Moreover, two rearrangements positioned V_β and J_β segments in an open reading frame that could potentially encode TCR-$V_\beta DJ_\beta$/Ig-C_μ hybrid proteins (data not shown).

The low frequency of V to D versus V to DJ joinings coupled with the evidence for D region sequences in most VDJ joinings indicates that, within the transgenic construct, formation of a complete VDJ gene in T cells usually involves an intermediate DJ step. This ordered rearrangement pathway was confirmed by the finding that direct V_β to D_β construct rearrangements were extremely rare in transgenic T-cell lines compared with DJ_β and $V_\beta DJ_\beta$ joinings (see below). Thus, within the limited confines of the transgenic construct, we see ordered joining reminiscent of the ordered assembly of endogenous murine H chain V, D, and J segments that are separated by large distances (Alt et al. 1984). The ordered assembly sequence may be effected by sequential activation of regulatory elements controlling the DJ_β and V_β joining steps (Ferrier et al. 1989), a linear tracking of the VDJ recombinase after binding the J region (Wood and Tonegawa 1980), or some combination of the two mechanisms. TCR V gene segments, as opposed to the IgH V gene segments, are capable of joining directly to J segments within the context of the 12/23 rule. However, our results indicate that other constraints may limit the relative frequency of such direct joinings, but as long as such joinings occur, even infrequently, cellular selection may allow them to contribute to TCR diversity.

T-cell-specific Rearrangements of the Introduced V_β Gene Segments

The relative intensities of the $V_\beta DJ_\beta$- and DJ_β-containing fragments varied greatly among different lymphoid tissues. In the thymus DNA, both types of rearrangements appeared at approximately equal levels (Fig. 2B; lanes 7 and 15). In lymph nodes and the spleen, $V_\beta DJ_\beta$ rearrangements were less abundant than DJ_β rearrangements (Fig. 2B, lanes 2 and 10 and 4 and 12); this difference was even more notable in bone marrow (Fig. 2B, lanes 9 and 17). Thus, the ratio of VDJ to DJ joinings in DNA from various tissues varied in rough proportion to the T-cell versus B-cell content of the tissues (Hokama and Nakamura 1982). This finding suggested that substrate D_β to J_β rearrangements occurred at about the same frequency in both cell types but that V_β to DJ_β rearrangements occurred preferentially in T cells. Accordingly, similar analyses of purified peripheral B and T lymphocyte populations from the spleen and lymph nodes of those two transgenic lines showed that purified T cells had similar levels of construct $V_\beta DJ_\beta$ to DJ_β rearrangements as observed in DNA from the transgenic thymus; in contrast, $V_\beta DJ_\beta$ rearrangements were essentially absent in genomic DNA from the B-cell-enriched populations, but high levels of DJ_β rearrangements were still observed (not shown).

To derive a system in which V gene rearrangements within the transgenes could be analyzed in clonal cell populations and compared directly with the endogenous TCR and immunoglobulin rearrangements, we produced Ab-MLV-transformed T-cell and B-cell-lines by infecting cells from the thymus and fetal liver of the E_μ^+ transgenic lines. Ab-MLV transformation of the transgenic fetal liver yielded multiple independent cell lines; five were chosen at random for analysis of lineage-specificity and construct rearrangements. Ab-MLV can infect and transform immature cells of the B lineage and under certain circumstances myeloid and mast cell lineages as well (Cook 1985; Pierce et al. 1985). Accordingly, three fetal liver transformants were found by multiple criteria to be B-lineage cells, and two others were found to be nonlymphoid cells—

probably mast cells (not shown). No rearrangements of the construct were detected in the Ab-MLV-transformed nonlymphoid cells (Fig. 3, lanes 7 and 8). However, in agreement with the results on purified cell populations, the Ab-MLV-transformed pre-B-cell lines showed substantial levels of construct DJ_β rearrangements but barely detectable levels of construct $V_\beta DJ_\beta$ rearrangements, which were apparent only after very long exposures (Fig. 4B, lanes 5 and 6). Of 24 independent thymus infections, 5 animals (one each in lines 379, 382, 390 and two in line 392) developed thoracic tumors, two of which (T3 and T7) were adapted to growth in tissue-culture. All of these tumors were T lymphoid in origin as determined by a variety of different criteria (not shown). Genomic DNA from all individual tumors or T-cell lines (two tumors are shown in Fig. 3, lanes 1 and 2; other data not shown) showed the characteristic $V_\beta DJ_\beta$ and DJ_β construct rearrangements, whereas in agreement with tissue analyses none had readily detectable $V_\beta D_\beta$ rearrangements.

All of the Ab-MLV-transformed transgenic T-cell lines had formed VDJ rearrangements within the construct at or shortly after the time of transformation; likewise, these lines also had formed rearrangements of their endogenous γ and β, but only two had rearranged TCRα genes (not shown). Together, these results indicate that DJ and VDJ rearrangements within the construct occurred as early events in pre-T-cell differentiation. Furthermore, densitometric analyses indicated similar relative levels of construct $V_\beta DJ_\beta$ and DJ_β rearrangements in normal purified T-cell populations compared with the various clonal transgenic T-cell lines (not shown); this result indicates that most normal T cells have rearranged some copies of the transgenic construct.

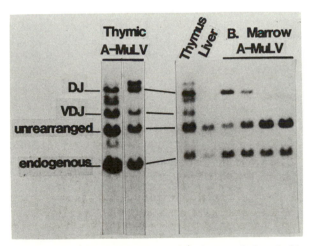

Figure 3. Rearrangements of the E_μ^+ construct in lymphoid cells of the transgenic mice. Genomic DNA from various Ab-MLV-transformed cells was assayed for rearrangements of the construct as described in Fig. 2. (Lanes *1* and *2*) Tumors T2 (290) and T7 (279); (lanes *3* and *4*) transgenic thymus and liver (382); (lanes *5* and *6*) Ab-MLV-transformed pre-B; and (lanes *7* and *8*) nonlymphoid cells from transgenic (379) bone marrow.

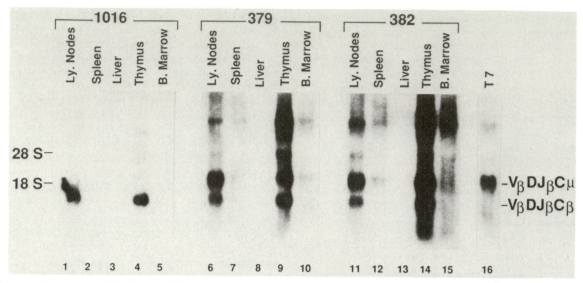

Figure 4. Expression of the functionally rearranged construct in transgenic mice. Total RNA was isolated from tissues of a 4-week-old transgenic female in the lines indicated and cell line T7, fractionated through formaldehyde agarose gels, transferred to nitrocellulose filters, and hybridized with the $V_\beta 14$-specific probe. The positions of the normal TCRβ mRNA and predicted hybrid TCRβ/Ig-C_μ transcripts are indicated.

To assess the relative efficiency with which the pre-B lines rearranged endogenous IgH versus the transgenic TCR$_\beta$ genes, we determined the rearrangement status of these genes in a series of 14 subclonal derivatives of two transgenic pre-B lines (Table 1, F_{12} and F_{18}). Like other Ab-MLV-transformed fetal liver lines (Alt et al. 1984), these lines had endogenous immunoglobulin J_H rearrangements on both chromosomes; the F_{12} line had $V_H DJ_H$ and DJ_H rearrangements, whereas F_{18} had a $V_H DJ_H$ rearrangement at its single detectable J_H allele (Table 1). Thus, these cells have already formed endogenous immunoglobulin $V_H DJ_H$ rearrangements and DJ_β rearrangements of the construct before or shortly after transformation but had not formed construct $V_\beta DJ_\beta$ rearrangements. Like many other Ab-MLV transformants with $V_H DJ_H$ rearrangements, the J_H rearrangements were relatively stable in subclones of these lines although several underwent apparent D_H or V_H replacement events. With respect to the transgenic construct, many subclones showed evidence of continuing D to J_β rearrangements, and a few contained V_β to DJ_β rearrangements (Table 1). These results indicate that, at least in cultured transformed pre-B-cell lines, this rearrangement can occur in B-lineage cells but at a low frequency. Finally, densitometric analyses of the relative level of construct DJ_β rearrangements in the pre-B-cell lines versus purified pre-B cells indicates that most differentiating normal pre-B cells form some construct DJ_β rearrangements (not shown).

Expression of the Microinjected V_β Gene

The flanking sequences of the various exons of the constructs contained elements such as the V_β-associated promotor elements and the V_β-, J_β-, C_μ-associated processing signals that are theoretically suf-

ficient to produce TCRβ/Ig-C_μ hybrid RNA transcripts. Thus, because of the larger size of the C_μ versus C_β coding region, we anticipated that $V_\beta DJ_\beta$ construct rearrangements should generate approximately 2.7-kb and 2.4-kb $V_\beta DJ_\beta C_\mu$ transcripts that are readily distinguishable from the 1.3-kb endogenous $V_\beta DJ_\beta C_\beta$ transcripts. To test for transgene expression, total RNA was prepared from various tissues of transgenic mice and assayed for hybridization to a $V_\beta 14$-specific probe. This probe detected only the endogenous 1.3-kb TCRβ transcript (and probable precursors) in the thymus, lymph nodes (T-cell-rich lymphoid organs), and (at a lower level) in the spleen of normal (C57Bl/ $6 \times$ CBA/J)F_2 mice (not shown) or E_μ^- transgenic mice (for example, see Fig. 4, line 1016, lanes 4, 1, and 2, respectively). In contrast, additional V_β-hybridizing transcripts that had the size predicted for the $V_\beta DJ_\beta C_\mu$ transcripts were present in RNA from the thymus, spleen, and lymph nodes, but generally not in bone marrow and not in nonlymphoid tissues, of all E_μ^+ transgenic lines (Fig. 4, lines 379 and 382 and lanes 6–15). These transcripts were also produced in cell lines that had formed a complete V region within the transgene including the T7 Ab-MLV-transformed T cells (lane 16) and at a lower level in subclones of the Ab-MLV-transformed pre-B-cell lines F_{12} and F_{18} (not shown). Notably, the relative abundance of the transgene transcripts as compared with endogenous V_β-hybridizing transcripts was higher in RNA from peripheral lymphoid organs (lymph nodes and spleen) than in the thymus (Fig. 4, compare lanes 6 and 11 and 7 and 12 with lanes 9 and 14).

These results indicate that, similar to the assembly of normal endogenous TCR genes, assembly of complete $V_\beta DJ_\beta$ genes in transgenic T cells led to accumulation of complete TCRβ V-region-containing transcripts.

Table 1. Construct TCRβ and Endogenous IgH Rearrangements in the Ab-MLV Pre-B-cell Lines

Ab-MLV pre-B cell lines and subclones	DJ_β rearrangement[a]	Continued DJ_β rearrangement[b]	$V_\beta DJ_\beta$ rearrangement[a]	J_H rearrangement[c]	Continued J_H rearrangement[c]	5' D probe[d]	Interpretation of the rearrangements[e] construct	endogenous
$F_{12.p}$	+		−	+/+		+/−	DJ_β	DJ_H–$V_H DJ_H$
$11 \times F_{12}$ subclone	+	+	−	+/+	−	+/−	add. DJ_β	DJ_H–$V_H DJ_H$
$1 \times F_{12}$ subclone	+	−	+	+/+	−	+/−	V_β	DJ_H–$V_H DJ_H$
$1 \times F_{12}$ subclone	+	+	−	+/+	+	+/−	add. DJ_β	DJ_H–V_H repla.
$1 \times F_{12}$ subclone	+	−	−	+/+	+	+/−	DJ_β	D_H repla.-$V_H DJ_H$
$F_{18.p}$	+		−	+		−	DJ_β	$V_H DJ_H$
$10 \times F_{18}$ subclone	+	−	−	+	−	−	DJ_β	$V_H DJ_H$
$1 \times F_{18}$ subclone	+	+	−	+	−	−	add. D_β	$V_H DJ_H$
$2 \times F_{18}$ subclone	+	−	+	+	−	−	V_β	$V_H DJ_H$
$1 \times F_{18}$ subclone	+	−	−	+	+	−	DJ_β	V_H repla.

[a] Construct rearrangements were determined as in Fig. 2.

[b] Continued DJ_β rearrangements were determined by comparing the intensities of the unrearranged and DJ_β-containing BglII fragments in the parent lines ($F_{12.p}$ and $F_{18.p}$) and in the derived subclones.

[c] J_H rearrangements were determined by Southern analysis transfers of EcoRI-restricted genomic DNA with a J_H probe; only one IgH allele was detectable in cell line F_{18}.

[d] 5' DSP.2 and 5' DFL.16 probes were hybridized to the Southern blots described in the third footnote to distinguish DJ rearrangements from VDJ rearrangements (Alt et al. 1984).

[e] (DJ_β and V_β) Constructs DJ_β and $V_\beta DJ_\beta$ joinings respectively, were determined as in the first footnote. (Add DJ_β) Additional DJ_β joinings within the construct as determined in the second footnote (DJ_H and VDJ_H) DJ and VDJ joinings, respectively, at the endogenous IgH locus were determined as in the third and fourth footnotes. (D_H repla., V_H replac.) D and V replacements, respectively, at one of the rearranged endogenous IgH alleles as determined in the third footnote and the fourth footnote.)

197

$V_\beta 14$ is the sole member of a proximal TCR V_β gene family that actually lies in inverted orientation downstream from the C_β locus (Malissen et al. 1986); proximal IgH V genes are preferentially expressed (because of preferential rearrangement) in primary B-cell differentiation organs, but their expression levels are normalized in the periphery (Yancopoulos et al. 1988). Correspondingly, relative to the transgenic $V_\beta 14$-containing transcripts, endogenous $V_\beta 14$-containing transcripts occurred at lower abundance in peripheral lymphoid tissue than in thymus tissue (Fig. 4). One explanation for this phenomenon is that mechanisms that work to normalize the normal TCR repertoire do not operate with respect to the hybrid transcript, suggesting that this transcript is innocuous regarding normal T-cell physiology. Although we found that productive $V_\beta DJ_\beta$ rearrangements are formed in the thymus of the transgenic mice (see above), we are so far unable to detect the corresponding proteins in either transgenic tissues or cell lines. It is possible that the hybrid protein may be actively degraded. In general, no expression or very low expression of the transgenic construct was observed in bone marrow, consistent with the inability of B cells to form complete V_β to DJ_β rearrangements. In addition, the V_β promoter may not

work efficiently in B cells (see below), reducing accumulation of transcripts even in rare B cells that do assemble complete TCRβ V region genes within the construct.

Expression of the Unrearranged $V_\beta 14$ Segment

Expression of germ-line V_H gene segments and the germ-line C_κ locus occurs at or prior to the time of the rearrangement of these loci in a manner consistent with a cause/effect relationship (Van Ness et al. 1981; Yancopoulos and Alt 1985). To assay for the potential expression of the endogenous and transgenic unrearranged $V_\beta 14$ gene segments, total RNA from various tissues of transgenic or control mice and transgenic cell lines was assayed for $V_\beta 14$ RNA expression by S1 nuclease protection assays. The probe employed was composed of 80 bp of the 3' end of the $V_\beta 14$ coding sequence plus 280 bp of adjacent downstream flanking sequences; thus, RNA transcripts from the unrearranged $V_\beta 14$ gene segment should protect 80 bp of the probe from S1 nuclease digestion, whereas transcripts from the unrearranged gene should protect up to 360 bp of this probe (Fig. 5, top and right panel). Hybridization to RNA from the thymus tissues but not bone

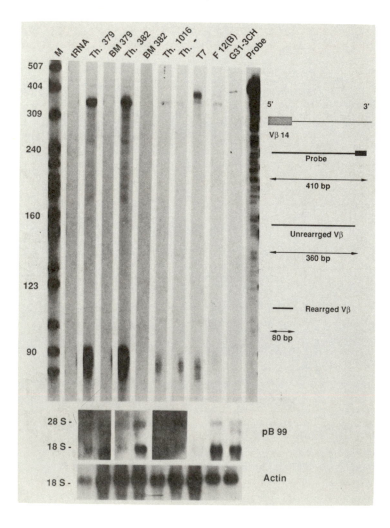

Figure 5. Expression of the $V_\beta 14$ gene. (*Top*) Total RNA (15 μg) from tissues of transgenic mice and from various cell lines was assayed for hybridization to a $V_\beta 14$-specific probe (that comprises 80 bp at the 3' end of the $V_\beta 14$ gene, 280 bp of adjacent downstream sequences, and 50 bp of polylinker plasmid sequences (■) by treatment with S1 nuclease and fractionation on 5% polyacrylamide 7 M urea gels. (*Bottom*) Total RNA was assayed as in Fig. 4 for hybridization to pB99 or actin probes (see text). (Lane *M*) ^{32}P-labeled pBR *Msp*I digest was used as a marker; (lane *tRNA*) 15 μg of yeast tRNA was used as a negative control; (lanes *Th.* and *BM*) total RNA from thymus or bone marrow of transgenic lines 379, 382, 1016, and of nontransgenic (−) mice; (lanes *T7* and *F12[B]*) total RNA from transgenic cell lines T7 (pre-T cell) and F$_{12}$ (pre-B cell); (lane *G31-3CH*) total RNA from an Ab-MLV-transformed cell line transfected with a construct similar to the E$_\mu^+$ construct (Ferrier et al. 1989).

marrow of two separate lines (379 and 382) containing the E_μ^+ construct protected high levels of fragments corresponding to germ-line $V_\beta 14$ transcripts and protected fragments corresponding to the rearranged $V_\beta 14$ gene as well. Significantly, RNA from the thymus of a transgenic line containing the E_μ^- construct (TH.1016) or from the thymus of a nontransgenic line (TH.$^-$) protected very low levels of similar probe fragments (Fig. 5, top and left).

To estimate roughly the relative levels of pre-B cells in the different tissues examined, we assayed each total RNA preparation for hybridization to a DNA probe complementary to a lymphoid-specific RNA sequence preferentially expressed in pre-B as opposed to pre-T cells (pB99, G.D. Yancopoulos et al., in prep.). This analysis indicated that the bone marrow preparations contained substantial amounts of RNA derived from pre-B cells; each preparation was also assayed for hybridization to a β-actin probe to control the amount of RNA assayed (Fig. 5, bottom). Together, these data demonstrate that the unrearranged $V_\beta 14$ gene in the transgenic construct generates substantial levels of steady-state $V_\beta 14$-containing RNA sequences in pre-T- but not pre-B-rich tissues. Germ-line $V_\beta 14$ transcripts are also present at similar low levels in RNA from thymus tissues of nontransgenic animals or transgenic mice containing the E_μ^- construct; thus, the transcripts in both of these types of animals probably arise primarily from the endogenous $V_\beta 14$ gene. Consistent with these results, we found high levels of germ-line $V_\beta 14$ transcripts in T-cell lines from mice harboring the E_μ^+ construct (Fig. 5, T7), but generally we did not detect germ-line $V_\beta 14$ transcripts in pre-B-cell lines (Fig. 5, lane G31-3CH). Also of note, we did detect low levels of germ-line $V_\beta 14$ transcripts in RNA from a pre-B line that generated subclones with a rearranged construct V gene (see Table 1 and Fig. 5, F_{12}).

Initiation of the Rearrangement Process

The accessibility model for control of V region gene assembly predicted existence of *cis*-acting regulatory elements that modulate access of the different antigen receptor loci to the common VDJ recombinase. We now demonstrate that a DNA fragment containing the IgH-chain transcriptional enhancer can serve as a recombinational enhancer. In both B and T lymphoid cells, the presence of this element within transgenic constructs randomly integrated into the mouse genome dominantly targeted associated TCR D_β and J_β gene segments for rearrangement in the majority of normal B and T lymphoid cells. The dominant control exerted by this element was evident by the observation that the E_μ-containing transgene D_β and J_β segments were accessible for recombination in nearly 100% of lymphoid cells, whereas with the construct lacking the E_μ-containing fragment no rearrangements were detected in any cell type. The segment of DNA containing the E_μ element is a complex region of DNA (for review, see Sen and Baltimore 1989). We have not defined the

exact sequences in the E_μ-containing fragment that generate the strong recombinational enhancing activity. However, the E_μ element is functional in both B and T cells (Grosschedl et al. 1984), and it also becomes active early in pre-B-cell development. Thus, the transcriptional enhancing activities of the E_μ element are consistent with the recombinational enhancing activities of the E_μ-containing fragment, suggesting a role for the E_μ element itself in targeting recombination.

Activation of the E_μ element early in B-cell development before the assembly of immunoglobulin V region genes is consistent with the possibility that this element may serve the physiological role of initiating rearrangement at the immunoglobulin J_H locus; other enhancers associated with the IgL and TCR loci may fulfill the enhancement requirements for the normal activation of rearrangement of those gene families. In the latter context, it is notable that the immunoglobulin κ-light-chain enhancer appears to become active during pre-B-cell differentiation at a time corresponding to the onset of κ-light-chain gene rearrangement (Van Ness et al. 1983; Sen and Baltimore 1986; Atchison and Perry 1987). Furthermore, the recombinational enhancing activities that we observe for the E_μ element in T-lineage cells are consistent with the frequent occurrence of immunoglobulin DJ_H joining in cells of this lineage. On the other hand, TCRβ V region gene rearrangements occur less frequently in B-lineage cells (Kronenberg et al. 1986), perhaps reflecting inactivity of the TCRβ enhancer element within B cells (McDougall et al. 1988). However, we clearly demonstrate that direct association of TCRβ D and J segments with an E_μ-containing DNA segment can dominantly abrogate the relative T-cell specificity of this joining event.

Like the mechanism(s) by which the E_μ element activates transcription, the mechanism by which the E_μ-containing DNA fragment enhances recombination remains to be determined. Previous transfection experiments demonstrated that the IgH-chain enhancer (or other known enhancers) need not be present to achieve V gene segment assembly within recombination substrates transfected into pre-B cell lines that express VDJ recombinase activity but only as long as the segments were associated with a transcriptionally active gene. Such experiments exploited recombination substrates that employed immunoglobulin λ-light-chain V and J segments (Fig. 6, construct 1) (Blackwell et al. 1986) or TCRβ D and J segments (Yancopoulos et al. 1986) in association with a transcriptionally activatable (by selection for expressing cells) herpes simplex virus thymidine kinase gene (HSV tk). These findings led to the suggestion that transcriptional activation of a flanking gene may constitute, either directly or indirectly, a recombinational enhancing activity. In this context, a recombination substrate that included the IgH-chain enhancer was not frequently rearranged in pre-B-cell lines except in derivatives in which an associated downstream HSV tk gene was transcribed (Fig. 6, construct

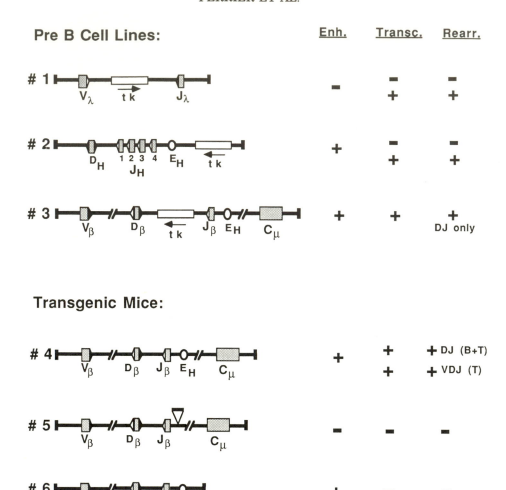

Figure 6. Summary of transfected and transgenic construct rearrangement activities. This figure is described in the text. Details of the analysis of constructs *1* and *2* were described by Blackwell et al. (1986), details of the analysis of construct *3* were described by Ferrier et al. (1989), and details of constructs *4–6* are in this paper.

2) (Blackwell et al. 1986). The latter construct did not contain significant amounts of sequence upstream of or downstream from the enhancer. Together with our current results, this observation may suggest that interaction of the enhancer with other sequences (possibly promoter elements leading to transcription, see below) is required for recombination enhancement activity. In addition, it is possible that these elements must go through normal developmental processes to be activated.

Tissue-specific Control of VDJ Recombinase Activity

We have demonstrated previously that an HSV-*tk*-based recombination substrate otherwise nearly identical in structure to the E_μ-containing transgenic construct (Fig. 6, construct 3) would undergo high-frequency D_β to J_β joining but not V_β to DJ_β joining when transfected into VDJ-recombinase-positive pre-B-cell lines (Ferrier et al. 1989). Because this construct contained both an E_μ element as well as an actively

transcribed *tk* gene, their relative contributions could not be assessed. However, in correlation with their rearrangement activities, the D_β to J_β portion of this construct was in a relatively DNase-I-sensitive region of chromatin when integrated within the pre-B genome, whereas the V_β portion of the construct was in a relatively DNase-I-insensitive region (Ferrier et al. 1989). This finding suggested that pre-B-cell lines may lack factors necessary to activate the V_β portion of the construct for rearrangement. Our current studies have confirmed and extended these observations. Thus, we now show that, although DJ_β rearrangements of E_μ-containing transgenic constructs occur at about equal frequency in T and B cells, V_β to DJ_β rearrangements of the construct are found at high frequency in T-lineage cells but are not found in B cells. Together, our findings indicate that elements other than the IgH enhancer, apparently associated with the TCR V_β region of the construct, can effect V_β to DJ_β joining and thus provide the lineage specificity of $V_\beta DJ_\beta$ assembly. These findings are in accord with the suggestion that the V to DJ joining step is the regulated step in the context of VDJ assembly (Alt et al. 1984, 1987; Uematsu et al. 1988).

Regarding known T-cell-specific elements, the TCRβ enhancer element was not contained within the sequences of the transgenic recombination substrate; therefore, it could not have provided the tissue-specific recombination targeting. Because no V_β rearrangements were detected within the construct lacking the IgH enhancer, the activity of the V_β-specific rearrangement elements appear to be dependent in some way on the presence of the enhancer or the occurrence of the DJ_β-joining event that it promotes. TCRβ promoter elements have also been observed to have relative T-cell specificity (Diamond et al. 1989), suggesting this element as a potential candidate for a recombination control element. In this context, we find transcripts from the unrearranged $V_\beta 14$ gene of the E_μ^+ construct in thymus cells but not in bone marrow of transgenic mice harboring this construct; this transcription pattern directly correlates with the rearrangement of the construct $V_\beta 14$ segment in these tissues (Fig. 6, construct 4). Likewise, we detected no significant level of unrearranged $V_\beta 14$ transcripts in the thymus tissues of mice harboring the E_μ^- construct versus normal control mice; therefore, the activity of the unrearranged $V_\beta 14$ gene segment in the transgenic construct also appears to depend on the presence of the E_μ element or the DJ_β rearrangement it promotes, again directly paralleling the rearrangement activity of the $V_\beta 14$ segment in this construct (Fig. 6, construct 5). The strong correlation between the two activities further suggests that transcriptional activation of the $V_\beta 14$ segment is either directly or indirectly related to its activation for recombination. Transcription and recombination activity have now been associated in the context of site-specific or homologous recombination events in a number of different systems (for review, see Lutzker and Alt 1989).

FUTURE STUDIES

The transgenic recombination substrate system that we have described has certain advantages over the previous cell-culture systems used for analyzing aspects of VDJ recombinase activity. Thus, no selection was employed to introduce the construct into the mouse genome, and no selection for transcription of associated genes was required to activate recombination. In addition, the various regulatory elements included appear to undergo the normal sequence of physiological activation events. Other transgenic substrates that employed murine V_H and DJ_H segments (B. Krippl et al., unpubl.) or rabbit V_κ and J_κ segments (Goodhardt et al. 1987) were rearranged in both B cells and T cells. Transgenic chicken V_λ and J_λ segments were rearranged specifically in murine B cells, but identical constructs present at a higher copy number (20 copies) were rearranged in T cells as well (Bucchini et al. 1987). The difference in specificity between the construct that we now describe and the others probably depends on the structure of individual constructs.

Modifications of our current construct should allow a more precise elucidation of the potential activities of the IgH enhancer and enhancer-associated elements in the initiation of the rearrangement process. For example, preliminary experiments (3 transgenic lines) suggest that deletion of all sequences starting just downstream from the enhancer element from the E_μ-containing construct abrogates the ability of the construct to rearrange in transgenic B or T cells, despite the presence of the E_μ element itself (Fig. 6, construct 6). Additional modifications should also allow definition of the activity of other known elements such as enhancers or transcriptional promoters in promoting this recombination process, perhaps in a tissue- or stage-specific manner. Finally, we note that we have described the IgH enhancer element as necessary to initiate the rearrangement process within the transgenic construct with additional element(s) controlling lineage-specific rearrangement. Clearly, regarding endogenous gene segments, such distinctions may not be as clear. Combinations of various elements likely interact to effect the complex rearrangement patterns observed.

ACKNOWLEDGMENTS

P.F. was a European Molecular Biology Organization fellow and is currently a fellow of the Howard Hughes Medical Institute. T.K.B. was a fellow of the Howard Hughes Medical Institute, and A.J.W.F. is a Jane Coffin Childs fellow. This work was supported by the Howard Hughes Medical Institute and grants from the National Institutes of Health (AI-20047 and CA-40427) to F.W.A. and a P.E.W. Scholars Award to F.C.

REFERENCES

Alt, F.W., T.K. Blackwell, and G.D. Yancopoulos. 1987. Development of the primary antibody repertoire. *Science* **238:** 1079.

Alt, F.W., N. Rosenberg, S. Lewis, E. Thomas, and D. Baltimore. 1981. Organization and reorganization of immunoglobulin genes in A-MuLV-transformed cells: Rearrangement of heavy but not light chain genes. *Cell* **27:** 381.

Alt, F.W., G.D. Yancopoulos, T.K. Blackwell, C. Wood, E. Thomas, M. Boss, R. Coffman, N. Rosenberg, S. Tonegawa, and D. Baltimore. 1984. Ordered rearrangement of immunoglobulin heavy chain variable region segments. *EMBO J.* **3:** 1209.

Atchison, M.L. and R.P. Perry. 1987. The role of the κ enhancer and its binding factor NF-κB in the developmental role of κ gene transcription. *Cell* **48:** 121.

Blackwell, T.K., M.W. Moore, G.D. Yancopoulos, H. Suh, S. Lutzker, E. Selsing, and F.W. Alt. 1986. Recombination between immunoglobulin variable region gene segments is enhanced by transcription. *Nature* **324:** 585.

Bucchini, D., C.-A. Reynaud, M.-A. Ripoche, H. Grimal, J. Jami, and J.-C. Weill. 1987. Rearrangement of a chicken immunoglobulin gene occurs in the lymphoid lineage of transgenic mice. *Nature* **326:** 409.

Cook, W.D. 1985. Thymocyte subsets transformed by Abelson murine leukemia virus. *Mol. Cell. Biol.* **5:** 390.

Costantini, F. and E. Lacy. 1981. Introduction of rabbit β-globin gene into the mouse germ line. *Nature* **294:** 92.

Davis, M.M. and P.J. Bjorkman. 1988. T-cell antigen receptor genes and T-cell recognition. *Nature* **334:** 395.

Desiderio, S.V. and K.R. Wolff. 1988. Rearrangement of exogenous immunoglobulin V_H and DJ_H gene segments after retroviral transduction into immature lymphoid cell lines. *J. Exp. Med.* **167:** 372.

Diamond, D.J., F.B. Nelson, and E.L. Reinherz. 1989. Lineage-specific expression of a T cell receptor variable gene promotor controlled by upstream sequences. *J. Exp. Med.* **169:** 1213.

Early, P., H. Huang, M. Davis, K. Calane, and L. Hood. 1980. An immunoglobulin heavy chain variable region gene is generated from three segments of DNA: V_H, D, J_H. *Cell* **19:** 981.

Ferrier, P., L.C. Covey, H. Suh, A. Winoto, L. Hood, and F.W. Alt. 1989. T cell receptor DJ but not VDJ rearrangement within a recombination substrate introduced into a pre-B cell line. *Int. Immunol.* **1:** 66.

Foster, A., M. Hobart, H. Hengartner, and T.H. Rabbitts. 1980. An immunoglobulin heavy chain gene is altered in two T cell clones. *Nature* **286:** 897.

Gascoigne, N.R.J., Y. Chien, D.M. Becker, J. Kavaler, and M.M. Davis. 1984. Genomic organization and sequence of T-cell receptor β-chain constant- and joining-region genes. *Nature* **310:** 387.

Goodhardt, M., P. Cavelier, M.A. Akimenko, G. Lutfalla, G. Babinet, and F. Rougeon. 1987. Rearrangement and expression of rabbit immunoglobulin κ light chain gene in transgenic mice. *Proc. Natl. Acad. Sci.* **84:** 4229.

Grosschedl, R., D. Weawer, D. Baltimore, and F. Costantini. 1984. Introduction of a μ immunoglobulin gene into the mouse germ line: Specific expression in lymphoid cells and synthesis of functional antibody. *Cell* **38:** 647.

Hokama, Y. and R. Nakamura, eds. 1982. The immune system: Cellular basis. In *Immunology and immunopathology*, p. 1. Little Brown, Boston.

Kemp, D.J., A.W. Harris, S. Cory, and J.M. Adams. 1980. Expression of the immunoglobulin C_μ gene in mouse T and B lymphoid and myeloid cell lines. *Proc. Natl. Acad. Sci.* **77:** 2876.

Kincade, P.W. 1987. Experimental models for understanding B lymphocyte formation. *Adv. Immunol.* **41:** 181.

Krimpenfort, P., R. de Jong, Y. Uematsu, Z. Dembic, S. Ryser, H. von Boehmer, M. Steinmetz, and A. Berns. 1988. Transcription of T cell receptor β-chain genes is controlled by a downstream regulatory element. *EMBO J.* **7:** 745.

Kronenberg, M., G. Siu, L. Hood, and N. Shastri. 1986. The molecular genetics of the T-cell antigen receptor and T-cell antigen recognition. *Annu. Rev. Immunol.* **4:** 529.

Kurosawa, Y., H. von Boehmer, W. Hass, and J.M. Adams. 1981. Identification of D segments of immunoglobulin heavy chain genes and their rearrangements in T lymphocytes. *Nature* **290:** 565.

Lenon, G.G. and R.P. Perry. 1986. C_μ-containing transcripts initiate heterogeneously within the IgH enhancer region and contain a novel 5'-nontranslatable exon. *Nature* **318:** 475.

Lieber, M.R., J.E. Hesse, K. Mizuuchi, and M. Gellert. 1987. Developmental stage specificity of the lymphoid V(D)J recombination activity. *Genes Dev.* **1:** 751.

Lutzker, S. and F.W. Alt. 1989. Immunoglobulin heavy chain class switching. In *Mobile DNA* (ed. D.E. Berg and M.M. Howe), p. 691. American Society for Microbiology, Washington, D.C.

Malissen, M., C. McCoy, D. Blanc, J. Trucy, C. Devaux, A.M. Schmitt-Verhulst, F. Fitch, L. Hood, and B. Malissen. 1986. Direct evidence for chromosomal inversion during T-cell receptor β-gene rearrangements. *Nature* **319:** 28.

McDougall, S., C.L. Peterson, and K. Calame. 1988. A transcriptional enhancer 3' of the $C_{\beta 2}$ in the T cell receptor β locus. *Science* **241:** 205.

Okazaki, K., D.D. Davis, and H. Sakano. 1987. T cell receptor β gene sequences in the circular DNA of thymocyte nuclei: Direct evidence for intramolecular DNA deletion in V-D-J joining. *Cell* **49:** 477.

Pierce, J.H., P.P. Di Fiore, S.A. Aaronson, M. Potter, J. Pumphrey, A. Scott, and J.N. Ihle. 1985. Neoplastic transformation of mast cells by Abelson-MuLV: Abrogation of IL-3 dependence by an non-autocrine mechanism. *Cell* **41:** 685.

Rosenberg, N. and D. Baltimore. 1976. A quantitative assay for transformation of bone marrow cells by A-MuLV. *J. Exp. Med.* **143:** 1453.

Sakano, H., R. Maki, Y. Kurosawa, W. Roeder, and S Tonegawa. 1980. Two types of somatic recombination are necessary for the generation of complete immunoglobulin heavy chain genes. *Nature* **286:** 676.

Shatz, D.G. and D. Baltimore. 1988. Stable expression of immunoglobulin gene V(D)J recombinase activity by gene transfer into 3T3 fibroblasts. *Cell* **53:** 107.

Sen, R. and D. Baltimore. 1986. Inducibility of κ immunoglobulin enhancer-binding protein NF-κB by a posttranslational mechanism. *Cell* **47:** 921.

———. 1989. Factors regulating immunoglobulin gene transcription. In *Immunoglobulin genes* (ed. T. Honjo et al.), p. 327. Academic Press, New York.

Siu, G., M. Kronenberg, E. Strauss, R. Haars, T.W. Mak, and L. Hood. 1984. The structure, rearrangement and expression of D_β gene segments of the murine T-cell antigen receptor. *Nature* **311:** 344.

Tonegawa, S. 1983. Somatic generation of antibody diversity. *Nature* **302:** 575.

Uematsu, Y., S. Ryser, Z. Dembic, P. Borgulya, P. Krimpenfort, A. Berns, H. von Boehmer, and M. Steinmetz. 1988. In transgenic mice the introduced functional T cell receptor β gene prevents expression of endogenous β genes. *Cell* **52:** 831.

Van Ness, B.G., M. Weigert, C. Coleclough, E.L. Mather, D.E. Kelley, and R.P. Perry. 1981. Transcription of the unrearranged mouse C_κ locus: Sequence of the initiation region and comparison of activity with a rearranged V_κ-C_κ gene. *Cell* **27:** 593.

von Boehmer, H. 1988. The developmental biology of T lymphocytes. *Annu. Rev. Immunol.* **6:** 309.

Winoto, A. and D. Baltimore. 1989. A novel, inducible and T cell-specific enhancer located at the 3' end of the T cell receptor α locus. *EMBO J.* **3:** 729.

Wood, C. and S. Tonegawa. 1980. Diversity and joining segments of mouse Ig H genes are closely linked and in the same orientation. *Proc. Natl. Acad. Sci.* **80:** 3030.

Yancopoulos, G.D. and F.W. Alt. 1985. Developmentally controlled and tissue-specific expression of unrearranged V_H gene segments. *Cell* **40:** 271.

Yancopoulos, G.D., B. Malynn, and F.W. Alt. 1988. Developmentally regulated and strain-specific expression of murine V_H gene families. *J. Exp. Med.* **168:** 417.

Yancopoulos, G.D., T.K. Blackwell, H. Suh, L. Hood, and F.W. Alt. 1986. Introduced T cell receptor variable region gene segments recombine in pre-B cells: Evidence that B and T cells use a common recombinase. *Cell* **44:** 251.

The Role of Idiotypic Interactions and B-cell Subsets in Development of the B-cell Repertoire

J.F. Kearney, M. Vakil, and N. Solvason
Division of Developmental and Clinical Immunology, Department of Microbiology and the Comprehensive Cancer Center, University of Alabama at Birmingham, Birmingham, Alabama 35294

In mammals, T and B lymphocytes develop from precursor pluripotent stem cells along separate lineages. As they differentiate, they express lineage as well as differentiation stage-specific surface markers. T and B cells recognize antigen via T-cell receptor (TCR) or immunoglobulin (Ig) molecules, respectively. Both of these consist of two distinct polypeptide chains, which in turn contain variable (V) and constant (C) domains. The genes encoding the V and C domains are separate and occur in clusters in the germ line. During differentiation, the rearrangement and juxtaposition of two or three of such genetic elements results in the expression of functional mRNA for individual polypeptides. Although a large number of gene segments encoding V, diversity (D), and joining (J) region of the polypeptides are available in the germ line for each polypeptide, only one functional immunoglobulin or TCR molecule is synthesized in a lymphocyte. This leads to diversity in the lymphocyte receptor repertoire.

Analysis of V region gene usage in the immunoglobulin heavy chains in the expressed B-cell repertoire in inbred strains of mice suggests that the recombination of V region elements occurs in a random manner. This mechanism ensures the availability of a highly diverse B-cell repertoire in adult mice. However, in recent studies, it has become clear that early on during development the mouse B-cell repertoire is highly restricted owing to the predominant expression of D_H proximal V_H genes, i.e., those contained in the V_H7183 and V_H Q52 families (Yancopoulis et al. 1987, 1988; Perlmutter et al. 1985). A similar preponderance of genes from the V_HIII family has been detected in cDNA libraries made from human fetal livers of 15 and 18 weeks of gestation. Although this V_H gene family is not the most D_H proximal on human chromosome 14, the gene segments exhibit a high degree of homology ($>90\%$) with the mouse V_H7183 genes. Preliminary studies on the immunoglobulin κ-light-chain genes have revealed that certain V_κ genes are selectively and frequently expressed early in development in both mice and humans (LeJeune et al. 1982; Hillson et al. 1989; Lawler et al. 1989).

Diversity in the TCR$\alpha\beta$-bearing T cells as a function of age has not been analyzed to date. However, the TCR$\gamma\delta$-bearing T cells depict a much more regulated pattern of expression for each of the various γ and δ V genes elements (see Tonegawa et al., this volume). Furthermore, sequence analysis of TCRγ and δ genes

rearranged and expressed during the first wave of thymocyte development in mice (13–15 days of embryogenesis) suggests that the joining sites of these genes lack the N segments, which are formed by extra nucleotides, a characteristic of all $\alpha\beta$ and adult $\gamma\delta$ T cells in humans and mice (Gregoire et al. 1978; Asarnow et al. 1988; McConnell et al. 1989). Similarly, although there is not yet sizable sequence data on immunoglobulin heavy- and light-chain genes expressed early during ontogeny, limited analysis suggests that N-region diversity and somatic hypermutation may also be absent in B cells during this stage of development (see Coutinho et al., this volume). Thus, there appears to be a bias in the molecular events at the immunoglobulin and TCR gene loci during lymphocyte ontogeny, which ensures limited heterogeneity in the expressed repertoire.

A careful and detailed analysis of the expressed B-cell repertoire in fetal and newborn mice was conducted following construction of B-cell hybridomas. It was found that a high proportion of perinatal B cells produce immunoglobulin with reactivity to self-antigens, among them immunoglobulin idiotypes (Holmberg et al. 1984; Vakil and Kearney 1986). A correlation between expression of V_H genes from V_H7183 family and autoreactivity was arrived at in two different laboratories (Holmberg et al. 1984; Vakil et al. 1986). Much of the autoreactivity appears to be idiotype-directed, and therefore the perinatal B-cell repertoire is notably restricted but highly interconnected.

Another characteristic of the perinatal B cells is that a large number of these express the CD5 antigen characteristic of a putative subset of B cells described by Herzenberg and Stall (this volume). Whereas CD5$^+$ B cells predominate early in development, it is the CD5$^-$ "conventional" B cells that appear to expand rapidly with increasing age. In adult mice, CD5$^+$ B cells localize predominantly in the peritoneal cavity ($>50\%$ of B cells) and may be found in the spleen ($<2–3\%$ of B cells), and they are absent from lymph nodes and blood.

We and other investigators have proposed that the conserved nature of the early B-cell repertoire serves a function other than defense against environmental pathogens. Our hypothesis contends that the mutual interactions observed between the early appearing subset of CD5$^+$ B cells and later appearing "conventional" B cells via immunoglobulin idiotypes serves to prime the development of B cells and that such interactions are essential to the acquisition of a mature B-cell repertoire. It follows therefore that either positive or negative interference with these CD5$^+$ B cells early in development will have long-lasting effects on the specificity repertoire that are not overcome by new B cells generated from the bone marrow at later stages. In essence, the developing immune system appears to undergo a process of learning whereby interactions through immunoglobulin receptors are involved in the development of the B-cell repertoire at this early stage. It is much more difficult to alter permanently or to modify the imprinted repertoire of adult mice by extraneous agents.

Interconnectivity

Idiotype-directed B-cell cascades. We and other investigators have constructed hybridomas from perinatal B cells of BALB/c mice and have shown that they represent B cells that are highly connected via idiotypic interactions (Holmberg et al. 1984; Vakil and Kearney 1986). Similar reactivities are rarely detected in hybridomas made from unstimulated splenic B cells from adult mice. Thus, this specificity repertoire is characteristic of the early perinatal period. We also noted that a certain idiotope defined by an IgG antibody (FD5-1) previously made against the DNP-binding plasmacytoma protein M460 is expressed by a large number of perinatal IgM antibodies (Vakil and Kearney 1986). Although the structural correlates of this idiotope have not been determined, administration of this IgG1 antibody in utero or early in perinatal life permitted the functional inactivation of certain of the early B cells. We were then able to analyze the effects of this treatment on the overall development of B cells, as well as the specific effects on the repertoire, in particular the clonally dominant responses induced by thymus-independent antigens such as phosphorylcholine (PC) and $\alpha 1 \rightarrow 3$ dextran (DEX) (Blomberg et al. 1972; Lieberman et al. 1974).

Two findings were notable. First, treatment in utero with FD5-1 antibody had a permanent effect on the number of clonable B cells (Kearney et al. 1989). These results suggest that there has been a functional deletion of a subset of B cells, which apparently is not replaced by B-cell lymphopoiesis in bone marrow as the mice mature. Similar results have been obtained by early treatment of F$_1$ mice with an antiallotype antibody specific for one of the parental allotypes that results in permanent depletion of CD5$^+$ B cells of the allotype (L. Herzenberg and A. Stall, this volume). Our results may be due to a permanent depletion of a population of CD5$^+$ B cells expressing the FD5-1 idiotope early in life, which are not replenished by the bone marrow.

More striking effects were seen in specific antibody responses to PC and DEX following treatment with this particular antibody. These results have been published previously and showed that administration of FD5-1

antibody in utero or at times after birth indirectly affected the responses to PC and DEX in an idiotype-specific manner. The timing of administration was critical and related to the normal developmental appearance of precursors specific for PC and DEX (Vakil et al. 1986). As discussed previously, we propose that the early appearing set of B cells (expressing the FD5-1 idiotype) are involved in activation and/or expansion of subsets of T15$^+$-PC- and J558$^+$-DEX-specific B cells that arise later in development. In related experiments, IgM antiidiotype antibodies were also isolated from hybridomas made from unstimulated perinatal B cells. In contrast with IgG antibodies, the IgM antibody, if administered at appropriate times, produced a direct effect of expansion of these PC- and DEX-specific precursors. B cells expressing these IgM antiidiotype antibodies themselves appeared to depend on normal development of the early FD5$^+$ subset of B cells (Vakil and Kearney 1986).

These results were the first to demonstrate that the extensive interconnectivity observed in the perinatal B-cell repertoire plays a functional role in establishing the adult B-cell repertoire (Vakil and Kearney 1986; Vakil et al. 1986). Interference with this proposed interconnectivity by functional inactivation of the earliest appearing B cells results in a permanent loss of specific clones of B cells, and the deficit does not appear to be made up as the animal matures.

Effects of passive administration of idiotype. It has been shown previously in many laboratories that neonatal exposure to antiidiotypic monoclonal antibodies made by conventional immunization procedures and specific for known germ-line-encoded idiotypes such as J558 and TEPC-15 will permanently deplete B cells expressing those idiotypes from the adult B-cell repertoire (Weiler et al. 1977; Pollok et al. 1984; Köhler et al. 1985). This has been shown to occur by a depletion of those cells (Pollok et al. 1984), and it seems likely that the mechanism involved is the exquisite sensitivity of neonatal B cells to cross-linking of their immunoglobulin receptors by IgG antiidiotype antibodies (Raff et al. 1975; Cambier et al. 1976).

If, as proposed above, idiotype interactions between secreted IgM and/or receptor IgM is the driving force behind expansion of certain B-cell clones, then administration of idiotype-bearing immunoglobulin may be expected to interfere with these interactions. Neonatal administration of immunoglobulin bearing the T15 idiotype at critical periods of perinatal life produced a subsequent severe depression of that idiotype in adult mice immunized with PC. This effect could also be transferred transplacentally to some degree by T15$^+$ IgG antibodies. More importantly, the same effect was produced by a mutant molecule of T15 (U10) that has a change in one amino acid in the V$_H$ so that the antibody no longer binds to PC but still expresses the T15 idiotype (M. Vakil et al., in prep.). These observations add to the findings from experimental manipulations of the developmental B-cell cascade outlined above. Administration of purified idiotype-bearing immunoglobulin interferes with the idiotype-related interactions, prevents the normal expansion or selection of these B-cell clones, and results in greatly depressed responses to these antigens both with respect to antigen-specific and T15-idiotype-bearing antibody. These results appear to contrast with those described previously in another idiotype-antigen system where administration of idiotype A48 or anti-Id A48 promotes the development of levan-specific B-cell clones expressing this idiotype. This situation is different in that the A48-positive clones of B cells are not normally expressed in the B-cell repertoire, a so-called silent idiotype (Hiernaux et al. 1981; Rubinstein et al. 1982). The mechanisms of induction of A48 Id may thus be much different from mechanisms involved in expression of dominant idiotypes such as T15 and J558.

Effects of perinatal-antigen-administration and B-cell repertoire development. Mice and humans show a characteristic programmed ability to respond to certain antigens. This paradoxical temporal acquisition of the ability to respond to different antigens is particularly evident when antibody responses to certain bacterial antigens are studied. The ability to respond to haptens, such as oxazalone and dinitrophenol, occurs during fetal development, whereas the ability to respond to PC, DEX, and levan does not appear until after birth (Klinman and Press 1975; Peltola et al. 1977; Sigal and Klinman 1978; Pincus et al. 1982 Stohrer and Kearney 1984). This is of interest as a paradox in relation to the ability of the V_H and V_L genes involved in these responses to undergo much earlier rearrangements and expression as B-cell receptors. It is also of practical importance since this delay in ability to respond to polysaccharide antigens makes the human infant particularly vulnerable to certain bacterial infections, such as *Hemophilus influenzae*, and staphylococcal infections. It was of interest then to determine whether administration of antigens in the early perinatal period would modulate the developmental patterns we have observed and whether in fact neonatal administration of antigen would be an effective way of hastening the development of B-cell clones able to respond to these antigens and hence provide protective immunity.

Newborn mice were treated with PC in the form of heat-killed bacterial vaccine R36A or purified C-polysaccharide and, after a rest period, were challenged with PC or DEX. Mice treated with PC at 2 days of age had a greatly increased response to vaccine when challenged as adults. However, the response largely lacked the T15 idiotype, which is normally dominant in BALB/c mice. Thus, neonatal treatment with PC dramatically increases the PC response but at the expense of the T15 idiotype. It has been shown previously that T15-idiotype-bearing antibody is much more highly protective against infections with virulent *Streptococcus pneumoniae*. These experiments suggest that attempts to hasten the development of protective immunity in neonates should be directed toward expanding or selecting the clones of B cells that express idiotypes of protective immunoglobulin, rather than indiscriminately expanding all PC-specific B-cell clones. On the basis of the observed interconnectivity and cascade of interactions between B cells, which we propose shapes the adult B-cell repertoire, we sought means to promote or exaggerate the idiotype-directed expansion of T15 B cells by deliberately immunizing with the hapten oxazalone coupled to type-I T-independent antigen brucella abortus (BA). B cells with natural anti-Id activity bind oxazalone (as do many of the first appearing B cells) (Kearney and Vakil 1986). Accordingly, mice were injected with OX-BA at 2 days after birth and then rested for 6 weeks and then were challenged with the heat-killed R36A. Mice treated this way had greatly elevated total anti-PC responses nearly all of which expressed the normally dominant idiotype T15. These results stand in marked contrast with the results obtained by neonatal exposure to PC vaccine and suggest that by appropriate deliberate manipulation of the idiotype-directed interactions that we propose normally occur during development, it is possible to enhance selectively the development of B cells expressing the protective idiotype T15. These results have a bearing on the development of neonatal vaccines in humans and may eventually be a suitable way of enhancing neonatal immunity to certain polysaccharides since the perinatal repertoire of antibodies of fetal and neonatal humans appears to be extremely restricted in the V_H and V_L genes used (Schroeder et al. 1988), and it may be possible to identify the specificities of these interconnected human immunoglobulin.

These experiments also revealed another phenomenon that would have been predicted from in vitro demonstrations of connectivity. Mice that were treated at 2 days of age with R36A and challenged with DEX as adults showed a complete ablation of the response to DEX, which is normally a strong antigen and induces large amounts of λ-bearing antibody expressing the J558 idiotype. Thus, it can be seen that not only did immunization with R36A or pneumococcal C-polysaccharide fail to induce T15-positive protective antibody-producing B cells but, by virtue of the interconnectivity described in the neonatal period, eliminated functional anti-DEX B cells.

These experiments augment the findings of the previously described experiments where various manipulations of the neonatal mice produced long-lasting effects on the target B-cells and support our hypothesis that certain early appearing B-cell clones are essential elements in shaping the adult repertoire. These B cells are characterized by restricted heterogeneity and specificities and appear to be essential components of the developing immune system.

Developmental Aspects of B Cells

Most of the developing B cells in the fetal liver and neonatal spleen express the CD5 antigen that is expressed not only on T cells, but also by a subset of B cells developmentally distinct from CD5$^-$ B cells (Kearney et al. 1989; Kerr et al., this volume). There is considerable evidence, summarized in this volume by L. Herzenberg and colleagues (Kerr et al.), which supports a separate lineage for these cells and, more pertinent to this discussion, which suggests that they have different functional characteristics among which is a high degree of autoreactivity of antibodies secreted by these cells. Since we propose that such self-interactions between idiotypes shape the B-cell repertoire, we have sought to determine the developmental sites of origin of this apparent separate lineage of CD5$^+$ B cells, with the eventual goal of analyzing V_H and V_L genes and all specificities of IgM produced by the first B cells developing in the fetus during in utero life.

To this end, we have transplanted a variety of fetal tissues and examined their capacity to reconstitute Ly-1 B cells. Thirteen-day gestation, fetal (C57BL/6 × BALB/c) F$_1$ liver, spleen, thymus, bone (femur and tibia), or omentum were transplanted into CB17 mice with the SCID defect (Bosma et al. 1983). These mice were selected as recipients because they carry a heritable defect exemplified by a complete lack of T and B lymphocytes. Omentum was included in this list since previous studies have shown that the omentum in both mice and humans contains organized lymphoid tissue (Holub et al. 1971). These lymphoid aggregates, called milk spots, within the omentum are barely visible in unimmunized mice. However, intraperitoneal injections of certain antigens cause a dramatic increase in cellularity of the milk spots, and antigen-specific antibody responses have been demonstrated in omental tissue (Dux et al. 1977). In addition, transplantation of 13-day-gestation fetal omentum into the anterior eye chamber of mice gave rise to donor-derived, dull Thy-1$^+$ lymphocytes (Kubai and Auerbach 1983). In these studies, it was not possible to identify the Thy-1$^+$ lymphocytes as B and/or T cells since no lineage-specific markers stained these cells. Interestingly, it was also reported that a small but consistent population of the cells was CD5$^+$ (Kubai and Auerbach 1983). Because of the anatomical location of the omentum within the peritoneal cavity where the largest numbers of CD5$^+$ B cells are found and the precedence of the omentum as a potential source of lymphocytes, we included the omentum in the transplantation experiments.

After transplant (4 months) of the various fetal primordia, the transplant recipient SCID mice were sacrificed, and the spleen, lymph nodes, and peritoneal cells were analyzed by flow cytometry for the presence of donor-derived T and B cells using anti-H2 antibodies in conjunction with anti-T3 and anti-IgM, respectively. Antiallotype antibodies were also used to identify donor-derived B cells and to quantitate donor IgM in the serum.

Liver-transplanted mice, as expected, had normal proportions of B and T cells in all lymphoid organs tested. The mouse that received the omentum transplant had donor-derived B cells, however, no T-cell reconstitution was evident. The mice with fetal spleen and bone had no detectable donor-derived lymphocytes. Additionally, in the peritoneal cavity of the mice with liver and omentum transplants almost 95% of the cells were donor in origin, and in each mouse approximately 40% of the B cells were clearly CD5$^+$. This is in contrast with the spleen of these same mice with liver and omentum transplants where CD5$^+$ B cells were essentially undetectable (Kearney et al. 1989; Solvason and Kearney 1989).

Serum analysis demonstrated the presence of donor-derived IgM in the mice with omentum and liver transplants. Interestingly, the mouse with omentum transplants had no detectable IgG1, however IgG2a, IgG2b, and IgG3 were present. This is in contrast with the mouse with the liver transplant that had high levels of IgG1, IgG2a, IgG2b, and IgG3.

These results clearly demonstrate that the omentum is a source of B cells, some of which are CD5$^+$, and that these B cells can migrate into the host lymphoid system. It should be stressed that CD5$^+$ B cells were found only in the peritoneal cavity, and it is interesting that the same percentage of CD5$^+$ B cells were found in the mouse that received the fetal omentum as the mouse that received the fetal liver. The spleen and lymph nodes of the mouse with omentum contained donor B cells that were all CD5$^-$, therefore it would be incorrect to think of the omentum as a source of exclusively CD5$^+$B cells. It will be of great interest to compare the functional characteristics of the splenic B cells derived from omentum to that in a normal adult mouse.

The fact that the fetal liver as well as omentum reconstitutes CD5$^+$ B cells raises the question as to the significance of the omentum in terms of its contribution to the developing repertoire in vivo. It is of interest that the omentum is a serous membrane formed by the back-to-back fusion of the mesodermally derived lining of the peritoneal cavity. Several reports have now documented the presence of an early intraembryonic source of lymphocytes (Dieterlen-Lievre 1987; Ogawa et al. 1988). In chickens, the presence of diffuse hematopoiesis in the intraembryonic mesoderm has been documented, and, furthermore, chicken-quail yolk sac chimera experiments have demonstrated the intraembryonic source of these cells. Thus, in our experiments, the omentum may represent a site in the peritoneal cavity where it is possible to isolate this mesodermal tissue. This lining also surrounds the liver so that transplantation of liver fragments probably also results in transfer of tissue similar or identical to the omentum. Although it seems initially that there are two sources of CD5$^+$B cells (the fetal liver and omentum), it may be in fact that this B-cell subset originates from the mesodermally derived lining of the peritoneal cavity, which is always transplanted in fetal liver fragments or cell suspensions. It will now be of great interest to determine if and how the omentally derived B cells differ from bone-marrow-derived B cells and perhaps to understand further how this B-cell subset interacts with conventional B cells to form an intact immune system.

ACKNOWLEDGMENTS

We acknowledge the patience of Ann Brookshire for the preparation of this manuscript and Peter Burrows for his criticisms. This work has been supported by National Institutes of Health grants CA-16673, CA-13148, and AI-14782.

REFERENCES

Asarnow, D.M., W.A. Kuziel, M. Bonyhadi, R.E. Tigelaar, P.W. Tucker, and J.P. Allison. 1988. Limited diversity of $\gamma\delta$ antigen receptor genes of Thy-1$^+$ dendritic epidermal cells. *Cell* **55**: 837.

Blomberg, B., W.R. Geckler, and M. Weigert. 1972. Genetics of the antibody response to dextran in mice. *Science* **177**: 178.

Bosma, G.C., R.P. Custer, and M.J. Bosma. 1983. A severe combined immunodeficiency mutation in the mouse. *Nature* **301**: 527.

Cambier, J.C., J.R. Kettman, E.S. Vitetta, and J.W. Uhr. 1976. Differential susceptibility of neonatal and adult murine spleen cells to *in vitro* induction of B cell tolerance. *J. Exp. Med.* **144**: 293.

Dieterlen-Lievre, F. 1987. Hemopoietic cell progenitors in the avian embryo: Origin and migrations, part II. Genes, development, and differentiation. *Ann. N.Y. Acad. Sci.* **511**: 77.

Dux, K., P. Janik, and B. Szavriawska. 1977. Kinetics of proliferation cell differentiation and IgM secretion in the omental lymphoid organ of B10/Sn mice following intraperitoneal immunization with sheep erythrocytes. *Cell. Immunol.* **32**: 97.

Gregoire, K.E., I. Goldschneider, R.W. Barton, and F.J. Bollum. 1978. Ontogeny of terminal deoxynucleotidyl transferase positive cells in lymphohemopoietic tissues of rat and mouse. *J. Immunol.* **123**: 1347.

Hillson, J.L., H.W. Schroeder, and R.M. Perlmutter. 1989. Development of the human antibody light chain repertoire. *J. Immunol.* (in press).

Hiernaux, J., C. Bona, and P.J. Baker. 1981. Neonatal treatment with low doses of anti-idiotypic antibodies leads to the expression of a silent clone. *J. Exp. Med.* **153**: 1004.

Holmberg, D., S. Forsgren, L. Forni, F. Ivars, and A. Coutinho. 1984. Reactions among IgM antibodies derived from normal neonatal mice. *Eur. J. Immunol.* **14**: 435.

Holub, M., I. Hadju, I. Trebichavsky, and L. Jaroskova. 1971. Formation of lymphoid cells from local precursors in irradiated mouse omenta. *Eur. J. Immunol.* **1**: 465.

Kearney, J.F., N. Solvason, and M. Vakil. 1989. Idiotypes and B cells development. *Prog. Allergy* **48**: (in press).

Klinman, N.R. and J.L. Press. 1975. The characterization of the B cell repertoire specific for the 2,4-dinitrophenol and 2,4,6-trinitrophenol determinants in neonatal BALB/c mice. *J. Exp. Med.* **141**: 1133.

Köhler, H., B.C. Richardson, D.A. Rowley, and S. Smyk. 1985. Immune response to phosphorylcholine. III. Requirement of the Fc portion and equal effectiveness of IgG subclasses in anti-receptor antibody-induced suppression. *J. Immunol.* **119**: 1979.

Kubai, L. and R. Auerbach. 1983. A new source of embryonic lymphocytes in the mouse. *Nature* **301**: 154.

Lawler, A.M., J.F. Kearney, M. Kuehl, and P.J. Gearhart. 1989. Early rearrangements of early immunoglobulin κ genes unlike heavy genes show no positional bias. *Proc. Natl. Acad. Sci.* (in press).

LeJeune, J.M., D.E. Briles, A.R. Lawton, and J.F. Kearney. 1982. Estimate of the light chain repertoire of fetal and adult BALB/cJ and CBA/J mice. *J. Immunol.* **129**: 673.

Lieberman, R., M. Potter, E.B. Mushinski, W. Humphrey, Jr., and S. Rudikoff. 1974. Genetics of a new immunoglobulin V$_H$ (T15 idiotype) marker in the mouse regulating natural antibody to phosphorylcholine. *J. Exp. Med.* **139**: 983.

McConnell, J., W.M. Yokoyama, G.E. Kikuchi, G.P. Einhorn, G. Stingl, E.M. Shevach, and J.E. Coligan. 1989. δ-chains of dendritic epidermal T cell receptors are diverse but pair with γ chains in a restricted manner. *J. Immunol.* **142**: 2924.

Ogawa, M., S. Nishikawa, K. Ikuta, F. Yamamura, M. Naito, K. Takahashi, and S.-I. Nishikawa. 1988. B cell ontogeny in murine embryo studied by a culture system with the monolayer of a stromal cell clone, ST2: B cell progenitor develops first in the embryonal body rather than in the yolk sac. *EMBO J.* **7**: 1337.

Peltola, H., H. Kayhty, A. Sivonen, P.H. Makela. 1977. Hemophilus influenzae in children: A double blind filed study of 100,000 vaccines 3 months to 5 years of age in Finland. *Pediatrics* **60**: 730.

Perlmutter, R.M., J.F. Kearney, S.P. Chang, and L.E. Hood. 1985. Developmentally controlled expression of immunoglobulin V$_H$ genes. *Science* **227**: 597.

Pincus, D.J., D. Morrison, C. Andrews, E. Lawrence, S.H. Sell, and P.F. Wright. 1982. Age-related response to two hemophilus influenzae type b vaccines. *J. Pediatr.* **100**: 197.

Pollok, B.A., J.F. Kearney, and R.S. Stohrer. 1984. Selective alteration of the humoral response to alpha-1→3 dextran and phosphorylcholine by early administration of monoclonal anti-idiotype. In *Idiotypy in biology and medicine* (ed. H. Köhler et al.), p. 187. Academic Press, New York.

Raff, M.C., J.J.T. Owen, M.D. Cooper, A.R. Lawton, M. Megson, and W.E. Gathings. 1975. Differences in susceptibility of mature and immature mouse B lymphocytes to anti-immunoglobulin induced suppression *in vitro*. Possible implications for B cell tolerance to self. *J. Exp. Med.* **142**: 1052.

Rubinstein, L., Y. Ming, and C. Bona. 1982. Idiotype-anti-idiotype regulation. II. Activation of A48Id silent clone by administration at birth of idiotopes is related to activation of A48Id specific helper T cells. *J. Exp. Med.* **156**: 506.

Schroeder, H.W., Jr., J.L. Hillson, and R.M. Perlmutter. 1988. Early restriction of the human antibody repertoire. *Science* **238**: 791.

Sigal, N.H. and N.R. Klinman. 1978. The B-cell clonotypic repertoire. *Adv. Immunol.* **26**: 255.

Solvason, N.W. and J.F. Kearney. 1989. Reconstitution of lymphocyte subsets in scid mice by transplantation of fetal primordia. In *The scid mouse* (ed. M. Bosma and R.A. Phillips). Springer-Verlag, Heidelberg. (In press.)

Stohrer, R. and J.F. Kearney. 1984. Ontogeny of B cell precursors responding to a1→3 dextran in BALB/c mice. *J. Immunol.* **133**: 2323.

Vakil, M. and J.F. Kearney. 1986. Functional characterization of monoclonal autoanti-idiotype antibodies from the early B cell repertoire of BALB/c mice. *Eur. J. Immunol.* **16**: 1151.

Vakil, M., H. Sauter, C. Paige, and J.F. Kearney. 1986. In vivo suppression of perinatal multispecific B cells results in a distortion of the adult B cell repertoire. *Eur. J. Immunol.* **16**: 1159.

Weiler, I.J., E. Weiler, R. Springer, and H. Cosenza. 1977. Idiotype suppression by maternal influence. *Eur. J. Immunol.* **7**: 591.

Yancopoulos, G.D., B.A. Malynn, and F.W. Alt. 1988. Developmentally regulated and strain-specific expression of murine V$_H$ gene families. *J. Exp. Med.* **168**: 417.

Yancopoulos, G.D., S.V. Desiderio, M. Paskind, J.F. Kearney, D. Baltimore, and F.N. Alt. 1984. Preferential utilization of the most J$_H$-proximal gene segments in pre-B cell lines. *Nature* **311**: 727.

Growth and Selection of B Cells In Vivo

K. Rajewsky, H. Gu, P. Vieira,* and I. Förster

Institute for Genetics, University of Cologne, D-5000 Cologne 41, Federal Republic of Germany

B lymphocytes are continuously generated in the organism from stem cells in the bone marrow. Each cell expresses a particular antibody specificity, and this specificity determines the fate of the cell. In this paper, we discuss ways in which this happens: the selection of a stable set of peripheral B cells from newly arising cells, the generation of memory B cells, and the growth and selection of Ly-1 B cells.

METHODS

Analysis of BrdU incorporation. Feeding of mice with 5-bromo-2'-deoxyuridine (BrdU) and flow cytometric detection of BrdU-labeled cells have been described previously (Förster et al. 1989).

Bone marrow chimeric mice. For bone marrow transfer, CB-20 mice were irradiated with 600 rads and reconstituted with 5×10^6 BALB/c bone marrow cells on the following day. Feeding with BrdU (1 mg of BrdU/ml of drinking water) started right after cell transfer.

V_H gene amplification, cloning, and hybridization. Total cellular RNA from 0.5×10^5 to 2×10^5 cells isolated by a fluorescence-activated cell sorter (FACS) was used for cDNA synthesis. Heavy chain variable (V_H) region cDNA was amplified as described by Loh et al. (1989) with modifications, using a primer specific for the μ constant region (C_μ). The amplified cDNA was cloned into a pTZ19(R) vector (Pharmacia). V_H gene hybridization was performed as described by Winter et al. (1985). For detection of V_H genes belonging to the J558 or the 7183 V_H gene family, a 220-bp *Eco*RI/*Sac*I fragment of the VH81X gene (Yancopoulos et al. 1984) or a 254-bp *Hin*fI/*Pst*I fragment of the V186.2 gene (Bothwell et al. 1981) were used as probes. V_H gene sequences were obtained by direct plasmid sequencing using the Sequenase kit (USB Corporation).

RESULTS AND DISCUSSION

Selection of B cells into the Peripheral Immune System

Although there is general agreement that the population of conventional B cells (as opposed to Ly-1 B cells; see below) consists of both short-lived and long-lived

cells, the frequencies of B cells with differing life spans have been a matter of debate over the last decades. Experiments by Röpke and colleagues (Röpke and Everett 1975; Röpke et al. 1975) and other investigators (Robinson et al. 1965; Sprent and Basten 1973), based on the incorporation of [³H]thymidine into the DNA of dividing cells, indicated that the majority of B cells in the spleen, blood, and thoracic duct lymph are long-lived with an estimated life span of weeks or months. Data compatible with this theory have been recently obtained by Gray (1988), who analyzed splenic B cells of rats that had been fed with the thymidine analog BrdU for up to 10 days. In contrast, Press et al. (1977) found that more than half of the splenic B cells of CBA/J mice could be labeled with [³H]thymidine within 4 days. Furthermore, Freitas et al. (1982, 1986) reported that they could deplete most splenic B cells within a couple of days by treating mice with the cytotoxic drug hydroxyurea. A similar depletion was seen in mice transgenic for the herpes simplex thymidine kinase gene under immunoglobulin κ-chain promoter and heavy-chain enhancer control when they were treated with the drug ganciclovir (Heyman et al. 1989). These data suggest that the majority of peripheral B cells are constantly renewed from B-cell precursors in the bone marrow.

In view of this controversy, we have made an attempt to obtain insight into the problem by measuring life spans of various B-cell subsets separately. For this purpose, we used in vivo BrdU-labeling in combination with a technique that allows simultaneous flow cytometric detection of cell-surface markers and BrdU incorporation (Förster et al. 1989). We showed that the bone marrow contains two populations of B cells as defined by differential expression of the pan-B-cell marker B220 (Coffman and Weissman 1981), surface μ and surface δ (Fig. 1). Whereas $B220^{dull}\mu^+\delta^-$ B cells appeared to have a rapid turnover and probably represent B cells newly generated from $B220^{dull}\mu^-$ pre-B cells, $B220^{bright}\mu^+\delta^+$ B cells hardly showed any BrdU incorporation over a period of 1 week. A similar result was obtained for $B220^+\delta^+$ B cells in the spleen, where less than 20% of these cells were labeled within 1 week. This indicates that most splenic B cells are long-lived cells (Förster et al. 1989).

To make sure that the low numbers of BrdU-labeled δ^+ B cells are not due to an artifact in the labeling procedure, it was necessary to confirm that (1) feeding mice with BrdU allows one to label all dividing cells and (2) resting BrdU-labeled cells do not lose the

---

*Present address: DNAX Research Institute, Palo Alto, California 94304-1104.

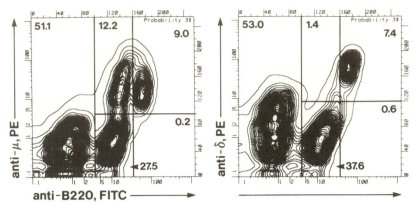

Figure 1. Flow cytometric analysis of normal BALB/c bone marrow cells. Shown are only cells that by light-scatter analysis fell into the "lymphocyte gate" (see Förster et al. 1989). Staining was done with RA3.3A1 fluorescein-isothyocyanate (FITC)-conjugated (anti-B220) and R33-24-12 phycoerythrin (PE) (anti-μ) or 10-4.22 (anti-δ) biotin plus streptavidin-PE. Percentages of cells within the different fluorescence windows are given in the figure. (Modified, with permission, from Förster et al. 1989.)

incorporated BrdU. For this purpose, CB-20 mice were sublethally irradiated and reconstituted with bone marrow cells from normal BALB/c donors. During the time of reconstitution, the mice were continuously fed with BrdU in their drinking water. Under these conditions, all donor-derived lymphocytes, progeny of the grafted bone marrow cells, should be labeled with BrdU. Once BrdU-labeling is stopped, long-lived cells should remain labeled, whereas dividing cells should lose the label.

Figure 2 shows representative fluorescence stainings of bone marrow cells from reconstituted mice that were either continuously treated with BrdU from the time of bone marrow grafting (Fig. 2, middle, weeks 0–15), treated with BrdU for the last 4 weeks before analysis (Fig. 2, left, weeks 11–15), or treated with BrdU for 11 weeks after bone marrow transplantation followed by a chase period of 4 weeks (Fig. 2, right). The stainings

shown in Figure 2 were performed with anti-B220 and anti-BrdU monoclonal antibodies. It is evident from the data that virtually all lymphocytes can be labeled with BrdU following bone marrow reconstitution (Fig. 2., middle) and that the majority of the long-lived B220^{bright} B cells remain BrdU-labeled over a chase period of 4 weeks. A similar result was obtained by staining with a monoclonal antibody specific for immunoglobulin D (IgD) of the donor-allotype (donor-derived IgD-bearing B cells represented 88–96% of all B cells in the chimeric mice with the exception of one mouse that possessed only 71% donor-derived B cells [data not shown]). In contrast, almost all of the B220^{dull} (pre-B and B) cells are unlabeled after the 4-week chase.

In the spleen, about 70% of the B220$^+$ B cells remained labeled with BrdU after the 4-week chase, corresponding to a mean of 34% labeled splenic B cells

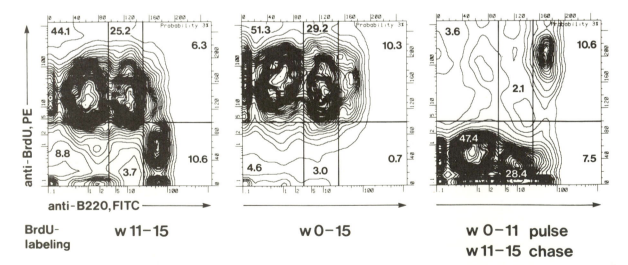

BrdU-labeling   w 11–15   w 0–15   w 0–11 pulse
                                                                 w 11–15 chase

Figure 2. Flow cytometric analysis of BrdU-incorporation in bone marrow cells of CB-20 mice that had been reconstituted with BALB/c bone marrow cells 15 weeks earlier. The periods of treatment of the mice with BrdU are indicated in the figure. Staining was performed with anti-BrdU (PE) (see Förster et al. 1989) and RA3.3A1 FITC (anti-B220). Percentages of cells within the different fluorescence windows refer to cells within the "lymphocyte gate."

after direct BrdU-labeling of the bone-marrow-reconstituted mice over 4 weeks (I. Förster and K. Rajewsky, in prep.). This is in line with the percentage of BrdU-labeled splenic B cells in normal 2–4-month-old BALB/c mice as shown in Figure 3. Taken together, the BrdU-labeling data indicate that the majority of peripheral B cells in the mouse are not rapidly renewed by newcomers from the bone marrow. The argument is particularly strong since we have shown in our previous investigations (Förster et al. 1989) that the pre-B and B cells in the bone marrow from which splenic B cells are derived have a turnover time of only a few days. Accordingly, in the reconstitution experiment described above, these cells are found unlabeled already after a 1-week chase (I. Förster, unpubl.).

Our experiments do not exclude a minor proliferative activity among the cells that exhibit BrdU-labeling throughout the 4-week chase period, but it is clear that essentially these cells represent a compartment of long-lived, stable lymphocytes. Consequently, the dramatic loss of B cells from the spleen of mice treated with cytotoxic drugs (Freitas et al. 1982; Heyman et al. 1989) cannot be explained by rapid B-cell renewal but rather reflects a major distortion of the peripheral immune system, perhaps in response to the massive cell death in the animal.

Does the entry of newly generated B cells into the stable peripheral B-cell pool occur at random, or does it involve selection? Data reported by Malynn et al. (1987) and Freitas et al. (1989) suggest that the V_H gene usage in bone marrow B cells is different from that of splenic B cells. These investigators describe a relative overrepresentation of V_H genes from the 7183 family over members from the J558 gene family (see Brodeur and Riblet 1984; Dildrop 1984) in bone marrow B cells, which correlated to the V_H gene usage in

fetal B cells (Alt et al. 1987). This overrepresentation of 7183 V_H genes in early B cells could be due to preferential rearrangement of V_H genes located most proximal to the diversity (D) region elements in the heavy-chain locus.

On the basis of these findings, we investigated whether V_H gene usage in the two different bone marrow B-cell populations described above, namely the rapidly renewing $B220^{dull}\mu^+\delta^-$ and the long-lived $B220^{bright}\mu^+\delta^+$ B cells, is different in terms of J558 and 7183 V_H gene expression. For this purpose, we isolated $\mu^+\delta^-$ and $\mu^+\delta^+$ B cells from the bone marrow of normal adult BALB/c mice by cell sorting (see Fig. 4). cDNA complementary to rearranged V_H regions transcribed into the mRNA of the cells was then prepared using a primer specific for the C_μ region and amplified with the help of the polymerase chain reaction. The amplified cDNA was used to construct a cDNA library in which the representation of J558 and 7183 V_H genes was determined by hybridization with J558- and 7183-specific probes. We found that the ratio of J558/7183 is more than twofold lower in δ^- compared with δ^+ B cells (Fig. 4). This result suggests that the shift in V_H gene usage observed earlier by others can be traced to the transition from short-lived ($\mu^+\delta^-$) to long-lived ($\mu^+\delta^+$) cells.

Although a more detailed analysis of the V_H gene repertoires expressed in the two cell populations is needed, it appears from the present data that the gener-

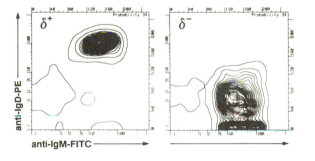

	no. of positive clones		
	V186.2 (J558)	VH81X (7183)	J558/7183
δ^+	30	12	2.5
δ^-	24	22	1.1

Figure 4. Representation of J558 and 7183 V_H genes in δ^+ and δ^- bone marrow B cells. Bone marrow cells from a pool of three 14-week-old BALB/c mice were stained with anti-δ (10-4.22) and anti-μ (R33-24.12). $\mu^+\delta^-$ and $\mu^+\delta^+$ cells were sorted out, partly used for V_H gene cDNA amplification, and partly reanalyzed as shown in the figure. The sorted cells did not contain IgM-plasma cells ($<2 \times 10^{-5}$ to 5×10^{-5}) as tested by cytoplasmic staining with anti-IgM. The results of hybridization with the V186.2 (J558 family) or VH81X probe (7183 family) are given in the table below the graphs. From each library, a total of 110 clones were analyzed, some of which might have contained only DJ rearrangements.

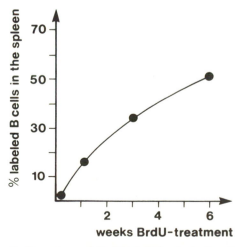

Figure 3. Percentage of BrdU-labeled splenic B cells as a function of time. All data were obtained from BALB/c mice that were 2–4 months of age at the beginning of treatment. At each time point, 2–3 individual mice were analyzed of which mean values are given in the figure (individual values varied by less than 15% from each other).

ation of long-lived B cells involves selection. The mechanism of this selection is obscure at the moment, but, since long-lived B cells are also generated in germ-free animals (Claesson et al. 1974), it may involve recognition of autologous ligands through the antigen receptor in analogy with the selection of T cells in the thymus.

B-cell Selection in Immune Responses: Somatic Hypermutation and Affinity Maturation in the Establishment of B-cell Memory

The processes of B-cell growth and selection discussed in the previous section generate the antibody repertoire from which immune responses evolve. In the course of such responses, subsets of these antibodies are selected on the basis of their specificity for the immunizing antigen.

This selection follows, in primary and secondary antibody responses, the rules of clonal selection (Burnet 1959) in that the repertoire of antibodies expressed in the response preexists at the level of the precursor cells. However, in a particular pathway of differentiation, namely that of memory B-cell generation, a new antibody repertoire is generated through somatic hypermutation and selection of cells expressing antibody mutants with a high affinity for the antigen. We concentrate on this latter pathway below (for review, see Kocks and Rajewsky 1989).

Although the molecular mechanism of somatic hypermutation of antibodies is still unresolved, some basic features of mutant generation and selection have been established: Point mutations are introduced at a high rate (in the order of 1 mutation per cell division) specifically into rearranged V region genes by a mechanism that is induced in B cells responding to a T-cell-dependent antigenic stimulus. This process continues over several, probably many, rounds of cell division. Because of the high mutation rate, the V regions of the antibodies expressed by cells in this differentiation pathway rapidly accumulate heavy loads of mutations.

The process of mutant generation goes hand-in-hand with mutant selection. Selection seems to depend stringently on antigenic stimulation since, in general, only cells expressing high-affinity antibodies "make it" in the selection process. There is direct evidence that somatic mutation accounts for increased antigen-binding affinity. Affinity maturation may be due to a single point mutation (Allen et al. 1987, 1988) or may occur stepwise in the course of clonal expansion, through the stepwise introduction of mutations (Kocks and Rajewsky 1988). As a rule, however, only a fraction of the mutations carried by an antibody contributes to its enhanced antigen-binding affinity.

Affinity Maturation Reflects a General Defense Mechanism against Microbial Infection

What is the physiological significance of antibody mutant generation in the establishment of immunological memory? Clearly, it must be advantageous to generate a set of high-affinity antibodies to come into action in the secondary response. However, affinity matura-

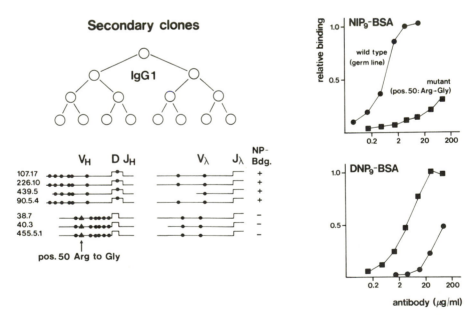

Figure 5. Somatic antibody mutants with changed antigen-binding specificity. The left side of the figure (modified, with permission, from Siekevitz et al. 1987) shows schematically the clonal expansion of a memory B cell in the secondary response. Progeny picked from two such clones exhibit identical patterns of somatic mutations (●, ▲) throughout the heavy- and light-chain variable regions (*left, bottom*). The antibody expressed by the cells of one of the two clones, although generated in response to the hapten NP, does not bind the hapten. It carries an arginine to glycine exchange in position 50 of the heavy chain, which essentially eliminates NP binding and causes enhanced binding to a dinitrophenyl/bovine serum albumin conjugate, when introduced into the germ-line sequences (*right*); NIP = 4-hydroxy-3-nitro-5-iodophenylacetyl behaves like NP in these assays. (Right side of figure modified, with permission, from Brüggemann et al. 1986.)

tion is only one facet of the biological process at which we are looking. Its first principle is the rapid generation of a population of activated B lymphocytes expressing a wide range of somatically mutated antibodies whose wild-type specificity was for the immunizing antigen. This population of cells responds to ligands to which its antibodies best fit, and, consequently, the response to the immunizing antigen is dominated by high-affinity antibodies. Likewise, however, if the antigen itself also undergoes structural changes in the course of the response, the antibody system will be able to adapt rapidly to this situation because the appropriate somatic antibody mutants are generated as well. The generation of somatic antibody mutants is thus the basis of a defense mechanism by which the immune system attempts to cope with microbial mutants, which often arise rapidly in the course of an infection because of the short generation time of the invading microbes. Affinity maturation reflects a key feature of this mechanism, namely the efficiency by which appropriate antibody mutants are recruited and selected.

A model experiment that argues the case is available. In 1987, our group identified within a population of somatic antibody mutants generated, upon immunization with the hapten 4-hydroxy-3-nitrophenylacetyl (NP), a mutant that had lost its NP-binding specificity. This was achieved by transferring NP-primed B cells into irradiated syngeneic recipients and stimulating the transferred cells with an appropriate antiidiotypic antibody instead of NP itself. In this experimental situation, transferred memory cells reactive with the antiidiotype expand to large clones in the absence of further somatic hypermutation. Thus, clonal progeny consisting of identically mutated cells can be isolated from the recipients in the form of hybridomas. It turned out that the cells of one of two clones isolated produced a somatically mutated antibody that, with respect to V region gene usage and the structure of the third complementarity-determining region of the heavy chain, looked like a typical anti-NP antibody but did not bind NP (Siekevitz et al. 1987). Significantly, one of the point mutations carried by the antibodies (an arginine to glycine exchange in position 50 of the heavy chain) had been shown in earlier work to eliminate NP-binding specificity when introduced into the germ-line-encoded V region. At the same time, it generated binding specificity for protein conjugates of a related hapten, 2,4-dinitrophenyl (Brüggemann et al. 1986). These results are summarized in Figure 5. Taken together, they indicate that upon immunization the immune system indeed generates and retains antibody mutants that have lost binding specificity for the immunizing antigen and acquired specificity for a related one.

B-cell Growth and Selection in the Ly-1 B Compartment

The major feature distinguishing growth and selection of conventional and Ly-1 B cells is that the latter

appear to be seeded into the immune system during the first weeks of life and then propagated as mature B cells over the lifetime of the mouse (Herzenberg et al. 1986; Rajewsky et al. 1987; Hayakawa and Hardy 1988). This implies that if the antibodies expressed by Ly-1 B cells do not somatically hypermutate, their repertoire should become more and more restricted in ontogeny. One could imagine a continuous process of cellular selection, at the end of which only a few specificities would persist. Since Ly-1 B cells often give rise to chronic B-cell leukemia (B-CLL) at later stages of life, these specificities should also be found at the level of B-CLLs.

This scenario has been largely verified by experimental results. In our laboratory, the V regions of 17 randomly picked hybridomas, which originated from Ly-1 B cells, were sequenced. These Ly-1 B cells originated from 6–10-month-old CB-20 mice and had been propagated over 9 months in allotype-congenic recipients (Förster et al. 1988). The sequences, part of which are schematically shown in Figure 6 and which include the antibody expressed by a spontaneous arising B-CLL, demonstrated clonal expansion of certain specificities, marked selection of certain V_H and V_κ genes in the population, and the virtual absence of somatic mutation in the antibody V regions (Förster et al. 1988). In an independent study, Haughton and colleagues (Pennell et al. 1988) had finished, almost at the same time, the structural analysis of the antibodies expressed by a set of 10 Ly-1 B-cell-derived B-CLLs from a related mouse strain also bearing the immunoglobulin heavy-chain (IgH^b) haplotype. Strikingly, in several cases the V regions identified in our study were also identically or almost identically represented in the B-CLL collection of Haughton's group. This pattern, which in some instances extended even to certain V_H-V_κ combinations, is schematically depicted in Figure 6.

We were curious at which stage of ontogeny the V genes repeatedly identified in the above collections begin to dominate in the Ly-1 B population. Therefore, Ly-1 B cells were sorted from the peritoneal cell population of 4-week-old CB-20 mice, a cDNA library was produced by C_μ-specific priming and subsequent cDNA amplification. Of the clones, 11 were randomly picked on the basis of hybridization with a V_H probe specific for the J558 V_H family and were sequenced. To our surprise, 7 of the 11 V_H genes were very similar or identical to V_H sequences contained in our original sequence collection (some of the sequence differences may represent artifacts of the cDNA amplification procedure). Two other genes were identical to each other, joining to the same D and joining (J_H) elements, but differed in N sequences (Fig. 7). In addition to the data in Figure 7, we have found that of six V_H genes randomly picked from a cDNA library of Ly-1 B cells from as early as day 4 of life, one was V165.1 and two were V6C7S, both repeatedly seen in the sequences listed in Figures 6 and 7 (see also legend to Fig. 6).

These data establish that certain V genes are predominantly expressed in the Ly-1 B-cell population

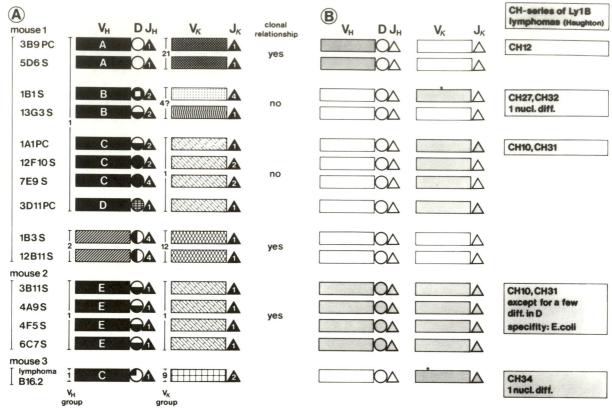

Figure 6. Comparison of antibody V regions expressed in hybridoma lines derived from long-term selected Ly-1 B cells and the Ly-1 B lymphoma B16.2 (Förster et al. 1988) to those expressed in the CH-series of Ly-1 B lymphomas (Pennell et al. 1988). (*A*) Different genes of the J558 family (V$_H$ group 1) are distinguished by different characters. V$_H$ genes designated B are identical to the V$_H$ gene V205.12 (Sablitzky et al. 1985), and those designated C are identical to the V$_H$ gene V165.1 (Siekevitz et al. 1987). In all other cases, identical shadings represent identical V genes. J elements are designated by their numbers. Differences at the VD and DJ borders have not been taken into account. (Modified, with permission, from Förster et al. 1988.) (*B*) V region genes expressed identically in one or two of the CH-lymphomas (as indicated in the figure) and one or several of the Ly-1 B-derived cell lines shown in *A* are marked by shading. In the case of the V$_κ$ gene of 1B1S compared with CH27/CH32 and the V$_κ$ gene of the lymphoma B16.2 compared with CH34, we found a single nucleotide difference in codon 47 and codon 26, respectively.

already very early in ontogeny. In some cases, these genes appear to be overrepresented also in conventional B cells (this is particularly clear for the V$_H$ gene 165.1, the V$_H$ genes similar to V205.12, and the V$_κ$1 gene K1A5; see Förster et al. [1988] and H.Gu, unpubl.). In others, they have so far been found expressed predominantly in the Ly-1 B compartment (the V$_H$ genes V6C7S and V10B10S [see Fig. 7]). Another example of a V$_H$ gene dominantly expressed in the Ly-1 B-cell population is VCP12, which is often rearranged in B cells specific for bromelain-treated mouse red blood cells (Reininger et al. 1988). Cells with this specificity and especially cells expressing the VCP12 gene have been found at high frequency among Ly-1 B cells of adult as well as 2–4-week-old mice but much less frequently among neonatal B cells (Mercolino et al. 1988; Andrade et al. 1989). Compared with our findings, this indicates that the overrepresentation of particular V genes within the Ly-1 B-cell population is established at varying time points during ontogeny.

We believe that the predominant expression of these genes is due to cellular selection, but it is very well

possible that this goes hand-in-hand with preferential V gene rearrangement. However, it should be noted in this context that most V$_H$ genes dealt with in this paper belong to the J558 V$_H$ family, whereas preferential V$_H$ gene rearrangement has been invoked so far for the 7183 V$_H$ genes that are most proximal to the D elements in the IgH locus. The possibility of preferential V gene rearrangement can be directly addressed in the pre-B-cell compartment, and studies in this direction are underway.

The mechanism and physiological role of Ly-1 B-cell selection is at present a matter of speculation. Selection could be initiated by idiotypic networks as the experiments of Kearney and colleagues (Vakil and Kearney 1986; Vakil et al. 1986) suggest, but other self-antigens and bacterial antigens could also play a role. Screening our set of Ly-1 B-cell-derived antibodies for self-reactivity, C. Bona (pers. comm.) found that six of them (5D6S/3B9PC, 1A1PC, 12F10S, 3D11PC, 10B10S, and 10H12S) showed some binding to double-stranded DNA. (Using a different assay, we had not detected DNA-binding specificity in our own analysis [Förster et

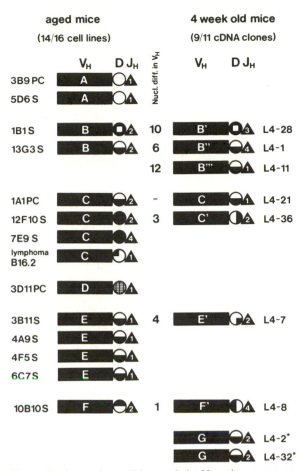

aged mice (14/16 cell lines)				4 week old mice (9/11 cDNA clones)		
	V_H	D J_H	Nucl. diff. in V_H	V_H	D J_H	
3B9 PC	A	◯△1				
5D6 S	A	◯△1				
1B1 S	B	◯□△2	10	B'	◐△3	L4-28
13G3 S	B	◐△2	6	B''	◐△1	L4-1
			12	B'''	◐△1	L4-11
1A1 PC	C	◯△2	–	C	◯△1	L4-21
12F10 S	C	◐△2	3	C'	◐△2	L4-36
7E9 S	C	◐△4				
lymphoma B16.2	C	◑△1				
3D11 PC	D	⬤△1				
3B11 S	E	◐△1	4	E'	◐△2	L4-7
4A9 S	E	◐△1				
4F5 S	E	◐△1				
6C7 S	E	◐△1				
10B10 S	F	◐△2	1	F'	◐△4	L4-8
				G	◐△2	L4-2*
				G	◐△2	L4-32*

Figure 7. Comparison of heavy-chain V region genes expressed in long-term selected Ly-1 B cells (14 of 16 sequences; see also Fig. 6) and those expressed in peritoneal Ly-1 B cells of 4-week-old CB-20 mice (9 of 11 randomly picked cDNA clones). Shown are only V regions containing V_H genes of the J558 family. For further details, see legend to Fig. 6. Numbers of nucleotide differences between the V_H genes compared are given in the figure. Differences at the VD and DJ borders have not been taken into account. Although the cDNA clones L4-2 and L4-32 bear the same V_H, D, and J_H elements, they are not derived from clonally related cells since they differ in N-sequences.

al. 1988].) 1A1PC and 10H12S, in addition, react with topoisomerase I, which is also recognized by 7E9S. Antibody 3D11PC appears to be multireactive, binding to DNA as well as to histone H2B and thyroglobulin. Remarkably, antibodies 1A1PC, 12F10S, 7E9S, as well as the light chain of 3D11PC, share 96–97% sequence homology with antibody MRL-DNA10 (Kofler et al. 1985) isolated from an autoimmune mouse strain and specific for single-stranded DNA (see also Förster et al. 1988). The $V_\kappa 1$ gene expressed in these antibodies is also frequently expressed in rheumatoid factor antibodies as described by Shlomchik et al. (1986).

The self-reactivity of the antibodies described above and the known reactivity of other Ly-1 B-cell-derived antibodies with self- or bacterial antigens (for review, see Hayakawa and Hardy 1988) are likely of physiological importance, considering that these antibodies

account for a major fraction of serum immunoglobulin (Herzenberg et al. 1986; Förster and Rajewsky 1987). As discussed elsewhere (Rajewsky et al. 1987; Kocks and Rajewsky 1989), Ly-1 B cells may represent an evolutionarily selected system of "natural" immunity against common pathogens in the environment.

CONCLUSIONS

In this paper, we have dealt with the in vivo growth and selection of B cells at three different levels. We provide evidence that most conventional B cells in the peripheral immune system are stable, long-lived cells selected by an unknown mechanism from a continuous supply of newborn cells that arise from stem cells in the bone marrow. The majority of the peripheral B cells is thus not subject to rapid renewal from precursor cells. The acquisition of longevity may coincide with the expression of surface IgD in addition to the initially expressed surface IgM. The continuous supply of (mostly short-lived) newborn cells together with a nucleus of stable, selected cells allows for the expression of a diverse and yet biased antibody repertoire.

In contrast, in the compartment of Ly-1 B cells where mature B cells are propagated from their time of generation in early ontogeny, an antibody repertoire is expressed in which a restricted set of germ-line V_H and V_L genes dominates. Although this dominance is presumably becoming more accentuated with increasing age because of the progressive loss of specificities (see also Lalor et al. 1989) and is particularly drastic at the level of B-CLL, it can be traced back to early ontogeny. Although the mechanisms of selection in this cellular compartment are still a matter of debate, their likely function is the generation of an efficient system of "natural immunity."

Germ-line-encoded antibody repertoires, expressed in natural immunity as well as in primary antibody responses, have evolved in phylogeny. In contradistinction, a process of somatic evolution operates in the generation of B-cell memory in T-cell-dependent immune responses. Here, a new repertoire of antibody-binding sites is generated through somatic hypermutation and cellular selection, resulting in antibody-affinity maturation. It is argued that these processes represent an efficient defense mechanism by which the immune system is able to deal efficiently with microbial mutants arising in the course of infection.

ACKNOWLEDGMENTS

We thank Dr. T. Ternynck for kind gifts of the anti-BrdU antibody 76.7, B. Mechtold and C. Göttlinger for technical help, A. Belyavsky, C. Kocks, W. Müller, A. Radbruch, J. Roes, B. Schitteck, and T. Simon for advice and discussion, U. Ringeisen for graphical work, and E. Siegmund for typing the manuscript. This work was supported by the Deutsche Forschungsgemeinschaft through SFB 243 and the Fazit Foundation.

REFERENCES

Allen, D., T. Simon, F. Sablitzky, K. Rajewsky, and A. Cumano. 1988. Antibody engineering for the analysis of affinity maturation of an anti-hapten response. *EMBO J.* **7:** 1995.

Allen, D., A. Cumano, R. Dildrop, C. Kocks, K. Rajewsky, N. Rajewsky, J. Roes, F. Sablitzky, and M. Siekevitz. 1987. Timing, genetic requirements and functional consequences of somatic hypermutation during B-cell development. *Immunol. Rev.* **96:** 5.

Alt, F.W., T.K. Blackwell, and G.D. Yancopoulos. 1987. Development of the primary antibody repertoire. *Science* **238:** 1079.

Andrade, L., A.A. Freitas, F. Huetz, P. Poncet, and A. Coutinho. 1989. Immunoglobulin V_H gene expression in Ly-1[+] and conventional B lymphocytes. *Eur. J. Immunol.* **19:** 1117.

Bothwell, A.L.M., M. Paskind, M. Reth, T. Imanishi-Kari, K. Rajewsky, and D. Baltimore. 1981. Heavy chain variable region contribution to the NP[b] family of antibodies: Somatic mutation evident in a γ2a variable region. *Cell* **24:** 625.

Brodeur, P.H. and R. Riblet. 1984. The immunoglobulin heavy chain variable region (Igh-V) in the mouse. I. One hundred Igh V genes comprise seven families of homologous genes. *Eur. J. Immunol.* **14:** 922.

Brüggemann, M., H.-J. Müller, C. Burger, and K. Rajewsky. 1986. Idiotypic selection of an antibody mutant with changed hapten binding specificity, resulting from a point mutation in position 50 of the heavy chain. *EMBO J.* **5:** 1561.

Burnet, M.F. 1959. *The clonal selection theory of immunity.* Cambridge University Press, Cambridge, England.

Claesson, M.H., C. Röpke, and H.P. Hougen. 1974. Distribution of short-lived and long-lived small lymphocytes in the lymphomyeloid tissues of germ-free NMRI mice. *Scand. J. Immunol.* **3:** 597.

Coffman, R.L. and I.L. Weissman. 1981. B220: A B cell specific member of the T200 glycoprotein family. *Nature* **289:** 681.

Dildrop, R. 1984. A new classification of mouse V_H sequences. *Immunol. Today* **5:** 85.

Förster, I. and K. Rajewsky. 1987. Expansion and functional activity of Ly-1[+] B cells upon transfer of peritoneal cells into allotype-congenic, newborn mice. *Eur. J. Immunol.* **17:** 521.

Förster, I., H. Gu, and K. Rajewsky. 1988. Germline antibody V regions as determinants of clonal persistence and malignant growth in the B cell compartment. *EMBO J.* **7:** 3693.

Förster, I., P. Vieira, and K. Rajewsky. 1989. Flow cytometric analysis of cell proliferation dynamics in the B cell compartment of the mouse. *Int. Immunol.* **1:** (in press).

Freitas, A.A., M.-P. Lambezat, and A. Coutinho. 1989. Expression of antibody V-regions is genetically and developmentally controlled and modulated by the B lymphocyte environment. *Int. Immunol.* (in press).

Freitas, A.A., B. Rocha, and A.A. Coutinho. 1986. Lymphocyte population kinetics in the mouse. *Immunol. Rev.* **91:** 5.

Freitas, A.A., B. Rocha, L. Forni, and A. Coutinho. 1982. Population dynamics of B lymphocytes and their precursors: Demonstration of high turnover in the central and peripheral lymphoid organs. *J. Immunol.* **128:** 54.

Gray, D. 1988. Population kinetics of rat peripheral B cells. *J. Exp. Med.* **167:** 805.

Hayakawa, K. and R.R. Hardy. 1988. Normal, autoimmune and malignant CD5[+] B cells: The Ly-1 B lineage? *Annu. Rev. Immunol.* **6:** 197.

Herzenberg, L.A., A.M. Stall, P.A. Lalor, C. Sidman, W.A.

Moore, D.R. Parks, and L.A. Herzenberg. 1986. The Ly-1 B cell lineage. *Immunol. Rev.* **93:** 81.

Heyman, R.A., E. Borrelli, J. Lesley, D. Anderson, D.D. Richman, S.M. Baird, R. Hyman, and R.M. Evans. 1989. Thymidine kinase obliteration (TKO): Creation of transgenic mice with controlled immune-deficiency. *Proc. Natl. Acad. Sci.* **86:** 2698.

Kocks, C. and K. Rajewsky. 1988. Stepwise intraclonal maturation of antibody affinity through somatic hypermutation. *Proc. Natl. Acad. Sci.* **85:** 8206.

———. 1989. Stable expression and somatic hypermutation of antibody V regions in B-cell developmental pathways. *Annu. Rev. Immunol.* **7:** 537.

Kofler, R., D.J. Noonan, D.E. Levy, M.C. Wilson, N.P.H. Muller, F.J. Dixon, and A.N. Theofilopoulos. 1985. Genetic elements used for a murine lupus anti-DNA autoantibody are closely related to those for antibodies to exogenous antigens. *J. Exp. Med.* **161:** 805.

Lalor, P.A., L.A. Herzenberg, S.A. Adams, and A.M. Stall. 1989. Feedback regulation of murine Ly-1 B cell development. *Eur. J. Immunol.* **19:** 507.

Loh, E.Y., J.F. Elliott, S. Cwirla, L.L. Lanier, and M.M. Davis. 1989. Polymerase chain reaction with single-sided specificity: Analysis of T cell receptor δ chain. *Science* **243:** 217.

Malynn, B.A., J.E. Berman, G.D. Yancopoulos, C.A. Bona, and F.W. Alt. 1987. Expression of the immunoglobulin heavy-chain variable gene repertoire. *Curr. Top. Microbiol. Immunol.* **135:** 75.

Mercolino, T.J., L.W. Arnold, L.A. Hawkins, and G. Haughton. 1988. Normal mouse peritoneum contains a large population of Ly-1[+] (CD5) B cells that recognize phosphatidyl choline. *J. Exp. Med.* **168:** 687.

Pennell, C.A., L.W. Arnold, G. Haughton, and S.H. Clarke. 1988. Restricted immunoglobulin variable region gene expression among Ly-1[+] B cell lymphoma. *J. Immunol.* **141:** 2788.

Press, O.W., C. Rosse, and J. Clagett. 1977. The distribution of rapidly and slowly renewed T, B, and "Null" lymphocytes in mouse bone marrow, thymus, lymph nodes, and spleen. *Cell. Immunol.* **33:** 114.

Rajewsky, K., I. Förster, and A. Cumano. 1987. Evolutionary and somatic selection of the antibody repertoire in the mouse. *Science* **238:** 1088.

Reininger, L., A. Kaushik, S. Izui, and J.-C. Jaton. 1988. A member of a new V_H gene family encodes anti-bromelinized mouse red blood cell autoantibodies. *Eur. J. Immunol.* **18:** 1521.

Robinson, S.H., G. Brecher, I.S. Lourie, and J.E. Haley. 1965. Leukocyte labeling in rats during and after continuous infusion of tritiated thymidine: Implications for lymphocyte longevity and DNA reutilization. *Blood* **26:** 281.

Röpke, C. and N.B. Everett. 1975. Life span of small lymphocytes in the thymolymphatic tissues of normal and thymus-deprived BALB/c mice. *Anat. Rec.* **183:** 83.

Röpke, C., H.P. Hougen, and N.B. Everett. 1975. Long-lived T and B lymphocytes in the bone marrow and thoracic duct lymph of the mouse. *Cell. Immunol.* **15:** 82.

Sablitzky, F., G. Wildner, and K. Rajewsky. 1985. Somatic mutation and clonal expansion of B cells in an antigen-driven immune response. *EMBO J.* **4:** 345.

Shlomchik, M.J., D.A. Nemazee, V.L. Sato, J. Van Snick, D.A. Carson, and M.G. Weigert. 1986. Variable region sequences of murine IgM anti-IgG monoclonal autoantibodies (rheumatoid factors). *J. Exp. Med.* **164:** 407.

Siekevitz, M., C. Kocks, K. Rajewsky, and R. Dildrop. 1987. Analysis of somatic mutation and class switching in naive and memory B cells generating adoptive primary and secondary responses. *Cell* **48:** 757.

Sprent, J. and A. Basten. 1973. Circulating T and B lymphocytes of the mouse. II. Lifespan. *Cell. Immunol.* **7:** 40.

Vakil, M. and J.F. Kearney. 1986. Functional characterization of monoclonal auto-anti-idiotype antibodies isolated from the early B cell repertoire of BALB/c mice. *Eur. J. Immunol.* **16:** 1151.

Vakil, M., H. Sauter, C. Paige, and J.F. Kearney. 1986. In vivo suppression of perinatal multispecific B cells results in a distortion of the adult B cell repertoire. *Eur. J. Immunol.* **16:** 1159.

Winter, E., A. Radbruch, and U. Krawinkel. 1985. Members of novel V_H gene families are found in VDJ regions of polyclonally activated B-lymphocytes. *EMBO J.* **4:** 2861.

Yancopoulos, G.D., S.V. Desiderio, M. Paskind, J.F. Kearney, D. Baltimore, and F.W. Alt. 1984. Preferential utilization of the most J_H-proximal V_H gene segments in pre-B-cell lines. *Nature* **311:** 727.

Conventional and Ly-1 B-cell Lineages in Normal and μ Transgenic Mice

L.A. Herzenberg and A.M. Stall

Department of Genetics, Stanford University, Stanford, California 94305

Although Ly-1 B cells represent only a small percentage of the overall murine B-cell population, they produce much of the serum immunoglobulin M (IgM) and many of the commonly studied autoantibodies in autoimmune and normal animals (Hayakawa et al. 1984, 1986a; Herzenberg et al. 1986; Stall et al. 1988; Mercolino et al. 1988). These cells express typical B-cell surface markers and have much in common with conventional B cells. Nevertheless, when contrasted carefully with conventional B cells, they show key differences in cell-surface phenotype (Herzenberg et al. 1986), cell size and granularity (Herzenberg et al. 1986), tissue localization (Hayakawa et al. 1986a; Herzenberg et al. 1986), strain distribution (Hayakawa et al. 1983; Herzenberg et al. 1986; Sidman et al. 1986), and relative frequencies of expressed variable (V_H) genes (Förster et al. 1988; Pennell et al. 1988; Tarlington et al. 1988; Hardy et al. 1989). Furthermore, they tend to be substantially longer lived and to display a characteristic growth and generalization pattern when they become neoplastic (Stall et al. 1988). A series of studies (Hayakawa et al. 1985, 1986b; Herzenberg et al. 1986, 1987; Hardy et al. 1987; Lalor et al. 1987, 1988; Davidson et al. 1988; Hanecak et al. 1989; Palacios et al. 1989), culminating in the elegant experiments reported by J. Kearney and colleagues (this volume), support the placement of Ly-1 B cells in a separate developmental lineage. Collectively, these studies demonstrate the following:

1. Ly-1 B-cell progenitors are distinct from conventional B-cell progenitors (Hayakawa et al. 1985, 1986b; Herzenberg et al. 1986; Kearney et al., this volume) (e.g., progenitors for Ly-1 B cells are present in fetal omentum but are largely missing in adult bone marrow, whereas progenitors for conventional B cells are abundant in adult bone marrow but missing in fetal omentum).

2. Ly-1 B cells are more closely related to macrophages and monocytes than conventional B cells. That is, Ly-1 B cells tend to be adherent (A.M. Stall, unpubl.). They inhabit serosal cavities, such as the peritoneal (Hayakawa et al. 1986a) and pleural (F.M.G. Kroese, unpubl.) cavities and other sites frequented by macrophages. In addition, peritoneal (although not splenic) Ly-1 B cells express a classical macrophage surface marker, CD11/MAC-1 (Herzenberg et al. 1987; A.M. Stall, unpubl.) and look "macrophage-like" in electron micrographs (F.M.G. Kroese et al., in prep.).

3. The Ly-1 B-cell developmental pathway appears to contain pre-B cells that can differentiate either to Ly-1 B cells or to monocytes/macrophages (e.g., several pre-B cell lines have been recognized that develop in this way) (Davidson et al. 1988; Hanecak et al. 1989; Palacios et al. 1989).

4. Ly-1 B-cell developmental mechanisms differ from conventional B-cell mechanisms (e.g., conventional B cells arise later in ontogeny and are replenished from Ig$^-$ progenitors throughout life, whereas Ly-1 B cells are derived from Ig$^-$ progenitors only during the first few weeks of life and persist thereafter as self-replenishing B cells that readily reconstitute the Ly-1 B population in irradiated recipients (Hayakawa et al. 1986b; Lalor et al. 1987, 1988).

Figure 1 summarizes our concept of the lineage distinction between conventional B cells and Ly-1 B cells. We assign the Ly-1 B cells to an evolutionarily primitive, self-replenishing lineage whose development from Ig$^-$ stem cells is regulated by a feedback mechanism that becomes effective shortly after weaning. The stem-cell population in this view differentiates further during early postnatal life and gives rise to the more highly evolved stem cells that replenish the conventional B-cell lineage throughout life.

We focus on B-cell development in Figure 1; however, the stem cells that we show are meant to be pluripotent stem cells that also give rise to lymphoid and myeloid cells. For example, if we were to extend this model to specify which T-cell and macrophage subsets derive from each of the stem cells, we would probably assign the $\gamma\delta$ T cells that pass through the thymus during fetal life to the primitive lineage and the $\alpha\beta$ T cells that emerge later in life to the conventional lineage.

This model differs from earlier (current) concepts of B-cell development, which view B cells as deriving from self-replenishing hematopoetic stem cells that start populating the immune system early in life and provide a steady flow of cells thereafter. In essence, it states that successive stem cells give rise to progressively more advanced lymphocyte lineages whose characteristics recapitulate evolutionary advances in lymphoid and myeloid development. This idea is clearly novel; however, it is consistent with many of the known prop-

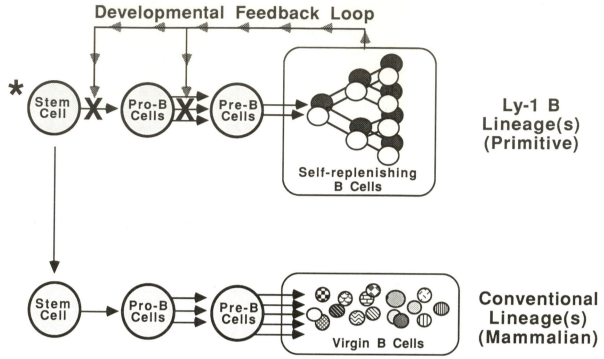

Figure 1. A model of B-cell development in the mouse. See text for explanation.

erties of the B-cell (lymphocyte) lineages as we have drawn them.

For example, the tendency for Ly-1 B cells to inhabit the peritoneal and pleural cavities and to participate extensively in mucosal immunity (Kroese et al. 1989) suggests that these cells may have a longer "biological history" than conventional B cells, which predominate in the more highly evolved lymphoid areas such as the B-cell follicles in spleen and lymph nodes, and tend to contribute more heavily to the immune responses that originate in these follicles. Similarly, the feedback regulation of Ly-1 B development and the maintenance of the Ly-1 B population by self-replenishment in adults approximates the more primitive B-cell development and maintenance mechanisms that operate in avian species (Pink et al. 1985; Ratcliff et al. 1986).

Feedback Regulation of Ly-1 B Development

The feedback mechanism that controls the development of Ly-1 B-lineage cells (see Fig. 1) was recently defined by P. Lalor in our laboratory. Lalor charted the recovery of conventional B cells and Ly-1 B cells in animals that had been treated during the first few weeks of life with anti-IgM allotype antibodies that deplete all B cells (in allotype homozygotes) or half of the B cells (in allotype heterozygotes). In essence, he found that conventional B cells recovered rapidly after the treatment antibody disappeared, regardless of whether the initial B-cell depletion was complete or partial. Ly-1 B-cell recovery, however, failed unless all B cells were removed initially. Thus, the neonatal depletion of paternal allotype Ly-1 B cells in allotype heterozygotes resulted in the lifelong depletion of these Ly-1 B cells with the consequent persistence of a Ly-1 B-cell population consisting only of B cells that express the maternal allotype. (These studies are summarized in Table 1.)

Lalor reproduced this selective failure of the depleted Ly-1 B cells to recover in the presence of Ly-1 B cells by depleting all of the B cells in allotype homozygotes and injecting Ly-1 B cells whose IgM allotype

Table 1. Feedback Inhibition of Ly-1 B Development

IgH allotype	Neonatal depletion of Ly-1 B[a]	Recovery of depleted Ly-1 B[b]
a/b	partial: paternal (b) allo in heterozygotes	no
b/b	complete: all B in homozygotes	yes
b/b (+ a/a)	complete: neonates restored with allotype-congenic Ly-1 B	no

Data summarized from Lalor et al. (1987, 1988).

[a]Mice were injected with 2 mg of anti-IgH-6b during the first 4 weeks of life. No IgH-6b[+] cells were detected for the first 6 weeks of age.

[b]Peritoneal cells were analyzed from mice up to 8 months of age. Conventional B cells are depleted and always completely recover.

did not react with the treatment antibody (like the maternal allotype Ly-1 B cells in the allotype heterozygotes). This procedure permanently established an allotype-congenic Ly-1 B-cell population derived from the injected cells and, by so doing, permanently prevented the recovery of the endogenous Ly-1 B population.

Without the injected (allotype-congenic) Ly-1 B cells, the endogenous Ly-1 B population recovered fully within a few weeks of the disappearance of the treatment antibody, no matter how long the antibody treatment was maintained after weaning. On the other hand, if the treatment antibody was allowed to fall below detectable levels during the neonatal period (3–5 weeks), the endogenous Ly-1 B population recovered despite the presence of a nondepletable (maternal allotype) Ly-1 B population. Thus, Ly-1 B cells differentiate de novo for the first few weeks of life without regard to the presence of other Ly-1 B cells; however, if sufficient numbers of Ly-1 B cells are present after this time, further de novo Ly-1 B-cell differentiation is blocked and the existent Ly-1 B population moves into its self-replenishing phase (which persists for the life of the animal).

The early termination of de novo Ly-1 B-cell development forces definition of the basic Ly-1 B repertoire during the first few weeks of life when newly emerging Ly-1 B cells committed to the production of particular antibody molecules are either accepted or depleted from the incoming pool. Once the feedback mechanism is triggered and de novo differentiation terminates, changes in the repertoire are limited to the expansion or depletion of existent clones. Thus, the neonatal repertoire continues to be expressed throughout life but tends to become progressively more narrow, particularly in older animals where dominant (faster-growing) clones and Ly-1 B tumors tend to take over the available "living space" (Stall et al. 1988).

This unique developmental pattern, coupled with the relatively large contribution Ly-1 B cells make to serum IgM and other serum immunoglobulin levels, means that factors that influence immunoglobulin V_H and V_L rearrangement and expression in Ly-1 B cells during neonatal life have a continuing effect on the antibodies produced by the animal. Similarly, antigenic stimulation, idiotypic network interactions, and environmental conditions that alter the Ly-1 B-cell repertoire in neonates or in young adults are reflected in the serum antibodies produced many months hence. In this sense, Ly-1 B cells provide a kind of primitive immunologic memory that keeps elements of the neonatal immunologic experience active throughout life.

B-cell Lineages, Antibody Responses, and Affinity Maturation

Although Ly-1 B cells play key role(s) in the mammalian immune system, they tend not to participate in high-affinity IgG antibody responses to haptens and proteins. These responses are mainly produced by conventional B cells which, according to our view, emerged later in evolutionary time and are more suited developmentally to producing such high-affinity responses (Herzenberg et al. 1986; P.A. Lalor, unpubl.).

Almost nothing is known about the mechanisms that determine which lineage responds to a given antigen. The neonatal mechanisms that control the antibody specificities present in the Ly-1 B repertoire probably contribute to these decisions. Physical characteristics of the antigen also appear to be important. Similarly, the anatomical habitat of the lineages may be a significant factor.

The high-turnover rate of the conventional B cells probably gives them a different type of advantage in high-affinity responses since the continual input of the newly rearranged cells into the "virgin" pool and the larger overall number of these cells in the pool in adult animals provides a wider range of antibody-combining site structures than can be provided in the Ly-1 B repertoire. Therefore, immunizing antigens are more likely to find a good (higher affinity) initial fit among combining sites expressed by conventional B cells and hence to trigger preferentially those B cells.

Somatic mutation, of course, plays a major role in increasing the affinity of the antibody produced by a B-cell clone once it is triggered. Conventional B cells are clearly capable of diversifying their combining sites by this mechanism (for review, see Rajewsky et al. 1987). Ly-1 B cells, in contrast, may not have a functional somatic mutation mechanism. Studies completed thus far favor this view since all of the Ly-1 B immunoglobulin V regions sequenced to date have germ-line encoded sequences (Förster et al. 1988; Pennell et al. 1988; Tarlington et al. 1988; Hardy et al. 1989). However, further work is required to determine whether these findings merely reflect the criteria used to select Ly-1 B immunoglobulins for sequencing or whether they are indicative of a more profound difference between the lineages, i.e., that the Ly-1 B lineage uses a simpler (more primitive?) mechanism for antibody diversification than the conventional lineage.

Developmental Changes in B-cell Lineages in μ Transgenic Mice

Given the major functional and developmental differences between the B-cell lineages outlined above, it is not surprising that these lineages are affected quite differently by the introduction of a μ (IgM) heavy-chain transgene. Conventional pre-B cells and B cells are often drastically depleted, particularly in older animals in certain strains (Herzenberg et al. 1987) (See Fig. 2 and Table 2). Furthermore, this defect in conventional B-cell development is accompanied by (or results in) a severe interference in the rearrangement and/or expression of endogenous immunoglobulin heavy (IgH) chains. In essence, those conventional B cells that manage to survive express the transgenic μ heavy chain (combined with a successfully rearranged

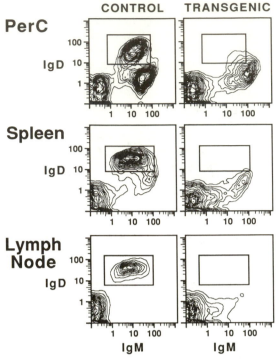

Figure 2. Development of conventional B cells is impaired in μ transgenic mice. Cells prepared from M54 peritoneum, spleen, and lymph nodes were stained with anti-IgM (331) and anti-IgD (AF6-122) and analyzed by a fluorescence-activated cell sorter (FACS) as described previously (Herzenberg et al. 1987). In each panel, the conventional B cells (dull IgM and bright IgD) are delineated by a box. (Data taken, with permission, from Herzenberg et al. 1987.)

light chain) and do not express detectable levels of endogenous μ (Stall et al. 1987; A.M. Stall, in prep.).

Ly-1 B cells, in contrast, are found in essentially normal numbers in μ transgenic animals and almost always rearrange and express endogenous μ chains (Herzenberg et al. 1987; Stall et al. 1987; A.M. Stall, in prep.). Surprisingly, however, many of these cells also express the μ transgene and can be triggered to secrete pentameric IgM molecules with "mixed" heavy chains (Herzenberg et al. 1987). Such "double-expressing" Ly-1 B cells predominate in certain transgenic strains,

e.g., M54, whereas other strains mainly have Ly-1 B cells that express endogenous μ and do not express detectable levels of transgenic μ (see Fig. 3 and Table 2). Some transgene-only Ly-1 B cells can be found; however, they are relatively rare and appear to be restricted to a particular (sister) subset of the Ly-1 B lineage (A.M. Stall, unpubl.).

The characterization of the immunoglobulin-expression pattern in the relatively few conventional B cells that survive in the transgenic mice was complicated by the presence of a normal-sized large population of Ly-1 B cells expressing both endogenous and transgenic μ in these mice. The conclusion (stated above) that the transgenic conventional B cells do not express endogenous μ required extension of our earlier studies to include the examination of these cells in lethally irradiated recipients reconstituted with transgenic bone marrow carrying a surface marker (Ly-5) that distinguishes donor-derived cells from surviving host cells. As expected (Hayakawa et al. 1985; Herzenberg et al. 1986), essentially all of the B cells in these reconstituted mice are conventional B cells that derive from progenitors in the donor (transgenic) bone marrow. Furthermore, as our earlier studies predicted (Herzenberg et al. 1987), essentially all of these donor-derived conventional B cells express the transgenic μ and virtually none express endogenous μ (see Fig. 4).

Taken together, the studies cited above demonstrate the following: (1) In Ly-1 B-lineage cells, the μ transgene is readily expressed but rarely interferes with endogenous IgH rearrangement and expression; and (2) in conventional lineage B cells, the μ transgene blocks expression (and most likely rearrangement) of endogenous μ and is the only surface immunoglobulin expressed on these B cells. These findings suggest a major difference between the two lineages in the way that they respond to the presence and activity of the μ transgene.

Transgenic μ, Endogenous μ, and Allelic Exclusion

B cells normally express IgH gene products encoded on only one of the two IgH chromosomes in the cell.

Table 2. B-cell Development and μ Gene Expression in μ Transgenic Mice

Mice	Transgene	Splenic B cells (% of sib control)	Peritoneal B cells detected			Background
			endogenous only	transgene only	double positive	
M54[a]	μ[a]	<20	+	+	+	C57BL
M95[a]	μ[a]	<20	+	+	+	C57BL
M52[a]	μ[a]	<20	+	+	+	C57BL
M94[a]	μ[a]	100[c]	+	−	−	C57BL
207-4[b]	μ[a], κ (αPC)	50–80	+	+	+	(C57BL × SJL)F₂ back-crossed to C57BL
243-4[b]	μ[a]	>90	+	+	+	(C57BL × SJL)F₂
254-3[b]	μ[a], Δ mem	100[c]	+	−	−	(C57BL × SJL)F₂

[a]Lines developed by Baltimore and Costantini (Grosschedl et al. 1984).
[b]Lines developed by Storb and Brinster (Storb et al. 1986).
[c]No difference could be detected between transgene-positive mice and transgene-negative sibs.

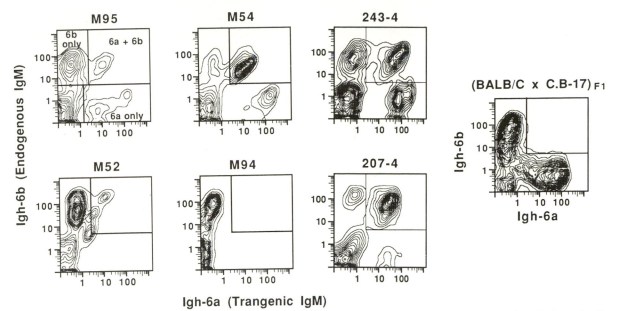

Igh-6a (Trangenic IgM)

Figure 3. Independent transgenic lines have characteristic patterns of endogenous and transgenic μ expression. Peritoneal cells from the μ transgenic indicated were stained with anti-IgH-6a (DS-1) (transgenic μ) and anti-IgH-6b (AF6-78) (endogenous μ) and analyzed by FACS as described previously (Stall et al. 1987). In the M95 panel, cells expressing endogenous (6b)-only, transgene (6a)-only or double expressors (6a + 6b) are boxed. The stippled areas in each contour plot show the 6a + 6b "double-producer" region. The transgenic lines are more fully described in Table 2. An IgH-6a/IgH-6b contour plot of the allotypic heterozygous F_1 strain (BALB/c × C.B17)F_1 demonstrates allelic exclusion in nontransgenic mice.

The mechanism that mediates this allelic (IgH haplotype) exclusion appears to be triggered by the occurrence of a successful μ heavy-chain rearrangement and/or the production of a functional μ chain. Thus, the expression of a μ heavy-chain transgene prior to the successful rearrangement of an endogenous μ chain would be expected to block endogenous μ-chain production.

The failure to express endogenous μ in conventional B cells in M54 mice is consistent with this hypothesis,

i.e., that the transgene product is mistaken for a successfully rearranged endogenous μ gene and that this "error" terminates IgH rearrangement before the endogenous genes can be rearranged. However, the unimpaired expression of endogenous μ in Ly-1 B cells in these animals challenges the generality (if not the very validity) of this commonly accepted hypothesis.

Can the Ly-1 B-cell data be reconciled with the current paradigm? We can dispense rapidly with the idea that the transgene product does not mediate the

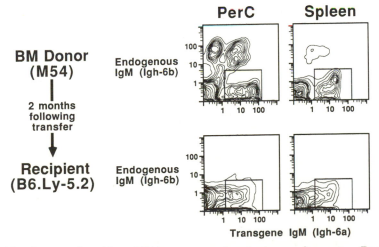

Figure 4. Conventional B cells reconstituted from M54 bone marrow do not express endogenous μ. Bone marrow cells from M54 mice were used to reconstitute a B6.Ly-5.1. These two strains are congenic, differing only with respect to their Ly-5 alleles and the μ transgene of the M54. After 2 months following reconstitution, the recipient mice were sacrificed and analyzed by FACS for donor-derived (Ly-5.2$^+$) B cells as described in Fig. 3. Only donor-derived (Ly-5.2$^+$) B cells are shown in the recipient plots. The donor-derived peritoneal B cells expressed no Ly-1 or MAC-1 antigens confirming that they are of the conventional lineage (not shown). Although the donor peritoneal B cells had a high frequency of endogenous μ-expressing cells, this population is missing in the recipient mice.

allelic exclusion mechanism to terminate IgH rearrangement in Ly-1 B cells because the allelic exclusion mechanism does not function in these cells. Data from multiple FACS analyses taken over the last several years demonstrate clearly that, like conventional B cells, Ly-1 B cells in allotype heterozygotes always express either one parental μ heavy chain or the other, not both (Stall et al. 1987; Palacios et al. 1989). Thus, these cells definitely have a functional allelic exclusion mechanism.

Can the long-term survival of Ly-1 B cells, and hence their susceptibility to selection, account for their endogenous immunoglobulin expression? Perhaps. Ly-1 B cells develop early and persist thereafter by self-replenishment. Conventional B cells, in contrast, turn over rapidly throughout life. Therefore, a few successful rearrangements of endogenous genes in conventional B cells might tend to be lost rapidly, whereas the same number of successful rearrangements in the Ly-1 B population might tend to be "trapped" and expanded into a normal-sized population expressing the endogenous μ with or without transgene accompaniment. In essence, this hypothesis views the transgene as having the same effect in Ly-1 B cells and conventional B cells, and it relegates the observed difference factors that affect the survival rather than the development of cells expressing endogenous μ.

Differential Selection of Ly-1 B and Conventional B Cells

A selection-based hypothesis is particularly attractive since selective forces that operate on the Ly-1 B population in neonates would certainly favor the expansion of those cells that rearrange endogenous μ and enter the population at this time. Nevertheless, evidence from current studies suggests that such differential survival does not account for the lineage differences (A.M. Stall et al., unpubl.). For example, if the success rate for IgH rearrangements were as low in Ly-1 B cells as it is in conventional B cells, the development of the Ly-1 B population should be retarded in neonates (since the input rate to the population should be greatly reduced). Preliminary frequency estimates of Ly-1 B cells in transgenic and normal neonates, however, suggest that the Ly-1 population increases at the same rate in both kinds of animals.

Similarly, if the Ly-1 B population is being generated from a smaller number of successfully rearranged cells, its repertoire should tend to be more restricted and clonal populations of chronic-lymphocytic-leukemia-like tumors should develop earlier than in normal animals. However, such a dramatic change in the frequency or age of onset of clonal populations does not occur in the transgenic animals. Furthermore, preliminary studies indicate that the Ly-1 B repertoire in these animals is relatively normal, at least with respect to the specificities tested so far (A.M. Stall, in prep.).

Finally, a differential survival model would predict the presence of many more Ly-1 B cells that express the transgene in combination with a light chain that makes the cells desirable from a selective standpoint. The occurrence of such cells should easily be as frequent as the occurrence of cells in which a successfully rearranged endogenous μ gene product is coupled with an appropriate light chain to create a desirable (and hence selectable) antibody specificity. However, as we have indicated, transgene-only cells are very rare in the Ly-1 B population. Thus, although the evidence is still not conclusive, we feel that differential survival of successfully rearranged Ly-1 B cells is not likely to account for the observed differences between conventional and Ly-1 B cells in μ transgenic mice.

If we rule out the selection hypothesis, then the lineage differences must be explained by intrinsic developmental differences that allow endogenous rearrangement to proceed successfully in Ly-1 B cells but prevent it in conventional B cells. A variety of such differences can be proposed, e.g., the transgene might be expressed at lower levels or too late in development to be effective in Ly-1 B cells; the Ly-1 B-lineage allelic exclusion mechanism might be qualitatively different and be insensitive to the presence of the transgene or its product; or, the basic assumption that the transgene controls endogenous rearrangement via the allelic exclusion route might be incorrect and the differences between the lineages may result from the operation of entirely unsuspected mechanisms.

These kinds of hypotheses are difficult to evaluate and even more difficult to test; however, that does not necessarily deny their validity. Given the striking series of physical, functional, and developmental differences that have already been recognized between the Ly-1 B-cell and the conventional B-cell lineages (see above), there are good reasons for suspecting that intrinsic developmental differences lie at the heart of the differences in immunoglobulin expression in these lineages in μ transgenic mice. Future studies hopefully will resolve these questions.

ACKNOWLEDGMENTS

This work was supported by grant HD-01287. A.M.S. is a special fellow of the Leukemia Society of America. We thank Drs. R. Grosschedl, U. Storb, and J. Kenney for generously providing transgenic mice. We wish to thank Dr. Leonard Herzenberg for helpful discussions and F. Timothy Gadus and Sharon Adams for expert technical assistance.

REFERENCES

Davidson, W.F., J.H. Pierce, S. Rudikoff, and H.C. Morse III. 1988. Relationship between B cell and myeloid differentiation. Studies with a B lymphocyte precursor. *J. Exp. Med.* **168:** 389.
Förster, I., H. Gu, and K. Rajewsky. 1988. Germline anti-

body V regions as determinants of clonal persistence and malignant growth in the B cell compartment. *EMBO J.* **7:** 3693.

Grosschedl, R., D. Weaver, D. Baltimore, and F. Costantini. 1984. Introduction of a μ immunoglobulin gene into the mouse germ line: Specific expression in lymphoid cells and synthesis of functional antibody. *Cell* **38:** 647.

Hanecak, R., D.C. Zovich, P.K. Pattengale, and H. Fan. 1989. Differentiation in vitro of a leukemia virus-induced B-cell lymphoma into macrophages. *Mol. Cell. Biol.* **9:** 2264.

Hardy, R.R., R. Kishimoto, and K. Hayakawa. 1987. Differentiation of B cell progenitors *in vitro*: Generation of surface IgM$^+$ B cells including Ly-1 B cells, from Thy-1$^-$ Asialo-GM$_1^+$ cells in newborn liver. *Eur. J. Immunol.* **17:** 1769.

Hardy, R.R., C.E. Carmack, S.A. Shinton, R.J. Riblet, and K. Hayakawa. 1989. A single VH gene is utilized predominately in anti-BrMRBC hybridomas derived from purified Ly-1 B cells. Definition of the VH11 family. *J. Immunol.* **142:** 3643.

Hayakawa, K., R.R. Hardy, and L.A. Herzenberg. 1986a. Peritoneal Ly-1 B cells: Genetic control, autoantibody production, increased lambda light chain expression. *Eur. J. Immunol.* **16:** 450.

Hayakawa, K., R.R. Hardy, L.A. Herzenberg, and L.A. Herzenberg. 1985. Progenitors for Ly-1 B cells are distinct from progenitors from other B cells. *J. Exp. Med.* **161:** 1554.

Hayakawa, K., R.R. Hardy, D.R. Parks, and L.A. Herzenberg. 1983. The "Ly1 B" cell subpopulations in normal, immunodefective and autoimmune mice. *J. Exp. Med.* **157:** 202.

Hayakawa, K., R.R. Hardy, A.M. Stall, L.A. Herzenberg, and L.A. Herzenberg. 1986b. Immunoglobulin-bearing B cells reconstitute and maintain the murine Ly-1 B cell lineage. *Eur. J. Immunol.* **16:** 1313.

Hayakawa, K., R.R. Hardy, M. Honda, L.A. Herzenberg, A.D. Steinberg, and L.A. Herzenberg. 1984. Ly-1 B cells: Functionally distinct lymphocytes that secrete IgM autoantibodies. *Proc. Natl. Acad. Sci.* **81:** 2494.

Herzenberg, L.A., A.M. Stall, J. Braun, D. Weaver, D. Baltimore, L.A. Herzenberg, and R. Grosschedl. 1987. Depletion of the predominant B cell population in immunoglobulin mu heavy chain transgenic mice. *Nature* **329:** 71.

Herzenberg, L.A., A.M. Stall, P.A. Lalor, C. Sidman, W.A. Moore, D.R. Parks, and L.A. Herzenberg. 1986. The Ly-1 B cell lineage. *Immunol. Rev.* **93:** 81.

Kroese, F.G.M., E.C. Butcher, A.M. Stall, P.A. Lalor, S. Adams, and L.A. Herzenberg. 1989. Many of the IgA producing plasma cells in murine gut are derived from self-replenishing precursors in the peritoneal cavity. *Int. Immunol.* **1:** 75.

Lalor, P.A., A.M. Stall, S. Adams, L.A. Herzenberg, and L.A. Herzenberg. 1987. Feedback regulation of murine Ly-1 B cell development. *Eur. J. Immunol.* **19:** 507.

———. 1988. Permanent alteration of the murine Ly-1 B repertoire due to selective depletion of Ly-1 B cells in neonatal animals. *Eur. J. Immunol.* **19:** 501.

Mercolino, T.J., L.W. Arnold, L.A. Hawkins, and G. Haughton. 1988. Normal mouse peritoneum contains a large population of Ly-1$^+$ (CD5) B cells that recognize phosphatidyl choline. Relationship to cells that secrete hemolytic antibody specific for autologous erythrocytes. *J. Exp. Med.* **168:** 687.

Palacios, R., S. Stuber, and A. Rolink. 1989. The epigenetic influences of bone marrow and fetal liver stroma cells on the developmental potential of Ly-1$^+$ pro-B lymphocyte clones. *Eur. J. Immunol.* **19:** 347.

Pennell, C.A., L.W. Arnold, G. Haughton, and S.H. Clarke. 1988. Restricted Ig variable region expression among Ly-1$^+$ B cell lymphomas. *J. Immunol.* **141:** 2788.

Pink, J.R.L., M.J.H. Ratcliff, and O. Vainig. 1985. Immunoglobulin-bearing stem cells for clones of B (bursa-derived) lymphocytes. *Eur. J. Immunol.* **15:** 617.

Rajewsky, K., I. Förster, and A. Cumano. 1987. Evolutionary and somatic selection of the antibody repertoire in the mouse. *Science* **238:** 1088.

Ratcliff, M.J.H., J.R.L. Pink, and O. Vainig. 1986. Avian B cell precursors: Surface-immunoglobulin expression is an early, possibly bursa-independent event. *Eur. J. Immunol.* **16:** 129.

Sidman, C.L., L.D. Shultz, R.R. Hardy, K. Hayakawa, and L.A. Herzenberg. 1986. Production of immunoglobulin isotypes by Ly-1($^+$) B cells in viable motheaten and normal mice. *Science* **232:** 1423.

Stall, A.M., P.A. Lalor, L.A. Herzenberg, and L.A. Herzenberg. 1986. Ly-1 B cells and autoantibodies. *Ann. Immunol. Inst. Pasteur* **137D:** 173.

Stall, A.M., F.G.M. Kroese, D.G. Sieckmann, F.T. Gadus, L.A. Herzenberg, and L.A. Herzenberg. 1987. Rearrangement and expression of endogenous immunoglobulin genes occurs frequently in murine B cells expressing transgenic membrane IgM. *Proc. Natl. Acad. Sci.* **85:** 3546.

Stall, A.M., M.C. Farinas, D.M. Tarlington, P.A. Lalor, L.A. Herzenberg, S. Strober, and L.A. Herzenberg. 1988. Ly-1 B cell clones similar to human chronic lymphocytic leukemias (B-CLL) routinely develop in older normal mice and young autoimmune (NZB-related) animals. *Proc. Natl. Acad. Sci.* **85:** 7312.

Storb, U., C. Pinkert, B. Arp, P. Engler, K. Gollohan, J. Manz, W. Brady, and R. Brinster. 1986. Transgenic mice with μ and κ genes encoding antiphosphorylcholine antibodies. *J. Exp. Med.* **164:** 627.

Tarlington, D., A.M. Stall, and L.A. Herzenberg. 1988. Repetitive usage of immunoglobulin V$_H$ and D gene segments in CD5$^+$ Ly-1 B clones of (NZB × NZW)F1 mice. *EMBO J.* **7:** 3705.

Templated, Targeted Sequence Diversification Displays a Similar Choreography in Different Organisms

V. David and N. Maizels

Department of Molecular Biophysics and Biochemistry, Yale University School of Medicine, New Haven, Connecticut 06510

We have begun a systematic investigation of the role of templated mutation, or gene conversion, in hypermutation of mammalian immunoglobulin (Ig) genes. The notion that some sort of segmental recombination might contribute to antibody structure is not a new one but rather has its origins in proposals made by Smithies (1967a,b) and by Edelman and Gally (1967, 1970). With the advent of DNA sequence analysis, Seidman et al. (1978) suggested that shared regions of homology might facilitate variable (V) region recombination in somatic cells, and Baltimore (1981) noted that multiple rounds of segmental recombination would produce the patchy sequence homology shared by different germ-line V regions.

Sequence analysis has provided abundant information about the products of somatic hypermutation during the murine immune response (recently reviewed by Allen et al. 1987; Berek and Milstein 1987; Malipiero et al. 1987; Manser et al. 1987; Rajewsky et al. 1987; Scharff et al. 1987; Wabl et al. 1987). As discussed in detail elsewhere (Maizels 1989), templating best explains a number of features of hypermutated sequences, including the repeated occurrence of identical silent mutations, the repeated use of particular codons at replacement mutations, and the apparent linkage of mutations in neighboring codons. Additionally, no bias in the ratio of transition to transversion mutations is apparent in the sequences of hypermutated V regions; since a pronounced transition:transversion bias characterizes the products of mutagenic polymerases (for review, see Kunkel 1988), it is unlikely that such an enzyme plays a role in the hypermutation process.

We have recently obtained experimental evidence (V. David and N. Maizels, in prep.) that germ-line template sequences direct somatic hypermutation of murine immunoglobulin genes. In mismatch-sensitive hybridization experiments, we used oligonucleotide probes to assay germ-line DNA for sequences identical with short hypermutated segments of expressed murine V regions. Not only have we found evidence that hypermutation is templated, but we have also been able to ascribe the entire mutational history of certain V regions to a process of segmental gene conversion. We would argue that this mechanism alone may account for all hypermutation at the mammalian immunoglobulin loci.

Targeted, regulated sequence diversification by gene conversion is not unique to the mammalian immune response. Rather than reiterate our experimental observations here, we will instead highlight the similarities in the choreography of sequence diversification by gene conversion in several organisms, both unicellular and multicellular. A recurrent theme in the contest between pathogen and host is the ability of the invader to modulate the structure of its cell-surface proteins. This phenomenon, known as antigenic variation, is a common strategy by which microorganisms evade the host immune system. In certain instances, gene conversion has been shown to be the mechanism of this alteration in primary structure, and we speculate that it may also be the mechanism of antigenic variation in other instances that await detailed molecular characterization. The observation that both antigen and antibody are diversified by templated processes implies that there is reciprocity in the relationship between host and pathogen and that each side has devised similar genetic armaments during generations of interaction.

Templated Diversification of Immunoglobulin Variable Regions in Chickens and Mammals

Somatic hypermutation is one of several mechanisms for diversifying the mammalian antibody repertoire. Combinatorial and junctional diversity shape the pre-immune repertoire, and these sources of diversity depend largely on the multiplicity of germ-line V, diversity (D), and joined (J) regions. Only after challenge with antigen does the templated, targeted process of somatic hypermutation diversify sequences at the immunoglobulin loci. Because somatic hypermutation is templated, it too depends on a preexisting repertoire, suggesting the intriguing possibility that sequences that are not explicitly expressed in each individual might still be under selection. One result of somatic hypermutation is the production of some antibodies with increased affinity for antigen, thereby enhancing the efficiency of the immune response. Hypermutation may also permit antibody specificity to keep pace with ongoing mutational processes in infecting microorganisms and parasites (Milstein and Svasti 1971; Berek and Milstein 1988).

In contrast with mammals, the chicken has only one functional light-chain V region and one functional heavy-chain V region; gene conversion templated by pseudo-V regions upstream of each functional V region is necessary to diversify the immunoglobulin repertoire before any encounter with an antigen (Reynaud et al. 1987, 1989). The λ light chain undergoes rearrangement during a limited period of embryonic development, and cells in which productive rearrangement has occurred undergo clonal expansion in the bursa, where targeted sequence diversification also takes place (Thompson and Neiman 1987; McCormack et al. 1989). Most of the mutations in the λ-light chain are templated by a family of 25 pseudo-V regions located just upstream of the functional gene (Reynaud et al. 1987); a few percent of the observed mutations have no obvious donors in the upstream pseudo-V family (Reynaud et al. 1987). These mutations may occur spontaneously as a consequence of heteroduplex formation and resolution during the process of gene conversion (e.g., see Thomas and Capecchi 1986), or they may be templated by sequences elsewhere in the genome that have not yet been identified.

The striking difference between templated diversification of chicken and mammalian immunoglobulin genes is that gene conversion diversifies the preimmune repertoire in chickens, whereas in mammals it only affects activated V regions subsequent to challenge with antigen. This difference appears to be one of regulation, however, rather than one of mechanism, and the two processes are otherwise quite similar. Both processes concentrate mutations in V regions with some mutations also evident in J regions and the J-C intron (recently tabulated for the mouse by Steele and Pollard 1987). Within V regions, most mutations affect complementarity-determining regions; in the mouse this has been ascribed to the demands of antigen-binding, but as we accumulate knowledge of template sequences this bias may turn out to reflect the library of sequences that template diversification as appears to be the case in the chicken (Reynaud et al. 1987). Hypermutation in mammals has been measured in units of single-base changes per generation in a calculation that assumes that mutation at each position is independent (e.g., see McKean et al. 1984; Sablitzky et al. 1985; Allen et al. 1987; Berek and Milstein 1987, 1988). We now must question this assumption: Hypermutation mediated by gene conversion will produce linked mutations, and a more appropriate rate measurement would reflect the number of rounds of gene conversion, counting the use of each separate donor as a new round. Nevertheless, it is interesting that a calculation based on the published data for the chicken λ light chain (Reynaud et al. 1987) produces the same rate of diversification of 10^{-3} per base per cell generation at that locus as was calculated for diversification of activated V regions in the mouse (see Maizels 1989).

Variation in surface antigens can enable pathogenic microorganisms to escape immune surveillance in their hosts. In many instances, variation in the major antigenic components of microbes does not reflect selection and outgrowth of spontaneous mutants but results instead from a regulated genetic event that uses germline sequences to diversify surface antigen genes. This process may be echoed by the mammalian B cell, which targets its own surface molecule, the antibody, for templated diversification. Below, we consider several examples of such templated variation, beginning with mating-type (or "homothallic") switching in the yeasts *Saccharomyces cerevisiae* and *Schizosaccharomyces pombe* as the paradigm for molecular analysis.

Binary Switches: Mating-type Switching in Yeasts

Although the yeasts *S. cerevisiae* and *S. pombe* are not pathogenic, they figure in this discussion both because the molecular and genetic process of templated diversification is better defined for homothallic switching than for any other system and also because other pathogenic yeasts may diversify sequences in an analogous fashion. The best-studied of the pathogenic yeasts, *Candida albicans*, lives commensally in healthy individuals but can also cause infections, especially in immunocompromised individuals. *Candida* switches frequently between the budding form and the virulence-associated hyphal form (Soll 1988); additionally, some members of a dispersed gene family in *Candida* appear to migrate within the genome by a conversion-like mechanism although migration of these particular sequences has not been correlated with the switching process (Scherer and Stevens 1988).

Mating-type switching in *S. cerevisiae* and *S. pombe* may be a paradigm for other important regulatory switches. In *S. cerevisiae* and *S. pombe*, mating type is determined by sequence information residing at a mating-type locus known as *MAT* in *S. cerevisiae* and *mat1* in *S. pombe* (for review, see Herskowitz and Oshima 1981; Klar 1987; Strathern 1988). The protein products of the mating-type locus regulate a variety of genes involved in determining mating type. These yeasts can undergo frequent and efficient mating-type "switching" mediated by a regulated, targeted gene conversion event in which the resident sequence at the mating-type locus is replaced by new sequence information derived from either of two nearby chromosomal sequences. Because there are only two possible donor sequences, switching is binary and yeast cells alternate between the two different mating types. Sequence information transfer is unidirectional, and the donor sequence remains unchanged after templating conversion (Fogel et al. 1981).

A variety of controls regulate the switching process, which can occur only in rapidly growing cells and during a specific stage in the cell cycle. A sequence-specific double-strand break within the mating-type locus initiates gene conversion (Strathern et al. 1982; Beach 1983; Kostriken et al. 1983; Egel et al. 1984), after which DNA on either side of the cleavage site participates in heteroduplex formation (McGill et al. 1989).

Unlike meiotic gene conversion in yeast, which exhibits a gradient of conversion away from the initiation site (Nicolas et al. 1989; Sun et al. 1989), the process of gene conversion responsible for homothallic switching respects strict boundaries distal to the initiation site (McGill et al. 1989).

There are some remarkable similarities between the yeast mating-type switch and *vir* locus variation *Bordetella pertussis*, the etiological agent of whooping cough. Although the mechanism of *vir* variation in this bacterium has yet to be defined, this locus plays a regulatory role not unlike that of the yeast mating-type locus, controlling coordinate synthesis of a group of virulence-associated determinants including toxins, hemagglutinin, and hemolysin. *B. pertussis* undergoes frequent transitions between *vir*$^+$ and *vir*$^-$ phenotypes with a rate as high as 10^{-3} per cell per generation in certain stains. Insertion of a C residue at a specific site in the *vir* locus is consistently associated with the *vir*$^+$ to *vir*$^-$ conversion (Stibitz et al. 1989). The mechanism of this genetic variation is unknown, but the high frequency and reversibility of the process suggest a targeted, regulated event.

Diversification of a Sequence at an Expression Site: Variable Surface Glycoprotein Diversification in Trypanosomes

African trypanosomes are unicellular parasitic flagellates that depend on antigenic variation to evade the immune response of the mammalian host (for review, see Donelson and Rice-Ficht 1985). In contrast with targeted gene conversion in yeasts, where only two donor sequences template binary diversification of a specific locus, trypanosomes possess a large repertoire of donor sequences that enables them to use targeted gene conversion to generate an enormous range of diversity in the major variable surface glycoprotein (VSG). Tsetse flies transmit trypanosomes to the mammalian bloodstream where the host immune system immediately begins to combat the infection by producing antibodies directed against the coat of the infecting microorganism. The major antigenic determinant of the parasite coat is VSG, and this 55–65-kD glycoprotein contains a variable region of amino-terminal sequences linked to a carboxy-terminal constant region. The initial stages of trypanosome infection are characterized by expression of a single VSG gene typical of the metacyclic (insect-borne) form of the parasite. As the host immune system combats this version of the parasite coat, the variable region of the VSG sequence undergoes sequence changes, which enable the parasite to evade the immune response. Subsequent rounds of diversification in the VSG sequence are manifest as successive waves of parasitemia in the host with each change in the VSG antigen parried by new specificities of host antibodies.

The active copies of VSG genes are located at specific sites, called expression sites, which are usually telomeric. Transcription is generally restricted to VSG genes at telomeric expression sites, called expression-linked copies (ELCs), although movement to an expression site is not sufficient for expression, and additional signals regulate VSG transcription (Hoejimakers et al. 1980; Pays et al. 1981; De Lange and Borst 1982; Longacre et al. 1983; Young et al. 1983; Bernards et al. 1984; Buck et al. 1984). Early in infection, variation of the expressed sequence is accomplished by transfer of a complete copy of coding information from a repertoire of silent genes (basic copies [BCs]) to the ELC (Longacre and Eisen 1986). The expression site to which a BC contributes information need not be on the same chromosome as the BC itself (Van der Ploeg et al. 1984). Later in infection, diversification of the expressed sequence is accomplished by further rounds of targeted gene conversion, which produce mosaic genes whose 5′ ends represent a patchwork of sequences derived from different donor BCs (Pays et al. 1983; Longacre and Eisen 1985; Roth et al. 1986).

Diversification of expression site sequences may also occur in *Borrelia hermsii*, the etiological agent of relapsing fever in mice. After infection, *B. hermsii* produces a pattern of variation in serotype-specific antigens called variable major proteins (VMPs); the common name of the disease caused by these organisms reflects the characteristic cycles of parasitemia (Meier et al. 1985). As described for trypanosomes, outgrowth of variants expressing a new VMP sequence correlates with the appearance of a second copy of the VMP gene at a putative expression site (Meier et al. 1985).

Antigenic variation also occurs during *Neisseria gonorrhoeae* infection, with both pilin, the major component of the pilus, and the outer membrane opacity protein undergoing diversification (Stern et al. 1984; Haas and Meyer 1986). Pilus variation has been reported to involve templated diversification of a sequence at an expression site (Haas and Meyer 1986; Segal et al. 1986; Swanson et al. 1986); however, a recent report ascribes diversification to a transformation-mediated pathway (Gibbs et al. 1989).

Gene Conversion Targets Sequences at Expression Sites

The instances of regulated gene conversion described above all display a similar choreography: In each case, gene conversion targets a sequence at an expression site. Although expression sites were originally described in studies of trypanosome VSG diversification, it is now clear that the concept can be naturally extended to other organisms. In particular, the yeast mating-type locus can be considered an expression site since mating-type information can be transcribed only when it is located at this site. We now discuss why templated diversification at the immunoglobulin loci can be usefully regarded as targeting sequences at expression sites.

One critical role of V region rearrangement is the juxtaposition of the promoter, just upstream of V, with the enhancer in the J-C intron. Thus V region rearrangement generates an expression site where transcription at the promoter can be activated by enhancer-specific DNA-binding proteins. During B-cell development, two expression sites are created, one for the heavy chain and one for the light chain.

Only rearranged V regions, V regions at expression sites, undergo diversification by gene conversion. In the chicken, sensitive restriction site analyses have shown that sequence diversification does not occur in the unrearranged allele (Thompson and Neiman 1987). In the mouse, sequence analysis has revealed that only the rearranged V region undergoes hypermutation; the unrearranged allele of the same V region is not a target for hypermutation (Pech et al. 1981; Gorski et al. 1983). Furthermore, rearranged transgenes can undergo hypermutation, albeit at lower levels than the endogenous gene, implying that rearrangement, not chromosomal location, is the critical factor in targeting the mutational process (O'Brien et al. 1987).

Although templated diversification targets sequences at expression sites, it is important to emphasize that there is no evidence that the process of transcription per se is essential to render a recipient sequence competent for diversification. It has been proposed that transcriptional activity is the determining factor in increasing the accessibility of a region of DNA in a developing lymphocyte and thus rendering it active as a substrate for recombination (Alt et al. 1986). It is also possible that specific signals at the expression sites, rather than the actual process of transcription, stimulate targeted gene conversion. It is interesting in this regard that Szostak and his colleagues (Nicolas et al. 1989; Sun et al. 1989) have mapped an initiation site for meiotic gene conversion in S. cerevisiae to the arg4 promoter region. These investigators suggest that, since transcriptional regulatory elements are under strong selective pressure, the coupling of recombinational with transcriptional signals would extend that selection to a recombination process as well (Nicolas et al. 1989).

Implications of Diversification by Targeted Gene Conversion

Although it has become fashionable to focus on somatic hypermutation of mammalian immunoglobulins genes as a mechanism for increasing antibody affinity, another role of the hypermutation process is to modulate the specificity of the immune response. Implicit in any process of templated diversification is the potential for donor sequences that contribute to variation to undergo selection along with the rest of the genetic complement. Antigenic variation is a survival strategy, and the templating of variation means that a pathogen can present the host with a *tested* repertoire of antigenic variants that have been successful in its progenitors. Templating of hypermutation in mammals implies that the host, in turn, can respond to infection with a similarly tested repertoire of its own.

REFERENCES

Allen, D., A. Cumano, R. Dildrop, C. Kocks, K. Rajewsky, N. Rajewsky, J. Roes, F. Sablitzky, and M. Siekevitz. 1987. Timing, genetic requirements and functional consequences of somatic hypermutation during B-cell development. *Immunol. Rev.* **96:** 5.

Alt, F.W., T.K. Blackwell, R.A. DePinho, M.G. Reth, and G.D. Yancopoulos. 1986. Regulation of genome rearrangement events during lymphocyte differentiation. *Immunol. Rev.* **89:** 5.

Baltimore, D. 1981. Gene conversion: Some implications for immunoglobulin genes. *Cell* **24:** 592.

Beach, D.H. 1983. Cell type switching by DNA transposition in fission yeast. *Nature* **305:** 682.

Berek, C. and C. Milstein. 1987. Mutation drift and repertoire shift in the maturation of the immune response. *Immunol. Rev.* **96:** 23.

———. 1988. The dynamic nature of the antibody repertoire. *Immunol. Rev.* **105:** 5.

Bernards, A., T. De Lange, P.A.M. Michels, A.Y.C. Liu, M.J. Huisman, and P. Borst. 1984. Two modes of activation of a single surface antigen gene of *Trypanosoma brucei*. *Cell* **36:** 163.

Buck, G., S. Longacre, A. Raibaud, U. Hibner, C. Giroud, T. Baltz, D. Baltz, and H. Eisen. 1984. Stability of expression-linked surface antigen genes in *Trypanosoma equiperdum*. *Nature* **307:** 563.

De Lange, T. and P. Borst. 1982. Genomic environment of the expression-linked extra copies of genes for surface antigens of *Trypanosoma brucei* resembles the end of a chromosome. *Nature* **299:** 451.

Donelson, J.E. and A.C. Rice-Ficht. 1985. Molecular biology of trypanosome antigenic variation. *Microbiol. Rev.* **49:** 107.

Edelman, G.M. and J.A. Gally. 1967. Somatic recombination of duplicated genes: An hypothesis on the origin of antibody diversity. *Proc. Natl. Acad. Sci.* **57:** 353.

———. 1970. Arrangement and evolution of eukaryotic genes. In *The neurosciences: Second study program* (ed. F.O. Schmitt), p. 962. Rockefeller University Press, New York.

Egel, R., D.H. Beach, and A.J.S. Klar. 1984. Genes required for initiation and resolution steps of mating-type switching in fission yeast. *Proc. Natl. Acad. Sci.* **81:** 3481.

Fogel, S., R. Mortimer, and K. Lusnak. 1981. Mechanisms of meiotic gene conversion, or "wanderings on a foreign strand." In *The molecular biology of the yeast, Saccharomyces* (ed. J.N. Strathern et al.), p. 289. Cold Spring Harbor Laboratory Press, Cold Spring Harbor, New York.

Gibbs, C.P., B.-Y. Reimann, E. Schultz, A. Kaufmann, R. Haas, and T.F. Meyer. 1989. Reassortment of pilin genes in *Neisseria gonorrhoeae* occurs by two distinct mechanisms. *Nature* **338:** 651.

Gorski, J., P. Rollini, and B. Mach. 1983. Somatic mutations of immunoglobulin variable genes are restricted to the rearranged V gene. *Science* **220:** 1179.

Haas, R. and T.F. Meyer. 1986. The repertoire of silent pilus genes in *Neisseria gonorrhoeae*: Evidence for gene conversion. *Cell* **44:** 107.

Herskowitz, I. and Y. Oshima. 1981. Control of cell type in *Saccharomyces cerevisiae*: Mating type and mating-type interconversion. In *The molecular biology of the yeast, Saccharomyces* (ed. J.N. Strathern et al.), p. 181. Cold Spring Harbor Laboratory Press, Cold Spring Harbor, New York.

Hoeijmakers, J.H.J., A.C.C. Frasch, A. Bernards, P. Borst, and G.A.M. Cross. 1980. Novel expression-linked copies of the genes for variant surface antigens in trypanosomes. *Nature* **284:** 78.

Klar, A.J.S. 1987. Differentiated parental DNA strands confer developmental asymmetry on daughter cells in fission yeast. *Nature* **32:** 466.

Kostriken, R., J.N. Strathern, A.J.S. Klar, J.B. Hicks, and F. Heffron. 1983. A site-specific endonuclease essential for mating-type switching in *Saccharomyces cerevisiae*. *Cell* **35**: 167.

Kunkel, T.A. 1988. Exonucleolytic proofreading. *Cell* **53**: 837.

Longacre, S. and H. Eisen. 1986. Expression of whole and hybrid genes in *Trypanosoma equiperdum* antigenic variation. *EMBO J.* **5**: 1057.

Longacre, S., U. Hibner, A. Raibaud, H. Eisen, T. Baltz, C. Giroud, and D. Baltz. 1983. DNA rearrangements and antigenic variation in *Trypanosoma equiperdum*: Multiple expression-linked sites in independent isolates of trypanosomes expressing the same antigen. *Mol. Cell. Biol.* **3**: 399.

Maizels, N. 1989. Might gene conversion be the mechanism of somatic hypermutation of mammalian immunoglobulin genes? *Trends Genet.* **5**: 4.

Malipiero, U.V., N.S. Levy, and P.J. Gearhart. 1987. Somatic mutation in anti-phosphorylcholine antibodies. *Immunol. Rev.* **96**: 59.

Manser, T., L.J. Wysocki, M.N. Margolies, and M.L. Gefter. 1987. Evolution of antibody variable region structure during the immune response. *Immunol. Rev.* **96**: 141.

McCormack, W.T., L.W. Tjoelker, C.F. Barth, L.M. Carlson, B. Petryniak, E.H. Humphries, and C.B. Thompson. 1989. Selection for B cells with productive IgL gene rearrangements occurs in the bursa of Fabricius during chicken embryonic development. *Genes Dev.* **3**: 838.

McGill, C., B. Shafer, and J. Strathern. 1989. Coconversion of flanking sequences with homothallic switching. *Cell* **57**: 459.

McKean, D., K. Huppi, M. Bell, L. Staudt, W. Gerhard, and M. Weigert. 1984. Generation of antibody diversity in the immune response of BALB/c mice to influenza virus hemagglutinin. *Proc. Natl. Acad. Sci.* **81**: 3180.

Meier, J.T., M.I. Simon, and A.G. Barbour. 1985. Antigenic variation is associated with DNA rearrangements in a relapsing fever Borrelia. *Cell* **41**: 403.

Milstein, C. and J. Svasti. 1971. Expansion and contraction in the evolution of immunoglobulin gene pools. In *Progress in immunology* (ed. B. Amos), p. 33. Academic Press, New York.

Nicolas, A., D. Treco, N.P. Schultes, and J.W. Szostak. 1989. An initiation site for meiotic gene conversion in the yeast *Saccharomyces cerevisiae*. *Nature* **338**: 35.

O'Brien, R.L., R.L. Brinster, and U. Storb. 1987. Somatic hypermutation of an immunoglobulin transgene in kappa transgenic mice. *Nature* **326**: 405.

Pays, E., M. Lheureux, and M. Steinert. 1981. The expression-linked copy of surface antigen gene in *Trypanosoma* is probably the one transcribed. *Nature* **292**: 262.

Pays, E., S. Van Assel, M. Laurent, M. Darville, T. Vervoort, N. Van Meirvenne, and M. Steinert. 1983. Gene conversion as a mechanism for antigenic variation in Trypanosomes. *Cell* **34**: 371.

Pech, M., J. Hochtl, H. Schnell, and H.G. Zachau. 1981. Differences between germ-line and rearranged immunoglobulin Vκ coding sequences suggest a localized mutation mechanism. *Nature* **291**: 668.

Rajewsky, K., I. Forster, and A. Cumano. 1987. Evolutionary and somatic selection of the antibody repertoire in the mouse. *Science* **238**: 1088.

Reynaud, C.-A., V. Anquez, H. Grimal, and J.-C. Weill. 1987. A hyperconversion mechanism generates the chicken light chain preimmune repertoire. *Cell* **48**: 379.

Reynaud, C.-A., A. Dahan, V. Anquez, and J.-C. Weill. 1989. Somatic hyperconversion diversifies the single V_H gene of the chicken with a high incidence in the D region. *Cell* **59**: 171.

Roth, C., S. Longacre, A. Raibaud, T. Baltz, and H. Eisen. 1986. The use of incomplete genes for the construction of a

Trypanosoma equiperdum variant surface glycoprotein gene. *EMBO J.* **5**: 1065.

Sablitzky, F., G. Wildner, and K. Rajewsky. 1985. Somatic mutation and clonal expansion of B cells in an antigen-driven immune response. *EMBO J.* **4**: 345.

Scharff, M.D., H.L. Aguila, S.M. Behar, N.C. Chien, R. DePinho, D.L. French, R.R. Pollock, and S.-U. Shin. 1987. Studies on the somatic instability of immunoglobulin genes in vivo and in cultured cells. *Immunol. Rev.* **96**: 75.

Scherer, S. and D.A. Stevens. 1988. A *Candida albicans* dispersed, repeated gene family and its epidemiologic applications. *Proc. Natl. Acad. Sci.* **85**: 1452.

Segal, E., P. Hagblom, H.S. Seifert, and M. So. 1986. Antigenic variation of gonococcal pilus involves assembly of separated silent gene segments. *Proc. Natl. Acad. Sci.* **83**: 2177.

Seidman, J.G., A. Leder, M. Nau, B. Norman, and P. Leder. 1978. Antibody diversity. *Science* **202**: 11.

Smithies, O. 1967a. Antibody variability. *Science* **157**: 267.

———. 1967b. The genetic basis of antibody variability. *Cold Spring Harbor Symp. Quant. Biol.* **32**: 161.

Soll, D. 1988. High-frequency switching in *Candida albicans*. In *Mobile DNA* (ed. M. Howe and D. Berg), p. 789. American Society for Microbiology, Washington, D.C.

Steele, E.J. and J.W. Pollard. 1987. Hypothesis: Somatic hypermutation by gene conversion via the error prone DNA → RNA → DNA information loop. *Mol. Immunol.* **24**: 667.

Stern, A., P. Nickel, T.F. Meyer, and M. So. 1984. Opacity determinants of *Neisseria gonorrhoeae*: Gene expression and chromosomal linkage to the gonococcal pilus gene. *Cell* **37**: 447.

Stibitz, S., W. Aaronson, D. Monack, and S. Falkow. 1989. Phase variation in *Bordetella pertussis* by frameshift mutation in a gene for a novel two-component system. *Nature* **338**: 266.

Strathern, J.N. 1988. Control and execution of homothallic switching in *Saccharomyces cerevisiae*. In *Genetic recombination* (ed. R. Kucherlapati and G.R. Smith), p. 445. American Society for Microbiology, Washington, D.C.

Strathern, J.N., A.J. Klar, J.B. Hicks, J.A. Abraham, J.M. Ivy, K.A. Nasmyth, and C. McGill. 1982. Homothallic switching of yeast mating type cassettes is initiated by a double-stranded cut in the *MAT* locus. *Cell* **31**: 183.

Sun, H., D. Treco, N.P Schultes, and J.W. Szostak. 1989. Double-strand breaks at an initiation site for meiotic gene conversion. *Nature* **338**: 87.

Swanson, J., S. Bergstrom, K. Robbins, O. Bariera, D. Corwin, and J.M. Coomey. 1986. Gene conversion involving the pilin structural gene correlates with pilus⁺-pilus⁻ changes in *Neisseria gonorrhoeae*. *Cell* **47**: 267.

Thomas, K.R. and M.R. Capecchi. 1986. Introduction of homologous DNA sequences into mammalian cells induces mutations in the cognate gene. *Nature* **324**: 34.

Thompson, C.B. and P.E. Neiman. 1987. Somatic diversification of the chicken immunoglobulin light chain gene is limited to the rearranged variable gene segment. *Cell* **48**: 369.

Van der Ploeg, L.H.T., D.C. Schwartz, C.R. Cantor, and P. Vorst. 1984. Antigenic variation in *Trypanosoma brucei* analyzed by electrophoretic separation of chromosome-sized DNA molecules. *Cell* **37**: 77.

Wabl, M., H.-M. Jack, J. Meyer, G. Beck-Engeser, R.C. von Borstel, and C.M. Steinberg. 1987. Measurements of mutation rats in B lymphocytes. *Immunol. Rev.* **96**: 91.

Young, J.R., J.S. Shah, G. Matthyssens, and R.O. Williams. 1983. Relationship between multiple copies of a *T. brucei* variable surface glycoprotein gene whose expression is not controlled by duplication. *Cell* **24**: 287.

Comparative Study of Two Fab-lysozyme Crystal Structures

D.R. DAVIES, S. SHERIFF, AND E. PADLAN

National Institutes of Health, National Institute of Diabetes and Digestive and Kidney Diseases,
Laboratory of Molecular Biology, Section on Molecular Structure, Bethesda, Maryland 20892

The investigation of the three-dimensional structure of antibodies complexed to their protein antigens has been carried out on several different antibody-antigen pairs (for review, see Alzari et al. 1988; Colman 1988; Davies et al. 1988). These studies considerably enlarge the scope of previous investigations that made use of myeloma proteins with hapten binding specificities. However, many of the basic questions remain the same, e.g., whether there are conformational changes upon binding, and what the nature is of the complementarity between the antibody and antigen. However, there were a number of additional questions that related to proteins as antigens. These had to do with the nature of the epitope, i.e., whether it was a continuous piece of polypeptide chain or whether it consisted of several pieces brought together by the folding of the protein. Also in question was the role of mobility in defining the epitope, i.e., whether the most mobile regions were those that were the most antigenic. These questions could only be answered by a direct study of antibodies complexed to protein antigens.

We have determined by X-ray analysis the crystal structures of two monoclonal antibody Fabs to lysozyme, HyHEL-5 and HyHEL-10, complexed with their antigen (Sheriff et al. 1987; Padlan et al. 1989). One of these, HyHEL-5, has been examined in two crystal forms. Here, we briefly summarize the results of these analyses and compare them with the data obtained from other antibody-antigen complexes.

The HyHEL-5/Lysozyme Complex

Experimental. Crystals of the HyHEL-5 Fab lysozyme complex were grown from 20% polyethylene glycol (PEG) 3400 in 0.1 M imidazole hydrochloride (pH 7.0), 10 mM spermine with an initial protein concentration of 7 mg/ml. The crystals were polymorphic, with the different forms differing principally in the b-axis dimension. X-ray data were measured from two forms with cell dimensions $a = 54.9$ A, $b = 65.2$ A, $c = 78.6$ A, and $\beta = 102.4°$, to 3 A resolution; and $a = 54.8$ A, $b = 74.8$ A, $c = 79.0$ A, and $\beta = 101.8°$, to 2.6 A resolution.

The structures were determined by molecular replacement (Rossmann 1972) using the program package assembled by Fitzgerald (1988). The three probes used were (1) tetragonal lysozyme (Diamond 1974), (2) C_H1 and C_L of McPC603 Fab (Satow et al. 1986),

and (3) V_L and V_H of McPC603 Fab with those hypervariable loops removed that have sequences differing from HyHEL-5. The structures have been refined, and the coordinates have been deposited in the Protein Data Bank (Bernstein et al. 1977).

Description of the complex. The complex formed between HyHEL-5 and lysozyme (Fig. 1a) produces a buried surface area of about 750 A^2 on the Fab and the lysozyme. The shape complementarity of the two surfaces is very close, and the refined structure indicates that only two water molecules remain in the interface.

On the antibody (Fig. 1b), all six complementarity determining regions (CDRs) are involved in the contact with lysozyme. Contacting residues are Asn-31, Tyr-32, Asp-40, Trp-91, Gly-92, Arg-93, and Pro-95 from the light chain, and Trp-33, Glu-35, Glu-50, Ser-54, Ser-56, Tyr-57, Asn-58, Gly-95, and Tyr-97 from the heavy chain. One framework residue, Trp-47, is also contacting. Additional residues partly buried in the interface are Ser-29, Val-30, Tyr-34, and Arg-46 from the light chain and Ser-30, Asp-31, Tyr-32, Leu-52, Gly-55, Asn-96, and Asp-98 from the heavy chain. The residues affected by the interaction make up 48% of the total CDRs, although only 30% are contacting.

The lysozyme epitope (Fig. 1c) involves three discrete segments of polypeptide chain: (1) Gln-41, Thr-43, Asn-44, Arg-45, Asn-46, Thr-47, Asp-48, Gly-49, and Tyr-53, which are in contact, and Thr-51 and Asp-52, which are partly buried; (2) Gly-67, Arg-68, Thr-69, and Pro-70, and the partly buried residues Asn-65, Asp-66, Gly-71, and Ser-72; and (3) Leu-84 in contact and the partly buried Pro-79, Ser-81, and Ser-85.

The epitope surface is relatively flat except for a protruding ridge that contains the two arginine side chains, Arg-45 and Arg-68. This ridge fits into a corresponding groove in the antibody, at the back of which are the carboxylates of the two side chains of Glu-35 and Glu-50. Salt bridges are formed between Glu-50 and the two arginines and between Glu-35 and Arg-68. There are altogether 74 van der Waals contacts in the interface.

Table 1 shows the hydrogen bonds and salt bridges that can be identified. The large difference in affinity that is observed between chicken lysozyme and bobwhite quail lysozyme (attributed to Arg-68→Lys-68; Smith-Gill et al. 1982) can be accounted for by the cavity created by the smaller lysine side chains and by

Table 1. Salt Links and Hydrogen Bonds from HyHEL-5 Fab to Lysozyme

Salt links
  H-Glu 350E1 . . . Arg 68NH1
  H-Glu 500E1 . . . Arg 45NH1
  H-Glu 500E1 . . . Arg 68NH2

Hydrogen bonds
  L-Gly 920   . . . Arg 45NE
  L-Arg 93NH1 . . . Arg 450
  L-Arg 93NH2 . . . Asn 460D1
  L-Arg 93NE   . . . Arg 450
  H-Trp 33NE1 . . . Tyr 530H
  H-Asn 58ND2 . . . Thr 430G1
  H-Asn 58ND2 . . . Thr 430
  H-Asn 580D1 . . . Thr 430G1
  H-Tyr 970H   . . . Pro 700

the disruption of the system of salt bridges and hydrogen bonds.

Comparison of the lysozyme complexed and uncomplexed to the antibody reveals that relatively small conformational changes occur in the region of the epitope. The rms difference in position for 96 main-chain atoms is 0.64 Å. The C_α of Pro-70 has moved by about 1.7 Å, probably as a result of contact with Tyr-97. In the side chains, relative to tetragonal lysozyme, some changes occur, the largest of which involves the indole of Trp-63, which rotates by 180° about the $C_\beta C_\gamma$ bond, despite the fact that this residue is outside the epitope.

Although a direct examination of the uncomplexed Fab conformation has not been made, the success of the molecular replacement procedure provides clear indication that no major conformational change has occurred either in the individual domains or in the positions of the domains relative to each other.

Comparison of the two crystal forms shows that the relative positions of lysozyme and the antibody V_H:V_L are the same in both. However, the relative positions of C_H1:C_L are not the same, and the difference can be accounted for by a change in the elbow bend of 8°, from 154° in the short b-axis form to 162° in the long b-axis form. This change is presumably due to the crystal packing forces in the two forms and indicates flexibility in the connecting region between V_H:V_L and C_H1:C_L.

The HyHEL-10/Lysozyme Complex

Experimental. The crystals of the complex were grown as described by Silverton et al. (1984) from solutions containing 5% PEG, 5% methylpentane diol, 0.1 M imidazole (pH 7.0). X-ray data were collected to 3.0 Å resolution. The crystal structure was determined by molecular replacement (Rossmann 1972), using the program package of Fitzgerald (1988). The search for the solution to the molecular replacement was more difficult than in the case of HyHEL-5, and it was only when the C_H1:C_L domain pair from HyHEL-5 was used as a probe that a satisfactory solution was obtained. The structure has been refined to an R-factor of 0.24 with deviations from ideality of 0.011 Å in bond

lengths and 0.034 Å in angle distances. Coordinates are available from the Protein Data Bank (Bernstein et al. 1977).

Description of the complex. As in HyHEL-5, there is very strong shape complementarity between the lysozyme epitope and the HyHEL-10 combining site (Fig. 1d). In the interface, there is no evidence that any water molecules remain. The area of lysozyme that is buried in the interface is 770 Å^2, and the corresponding area of the antibody is 720 Å^2.

The antibody combining site (Fig. 1e) has at least one contacting residue from each CDR. These include Gly-30, Asn-31, Asn-32, Tyr-50, Gln-53, Ser-91, Asn-92, and Tyr-96 from V_L, and Thr-30, Ser-31, Asp-32, Tyr-33, Tyr-50, Ser-52, Tyr-53, Ser-54, Ser-56, Tyr-58, and Trp-98 from V_H. Also contacting is Thr-30 of V_H, which is a framework residue. A striking feature of this site is the presence of seven aromatic residues, one tryptophan and six tyrosines. Disproportionate numbers of aromatic residues, particularly tyrosines, have also been noted in the combining site of McPC603 (Satow et al. 1986), D1.3 (Amit et al. 1986), and in the combining site of HLA (Bjorkman et al. 1987). Tyrosine side chains have properties that might favor their use in complex formation: (1) They are neutral residues with a capacity for hydrogen bonding through the terminal hydroxyl group as well as being capable of accepting hydrogen bonds directed at the center of the aromatic ring; (2) they have an aromatic component that is quite capable of large packing adjustments by a small rotation about single bonds; and (3) they have low conformational entropy that would minimize the decrease in entropy as a result of complex formation.

The surface of HyHEL-10 in contact with the lysozyme is unusual in that it is not particularly concave and does not contain deep grooves or cavities. On the contrary, it has a protrusion that fits into the active-site cleft of the lysozyme molecule. The residues that form this protrusion are mainly Tyr-33 and Tyr-53 from the heavy chain.

The lysozyme epitope (Fig. 1f) is dominated by a central α helix, residues 88–99, and can best be described as consisting of this helix together with some amino acids on either side of the helix. These are His-15, Gly-16, Tyr-20, and Arg-21 on one side of the helix; Thr-98, Asn-93, Lys-96, Lys-97, and Ile-98 in the helix; Ser-100, Asp-101, and Gly-102 extending beyond the helix; Trp-63 in the active-site cleft of lysozyme; and Arg-73 and Leu-75 on the other side of the cleft. Partly buried, but noncontacting residues include Asn-19, Asn-103, and Ala-107. Most of the contacting residues are polar, and five are charged, i.e., this is a representative selection of protein surface residues.

The principal interactions between the two proteins involve van der Waals contacts, of which there are 111. In addition, there are 14 hydrogen bonds (Table 2). Despite the fact that six of the contacting residues are charged, only one rather weak salt bridge is formed between Asp-32 of HyHEL-10 and Lys-97 of lysozyme.

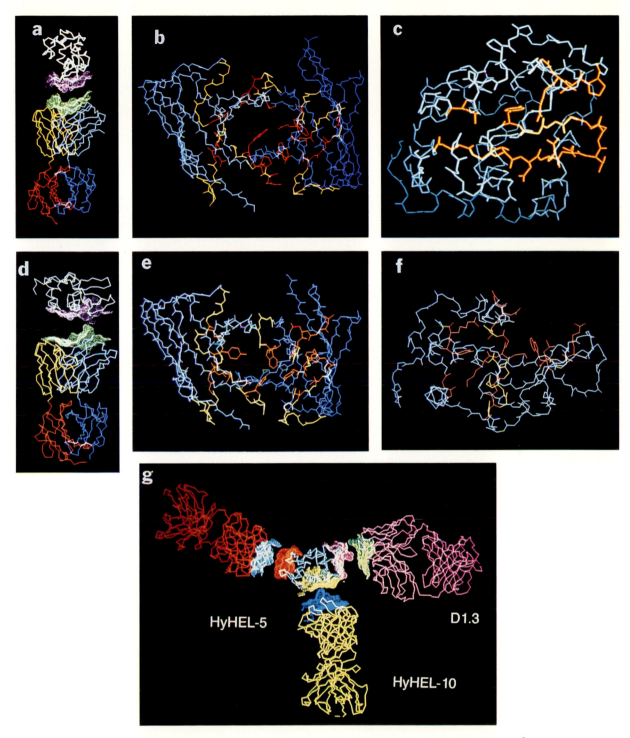

Figure 1. (*a*) Complex of HyHEL-5 Fab and lysozyme. The two molecules have been displaced by 14 Å from the positions observed in the crystal structure. The dot surface indicates the epitope on the lysozyme and the contacting surface on the Fab. V_H is blue, V_L is yellow, C_H1 is dark blue, and C_L is red. (*b*) HyHEL-5 combining site. CDR main chains in yellow, with the contacting residues in red. The light and heavy chains are blue and purple, respectively. (*c*) Lysozyme structure with the epitope highlighted in red (contacting residues) and yellow (buried noncontacting residues). (*d*) Same as *a*, but for HyHEL-10; (*e*) same as *b*, but for HyHEL-10; (*f*) same as *c*, but for HyHEL-10. (*g*) Lysozyme molecule together with the Fabs of HyHEL-5, HyHEL-10, and D1.3 (Amit et al. 1986). The Fabs have been displaced 12.5 A from the positions observed in the crystal structures. The dot surface on lysozyme shows the three epitopes that together cover over 40% of the lysozyme surface. (Reprinted, with permission, from Davies et al. 1989.)

Table 2. Hydrogen Bonds between HyHEL-10 and Lysozyme

HyHEL-10		Lysozyme
	Asn 31	His 15
VL:	Asn 31 OD1	Lys 96 NZ
	Asn 32 ND2	Gly 16 O
	Gln 53 OE1	Asn 93 ND2
	Gln 53 NE2	Asn 93 OD1
	Ser 91 O	Tyr 20 OH
	Asn 92 O	Arg 21 N
	Tyr 96 OH	Arg 51 NH1
VH:	Thr 30 O	Arg 73 NH1
	Ser 31 OG	Arg 73 NH1
	Tyr 33 OH	Lys 97 O
	Tyr 50 OH	Arg 21 NH1, Ser 100 O
	Tyr 53 O	Asp 101 OD1
	Tyr 58 OH	Gly 102 N

Small conformational changes in the lysozyme as a result of binding are observed in the C_α coordinates of residues 47 (1.44 A), 101 (1.80 A), and 102 (213 A). The side chain of Trp-62 appears to have been rotated by 150° about the C_β-C_γ bond. The close similarity of the V_L of HyHEL-10 to REI (Epp et al. 1974) and of the V_H CDRs to those of D1.3 and New strongly suggests that no major conformational change has occurred in the antibody.

DISCUSSION

There are now three lysozyme epitopes that have been defined by crystallographic analyses. HyHEL-5 and HyHEL-10 have been described above, and D1.3 has been described by Amit et al. (1986). These three epitopes (Fig. 1g), which are almost entirely nonoverlapping, provide an opportunity to address a number of questions concerning antibody-antigen interactions (Davies et al. 1988).

In all three cases, the epitope consists of several segments of polypeptide chain brought into proximity by the folding of the antigen. The HyHEL-5 and D1.3 epitopes are dominated by two segments of chain, whereas the HyHEL-10 epitope can be regarded as the external surface of an α helix together with surrounding residues. For NC41, an anti-neuraminidase monoclonal antibody, the epitope is discontinuous, consisting of at least four segments of polypeptide chain (Colman et al. 1987).

The three antibody-lysozyme interfaces are characterized by a strong shape complementarity between the two surfaces so that the packing density within the interface resembles that of protein interiors and the interface is devoid of water molecules. The areas of the interacting surface are rather similar, about 700–800 A^2, and the interaction involves a large number of van der Waals contacts together with about a dozen hydrogen bonds. Although the formation of ion pairs seems to be an important part of the HyHEL-5 interaction, strong salt bridges are not observed in the other complexes.

Correlation between antigenicity and the physical properties of the antigenic surface has been suggested previously, with mobility and protrusion being the two principal correlates (for a more detailed discussion of this point, see Davies et al. 1988). An analysis of the crystallographic B factors, which are a measure of mobility, in these three lysozyme epitopes shows no strong correlation between mobility and antigenicity. Accessibility, on the other hand, provides a better correlation. The observation that the three lysozyme epitopes constitute greater than 40% of the total surface of the lysozyme, together with the known existence of other antibodies to different regions of lysozyme, provides support for the conclusion that all accessible parts of the molecule are potentially antigenic (Benjamin et al. 1984).

In the HyHEL-5 and HyHEL-10 complexes, only small conformational changes are observed in the lysozyme upon binding to the antibody. The same has been reported for D1.3. To the extent that it is possible to generalize from these three examples, it would seem unlikely that gross conformational changes will occur. However, lysozyme is a small, compact, and rather rigid protein not subject to large changes as a result of external stimulus (Kundrot and Richards 1987) so that these results could be misleading for other more flexible proteins. Indeed, Colman et al. (1987) have reported significant changes in the neuraminidase upon binding to NC41.

Conformational change in the antibody is more difficult to assess on the basis of the data presented here. However, for HyHEL-5 and HyHEL-10, there is good similarity between the secondary structure of the domains and that observed in other uncomplexed Fab structures. Also, the relationship of V_H and V_L falls within the range of values observed for other Fabs, leading us to conclude that no gross conformational change has occurred. In some CDRs, however, e.g., CDR1 of the light chain of McPC603, the insertion of additional residues results in a long and highly flexible loop that extends into the solvent and cannot be uniquely located in the electron density map. In such cases, it is not meaningful to ask whether conformational change takes place. Other CDRs might move in a hinged motion, with the whole CDR swinging as a unit about a few bonds. An example of this kind of motion may occur in HyHEL-5 (Hartman et al. 1988).

One curious feature of the HyHEL-10 structure in the complex is the extent to which the aromatic residues stick out from the antibody surface and penetrate parts of the antigen. It is pertinent to ask whether these side chains adopt the same conformation in the absence of antigen, which would drastically expose them to solvent. However, in several of the previous Fab structures, such as McPC603 (Satow et al. 1986), J539 (Suh et al. 1986), and R19.9 (Lascombe et al. 1989), in which the Fab is not complexed to antigen, many of the aromatic residues in the CDRs are quite exposed to solvent in a manner not usually seen on protein surfaces, raising the possibility that they do not undergo a

Table 3. Comparison of Elbow Bend Angles in Fab Fragments

Fab fragment	Elbow bend angle	Reference
New	132	Saul et al. (1978)
McPC603	133	Satow et al. (1986)
S10/1	~135	Colman and Webster (1987)
J539	145	Suh et al. (1986)
Dob	147	Silverton et al. (1977)
HyHEL-10[a]	147	Padlan et al. (1989)
NC41[a]	~150	Colman et al. (1987)
HyHEL-5	154	Sheriff et al. (1987)
Jel 42 (molecule 1)	159	Prasad et al. (1988)
HyHEL-5 (b = 74.8 A)[a]	162	Sheriff et al. (1987)
HED10	162	Cygler et al. (1987)
CF4C4	164	Vitali et al. (1987)
Jel 42 (molecule 2)	167	Prasad et al. (1988)
Kol	167	Marquart et al. (1980)
D1.3[a]	172	Amit et al. (1986)
R19.9	178	Lascombe et al. (1989)

[a]Fab-protein antigen complexes.

large change upon binding. However, direct proof of conformational change in the antibody will necessitate the X-ray analysis of crystals of the uncomplexed Fab.

Fab structures show variation in the elbow bend angle relating the orientation of the $V_H:V_L$ pair to the $C_H1:C_L$ pair. This angle, between the pseudo dyad axes of the two domain pairs, is observed to vary between 135° and 180°. In the two crystal forms of the HyHEL-5/lysozyme complex, the principal difference between the two Fab structures lies in an 8° difference in the elbow bends, despite the fact that the two forms contain the same Fab complexed to the same antigen. The data in Table 3 show the Fab elbow bends in published crystal structures. It is clear that there is a lack of correlation with the liganded state of the antigen. The large range of angles observed demonstrates that there is considerable flexibility in this region of the antibody molecule.

REFERENCES

Alzari, P.M., M.B. Lascombe, and R.J. Poljak. 1988. Three-dimensional structure of antibodies. *Annu. Rev. Immunol.* **6:** 555.

Amit, A.G., R.A. Mariuzza, S.E.V. Phillips, and R.J. Poljak. 1986. Three-dimensional structure of an antigen-antibody complex at 2.8 Å resolution. *Science* **233:** 747.

Benjamin, D.C., J.A. Berzofsky, I.J. East, F.R.N. Gurd, C. Hannum, S.J. Leach, E. Margoliash, J.G. Michael, A. Miller, E.M. Prager, M. Reichlin, E.E. Sercarz, S.J. Smith-Gill, P.E. Todd, and A.C. Wilson. 1984. The antigenic structure of proteins: A reappraisal. *Annu. Rev. Immunol.* **2:** 67.

Bernstein, F.C., T.F. Koetzle, G.J.B. Williams, E.F. Meyer, Jr., M.D. Brice, J.R. Rodgers, O. Kennard, T. Shimanouchi, and M. Tasumi. 1977. The Protein Data Bank: A computer-based archival file for macromolecular structures. *J. Mol. Biol.* **112:** 535.

Bjorkman, P.I., M.A. Saper, B. Samroui, W.S. Bennett, J.L. Strominger, and D.C. Wiley. 1987. Structure of the human class I histocompatibility antigen, HLA-A2. *Nature* **329:** 506.

Colman, P.M. 1988. Structure of antibody-antigen complexes: Implications for immune recognition. *Adv. Immunol.* **43:** 99.

Colman, P.M. and R.G. Webster. 1987. The structure of an antineuraminidase monoclonal Fab fragment and its interaction with the antigen. In *Biological organization: Macromolecular interactions at high resolution* (ed. R. Burnett and H.J. Vogel), p. 125. Academic Press, Orlando, Florida.

Colman, P.M., W.G. Laver, J.N. Varghese, A.T. Baker, P.A. Tulloch, G.M. Air, and R.G. Webster. 1987. Three-dimensional structure of a complex of antibody with influenza virus neuraminidase. *Nature* **326:** 358.

Cygler, M., A. Boodhoo, J.S. Lee, and W.F. Anderson. 1987. Crystallization and structure determination of an autoimmune anti-poly (dT) immunoglobulin Fab fragment at 3.0 Å resolution. *J. Biol. Chem.* **262:** 643.

Davies, D.R., S. Sheriff, and E.A. Padlan. 1988. Antibody-antigen complexes. *J. Biol. Chem.* **263:** 10541.

Davies, D.R., S. Sheriff, E.A. Padlan, E.W. Silverton, G.H. Cohen, and S.J. Smith-Gill. 1989. Three-dimensional structures of two Fab complexes with lysozyme. In *The immune response to structurally defined proteins: The lysozyme model* (ed. S.J. Smith-Gill and E.E. Sercarz), p. 125. Adenine Press, Schenectady, New York.

Diamond, R. 1974. Real-space refinement of the structure of hen egg-white lysozyme. *J. Mol. Biol.* **82:** 371.

Epp, O., P. Colman, H. Fehlhammer, W. Bode, M. Schiffer, R. Huber, and W. Palm. 1974. Crystal and molecular structure of a dimer composed of the variable portions of the Bence-Jones protein REI. *Eur. J. Biochem.* **45:** 513.

Fitzgerald, P.M.D. 1988. Merlot, an integrated package of computer programs for the determination of crystal structures by molecular replacement. *J. Appl. Crystallogr.* **21:** 273.

Hartman, A.B., C.P. Mallett, S. Sheriff, and S.J. Smith-Gill. 1988. Unusual joining sites in the H and L chains of an anti-lysozyme antibody. *J. Immunol.* **141:** 932.

Kundrot, C.E. and F.M. Richards. 1987. Crystal structure of hen egg white lysozyme at a hydrostatic pressure of 1000 atmospheres. *J. Mol. Biol.* **193:** 157.

Lascombe, M.B., P.M. Alzari, G. Boulot, P. Saludjian, P. Tougard, C. Berek, S. Haba, E.M. Rowen, A. Nisonoff, and R.J. Poljak. 1989. Three-dimensional structure of Fab R19.9, a monoclonal murine antibody specific for the p-azobenzenearsonate group. *Proc. Natl. Acad. Sci.* **86:** 607.

Marquart, M., J. Deisenhofer, R. Huber, and W. Palm. 1980. Crystallographic refinement and atomic models of the intact immunoglobulin molecule Kol and its antigen-binding fragment at 3.0 Å and 1.9 Å resolution. *J. Mol. Biol.* **141:** 369.

Padlan, E.A., E.W. Silverton, S. Sheriff, G.H. Cohen, S.J. Smith-Gill, and D.R. Davies. 1989. Structure of an antibody:antigen complex: Crystal structure of the HyHEL-10 Fab:lysozyme complex. *Proc. Natl. Acad. Sci.* **86:** 5938.

Prasad, L., M. Vandonselaar, J.S. Lee, and L.T.J. Delbaere. 1988. Structure determination of a monoclonal Fab fragment specific for histidine-containing protein of the phosphoenolpyruvate: Sugar phosphoesterase system of *Escherichia coli. J. Biol. Chem.* **263:** 2571.

Rossmann, M.G., ed. 1972. *The molecular replacement method.* Gordon and Breach, New York.

Satow, Y., G.H. Cohen, E.A. Padlan, and D.R. Davies. 1986. Phosphocholine binding immunoglobulin Fab McPC603. An X-ray diffraction study at 2.7 Å. *J. Mol. Biol.* **190:** 593.

Saul, F., L.M. Amzel, and R.J. Poljak. 1978. Preliminary refinement and structural analysis of the Fab fragment from human immunoglobulin new at 2.0 Å resolution. *J. Biol. Chem.* **253:** 585.

Sheriff, S., E.W. Silverton, E.A. Padlan, G.H. Cohen, S.J. Smith-Gill, B.C. Finzel, and D.R. Davies. 1987. Three-dimensional structure of an antibody-antigen complex. *Proc. Natl. Acad. Sci.* **84:** 8075.

Silverton, E.W., E.A. Padlan, D.R. Davies, S.J. Smith-Gill, and M. Potter. 1984. Crystalline monoclonal antibody Fabs complexed to hen egg white lysozyme. *J. Mol. Biol.* **180:** 761.

Silverton, E.W., M.A. Navia, and D.R. Davies. 1977. Three-dimensional structure of an intact human immunoglobulin. *Proc. Natl. Acad. Sci.* **74:** 5140.

Suh, S.W., T.M. Bhat, M.A. Navia, G.H. Cohen, D.R. Rao, S. Rudikoff, and D.R. Davies. 1986. The galactan-binding immunoglobulin Fab J539. An X-ray diffraction study at 2.6-Å resolution. *Proteins Struct. Funct. Genet.* **1:** 74.

Smith-Gill, S.J., A.C. Wilson, M. Potter, E.M. Prager, R.M. Feldmann, and C.R. Mainhart. 1982. Mapping the antigenic epitope for a monoclonal antibody against lysozyme. *J. Immunol.* **128:** 314.

Vitali, J., W.W. Young, V.B. Schatz, S.E. Sabottka, and R.H. Kretsinger. 1987. Crystal structure of an anti-Lewis *a* Fab determined by molecular replacement methods. *J. Mol. Biol.* **198:** 351.

Immunochemical and Crystallographic Studies of Antibody D1.3 in Its Free, Antigen-liganded, and Idiotope-bound States

G.A. BENTLEY, T.N. BHAT, G. BOULOT, T. FISCHMANN, J. NAVAZA, R.J. POLJAK, M.-M. RIOTTOT, AND D. TELLO

Unité d'Immunologie Structurale, Département d'Immunologie (URA 359, Centre National de la Recherche Scientifique), Institut Pasteur, 75724 Paris, France

The three-dimensional structure of several Fab fragments from human immunoglobulins and murine monoclonal antibodies (MAbs) have been determined by X-ray crystallography (for review, see Amzel and Poljak 1979; Davies and Metzger 1983; Alzari et al. 1988). Further analyses of the steric structure of the antigen-combining site of antibodies were made possible by the X-ray diffraction studies of two Fab complexes with the haptens phosphorylcholine (Segal et al. 1974) and vitamin K_1OH (Amzel et al. 1974). Although these studies have contributed much to our current understanding of antibody structure and specificity, several questions relating to antigen-antibody reactions remained unanswered until the recent structural studies of Fab-antigen complexes by X-ray crystallographic techniques (Amit et al. 1986; Colman et al. 1987; Sheriff et al. 1987). These studies converged in defining the topographical or discontinuous nature of antigenic determinants (or epitopes), the area of the antigen-antibody interface, and the chemical nature of their interactions (for review, see Colman 1988; Davies et al. 1988). A question that has remained unresolved, however, concerns the possibility of conformational changes in the antibody molecule upon binding to antigen. This has been largely due to the lack of success in crystallizing unliganded Fabs to provide the necessary structural comparison between their free and antigen-bound forms.

A model antigen, hen egg white lysozyme (HEL), has been used in our laboratory to obtain monoclonal antibodies produced during the course of a secondary response in BALB/c mice (Harper et al. 1987). These antibodies have been systematically employed to explore possible crystallization conditions of Fab-HEL complexes. Several crystalline antigen-antibody complexes have now been obtained (Mariuzza et al. 1983; Fischmann et al. 1988), including one with a cross-reacting antigen, pheasant egg white lysozyme (Guillon et al. 1987). The successful X-ray crystallographic analysis of one of these, the FabD1.3-HEL complex (Amit et al. 1985, 1986), prompted us to intensify efforts to crystallize the unliganded FabD1.3 to establish whether significant conformational changes do occur in the antibody upon binding antigen. In this paper, we report the crystallization of FabD1.3 and the current progress of the determination of its three-dimensional structure. We also review progress in the crystallographic refinement of the complex FabD1.3-HEL.

Our investigations of D1.3 have also included an examination of idiotope–anti-idiotope interactions of this antibody. Particular interest surrounds those anti-idiotopic antibodies recognizing idiotopes located on the paratope of an antibody, because evidence suggests that these can mimic the original antigen (Gaulton and Greene 1986). With this end in view, we have obtained monoclonal anti-idiotopic antibodies to D1.3 for crystallization trials of Fab-Fab idiotope–anti-idiotope complexes. We have previously reported the crystallization of FabD1.3 as a complex with the Fab of one of its anti-idiotopic antibodies, E225 (Boulot et al. 1987); although its structural analysis is not yet complete, we show results here that provide some preliminary answers concerning antigen mimicry by antibodies. Finally, we give immunochemical evidence using polyclonal and monoclonal anti-E225 antibodies that E225 does mimic HEL in some way; i.e., it carries an *internal image* of the external antigen.

EXPERIMENTAL PROCEDURES

Crystallization of FabD1.3. The crystallization conditions for the FabD1.3-HEL (Mariuzza et al. 1983) and the FabD1.3-FabE225 (Boulot et al. 1987) complexes have been described. FabD1.3 was crystallized from 1.9 M ammonium sulfate, 0.1 M sodium acetate buffer (pH 4.2), by microdialysis. The crystals belong to the space group $P2_1$, with a = 79.6 Å, b = 42.2 Å, c = 72.2 Å, and β = 113.7°.

X-ray intensity measurements. Diffraction data from crystals of FabD1.3, FabD1.3-HEL, and FabD1.3-FabE225 were recorded at the Multiwire Area Detector Facility, University of Virginia, Charlottesville (Sobottka et al. 1984), using a rotating anode generator operated at 42 kV, 150 mA, with CuKα radiation passing through a graphite monochromator. Details concerning the measurement and processing of the intensity data are summarized in Table 1.

Monoclonal antibodies. The techniques for cell hybridization, propagation and production, and the

Table 1. Details of Collection and Processing of Diffraction Data

	D1.3	D1.3-HEL	D1.3-E225
No. of crystals used	1	3	1
Detector distance (cm)	64	113	83
No. of detectors	2	2	2
Resolution range (Å)	8–2.6	5–2.5	13.7–2.5
No. of independent reflexions	12870	17346	33500
R_{sym}	0.134	0.102	0.065

$R_{sym} = \Sigma(|I - \langle I \rangle|)/\Sigma\langle I \rangle$, where I is the intensity of an X-ray reflexion.

characterization of anti-HEL monoclonal antibodies and their fragments have been reported previously (Harper et al. 1987). E225 is an anti-idiotopic monoclonal antibody (IgG2b[κ]), obtained by immunization of syngeneic (BALB/c) mice with the anti-HEL MAb D1.3 (Boulot et al. 1987). MAb E225 was used, in turn, as an antigen to immunize BALB/c mice subcutaneously with 100 μg E225-conjugated keyhole limpet hemocyanin. Complete Freund's adjuvant was used for the first immunization, and incomplete adjuvant was used for booster injections at days 17 and 28. A last peritoneal antigen injection without adjuvant was performed 3 days before fusion.

Sera from the polyclonal primary and secondary anti-E225 response thus produced were assayed for anti-HEL and anti-E225 activities by direct enzyme-linked immunosorbent assay (ELISA), using HEL and FabE255, respectively, coupled to the solid phase. The threshold serum dilution still capable of producing a positive ELISA reaction was measured as a function of the number of days after immunization. The preparation of ELISA plates was carried out as described previously (Harper et al. 1987).

A third assay was used to monitor the binding of MAb E225 to anti-E225 serum in the liquid phase as a function of time after immunization. In this procedure, a fixed quantity of MAb E225 was preincubated with anti-E225 serum at different dilutions. The mixture was then tested for binding to FabD1.3, coupled to the solid phase, using ELISA. The percentage of inhibition of MAb E225 binding to FabD1.3 by anti-E225 serum was also measured by reference to control runs made in the absence of added serum.

RESULTS

Structural Analysis of FabD1.3

The crystal structure of FabD1.3 was determined by the molecular replacement technique, using the VH-VL and CH1-CL dimers of D1.3 from the D1.3-HEL complex (Amit et al. 1986) as two independent search models. The correct solutions proved to be those that gave the highest coincidence peaks in the rotation and translation functions. The problem of arbitrary origin along the b axis in the space group $P2_1$ was solved by a minimum R-factor search (agreement index between calculated and observed structure factors) in which the CH1-CL dimer was moved systematically in the y direc-

tion while holding the VH-VL dimer fixed. This gave a plausible assembly of the dimers to produce a Fab molecule. The initial model was refined by use of the constrained-restrained refinement method (CORELS; Sussmann 1985) and subsequently by XPLOR (Brunger et al. 1987). The current R-factor is 0.27, with a root mean square deviation of bond lengths from their ideal values of 0.021 Å.

Structural Analysis of the FabD1.3-HEL Complex

Using the area detector data set from 5.0 to 2.5-Å resolution and the previously measured diffractometer intensity data from 10.0 to 5.0 Å, refinement of atomic parameters of this complex, as obtained from the isomorphously phased electron density maps, was begun. Corrections to the previous model were mainly introduced in the CL and CH1 domains and residues near the amino terminus of the VL domain. After several cycles of refinement of coordinates by PROLSQ (Hendrickson 1985), alternated by manual correction on a graphics display using the program FRODO (Jones 1985), the R-factor between calculated and observed structure factors was 0.28. Further refinement, accomplished by use of the program XPLOR, reduced the R-factor to 0.23, with a root mean square deviation from ideality of bond lengths of 0.021 Å. Further refinement and corrections to the structure are still in progress.

Structural Analysis of the FabD1.3-FabE225 Complex

The crystal structure of FabD1.3-FabE225 was solved by a combination of the isomorphous replacement and molecular replacement techniques. Two heavy atom derivatives were prepared from $K_3UO_2F_5$ and tetrakis(acetoxymercuri)methane. Patterson syntheses readily provided solutions to the heavy atom positions, but subsequent heavy atom parameter refinement and phase determination showed a serious lack of isomorphism in both derivatives at high resolution, and the phases were not used beyond 4.0-Å resolution. Interpretation of the molecular boundaries of the two Fabs was unclear upon preliminary inspection of the low-resolution electron density map.

An analysis of the structure by molecular replacement was followed in parallel using the variable and constant dimers as search models in the same way as described above for the unliganded FabD1.3 structure.

The rotation and translation functions gave solutions for four independent components, as expected (a variable dimer and a constant dimer for each of the two Fabs in the complex), which were subsequently referred to a common crystallographic origin using the isomorphous phase information in the phased translation function (Colman et al. 1976). This produced an acceptable model of two Fabs interacting by way of their hypervariable regions. The results of the phased translation function, in fact, confirmed the correctness of the model, as it showed concordance between the two independent methods, isomorphous replacement and molecular replacement. Having thus placed the complex in the unit cell, the low-resolution details of the structure could be readily interpreted in the 4.0-Å electron density map phased by isomorphous replacement.

The preliminary model of the complex assumed the D1.3 structure for both Fab components, because, initially, we had no unambiguous indications as to their identity in the crystal structure. The first cycles of refinement used the program CORELS to treat each of the eight domains (VL, VH, CL, CH1, for each Fab) as rigid bodies. Subsequent cycles of refinement were performed using the program PROLSQ, followed by extensive manual corrections on a graphics display. At this stage, one round of refinement using XPLOR reduced the R-factor from 0.40 to 0.24, with the model having a 0.021 Å root mean square departure from ideal bond lengths. The electron density map subsequently calculated showed that the E225 amino acid sequence (H. Souchon et al., in prep.) could be fitted very well into the density of one of the Fabs. The clearest indications were given by the difference in structure of complementarity-determining region (CDR)2 and CDR3 of the heavy chain from that of D1.3, although several differences in side-chain density in the framework regions, where main-chain conformation is largely conserved, could also be perceived. Crystallographic refinement of the atomic positions of this structure is still in progress.

Anti-E225 Antibodies

As shown in Table 2, immunizing syngeneic BALB/c mice with the anti-idiotope E225 resulted in the production of immune responses exhibiting anti-HEL activity in addition to anti-E225 activity. The activity increased with boosting injections of the immunogen, as evidenced by the decreasing threshold of serum dilution capable of producing a positive ELISA reaction. Furthermore, as shown in Table 3, IgG and IgM monoclonal antibodies that recognized both HEL and the anti-idiotopic MAb E225 were obtained.

DISCUSSION

The results described above show the Fab fragment of D1.3 in three states: unliganded, bound to its specific antigen HEL, and engaged by an anti-idiotopic antibody. The first two undoubtedly correspond to physiological states of antibody molecules. It has been postulated that the third state, involving idiotope–anti-idiotope interactions, is also part of a physiological process that regulates antibody levels and specificity (Jerne 1974).

The three-dimensional structure of FabD1.3 shows that the relative disposition (quaternary structure) of the VH-VL and CH1-CL homology subunits, as expressed by the *elbow* angle (made by the two approximate twofold axes, one relating VL to VH and the other CL to CH1), cannot be easily correlated with an antigen-bound or unbound state of the combining site. The value for this angle is 138° in FabD1.3 alone, 172° in the FabD1.3-HEL complex, and 140° in its complex with E225. This variability is consistent with the idea that the different elbow angles observed in Fab structures result from intrasegmental flexibility in antibody molecules.

Although a detailed structural comparison of Fab-D1.3 in its free state and in its complexes with HEL or E225 requires completion of the structural refinement, present indications suggest that no significant change in

Table 2. Kinetics of BALB/c Response to Immunization with the Syngeneic Anti-idiotope MAb E225

Days after immunization	Anti-HEL[a]	Anti-FabE225[b]	Inhibition of MAb E225 binding[c]	
14	2.5×10^{-2}	n.d.	n.d.	n.d.
24	2.5×10^{-2}	5×10^{-2}	5×10^{-2}	59%
32	5×10^{-3}	$\geq 10^{-3}$	5×10^{-3}	47%
35	$\geq 5 \times 10^{-3}$	$\geq 2.5 \times 10^{-4}$	7.4×10^{-4}	44%

Anti HEL, anti-FabE225, and anti-IgG E225 activities were measured by the threshold serum dilution which produced a positive ELISA reaction.

n.d. indicates not determined.

[a]Binding of serum to solid-phase-coupled HEL. Only the IgM was measured; no IgG activity was detected.

[b]Binding of serum to solid-phase-coupled FabE225. Only the IgG activity was determined.

[c]Inhibition of IgG E225 binding to solid-phase-coupled FabD1.3, the IgG E225 being preincubated with the anti-E225 serum. The first column gives the serum dilution for a positive ELISA reaction, and the second column gives the percentage inhibition of binding to FabD1.3. Only the IgG activity was measured.

Table 3. Specificity of Anti-E225 Hybridomas

Hybridomas	Isotype	Anti-FabE225 only	Anti-HEL only	Combined anti-FabE225 and anti-HEL
Uncloned	IgG	1	0	4
	IgM	n.d.	6	7
Cloned	IgG	0	0	2
	IgM	0	0	4

Number of different hybridomas expressing exclusively anti-FabE225 activity, exclusively anti-HEL activity, and activity against both HEL and FabE225. The antibody activities were determined by ELISA (see text). n.d. indicates not determined.

the relative orientation of the VH and VL domains has occurred.

The more important conclusions concerning interaction between antigen and antibody in the FabD1.3-HEL complex remain essentially unchanged from a previous report (Amit et al. 1986). Although some modifications have been made in CDR1 of the heavy chain and CDR3 of the light chain during the course of the crystallographic refinement, these modifications have not altered the particular residues involved in contacts at the antigen-antibody interface. Specifically, these changes are at (1) Leu-29 of the heavy chain which, while exposed to the solvent in the old model, is now buried and (2) the peptide link between Thr-94 and Pro-95, which is now *cis*.

In the FabD1.3-FabE225 complex, the two Fabs are roughly aligned along their major lengths (see Fig. 1). They differ in their elbow bending angles, which are of 140° for D1.3 and 158° for E225. The complex is formed by interactions mostly between the hypervariable regions of the two Fabs. Although a definitive and detailed description of these contacts must await completion of the crystallographic refinement of the atomic coordinates, a summary of the regions implicated in the formation of the complex is shown in Table 4; these general conclusions are not expected to change in the final model. Thus, we see that although all CDRs of E225 make contact with D1.3, only five CDRs of D1.3 make contact, in turn, with E225. Of particular note, it seems that CDR3 of the E225 light chain makes the most important contribution, as residues 91, 92, 93, and 94 interact with D1.3. In addition, VL residues 65–67 from a framework loop of D1.3 occur at the interface between the two Fabs (in this complex, D1.3 is the antigen), forming contacts with the heavy chain CDR2 of E225 and some of its adjacent framework residues.

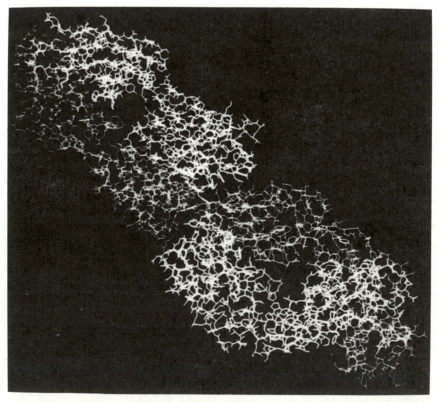

Figure 1. Skeletal model of the structure of the complex, FabD1.3-FabE225. (*Top left*) Anti-idiotope FabE225. Light chains are shown in faint tracing; heavy chains are shown in heavy tracing.

Table 4. Contacts between D1.3 and E225

E225	Contacts with D1.3	D1.3	Contacts with E225
CDR1 (L)	CDR2 (H), CDR3 (H)	CDR1 (L)	CDR3 (L), CDR1 (H), CDR2 (H)
CDR2 (L)	CDR3 (H)	CDR2 (L)	CDR3 (L), CDR2 (H), CDR3 (H)
CDR3 (L)	CDR1 (L), CDR2 (L), CDR3 (L)	CDR3 (L)	CDR3 (L)
CDR1 (H)	CDR1 (L)	CDR1 (H)	None
CDR2 (H)	CDR1 (L) CDR2 (L) Fw (L), residues 65, 66, 67	CDR2 (H)	CDR1 (L)
CDR3 (H)	CDR2 (L), CDR3 (H)	CDR3 (H)	CDR1 (L), CDR2 (L), CDR3 (H)

Contacts made by E225 and D1.3 CDRs. L and H indicate their location on the light or heavy chain, respectively. Fw indicates framework region.

Thus, as has been observed in other antigen-antibody complexes, including D1.3-HEL, the proposed division between the generally accepted CDRs and framework regions (Kabat et al. 1987) is not rigidly adhered to in E225.

No significant difference in conformation of the VH-VL dimer of D1.3, whether complexed with lysozyme or E225, exists in the models of the D1.3-HEL and the E225-D1.3 complexes at the current state of analysis. This holds true both for the quaternary and the tertiary structures and, in particular, for the conformation of all six CDRs of D1.3. Again, no major changes are expected in these conclusions upon completion of the refinement of these two complexes. The accuracy of the model of the unliganded D1.3 is not yet sufficient to make detailed comparisons with this Fab in the free state.

In the idiotope–anti-idiotope complex, the axes of approximate twofold symmetry relating the VH to the VL subunit of each Fab do not coincide. They form an angle of 168° and are displaced from each other such that their distance of closest approach is about 8 Å; this distance corresponds approximately to the separation between the centers of the antigen-binding sites of D1.3 and E225. Thus, the idiotope of D1.3 recognized by E225 is largely centered on the VL domain but with CDR3 and, to a lesser extent, CDR2 of the VH domain contributing as well. Consequently, the idiotope and the anti-HEL paratope of D1.3 do not entirely overlap in this example of an idiotope–anti-idiotope interaction. Indeed, if this displacement is examined from the point of view of D1.3, it is remarkable how closely the volume occupied by lysozyme in the complex of D1.3-HEL coincides with that occupied by the VL domain of E225 in the idiotope–anti-idiotope complex. The fact that E225 makes more contacts with VL on D1.3 is probably dictated by the surface topology of the antigen-binding sites of D1.3 and E225. Although individual amino acid residues modulate the surface of each antigen-binding site with small-scale hollows and protrusions, the overall shape is characteristically concave, with its center at the bottom of the depression between VL and VH. Thus, a strictly face-to-face interaction where the approximate twofold symmetry axes of the two Fabs coincide would lead to poor complementary contacts between them. Because most antibodies generally have a concave surface topology between the VL and VH domains centered approximately on their antigen-binding sites, a displacement of the type we have observed in the D1.3-E225 complex seems to be the most natural way of assembling an idiotope–anti-idiotope complex. Thus, we might predict that an idiotope is largely associated with either the VL or the VH domain. This conclusion could also apply to idiotopes that are not associated with the antigen-binding site.

MAb E225 recognizes a private idiotope of D1.3, not present in other anti-HEL monoclonal antibodies obtained in this laboratory (> 25). This fact was further confirmed by its binding to Fv46, a *humanized* Fv D1.3 construct (Verhoeyen et al. 1988), consisting of the CDRs of MAb D1.3 and a human immunoglobulin framework. Although E225 is in contact with the framework residues 65–67 of the D1.3 light chain, we note that the corresponding residues in Fv46, which are derived from the Bence-Jones dimer REI, are the same. The idiotope is heavy- and light-chain-dependent because, in the complex, the D1.3 CDRs from both chains are in contact with the E225-combining site even though it is largely centered on the VL domain. In particular, the VH CDR3 of D1.3 makes important contacts with the anti-idiotope. The heavy chain CDR3s, partially encoded by the diversity (D) genetic segments, are known to be the most variable parts of antibodies. This implies that the determinant recognized by E225 is very idiosyncratic to D1.3 and uniquely determined by the particular association of VH and VL. The idiotope of D1.3, as defined by its reaction with E225, shares distinctive features of epitopes as determined for antigens such as HEL (Sheriff et al. 1987) and the influenza virus neuraminidase (Colman et al. 1987). It is, for example, discontinuous (see Table 4) and involves a considerable contact area with the specific antibody.

An important question that remains to be answered by the crystal structure of the D1.3-E225 complex is whether or not E225 carries an *internal image* of the antigen HEL and, if so, what is its nature. The results presented here show conclusively that the idiotope of D1.3 recognized by E225 is related to the HEL-combining site, as would be required for such an anti-idiotopic antibody. The structural similarity between the combining site of E225 and the HEL epitope recognized by D1.3 appears sufficient to confer anti-HEL properties upon some of the anti-E225 monoclonal antibodies obtained. Table 2 shows that attempts to obtain anti-HEL antibodies in the polyclonal immune response of syngeneic BALB/c mice, using MAb E225 as an immunogen, were successful. Furthermore, monoclonal antibodies displaying anti-HEL activity have been isolated (Table 3). Thus, the anti-idiotopic antibody E225 can be considered to be one of an internal image set, which mimics the external antigen in its binding reaction with MAb D1.3.

Because the molecular structure of the HEL epitope bound by D1.3 is well known (Amit et al. 1986), a comparison between this and the paratope of E225 can readily be made. Perfect mimicry of epitopes by anti-idiotopic antibodies is not necessary at the level of tertiary structure; it only requires duplication, both in sequence and in placement, of those antigen residues in contact with the idiotope. We are now in a position to observe that this is not even approximately achieved in E225. A visual comparison shows that there is no correlation between the E225 paratope and the HEL epitope in amino acid type and position. We should rather examine epitope mimicry in terms of equivalence of surface topology and hydrophilic and hydrophobic character. E225 can be said to mimic HEL at least to the extent that it is also recognized by D1.3, with the binding sites for E225 and HEL having a significant area in common. Taken together, with the conserved conformation of the D1.3 CDRs in the two complexes, this observation might naturally lead us to expect some equivalence between E225 and HEL in the regions of common D1.3 interaction. This equivalence may not be closely adhered to because small imperfections of fit are already present at the D1.3-HEL interface. These imperfections take the form of small cavities, in one case being sufficiently large to accommodate a hypothetical water molecule (Amit et al. 1986). The fidelity with which E225 reproduces the character of the HEL epitope will only become evident in the final model of the E225-D1.3 complex upon completion of the crystallographic refinement of the atomic coordinates currently in progress.

ACKNOWLEDGMENTS

This research was supported by grants from the Institut Pasteur, Centre National de la Recherche Scientifique, grant AI-25369 from the National Institutes of Health, and contract BAP-0221(DC) from the European Economic Community. We thank our laboratory colleagues for advice and discussion, Dr. R.J. Chandross for help and advice during data collection, Dr. G. Taylor for advice and help in using the program X-PLOR on a Convex C210 computer at the Laboratory of Molecular Biophysics, University of Oxford, Dr. G. Winter and colleagues for making available the *humanized* construct Fv46, and H. Souchon, N. Doyen, and F. Rougeon for making the E225 VH and VL nucleotide sequences available to us before publication.

REFERENCES

Alzari, P.M., M.-B. Lascombe, and R.J. Poljak. 1988. Three-dimensional structure of antibodies. *Annu. Rev. Immunol.* **6:** 555.

Amit, A.G., R.A. Mariuzza, S.E.V. Phillips, and R.J. Poljak. 1985. The three-dimensional structure of an antigen-antibody complex at 6 Å resolution. *Nature* **133:** 156.

———. 1986. The three-dimensional structure of an antigen-antibody complex at 2.8 Å resolution. *Science* **233:** 747.

Amzel, L.M. and R.J. Poljak. 1979. Three-dimensional structure of immunoglobulins. *Annu. Rev. Biochem.* **48:** 961.

Amzel, L.M., R.J. Poljak, F. Saul, J.M. Varga, and F.F. Richards. 1974. The three-dimensional structure of a combining region-ligand complex of immunoglobulin New at 3.5 Å resolution. *Proc. Natl. Acad. Sci.* **71:** 1427.

Boulot, G., C. Rojas, G.A. Bentley, R.J. Poljak, E. Barbier, C. Le Guern, and P.A. Cazenave. 1987. Preliminary crystallographic study of a complex between the Fab fragment of a monoclonal anti-lysozyme antibody (D1.3) and the Fab fragment from an anti-idiotypic antibody against D1.3. *J. Mol. Biol.* **194:** 577.

Brunger, A.T., J. Kurian, and M. Karplus. 1987. Crystallographic R-factor refinement by molecular dynamics. *Science* **235:** 458.

Colman, P.M. 1988. Structure of antibody-antigen complexes. *Adv. Immunol.* **43:** 99.

Colman, P.M., H. Fehlammer, and K. Bartels. 1976. Patterson search methods in protein structure determination: β-trypsin and immunoglobulin fragments. In *Crystallographic computing techniques* (ed. F.R. Ahmed, et al.), p. 248. Munksgaard, Copenhagen.

Colman, P.M.., W.G. Laver, J.N. Varghese, A.T. Baker, P.A. Tulloch, G.M. Air, and R.G. Webster. 1987. Three-dimensional structure of a complex of antibody with influenza virus neuraminidase. *Nature* **326:** 358.

Davies, D.R. and H. Metger. 1983. Structural basis of antibody function. *Annu. Rev. Immunol.* **1:** 87.

Davies, D.R., S. Sheriff, and E.A. Padlan. 1988. Antibody-antigen complexes. *J. Biol. Chem.* **263:** 10541.

Fischmann, T., H. Souchon, M.-M. Riottot, D. Tello, and R.J. Poljak. 1988. Crystallization and preliminary X-ray diffraction studies of two antigen-antibody (lysozyme-Fab) complexes. *J. Mol. Biol.* **203:** 527.

Gaulton, G.N. and M.I. Greene. 1986. Idiotypic mimicry of biological receptors. *Annu. Rev. Immunol.* **4:** 253.

Guillon, V., P.M. Alzari, and R.J. Poljak. 1987. Preliminary crystallographic study of a complex between an heteroclitic anti-hen egg-white lysozyme antibody and the heterologous antigen pheasant egg-white lysozyme. *J. Mol. Biol.* **197:** 375.

Harper, M., F. Lema, G. Boulot, and R.J. Poljak. 1987. Antigen specificity and cross-reactivity of monoclonal anti-lysozyme antibodies. *Mol. Immunol.* **2:** 97.

Hendrickson, W.A. 1985. Stereochemically restrained refinement of macromolecular structures. *Methods Enzymol.* **115:** 253.

Jerne, N.K. 1974. Towards a network theory of the immune system. *Ann. Immunol. Inst. Pasteur* **C125:** 373.

Jones, T.A. 1985. Interactive computer graphics: FRODO. *Methods Enzymol.* **115:** 197.

Kabat, E.A., T.T. Wu, H. Bilofsky, M. Reid-Milner, and H. Perry, eds. 1987. *Sequences of proteins of immunnological interest.* U.S. Public Health Service, Washington, D.C.

Mariuzza, R.A., D. L. Jankovic, G. Boulot, A.G. Amit, P. Saludjian, A. Le Guern, J.C. Mazié, and R.J. Poljak. 1983. Preliminary crystallographic study of the complex between the Fab fragment of a monoclonal anti-lysozyme antibody and its antigen. *J. Mol. Biol.* **170:** 1055.

Segal, D.M., E.A. Padlan, G.H. Cohen, S. Rudikoff, M. Potter, and D.R. Davies. 1974. The three-dimensional structure of a phosphoryl-choline-binding mouse immunoglobulin Fab and the nature of the antigen binding site. *Proc. Natl. Acad. Sci.* **71:** 4298.

Sheriff, S., E.W. Silverton, E.A. Padlan, G.H. Cohen, S.J. Smith-Gill, B.C. Finzel, and D.R. Davies. 1987. Three-dimensional structure of an antibody-antigen complex. *Proc. Natl. Acad. Sci.* **84:** 8075.

Sobottka, S.F., G.G. Cornick, R.H. Kretsinger, R.G. Rains, W.A. Stephens, and L.J. Weissman. 1984. A MWPC X-ray diffractometer facility for protein crystallography. *Nucl. Inst. Methods Phys. Res.* **220:** 575.

Sussman, J. 1985. Constrained-restrained least-squares (CORELS) refinement of proteins and nucleic acids. *Methods Enzymol.* **115:** 271.

Verhoeyen, M., C. Milstein, and G. Winter. 1988. Reshaping human antibodies: Grafting an anti-lysozyme activity. *Science* **239:** 1534.

Antibody Recognition of the Influenza Virus Neuraminidase

G.M. AIR,* W.G. LAVER,† R.G. WEBSTER,‡ M.C. ELS,* AND M. LUO*

*Department of Microbiology, University of Alabama at Birmingham, Birmingham, Alabama 35294; †Australian National University, Canberra, ACT 2601, Australia; ‡St. Jude Childrens Research Hospital, Memphis, Tennessee 38101

Influenza virus neuraminidase (NA) was the first enzyme found to be an integral part of a virus and coded by the viral genome. It remains one of the best-characterized viral enzymes at the molecular level, although its role in viral infection is still not well understood. NA cleaves terminal N-acetyl neuraminic acid (sialic acid) from glycoconjugates on the cell surface. Because sialic acid is the receptor to which influenza virus hemagglutinin (HA) initially binds on the host cell, NA is a receptor-destroying enzyme. It allows virus to be released from the surface of infected cells and prevents self-aggregation by cleaving sialic acid from the complex carbohydrates on the HA (Palese et al. 1974; Basak et al. 1985). NA may also assist in virus spread and access to new cells by cleaving sialic acid from the mucins that overlie the epithelial cells of the respiratory tract. Although the relative importance of these functions of NA are not well understood, NA induces antibodies that protect against lethal influenza viruses (Webster et al. 1988).

NA is one of two surface glycoprotein spikes (the other being the receptor-binding moiety, HA) embedded in the lipid envelope of the virion. NA accounts for about 5–10% of the virus protein and is seen in the electron microscope as a mushroom-shaped protrusion. It is a tetramer with a box-shaped head, $100 \times 100 \times 60$ Å, made of four coplanar, roughly spherical identical subunits with a centrally attached stalk anchored in the virus membrane by a hydrophobic region near the amino-terminal end of the polypeptide (Fig. 1). This contrasts with the influenza HA, which is anchored by a hydrophobic sequence near the carboxyl terminus. No posttranslational cleavage of the NA polypeptide occurs, no signal peptide is split off, and even the initiating methionine is retained (Blok et al. 1982). Nor is there processing at the carboxyl terminus; the carboxy-terminal sequence Met-Pro-Ile, predicted from the gene sequence for N2 NA, is found in intact NA molecules isolated from the virus. A sequence of six polar amino acids at the amino terminus of the NA polypeptide, which are totally conserved in each of the nine different influenza A NA subtypes (Blok and Air 1982; Air et al. 1985a) but not in influenza B (Shaw et al. 1982), is followed by a sequence of hydrophobic amino acids that must represent the transmembrane regions of the NA (Fields et al. 1981). This sequence is not conserved at all between subtypes (apart from conservation of hydrophobicity). For biochemical studies, a soluble form of the NA can be released from the virus particles by treatment with proteinases, which cleave the polypeptide in the positions shown (Fig. 1), removing the stalk and releasing the enzymatically and antigenically active head of the NA, which can be crystallized in some cases (Laver 1978). Viruses have been obtained with "stubby" NA molecules in which the stalk is shortened by deletions of up to 18 amino acids, which is nearly 50% of the length (Els et al. 1985). The three-dimensional structures of two influenza NAs have been determined by X-ray crystallography and published at 3 Å resolution (Varghese et al. 1983; Baker et al. 1987). Further refinement has since been done (Tulip et al., this volume).

The genome of the influenza A and B viruses consists of single-stranded RNA of negative sense existing in eight pieces, packaged in orderly fashion within the virion by some as yet unknown mechanism. Each piece codes for one of the major viral proteins, and in some cases, minor proteins are also coded, using overlapping reading frames (for review, see Lamb and Choppin 1983). NA is coded by the sixth largest RNA segment. Each of the viral genes has been sequenced completely, some from many isolates of different virus subtypes, and the three-dimensional structures of the two surface glycoproteins have been determined (Wilson et al. 1981; Varghese et al. 1983).

Despite this wealth of information, influenza remains a potentially devastating disease of man, lower mammals, and birds. No effective vaccine exists, and no cure is available once infection has set in.

Antigenic Variation in Influenza Virus NA

Influenza viruses are classified into three types: A, B, and C. Influenza virus type C is rather different from the other two types and has a different receptor-destroying enzyme; only types A and B will be discussed here. Influenza viruses of types A and B continually undergo antigenic variation in the two surface antigens (HA and NA) toward which neutralizing antibodies are directed. Because of this rapid evolution, vaccines have not been very effective.

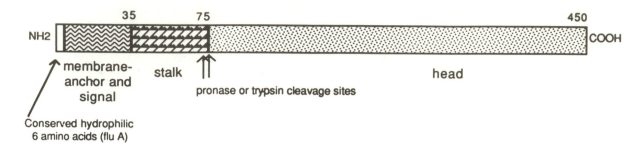

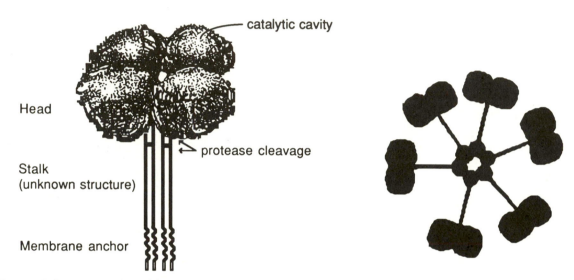

Figure 1. Influenza NA polypeptide and its folding into domains. Intact NA can be released by detergent; when the detergent is removed, the tetramers aggregate by their hydrophobic anchor sequences. Isolated tetrameric heads are obtained by proteinase treatment.

Two forms of antigenic variation have been characterized in type-A influenza: antigenic drift and major antigenic shifts. Antigenic shift involves a sudden and dramatic change in antigenic properties, usually of the HA but sometimes also the NA. Thus, nine subtypes of NA, which lack any antigenic cross-reactivity, have been classified (WHO Memorandum 1980). N1 and N2 have been found in viruses infecting man and N1–N9 in viruses infecting other animals, mainly wild birds.

Antigenic drift in influenza A is a progressive alteration in antigenic properties over time, with each new epidemic being caused by a virus that is more unlike the prototype virus than the previous epidemic. This incremental change in antigenic structure is the result of incremental changes in the protein sequence; there is an accumulation of amino acid sequence changes over time. We believe that the rather high mutation rate in influenza viruses is the result of errors by the RNA polymerases, which do not have the editing capacity of DNA polymerases, but that the vast majority of such errors are only detected after some force of positive selection has been applied, such as by neutralizing antibodies (Hall and Air 1981).

Influenza B viruses do not undergo antigenic shift,

and there are no subtype divisions in influenza B. It is still debatable whether they undergo antigenic drift. They certainly show antigenic variation, but the antigenic properties change erratically rather than progressively (Lu et al. 1983; Oxford et al. 1984). The limited sequence data available to date show considerably fewer changes than are seen during influenza A antigenic drift, and a sequential accumulation of changes is not so obvious (Krystal et al. 1983; Yamashita et al. 1988). The impressive correlation between antigenic properties and sequence changes in influenza A does not apply to influenza B.

We have been studying the mechanisms of antigenic variation in influenza A and B. We are interested in how the amino acid sequence changes affect individual epitopes, what constitutes an epitope, why a single amino acid sequence change is sufficient to destroy an epitope (in the sense that antibody can no longer bind), and why, particularly in the case of influenza B, so very few amino acid sequence changes are required to start a new epidemic.

The enzyme activity of the NA protein is conserved among all the different strains and subtypes of influenza virus and depends on conservation of the amino acid side chains lining the active-site pocket. Thoughts of using this conserved region to develop a (universal) vaccine against all influenza strains are dashed by the knowledge from the three-dimensional structure that it is inaccessible to antibodies. A similar situation of conserved amino acids inaccessible to antibody surrounded by variable amino acids was noted in rhinoviruses and has become known as the "canyon hypothesis" (Rossmann et al. 1985). Detailed information about the activity and structure of the active site of influenza NA may enable the design of new inhibitors to control the virus effectively, regardless of its antigenic structure.

Monoclonal Antibody Escape Mutants

Antibodies to the NA do not neutralize virus infectivity, but some antibodies do inhibit the enzyme. Thus, newly formed virus cannot leave the infected cell and the infection is terminated effectively. Escape mutants (Gerhard and Webster 1978; Rossmann and Rueckert 1987) of N2 and N9 NA were obtained by growing the viruses in the presence of high concentrations of monoclonal antibodies to NA (Webster et al. 1982, 1987). The NA genes of a number of the escape mutants have been sequenced. Almost all of the escape mutants have single nucleotide changes that result in single amino acid sequence changes in the NA polypeptide (Lentz et al. 1984; Air et al. 1985b). Most of these sequence changes are located on the top of the tetrameric NA head, on the rim around the active-site crater, suggesting that the neutralizing antigenic determinants (epitopes) are located in this region. Other epitopes almost certainly exist at the base of the tetramer, but escape mutants have not been isolated, presumably because antibodies binding in this region do not neutralize NA activity. The analysis of escape mutants, together with knowledge of the three-dimensional structure of NA alone and in complex with antibodies (Colman et al. 1987b; Tulip et al., this volume), has enabled characterization of epitopes on the NA.

What Is an Epitope?

We define an epitope as the region on the surface of a protein that binds a particular monoclonal antibody molecule. Regions on unfolded proteins that bind antibodies are not considered to be epitopes by this definition. The best evidence that an antibody is binding to native protein is that the biological activity of the protein is affected by antibody in a measurable way. Antibodies that affect biological activity presumably must be binding to the native (biologically active) form. However, it is almost certain that not all antibodies that bind to native protein affect biological activity.

It has been proposed that there are two kinds of epitopes on proteins: sequential and conformational (Sela 1969). Of the five epitopes characterized so far by X-ray crystallography (Amit et al. 1986; Colman et al. 1987b, 1989; Sheriff et al. 1987; Padlan et al. 1989), all are conformational (i.e., made up of several short amino acid sequences, close together in the three-dimensional structure but, perhaps, widely separated in the primary sequence).

We believe that sequential epitopes on proteins may be very rare and that most of the continuous epitopes described so far reside on unfolded, denatured protein molecules. In any case, it is doubtful that even segments of unfolded protein are truly continuous, with all amino acid side chains in contact with antibody.

Here, we describe some of the properties of epitopes on influenza virus NA of type A (subtypes N2 and N9) and type B.

N2 NA

The three-dimensional structure of N2 NA heads, determined from an electron density map at 2.9 Å resolution, shows that each monomer is composed of six topologically identical β sheets arranged in a propeller formation (Varghese et al. 1983). The tetrameric enzyme has circular fourfold symmetry, with the catalytic sites located in deep pockets that occur on the upper corners of the box-shaped tetramer. Sugar residues are attached to four of the five potential glycosylation sequences, and in one case, the carbohydrate contributes to the interaction between subunits in the tetramer. The enzyme catalytic site is contained within a deep crater on the top surface of the NA and is lined with amino acid side chains that are conserved in all NAs that have been sequenced. Site-directed mutagenesis of some of these conserved amino acids has tentatively identified the catalytic center (Lentz et al. 1987).

Neutralizing monoclonal antibodies raised against the N2 NA (Webster et al. 1982, 1984) do not recognize unfolded protein. Almost all of them select escape mutants with amino acid sequence changes in the loops that protrude from the β sheets on the top surface of the molecule (i.e., farthest from the viral membrane) and that surround the active-site crater (Fig. 2) (Colman et al. 1983). Some nonneutralizing antibodies may recognize other regions of the monomer, but without biological activity, it is hard to be sure that these are binding to native protein. A high proportion of neutralizing monoclonal antibodies from BALB/c mice to two strains of N2 virus select or recognize escape mutants with changes in the region around amino acid 344 (Fig. 2). Antibodies to epitopes in this region do not, however, predominate in rabbit antiserum.

Structure of Escape Mutants

No crystals of X-ray diffraction quality have been obtained of antibody molecules (or Fab fragments) bound to N2 NA, and the question is raised of how single amino acid sequence changes in the loops abolish antibody binding. Only 1 out of perhaps 20 contact residues is altered in each mutant. One possible mechanism is that a single sequence change can drastically

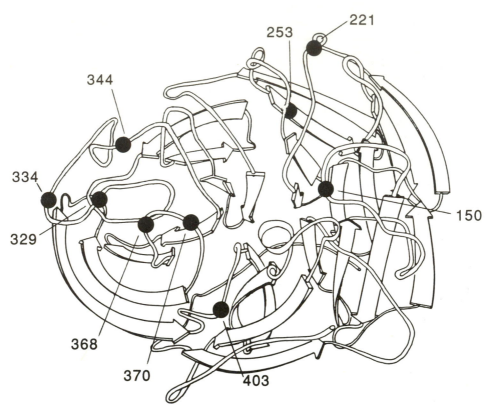

Figure 2. Location of escape mutants of N2 NA on the three-dimensional structure of the NA monomer. The structure has been revised from that published (Colman et al. 1983) in the region involving amino acids 329–344. (Kindly provided by W. Tulip, this volume.)

alter the conformation of the whole epitope, so that it is no longer recognized by antibody.

Varghese et al. (1988) reported the structure of an escape mutant of influenza virus N2 NA (A/Tokyo/3/67), which was selected with monoclonal antibody S10/1. Residue 368, which is lysine in the wild type, changed to glutamic acid in the mutant (Laver et al. 1982). This change abolished S10/1 antibody binding. The difference Fourier map showed clear difference peaks resulting from a shift of electrons from the lysine side chain to a new position of glutamic acid in the mutant, but no other differences between the structures are indicated in the difference electron density map.

This experiment shows that the S10/1 epitope does indeed include amino acid residue 368 and that the change in the side chain has sufficed to effectively abolish binding of the antibody to the epitope. Similar results have been obtained with the influenza HA, where substitution of an aspartic acid for a glycine residue also caused only local structural alterations on the surface of the molecule (Knossow et al. 1984).

A survey of single amino acid changes in escape mutants of influenza antigens (Wiley et al. 1981; Caton et al. 1982; Lentz et al. 1984; Air et al. 1985b; Webster et al. 1987) does not show any preference for size or character of the replacing or the replaced residue in the antigen and indicates that even very subtle changes can abolish the binding of an antibody for an antigen.

Although the possibility of some escape mutants influencing antibody binding at a distance cannot be ruled out, the two influenza virus surface antigens studied so far both show that local structural changes suffice to effectively abolish antibody binding to an antigen.

N9 NA

The three-dimensional structure of an NA of subtype N9 from an avian influenza virus (A/tern/Australia/G70c/75), which shares 50% sequence identity with the human N2 influenza virus NA, has been determined by X-ray crystallography (Baker et al. 1987) and shown to be folded similarly to N2 NA. Differences occur in the way in which the subunits are organized around the molecular fourfold axis, and insertions and deletions with respect to subtype N2 NA occur in four regions.

Neutralizing monoclonal antibodies raised in BALB/c mice again showed a dominant region in the loops surrounding the enzyme active site (Webster et al. 1987), with most escape mutants (32 out of 33, selected with 16 antibodies) mapping in the loops around residues 329, 368, 400, and 432 (Fig. 3). Although almost all of the monoclonal antibodies recognize changes in this region, the epitopes are distinct both in area and in selection of loops, as summarized in Table 1. As in the case of N2 NA, heterogeneous rabbit antisera did not contain a preponderance of antibodies against this re-

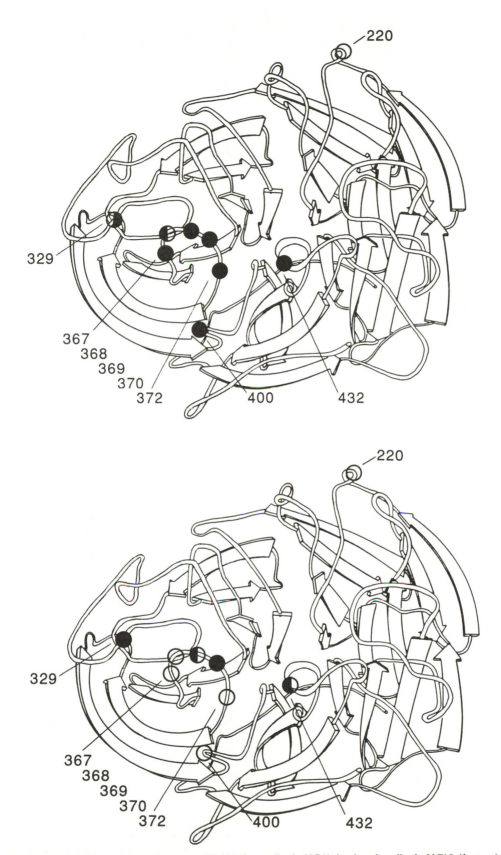

Figure 3. Serological definition of the epitopes on N9 NA for antibody NC41 (*top*) and antibody NC10 (*bottom*). Shown are amino acid positions that change in escape mutants selected with these and other antibodies. Although the NC41 and NC10 epitopes overlap extensively, they are quite distinct. (●) Amino acid changes that abolish binding; (○) amino acid substitutions that have no effect on antibody binding. Half circles are intermediate.

Table 1. Binding of Monoclonal Antibodies to N9 Escape Mutants

Antibody	Variant (and site of change)								
	V38 (220)	V35 (329)	V41 (367)	V24 (368)	V20 (369)	V32/3 (370)	V44 (372)	V42 (400)	V34 (432)
NC41		(0)	0	(0)	0	0	0	0	0
NC66		0		0	(0)	0			0
NC35		0	0		0		(0)		0
NC10		0			(0)	0			(0)
NC24		0		0		0	0		0
NC34		(0)			(0)				(0)
NC17		0		0	(0)	0			
NC45			0		0		0	0	0
NC47		0			0		0	0	
NC42			0		0		0	0	
NC31				0	0				
NC20				0	0				
NC11				0	0				
NC38	0								

gion and did not distinguish any of the escape mutants selected with monoclonal antibodies.

Influenza Type-B NA

Influenza B/Lee/40 NA has less than 25% sequence identity when compared with either N2 or N9 NA in the head region. Conservation of 16 cysteine residues, which form disulfide bonds in N2 and N9 NAs, and of several amino acid side chains, which line the active-site pocket, and the results of site-directed mutations (Wei et al. 1987) suggest that the polypeptides may be similarly folded, but this can only be confirmed by a complete structure determination. No subtypes of influenza B virus exist, and influenza B has so far been found only in the human population, in marked contrast to influenza A.

Crystals of NA heads from two different influenza B virus strains, B/Lee/40 and B/Hong Kong/8/73, have been grown, and unit cell parameters have been determined (Bossart et al. 1988). On further analysis, these crystals showed disorder, making the solution of the structure difficult, if not impossible. However, when the B/Lee/40 NA is complexed with Fab fragments of a monoclonal antibody, well-ordered crystals are obtained, and the route to the structure determination of influenza B NA may be through its complex with antibody (Laver et al. 1988).

The observation that proteins that do not crystallize or that form disordered crystals may yield better-quality crystals when complexed with Fab fragments of monoclonal antibodies has now been made three times. As well as influenza B NA described above, an N9 NA isolated from a whale formed good crystals only in complex with Fabs (Air et al. 1987), and the hemagglutinin neuraminidase (HN) protein from Sendai virus has been crystallized only in complex with Fabs (Laver et al. 1989).

Because the major crystal contacts in the NA-Fab complexes studied so far are mediated by the conserved region of the Fabs (Tulloch et al. 1986; Colman et al.

1987b; Tulip et al., this volume) and because the Fab elbow is known to be flexible, this way of obtaining crystals may be more widespread than just for NA and HN. However, it is obvious that the antibody chosen must bind to native protein. A monoclonal antibody that binds in a Western blot, for example, is not a good candidate for these experiments.

Crystals of NA-Fab Complexes

The first crystals of an NA-antibody complex, between N9 NA and antibody 32/3 Fab, could be grown as extremely thin, extensive two-dimensional platelet microcrystals, but all attempts to grow three-dimensional crystals suitable for X-ray diffraction analysis have failed (Tulloch et al. 1986). However, recent advances in high-resolution electron microscopy suggest that considerable structural information may be gleaned from such crystals. Using new methods for electron imaging, which cut down the effects of radiation-induced specimen movements (Bullough and Henderson 1987), and sophisticated methods of computer processing (Henderson et al. 1986), Bullough and Tulloch were able to extract phases from images to relatively high resolution (Bullough 1988). Despite the large unit cell dimensions of these crystals ($a = b = 159.5$ Å) and the large solvent content ($\sim 70\%$ by volume), a projection structure was determined to 6 Å resolution.

The N9 NA-NC41 complex, which has been solved to atomic resolution, is discussed by Tulip et al. (this volume). Comparison of the N9 NA-NC41 and N9 NA-32/3 complexes has suggested that the 32/3 Fab binds to the NA in the same general antigenic region as the NC41 Fab. This is entirely consistent with the known serology (Webster et al. 1987), because 32/3 can select NA escape mutants with amino acid substitutions at 329 and 370 (Table 1).

So far, crystals of five complexes involving N9 NA complexed with antibody, which diffract X-rays to beyond 3 Å, have been obtained: NC41 Fab complexed

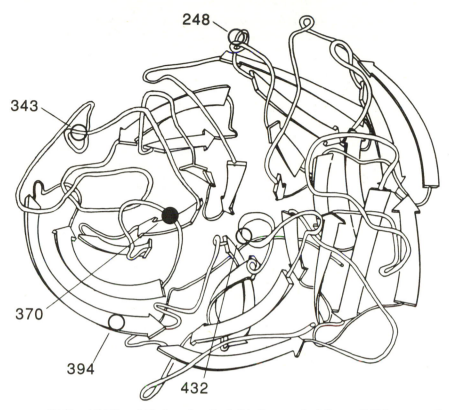

Figure 4. Escape mutants of B/Lee/40 NA and binding of antibody B1. Because the influenza B NA structure is not yet solved, the mutant positions are plotted on the N2 structure. (●) Amino acid changes that abolish binding; (○) amino acid substitutions that have no effect on antibody binding.

with N9 NA from tern and whale viruses and with two variants of tern virus NA with sequence changes that reduce but do not abolish binding, and whale virus N9 NA with another antibody, NC10 Fab. The structures of some of these complexes are discussed elsewhere in this volume (Tulip et al.).

Fab fragments from four different monoclonal antibodies have also been complexed with influenza B virus NA (B/Lee/40), and the complexes have been crystallized. Three of the complex crystals are not suitable for X-ray diffraction studies so far, but the fourth (B/Lee/40 NA-B1 Fab) forms large crystals that diffract X-rays to 3 Å resolution (Laver et al. 1988), and structure analysis is under way.

Escape mutants of the influenza B/Lee/40 NA have been selected with monoclonal antibodies. As in the case of influenza B HA (Berton et al. 1984), escape mutants are obtained with lower frequency when compared with influenza A, and the data base for defining the B1 epitope is sparse. However, it appears to involve the same region on B/Lee/40 NA as NC41 on N9 (see Fig. 4).

Mechanism of Inhibition of NA Activity by Antibody

Many monoclonal antibodies to the NA inhibit enzyme activity toward large substrates, such as fetuin (m.w. 50,000), presumably by blocking access of this large molecule to the active site. Enzyme activity toward small substrates such as N-acetyl neuraminyl lactose (NANL; m.w. 500) is not inhibited at all by some of these monoclonal antibodies, even at the highest concentration obtained (Colman et al. 1987a). Other antibodies, however, do inhibit enzyme activity toward the small substrate. NC41 antibody belongs in this category. Both the intact antibody and Fab fragments reduce the enzyme activity toward NANL by 75%. What is the mechanism of this inhibition?

In the published structure of the N9 NA-NC41 Fab complex (Colman et al. 1987b), it appears that the active site is still accessible to small substrates and that inhibition of enzyme activity by NC41 Fab is not due to steric hindrance. The crystal structure does show a small shift in the position of an active-site residue, Arg-371, which is known to be critical for enzyme activity because mutation to lysine resulted in loss of enzyme activity (Lentz et al. 1987). It is possible that this shift causes the lower enzyme activity. However, a more likely explanation may be formulated based on the knowledge that enzyme active sites need to be mobile to carry out catalytic function, because the conformations binding substrate, transition state(s), and product are different. It is possible that binding of NC41 antibody freezes the NA in an unfavorable configuration. If this is correct, then there may be two classes of antibodies with biological effects: those that physically block access of an interacting molecule and those that freeze the antigen into an inactive form. The latter class may well be required to have multiple contact points. In poliovirus, only intact (divalent) antibody molecules, and not Fabs, will neutralize infectivity (Emini et al. 1983; Icenogle et al. 1983), and Fabs that neutralize influenza virus by inhibition of the NA contact several loops of the structure.

CONCLUSIONS

NA molecules from two influenza virus A subtypes and from influenza B virus have been crystallized, and the three-dimensional structures of the type-A NAs have been determined by X-ray crystallography, whereas that of type B is under way. Influenza virus NA is being used in experiments aimed at understanding the structure of epitopes on protein molecules, how single amino acid sequence changes are able to abolish antibody binding, and how antibody molecules block infectivity of the virus. Seven crystalline complexes, involving NA with Fab fragments, are currently being analyzed. These complexes are NC41 Fab complexed with N9 NA from tern and whale viruses and with two variants of tern virus NA, with sequence changes that reduce, but do not abolish, binding. The other three complexes are N9 NA-NC10 Fab, N9 NA-32/3 Fab (thin crystals only), and type-B influenza virus NA complexed with antibody B1 Fab.

Studies on the influenza virus NA are thus yielding a wealth of information about its structure, enzymatic activity, antigenic properties, and ways in which the enzyme interacts with substrates, inhibitors, and antibodies. Moreover, the work is being done on a component of an important human pathogen; therefore, some of the results obtained with this protein, while yielding information of great general interest, may also be directly applicable to alleviating a widespread and potentially devastating human disease.

ACKNOWLEDGMENTS

This work was supported, in part, by grants AI-19084, AI-18203, AI-08831, and AI-21659 from the National Institutes of Health. We thank Per Bullough and Richard Henderson for making unpublished results available, and the Australian Overseas Telecommunications Commission for provision of international telephone facilities. P.M. Colman, J.N. Varghese, and W.R. Tulip contributed unpublished information, but chose not to be coauthors.

REFERENCES

Air, G.M., L.R. Ritchie, W.G. Laver, and P.M. Colman. 1985a. Gene and protein sequence of an influenza neuraminidase with hemagglutinin activity. *Virology* **145**: 117.

Air, G.M., R.G. Webster, P.M. Colman, and W.G. Laver. 1987. Distribution of sequence differences in influenza N9 neuraminidase of tern and whale viruses and crystallization of the whale neuraminidase complexed with antibodies. *Virology* **160**: 346.

Air, G.M., M.C. Els, L.E. Brown, W.G. Laver, and R.G. Webster. 1985b. Location of antigenic sites on the three-dimensional structure of the influenza N2 virus neuraminidase. *Virology* **145**: 237.

Amit, A.G., R.A. Mariuzza, S.E.V. Phillips, and P.J. Poljak. 1986. Three dimensional structure of an antigen-antibody complex at 2.8 Å resolution. *Science* **233**: 747.

Baker, A.T., J.N. Varghese, W.G. Laver, G.M. Air, and P.M. Colman. 1987. Three-dimensional structure of neuraminidase of subtype N9 from an avian influenza virus. *Proteins* **2**: 111.

Basak, S., M. Tomana, and R.W. Compans. 1985. Sialic acid is incorporated into influenza hemagglutinin glycoproteins in the absence of viral neuraminidase. *Virus Res.* **2**: 61.

Berton, M.T., C.T. Naeve, and R.G. Webster. 1984. Antigenic structure of the influenza B hemagglutinin: Nucleotide sequence analysis of antigenic variants selected with monoclonal antibodies. *J. Virol.* **52**: 919.

Blok, J. and G.M. Air. 1982. Sequence variation at the 3' end of the neuraminidase gene from 39 influenza A type viruses. *Virology* **121**: 211.

Blok, J., G.M. Air, W.G. Laver, C.W. Ward, G.G. Lilly, E.F. Woods, C.M. Roxburgh, and A.S. Inglis. 1982. Studies on the size, chemical composition and partial sequence of the neuraminidase (NA) from type A influenza viruses show that the N-terminal region of the NA is not processed and serves to anchor the NA in the viral membrane. *Virology* **119**: 109.

Bossart, P.J., Y.S. Babu, W.J. Cook, G.M. Air, and W.G. Laver. 1988. Crystallization and preliminary X-ray analyses of two neuraminidases from influenza B virus strains B/Hong Kong/8/73 and B/Lee/40. *J. Biol. Chem.* **263**: 6421.

Bullough, P. 1988. "High resolution electron microscopy of thin crystals." Ph.D. thesis, University of Cambridge.

Bullough, P. and R. Henderson. 1987. Use of spot-scan procedure for recording low-dose micrographs of beam-sensitive specimens. *Ultramicroscopy* **21**: 223.

Caton, A.J., G.G. Brownlee, J.W. Yewdell, and W. Gerhard. 1982. The antigenic structure of the influenza virus A/PR/8/34 hemagglutinin (H1) subtype. *Cell* **31**: 417.

Colman, P.M., J.N. Varghese, and W.G. Laver. 1983. Structure of the catalytic and antigenic sites in influenza virus neuraminidase. *Nature* **303**: 41.

Colman, P.M., W.G. Laver, J.N. Varghese, A.T. Baker, P.A. Tulloch, G.M. Air, and R.G. Webster. 1987a. The three-dimensional structure of a complex of antibody with influenza virus neuraminidase. *Nature* **326**: 358.

Colman, P.M., G.M. Air, R.G. Webster, J.N. Varghese, A.T. Baker, M.R. Lentz, P.A. Tulloch, and W.G. Laver. 1987b. How antibodies recognize virus proteins. *Immunol. Today* **8**: 323.

Colman, P.M., W. Tulip, J.N. Varghese, P.A. Tulloch, A.T. Baker, W.G. Laver, G.M. Air, and R.G. Webster. 1989. Three-dimensional structures of influenza virus neuraminidase-antibody complexes. *Philos. Trans. R. Soc. Lond. B. Biol. Sci.* **323**: 511.

Els, M.C., G.M. Air, K.G. Murti, R.G. Webster, and W.G. Laver. 1985. An 18 amino acid deletion in an influenza neuraminidase. *Virology* **142**: 241.

Emini, E.A, P. Ostapchuk, and E. Wimmer. 1983. Bivalent attachment of antibody onto poliovirus leads to conformational alteration and neutralization. *J. Virol.* **48**: 547.

Fields, S., G. Winter, and G.G. Brownlee. 1981. Structure of the neuraminidase gene in human influenza virus A/PR/8/34. *Nature* **290**: 213.

Gerhard, W. and R.G. Webster. 1978. Antigenic drift in influenza A viruses. Selection and characterization of antigenic variants of A/PR/8/34 (HON1) influenza virus with monoclonal antibodies. *J. Exp. Med.* **148**: 383.

Hall, R.M. and G.M. Air. 1981. Variation in nucleotide sequences coding for the N-terminal regions of the matrix and nonstructural proteins of influenza A viruses. *J. Virol.* **38**: 1.

Henderson, R., J.M. Baldwin, K.H. Downing, J. Lepault, and F. Zemlin. 1986. Structure of purple membrane from *Halobacterium halobium*: Recording, measurement and evaluation of electron micrographs at 3.5 Å resolution. *Ultramicroscopy* **19**: 147.

Icenogle, J., H. Shiwen, G. Duke, S. Gilbert, R. Rueckert, and J. Anderegg. 1983. Neutralization of poliovirus by a monoclonal antibody: Kinetics and stoichiometry. *Virology* **127**: 412.

Knossow, M., R.S. Daniels, A.R. Douglas, J.J. Skehel, and D.C. Wiley. 1984. Three-dimensional structure of an antigenic mutant of the influenza virus hemagglutinin. *Nature* **311**: 678.

Krystal, M., J.F. Young, P. Palese, I.A. Wilson, J.J. Skehel, and D.C. Wiley. 1983. Sequential mutations in hemagglutinins of influenza B virus isolates: Definition of antigenic domains. *Proc. Natl. Acad. Sci.* **80**: 4527. Correction: *Proc. Natl. Acad. Sci.* **81**: 1261 (1984).

Lamb, R.A. and P.W. Choppin. 1983. The gene structure and replication of influenza virus. *Annu. Rev. Biochem.* **52**: 467.

Laver, W.G. 1978. Crystallization and peptide maps of neuraminidase "heads" from H2N2 and H3N2 influenza virus strains. *Virology* **86**: 78.

Laver, W.G., G.M. Air, R.G. Webster, and L.J. Markoff. 1982. Amino acid sequence changes in antigenic variants of type A influenza virus N2 neuraminidase. *Virology* **122**: 450.

Laver, W.G., S.D. Thompson, K.G. Murti, and A. Portner. 1989. Crystallization of Sendai virus HN protein complexed with monoclonal antibody Fab fragments. *Virology* **171**: 291.

Laver, W.G., M. Luo, P.J. Bossart, Y.S. Babu, C. Smith, M.A. Accavitti, P.A. Tulloch, and G.M. Air. 1988. Crystallization and preliminary X-ray analysis of type B influenza virus neuraminidase complexed with antibody Fab fragments. *Virology* **167**: 621.

Lentz, M.R., R.G. Webster, and G.M. Air. 1987. Site-directed mutation of the active site of influenza neuraminidase and implications for the catalytic mechanism. *Biochemistry* **26**: 5351.

Lentz, M.R., G.M. Air, W.G. Laver, and R.G. Webster. 1984. Sequence of the neuraminidase gene of influenza virus A/Tokyo/3/67 and previously uncharacterized monoclonal variants. *Virology* **135**: 257.

Lu, B.L., R.G. Webster, L.E. Brown, and K. Nerome. 1983. Heterogeneity of influenza B viruses. *Bull. WHO* **61**: 681.

Oxford, J.S., A.I. Klimov, T. Corcoran, Y.Z. Ghendon, and G.C. Schild. 1984. Biochemical and serological studies of influenza B viruses: Comparisons of histological and recent isolates. *Virus Res.* **1**: 241.

Padlan, E.A., E.W. Silverton, E. Sheriff, G.H. Cohen, S.J. Smith-Gill, and D.R. Davies. 1989. Structure of an antibody-antigen complex: Crystal structure of the HyHEL-10 Fab:lysozyme complex. *Proc. Natl. Acad. Sci.* **86**: 5938.

Palese, P., K. Tobita, M. Ueda, and R.W. Compans. 1974. Characterization of temperature-sensitive influenza virus mutants defective in neuraminidase. *Virology* **61**: 397.

Rossmann, M.G. and R.R. Rueckert. 1987. What does the molecular structure of viruses tell us about viral functions? *Microbiol. Sci.* **4**: 206.

Rossmann, M.G., E. Arnold, J.W. Erickson, E.A. Frankenberger, J.P. Griffith, H.J. Hecht, J.E. Johnson, G. Kamer, M. Luo, A.G. Mosser, R.R. Rueckert, B. Sherry, and G. Vriend. 1985. Structure of a human common cold virus and functional relationship to other picornaviruses. *Nature* **317**: 145.

Sela, M. 1969. Antigenicity: Some molecular aspects. *Science* **166**: 1365.

Shaw, M.W., R.A. Lamb, B.W. Erickson, D.J. Breidis, and P.W. Choppin. 1982. Complete nucleotide sequence of the neuraminidase gene of influenza B virus. *Proc. Natl. Acad. Sci.* **79**: 6817.

Sheriff, S., E.W. Silverton, E.A. Padlan, G.H. Cohen, S.J. Smith-Gill, B.C. Finzel, and D.R. Davies. 1987. Three-dimensional structure of an antibody-antigen complex. *Proc. Natl. Acad. Sci.* **84**: 8075.

Tulloch, P.A., P.M. Colman, P.C. Davis, W.G. Laver, R.G. Webster, and G.M. Air. 1986. Electron and X-ray diffraction studies of influenza neuraminidase complexed with monoclonal antibodies. *J. Mol. Biol.* **190**: 215.

Varghese, J.N., W.G. Laver, and P.M. Colman. 1983. Structure of the influenza virus glycoprotein antigen neuraminidase at 2.9 Å resolution. *Nature* **303**: 35.

Varghese, J.N., R.G. Webster, W.G. Laver, and P.M. Colman. 1988. Structure of an escape mutant of glycoprotein N2 neuraminidase of influenza virus A/Tokyo/3/67 at 3Å. *J. Mol. Biol.* **200**: 201.

Webster, R.G., L.E. Brown, and W.G. Laver. 1984. Antigenic and biological characterization of influenza virus neuraminidase (N2) with monoclonal antibodies. *Virology* **135**: 30.

Webster, R.G., V.S. Hinshaw, and W.G. Laver. 1982. Selection and analysis of antigenic variants of the neuraminidase of N2 influenza viruses with monoclonal antibodies. *Virology* **117**: 93.

Webster, R.G., P.A. Reay, and W.G. Laver. 1988. Protection against lethal influenza with neuraminidase. *Virology* **164**: 230.

Webster, R.G., G.M. Air, D.W. Metzger, P.M. Colman, J.N. Varghese, A.T. Baker, and W.G. Laver. 1987. Antigenic structure and variation in an influenza N9 neuraminidase. *J. Virol.* **61**: 2910.

Wei, X., M.C. Els, R.G. Webster, and G.M. Air. 1988. Effects of site-specific mutation on structure and activity of influenza virus B/Lee/40 neuraminidase. *Virology* **156**: 253.

WHO Memorandum. 1980. A revision of the system of nomenclature for influenza viruses. *Bull. WHO* **58**: 585.

Wiley, D.C., I.A. Wilson, and J.J. Skehel. 1981. Structural identification of the antibody-binding sites of Hong Kong influenza hemagglutinin and their involvement in antigenic variation. *Nature* **289**: 373.

Wilson, I.A., J.J. Skehel, and D.C. Wiley. 1981. Structure of the hemagglutinin membrane glycoprotein of influenza virus at 3 Å resolution. *Nature* **289**: 366.

Yamashita, M., M. Krystal, W.M. Fitch, and P. Palese. 1988. Influenza B virus evolution: Co-circulating lineages and comparison of evolutionary pattern with those of influenza A and C viruses. *Virology* **163**: 112.

Crystal Structures of Neuraminidase-Antibody Complexes

W.R. Tulip,* J.N. Varghese,* R.G. Webster,** G.M. Air,† W.G. Laver,‡ and P.M. Colman*

*C.S.I.R.O. Division of Biotechnology, Parkville 3052, Australia; **St. Jude Children's Research Hospital, Memphis, Tennessee 38101; †Department of Microbiology, University of Alabama, Birmingham, Alabama 35294; ‡John Curtin School of Medical Research, Australian National University, Canberra 2601, Australia

The nature of antigen-antibody interactions has become clearer in the last few years as crystal structures of antigen-antibody complexes have been elucidated. Such structures have permitted a visualization of the interface between antigen and antibody. Three-dimensional structures of five complexes have now been reported, two containing the influenza virus neuraminidase as antigen and the Fabs NC41 and NC10 (Colman et al. 1987, 1989), and three with hen egg-white lysozyme and the Fabs D1.3, HyHEL-5, and HyHEL-10 (Amit et al. 1986; Sheriff et al. 1987b; E.A. Padlan et al., in prep.). The major parameters that define the scope of the antigen-antibody interface are emerging as more structures are solved and refined to greater precision. Several reviews have dealt with this topic (Mariuzza et al. 1987; Colman 1988; Davies et al. 1988).

Influenza is an orthomyxovirus and possesses an outer lipid membrane. Embedded in this membrane are two protein antigens, a hemagglutinin and a neuraminidase, the latter being a tetrameric glycoprotein comprising a head and an amino-terminal stalk that provides the attachment to the virus. Heads with full enzymatic and antigenic properties may be removed from the stalk with pronase and thus made soluble. Such heads have been used in all crystallographic investigations of the enzyme. The structure of neuraminidase of N2 subtype is known (Varghese et al. 1983) and has a structure similar to that of subtype N9 (Baker et al. 1987). N9 neuraminidase is the antigen in both of the complexes discussed here.

In this paper, we describe the crystal structure of the neuraminidase–NC41 Fab complex as refined at 2.9 Å resolution and give a structural basis for the observed lack of binding of NC41 antibody with escape mutants of N9 neuraminidase. The main features of this complex and the neuraminidase–NC10 Fab complex are also compared with those of the lysozyme complexes.

METHODS

The isolation (Laver et al. 1984) and sequencing (Air et al. 1985) of N9 neuraminidase, production of monoclonal antibodies, and properties of the neuraminidase-antibody complexes (Tulloch et al. 1986; Webster et al. 1987) have all been reported previously. Sequences of antibodies were obtained from RNA (G.M. Air, un-

publ.). The crystallization and structure determination were described for complexes containing two of these antibodies, namely, NC41 (Colman et al. 1987; Laver et al. 1987) and NC10 (Air et al. 1987; Colman et al. 1989). Diffraction data sets extending to resolutions of 2.9 Å and 3.0 Å, respectively, were collected on film from a rotating anode source, and a 2.5 Å synchrotron data set was obtained for the NC41 complex. Refinement of these two crystal structures proceeded initially by the stereochemically restrained least-squares program PROLSQ (Hendrickson and Konnert 1981). In later stages, the molecular dynamics program X-PLOR (Brunger 1988) was used. The NC41 structure will be further refined against the 2.5 Å resolution data, and full details of the refinements will be presented elsewhere. Between successive rounds of refinement, the atomic models were rebuilt on an Evans and Sutherland PS300, using FRODO (Jones 1985) and displaying a $2F_o - F_c$ electron density map (where F_o is the observed structure factor and F_c is the calculated structure factor). The mean positional error of the models was estimated by a statistical method (Luzzati 1952). In the description of the structure, maximum distances for van der Waals contacts, hydrogen bonds, and salt links were as defined in Table 1 (see also Sheriff et al. 1987a). The molecular surface program MS (Connolly 1983) was used to calculate buried surface area with a probe radius of 1.7 Å. MS calculates the molecular surface area, rather than the solvent-accessible surface area (Lee and Richards 1971; Connolly 1983). Kabat numbering was used for the antibodies (Kabat et al. 1987). Amino acid residue numbers are prefixed by L (light chain) and H (heavy chain). Complementarity-determining regions (CDRs) were defined as in Kabat et al. (1987), and their sequence numbers are light chain 24–34, 50–56, and 89–97 and heavy chain 31–35, 50–65, and 95–102.

RESULTS

NC41 Complex

The R-factor ($\Sigma \|F_o| - |F_c\| / \Sigma |F_o|$) for 20,065 reflections from 6.0 to 2.9 Å resolution is 0.187 for the current model. Virtually all of the main-chain is observed in continuous electron density, as are most of the side-chains, but the orientations of only about half

Table 1. Contact Residues in the Interface between Neuraminidase and NC41 Fab

N9 neuraminidase	NC41 Fab																			
	light chain										heavy chain									
	Y49	W50	S52	T53	H55	I56	Y92	S93	P94	W96	N31	Y32	N52	N53	E96	D97	N98	F99	S100A	L100B
P326		X																		
R327	X																			
P328	X			X																
N329					X	X														
G343		X		X																
N344		X	X	X																
N345			X																	
N347		X																		
I366											X				X					
S367												X			X	X				
I368	X	X													X					
A369		X													X	X				
S370																X				
S372																	X			X
L399											X			X						
N400											X	X					X			
T401													X	X						
D402																X	X			
W403																	X	X		
P431							X	X												
K432									X	X						X			X	
D434								X	X	X										

Residues are grouped in segments of polypeptide chain. Crosses indicate residue pairs that have at least one pair of atoms within van der Waals contact distance. Maximum contact distances (Sheriff et al. 1987a) are as follows, where C = carbon, N = nitrogen, O = oxygen: (CC) 4.107 Å; (NN) 3.441 Å; (OO) 3.33 Å; (CN) 3.774 Å; (CO) 3.719 Å; (NO) 3.386 Å. Residues partially buried from solvent by the interaction, but not in direct contact, are Thr-L31, Arg-L54, His-L91, Pro-L95, Thr-H28, Thr-H30, Gly-H33, Trp-H50, Thr-H52A, Thr-H54, Glu-H56, and Asp-H101 on the Fab, and Ile-149, Asp-330, Asn-346, Thr-396, Arg-430, Glu-433, Asp-457, Pro-459, Lys-463, and Ile-464 on the neuraminidase. In addition, two mannose residues, designated 200D and 200F, which are in the carbohydrate attached to Asn-200 of a neighboring neuraminidase subunit, are partially buried.

of the peptide carbonyl oxygen atoms are unambiguously determined in electron density at this resolution. Six water molecules were included in the model with full occupancy. The root mean square difference between ideal and observed values is 0.022 Å for bonds and 4.5° for angles, whereas the mean positional error of the atoms was estimated to be 0.3 Å.

Atoms at the interface between neuraminidase and antibody are all in convincing electron density, with the exception of side-chains in the neuraminidase segment 431–435. There appear to be no water molecules buried from solvent in the interface, but at least one water molecule is in contact with both antigen and antibody. The outline of the buried surface resembles a three-leaf clover in shape, as shown in Figure 1, with the active site in between two of the "leaves." A remarkable shape complementarity exists over most of the interface, with protuberances on one protein matched by depressions on the other. There is a large groove between the variable domains of the light and heavy chains (V_L and V_H) that accommodates a large ridge traversing the epitope made up of residues Asp-434, Lys-432, Ser-370, Ala-369, Ile-368, and Asn-329. Distances of 27 Å, 30 Å, and 27 Å separate the tips of the three parts of the interface.

Interactions between antigen and antibody include 1 salt link from Lys-432 to Asp-H97, 10 hydrogen bonds, and 115 additional van der Waals contacts, although these latter numbers may change slightly after the high-angle refinement. The buried surface area was calculated to be about 878 Å^2 on the surface of neuraminidase and 885 Å^2 on the Fab. The nonpolar (carbon and sulfur) components of the total buried surface area of neuraminidase and the NC41 variable module are 61% and 53%, respectively. These numbers are not significantly different from those of the exposed surfaces of the two proteins (58% and 59%), which implies that the epitope and paratope are not particularly hydrophobic or hydrophilic.

The epitope on neuraminidase is extensive (see Fig. 1; Table 1). It involves 5 segments on the upper surface of the enzyme, which contribute 22 residues in direct contact and 5 that are partially buried. In addition, there are partially buried atoms in 5 residues from 2 other segments and in 2 sugar residues from the carbohydrate of a neighboring subunit.

The binding site of the Fab is composed of 20 contact residues and 12 partially buried residues (see Fig. 1; Table 1). As CDR L1 is at least 5 Å from neuraminidase, only 5 of the 6 CDRs are in direct contact; as a

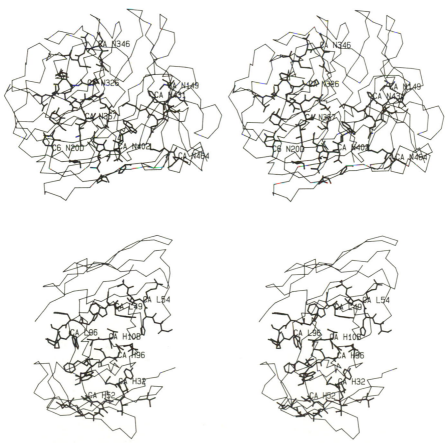

Figure 1. Stereoviews of the NC41 complex. (*Top*) N9 neuraminidase; (*bottom*) the NC41 $V_L V_H$ dimer (light chain uppermost). The two proteins are shown opened out from a view, with the neuraminidase at left and the Fab at right, so that the interfaces are viewed *en face*. A Ca trace is drawn in thin lines for noninteracting residues. Contact and partially buried residues are shown *in toto* by bold lines. (For pairs of residues in contact, see Table 1.)

result, the heavy chain has more interaction than the light chain. The comparative data for heavy and light chains, respectively, are 506 Å^2 and 383 Å^2 for the buried surface area; 6 and 5 for the number of ion pairs and hydrogen bonds; and 72 and 43 for the number of other contacts. Among the hypervariable loops, CDR H3 has the most buried surface area (267 Å^2), representing 30% of the total, and it also has the greatest number of contacts (60). There are three framework region (FR) residues in the paratope, namely, Tyr-L49, Thr-H28, and Thr-H30, all of which are in segments adjacent to CDRs.

Possible Conformational Changes in Antigen and Antibody

Colman et al. (1987) reported that the structure of both the antigen and NC41 antibody may have changed as a result of antibody binding (for review, see Colman 1988). The refinement of the NC41 complex is essentially complete, whereas the refinement of uncomplexed N9 neuraminidase (Baker et al. 1987) at 2.2 Å resolution has not yet converged. A detailed comparison of the free and liganded neuraminidase structures will be possible in the near future. On the other hand, the structure of the free Fab has not been determined; hence, there can be no direct comparison with the uncomplexed antibody. Comparisons with other Fab structures may suggest possibilities.

At the level of local change, it appears that the main-chain conformations of five CDRs follow the canonical structures as predicted (Chothia and Lesk 1987; C. Chothia et al., in prep.). Hence, the local fold of each of these five loops is unlikely to have changed substantially upon the formation of a complex. However, CDRs can be flexible, for example, CDR L1 in Fab McPC603 (Satow et al. 1986) and CDR H3 in Fab 19.9 (Lascombe et al. 1989). As the Fab engages antigen, structural rearrangements might take place in both proteins. Such changes could be similar to those seen in the regions of crystal contacts (Wlodawer et al. 1987) or in enzyme-inhibitor interactions (Greenblatt et al. 1989).

On the basis of observed variability in $V_L V_H$ interactions in antibodies (Davies and Metzger 1983), it has been suggested that antigen might cause small rearrangements in the $V_L H_H$ interface (Colman et al. 1987). Whether or not this has happened in the NC41 complex remains unclear. The analysis of that complex showed that its $V_L V_H$ pairing was an outlier among other uncomplexed Fab structures. The angular differences in the $V_L V_H$ pairing (see Table 1 in Colman et al. 1987) of NC41 relative to New, McPC603, Kol, and J539 are currently 7.4°, 7.7°, 10.3°, and 11.5°. Given that such differences of up to 12.8° have since been found between uncomplexed Fabs (Lascombe et al. 1989), NC41 can no longer be considered as an outlier. Direct evidence for this putative quaternary change can only come from comparison of complexed and uncom-

plexed antibodies. A reported rotation of the side-chain of Trp-H47 (Colman et al. 1987) has not been substantiated by the structure refinement. That tryptophan now appears to have a canonical structure.

Escape Mutants of N9 Neuraminidase

Monoclonal antibodies directed against neuraminidase have selected a number of escape mutants of N9 (see Tables 2 and 3 in Webster et al. 1987). Nine different mutants have been so selected, eight of them possessing single-site sequence changes in the contact surface with NC41. Figure 2 shows the positions of the nine mutants on a schematic diagram of neuraminidase. Several of these mutants crystallize isomorphously with wild-type N9, and their structures are being analyzed. Two, in particular, Ox1 (370 Ser → Leu) and Ox2 (329 Asn → Asp), have now been studied by difference Fourier methods, and preliminary results indicate local changes only for the Ox1 substitution, and no structural change associated with the Ox2 substitution.

The possible effect of the nine substitutions on the binding of NC41 antibody can be considered now that the structure of the interface is known in detail. The inhibition of neuraminidase activity by NC41 antibody was measured for these nine substitutions (see Fig. 2 in Colman et al. 1987). Wild-type neuraminidase is inhibited, but there is no loss of activity for most of the mutants, indicating that the mutation has lowered the binding affinity of NC41. A decrease in activity, as a result of antibody binding, could be explained by two mechanisms. First, the access of substrate to and/or release of product from the enzyme's active site may be sterically hindered. Second, the active site could be

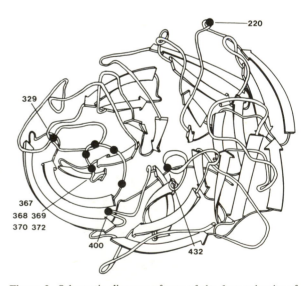

Figure 2. Schematic diagram of one of the four subunits of neuraminidase viewed down the molecular fourfold rotation axis (*bottom right*). Arrows represent β-sheet strands. Sites of mutation in N9 neuraminidase are numbered. All of the mutations except 220 occur at residues that lie in the epitope recognized by NC41 Fab and reduce its binding affinity.

deformed statically or dynamically. Recent studies (J.N. Varghese, unpubl.) have shown the orientation of sialic acid in the active site, which implies that the approach of substrate into the site requires the aglycon part of the substrate to be in the vicinity of the epitope recognized by NC41.

Six of the nine substitutions replace smaller side chains by larger ones, namely, 367 Ser→Asn, 368 Ile→Arg, 369 Ala→Asp, 370 Ser→Leu, 372 Ser→Tyr, and 400 Asn→Lys. All of these substitutions would be expected to diminish the shape complementarity of the antigen-antibody interface leading to low binding affinity, and the results indicate that this is true for all but the 368 substitution, designated NC24V1. Ile-368 is spatially near the middle of the epitope, and yet the mutation has little effect on the binding of NC41. An inspection shows that it is sitting at the base of a solvent-accessible pocket, which has both Fab and neuraminidase residues on its sides, and that an arginine side-chain could be accommodated if it followed the CG2 path of the isoleucine. This would first entail the loss of contacts made by CG1 and CD1 of the isoleucine and the creation of a hole where those two atoms were, and then the possible disturbance of other interacting residues by the arginine side-chain, such as Asn-329 and mannose-200F. Tentative support for such a placement of the arginine side-chain is given by a difference Fourier with $(F_{obs}NC24V1 - F_{obs}Nati)$ as coefficients, but the data are sparse and only extend to 3.8 Å resolution.

One mutant, 432 Lys→Asn, involves a decrease in the size of the side-chain, and although this would not produce a clash as above, the inhibition result indicates that the affinity of NC41 for that mutant is very low. This is not surprising because two good contacts (< 3.0

Å) and two ordinary contacts (< 3.9 Å) would be lost, including the only ion pair in the interface. The charge on Asp-H97 would then be unbalanced, even if a water molecule were bound in the hole.

The only mutant that potentially preserves the shape complementarity but changes the chemical complementarity of the epitope is 329 Asn → Asp, designated Ox2. Its neuraminidase activity is decreased, indicating that NC41 does bind to Ox2 but not as strongly as to wild type. The complex between Ox2 and NC41 Fab crystallizes isomorphously to wild type, and a data set has been collected from the crystals, but the model has not as yet been refined against it. A difference map of the wild-type complex with the Ox2 complex confirms our earlier conclusion (Colman et al. 1987) that the binding of the antibody to these two antigenically distinct neuraminidases is isosteric. An X-ray refinement of the mutant complex is needed to confirm and clarify any small structural rearrangements that may be a consequence of accommodating the aspartate at 329 in the interface.

NC10 Complex

At this stage, the refinement has not progressed significantly since the structure was reported (Colman et al. 1989). The R-factor for 12,674 reflections in the resolution range 6.0–3.0 Å is 0.20, but segments of chain still remain out of density. In particular, the details of the interface, including buried surface area and numbers of contacts, are not clear. Nevertheless, it is apparent that the epitopes recognized by NC10 and NC41 are largely overlapping (Colman et al. 1989). In addition, the mode of attachment of the two antibodies is completely different. As shown in Figure 3, the

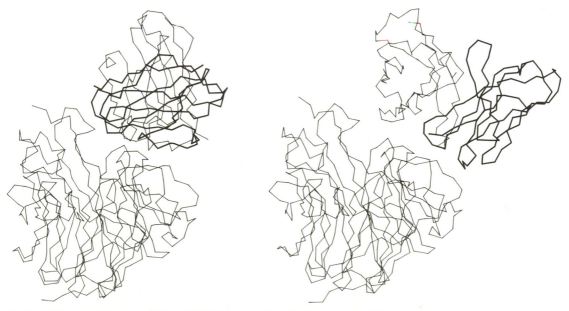

Figure 3. (*Left*) The tern N9 neuraminidase–NC41 Fab complex; (*right*) the whale N9 neuraminidase–NC10 Fab complex. On both diagrams, the neuraminidase (*lower left*) and the V_LV_H dimer (*upper right*) are shown, with the neuraminidases in the same orientation. Ca traces of neuraminidase and heavy chains are indicated by thin lines, and light chains, by bold lines.

relative positions of V_L and V_H place equivalent CDRs a long distance from each other with respect to the antigen, and only four of the six CDRs on NC10 are in contact with the antigen, namely, CDRs L1, L3, H2, and H3. The similarity of the shape and charge distribution of the surfaces of the NC10 and NC41 combining sites remains to be seen.

DISCUSSION

It appears that the neuraminidase–NC41 Fab interface is somewhat more extensive than the interfaces between lysozyme and the Fabs D1.3, HyHEL-5, and HyHEL-10. The surface area buried by complex formation is larger, and with the exception of HyHEL-10, there are more van der Waals contacts. However, the number of hydrogen bonds and salt bridges is about the same. The extent of the interacting surface is also reflected in the numbers of contacting and partially buried residues (see Table 2). This result is achieved through contact with only five antibody CDRs because more of CDR L2 and CDR H3 are used in this case than in the lysozyme examples.

There are two significant differences between the interfaces of the neuraminidase and lysozyme complexes. First, the NC41 and NC10 complexes demonstrate that an antibody does not require the use of all six CDRs in the interaction to achieve the number of contacts and buried surface area needed to bind effectively. In the NC41 complex, the only noncontacting CDR, L1, is "hanging over" the active site. In this position, it could possibly interfere with the access of substrate to the enzyme. Second, the outline of the interface of the NC41 complex has a peculiar trefoil shape, which is partly due to the presence of the active-site pocket and the fact that CDR L1 is not in contact. In contrast, the interfaces of the lysozyme complexes, which all have six CDRs in contact, have simpler outlines.

An important similarity between the neuraminidase and lysozyme complexes is the presence of FR residues in the paratope. Berek and Milstein (1987) reported that somatic hypermutation occurred at framework sites in the maturation of the immune response against a hapten. There is *a priori* no reason to exclude FR residues from the antigen-binding site of an antibody. Their capacity to participate in such binding remains a property of the adjacent CDR surface.

The epitopes in the two neuraminidase complexes are composed of more segments than the epitopes in the three lysozyme complexes, which is in contrast with the number of antibody CDRs in contact (Table 2). The highly discontinuous nature of the neuraminidase epitope is largely determined by the tertiary structure of the enzyme (Varghese et al. 1983; Baker et al. 1987), which has many short loops on its upper surface connecting the β-sheet strands. The lengths of the neuraminidase segments in contact are correspondingly shorter than in the lysozyme complexes.

Chothia et al. (1986) reported that in the lysozyme-D1.3 complex, the observed main-chain conformations of four of the CDRs were close to their predictions. Similarly, predictions were made for the NC41 CDRs. Five hypervariable loops follow the canonical structures and are close to the predicted conformations (C. Chothia et al., in prep.). However, there are errors between 0.4 Å and 3.0 Å in the predicted spatial arrangement of the CDRs with respect to each other.

ACKNOWLEDGMENTS

We thank Peter Tulloch for helpful discussions on the manuscript, Paul Davis for assistance with computing, and Bert van Donkelaar for technical support. Steven

Table 2. Number of Contacts and Buried Surface Areas in Antigen-antibody Complexes

	Antigen		Antibody		Buried surface area (Å^2)[a]
	segments	residues[b]	CDRs	residues[b]	antigen/antibody
Neuraminidase					
NC41[c]	5	22/34	5	20/32	878/885
NC10[c]	5 + 1 CHO	?	4	?	?
Lysozyme[d]					
D1.3	2	16/27	6	17/22	690/680
HyHEL-5	3	14/24	6	17/28	750/745
HyHEL-10	4	15/27	6	19/30	774/721

[a]In conjunction with S. Sheriff, who provided invaluable help, the buried surface areas were calculated with the same parameters so that the numbers of buried residues and surface areas are directly comparable.

[b]X/Y denotes that X residues are in direct contact and Y residues are fully or partially buried. Maximum contact distances are defined in Table 1 (also see Sheriff et al. 1987a), with the exception of the D1.3 complex in which a 4.0 Å cutoff was used.

[c]Only segments in direct contact are counted.

[d]References of structure reports: D1.3 (Amit et al. 1986); HyHEL-5 (Sheriff et al. 1987b; Davies et al. 1988; HyHel-10 (Davies et al. 1988). Additional data for HyHEL-10 were kindly provided by E.A. Padlan and D.R. Davies prior to publication (E.A. Padlan et al., in prep.).

Sheriff provided data for buried surface areas. This work was supported by a Commonwealth Postgraduate Research Award to W.R.T. and by U.S. Public Health Service research grants AI-21659, AI-08831, AI-20591, and AI-19084 from the National Institute of Allergy and Infectious Diseases.

REFERENCES

Air, G.M., L.R. Ritchie, W.G. Laver, and P.M. Colman. 1985. Gene and protein sequence of an influenza neuraminidase with haemagglutinin activity. *Virology* **145:** 117.

Air, G.M., R.G. Webster, P.M. Colman, and W.G. Laver. 1987. Distribution of sequence differences in influenza N9 neuraminidase of tern and whale viruses and crystallization of the whale neuraminidase complexed with antibodies. *Virology* **160:** 346.

Amit, A.G., R.A. Mariuzza, S.E.V. Phillips, and R.J. Poljak. 1986. Three-dimensional structure of an antigen-antibody complex at 2.8 Å resolution. *Science* **233:** 747.

Baker, A.T., J.N. Varghese, W.G. Laver, G.M. Air, and P.M. Colman. 1987. Three-dimensional structure of neuraminidase of subtype N9 from an avian influenza virus. *Proteins* **2:** 111.

Berek, C. and C. Milstein. 1987. Mutation drift and repertoire shift in the maturation of the immune response. *Immunol. Rev.* **96:** 23.

Brunger, A.T. 1988. Crystallographic refinement by simulated annealing. Application to a 2.8 Å resolution structure of aspartate aminotransferase. *J. Mol. Biol.* **203:** 803.

Chothia, C. and A.M. Lesk. 1987. Canonical structures for the hypervariable regions of immunoglobulins. *J. Mol. Biol.* **196:** 901.

Chothia, C., A.M. Lesk, M. Levitt, A.G. Amit, R.A. Mariuzza, S.E.V. Phillips, and R.J. Poljak. 1986. The predicted structure of immunoglobulin D1.3 and its comparison with the crystal structure. *Science* **233:** 755.

Colman, P.M. 1988. Structure of antibody-antigen complexes: Implications for immune recognition. *Adv. Immunol.* **43:** 99.

Colman, P.M., W.G. Laver, J.N. Varghese, A.T. Baker, P.A. Tulloch, G.M. Air, and R.G. Webster. 1987. Three-dimensional structure of a complex of antibody with influenza virus neuraminidase. *Nature* **326:** 358.

Colman, P.M., W.R. Tulip, J.N. Varghese, A.T. Baker, W.G. Laver, G.M. Air, and R.G. Webster. 1989. 3-D structures of influenza virus neuraminidase-antibody structures. *Philos. Trans. R. Soc. Lond. B* **323:** 511.

Connolly, M.L. 1983. Analytical molecular surface calculation. *J. Appl. Crystallogr.* **16:** 548.

Davies, D.R. and H. Metzger. 1983. Structural basis of antibody function. *Annu. Rev. Immunol.* **1:** 87.

Davies, D.R., S. Sheriff, and E.A. Padlan. 1988. Minireview: Antigen-antibody complexes. *J. Biol. Chem.* **263:** 10541.

Greenblatt, H.M., C.A. Ryan, and M.N.G. James. 1989. Structure of the complex of *Streptomyces griseus* protein-ase B and polypeptide chymotrypsin inhibitor-1 from Russet Burbank potato tubers at 2.1 Å resolution. *J. Mol. Biol.* **205:** 201.

Hendrickson, W.A. and J.H. Konnert. 1981. Stereochemically restrained crystallographic least-squares refinement of macromolecule structures. In *Biomolecular structure, conformation, function, and evolution* (ed. R. Srinivasan), vol. 1, p. 43. Pergamon Press, Oxford.

Jones, T.A. 1985. Interactive computer graphics: FRODO. *Methods Enzymol.* **115:** 157.

Kabat, E.A., T.T. Wu, M. Reid-Miller, H.M. Perry, and K.S. Gottesman. 1987. *Sequences of proteins of immunological interest*, 4th edition. U.S. Public Health Service, National Institutes of Health, Washington, D.C.

Lascombe, M.-B., P.M. Alzari, G. Boulot, P. Saludjian, P. Tougard, C. Berek, S. Haba, E.M. Rosen, A. Nishonhoff, and R.J. Poljak. 1989. Three-dimensional structure of Fab R19.9, a monoclonal murine antibody specific for the *p*-azobenzenearsonate group. *Proc. Natl. Acad. Sci.* **86:** 607.

Laver, W.G., R.G. Webster, and P.M. Colman. 1987. Crystals of antibodies complexed with influenza virus neuraminidase show isosteric binding of antibody to wild-type and variant antigens. *Virology* **156:** 181.

Laver, W.G., P.M. Colman, R.G. Webster, V.S. Hinshaw, and G.M. Air. 1984. Influenza virus neuraminidase with haemagglutinin activity. *Virology* **137:** 314.

Lee, B. and F.M. Richards. 1971. The interpretation of protein structures: Estimation of static accessibility. *J. Mol. Biol.* **55:** 379.

Luzzati, V. 1952. Statistical treatment of errors in the determination of crystal structures. *Acta Crystallogr.* **5:** 802.

Mariuzza, R.A., S.E.V. Phillips, and R.J. Poljak. 1987. The structural basis of antigen-antibody recognition. *Annu. Rev. Biophys. Chem.* **16:** 139.

Satow, Y., G.H. Cohen, E.A. Padlan, and D.R. Davies. 1986. Phosphocholine binding immunoglobulin Fab McPC603. An X-ray diffraction study at 2.7 Å. *J. Mol. Biol.* **190:** 593.

Sheriff, S., W.A. Hendrickson, and J.L. Smith. 1987a. Structure of myohemerythrin in the azidomet state at 1.7/1.3 Å resolution. *J. Mol. Biol.* **197:** 273.

Sheriff, S., E.W. Silverton, E.A. Padlan, G.H. Cohen, S.J. Smith-Gill, B.C. Finzel, and D.R. Davies. 1987b. Three-dimensional structure of an antibody-antigen complex. *Proc. Natl. Acad. Sci.* **84:** 8075.

Tulloch, P.A., P.M. Colman, P.C. Davis, W.G. Laver, R.G. Webster, and G.M. Air. 1986. Electron and X-ray diffraction studies of influenza neuraminidase complexed with monoclonal antibodies. *J. Mol. Biol.* **190:** 215.

Varghese, J.N., W.G. Laver, and P.M. Colman. 1983. Structure of the influenza virus glycoprotein antigen neuraminidase at 2.9 Å resolution. *Nature* **303:** 35.

Webster, R.G., G.M. Air, D.W. Metzger, P.M. Colman, J.N. Varghese, A.T. Baker, and W.G. Laver. 1987. Antigenic structure and variation in an influenza virus N9 neuraminidase. *J. Virol.* **61:** 2910.

Wlodawer, A., J. Deisenhofer, and R. Huber. 1987. Comparison of two highly refined structures of bovine pancreatic trypsin inhibitor. *J. Mol. Biol.* **193:** 145.

Generating Binding Activities from *Escherichia coli* by Expression of a Repertoire of Immunoglobulin Variable Domains

D. Güssow, E.S. Ward, A.D. Griffiths, P.T. Jones, and G. Winter
MRC Laboratory of Molecular Biology, Cambridge CB2 2QH, United Kingdom

The immunoglobulin molecule consists of a string of domains, each consisting of about 100 amino acid residues. The antigen-binding site is fashioned by both heavy (V_H) and light (V_L; V_κ or V_λ) chain variable domains, as demonstrated by the solved crystallographic structures of antibody in association with antigen (Amit et al. 1986; Colman et al. 1987; Sheriff et al. 1987) or hapten (Satow et al. 1986). In the crystallographic structures of antibody-antigen complexes, the relative contributions of V_H and V_L domains to antigen binding appear to vary, although both domains make extensive interactions with the antigen. Light-chain dimers (Bence-Jones proteins) have also been crystallized, in which the two chains form a cavity that is able to bind to a single molecule of hapten (Edmundson et al. 1984).

We have been dissecting the interactions of the antilysozyme antibody, D1.3, with antigen (Amit et al. 1986) and have expressed the V_H and V_L domains individually, or in association as an Fv fragment by secretion into *Escherichia coli* periplasm (Skerra and Plückthun 1988). We find that both the Fv fragment and the V_H domain bind to antigen with a high affinity. This inspired us to generate a repertoire of V_H domains for the expression of binding activities in *E. coli*. Two approaches were used for the generation of a repertoire: (1) Residues in the third hypervariable region of a cloned V_H domain were mutated extensively, and (2) rearranged V_H genes were cloned from antibody-producing cells using the polymerase chain reaction (PCR) (Saiki et al. 1985; Orlandi et al. 1989). Each repertoire was cloned into vectors for expression of V_H domains in the periplasm of *E. coli* and screened for antigen-binding activity.

METHODS

Vectors. For expression of the V_H domain (V_HD1.3) of the D1.3 antibody, the vector pSW1-V_HD1.3 was built by cloning the gene into a pUC19 vector (Yanisch-Perron et al. 1985) with a synthetic oligonucleotide encoding a pelB signal sequence (Better et al. 1988) (Fig. 1). For expression of both domains, the vector pSW1-V_HD1.3-V_κD1.3 was built by cloning the V_κ domain and pelB signal into pSW1. For cloning and expression of the V_H repertoire, the vector pSW1-V_HPOLY was built by cloning a restriction enzyme polylinker sequence to replace the body of the V_HD1.3 gene. This vector was adapted further (pSW1-V_HPOLY-TAG1) by adding a synthetic oligonucleotide encoding a peptide tag (Glu-Gln-Lys-Leu-Ile-Ser–Glu-Glu-Asp-Leu-Asn) from c-*myc* (Evan et al. 1985; Munro and Pelham 1986) to the carboxy-terminal end.

PCR amplification of mouse genomic DNA. BALB/c mice were hyperimmunized with hen egg white lysozyme (100 μg antigen intraperitoneally day 1 in complete Freund's adjuvant, and 50 μg antigen intravenously day 35 in incomplete Freund's adjuvant; kill day 39) or similarly with keyhole limpet hemocyanin (KLH). DNA was prepared from the spleen (Maniatis et al. 1982), and the rearranged mouse V_H genes were amplified using PCR (Saiki et al. 1985; Orlandi et al. 1989) using the primers V_H1FOR-2 (5'-TGA GGA GAC GGT GAC CGT GGT CCC TTG GCC CC-3'. and V_H1BACK (5'-AGG T(C/G)(C/A) A(G/A)C TGC AG(G/C) AGT C(T/A)GG-3' (Fig. 2). The conditions for amplification were 50–200 ng DNA, 25 pmoles of each primer, 250 μM of each dNTP, 10 mM Tris-HCl (pH 8.8), 50 mM KCl, 1.5 mM MgCl$_2$, and 100 μg/ml gelatin. The sample was overlaid with paraffin oil and heated to 95°C for 2 minutes (denature), to 65°C for 2 minutes (anneal), and to 72°C. The *Taq* polymerase (2 units Cetus) was added after the sample had reached the elongation temperature (72°C), and the reaction was continued for 2 minutes at 72°C. The sample was then subjected to an additional 29 rounds of temperature cycling, using the Techne PHC-1 programmable heating block.

PCR mutagenesis. The V_HD1.3 gene cloned into M13mp19 was amplified with a mutagenic primer based in complementarity-determining region (CDR) 3 and a primer based in the M13 vector backbone (Fig. 2). The mutagenic primer 5'-GGA GAC GGT GAC CGT GGT CCC TTG GCC CCA GTA GTC AAG NNN NNN NNN NNN CTC TCT GGC-3' (where N is an equimolar mixture of T, C, G, and A) hypermutates the central four residues of CDR3 (Arg-Asp-Tyr-Arg). The PCR is the same as above, except a cycle of 95°C for 1.5 minutes, 25°C for 1.5 minutes, and 72°C for 3 minutes was used.

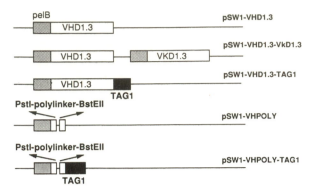

Figure 1. Expression vectors.

Cloning and expression of antigen-binding activities.
PCR-amplified DNA was digested with *Pst*I and *Bst*EII (encoded within the amplification primers) and fractionated on an agarose gel. A band of about 350 bp was extracted and cloned into the M13VHPCR1 vector (Orlandi et al. 1989) for sequencing or into the pSW1-V$_H$POLY or pSW1-V$_H$POLY-TAG1 vector for expression. The recombinant plasmids were transfected into *E. coli* BMH71-18 (Gronenborn 1976), and colonies were selected on TYE plates (Miller 1972) with 1% glucose and 100 μg/ml ampicillin and toothpicked into 200 μl of 2 × TY (Miller 1972), ampicillin, and glucose in wells of enzyme-linked immunosorbent assay (ELISA) plates. Colonies were grown at 37°C for 16 hours. Cells were pelleted and resuspended in 200 μl of 2 × TY, ampicillin, and 1 mM inducer isopropyl-thiogalactoside (IPTG) and grown for an additional 16–24 hours. The cells were cooled and pelleted, and supernatants were screened for secretion of V$_H$ domains (by Western blotting) or antigen-binding activity (by direct ELISA).

Western blotting was done according to the method of Towbin et al. (1979). Supernatant (10 μl) from the cultures was subjected to SDS-PAGE (Laemmli 1970), and the proteins were transferred electrophoretically to nitrocellulose. The V$_H$ domains were detected via the peptide tag with the 9E10 antibody (Evan et al. 1985; Munro and Pelham 1986), using horseradish peroxidase-conjugated rabbit anti-mouse antibody and 4-chloro-1-naphthol as the peroxidase substrate.

Wells of ELISA plates (Falcon) were coated with antigen in 50 mM NaHCO$_3$, pH 9.6, overnight (3 mg/ml lysozyme or 50 μg/ml KLH) and blocked with 2% skimmed milk powder in PBS for 2 hours at 37°C. Bacterial supernatant was added and incubated at 37°C for 2 hours. V$_H$D1.3 domains were detected with rabbit polyclonal antiserum raised against the D1.3 Fv fragment, using peroxidase-conjugated goat anti-rabbit immunoglobulin. Tagged V$_H$ domains were detected as described in Western blotting, except with 2,2'-azino-*bis* (3-ethylbenzthiazoline-6-sulfonic acid) as the peroxidase substrate. Three washes of 0.05% Tween 20 in PBS were followed by three washes of PBS between each step (only PBS washes before addition of blocker or bacterial supernatants).

Purification of Fv and V$_H$ domains binding to lysozyme.
Cultures (500 ml) were grown and induced as above, and the supernatant was passed through a 0.45-μm filter (Nalgene) and down a 5-ml column of lysozyme-Sepharose (Riechmann et al. 1988). After washing with PBS, the Fv fragment or V$_H$ domains were eluted with 50 mM diethylamine and analyzed by SDS-PAGE.

Affinity for lysozyme.
The purified D1.3 Fv fragment and V$_H$ domains were titrated with lysozyme using fluorescence quench (Perkin-Elmer LS 5B lumin-

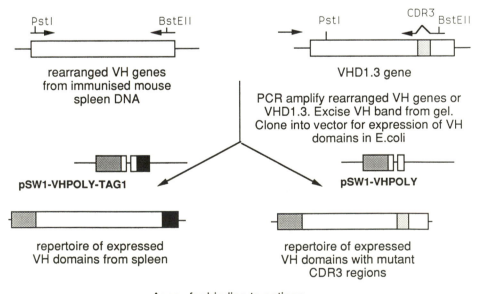

Assay for binding to antigen

Figure 2. Scheme for cloning V$_H$ gene repertoire.

Table 1. Binding Affinities of Immunoglobulin Fragments for Lysozyme

	Stoichiometry	Affinity (nM)	k_{on} $M^{-1} s^{-1}$	k_{off} s^{-1}	k_{off}/k_{on} nM
Fv-D1.3	n.d.	3	1.9×10^6	n.d.	n.d.
V_HD1.3	1.2	<40	3.8×10^6	0.075	19
V_H1	n.d.	<15	n.d.	n.d.	n.d.
V_H3	n.d.	n.d.	2.9×10^6	0.036	12
V_H8	n.d.	n.d.	3.3×10^6	0.088	27

n.d. indicates not determined. k_{on} = rate constant for association; units, moles^{-1} sec^{-1}; k_{off} = rate constant for dissociation; units, sec^{-1}.

escence spectrometer) to determine their affinities of binding (see Jones et al. 1986). The stoichiometry of binding of the V_HD1.3 domain was measured by fluorescence quench titration (to yield the total number of lysozyme-binding sites) and by amino acid hydrolysis (to yield the total amount of protein). The kinetics of lysozyme binding were determined by stopped-flow experiments (HI Tech Stopped Flow SHU) at 20°C under pseudo-first-order conditions with binding sites in five- to tenfold excess over lysozyme (Levison et al. 1970). The number of binding sites was determined by fluorescence quench titration with lysozyme in excess.

RESULTS

Expression and Activity of the V_H Domain of D1.3 Antibody

The Fv fragment of the D1.3 antibody was purified on a lysozyme affinity column and analyzed by SDS-PAGE. Two bands of about M_r 14,000 were revealed, and the amino-terminal sequences were checked by gas-phase protein sequencing after elution of the bands onto PVDF membranes (Matsudaira 1987; Fearnley et al. 1989). The V_H domain was purified the same way, and the binding affinity of the Fv fragment and V_HD1.3 to lysozyme was determined by fluorescence quench titration (Table 1). The affinity of the Fv fragment (3 nM) is similar to that of the parent antibody (2 nM). The affinity of the V_H domain for lysozyme was determined as less than 40 nM by fluorescence quench and as 19 nM by stopped-flow. Thus, the affinity of the V_H domain is only tenfold weaker than the complete antibody. The stoichiometry of binding of the V_H domain was determined as 1.2 mole V_H per mole of lysozyme, suggesting an equimolar complex.

Repertoire of V_H Sequences from Antibody-producing Cells

M13 clones from the mouse V_H repertoire generated from spleen DNA of a mouse immunized with lysozyme were sequenced. The complete sequences of 48 V_H gene clones were determined (Fig. 3). Three families of D segments, four families of J segments, and all but two of the mouse V_H gene families (Kabat et al. 1987) were represented (Table 2). The different sequences of CDR3 marked each of the 48 clones as unique. Nine pseudogenes and 16 unproductive rearrangements were identified: Of the clones sequenced, 27 have open reading frames. V_H gene libraries have also been generated from mRNA of human peripheral blood lymphocytes (J. Marks, unpubl.).

Repertoire of Antigen-binding Activities from Antibody-producing Cells

Amplified DNA from a mouse immunized with lysozyme was cloned for expression into a vector that incorporates a carboxy-terminal tag to facilitate detection of expressed V_H domains (Figs. 1 and 2). Bacterial supernatants were analyzed by SDS-PAGE, followed by Western blotting, and bands of the expected size ($\sim M_r$ 14,000) were detected for 14 of 17 clones by probing with antibody directed against the tag. To screen for lysozyme-binding activities, about 2000 colonies were toothpicked in groups of five into wells of ELISA plates, and the supernatants were tested for binding to lysozyme-coated plates. Of the supernatants, 21 were shown to have lysozyme-binding activity. As a control, the supernatants were tested for binding to KLH, and two supernatants were identified with KLH-binding activity. A second expression library was

Table 2. Usage of V_H gene D-segment and J-region Families in the Repertoire

V_H genes		D segments		J regions	
family	number	family	number	family	number
IA	4	SP2	14	J_H1	3
IB	12	FL16	11	J_H2	7
IIA	2	Q52	5	J_H3	14
IIB	17			J_H4	14
IIIA	3				
IIIB	8				
IIIC	1				
VA	1				

	FR1	CDR_1	FR2	CDR_2	FR_3	CDR_3	
KABAT IA							
A07	PGLVKPSQSLSLTCSVTGYSIT	SGYYWN	WIRQFPGNKLEWMG	YISYDGSNNYNPSLKN	RISITRDTSKNQFFIKINSVTTEDTATYYCAR	EGNWDGFAY	
A09	PGLVKPSQSLFLTCSITGFPIT	SGYYWI	WIRQSPGKPLEWMG	YITHSGETFYNPSLQS	PISITRETSKNQFFIQLNSVTTEDTAMYYCAG	DRDKLGPWFAY	
E03	PGLVKPSQSLSLTCSVTGYSIT	SGYYWN	WIRQFPGNKLEWMG	YISYDGSNNYNPSLKN	RISITRDTSKNQFFIQLNSVTTEDTATYYCAR	DSSGSMDY	
G01	PGLVKPSQSLSLTCSVTGYSIT	SGYYWN	WIRQFPGNKLEWMG	YISYDGSNNYNPSLKN	RISITRDTSKNQFFIKINSVTTEDTATYYCAR	VSSGYESMDY	
KABAT IB							
A06	PVLVAPSQSLSITCAVSDFSLT	NYGVL	WVRQPPGKGLEWLG	VITWAGGITNYNSALMS	RLSISKDTSKSQVFLKMNSLQTDDTAVYYCAK	HGDSSGYFDY	
25G07	PGLVQPSQSLSITCTVSGFSLT	SYGVH	WVRQPPGKGLEWLG	VIWSGGSTNYNAAFIS	RLSISKDNSKSQVFFKMNSLQADDTAIYYCAR	NDGYY	
B03	PGLVAPSQSLSITCTVSGFSLT	SYGVD	WVRQPPGKGLEWLG	VIWGGSTNYNSALMS	RLSISKDNSKSQVFLKMNSLQTDDTAMYYCAK	LGRGYAMDY	
G03	PGLVQPSQSLSITCTVSGFSLT	SYGVH	WVRQSPGKGLEWLG	VIWSGGSTDYNAAFIS	RLSISKDNSKSQVFFKMNSLQADDTAIYYCAR	KRDYDYDRGYYYAMDY	
H09	PVLVAPPQSLSITCTVSGFSLT	SYGVH	WVRQPPGKGLEWLG	VIWAGGSTNYNSALMS	RLSISKDNSKSQVFLKMNSLQTDDTAMYCAI	YYDGSFFAY	
25C10	PGLVAPSQSLSITCTVSGFSLT	SYAIS	WVRQPPGKGLEWLG	VIWTGGTNYNSALKS	RLSISKDNSKSQVFLKMNSLQTDDTARYYCAR	EGYYYFAY	
A12	PGLVAPSQSLSITCTVSGFSLT	SYAIS	WVRQPPGKGLEWLG	VIWTGGTNYNSALKS	RLSISKDNSKSQVFLKMNSLQTDDTARYYCAR	IYYDGSSDYYAMDY	
A08	PGLVAPSQSLSITCTVSGFSLT	SYGVH	WVRQPPGKGLEW**	*****GTTYNSALKS	*RLSISKDNSKSQVFLKMNSLQTDDTAMYYCAR*	13 nt.	Ps.gene/Unproductive
25G08	PGLVQPSQSLSITCTVSGFSLT	SYDVD	WVRQSPGKGLEWLG	VIWGGGSTNYNSALKS	RLSISKDNSKSQVFLKMNSLQTDDTAMYYCAR	21 nt.	Unproductive
A03	PGLVQPSQSLSITCTVSGFSLT	SYGVH	WVRQSPGKGLEWLG	VIWSGGSTDYNAAFIS	RLSISKDNSKSQVFFKMNSLQADDTAIYYCAR	28 nt.	Unproductive
C07	PVLVAPSQSLSITCTVSGFSLT	SYGVH	WVRQPPGKGLEWLG	VIWAGGSTNYNSALMS	RLSISKDNSKSQVFLKMNSLQTDDTAMYYCAK	37 nt.	Unproductive
H04	PGLVAPSQSLSITCTVSGFSLT	SYGVD	WVRQSPGKGLEWLG	VIWGVGSTNYNSALKS	RLSISKDNSKSQVFLKMNSLQTDDTAMYYCAS	32 nt.	Unproductive
KABAT IIA							
E04	PELVRPGVSVKISCKGSGYTFT	DYAMH	WVKQSHAKSLEWIG	VISTYYGDASYNQKFKD	KATMTVDKSSSTAYMELARLTSEDSAVYYCAR	40 nt.	Unproductive
H07	PELVRPGVSVKISCKGSGYTFT	DYAMH	WVKQSHAKSLEWIG	VISTYYGDASYNQKFKD	KATMTVDKSSSTAYMELARLTSEDSAVYYCAR	22 nt.	Unproductive
KABAT IIB							
A02	AELVMPGASVKLSCKASGYTFT	SYWMH	WVKQRPGQGLEWIG	EIDPSDSYTNYNQKFKG	KATLTVDKSSSTAYMQLSSLTSEDSAVYYCVR	RGLTYAMDY	
B04	AELVKPGASVKMSCKASGYTFT	SYWIT	WVKQRPGQGLEWIG	DIYPGSGSTNYNEKFKS	KATLTVDTSSSTAYMQLSSLTSEDSAVYYCAR	YYSNYFDY	
C05	AELVKPGASVKLSCKASGYTFT	SYWMH	WVKQRPGRGLEWIG	RIDPNSGGTKYNEKFKS	KATLTVDKPSSTAYMQLSSLTSEDSAVYYCAR	PNWDHYYYGMDV	
C09	AELVKPGASLKLSCKASGYTFT	SYWMH	WVKQRPGQGLEWIG	EINPSNGGTNYDEKFKS	KATLTVDKSSSTAYMQLSSLTSEDSAVYYCTL	LYYYAMDY	
D06	ASLVKPGASVKMSCKASGYTFT	SYWIT	WVKQRPGQGLEWIG	DIYPGSGSTNYNEKFKS	KATLTVDTSSSTAYMQLSSLTSEDSAVYYCAR	SSGYDY	
D08	PELVKPGASVKLTCKASGYTFT	SYWMH	WVKQRPGQGLEWIG	EINPSNGGTNYNEKFKS	KATLTVDKSSSTAYMQLSSLTSEDSAVYYCTI	GAARATNAY	
E07	AELVRPGASVKLSCKASGYTFT	DYEMH	WVKQTPVHGLEWIG	AIDPETGGTAYNQKFKG	KATLTVDKSSSTAYMQLSSLTSEDSAVYYCAR	GGFAY	
G08	PELVKPGASVKISCKASGYTFT	DYYIN	WVKQRPGQGLEWIG	WIYPGSGNTKYNEKFKG	KATLTVDTSSSTAYMQLSSLTSEDSAVYYCAR	SPMDY	
G10	AELVKPGASVKVSCKASGYTFT	SYWMH	WVKQNHGKSLEWIG	RIHPSDSDTNYNQKFKG	KATLTVEKSSSTVYLELSRLTSDDSAVYYCAI	EVPGGFYATDY	
25G09	AELVKPGASVKMSCKASGYTFT	TYPIE	WVKQRPGQGLEWIG	NFHPYNDDTKYNEKFKG	KATLTVEKSSSTVYLELSRLTSDDSAVYYCAR	MDYYGSSLWFAY	
F04	TELVKPGASVKLSCKASGYTFT	SYWMH	WVKQRPGQGLEWIG	NINPSNGGTNYNQKFKG	KATLTVDKSSSTAYMQLSSLTSEDSAVYYCAK	TTVAFDY	
H02	AELVKPGASVKLSCKASGYTFT	SYWMH	WVKQRPGQGLEWIG	NIDPSDSETHYNQKFKD	KATLTVDKSSSTAYMQLSSLTSEDSAVYYCAR	KRDYSTYFDH	

H01	AELVMPGASVKLSCKASGYTFT	SYMH	WVKQRPGQGLEWIG	EIDPSDSYTNYN*KVQG	KATLTVDKSSSTAYMQLSSLTSEDSAVYCAP	TGTEFAY	Ps.gene
25C05	PELVRPGTSVKMSCKASGYTFF	NYWMK	WV*QRPGQGLEWIG	QIFPASGSIYNEMHKD	KAAWAVDTSSSTAYMQLSSLTSEDTAVYFCL*	24 nt.	Ps.gene/Unproductive
B01	AELVKPGASVKMSCKASGYTFT	SYWIT	WVKQRPGQGLEWIG	DIYPGSGSTNYNEKFKS	KATLTVDKPSDTAYMQLSSLTSEDSASYYCAR	9 nt.	Unproductive
B05	AELVRPGSSVKLSCKDSYFAFM	RHAMH	WVKQRPGHGLEWIG	SFTMYSDATEYSENFKG	KATLTANTSSSTAYMELSSLTSEDSAVYYCAR	23 nt.	Unproductive
B11	AELVKPGASVKMSCKASGYTFT	SYWIT	WVKQRPGQGLEWIG	DIYPGSGSTNYNEKFKS	KATLTVDTSSSTSYMQLSSLTSEDSAVYYCAR	15 nt.	Unproductive

KABAT III A

25G05	GGLVQAWGSLSLSCAASGFTFT	DYYMS	WVRQPPGKALEWLG	FIRNKANGYTEYSASVKG	RFTISRDNSQSILYLQMNALRAEDSATYYCAR	YMILGAMDY	
C10	GGLVQPGGSLSLSCAASGFTFT	DYYMN	WVRQPPGKALEWLA	LIRHKANGYTMEYSASVKG	RFTISRDNSQSILYLQMNALRAEDSATYYCAR	GYYYDGSYYAMDY	
B07	GGLVQPGGSLSLSCAASGFTFT	DYYMS	WVRQPPGKALEWLA	LIRNKANGYTTEYSASVKG	RFTISRDNSQSILYLQMNALRAEDSATYYCAR	23 nt.	Unproductive

KABAT III B

G05	GGLVKPGGSLIKLSCAASGFTFS	DYGMH	WVRQAPEKGLEWVA	YISSGSSTIYYADTVKG	RFTISRDNAKNTLFLQMTSLRSEDTAMYYCAR	AKFHLYFDY	Ps.gene
B12	GGLVQPGESLIKLSCESNEYEFP	SHDMS	WVR********VA	AINSDGGSTYYPDTMER	RFIISRDNTKKTLYLQMSSLRSEDTALYYCAR	REGVESRLDGDV	Ps.gene
D04	GGLVQPGGSLRLSCAASGFTFS	SYAMS	WVA*APGKGLEWVS	AISGSGSTYYADSVKG	RFTISRDNSKNTLYLQMNSLRAEDTAVYYCAD	RGLHWFDP	Ps.gene
D05	GGLVQPGGSLRLSCAASGFTFS	SYAMS	WVA*APGKGLEWVS	AISGSGSTYYADSVKG	RFTISRDNSKNTLYLQMNSLRAEDTAVYYCAK	RNYGSSPFDY	Ps.gene
F12	GGLVQPGESWKLSCVIQQ****	*****	WVRQ*PEKRLELVA	AINSDGGSTYYPDTMER	RFIISRDNSKKTLYLQMSSLRSEDTALYYCAR	PPMMPSY	Ps.gene/Unproductive
F06	GGLVQPGGSLRLSCAASGFTFS	SYAMS	WVA*APGKGLEWVS	AISGSGSTYYADSAKG	RFTISRDNSKNTLYLQMNSLRAEDTAVYYCAK	43 nt.	Ps.gene/Unproductive
D02	GGLVQPGELKLSCESNEYVIP	*HDMS	WVRQDSGE*LELVA	AINSDGGSTYYPDTMER	RFIISRDNTKKTLYLQMSSLRSEDTALYYCAR	28 nt.	Ps.gene/Unproductive
F09	GDLVKPGGSLIKLSCAASGFTFS	SYGMS	WVRQTPDKRLEWVA	TISSGSSYTYYPDSVKG	RFTISRDNAKNTLYLQMSSLKSEDTAMYYCAR	35 nt.	Unproductive

KABAT III C

E06	GGLVQPGGSMKLSCAASGFTFS	DAWMD	WVRQSPEKGLEWVA	EIRNKANNHATYAESVKG	RFTISRDDSKSRVYLQMNSLRAEDTGIYCTG	30 nt.	Unproductive

KABAT V A

C04	AELVKPGASVKLSCKASGYTFT	EYTIH	WVKQRSGQGLEWIG	WFYPGSGSIKYNEKFKD	KATLTADKSSSTVYMELSRLTSEDSAVYFCAR	HEDRDSSGYAMDY	

Figure 3. Encoded amino acid sequences of V_H domain repertoire arranged as Kabat V_H gene families (Kabat et al. 1987). For unproductive rearrangements (stop codons, frameshifts in CDR3), the total number of nucleotides (nt.) in CDR3 is indicated. For pseudogenes, the positions of frameshifts or stop codons are indicated by asterisks (*), and the sequences downstream from these positions are translated as if no frameshift were present and are in italics.

prepared from a mouse immunized with KLH and screened as above. Of the supernatants, 14 had KLH-binding activities, and two supernatants had lysozyme-binding activity.

Characterization of Two Lysozyme-binding Clones

Two of the clones (V_H3 and V_H8) with lysozyme-binding activities were sequenced (Fig. 4). They belong to the same V_H gene (Kabat IIB) families and D-segment families (FL16) but have different J segments (J_H2 and J_H4) (Kabat et al. 1987). There are only six amino acid differences between the (unrearranged) V_H genes, but the sequences of CDR3 are completely different. The V_H domains were purified, and affinities for lysozyme were determined (Table 1). The affinities, in the 20 nM range, are similar to those of the V_H domain of the D1.3 antibody.

Repertoire of Binding Activities by Mutagenesis

The central four residues of CDR3 of the $V_HD1.3$ domain were mutated extensively, using a partly degenerate primer and PCR. The amplified DNA was cloned into an M13 vector for sequencing and also into pSW1-V_HPOLY for expression and secretion of the mutated domains. Sequencing confirmed that CDR3 had been mutated extensively. Supernatants from the expression library were screened for secretion of lysozyme- and KLH-binding activities, and 2000 clones were screened, as above, for lysozyme- and KLH-binding activities; 19 supernatants were identified with lysozyme-binding activities, and 4 were identified with KLH-binding activities.

One clone (V_H1) with lysozyme-binding activity was characterized further. The domain was purified on a lysozyme affinity column and titrated by fluorescence quench, and used in a competition ELISA with the $V_HD1.3$ domain. The titration suggested a binding affinity of less than 15 nM (Table 1), and the V_H1 also competed effectively in ELISA with $V_HD1.3$ for binding to lysozyme. The V_H1 gene was sequenced and shown to be identical to the $V_HD1.3$ gene, except for the central residues of CDR3 (Arg-Asp-Tyr-Arg); these were replaced by Thr-Gln-Arg-Pro.

DISCUSSION

The secretion of associated V_H and V_κ domains of the D1.3 antibody from *E. coli* confirms previous work of Skerra and Plückthun (1988), although our levels of expression are higher (10 mg/liter of active fragment in the supernatant compared with 0.5 mg/liter). However, the isolated V_H domain of the D1.3 antibody is expressed at much lower levels, suggesting that the presence of the V_κ domain may help the folding of the V_H domain or prevent its aggregation.

Our finding that the V_H domain of the D1.3 antibody binds to lysozyme in an equimolar complex and has a good affinity for the antigen is a new observation. In previous work, separated heavy and light chains were identified with antigen-binding (Fleischmann et al. 1963) or hapten-binding activities (Utsumi and Karush 1964), but the affinities were poor, with no evidence for binding by single chains (Jaton et al. 1968) rather than dimers (Edmundson et al. 1984). However, although our data suggest a complex of one V_H domain with one molecule of lysozyme, they do not rule out a complex of two V_H domains with two molecules of lysozyme.

In the D1.3 antibody, lysozyme makes extensive interactions to both domains, including three hydrogen bonds to the V_κ domain and nine hydrogen bonds to the V_H domain. Binding of lysozyme buries about 300 $Å^2$ of V_κ domain to solvent, and 400 $Å^2$ of the V_H domain (Amit et al. 1986; C. Chothia, unpubl.). Despite these interactions, the V_κ domain appears to make only a small net contribution to the energetics of binding. The V_H domain presumably binds to lysozyme in a similar way as the antibody, although it is possible that the whole surface of interaction might reorientate slightly, presumably by rocking on side chains to create a new set of contacts (Chothia et al. 1983), or that the loops of the V_H domain could adjust to binding of antigen (Getzoff et al. 1987).

The finding that a diverse library of V_H genes can be cloned from the chromosomal DNA of mouse spleen using the PCR and two "universal" primers extends our previous results in which V_H genes, corresponding to different V_H families, were cloned from cDNAs of mouse hybridomas (Orlandi et al. 1989). Clearly, we can generate a diverse repertoire of V_H genes using PCR, but we cannot rule out a systematic bias due to our choice of primers or hybridization conditions.

Furthermore, from the library of V_H genes, we show that V_H domains can be derived with binding activities to lysozyme and KLH (and presumably other antigens). Prior immunization facilitates the isolation of these activities. The affinities of the V_H domains for lysozyme (20 nM) lie within the range expected for monoclonal antibodies for protein antigens; thus, PCR cloning of V_H domains from immunized spleen may offer an alternative to hybridoma technology. Although we have used plasmid vectors for secretion of the V_H domains and assayed bacterial supernatants for binding activities, a variety of other vectors and formats for screening antigenic activities should also be possible. For example, bacterial colonies, lytic plaques from λ vectors or nonlytic plaques from M13 vectors, could in principle be transferred to nitrocellulose and screened for binding to antigen directly.

Hypermutation of CDR3 of V_H domains also appears to be a promising way of generating antigen-binding activities. CDR3 was chosen because it is the most diverse portion of sequence in antibodies, derived by the joining of three genetic elements, V, D, and J, and would be expected to carry major determinants for binding to antigen. For example, in the D1.3 antibody, the three residues Arg-99, Asp-100, and Tyr-101 make six of the nine hydrogen bonds of the heavy chain (Amit et al. 1986) and, presumably, have similar roles

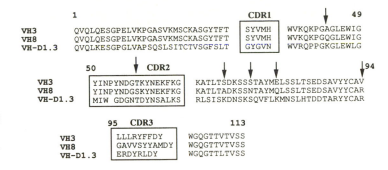

```
                        1                    CDR1              ↓      49
        VH3     QVQLQESGPELVKPGASVKMSCKASGYTFT  SYVMH   WVKQKPGAGLEWIG
        VH8     QVQLQESGPELVKPGASVKMSCKASGYTFT  SYVMH   WVKQKPGQGLEWIG
        VH-D1.3 QVQLKESGPGLVAPSQSLSITCTVSGFSLT  GYGVN   WVRQPPGKGLEWLG

               50          ↓  CDR2          ↓      ↓     ↓      ↓        ↓94
        VH3        YINPYNDGTKYNEKFKG   KATLTSDKSSSTAYMELSSLTSEDSAVYYCAV
        VH8        YINPYNDGSKYNEKFKG   KATLTADKSSNTAYMQLSSLTSEDSAVYYCAR
        VH-D1.3    MIW GDGNTDYNSALKS   RLSISKDNSKSQVFLKMNSLHTDDTARYYCAR

                    95  CDR3           113
        VH3        LLLRYFFDY    WGQGTTVTVSS
        VH8        GAVVSYYAMDY  WGQGTTVTVSS
        VH-D1.3    ERDYRLDY     WGQGTTLTVSS
```

Figure 4. Sequences of two V_H domains with lysozyme-binding activities. The sequences of the V_H domains are aligned with that of the D1.3 antibody. Arrows indicate differences between unrearranged V_H3 and V_H8 (see text).

in the isolated V_H domain. When these residues are changed en bloc by PCR mutagenesis, the vast majority of mutants lose affinity for lysozyme. However, of 2000 colonies screened, 19 retain high affinity for lysozyme and 4 acquire the ability to bind to KLH. One of the mutants (V_H1), which binds to lysozyme, has a completely different amino acid sequence in CDR3 and has a slightly improved affinity compared with the parent V_H domain. The interaction of lysozyme with this region (and perhaps also with CDR1 and CDR2) is also likely to differ, as the main chain now incorporates a proline at residue 102.

V_H domains with binding activities can be generated in a matter of days without recourse to tissue culture and may also have other advantages over monoclonal antibodies. For example, the smaller molecule should penetrate tissues more readily, could permit the blocking of "canyon" sites on viruses (Rossman et al. 1985; Weis et al. 1988), and could allow epitope mapping at higher resolution. However, we also envisage that V_H domains with binding activities could also serve as the building blocks for making Fv fragments or complete antibodies. For example, V_H domains could be coexpressed with a repertoire of V_κ domains, derived by PCR amplification of V_κ genes (Orlandi et al. 1989) and screened for association of the domains and antigen binding.

ACKNOWLEDGMENTS

We thank C. Milstein and L. Riechmann for invaluable discussions, T. Clackson for a V_H gene library, C. Chothia for surface area calculation, J.M. Skehel and I. Fearnley for protein hydrolysis and protein sequencing, J. Foote for help with fluorescence quench and stopped flow, G. Evan for the antibody 9E10, and M. Novak for donating a KLH-immunized mouse. A.D.G. was supported by Celltech, D.G. by Behringwerke, and E.S.W. by a Stanley Elmore Senior Medical Research Fellowship, Sidney Sussex College, Cambridge.

REFERENCES

Amit, A.G., R.A. Mariuzza, S.E.V. Phillips, and P.J. Poljak. 1986. Three-dimensional structure of an antigen-antibody complex at 2.8 Å resolution. *Science* **233:** 747.

Better, M., C.P. Chang, R.R. Robinson, and A.H. Horwitz. 1988. *Escherichia coli* secretion of an active chimeric antibody fragment. *Science* **240:** 1041.

Chothia, C., A.M. Lesk, G.G. Dodson, and D.C. Hodgkin. 1983. Transmission of conformational change in insulin. *Nature* **302:** 500.

Colman, P.M., W.G. Laver, J.N. Varghese, A.T. Baker, P.A. Tulloch, G.M. Air, and R.G. Webster. 1987. Three dimensional structure of a complex of antibody with influenza virus neuraminidase. *Nature* **326:** 358.

Edmundson, A.B., K.R. Ely, and J.N. Herron. 1984. A search for site-filling ligands in the Mcg Bence-Jones dimer: Crystal binding studies of fluorescent compounds. *Mol. Immunol.* **21:** 561.

Evan, G.I., G.K. Lewis, G. Ramsay, and J.M. Bishop. 1985. Isolation of monoclonal antibodies specific for human c-myc proto-oncogene product. *Mol. Cell. Biol.* **5:** 3610.

Fearnley, I.M., M.J. Runswick, and J.E. Walker. 1989. A homologue of the nuclear coded 49 kd subunit of bovine mitochondrial NADH-ubiquinone reductase is coded in chloroplast DNA. *EMBO J.* **8:** 665.

Fleischman, J.B., R.R. Porter, and E.M. Press. 1963. The arrangement of the peptide chains in γ-globulin. *Biochem. J.* **88:** 220.

Getzoff, E.D., H.M. Geyson, S.J. Rodda, H. Alexander, J.A. Tainer, and R.A. Lerner. 1987. Mechanisms of antibody binding to a protein. *Science* **235:** 1191.

Gronenborn, B. 1976. Overproduction of phage lambda repressor under the control of the *lac* promoter of *E. coli*. *Mol. Gen. Genet.* **148:** 243.

Jaton, J.-C., N.R. Klinman, D. Givol, and M. Sela. 1968. Recovery of antibody activity upon reoxidation of completely reduced polyalanyl heavy chain and its Fd fragment derived from anti-2,4-dinitrophenyl antibody. *Biochemistry* **7:** 4185.

Jones, P.T., P.H. Dear, J. Foote, M.S. Neuberger, and G. Winter. 1986. Replacing the complementarity-determining regions in a human antibody with those from a mouse. *Nature* **321:** 522.

Kabat, E.A., T.T. Wu, M. Reid-Miller, and K.S. Gottesman. 1987. *Sequences of proteins of immunological interest*. U.S. Department of Health and Human Services, U.S. Government Printing Office, Washington, D.C.

Laemmli, U.K. 1970. Cleavage of structural proteins during the assembly of the head of bacteriophage T4. *Nature* **227:** 680.

Levison, S.A., F. Kierszenbaum, and W.B. Dandliker. 1970. Salt effects on antigen-antibody kinetics. *Biochemistry* **9:** 322.

Maniatis, T., E.F. Fritsch, and J. Sambrook. 1982. *Molecular cloning: A laboratory manual*. Cold Spring Harbor Laboratory, Cold Spring Harbor, New York.

Matsudaira, P. 1987. Sequence from picomole quantities of proteins electroblotted onto polyvinylidene difluoride membranes. *J. Biol. Chem.* **262:** 10035.

Miller, J.H. 1972. *Experiments in molecular genetics*. Cold Spring Harbor Laboratory, Cold Spring Harbor, New York.

Munro, S. and H. Pelham. 1986. An Hsp-70-like protein in the ER: Identity with the 78 kd glucose-regulated protein and immunoglobulin heavy chain binding protein. *Cell* **46:** 291.

Orlandi, R., D.H. Güssow, P.T. Jones, and G. Winter. 1989. Cloning immunoglobulin variable domains for expression by the polymerase chain reaction. *Proc. Natl. Acad. Sci.* **86:** 3833.

Riechmann, L., J. Foote, and G. Winter. 1988. Expression of an antibody Fv fragment in myeloma cells. *J. Mol. Biol.* **203:** 825.

Rossman, M.G., E. Arnold, J.W. Erickson, E.A. Frankenberger, J.P. Griffith, H.-J. Hecht, J.E. Johnson, G. Kamer, M. Luo, A.G. Mosser, R.R. Rueckert, B. Sherry, and G. Vriend. 1985. Structure of a human common cold virus and functional relationship to other picornaviruses. *Nature* **317:** 145.

Saiki, R.K., S. Scharf, F. Faloona, K.B. Mullis, G.T. Horn, H.A. Erlich, and N. Arnheim. 1985. Enzymatic amplification of β-globin genomic sequences and restriction site analysis for diagnosis of sickle cell anemia. *Science* **230:** 1350.

Satow, Y., G.H. Cohen, E.A. Padlan, and D.R. Davies. 1986. Phosphocholine binding immunoglobulin Fab McPC603. An X-ray diffraction study at 2.7 Å. *J. Mol. Biol.* **190:** 593.

Sheriff, S., E.W. Silverton, E.A. Padlan, G.H. Cohen, S.J. Smith-Gill, B.C. Finzel, and D.R. Davis. 1987. Three dimensional structure of an antibody-antigen complex. *Proc. Natl. Acad. Sci.* **84:** 8075.

Skerra, A. and A. Plückthun. 1988. Assembly of a functional immunoglobulin Fv fragment in *Escherichia coli*. *Science* **240:** 1038.

Towbin, H., T. Staehelin, and J. Gordon. 1979. Electrophoretic transfer of proteins from polyacrylamide gels to nitrocellulose sheets: Procedure and some applications. *Proc. Natl. Acad. Sci.* **76:** 4350.

Utsumi, S. and F. Karush. 1964. The subunits of purified rabbit antibody. *Biochemistry* **3:** 1329.

Weis, W., J.H. Brown, S. Cusack, J.C. Paulson, J.J. Skehel, and D.C. Wiley. 1988. Structure of the influenza virus haemagglutinin complexed with its receptor, sialic acid. *Nature* **333:** 426.

Yanisch-Perron, C., J. Vieira, and J. Messing. 1985. Improved M13 phage cloning vectors and host strains: Nucleotide sequences of the M13mp18 and pUC19 vectors. *Gene* **33:** 103.

A Combinatorial System for Cloning and Expressing the Catalytic Antibody Repertoire in *Escherichia coli*

S.A. IVERSON,* L. SASTRY,* W.D. HUSE,* J.A. SORGE,†
S.J. BENKOVIC,‡ AND R.A. LERNER*

*Department of Molecular Biology and Chemistry, The Research Institute of Scripps Clinic,
La Jolla, California 92037; †Stratagene Inc., La Jolla, California 92037;
‡Department of Chemistry, Pennsylvania State University, University Park, Pennsylvania 16802

Hybridoma monoclonal antibody technology is one of the fundamental techniques for the study of biological macromolecules (Lerner 1984). Monoclonal antibodies are used for important applications such as clinical diagnosis, immunofluorescence, cell sorting, gene product analysis, and many other techniques. Recently, a new technology involving catalytic monoclonal antibodies has appeared. This quickly evolving field combines the programmable specificity of antibody binding with chemical catalysis (Lerner and Benkovic 1988). Several of the reactions catalyzed with antibodies are listed in Figure 1.

These applications benefit from the high binding constants and specificity inherent in antibody recognition and the production of homogeneous antibody via hybridoma technology. Although the production of monoclonal antibodies from hybridomas has become routine in many laboratories, the process remains very time-consuming, labor-intensive, and inefficient. In fact, the procedures involved have not been significantly modified since the original work of Kohler and Milstein (1975). In this paper, we describe a system designed to use the techniques of modern molecular biology to dramatically decrease the effort and increase the efficiency of producing homogeneous F_v regions of antibody molecules (Fig. 2). This system involves the immunological stimulation of an animal followed by the highly efficient expression of antibody gene products in a bacterium. This system will simplify the exploration of the incredible numbers of unique antibodies generated by a single animal following immunization with a given antigen.

The cloning and expression of antibody gene products is somewhat complicated by the fact that immunoglobulin molecules are composed of two chains that are encoded by separate genes (Hood et al. 1975; Alt et al. 1987). There is evidence to suggest that a significant amount of binding energy comes just from the heavy chain (V_H) (Fleischman et al. 1963; Roholt et al. 1963; Rockey 1966) in contrast to isolated light chains (V_L), which exhibit little antigen affinity (Spiegelberg and Weigle 1966; Yoo et al. 1967). Binding affinities of heavy chains can be increased to various degrees by recombination with nonspecific light chains (Fougereau et al. 1964; Hong and Nissonoff 1965; Roholt et al. 1965; Klinman 1971). This piece of evidence allows the

design of experiments in which large numbers of functional antibodies can be anticipated from the combination of a complete set of heavy chains with relatively few light chains. The dramatic increase in the number of clones that can be analyzed is necessary to compensate for any loss of binding affinity due to the use of nonspecific light chains (Kranz and Voss 1981; Kranz et al. 1982).

Initial experiments that have been recently published (Sastry et al. 1989) concentrated on the cloning of variable region heavy chains. In the present work, this system has been extended and modified to allow for expression and detection of heavy-chain sequences, as well as cloning and expression of the variable region light chains. In addition, a vector system has been designed to allow for expression of V_H and V_L sequences in tandem from the same promoter to increase the probability of recombination of a functional F_v molecule capable of catalysis.

EXPERIMENTAL PROCEDURES

General methods. Bacterial growth, restriction enzyme digestion, transformation of *Escherichia coli* and purification of plasmid and λ phage DNA were carried out according to the methods of Maniatis et al. (1982). DNA sequencing was performed according to the method of Sanger et al. (1977). Antibody screens and in vivo excision protocols were carried out according to the method of Short et al. (1988). Polyacrylamide gel electrophoresis and Western blot analysis were carried out as described previously (Laemmli 1970; Blake et al. 1984).

DNA synthesis. Oligonucleotides for construction of the heavy- and light-chain vectors and all primer sequences were purchased from Research Genetics, Huntsville, Alabama. These were then purified using polyacrylamide gel electrophoresis, phosphorylated with polynucleotide kinase, annealed, and ligated to the vector with T4 ligase according to procedures described previously (Maniatis et al. 1982).

RESULTS AND DISCUSSION

A key element to the success of this project is the ability to obtain several V_H and V_L sequences from

Antigen	Substrate	Rate Increase as k_{cat}/k_{uncat} or Effective Molarity	Ref.
		6,250,000	Tramantano et al. 1986
		770	Pollack et al. 1986
		167	Napper et al. 1987
		16 M	Benkovic et al. 1988
		4.2 M	Janda et al. 1988a
		1,000,000	Janda et al. 1988b

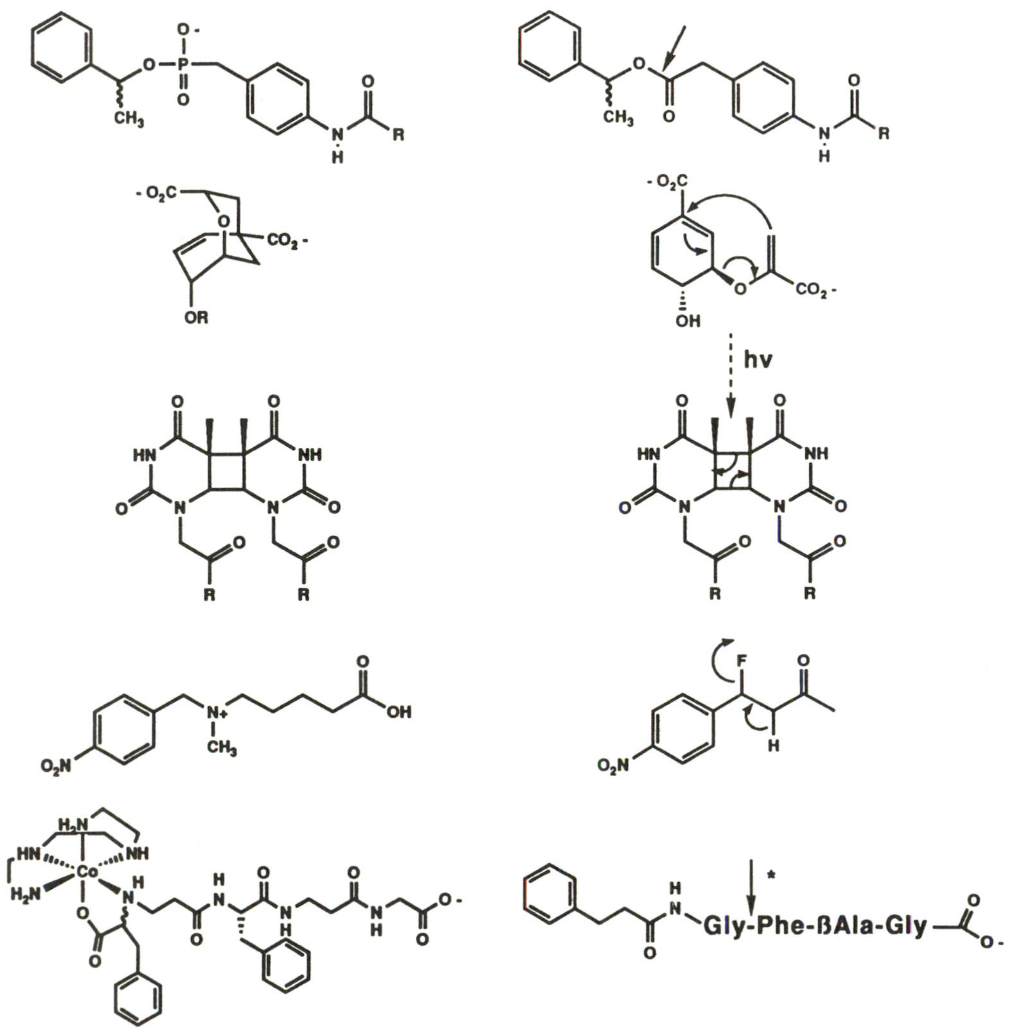

Janda et al. 1989

Hilvert and Nared 1988
Jackson et al. 1988

Cochran et al. 1988

Shokat et al. 1989

Iverson and
Lerner 1989

80,000

190
10,000

218

1500

20,000 **

* Metal cofactor required

** Simple ratio of turnover numbers for catalyzed and uncatalyzed reactions. Kahne and Still 1988

Figure 1. Reactions that have been catalyzed by antibodies.

275

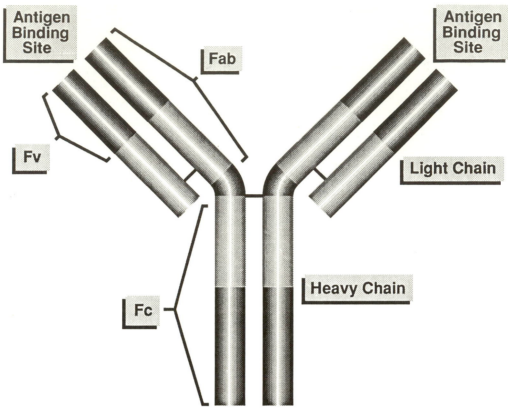

Figure 2. Schematic representation of an antibody molecule illustrating the heavy chain, light chain, and the location of interchain disulfide bonds. Alternating lighter and darker segments represent the individual domains of the molecule. The Fab, F_C, and F_V labels indicate which domains comprise those fragments.

spleen cells and hybridomas using the polymerase chain reaction (PCR). Although the design of primers may appear difficult due to the highly variable nature of the protein complementarity-determining regions (CDRs), one may take advantage of the regions of conserved sequence that flank the V_H and V_L domains (Early et al. 1980; Kabat et al. 1987). Amplification primers have been constructed for hybridization to these regions as well as incorporating the appropriate restriction sites for cloning the amplified fragment into an expression vector. This strategy of amplification by PCR followed by the force cloning of the fragment into a vector has also been described by Orlandi et al. (1989) for V_H sequences from hybridomas. In our initial experiments, several types of primers were designed in an effort to maximize amplification of V_H sequences. These primers were either a mixed pool of primers degenerate at several positions, primers that contained inosine at several degenerate positions, or unique primers. To achieve consistent results with both spleen and hybridoma mRNA, it was necessary to use unique primers for amplification of V_H and V_L sequences.

A heavy-chain library was constructed using the products from eight amplifications, each performed with a different unique primer at the 5′ end (as shown in Table 1). The products were digested with XhoI and EcoRI as these sites have been incorporated into the fragments during the amplification. These amplified

products were then cloned into Lambda Zap (Short et al. 1988) to produce a cDNA library of 9×10^5 pfu. The sequencing of the 120 amino-terminal bases of 18 clones chosen at random showed a diverse population of sequences that exhibited 80–90% homology with sequences of known heavy-chain origin. These results demonstrated that one may obtain a diverse population of V_H fragments by amplification using unique primers followed by cloning into a bacteriophage λ vector.

Since it has been shown that a diverse population of V_H fragments may be cloned by this method, expression vectors have been constructed for V_H, V_L, and F_V libraries. These vectors were constructed by modification of Lambda Zap by including synthetic oligonucleotides into the vector. These inserted sequences include the sequence for a leader peptide from the bacterial pelB gene, which has been used successfully to secrete Fab fragments expressed in E. coli (Lei et al. 1987; Better et al. 1988), a sequence to place a ribosome-binding site at the optimal distance for expression of the cloned sequences, and in the V_H expression vector, a sequence that codes for a decapeptide tag at the carboxyl terminus of the expressed V_H fragment. Monoclonal antibodies have been raised against this peptide and used successfully for immunoaffinity purification of fusion proteins (Field et al. 1988). Restriction endonuclease sites have also been included in each vector to allow for cloning of V_H and V_L fragments.

Table 1. Primers for Amplification of V_H Sequences

Heavy chain primers	Description
(1) 5'-AGGT(C/G)(C/A)A(G/A)CT(G/T)CTCGAGTC(T/A)GG-3'	degenerate 5' primer for the amplification of V_H
(2) 5'-AGGTCCAGCTGCTCGAGTCTGG-3'	unique 5' primer for the amplification of V_H
(3) 5'-AGGTCCAGCTGCTCGAGTCAGG-3'	unique 5' primer for the amplification of V_H
(4) 5'-AGGTCCAGCTTCTCGAGTCTGG-3'	unique 5' primer for the amplification of V_H
(5) 5'-AGGTCCAGCTTCTCGAGTCAGG-3'	unique 5' primer for the amplification of V_H
(6) 5'-AGGTCCAACTGCTCGAGTCTGG-3'	unique 5' primer for the amplification of V_H
(7) 5'-AGGTCCAACTGCTCGAGTCAGG-3'	unique 5' primer for the amplification of V_H
(8) 5'-AGGTCCAACTTCTCGAGTCTGG-3'	unique 5' primer for the amplification of V_H
(9) 5'-AGGTCCAACTTCTCGAGTCAGG-3'	unique 5' primer for the amplification of V_H
(10) 5'-AGGTIIAICTICTCGAGTC(T/A)GG-3'	degenerate 5' primer containing inosine at four degenerate positions
(11) 5'-CTATTAACTAGTAACGGTAACAGT-GGTGCCTTGCCCCA-3'	3' primer for the amplification of V_H

Underlined sequences represent restriction endonuclease sites; the 5' and 3' primers for PCR of V_H regions contain *Xho*I and *Eco*RI sites, respectively. For cloning into the V_H expression vector, an *Spe*I site replaces the *Eco*RI recognition sequence in the 3' primer.

Construction of V_H and V_L Expression Library

The vector for V_H expression was constructed as shown in Figure 3. This vector was used to create a library of V_H fragments from the PCR amplification of mRNA isolated from a BALB/c mouse previously immunized with a protein conjugate of fluorescein. This primary library, which contains 3×10^5 pfu, has been screened for the expression of the decapeptide tag. The sequence for this peptide is only in frame for expression following the cloning of a V_H fragment into the vector. At least 30% of the clones from this library are expressing V_H fragments, based on a screen using a monoclonal antibody raised against the decapeptide tag that has been coupled to alkaline phosphatase. Positive clones were screened again by Western blot analysis. These screens are shown in Figures 4 and 5.

The vector for expression of V_L fragments has been constructed as diagramed. As in the V_H expression vector, oligonucleotide sequences were inserted into Lambda Zap to create an optimal ribosome-binding site and the PelB leader peptide sequence in front of the cloned V_L fragment. The vector was characterized by restriction digest analysis as well as DNA sequencing. This V_L expression vector has been used to create two libraries of V_L sequences from the amplification products derived from the spleen of mice immunized with protein conjugates of fluorescein or a paranitroanaline compound. These fragments were amplified from mRNA isolated from the spleen of the immunized mouse with the primers shown in Table 2. A V_L fragment has also been amplified from the mRNA of a fluorescein-specific hybridoma and cloned into the V_L expression vector. Several clones from each library are being prepared for DNA sequence analysis to assess the diversity of the amplified fragments.

F_V Fragments: Combination of Heavy and Light Chains

The expression system has been designed to allow the combination of V_H and V_L libraries that have been constructed separately. These fragments will be co-expressed to obtain F_V fragments composed of several combinations of unique V_H and V_L sequences. This

Table 2. Primers for Amplification of V_L Sequences

Light chain primers	Description
(1) 5'-CCAGTTCCGAGCTCGTTGTGACTCAGGAATCT-3'	unique 5' primer for the amplification of V_L
(2) 5'-CCAGTTCCGAGCTCGTGTTGACGCAGCCGCCC-3'	unique 5' primer for the amplification of V_L
(3) 5'-CCAGTTCCGAGCTCGTGCTCACCCAGTCTCCA-3'	unique 5' primer for the amplification of V_L
(4) 5'-CCAGTTCCGAGCTCCAGATGACCCAGTCTCCA-3'	unique 5' primer for the amplification of V_L
(5) 5'-CCAGATGTGAGCTCGTGATGACCCAGACTCCA-3'	unique 5' primer for the amplification of V_L
(6) 5'-CCAGATGTGAGCTCGTCATGACCCAGTCTCCA-3'	unique 5' primer for the amplification of V_L
(7) 5'-CCAGTTCCGAGCTCGTGATGACACAGTCTCCA-3'	unique 5' primer for the amplification of V_L
(8) 5'-GCAGCATTCTAGAGTTTCAGCTCCAGCTTGCC-3'	unique 3' primer for the amplification of V_L

Underlined sequences represent restriction endonuclease sites; the 5' and 3' primers for PCR of V_L regions contain *Sac*I and *Xba*I sites, respectively.

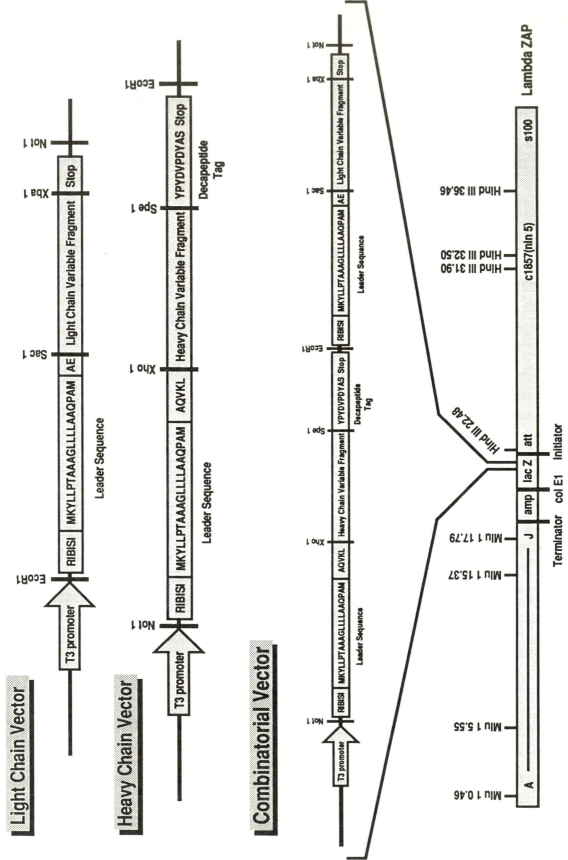

Figure 3. Diagram to illustrate the construction of V_H, V_L, and F_V expression vectors and their essential components.

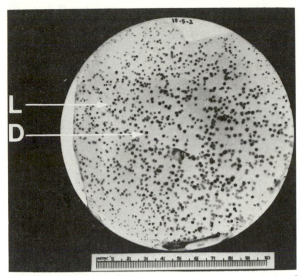

Figure 4. Expression of a diverse population of V_H fragments: The V_H-specific cDNA library constructed from the spleen of a mouse immunized with fluorescein isothiocyanate (FITC) was screened for expression by incubation with a mouse IgG2b that recognizes the decapeptide tag at the end of the variable regions. Plates containing approximately 2000 phage units of the library were overlaid with nitrocellulose filters coated with 10 mM isopropyl thiogalactoside (IPTG) for 3 hr at 37°C and were blocked with Tris-buffered saline (TBS) containing 1% BSA. The blocked filters were incubated for 1 hr with the anti-decapeptide antibody (28 μg/ml), and the unreacted antibody was removed by washing the filters with TBS containing 0.1% Tween 20. The filters were subsequently incubated with a secondary antibody (goat anti-mouse, ~1 μg/ml) conjugated to alkaline phosphatase for 1 hr, and washed with TBST. The primary binding was detected by the addition of the substrates, nitro blue tetrazolium (NBT, 200 μg/ml) and 5-bromo-4-chloro-3-indolyl phosphate (BCIP, 80 μg/ml). The enzymatic reaction resulted in dark purple spots (labeled *D* in the figure) that represent positive anti-decapeptide binding clones. The background reaction is indicated by the lighter spots (labeled *L* in the figure). According to this screening assay, approximately 30% of the V_H clones in the library are being expressed.

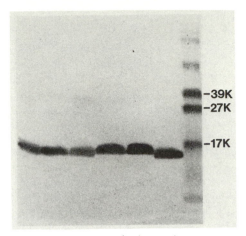

Figure 5. Western blot analysis of excised plasmids that were shown to give a positive signal with anti-decapeptide antibody (see Fig. 3). Single plaques were picked, and the plasmid was excised from anti-decapeptide-positive clones. Overnight cultures of plasmid clones were grown in 5 ml of L-broth at 37°C. Cells were spun down, the pellet was resuspended in 5 ml M9 with media 2 mM IPTG and allowed to grow at 37°C overnight. These cultures were spun down, and the pellet was resuspended in 100 μl protein gel sample buffer. From each of 6 clones, 25 μl was loaded onto a 12.5% SDS-PAGE. The samples were transferred to nitrocellulose, followed by Western blot analysis using anti-decapeptide antibody as the primary antibody and goat-anti-mouse alkaline phosphatase secondary antibody for color detection as described previously for Fig. 4. A band just below the 17K marker is apparent in each lane and corresponds to the expected size for the expressed region heavy chain.

combination of V_H and V_L sequences can be achieved quickly and efficiently by cleaving each separate library with *Eco*RI (refer to Fig. 3) and ligating the DNA to form a complete vector. Since the effect of combining particular V_H and V_L fragments cannot be predetermined, it is important that the system be flexible and allow one to combine, for example, an entire V_H library with one V_L sequence, several V_L sequences, or an entire V_L library to optimize binding that is sufficient for a catalytic F_V fragment.

Assay Systems for Leaving Groups of Biologically Active Molecules

In an effort to analyze the scope and limitations of this *E. coli*-based F_V expression system, experiments for the near future will involve convenient assay systems for the identification of any catalytic activity in the F_V proteins produced. Assays that will be investigated initially will focus on the use of chromogenic substrates

such as X-gal or paranitroanilides. These experiments will allow the screening of the expected large numbers of F_V clones for catalytic activity and allow a quantitative analysis of the very diverse repertoire of F_V fragments that can be produced in our system.

Another approach to identify catalytic activity screening will involve the cleavage of antibiotics to give a positive selection advantage for catalytic F_V clones. Along the same lines, one may also design molecules that, when cleaved, release a component necessary for cell growth, such as an essential amino acid, sugar, or nucleic acid. When used in conjunction with the appropriate auxotrophic strain, this assay will also produce a positive selection for those F_V clones capable of the desired catalytic activity.

The results of the near-term experiments just described will allow the critical analysis of this expression system for V_L, V_H, and F_V sequences in *E. coli*. This scrutiny will identify any modifications necessary to maximize the efficiency of this expression system for catalytically active molecules.

A longer-term goal will involve the production of a more universal assay system for different types of catalytic activity. Ideally, selection, not only screening, will be utilized. Such a universal assay will allow for the new field of catalytic antibodies to fully exploit the tremendous advantages of efficient expression of the immunological repertoire that our bacterial system promises.

Once catalytic clones are identified, the in vivo excision properties of the expression vectors allow them to be manipulated quite easily for site-directed mutagenesis DNA sequence analysis and protein production from the plasmid.

ACKNOWLEDGMENTS

We gratefully acknowledge Beverly Hay for technical assistance. We thank Jay Short, Michelle Alting-Mees, and Rebecca Mullinax for helpful discussions, and Brent Iverson for suggestions and assistance with graphics for this manuscript. S.A.I. is supported by a postdoctoral grant from the National Institutes of Health, F32 GM-12047-02.

REFERENCES

Alt, F.W., T.K. Blackwell, and G.D. Yancopoulos. 1987. Development of the primary antibody repertoire. *Science* **238:** 1079.

Benkovic, S.J., A.D. Napper, and R.A. Lerner. 1988. Catalysis of a stereospecific bimolecular amide synthesis by an antibody. *Proc. Natl. Acad. Sci.* **85:** 5355.

Better, M., C.P. Chang, R.R. Robinson, and A.H. Horwitz. 1988. *Escherichia coli* secretion of an active chimeric antibody fragment. *Science* **240:** 1041.

Blake, M.S., K.H. Johnson, G.J. Russel-Jones, and E.C. Gotschlich. 1984. A rapid sensitive method for detection of alkaline phosphatase-conjugated anti-antibody on western blots. *Anal. Biochem.* **36:** 175.

Cochran, A.G., R. Sugasawara, and P.A. Schultz. 1988. Photosensitized cleavage of a thymine dimer by an antibody. *J. Am. Chem. Soc.* **110:** 7888.

Early, P., H. Huang, M. Davis, K. Calame, and L. Hood. 1980. An immunoglobulin heavy chain variable region gene is generated from three segments of DNA: V_H, D and J_H. *Cell* **19:** 981.

Field, J., J.-I. Nikawa, D. Broek, B. MacDonald, L. Rodgers, I.A. Wilson, R.A. Lerner, and M. Wigler. 1988. Purification of a RAS-responsive adenyl cyclase complex from *Saccharomyces cerevisiae* by use of an epitope addition method. *Mol. Cell. Biol.* **8:** 2159.

Fleischman, J.B., R.R. Porter, and E.M. Press. 1963. The arrangement of the peptide chains in γ-globulin. *Biochem. J.* **88:** 220.

Fougereau, M., D.E. Olins, and G.M. Edelman. 1964. Reconstitution of antiphage antibodies from L and H polypeptide chains and the formation of interspecies molecular hybrids. *J. Exp. Med.* **120:** 349.

Hilvert, D. and K.D. Nared. 1988. Stereospecific claisen rearrangement catalyzed by an antibody. *J. Am. Chem. Soc.* **110:** 5593.

Hong, R. and A. Nisonoff. 1965. Heterogeneity in the complementation of polypeptide subunits of a purified antibody isolated from an individual rabbit. *J. Immunol.* **96:** 622.

Hood, L., J.H. Campbell, and S.C.R. Elgin. 1975. The organization, expression and evolution of antibody genes and other multigene families. *Annu. Rev. Genet.* **9:** 305.

Iverson, B.L. and R.A. Lerner. 1989. Sequence-specific peptide cleavage catalyzed by an antibody. *Science* **243:** 1184.

Jackson, D.Y., J.W. Jacobs, R. Sugasawara, S.H. Reich, P.A. Bartlett, and P.G. Schultz. 1988. An antibody-catalyzed Claisen rearrangement. *J. Am. Chem. Soc.* **110:** 4841.

Janda, K.D., S.J. Benkovic, and R.A. Lerner. 1989. Catalytic antibodies with lipase activity and R or S substrate selectivity. *Science* **244:** 437.

Janda, K.D., R.A. Lerner, and A. Tramontano. 1988a. Antibody catalysis of bimolecular amide formation. *J. Am. Chem. Soc.* **110:** 4835.

Janda, K.D., D. Schloeder, S.J. Benkovic, and R.A. Lerner. 1988b. Induction of an antibody that catalyzes the hydrolysis of an amide bond. *Science* **241:** 1188.

Kabat, E.A., T.T. Wu, M. Reid Muller, H.M. Perry, and U.S. Grottesman. 1987. *Sequences of proteins on immunological interest*, 4th edition. Department of Health and Human Services, Washington, D.C.

Klinman, N.R. 1971. Regain of homogeneous binding activity after recombination of chains of "monofocal" antibody. *J. Immunol.* **106:** 1330.

Köhler, G. and C. Milstein. 1975. Continuous cultures of fused cells secreting antibody of predefined specificity. *Nature* **256:** 495.

Kranz, D.M. and E.W. Voss. 1981. Restricted reassociation of heavy and light chains from hapten-specific monoclonal antibodies. *Proc. Natl. Acad. Sci.* **78:** 5807.

Kranz, D.M., J.N. Herron, and E.W. Voss. 1982. Mechanisms of ligand binding by monoclonal anti-fluorescyl antibodies. *J. Biol. Chem.* **257:** 6987.

Laemmli, U.K. 1970. Cleavage of structural proteins during the assembly of the head of bacteriophage T4. *Nature* **227:** 680.

Lei, S.-P., H.-C. Lin, S.-S. Wang, J. Callaway, and G. Wilcox. 1987. Characterization of the *Erwinia carotova* Pel B gene and its product pectate lyase. *J. Bacteriol.* **169:** 4379.

Lerner, R.A. 1984. Antibodies of predetermined specificity in biology and medicine. *Adv. Immunol.* **36:** 1.

Lerner, R.A. and S.J. Benkovic. 1988. Principles of antibody catalysis. *BioEssay* **9:** 107.

Maniatis, T., E.R. Fritsch, and J. Sambrook. 1982. *Molecular Cloning: A Laboratory Manual.* Cold Spring Harbor Laboratory, Cold Spring Harbor, New York.

Orlandi, R., D.H. Güssow, P.T. Jones, and G. Winter. 1989. Cloning immunoglobulin variable domains for expression by the polymerase chain reaction. *Proc. Natl. Acad. Sci.* **86:** 8333.

Napper, A.D., S.J. Benkovic, A. Tramontano, and R.A. Lerner. 1987. A stereospecific cyclization catalyzed by an antibody. *Science* **237:** 1041.

Pollack, S.J., J.W. Jacobs, and P.G. Schultz. 1986. Selective chemical catalysis by an antibody. *Science* **234:** 1570.

Rockey, J.H. 1966. Equine antihapten antibody. *J. Exp. Med.* **125:** 249.

Roholt, O.A., G. Radzimski, and D. Pressman. 1963. Antibody combining site: The B poly peptide chain. *Science* **141:** 726.

———. 1965. Preferential recombination of antibody chains to form effective binding sites. *J. Exp. Med.* **122:** 785.

Sanger, F., S. Nicklen, and A.R. Coulson. 1977. DNA sequencing with chain-terminating inhibitors. *Proc. Natl. Acad. Sci.* **74:** 5463.

Sastry, L., M. Alting-Mees, W. Huse, J.M. Short, J.A. Sorge, B.N. Hay, K.D. Janda, S.J. Benkovic, and R.A. Lerner. 1989. Cloning of the immunological repertoire in *E. coli* for generation of monoclonal catalytic antibodies. I. Construction of a V_H specific cDNA library. *Proc. Natl. Acad. Sci.* **86:** 5728.

Shokat, K.M., C.J. Leumann, R. Sugasawara, and P.G. Schultz. 1989. A new strategy for the generation of catalytic antibodies. *Nature* **338:** 269.

Short, J.M., J.M. Fernandez, J.A. Sorge, and W.D. Huse. 1988. Lambda Zap: A bacteriophage Lambda expression vector with in vivo excision properties. *Nucleic Acids Res.* **16:** 7583.

Spiegelberg, H.L. and W.O. Weigle. 1966. The in vivo formation and fate of antigen-antibody complexes formed by fragments and polypeptide chains of rabbit γG-antibodies. *J. Exp. Med.* **123:** 999.

Kahne, D. and C. Still. 1988. Hydrolysis of a peptide bond in neutral water. *J. Am. Chem. Soc.* **110:** 7529.

Tramontano, A., K.D. Janda, and R.A. Lerner. 1986. Chemical reactivity at an antibody binding site elicited by mech-

anistic design of synthetic antigen. *Proc. Natl. Acad. Sci.* **83:** 6736.

Yoo, T.J., O.A. Roholt, and D. Pressman. 1967. Hapten binding activity in isolated light polypeptide chain from rabbit antibody. *Cold Spring Harbor Symp. Quant. Biol.* **32:** 117.

A New Effector Mechanism for Antibodies: Catalytic Cleavage of Peptide Bonds

S. PAUL

Department of Pharmacology, University of Nebraska Medical Center, Omaha, Nebraska 68105

Antibodies have traditionally been held to mediate their function as immunological effector agents via specific recognition and binding of target antigens. The chemical and physical forces involved in antigen interactions with antibodies are very similar to those involved in enzyme interactions with substrates and receptor interactions with hormones and neurotransmitters, namely, hydrogen bonding, electrostatic interactions, van der Waals forces, and the hydrophobic effect. In recent years, it has become evident that antigen binding by antibodies can be followed by chemical transformation of the antigen. Antibodies have been designed that catalyze a variety of chemical reactions, including various forms of acyl group transfers (Tramantano et al. 1986a,b; Jacobs and Schultz 1987; Janda et al. 1988) and a pericyclic rearrangement (Jackson et al. 1988). The approaches used to design catalytic antibodies are (1) immunization against analogs of the presumed transition states of chemical reactions (Tramantano et al. 1986a,b; Hilvert et al. 1988), (2) introduction of charged reactive groups (e.g., a thiol moiety) in the active site of antibodies (Pollack et al. 1988), (3) induction of charge complementarity between antibody and antigen (Shokat et al. 1989), and (4) immunization against substrate-metal complexes, resulting in antibodies capable of metal ion-assisted catalysis (Iverson and Lerner 1989).

Amino acid residues in the complementarity-determining regions (CDRs) of antibody molecules are highly variable (French et al. 1989). This variability underlies, in part, the range of antibody specificities that the immune system can produce. Although the primary thrust of antibody evolution may be toward greater antigen-binding affinities, it is not difficult to conceive that a catalytic function can be acquired by antibodies, via mechanisms such as somatic hypermutation and junctional diversity. Substitution of chemically reactive amino acids in the antibody-combining site, e.g., aspartic acid, serine, and histidine, for relatively nonreactive residues, could confer catalytic activity to the antibody, provided such changes do not destroy antigen recognition. We have observed that some naturally occurring autoantibodies directed against a neuropeptide, vasoactive intestinal peptide (VIP), can hydrolyze VIP in a sequence-specific and catalytic fashion.

MATERIALS AND METHODS

Most materials and experimental techniques utilized in this study have been described elsewhere (Paul and Said 1988; Paul et al. 1989a,b). Immobilization of VIP on CNBr-Sepharose was done according to the manufacturer's instructions (Pharmacia). Values for the antibody-mediated hydrolysis of VIP labeled with ^{125}I at Tyr-10 ([Tyr-10-^{125}I]-VIP) are normalized for the trichloroacetic acid (TCA)-soluble radioactivity observed after incubation in assay diluent (Paul et al. 1989a).

RESULTS

Human subjects positive for plasma autoantibodies against VIP were identified by measuring binding of [Tyr-10-^{125}I]-VIP that was inhibited competitively by unlabeled VIP (Paul and Said 1988). Reversed-phase high-performance liquid chromatography (HPLC) of VIP treated with IgG purified from one such subject revealed two peptides that were absent in chromatograms of VIP incubated with buffer or VIP incubated with nonimmune IgG. These peptides were purified by a second round of HPLC (Fig. 1). Amino acid sequencing and fast atom bombardment–mass spectrometry showed that the two purified peptides were VIP(1-16) and VIP(17-28). The peptide bond between residues 16 and 17 (glutamine and methionine, respectively) was broken by treatment with the IgG. To characterize the hydrolysis of VIP by the IgG and study its kinetics, a rapid assay method was developed. The substrate used was [Tyr-10-^{125}I]-VIP. Precipitation with 10% TCA was used to separate intact VIP, which appeared in the pellet, from the radioactive fragment VIP(1-16), which appeared in the supernatant. The amount of radioactivity rendered TCA-soluble by the IgG correlated well with the amount of radioactivity in an early eluting fraction (retention time, 10 min) in reversed-phase HPLC of [Tyr-10-^{125}I]-VIP after treatment with the IgG. The retention time of intact [Tyr-10-^{125}I]-VIP was 25 minutes. Cleavage of VIP by the IgG was pH-dependent, with a pH optimum of about 8.0 (Fig. 2). The hydrolysis of VIP by the IgG was saturable, as seen in experiments in which the [Tyr-10-^{125}I]-VIP mixed with increasing concentrations of unlabeled VIP was

HIS-SER-ASP-ALA-VAL-PHE-THR-ASP-ASN-TYR-THR-ARG-LEU-ARG-LYS-GLN

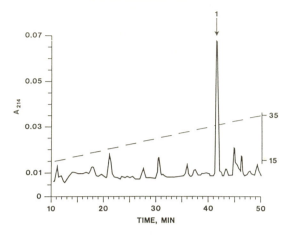

MET-ALA-VAL-LYS-LYS-TYR-LEU-ASN-SER-ILE-LEU-ASN

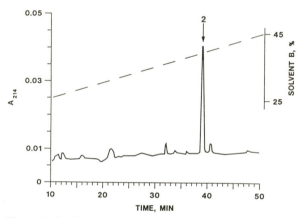

Figure 1. Purification by reversed-phase HPLC and amino acid sequences of two peptides (*1* and *2*) generated by treatment of VIP with immune IgG. Shown are the chromatographies performed to purify two A_{214}-absorbing peaks that were identified by an initial HPLC run (not shown). These peptides were not detected in a nonimmune IgG-treated VIP preparation.

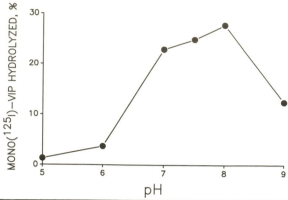

Figure 2. pH dependence of [Tyr-10-^{125}I]-VIP hydrolysis by immune IgG (17.5 μg per assay tube).

the IgG did not occur under these conditions (Paul et al. 1989a). The antibody concentration and affinity were determined by Scatchard analysis of the binding data. Compared to enzymes, the observed K_m and K_d values are low (Table 1), suggesting relatively tight binding of VIP by the antibody. For an antibody-catalyzed reaction, the observed turnover number k_{cat}: 15.6/min is impressive. This value is greater by two to three orders of magnitude than that observed for metal cofactor-assisted peptide bond hydrolysis by an antibody (Iverson and Lerner 1989).

The IgG fraction used in these experiments was prepared by ammonium sulfate precipitation of human plasma, chromatography on DEAE-cellulose columns, and chromatography on immobilized protein G. SDS-PAGE of the IgG, followed by silver staining, showed a single major band with a molecular weight of 150,000. Heavily overloaded IgG samples showed several silver-stained bands, in addition to the major band with molecular weight of 150,000, but each of these bands was stainable with anti-human IgG conjugated to peroxidase in immunoblotting experiments. These additional bands seen in overloaded IgG may be due to reduction of disulfide bonds and chain separation in the IgG molecule during sample handling (which included boiling for 5 min in 2.5% SDS) and SDS-PAGE. It is highly unlikely that the observed hydrolysis of VIP was due to an adventitiously associated proteinase, rather than the antibody. This conclusion is based on the following evidence: (1) The antibody Fab fragment, prepared by chromatography of papain-treated IgG on immobilized protein A, was able to hydrolyze VIP (Fig. 3); (2) gel filtration chromatography of the IgG

treated with the IgG. Curves of the reciprocal of the velocity of VIP hydrolysis versus the reciprocal of VIP concentration were linear, suggesting that the hydrolytic reaction followed Michaelis-Menten kinetics. Binding of VIP by the antibodies was studied in radioimmunoassay buffer at 4°C. Hydrolysis of VIP by

Table 1. Binding and Catalytic Characteristics of the Anti-VIP Autoantibody

Anti-VIP concentration (fmole/mg IgG)	K_d^a (nM)	K_m^b (nM)	k_{cat}^b (min^{-1})	k_{cat}/K_m (min/M)
73.4	0.4 ± 0.1	37.9 ± 5.5	15.6 ± 0.6	4.1×10^8

[a]Determined by Scatchard analysis of (Tyr^{10}-^{125}I)-VIP binding under conditions that did not lead to hydrolysis.

[b]Obtained from Lineweaver-Burke plots of (Tyr^{10}-^{125}I)-VIP hydrolysis by anti-VIP in the presence of increasing concentration of unlabeled VIP (7.5–480 nM).

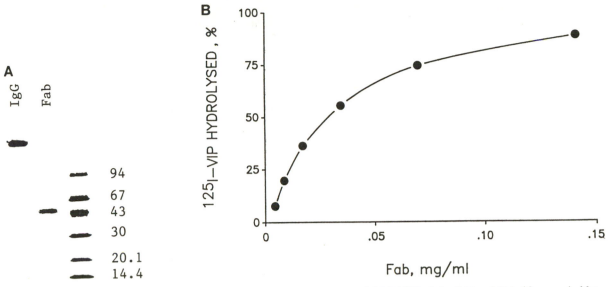

Figure 3. VIP hydrolysis by the Fab fragment of immune IgG. Shown are SDS-PAGE of the IgG and Fab (Coomassie-blue-stained) (*A*), and [Tyr-10-^{125}I]-VIP hydrolysis as a function of the Fab concentration, expressed as percentage of the total radioactivity (*B*).

under conditions that favored disruption of noncovalent protein interactions (pH 2.7) did not dissociate the VIP hydrolytic activity from the IgG; (3) an anti-IgG serum precipitated the majority of the hydrolytic activity present in the IgG (Fig. 4); (4) the VIP hydrolytic activity was present in antibodies purified by affinity chromatography on immobilized VIP; (5) the low K_m value observed is consistent with relatively tight binding, as expected for an antibody; and (6) the bond broken by the antibody (Gln-16–Met-17) is different from the peptidase-sensitive bonds in VIP (Caughey et al. 1988).

Little or no VIP hydrolytic activity was present in the IgG fraction when it was tested directly after its purifi-

cation on immobilized protein G. The VIP hydrolytic activity was observed after subjecting the IgG to the following treatments (Table 2): (1) two cycles of ultrafiltration, (2) extensive dialysis, (3) prolonged washing of the IgG at neutral pH when bound on protein G–Sepharose, and (4) chromatography on a VIP-Sepharose column. It appears that removal of a tightly bound inhibitor imparts VIP hydrolytic activity to the antibody.

DISCUSSION

Until now, antigen binding has been thought to be the sole function of the F_v portion of antibody molecules. Our studies point to a new effector function for antibodies—the catalytic cleavage of peptide bonds in target antigens. Although in this paper we describe the antibody present in a single individual, we have now identified three different individuals with catalytic anti-VIP antibodies. Our data show that these antibodies cleave VIP at different bonds, and the antibodies from

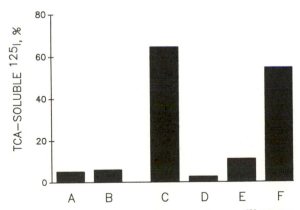

Figure 4. Evidence that the hydrolysis of [Tyr-10-^{125}I]-VIP is mediated by an IgG molecule. Shown are values of TCA-soluble radioactivity observed after treatment of [Tyr-10-^{125}I]-VIP with assay diluent (*A*), nonimmune IgG (*B*), immune IgG (*C*), boiled immune IgG (10 min) (*D*), the supernatant after precipitation of the immune IgG with anti-human IgG (*E*), and the ammonium sulfate precipitate of the immune IgG (*F*).

Table 2. Induction of VIP-hydrolytic Activity by Removal of a Putative Inhibitor from the Anti-VIP Preparation

IgG treatment[a]	(Tyr^{10}–^{125}I)VIP (cpm hydrolyzed ± s.m.)
None	−117 ± 156
Dialysis[b]	2461 ± 37
Ultrafiltration[c]	2346 ± 272
Washing on protein G-Sepharose[d]	2662 ± 77
Purification on VIP-Sepharose[e]	1660 ± 289

[a]75 μg IgG per assay tube in the first four sets.
[b]96 hr with three changes of buffer.
[c]Two cycles on a 10-kD YM-10 cutoff filter (Amicon).
[d]1 mg IgG immobilized on protein G-Sepharose, washed extensively with a neutral pH buffer, followed by elution at pH 2.7.
[e]100 ng anti-VIP antibody (obtained by acid elution) per assay tube.

one of the individuals cleave the molecule at multiple sites. It is unlikely that the observed antibody-mediated cleavage of VIP is an isolated phenomenon or one that is simply due to the presence of an unusually labile peptide bond in VIP. On the other hand, the generality of these findings is yet to be tested with autoantibodies directed against other peptides and proteins.

In general, the biological consequences of catalytic antipeptide antibodies are likely to be more profound than those of antibodies that are noncatalytic. First, cleavage of peptide bonds in most protein antigens by an antibody is likely to result in loss of biological activity. Second, catalytic antibodies, by definition, are reusable. Thus, low titers of catalytic antibodies would neutralize greater amounts of an antigen than an equivalent titer of antibodies that simply bind antigens. If directed against protein antigens of invading pathogens, catalytic antibodies that can cleave peptide bonds are likely to be highly efficient defender molecules. Catalytic antibodies offer exciting new therapeutic possibilities. For instance, passive immunization with small amounts of catalytic antibodies directed against viral and bacterial antigens could be used to treat infections. The antibodies we are examining are autoantibodies, directed against a putative neurotransmitter. The mechanisms responsible for the pathogenesis of many autoimmune disorders remain to be identified fully. Catalytic antibodies directed against self-constituents appear to possess a high potential to cause biological damage.

The catalytic VIP autoantibody described in this study was isolated from a healthy subject. The catalytic activity of this autoantibody was observed after it had been "activated" by procedures that removed relatively small-size molecular species. These data are consistent with the presence of an inhibitor, the removal of which confers catalytic activity on the autoantibody. The chemical nature of this putative inhibitor is not known. Chromatography on immobilized VIP resulted in an antibody preparation with VIP-hydrolytic activity, suggesting that the inhibitor may be active-site directed.

The autoantibodies we have observed are relatively efficient in their catalytic ability, compared to an engineered antibody that hydrolyzes a peptide bond when assisted by metal cofactors (Iverson and Lerner 1989). Hydrolysis of peptide bonds is considerably more difficult than other types of chemical reactions shown to be catalyzed by engineered antibodies with reasonably high efficiencies. An understanding of the mechanisms of peptide bond hydrolysis by naturally occurring au-toantibodies is likely to provide clues in designing antipeptide antibodies with greater catalytic efficiencies than hitherto possible.

ACKNOWLEDGMENTS

This work was supported, in part, by the National Institutes of Health and by Igen, Inc. Expert preparation of the manuscript was by Lori Swigart. I am grateful to R. Massey, T. Rees, M. Powell, D. Johnson, and A. Thompson for their helpful suggestions, and to D.J. Volle and C. Beach for discussions and experimental help.

REFERENCES

Caughey, G.H., F. Leidig, N.F. Viro, and J.A. Nadel. 1988. Substance P and vasoactive intestinal peptide degradation by mast cell tryptase and chymase. *J. Pharmacol. Exp. Ther.* **244:** 133.

French, D.L., R. Laskov, and M.D. Scharff. 1989. The role of somatic hypermutation in the generation of antibody diversity. *Science* **244:** 1152.

Hilvert, D., S.H. Carpenter, K.D. Nared, and M.-T.M. Auditor. 1988. Catalysis of concerted reactions by antibodies: The Claisen rearrangement. *Proc. Natl. Acad. Sci.* **85:** 4953.

Iverson, B.L. and R.A. Lerner. 1989. Sequence-specific peptide cleavage catalyzed by an antibody. *Science* **243:** 1184.

Jackson, D.Y., J.W. Jacobs, R. Sugasawara, S.H. Reich, P.A. Bartlett, and P.G. Schultz. 1988. An antibody-catalyzed Claisen rearrangement. *J. Am. Chem. Soc.* **110:** 4841.

Jacobs, J. and P.G. Schultz. 1987. Catalytic antibodies. *J. Am. Chem. Soc.* **109:** 2174.

Janda, K.D., D. Schloeder, S.J. Benkovic, and R.A. Lerner. 1988. Induction of an antibody that catalyzes the hydrolysis of an amide bond. *Science* **241:** 1188.

Paul, S. and S.I. Said. 1988. Autoantibodies to vasoactive intestinal peptide: Increased incidence of muscular exercise. *Life Sci.* **43:** 1079.

Paul, S., D.J. Volle, C.M. Beach, D. Johnson, M.J. Powell, and R.J. Massey. 1989a. Catalytic hydrolysis of vasoactive intestinal peptide by human autoantibody. *Science* **244:** 1158.

Paul, S., D.J. Volle, S.I. Said, A. Thompson, D.K. Agrawal, and S. de la Rocha. 1989b. Characterization of autoantibodies to VIP in asthma. *J. Neuroimmunol.* **23:** 133.

Pollack, S.J., G.R. Nakayama, and P.G. Schultz. 1988. Introduction of nucleophiles and spectroscopic probes into antibody combining sites. *Science* **242:** 1038.

Shokat, K.M., C.J. Leumann, R. Sugasawara, and P.G. Schultz. 1989. A new strategy for the generation of catalytic antibodies. *Nature* **338:** 269.

Tramontano, A., K.D. Janda, and R.A. Lerner. 1986a. Catalytic antibodies. *Science* **234:** 1566.

———. 1986b. Chemical reactivity at an antibody binding site elicited by mechanistic design of a synthetic antigen. *Proc. Natl. Acad. Sci.* **83:** 6736.

Proteolytic Processing in Endosomal Vesicles

J.S. Blum, R. Diaz, S. Diment, M. Fiani, L. Mayorga,
J.S. Rodman, and P.D. Stahl
Washington University School of Medicine, St. Louis, Missouri 63110

Molecules bound to specific receptors or taken up by fluid phase processes are transported inside cells via endocytic vesicles. In the case of receptor-mediated endocytosis, cell-surface receptors bind ligand, and these complexes cluster in coated pits. The receptor-ligand complexes are internalized via clathrin-coated vesicles, which give rise to endosomal vesicles. Shortly after their formation, the internal pH of endocytic vesicles drops to approximately pH 5.0–6.0 (Tycko and Maxfield 1982). Many receptor-ligand complexes dissociated upon acidification, with unoccupied receptors recycling back to the cell surface (Tietze et al. 1982). In some cases, the contents of endocytic vesicles are directed to lysosomes (Goldstein et al. 1979; Stahl et al. 1980; Mellman and Plutner 1984) or the Golgi network (Snider and Rogers 1985). Toxins and viruses have been shown to translocate from endocytic vesicles directly into the cytoplasm (Sandvig and Olsnes 1981; Marsh 1984). Thus, endosomal vesicles serve as a sorting and transport compartment from which molecules are recycled back to the cell surface or delivered to intracellular sites such as lysosomes, Golgi, or cytoplasm.

Endosomal vesicles also function as a processing compartment in that these vesicles contain active proteinases (Diment and Stahl 1985; Roederer et al. 1987). Susceptible proteins delivered into endocytic vesicles are rapidly proteolyzed. Endosomal proteolysis may be important in the processing of antigens, in the conversion of hormones to active or inactive forms, and in the activation of toxins. We have focused on identifying proteins processed in endosomes, as well as the enzymes responsible for proteolysis. In addition, studies have been undertaken to reconstitute the endocytotic pathway in vitro and to elucidate how proteinases are delivered into endosomal vesicles.

EXPERIMENTAL PROCEDURES

Proteolysis. Alveolar macrophages were harvested from adjuvant-induced rabbits, and mouse peritoneal macrophages were induced with thioglycollate medium. J774 E clone is a variant of the mouse macrophage cell line J774, which constitutively expresses high levels of the mannose receptor (Diment et al. 1987). The ligands β-glucuronidase and mannose-derivatized bovine serum albumin (mannose-BSA) are bound and internalized into macrophages via the mannose receptor (Wileman et al. 1984; Simmons et al.

1986). The macrophage Fc receptor was used to study the endocytosis and proteolysis of immune complexes of dinitrophenyl-derivatized bovine serum albumin (DNP-BSA) and the HDP-1 monoclonal antibody that recognizes DNP (Mayorga et al. 1989). Radiolabeled ligands were preincubated with cells at 4°C, followed by warming to 37°C. The amount of ligand taken up by the cells, as well as the proteolytic (trichloroacetic-acid-soluble) fragments of ligand released into the medium, was determined. Membrane fractionation studies to isolate endosomal vesicles have been described previously (Diment and Stahl 1985; Mayorga et al. 1989). Membrane vesicles were prepared and used to study endosomal proteolysis in vitro. Procedures to reconstitute vesicle fusion have been described (Diaz et al. 1988; Mayorga et al. 1989).

Purification and characterization of endosomal proteinases. Cathepsin D was isolated from rabbit alveolar macrophages, and a specific antibody was generated to this proteinase (Diment et al. 1988). A similar procedure was used to purify cathepsin D from mouse liver and to prepare antibodies against the mouse proteinase. Endosomal vesicles from rabbit or mouse macrophages were radiolabeled by incorporation of lactoperoxidase into these vesicles, followed by exposure to glucose oxidase and labeling with ^{125}I (Diment and Stahl 1985; Schmid et al. 1988). Alveolar macrophages were radiolabeled biosynthetically and used to study the synthesis and subcellular distribution of cathepsin D. The proteinase was further localized in macrophages by immunofluorescence and immunocytochemistry on frozen tissue sections (Rodman et al. 1987).

RESULTS

Proteolysis of Ligands Undergoing Endocytosis

The mannose receptor is expressed on the surface of macrophages and binds ligands with mannose terminal oligosaccharides. Ligands bound to the mannose receptor are delivered rapidly from the cell surface into endocytic vesicles. Depending on the ligand employed, differences in the amount of cell-associated ligand are observed (Fig. 1). Uptake of β-glucuronidase by cells is linear with time during incubation at 37°C. In contrast, internalization of mannose-BSA into cells appears to plateau after only 5–10 minutes. Examination of the medium surrounding the macrophages revealed

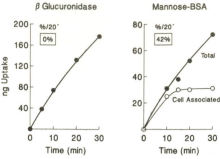

Figure 1. Uptake and degradation of protein ligands following receptor-mediated endocytosis. Macrophages were preincubated with radiolabeled ligands and shifted to 37°C for various times. For cells incubated with β-glucuronidase (*left*), the amount of cell-associated ligand is indicated (●). Uptake of mannose-BSA (*right*) is plotted as the amount of cell-associated ligand (○), as well as the sum of the cell-associated ligand and proteolyzed ligand present in the medium (●). Experiments were carried out using rat alveolar macrophages.

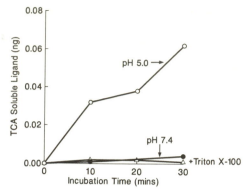

Figure 2. Endosomal proteolysis of mannose-BSA. Isolated endocytic vesicles containing radiolabeled mannose-BSA were incubated at 37°C in buffers at pH 5.0 or 7.4. Proteolysis at pH 5.0 was abolished when vesicle integrity was disrupted with Triton X-100. (Reprinted, with permission, from Diment and Stahl 1985.)

that proteolytic fragments of mannose-BSA are released rapidly by cells. By summing the cell-associated ligand with the degraded ligand released into the medium, it could be shown that the uptake of each ligand via the mannose receptor was a continuous, linear function. After 20 minutes, 42% of the total mannose-BSA incorporated into macrophages was degraded, suggesting that this ligand is very susceptible to proteolysis. In contrast, β-glucuronidase, a lysosomal enzyme, is resistant to proteolysis and is transported intact from endosomes to lysosomes (Wileman et al. 1984).

Membrane fractionation studies showed that mannose terminal ligands delivered into macrophages are localized in endocytic vesicles after 5–10 minutes of uptake (Wileman et al. 1984). To determine whether endosomal vesicles were indeed capable of ligand proteolysis, the following experiments were conducted. Macrophages were incubated with mannose-BSA for 20 minutes, and membrane fractions were isolated from these cells on Percoll density gradients. The ligand was found predominantly in light endosomal vesicles, suggesting that endosomes were the site of early ligand proteolysis. Further experiments showed that a substantial amount of proteinase activity was found in light, endosomal membrane fractions (Diment and Stahl 1985). Isolated endosomal vesicles containing ligand can be used to study proteolysis in vitro. Proteolysis of mannose-BSA in endosomal vesicles from alveolar macrophages was stimulated by ATP, which drives endosome acidification. Nigericin added to vesicles blocked proteolysis by dissipating the internal proton gradient. In the absence of added ATP, degradation of mannose-BSA was observed when vesicles were incubated in acidic medium (Fig. 2). Proteolysis of mannose-BSA was not observed when vesicles were incubated at neutral pH or in the presence of detergent, which disrupts vesicle integrity. Preliminary experiments using different ligands indicate that proteolysis can be observed at neutral pH using endosomal vesicles

(J. Blum et al., unpubl.). The different pH optimums observed for proteolysis may reflect differences in ligand susceptibility or the presence of several different proteinases in endosomal vesicles. Studies with specific proteinase inhibitors indicate that both pepstatin- and leupeptin-sensitive proteinases are present in macrophage endosomes. Endocytic vesicles gradually acidify as they are transported through the cells so that proteinases with different pH optimums may function in vivo in these vesicles.

Several proteins and peptides of biological importance appear to be proteolyzed in endosomal vesicles. The toxin ricin-A chain is cleaved rapidly following endocytosis (Fiani and Stahl 1988). Proteolysis may be required for toxin translocation across membranes as proteinase inhibitors block ricin-A chain cytotoxicity. Immunoglobulins undergoing endocytosis are generally directed to lysosomes for catabolism. However, some monoclonal antibodies are more sensitive to proteolysis and are cleaved shortly after internalization by cells (Ruud et al. 1988). A number of hormones are proteolytically processed in endocytic vesicles, including parathyroid hormone (Diment et al. 1989), insulin (Pease et al. 1985; Hamel et al. 1988), and epidermal growth factor (Schaudies et al. 1987). In the case of parathyroid hormone, endosomal proteolysis results in the generation of biologically active peptides.

Identification of Cathepsin D in Endosomes

Using rabbit alveolar macrophages, the aspartyl proteinase cathepsin D was localized in endocytic vesicles (Diment and Stahl 1985; Diment et al. 1988). Endosomal proteolysis of mannose-BSA was substantially reduced in the presence of pepstatin A, an inhibitor of cathepsin D. The contents of endosomal vesicles were radiolabeled and then passed over a column of pepstatin agarose. A 46-kD protein was isolated in these experiments and was identified as cathepsin D using specific antibodies. Experiments with mouse peritoneal macrophages have also shown that cathepsin D is present in endocytic vesicles. Endosomes from these cells were radiolabeled using lactoperoxidase, and both cathepsin D and the mannose receptor could be specifically immunoprecipitated from these vesicles (Fig. 3).

Cathepsin D is synthesized and transported through the Golgi to endosomes and lysosomes. The newly synthesized proteinase is tightly associated with membranes, and a significant proportion of the endosomal cathepsin D is still bound to membranes (Diment et al. 1988). Cathepsin D in the lysosomes exists as a soluble enzyme, suggesting that the proteinase is first transported to endosomes and then to lysosomes. Immunocytochemical analysis at the electron microscopy level has confirmed the biochemical localization of cathepsin D in endosomes (Rodman et al. 1987). Alveolar macrophages were incubated with mannose-BSA coated with gold for 5 minutes to label endocytic vesicles. Cathepsin D was detected in endocytic vesicles, using an antibody specific for this proteinase and protein A gold (Fig. 4). The majority of cathepsin D was present in lysosomes, but a significant percentage was found in small peripheral vesicles. These small vesicles may serve to shuttle proteinase from the Golgi to endosomes or from endosome to endosome.

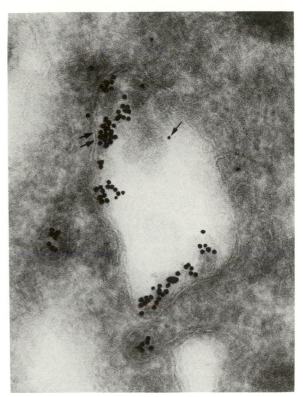

Figure 4. Immunocytochemical localization of cathepsin D in endocytic vesicles from alveolar macrophages. Endocytic vesicles were marked with mannose-BSA conjugated to colloidal gold (20-nm large gold, double arrows). Cathepsin D was localized with small gold (10-nm, single arrow) and is present in endosomes, as well as some small vesicles around endosomes.

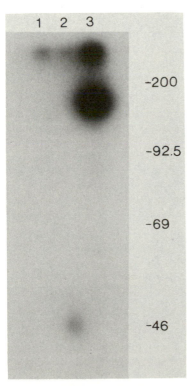

Figure 3. Presence of cathepsin D in endocytic vesicles from mouse macrophages. The contents of endosomal vesicles were radiolabeled using lactoperoxidase and ^{125}I. The vesicles were solubilized and immunoprecipitated using normal rabbit serum (lane *1*), an antibody specific for mouse cathepsin D (lane *2*), or an antibody specific for the mouse mannose receptor (lane *3*).

Reconstitution of Ligand Delivery to Proteolytic Endosomes

These biochemical and morphological studies indicated that in vivo ligands are transported from the plasma membrane into endocytic vesicles containing proteolytic enzymes. To better understand the early events that control this process, in vitro studies to reconstitute the transport of ligands into proteolytic endosomes were carried out (Mayorga et al. 1989). Immune complexes of DNP-BSA and an antibody directed against DNP undergo endocytosis into macrophages via cell-surface Fc receptors. Although the antibody itself is resistant to endosomal proteolysis, the antigen DNP-BSA is susceptible to endosomal proteinases. After 5 minutes of internalization, degradation of radiolabeled DNP-BSA is observed in endosomal vesicles (Fig. 5). Ligand bound to the plasma membrane is not proteolyzed, and proteolysis is minimal in early endosomes (1–2 min). Under the appropriate conditions, plasma-derived vesicles can be fused with endosomal vesicles such that the contents of these vesicles are mixed (Mayorga et al. 1988). Vesicles were prepared containing ligand after different times of internalization and incubated under conditions that promote

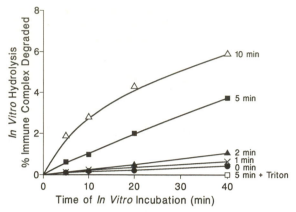

Figure 5. Degradation of IgG-^{125}I-DNP-BSA complexes in membrane vesicles isolated from J774 E macrophages. Macrophages were incubated with ligand for 2 hr at 4°C, followed by warming to 37°C for 0, 1, 2, 5, and 10 min. Membrane vesicles were prepared from these cells and incubated in buffer at pH 4.5 to permit internal ligand to be proteolyzed. The acid-soluble radioactivity was determined at each time and expressed as a percentage of the radioactivity initially bound to cells. Ligand proteolysis was prevented when the vesicles were disrupted with Triton X-100. (Reprinted, with permission, from Mayorga et al. 1989.)

into proteolytic endosomes was dependent on the presence of cytosolic factors and potassium, both of which are required for vesicle fusion (Diaz et al. 1988). A cytosolic factor, sensitive to *N*-ethylmaleimide (NEM) and required for fusion of vesicles derived from Golgi cisternae, has been identified and characterized (Block et al. 1988). This protein (NSF) is required for the fusion of endosomal vesicles (Diaz et al. 1989). An antibody directed against NSF, which inhibits fusion between endosomes, prevents the delivery of ligand into endosomes containing proteinases. These results indicate that the transport of ligand from plasma-membrane-derived vesicles to proteolytic endosomes is mediated by a vesicle fusion event.

DISCUSSION

The presence of proteolytic enzymes in endocytic vesicles may permit the specific and limited cleavage of molecules. Proteins that have undergone endocytosis are exposed to proteinases of different specificities as these molecules move along the endocytic pathway. In addition, the proteolytic fragments generated in endosomes can be shuttled back to the cell surface or to intracellular compartments such as Golgi, lysosomes, and, presumably, the cytoplasm. In contrast, lysosomes may be the site of more terminal protein processing and catabolism. Numerous proteinases and hydrolases are found in lysosomes, and the internal pH of lysosomes is more acidic than that of endosomes.

Biochemical and morphological studies have shown that cathepsin D is present in endosomes. The residence of cathepsin D in endosomal vesicles may be transient. Cathepsin D is tightly associated with endo-

or prevent membrane fusion (Fig. 6). Following a 30-minute incubation, the vesicles are diluted and incubated in buffer at pH 4.5 to permit proteolysis. The enhanced proteolysis observed in vesicles incubated under fusion conditions indicates that ligand is being delivered into endosomes containing proteinases. Membrane fractionation studies show that proteolysis occurs as the ligand is delivered into endosomal vesicles, rather than lysosomes (Fig. 7). Delivery of ligand

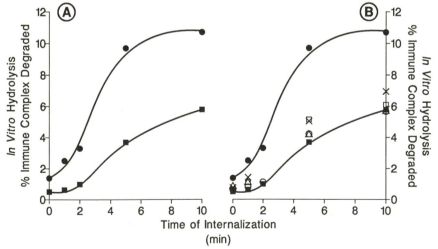

Figure 6. Enhancement of ligand proteolysis by vesicle fusion. Ligand was bound at 4°C and internalized into cells at 37°C for different times. Membrane vesicles were prepared and used to examine ligand proteolysis. (*A*) Ligand hydrolysis upon incubation in buffer at pH 4.5 alone (■); ligand hydrolysis in vesicles incubated first in fusion buffer for 30 min, followed by incubation at pH 4.5 (●). (*B*) Ligand hydrolysis upon incubation in buffer at pH 4.5 alone (■); ligand hydrolysis using vesicles first incubated in fusion buffer and then in buffer at pH 4.5 (●); ligand hydrolysis using vesicles first incubated in fusion buffer without cytosol (○), with NEM-treated cytosol (□), or without KCl (△), in each case followed by vesicle incubation at pH 4.5; ligand hydrolysis using trypsin-treated vesicles incubated under fusion conditions, followed by exposure to buffer at pH 4.5 (×). (Reprinted, with permission, from Mayorga et al. 1989.)

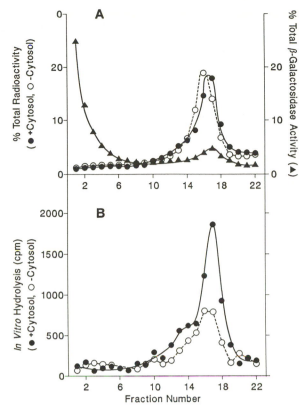

Figure 7. Distribution of fusion-dependent proteolytic compartment on Percoll density fractionation. IgG-^{125}I-DNP-BSA was bound to J774 E cells and internalized for 2.5 min. Membrane vesicles were prepared from these cells and incubated under complete fusion conditions (●) or under nonfusogenic conditions (○) for 30 min. These samples were then fractionated on Percoll density gradients. (*A*) Distribution of radiolabeled ligand in light endosomal vesicles. The enzyme β-galactosidase was assayed to show the position of lysosomes in these gradients. (*B*) In vitro hydrolytic activity of the vesicles from each portion of the gradient. Ligand proteolysis was observed only in light membrane fractions, both before and after fusion, indicating that lysosomes are not responsible for the hydrolysis observed. (Reprinted, with permission, from Mayorga et al. 1989.)

somal membranes that may serve to anchor the proteinase in these vesicles. Conversion of cathepsin D to a soluble form coincides temporally with its transit from endosomes to lysosomes. Using a cell-free system, it has been possible to reconstitute the delivery of ligand from the plasma membrane into vesicles containing proteinases. Future studies will focus on reconstituting the transport of proteinases from Golgi to endosomes and, finally, to lysosomes.

Endosomal vesicles and proteinases may play an important role in the processing and presentation of protein antigens. Receptor-mediated endocytosis has been shown to enhance class II antigen-dependent presentation by facilitating the uptake of antigens into B cells (Lanzavecchia 1988) and, in some cases, macrophages (Manca et al. 1988). Proteins that have undergone endocytosis are delivered into an intracellular compartment containing class II antigens associated with the invariant chain (Cresswell 1985). Proteinases that catalyze the proteolytic cleavage of the invariant chain and subsequent release of class II antigens are also found in this compartment (Blum and Cresswell 1988). These proteinases are similar to those involved in antigen processing and are sensitive to inhibitors, such as leupeptin, which block endosomal proteolysis. Thus, class II antigens and the invariant chain may be transported to endosomal vesicles, where the invariant chain is proteolytically cleaved and processed antigens are being formed. Cells defective in endosomal acidification have a reduced capacity to process antigen, supporting this idea that endosomal proteinases may function in antigen processing (McCoy and Schwartz 1988). In addition, chloroquine, which blocks the processing of bacterial and protein antigens (Ziegler and Unanue 1982; Allen and Unanue 1984), is known to inhibit the acidification of endosomes as well as lysosomes. The intracellular fusion and trafficking events that subserve the processing and presentation of antigen may exist in most cells for the normal trafficking of macromolecules through secretion and exocytotic pathways. Figure 8

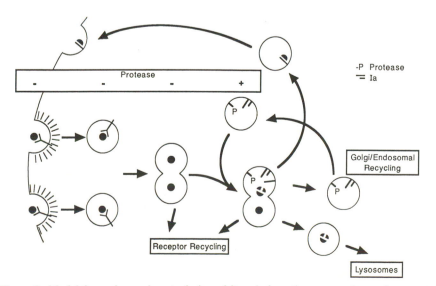

Figure 8. Model for endosomal proteolysis and its role in antigen processing and presentation.

outlines a model for the recycling of proteinases through endosomal vesicles, which permits their interaction with class II glycoproteins and protein antigens.

ACKNOWLEDGMENTS

This work was supported by grants from the Department of Health, Education, and Welfare. J.B. is a fellow of the Leukemia Society of America. L.M. was supported by a grant from CONICET (National Research Council of Argentina). We thank Marilyn A. Levy for her expertise with the electron microscopy studies.

REFERENCES

Allen, P.M. and E.R. Unanue. 1984. Differential requirements for antigen processing by macrophages for lysozyme-specific T cell hybridomas. *J. Immunol.* **132:** 1077.

Block, M.R., B.S. Glick, C.A. Wilcox, F.T. Wieland, and J.E. Rothman. 1988. Purification of an N-ethylmaleimide sensitive protein catalyzing vesicular transport. *Proc. Natl. Acad. Sci.* **85:** 7852.

Blum, J. and P. Cresswell. 1988. Role for intracellular proteases in the processing and transport of class II HLA antigens. *Proc. Natl. Acad. Sci.* **85:** 3975.

Cresswell, P. 1985. Intracellular class II HLA antigens are accessible to transferrin-neuraminidase conjugates internalized by receptor-mediated endocytosis. *Proc. Natl. Acad. Sci.* **82:** 8188.

Diaz, R., L. Mayorga, and P.D. Stahl. 1988. *In vitro* fusion of endosomes following receptor-mediated endocytosis. *J. Biol. Chem.* **263:** 6093.

Diaz, R., L.S. Mayorga, P.J. Weidman, J.E. Rothman, and P.D. Stahl. 1989. Vesicle fusion following receptor-mediated endocytosis requires a protein active in Golgi transport. *Nature* **339:** 398.

Diment, S. and P. Stahl. 1985. Macrophage endosomes contain proteases which degrade endocytosed protein ligands. *J. Biol. Chem.* **260:** 15311.

Diment, S., M. Leech, and P. Stahl. 1987. Generation of macrophage variants with 5-azacytidine: Selection for mannose receptor expression. *J. Leukocyte Biol.* **42:** 485.

———. 1988. Cathepsin D is membrane-associated in macrophage endosomes. *J. Biol. Chem.* **263:** 6901.

Diment, S., K. Martin, and P. Stahl. 1989. Cleavage of parathyroid hormone in macrophage endosomes illustrates a novel pathway for intracellular processing of proteins. *J. Biol. Chem.* **264:** 13403.

Fiani, M.L. and P.D. Stahl. 1988. Intracellular processing of ricin and ricin A chain by macrophages. *J. Cell Biol.* **107:** 114a.

Goldstein, J.L., R.G.W. Anderson, and M.S. Brown. 1979. Coated pits, coated vesicles and receptor-mediated endocytosis. *Nature* **279:** 679.

Hamel, F.G., B.I. Posner, J.J.M. Bergeron, B.H. Frank, and W.C. Duckworth. 1988. Isolation of insulin degradation products from endosomes derived from intact rat liver. *J. Biol. Chem.* **263:** 6703.

Lanzavecchia, A. 1988. Clonal sketches of the immune response. *EMBO J.* **7:** 2945.

Manca, F., D. Fenoglio, A. Kunkl, C. Cambiaggi, M. Sasso, and F. Celada. 1988. Differential activation of T cell clones stimulated by macrophages exposed to antigen complexed with monoclonal antibodies. *J. Immunol.* **140:** 2893.

Marsh, M. 1984. The entry of enveloped viruses into cells by endocytosis. *Biochem. J.* **218:** 1.

Mayorga, L.S., R. Diaz, and P.D. Stahl. 1988. Plasma membrane-derived vesicles containing receptor-ligand complexes are fusogenic with early endosomes in a cell-free system. *J. Biol. Chem.* **263:** 17213.

———. 1989. Reconstitution of endosomal proteolysis in a cell-free system. *J. Biol. Chem.* **264:** 5392.

McCoy, K.L. and R.H. Schwartz. 1988. The role of intracellular acidification in antigen processing. *Immunol. Rev.* **106:** 129.

Mellman, I.S. and H. Plutner. 1984. Internalization and degradation of macrophage Fc receptors bound to polyvalent immune complexes. *J. Cell Biol.* **98:** 1170.

Pease, R.J., G.D. Smith, and T.J. Peters. 1985. Degradation of endocytosed insulin in rat liver is mediated by low-density vesicles. *Biochem. J.* **228:** 137.

Rodman, J.S., M.A. Levy, S. Diment, and P.D. Stahl. 1987. Immunolocalization of cathepsin D in macrophage endosomes. *J. Cell Biol.* **105:** 248a.

Roederer, M., R. Bowser, and R.F. Murphy. 1987. Kinetics and temperature dependence of exposure of endocytosed material to proteolytic enzymes of low pH: Evidence for a maturation model for the formation of lysosomes. *J. Cell Physiol.* **131:** 200.

Ruud, E., G.M. Kindberg, H.K. Blomhoff, T. Godal, and T. Berg. 1988. Degradation of a monoclonal anti-μ chain antibody in a human surface IgM-positive B cell line starts in prelysosomal vesicles. *J. Immunol.* **141:** 2951.

Sandvig, K. and S. Olsnes. 1981. Rapid entry of nicked diphtheria toxin into cells at low pH. Characterization of the entry process and effect of low pH on the toxin molecule. *J. Biol. Chem.* **256:** 9068.

Schaudies, R.P., R.M. Gorman, C.R. Savage, and R.D. Poretz. 1987. Proteolytic processing of epidermal growth factor within endosomes. *Biochem. Biophys. Res. Commun.* **143:** 710.

Schmid, S.L., R. Fuchs, P. Male, and I. Mellman. 1988. Two distinct subpopulations of endosomes involved in membrane recycling and transport to lysosomes. *Cell* **52:** 73.

Simmons, B.M., P.D. Stahl, and J.H. Russell. 1986. Mannose receptor-mediated uptake of ricin toxin and ricin A chain by macrophages. *J. Biol. Chem.* **261:** 7912.

Snider, M.D. and O.C. Rogers. 1985. Intracellular movement of cell surface receptors after endocytosis: Resialylation of asialo-transferrin receptor in human erythroleukemia cells. *J. Cell Biol.* **100:** 826.

Stahl, P., P.H. Schlesinger, E. Sigardson, J.S. Rodman, and Y.C. Lee. 1980. Receptor-mediated pinocytosis of mannose glycoconjugates by macrophages: Characterization and evidence for receptor recycling. *Cell* **19:** 207.

Tietze, C., P. Schlesinger, and P. Stahl. 1982. Mannose-specific endocytosis receptor of alveolar macrophages: Demonstration of two functionally distinct intracellular pools of receptor and their roles in receptor recycling. *J. Cell Biol.* **92:** 417.

Tycko, B. and F.R. Maxfield. 1982. Rapid acidification of endocytic vesicles containing α-macroglobulin. *Cell* **28:** 643.

Wileman, T., R.L. Boshans, P. Schlesinger, and P. Stahl. 1984. Monensin inhibits recycling of macrophage mannose-glycoprotein receptors and ligand delivery to lysosomes. *Biochem. J.* **220:** 665.

Ziegler, K. and E.R. Unanue. 1982. Decrease in macrophage antigen catabolism caused by ammonia and chloroquine is associated with inhibition of antigen presentation to T cells. *Proc. Natl. Acad. Sci.* **79:** 175.

The Importance of Antigen Processing in Determinant Selection and of the Cell Membrane as a Reservoir of Processed Antigen

B. BENACERRAF, M.T. MICHALEK, L.H. DANG, AND K.L. ROCK

Dana-Farber Cancer Institute and Department of Pathology, Harvard Medical School, Boston, Massachusetts 02115

At the first Cold Spring Harbor Symposium concerned with immunology, 22 years ago, the existence of autosomal dominant genes (Ir genes) controlling specific immune recognition of synthetic polypeptide antigens with limited heterogeneity was reported (Benacerraf et al. 1967). It was concluded, at the time, that "Most probably, the PLL gene controls an initial process required for the subsequent induction of the immune response, and the stimulation of specifically sensitized cells. A limited number of such genes, specific for the processing of different antigens with different amino acid sequences, may indeed exist, and their activity could only be detected when polyamino acids of relatively simple structure are used."

The linkage of Ir genes to H-2 observed by McDevitt and Chinitz (1969) and the demonstration of major histocompatibility complex (MHC) restrictions in the reactivity of T lymphocytes, for class II molecules by Rosenthal and Shevach (1973) and Katz et al. (1973), and for class I molecules by Zinkernagel and Doherty (1974), provided the basis for an understanding of T-cell recognition.

These contributions, along with the early observations of Gell and Benacerraf (1959) and Unanue and Askonas (1968) that T-cell-dependent protein antigens needed to be processed by accessory cells to generate the immunogenic fragment recognized by T cells in association with MHC molecules, set the stage for the concept of determinant selection by MHC molecules as proposed independently by Rosenthal et al. (1977) and Benacerraf (1978). In the latter paper, one of us proposed that "specific Ir gene function dictates the ability of Ia molecules on macrophages and B cells to interact specifically with unique amino acid sequences on the antigen concerned. A limited number of such binding sites on a small number of Ia molecules can generate from the available antigens an almost unlimited number of determinants specific for T cells."

Direct evidence for such a specific interaction between class II MHC molecules and processed antigen, predicted on the basis of Ir gene activity, was provided by Babbitt et al. (1985). The recent elucidation of the crystalline structure of human class I MHC molecules by Bjorkman et al. (1987) has put the final nail in the coffin and has demonstrated the functional role of MHC molecules as peptide presenters.

After a short span of 22 years and three Cold Spring Harbor Conferences, some of us who were present at the beginning of this exciting and complex tale concerned with the mechanism of the recognition of immunogenicity can rejoice to see the light at the end of this long tunnel and marvel at the complicated mechanism that evolution has devised to distinguish self from non-self in complex organisms.

However, despite the considerable advances of the last 22 years, all the problems are not resolved and all the controversies are not behind us. To list some of the major unresolved issues: (1) A detailed knowledge of antigen processing, of the generation of the unfolded immunogenic determinants, and of their pathway to the cell membrane still eludes us. (2) Whether the processed peptides are capable of interaction with the cell membrane independently of their association with MHC molecules, and the postulated role of MHC molecules in the transport of processed antigen to the cell membrane are issues to be settled by further experimentation. (3) The mechanisms that govern the generation of antigenic determinants with specificity for class I or class II MHC molecules, respectively, need to be elucidated. (4) The contributions of cell interaction molecules, such as LFA-1, ICAM-1, ICAM-2, CD2, LFA-3, CD4, and CD8, to the association between specific T cells and antigen-presenting cells (APCs) needed to initiate T-cell activation must be better defined.

The Cell Membrane as a Reservoir of Processed Peptides

As an explanation for our observation that treatment of antigen-pulsed accessory cells with phospholipases caused the loss of surface antigen and decreased significantly the ability of the cells to stimulate antigen-specific T cells (Falo et al. 1986), we proposed that processed antigen is capable of association with the cell membrane independently of the MHC molecules. We discuss the rational basis for this hypothesis as well as the possible approaches to resolve this issue definitively.

Considering the limited number of distinct MHC molecules on an APC and the very large number of peptides capable of associating specifically with them, the ability of the cell membrane to act as a reservoir for processed peptides capable of reversible interaction with the MHC molecules would improve the efficiency of the system by increasing the probability of an interaction between an MHC molecule and an immunologically relevant peptide. Already there is evidence, albeit circumstantial, in favor of this hypothesis. Previous to the demonstration of the specific interaction of MHC molecules and processed peptide (Babbitt et al. 1985), such an interaction had been biologically documented by the phenomenon of antigen competition (Werdelin 1982; Rock and Benacerraf 1983). Such competition was demonstrated to occur at the level of the APC and to be MHC-restricted (Rock and Benacerraf 1984). Antigen competition is generally accepted today as reflecting in vivo competition of different peptides for the same or closely situated sites on the binding region of MHC molecules and is widely used to investigate the specificity of MHC/peptide interactions (Guillet et al. 1986). Such competition involving sets of processed antigens would function most effectively if they were membrane-bound rather than soluble in the water phase. The demonstration by DeLisi and Berzofsky (1985) that a significant fraction of immunogenic peptides have amphipathic properties is very much in favor of our hypothesis. Moreover, the membrane-associated properties that we propose for immunogenic peptides would not be unique to these molecules. There is an abundant literature concerning the binding properties of peptide toxins and hormones such as calcitonin, glucagon, parathyroid hormone (PTH), and β-endorphin, to phospholipids of cell membranes. For these hormones, the amphipathic sequence can be spatially distinct from the receptor (Kaiser and Kezdy 1987). Although we cannot now produce direct evidence for the MHC-independent processing of antigen and its direct membrane interaction, experiments are in progress in our laboratory to attempt to demonstrate that an

accessory cell mutant of the BALB/c B-cell lymphoma M12.4.1 lacking class II expression, M12.C3 (Glimcher et al. 1985), is capable of processing antigen and expressing it on its cell surface in a manner identical to the original M12.4.1 cell.

Leaving this very important problem aside, we shall address some of the other unresolved issues in antigen processing and presentation listed earlier, for which recent experiments from our laboratories have contributed definitive answers.

Antigen Processing and Determinant Selection

Antigen processing is essential to produce immunogenic peptides capable of specific association with MHC molecules. It is highly probable that genetically determined differences in antigen processing can affect the nature of the determinants recognized by T lymphocytes, and, as a consequence, the repertoire of immunogenic peptides. It is also possible that differences in antigen processing might be expressed in distinct accessory cells with identical genetic background. The existence of such differences would increase considerably the number and heterogeneity of T-cell-specific determinants generated from a given antigen and would contribute appreciably to immunity. In the course of our studies on antigen processing, we have observed that two genetically identical antigen-presenting cell clones display heterogeneity in antigen processing (Michalek et al. 1989).

These studies were carried out with two (BALB/c × BW5147) T-T hybridomas, DO-11.10.S4.4 and 3DO-54.8, specific for crystallized chicken ovalbumin (OVA) +I-A^d, kindly provided by J.W. Kappler and P. Marrack. In addition, two BALB/c B-lymphoblastoid, Ia-bearing accessory cells were used to present antigen: the A20.2J (A20) cell line supplied by J.W. Kappler and

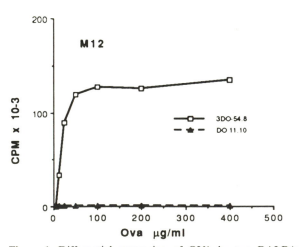
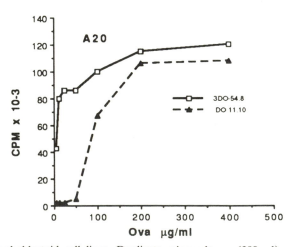

Figure 1. Differential processing of OVA by two BALB/c B-lymphoblastoid cell lines. Duplicate microcultures (200 μl) containing the indicated concentrations of antigen were prepared with T-cell hybridomas (10^5 cells) DO-11.10 and 3DO-54.8 and either 10^5 M12 or A20 antigen-presenting cells (APC), as indicated. Cultures were incubated for 18–24 hr at 37°C, after which 100 μl of the supernatant was removed, X-irradiated, and assayed for IL-2 content by incorporation of [^{3}H]thymidine by IL-2-dependent HT-2 cells, as described by Michalek et al. (1989).

P. Marrack and the M12.4.1 (M12) cell line kindly supplied by L. Glimcher.

Shimonkevitz et al. (1984) reported that both DO-11.10 and 3DO-54.8 are stimulated by the OVA peptide p323-339 in association with I-A^d. However, their fine specificity differs, since the shorter peptide p323-336 stimulates 3DO-54.8 but not DO-11.10. A more extensive analysis by Buus et al. (1987) revealed that DO-11.10 recognizes the p327-337 decapeptide, whereas 3DO-54.8 responds to the p326-336 decapeptide.

As shown by representative experiments, displayed in Figures 1 and 2, M12 cells, either in culture with ovalbumin or preincubated with ovalbumin, are able to stimulate 3DO-54.8 to secrete IL-2 far better than DO-11.10, whereas A20 cells do not display any appreciable difference in their ability to present ovalbumin to the same two T-T hybridomas. This difference in the presentation of ovalbumin between M12 and A20 must be ascribed solely to heterogeneity in processing by these two cell lines, since both M12 and A20 present tryptic digest of ovalbumin (Fig. 3) or the synthesized OVA peptide p323-339 to both 3DO-54.8 and DO-11.10 equally well.

Our results, however, could not define the difference in processing between M12 and A20 cells. As we proposed earlier (Michalek et al. 1989), the possibility should be considered that M12 cells may produce predominantly a processed form of OVA with a carboxy-terminal glutamic acid residue (Glu-336). Alternatively, it is also possible that M12 produces a fragment of OVA containing the 323-339 heptadecapeptide sequence as well as an epitope-specific hindering structure that interferes with the interaction between the peptide and DO-11.10 but not 3DO-54.8. Although we cannot identify the precise molecular species of OVA produced and presented by M12 cells, we can conclude that a large majority of the fragments produced by M12 and recognized by 3DO-54.8 do not have the exact amino acid sequence of p323-339. Therefore, this representative synthetic peptide generally used as the de-

terminant recognized in association with I-A^d cannot duplicate what is made in vivo by selected individual APCs, of which M12 is an example.

If the differences observed in the manner A20 and M12 process a model antigen are, indeed, representative of similar differences in antigen processing by individual accessory cells of a given individual, such diversity could very much increase the heterogeneity of processed determinants and the challenge for the T-cell repertoire.

The Role of Cell Adhesion Molecules in the Generation of Immune Responses

In some instances, APCs have been shown to be killed by the T-cell clones they stimulate (Tite and Janeway 1984). In a recent study carried out in our laboratory, we used this phenomenon to select mutants of the A20 APC cell line that expressed defects in their ability to present antigen to T-T hybridomas (L.H. Dang et al., in prep.). The general method used in the selection is described in Figure 4.

Several such mutants were selected. As expected, some of the mutant lines had defects in their expression of class II MHC molecules. Other mutants displayed normal levels of surface Ia molecules. Two of these cloned lines that expressed normal levels of class II MHC antigens, A20.M1 and A20.M2, were studied further.

As compared with the wild-type A20 cell line, both A20.M1 and A20.M2 displayed marked impairment in their capacity to present the terpolymer of L-glutamic acid, L-alanine, and L-tyrosine (GAT) to the GAT-specific T-T hybridoma (Fig. 5). A similar deficiency of the presentation of ovalbumin to 3DO.54.8 by A20.M1 and A20.M2 was also observed, although this defect was less severe than the impairment observed with the antigen GAT that had been used for the selection.

Experiments with these mutants were then carried out to identify the nature of the defect that was respon-

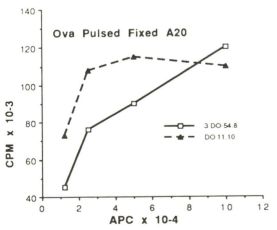

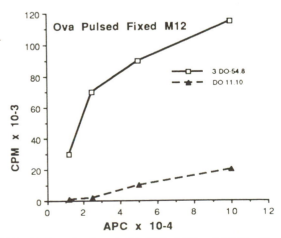

Figure 2. Stimulation of the T-cell hybridomas DO-11.10 and 3DO-54.8 by APCs preincubated with OVA. M12 and A20 B cells were preincubated with OVA (1 mg/ml for 18 hr at 37°C), washed extensively, and fixed with 1% paraformaldehyde. Duplicate microcultures were prepared as described in Fig. 1 with the indicated number of fixed APCs.

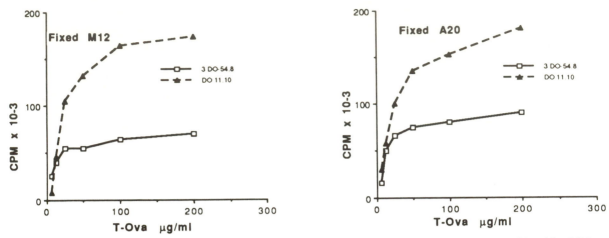

Figure 3. Stimulation of the T-cell hybridomas DO-11.10 and 3DO-54.8 by tryptic digests of OVA presented by either M12 or A20 APCs. Microcultures were prepared as described in Fig. 1.

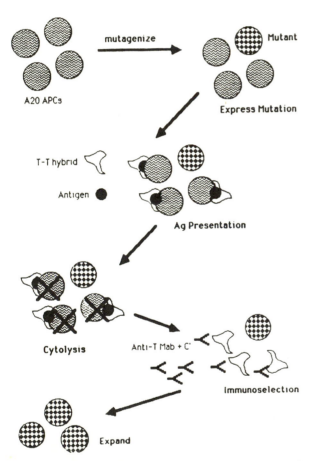

Figure 4. General method to derive antigen-presenting cell mutants. A20 cells were mutagenized with γ irradiation, and then cultured to allow mutations to be expressed. The mutagenized A20 cells were cocultured with the GAT + I-A^d-specific T-T hybrid, RF9.140.8, in the presence of antigen, for 18–24 hr, to allow antigen-specific killing to take place. After this period of selection, the viable A20 cells were isolated. This procedure was repeated until a population of A20 cells that was no longer susceptible to killing by the GAT-specific T-T hybrid was obtained. The selected A20 cells were cloned by limiting dilution.

sible for their decreased efficiency in presenting antigen to specific T cells. The results of these studies are summarized in Table 1.

To verify that the inability of the mutants A20.M1 and A20.M2 to present GAT and OVA, which are antigens presented in the context of I-A^d, could not be explained by a structural mutation in the I-A genes, we determined that the defective antigen presentation extended to the terpolymer of L-glutamic acid, L-lysine, and L-phenylalanine (GLPhe) that is recognized in association with I-E^d (Dorf and Benacerraf 1975).

It is clear also that the inability of the mutant APCs to present OVA at low concentration could not be attributed to defective antigen processing, since both A20.M1 and A20.M2 are poor presenters of the OVA peptide p323-339 to T cells, as compared with the native A20 cell line, even when the APCs are fixed.

Table 1. Properties of A20 Mutants Selected for Deficient Antigen Presentation

Phenotype	A20 +/+	A20. M1	A20. M2
Expresses class II MHC	++++	++++	++++
Presents GAT + I-A^d	++++	+/−	+
Presents OVA + I-A^d	++++	+	++
Presents GLPhe + I-E^d	++++	+	+
Presents OVA p323–339 to fixed cells	++++	+	++
Inhibited by anti-LFA-1	strong	weak	weak
Expresses MALA-2 murine homol. of ICAM-1	++++	+/−	+/−
Blocking of Ag. presentation by anti-MALA-2	++++	−	+/−

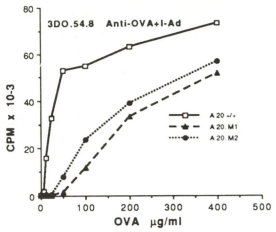
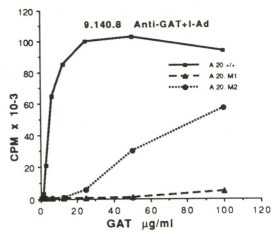

Figure 5. Presentation of GAT and OVA in association with I-A^d by A20 + / + , A20.M1, and A20.M2 cells. Wild-type A20 (+/ +), A20.M1, or A20.M2 were tested for their ability to present antigen to the T-T hybrids RF9.140.8 (Anti-GAT + I-A^d) and 3DO-54.8 (Anti-OVA + I-A^d). 2.5 × 10^4 APCs were cocultured with 5 × 10^4 T-T hybrids in the presence of the indicated concentration of antigen. After 18–24 hr at 37°C, 100 μl of the supernatant was removed, X-irradiated, and assayed for IL-2 content with HT-2 cells.

The data summarized in Table 1 illustrate that the defect in A20.M1 and A20.M2 responsible for their marked decreased ability to present antigen can be ascribed to a failure in the proper expression of the murine ligand for LFA-1. Immunofluorescence studies of A20, A20.M1, and A20.M2 with anti-MALA-2, which is a monoclonal antibody specific for the murine equivalent of ICAM-1 (Takei 1985), revealed that both mutants failed to stain with this antibody. Moreover, anti-MALA-2 antibody was able to block significantly the ability of A20 to present antigen, but failed to affect antigen presentation by A20.M1 or A20.M2. In agreement with this conclusion, antigen presentation was strongly inhibited by anti-LFA-1 monoclonal antibody only when A20 was used as APC. The same antibody had little effect on the ability of A20.M1 or A20.M2 to present antigen.

We can conclude from these experiments that "cell interaction molecules," such as LFA-1 on T cells and its ligand on APCs, are important, but not essential to antigen presentation, since the defect in the A20.M1 and A20.M2 mutants could be overcome by the use of considerably higher concentrations of antigen. However, since antigen is often presented at limiting dilution in vivo, a defect in this system of "interaction molecules" could have important consequences for immune function.

REFERENCES

Babbitt, B.P., P.M. Allen, G. Matsueda, E. Haber, and E. Unanue. 1985. Binding of immunogenic peptides to Ia histocompatibility molecules. *Nature* **317:** 359.

Benacerraf, B. 1978. A hypothesis to relate the specificity of T-lymphocytes and the activity of I region specific Ir genes in macrophages and B cells. *J. Immunol.* **120:** 1809.

Benacerraf, B., I. Green, and W.E. Paul. 1967. The immune response of guinea pigs to hapten-poly-L-lysine conjugates as an example of the genetic control of the recognition of antigenicity. *Cold Spring Harbor Symp. Quant. Biol.* **32:** 569.

Bjorkman, P.J., M.A. Saper, B. Samraoui, W.S. Bennett, J.L. Strominger, and D.C. Wiley. 1987. Structure of the human class I histocompatibility antigen, HLA-A2. *Nature* **329:** 506.

Buus, S., A. Sette, and H.M. Grey. 1987. The interaction between protein-derived immunogenic peptides and Ia. *Immunol. Rev.* **98:** 115.

DeLisi, C. and J.A. Berzofsky. 1985. T cell antigenic sites tend to be amphipathic structures. *Proc. Natl. Acad. Sci.* **82:** 7048.

Dorf, M.E. and B. Benacerraf. 1975. Complementation of H-2 linked Ir genes in the mouse. *Proc. Natl. Acad. Sci.* **72:** 3671.

Falo, L.D., B. Benacerraf, and K.L. Rock. 1986. Phospholipase pretreatment of antigen pulsed accessory cells selectively inhibits antigen specific MHC restricted but not allospecific stimulation of T lymphocytes. *Proc. Natl. Acad. Sci.* **83:** 6694.

Gell, P.G.H. and B. Benacerraf. 1959. Studies on hypersensitivity. II. Delayed sensitivity to denatured proteins in guinea pigs. *Immunology* **2:** 64.

Glimcher, L.H., D.J. McKean, E. Chol, and J.G. Seidman. 1985. Complex regulation of class II gene expression: Analysis with class II mutant cell lines. *J. Immunol.* **135:** 3542.

Guillet, J.G., M.Z. Lai, T.J. Briner, J.H. Smith, and M.L. Gefter. 1986. Interaction of peptide antigens and class II major histocompatibility complex antigens. *Nature* **324:** 260.

Kaiser, E.T. and F.J. Kezdy. 1987. Peptides with affinity for membranes. *Annu. Rev. Biophys. Biophys. Chem.* **16:** 561.

Katz, D.H., T. Hamaoka, M.E. Dorf, and B. Benacerraf. 1973. Cell interactions between histoincompatible T and B lymphocytes. III. Demonstration that H-2 gene complex determines successful physiologic lymphocyte interactions. *Proc. Natl. Acad. Sci.* **70:** 2624.

McDevitt, H.O. and A. Chinitz. 1969. Genetic control of antibody response: Relationship between immune response and histocompatibility (H-2) type. *Science* **163:** 1207.

Michalek, M.T., B. Benacerraf, and K.L. Rock. 1989. Two

genetically identical antigen-presenting cell clones display heterogeneity in antigen processing. *Proc. Natl. Acad. Sci.* **86:** 3316.

Rock, K.L. and B. Benacerraf. 1983. Inhibition of antigen-specific T cell activation by structurally related Ir gene controlled polymers. Evidence of specific competition for accessory cell antigen-presentation. *J. Exp. Med.* **157:** 1618.

——. 1984. Selective modification of a private I-A allo-stimulating determinant upon association of antigen with an antigen-presenting cell. *J. Exp. Med.* **159:** 1238.

Rosenthal, A.S. and E.M. Shevach. 1973. Function of macrophages in antigen recognition by guinea pig T lymphocytes. I. Requirement for histocompatible macrophages and lymphocytes. *J. Exp. Med.* **138:** 1194.

Rosenthal, A.S., M.A. Barcinski, and T.J. Blake. 1977. Determinant selection is an immune response gene function. *Nature* **267:** 156.

Shimonkevitz, R., S. Colon, J.W. Kappler, P. Marrack, and H.M. Grey. 1984. Antigen recognition by H-2 restricted cells. II. A tryptic ovalbumin peptide that substitutes for processed antigen. *J. Immunol.* **133:** 2067.

Takei, F. 1985. Inhibition of mixed lymphocyte response by a rat monoclonal antibody to a novel murine lymphocyte activation antigen (MALA-2). *J. Immunol.* **134:** 1403.

Tite, J.P. and C.A. Janeway, Jr. 1984. Cloned helper T cells can kill B-lymphoma cells in the presence of specific antigen: Ia-restriction and cognate vs. non-cognate interactions in cytolysis. *Eur. J. Immunol.* **14:** 878.

Unanue, E.R. and B.A. Askonas. 1968. Persistence of immunogenicity of antigen after uptake by macrophages. *J. Exp. Med.* **127:** 915.

Werdelin, O. 1982. Chemically related antigens compete for presentation by accessory cells to T cells. *J. Immunol.* **129:** 1883.

Zinkernagel, R.M. and P.C. Doherty. 1974. Restriction of in vitro T cell-mediated cytotoxicity in lymphocytic choriomeningitis within a syngeneic or semi-allogeneic system. *Nature* **248:** 701.

A Mutant Cell in Which Association of Class I Heavy and Light Chains Is Induced by Viral Peptides

A. TOWNSEND,* C. ÖHLÉN,† L. FOSTER,* J. BASTIN,* H.-G. LJUNGGREN,† AND K. KÄRRE†
*Institute of Molecular Medicine, John Radcliffe Hospital, Oxford OX3 9DU, England;
†Department of Tumour Biology, Karolinska Institute, S-104 01 Stockholm, Sweden

The majority of cytotoxic T lymphocytes (CTLs) recognize epitopes of viral proteins in association of class I molecules of the major histocompatibility complex (MHC) (Zinkernagel and Doherty 1979). Epitopes can be generated from protein antigens synthesized in the cytoplasm and are presented at the cell surface in a form that can be replaced in vitro with short synthetic peptides (for review, see Townsend and Bodmer 1989). These results imply that distinct mechanisms may control degradation of antigen, transport of peptides across a membrane, and association of peptides with the binding site of a class I molecule.

We have identified a mutant cell, RMA-S (see Ljunggren and Kärre 1985), that is not able to present an epitope of influenza nucleoprotein (NP) synthesized in the cytoplasm but can present the same epitope when exposed to it as a peptide in the extracellular fluid. This phenotype is consistent with a mutation disrupting transport of peptides from the cytoplasm to an organelle where association of class I molecules occurs. The cell also has a defect in the association of class I heavy chains with β_2-microglobulin, with reduced expression of assembled class I molecules at the cell surface (Ljunggren et al. 1989).

This led to the suggestion that the two traits were the result of the same mutation and that intracellular assembly of class I molecules is dependent on peptide binding. Consistent with this idea is the finding that exposure of the cells to a high concentration of specific peptides in the extracellular fluid induces association of class I heavy chains with β_2-microglobulin and restores expression of class I molecules at the cell surface (Townsend et al. 1989).

METHODS

RMA-S and RMA cells. The mutant cell line RMA-S was derived from the Rauscher-virus-induced H-2b lymphoma RBL-5 by exposure to the mutagen ethylmethane sulfonate (EMS) and repeated rounds of treatment with antisera to class I molecules and complement (Ljunggren and Kärre 1985; Kärre et al. 1986). It expressed about one-twentieth the amount of H-2D^b, K^b, and β_2-microglobulin at the cell surface as RBL-5 cells exposed to EMS but not selected with antibodies (referred to as RMA). RMA-S synthesizes both class I heavy chains and β_2-microglobulin, but the majority of the heavy chains bear high-mannose oligosaccharides, do not associate with β_2-microglobulin, and remain intracellular (Ljunggren et al. 1989).

Monoclonal antibodies. The H-2b-specific antibodies used were (1) B22.249, specific for the α_1 domain of H-2D^b (Hammerling et al. 1979; Allen et al. 1984, 1986); (2) 28148S, specific for the α_3 domain of H-2D^b (Ozato and Sachs 1980; Allen et al. 1984); (3) 271113S, specific for the α_1 domain of H-2D^b (Ozato and Sachs 1980; Allen et al. 1984); and (4) K10-56, specific for the α_1 and α_2 domains of H-2K^b (Hammerling et al. 1982; Allen et al. 1984). For immunoprecipitation and for indirect immunofluorescence, where stated, antibodies were purified by protein A–Sepharose chromatography, as described by Ey et al. (1978).

CTL clone F5 and ^{51}Cr release assay. Clone F5 was isolated from an influenza-infected C57BL/6 mouse, as described previously (Townsend et al. 1985). It was tested by ^{51}Cr release assay on influenza E61-13-H17 virus-infected or peptide-treated (5×10^{-5} moles/liter for 1 hr) RMA-S and RMA cells, as described previously (Townsend et al. 1986b) ^{51}Cr-labeled target cells (2×10^4) were exposed to varying numbers of CTL clone F5 to give the killer-to-target (K:T) ratios shown. After 4 hours of contact, the ^{51}Cr released from target cells into the supernatant was measured, and percentage of specific lysis was calculated as follows: Release by CTL – release in medium alone/(2.5% Triton X-100 release – release in medium alone). Spontaneous ^{51}Cr released in medium was 12–19% of that released by Triton X-100.

In Figure 2B, ^{51}Cr-labeled RMA-S cells were exposed continuously to the peptide NP(1968)366-379 at 10^{-7} M, either alone (Fig. 2B, no blocker) or in combination with the blocking peptides shown in Figure 2 at a fixed concentration of 10^{-4} M. The molar ratios of blockers to NP(1968)366-379 and clone F5 to targets were 10^3:1 and 4:1, respectively.

Peptides. The peptides shown in Table 1 were synthesized by solid-phase techniques on an Applied Biosystems synthesizer 430A, as described previously (Townsend et al. 1986b), and were kindly supplied by J. Rothbard.

Table 1. Peptides Synthesized by Solid-phase Techniques

Origin	Sequence	Known class I restriction
NP (1968) 366-379	I A S N E N M D A M E S S T L	D^b (Townsend et al. 1986b)
Retro-D 366-379		none (Bodmer et al. 1989)
NP (1934) 365-380	I A S N E N M E T M E S S T L E	D^b (Townsend et al. 1986b)
NP (1968) 50-63	S D Y E G R L I Q N S L T I	K^k (Bastin et al. 1987)
NP (1968) 147-158	T Y Q R T R A L V R T G	K^d (Taylor et al. 1987)
NP (1968) 345-360	S F I R G T K V S P R G K L S T	none (Townsend et al. 1986b)
D^b 171-182	Y L K N G N A T L L R T	none (Bodmer et al. 1989)

Induction of class I expression by peptides and measurement by indirect immunofluorescence. RMA-S cells (5×10^5) were exposed to medium alone (RPMI/10) or peptides at the concentrations stated and harvested and stained by indirect immunofluorescence, as described previously (Townsend et al. 1985). The first layer was one of the D^b-specific monoclonal antibodies described above, either as neat culture supernatant (C/S) or purified at 5 μg/ml, and the second layer was FITC-labeled affinity-purified goat anti-mouse antibody (Sigma) at 1:40 dilution. The samples were analyzed on an Orthocytofluorograf.

Immunoprecipitation. Figure 1C: RMA-S and RMA cells (6×10^6) were exposed to either 0.25 ml of infectious allantoic fluid containing egg-grown E61-13-H17 influenza A virus or 10 pfu/cell of a recombinant vaccinia that expresses a rapidly degraded ubiquitin-NP fusion protein (Ub-R-NP-VAC 7.5K [Townsend et al. 1988]) for 90 minutes at 37°C. The cells were then incubated at 37°C for 3 hours to establish viral protein synthesis. After washing twice in phosphate-buffered saline (PBS), the cells were resuspended at 5×10^6/ml in methionine-free medium for 1 hour, before adding 250 μCi [^{35}S]methionine and incubating at 37°C for 30 minutes. Cells were then diluted in RPMI/10% FCS/4 mmoles L-methionine to 10^6/ml, and an aliquot of 2×10^6 was taken for lysis. The remainder were incubated at 37°C for 90 minutes before taking a second aliquot of 2×10^6 cells for lysis. Immunoprecipitates were prepared with antibody 5/1 to NP and analyzed as described previously (Townsend et al. 1988).

Figure 5: RMA-S and RMA cells were resuspended at 10^6/ml in medium (RPMI 1640/10% FCS) alone or containing peptides at 10^{-4} moles/liter for 5 hours. They were then washed twice in warmed PBS and resuspended at 5×10^6/ml in methionine-free medium containing peptides at the same concentration for an additional hour. [^{35}S]Methionine (120 μCi) was then added, and the mixture was incubated for 40 minutes at 37°C. The labeled cells were then washed once in ice-cold PBS and resuspended in 0.5 ml lysis buffer (0.5% v/v NP-40, 0.5% mega 9 [Hildreth et al. 1982; Townsend et al. 1985], 150 mmoles/liter NaCl, 5 mmoles/liter EDTA, 50 mmoles/liter Tris at pH 7.5), containing 2 mmoles/liter phenylmethylsulfonyl fluoride (PMSF) and 5 mmoles/liter iodoacetamide. The lysates were precleared with *Staphylococcus aureus* or-

ganisms overnight at 4°C. Purified 28148S antibody was then added to a final concentration of 5 μg/ml, and the mixture was incubated on ice for 90 minutes. Immunoprecipitation was then performed as described previously (Townsend et al. 1985). Reduced immunoprecipitates were electrophoresed on a 12% SDS-polyacrylamide gel, which was then fixed, stained, treated with Amplify (Amersham), dried, and exposed to pre-flashed X-ray film.

Figure 6: RMA-S and RMA cells were resuspended at 5×10^6/ml in medium alone or containing peptides at 2×10^{-4} moles/liter for 4 hours. Aliquots of cells (2×10^7) were then washed and resuspended in 1 ml methionine-free medium containing peptides at the same concentration for 1 hour. [^{35}S]Methionine (250 μCi) was then added, and the mixtures were incubated at 37°C for 15 minutes. The cells were then washed once in 15 ml of ice-cold PBS containing 2 mmoles/liter of unlabeled L-methionine and lysed as described above. The lysates were divided into two equal parts, either 28148S or B22.249 was added to 10 μg/ml, and immunoprecipitates were prepared as described above.

Figure 7: RMA-S and RMA cells were prepared as described for Figure 5. After incubation in [^{35}S]methionine-containing medium for 15 minutes, each aliquot of 2×10^7 cells was diluted to 5×10^6/ml by the addition of 3 ml of RPMI/10% FCS (prewarmed) containing the relevant peptides at 2×10^{-4} M and unlabeled L-methionine at 4 mmoles/liter. Two milliliters (10^7 cells) was harvested immediately; the remaining cells were incubated at 37°C for 4 hours and then harvested. The cells were then processed as described for Figure 5, and the D^b heavy chains were immunoprecipitated with B22.249 at 10 μg/ml.

Figure 8: Aliquots of 1.8×10^7 RMA-S or RMA cells were resuspended in 1 ml of methionine-free medium alone or containing peptides at 2×10^{-4} moles/liter. After incubation for 1 hour, 250 μCi [^{35}S]methionine was added, and the mixtures were incubated for 5 hours at 37°C. The cells were lysed in 1 ml of lysis buffer (as above), and immunoprecipitates were prepared with the 28148S antibody at 10 μg/ml and divided into two equal portions. One portion was digested with 0.005 units of endo-β-N-acetylglucosaminidase H (endo H) (Boehringer), as described by Owen et al. (1980); the other was mock-digested. The samples were TCA-precipitated, with 50 μg Sigma SDS-7 molecular-weight markers as carrier, and analyzed as in Figure 4.

RESULTS

RMA-S Presents Extracellular Peptide but Not Intracellular Antigen

The mutant RMA-S was compared with RMA as a target for recognition by a cytotoxic T-cell clone (F5) specific for influenza NP in association with the class I molecule H-2D^b (Townsend et al. 1986b). RMA was efficiently recognized and killed by clone F5 after infection with influenza virus. RMA-S was resistant to lysis under identical conditions (Fig. 1A). The lack of recognition by the CTL clone of infected RMA-S cells was not due to inefficient infection by the virus, since synthesis of NP in infected RMA-S was not impaired (Fig. 1C, lanes B and G). In addition, degradation of an unstable ubiquitin-Arg-NP fusion protein (Townsend et al. 1988) was equivalent in RMA-S and the control (Fig. 1C, lanes D,E and I,J). RMA-S cells expressing this form of NP were also resistant to lysis by clone F5 (data not shown).

RMA-S and RMA cells were then compared as targets after treatment with the peptide epitope recognized by the CTL clone (amino acids 366–379 of NP, 1968 sequence [Townsend et al. 1986b]). We found that the two cells were recognized to the same extent after exposure to peptide at concentrations greater than 10^{-6} moles/liter (Fig. 1B), despite the fact that untreated RMA-S cells expressed about one-twentieth the number of H-2D^b molecules as RMA. At lower concentrations of peptide, RMA-S was killed less efficiently than RMA by the CTL clone F5, requiring approximately tenfold more peptide to obtain half-maximal lysis (data not shown).

Hypothesis

These results showed that the mutant RMA-S assembled sufficient functional D^b molecules to present extracellular peptide but not intracellular antigen. The mutant RMA-S may therefore have lost a function required for the transport of NP peptides from the cytoplasm to the outside of the infected cell. RMA-S also has a known defect in the association of class I heavy chains with β_2-microglobulin (Ljunggren et al.

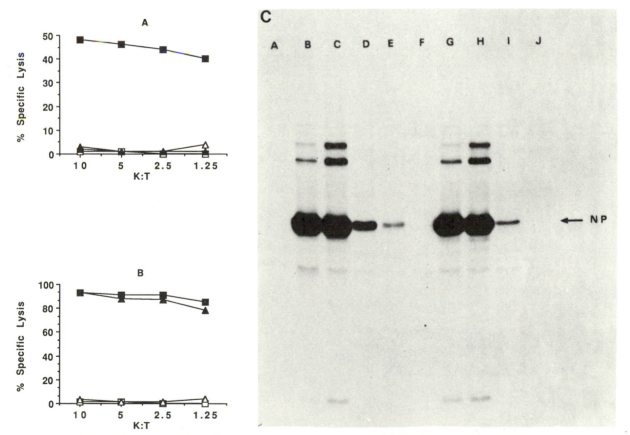

Figure 1. CTL clone F5 recognizes RMA-S cells treated with peptide NP(1968)366-379, but not infected with influenza A virus. (*A*) Target cells were RMA infected with influenza E61-13-H17 (■); RMA uninfected (□); RMA-S infected with E61-13-H17 (▲); RMA-S uninfected (△). (*B*) Target cells were RMA treated with NP(1968)366-379 (■); RMA untreated (□); RMA-S treated with NP(1968)366-379 (▲); RMA-S untreated (△). (*C*) Synthesis and degradation of influenza NP in RMA-S is not impaired. (*A–E*) Samples were from RMA; (*F–J*) from RMA-S. (*A* and *F*) Uninfected; (*B* and *G*) infected with influenza and labeled for 30 min; (*C* and *H*) infected with influenza, labeled for 30 min, and chased for 90 min; (*D* and *I*) infected with Ub-Arg-NP-VAC 7.5K and labeled for 30 min; (*E* and *J*) infected with Ub-Arg-NP-VAC 7.5K, labeled for 30 min, and chased for 90 min. (Fig. 1A and B reprinted, with permission, from Townsend et al. 1989.)

1989). Since the RBL-5 line (from which RMA-S was derived) is homozygous, it seemed likely that both of these traits were the result of a single mutation.

This led to the speculation that peptides derived from the degradation of proteins in the cytoplasm are involved in the assembly of class I molecules. If so, exposure of RMA-S to a high concentration of extracellular peptide might induce the class I heavy chains in RMA-S to associate with β_2-microglobulin and restore expression of assembled class I molecules at the cell surface.

Peptides Induce Expression of Class I Molecules at the Cell Surface

A comparison of RMA-S cells before and after exposure to 5×10^{-5} M NP(1968)366-379 for 5 hours revealed an increase in D^b expression at the cell surface of greater than twofold (Fig. 2A). This was detected with the antibody B22.249, which is specific for the α_1 domain of the D^b heavy chain (Allen et al. 1984).

We then tested three additional peptides known to prevent presentation of the sequence NP(1968)366-379 to the CTL clone F5 (Bodmer et al. 1989). The inhibitory effect of these peptides implied that they bound the D^b molecule, although this has not been demon-

strated directly. Two are derived from NP. One of these, NP(1934)365-380, is closely related in sequence and is also a D^b-restricted epitope (see Methods); the second is unrelated (residues 50–63), and the third is from a conserved region of the D^b molecule itself (residues 171–182). The latter was chosen for its homology with the equivalent sequence from HLA CW3, which has been shown to have similar inhibitory activity (Maryanski et al. 1988; Bodmer et al. 1989). To ensure that the D^b molecules on RMA-S (which had been exposed to a mutagen) retained their specificity for peptides, the inhibition assay was repeated with RMA-S cells (Fig. 2B; Methods).

The peptides that inhibited the recognition of RMA-S by the D^b-restricted clone F5 also induced expression of D^b at the surface of RMA-S cells (cf. Figs. 2,A and B). The three control peptides neither inhibited recognition by clone F5 nor induced expression of D^b. Therefore, a correlation exists between induction of D^b expression of RMA-S and inhibition of presentation of NP(1968)366-379 in the lysis assay, implying that only peptides that bind D^b induce its expression.

We used additional class-I-specific monoclonal antibodies to show that the effect of peptides on RMA-S cells is H-2 allele-specific (Fig. 3). Treatment with NP(1934)365-380 induced D^b but not K^b. In contrast, NP(1968)345-360 had the opposite effect and induced K^b but not D^b. The polyclonal cytotoxic T-cell response to influenza NP in H-2b mice is not restricted through K^b (Taylor et al. 1987). However, the induction of K^b by a peptide is not unexpected, since we have found other peptides that induce D^b on RMA-S cells (Fig. 2A), and block in the CTL lysis assay (Fig. 2B), but are not epitopes recognized by CTL from H-2b mice (Bodmer et al. 1989).

The class I molecule D^b is unusual because it can reach the cell surface in the absence of endogenous β_2 synthesis in the murine cell line R1E (Allen et al. 1986). The D^b molecules expressed on R1E were detected with the α_3 domain-specific antibody 28148S, but not with B22.249, which binds the α_1 domain of assembled heavy chains (Allen et al. 1984). This implied that the α_1 and α_2 domains of dissociated D^b molecules were denatured in R1E (Allen et al. 1986).

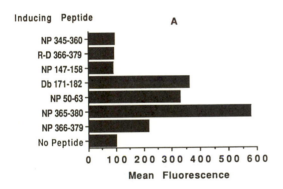

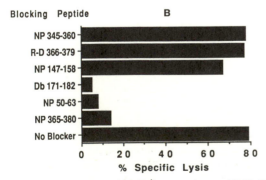

Figure 2. (*A*) Induction of H-2D^b expression on RMA-S by specific peptides. (*B*) The peptides that induce D^b expression also block recognition of NP(1968)366-379 by the D^b-restricted CTL clone F5.

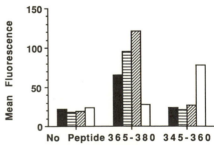

Figure 3. Induced expression of class I by peptides is allele-specific. Class I expression was detected with 28148S (α_3 of D^b) (closed box); 271113S (α_1 of D^b) (horizontal lines); B22.249 (α_1 of D^b) (hatched lines); K10.56 (α_1 and α_2 of K^b) (open box).

A comparison of binding by these two antibodies did not reveal an excess of free D^b heavy chains on the surface of RMA-S cells (Fig. 3). The increase in binding by B22.249 to peptide-treated RMA-S cells therefore could not be explained by denatured D^b molecules present at the cell surface acquiring the epitope detected by B22.249.

The time course and dose response characteristics of the induction of H-2D^b on RMA-S cells are shown in Figure 4, A and B. The effect is detected after 1 hour of exposure to peptide and increases over 6 hours. The maximum level of D^b induced was about one-fifth that on the RMA cell.

We have also observed that both RMA and L-cell fibroblasts, or the NS-0 myeloma transfected with the D^b gene, respond with a modest, but specific, increase in class I expression (33–235%) after exposure to appropriate peptides (data not shown). Normal cells may therefore exhibit a less exaggerated form of the phenomenon we have defined in RMA-S cells.

Association of D^b with β_2-Microglobulin

RMA-S cells were labeled with [^{35}S]methionine after exposure to peptides, and the D^b heavy chains (both free and β_2-associated) were immunoprecipitated with the antibody 28148S, which is specific for the α_3 domain. If class I assembly was stimulated by peptides, more ^{35}S-labeled β_2-microglobulin should be coprecipitated with D^b heavy chains.

Figure 5 (lane A) shows that the D^b heavy chains in RMA-S coprecipitated a low level of β_2-microglobulin, as described recently (Ljunggren et al. 1989). Figure 5 (lanes B and C) shows that treatment with two control peptides for 6 hours had no effect on chain association. In contrast, each of the four peptides thought to bind D^b increased the amount of coprecipitated β_2 labeled during a 40-minute pulse with [^{35}S]methionine (Fig. 5, lanes D–G and H, respectively). Of these, NP(1968) 50-63 (lane F) appeared to be the most effective. This correlates with the observation that NP(1968)50-63 was found to be a more potent inhibitor of recognition by D^b-restricted T cells (Bodmer et al. 1989). It may therefore have a higher affinity for D^b.

Not only assembly, but also folding of the D^b heavy chain is driven by peptide (Fig. 6). The antibody B22.249 reacts with a determinant on the α_1 domain of D^b that appears only when D^b is associated with β_2-microglobulin (Allen et al. 1986). Figure 6 (lanes A and B) defines a cohort of D^b molecules that were labeled in RMA-S cells during a 15-minute pulse with [^{35}S] methionine and precipitated with 28148S. The majority

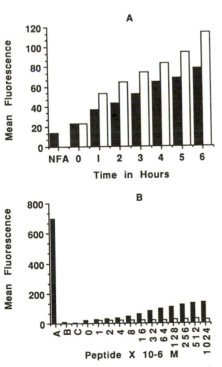

Figure 4. (*A*) Time course in response to 2.5×10^{-4} M (□) or 0.5×10^{-4} M (■) of NP(1934)365-380. (*B*) Dose response of D^b expression induced by NP(1934)365-380 (■) and NP(1968)345-360 (□), after 6 hr of exposure. (A) RMA control stained with B22.249 for comparison; (B) background staining of RMA with no first antibody; (C) background staining of RMA-S with no first antibody; (0) untreated RMA-S stained with B22.249. (Reprinted, with permission, from Townsend et al. 1989.)

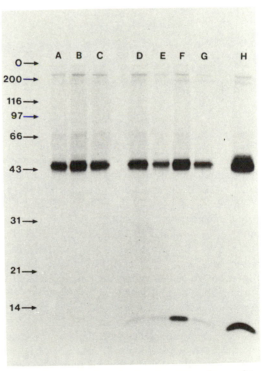

Figure 5. Coprecipitation of β_2-microglobulin with D^b heavy chains from RMA-S treated with peptides for 6 hr. (*A*) Untreated RMA-S; (*B*) RMA-S + NP(1968)345-360; (*C*) RMA-S + retro-D isomer NP(1968)366-379; (*D*) RMA-S + NP(1968)366-379; (*E*) RMA-S + NP(1934)365-380; (*F*) RMA-S + NP(1968)50-63; (*G*) RMA-S + H-2D^b 171-182; (*H*) RMA untreated. (Reprinted, with permission from Townsend et al. 1989.)

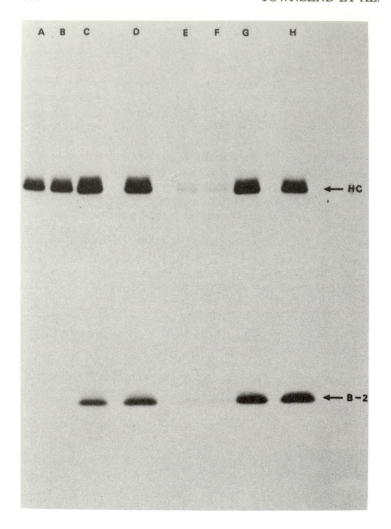

Figure 6. Peptide induces a conformational change in the α_1 domain of the D^b heavy chain in RMA-S cells. (*A* and *E*) RMA-S untreated cells; (*B* and *F*) RMA-S + NP(1968)345-360; (*C* and *G*) RMA-S + NP(1968)50-63; (*D* and *H*) RMA untreated. (*A–D*) Samples were immunoprecipitated with the antibody 28148S (specific for the α_3 domain); (*E–H*) samples were immunoprecipitated with B22.249 (specific for the α_1 domain). (Reprinted, with permission, from Townsend et al. 1989.)

of these molecules were neither associated with β_2-microglobulin (Fig. 6, lanes A and B) nor reactive with the α_1 domain-specific antibody B22.249 (Fig. 6, lanes E and F). However, in cells exposed to NP(1968)50-63 for 5 hours, the D^b heavy chains bound β_2 and folded into a conformation detected by B22.249, within 15 minutes of being made (cf. A,B,C with E,F,G in Fig. 6). We have also noted that the antibody 28148S (specific for the α_3 domain) precipitates D^b heavy chains more efficiently when they are associated with β_2-microglobulin (cf. A with C in Fig. 6). It may therefore bind to assembled class I molecules with higher affinity than to free heavy chains.

The fate of D^b molecules with time in cells exposed to peptide is shown in Figure 7. A cohort of D^b molecules was labeled for 15 minutes and then followed for 4 hours by incubating labeled cells in excess unlabeled L-methionine. B22.249 was used to immunoprecipitate selectively the assembled D^b molecules that had been influenced by exposure to NP(1968)50-63.

Figure 7 (lanes A and B) confirms that B22.249 detected a minimal level of assembled D^b molecules in RMA-S compared to the control RMA (Fig. 7, lanes G

and H). In RMA, the D^b molecules detected with B22.249 were associated with β_2-microglobulin within 15 minutes of synthesis, and the whole cohort migrated more slowly in the 12% polyacrylamide gel after the chase period (Fig. 7, lanes G and H). This change in migration rate of heavy chains with time correlates with conversion of their N-linked oligosaccharides from the high mannose (endo-H-sensitive) to the complex (endo-H-resistant) form as they pass through the Golgi stack (demonstrated below).

In RMA-S cells exposed to the peptide NP(1968)50-63, B22-249 precipitates as much D^b as in the control RMA (cf. E and G in Fig. 7), and these heavy chains also bound β_2 within 15 minutes of synthesis. However, in contrast to RMA cells, only a small proportion of them change their rate of migration during the 4-hour chase period (cf. F and H in Fig. 7). This difference was not due to a toxic effect of peptide on the transport of heavy chains, because the same concentration of peptide did not affect the rate maturation of heavy chains in the control cell RMA (Fig. 7, lanes I and J).

The decrease in intensity during the chase period of the band representing β_2-microglobulin is likely to be

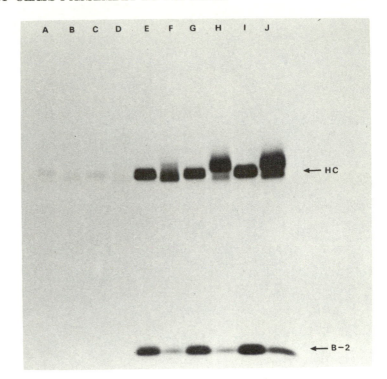

Figure 7. Transport of assembled D^b molecules induced by peptide NP(1968)50-63 is impaired in RMA-S cells. (*A, C, E, G, I*) Samples were from cells labeled for 15 min; (*B, D, F, H, J*) from cells labeled for 15 min and chased for 4 hr. (*A* and *B*) RMA-S untreated cells; (*C* and *D*) RMA-S + NP(1968)345-360; (*E* and *F*) RMA-S + NP(1968)50-63; (*G* and *H*) RMA untreated; (*I* and *J*) RMA + NP(1968)50-63. Samples were immunoprecipitated with B22.249 (specific for the α_1 domain).

due mainly to exchange at the surface of the cell with unlabeled bovine β_2-microglobulin (Bernabeu et al. 1984; for review see Hochman et al. 1988).

If the rate of transport of assembled D^b is slower in the mutant, the proportion converted to endo-H resistance during a long exposure to [^{35}S]methionine should be correspondingly reduced. RMA-S cells were labeled for 5 hours in the presence of peptides to allow accumulation of heavy chains that have passed through the Golgi and acquired endo-H resistance (Tarentino and Maley 1974; Krangel et al. 1979; Owen et al. 1980). Both free and β_2-associated D^b molecules were then immunoprecipitated with 28148S. Figure 8 (lanes A–D) shows that in untreated RMA-S cells and cells treated with a control peptide, D^b heavy chains were associated with a low level of β_2-microglobulin and acquired minimal endo-H resistance compared to those in RMA (Fig. 8, lanes I and J). The D^b heavy chains in RMA-S treated with two active peptides (Fig. 8, lanes E–H), bound more β_2-microglobulin and acquired a degree of endo-H resistance that was comparable with the level of D^b induced at the cell surface, within the same time period, relative to the RMA control (cf. A and B in Fig. 4).

DISCUSSION

Peptides Drive Assembly of Class I

We have shown that exposure of the RMA-S mutant cells to specific peptides partially restores association of D^b heavy chains with β_2-microglobulin and expression of D^b or K^b molecules at the cell surface. The results in

Figures 5–8 imply that extracellular peptides can reach a pre-Golgi compartment of RMA-S, where they induce newly synthesized D^b molecules to fold (acquire the epitope bound by B22.249), and associate with β_2-microglobulin. This compartment could be the endoplasmic reticulum (ER) or possibly an intermediate compartment between the ER and Golgi (Warren 1987). The assembled D^b molecules are then transported through the Golgi to the cell surface.

The effect on D^b is specific to peptides identified as either epitopes recognized by CTLs in association with D^b (Townsend et al. 1986b; Bastin et al. 1987) or sequences able to prevent the presentation of known epitopes to D^b-restricted CTLs (Bodmer et al. 1989) (Fig. 2). These functional criteria imply that only peptides that bind to D^b or K^b increase their expression at the surface of RMA-S cells.

The most likely site for peptides to bind on the class I heavy chain is the groove formed by the polymorphic α_1 and α_2 domains of the molecule (Bjorkman et al. 1987a). Deletion of these domains prevents binding of β_2-microglobulin to the α_3 domain of the D^b molecule (Allen et al. 1986). Furthermore, in the crystal structure of HLA-A2, β_2-microglobulin makes multiple contacts with both the α_1 and α_2 domains (Bjorkman et al. 1987b) but almost certainly would not make direct contact with bound peptide.

Chain association may therefore depend on correct folding of these domains. Our results suggest that folding depends on the availability of peptide ligands and that peptides form an integral part of the class I structure. The α_1 and α_2 domains of newly synthesized class I heavy chains may fold around the peptide to form a

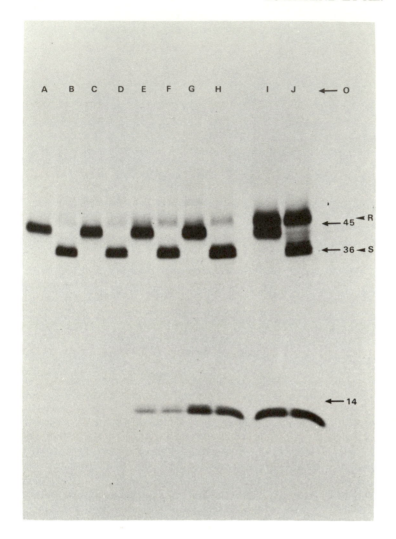

Figure 8. D[b] heavy chains in RMA-S acquire endo-H resistance after treatment with peptides. (*A, C, E, G, I*) Samples were mock-digested; (*B, D, F, H, J*) digested with endo H. (*Right*) Positions, after digestion, of resistant (R) and sensitive (S) heavy chains. (*A* and *B*) RMA-S untreated cells; (*C* and *D*) RMA-S + NP(1968)345-360; (*E* and *F*) RMA-S + NP(1934)368-380; (*G* and *H*) RMA-S + NP(1968)50-63; (*I* and *J*) RMA untreated. (Reprinted, with permission, from Townsend et al. 1989.)

three-dimensional structure with affinity for β_2-microglobulin. The assembled complex of heavy chain, peptide, and β_2-microglobulin is then transported through the Golgi by a mechanism that distinguishes between folded and unfolded heavy chains.

This concept does not rule out the exchange of one bound peptide for another, after the class I molecule has assembled, and is exposed at the cell surface. Peptide exchange is conceptually similar to β_2-microglobulin exchange (Bernabeu et al. 1984). The fact that fixed cells (Hosken et al. 1989) and cells treated with Brefeldin-A (Nuchtern et al. 1989; Yewdell and Bennink 1989) can present extracellular peptide to class-I-restricted T cells implies that peptide exchange can occur at the surface of nonmutant cells. However, the extremely low level of saturation (0.3%) of class I cells achieved with peptides in vitro argues that it is inefficient (Chen and Parham 1989). In addition, the observation that Brefeldin-A blocks antigen presentation in influenza-infected cells also suggests that epitopes derived from cytoplasmic antigens associate preferentially with newly synthesized class I molecules, in a pre-Golgi compartment of the cell (Nuchtern et al. 1989; Yewdell and Bennink 1989).

In RMA-S cells treated with the peptide NP(1968) 50-63, assembly of D[b] molecules is restored to a level close to that in the control cell (Fig. 5), but the proportion transported through the Golgi within 4 hours is less in mutant RMA-S than in control RMA cells. The transport of these peptide-induced complexes through the Golgi may be impaired (Figs. 6 and 7). This difference in transport of assembled complexes in RMA-S and RMA cells could be due either to the defect in the RMA-S cell or to a difference in the intrinsic properties of D[b]/β_2-microglobulin complexes induced by synthetic versus cell-derived peptides. The latter may play a role because the peptides NP(1968)50-63 and NP(1934)365-380 show some differences in their effects on RMA-S cells. NP(1968)50-63 appears to induce chain association more effectively than NP(1934)365-380 (Figs. 4 and 7) but induces the equivalent or slightly less D[b] at the cell surface (Fig. 2 and data not shown).

The Defect in RMA-S Cells

Our demonstration of the role of peptide in class I assembly could explain why class I heavy and light chains synthesized in vitro, in the absence of peptide, fail to associate (Ploegh et al. 1979). It also suggests the types of mutations that might have given rise to the RMA-S cell and others resembling it (DeMars et al. 1985; Salter and Cresswell 1986; Klar and Hammerling 1989). There are at least three alternatives.

Mutations in the heavy chain, or β_2-microglobulin, could interfere with class I assembly (Krangel et al. 1982; Santos-Aguado et al. 1987). However, this is unlikely in RMA-S cells because fusion with L-cell fibroblasts restores H-2b class I assembly, expression, and antigen presentation (C. Öhlén et al., in prep.).

Loss of peptide transport from the cytoplasm to a pre-Golgi compartment could account for the loss of class I assembly in RMA-S cells. If assembly of class I molecules is dependent on peptide binding, a defect that reduced the concentration of peptides available during folding could prevent chain association. We have argued previously that to bring peptides derived from the degradation of cytoplasmic proteins into contact with class I molecules, a specialized transport system must exist (Townsend et al. 1985, 1986a,b; Gould et al. 1989).

An additional explanation can be based on the possibility that impaired transport of assembled D^b/β_2-microglobulin complexes from the ER through the Golgi is the primary defect in RMA-S cells (Fig. 7). A factor may exist in the ER that stabilizes the complex (perhaps by binding to it) and is responsible for its transport through the Golgi. Loss of this factor would lead to the buildup of relatively unstable complexes and free heavy chains in the ER. The ratio of free to β_2-associated heavy chains would depend on the local concentrations and binding affinities of β_2-microglobulin and peptides. Under conditions where peptide concentration is limiting and the affinity for β_2 is low, the majority of class I heavy chains may not associate with β_2-microglobulin.

Finally, it is conceivable that a single mechanism, which is defective in RMA-S cells, mediates both movement of peptides into the ER and transport of assembled class I molecules from ER to Golgi.

SUMMARY

Association of the D^b heavy chain with β_2-microglobulin and expression of D^b and K^b at the surface of the cell are induced by specific peptides in the mutant RMA-S. Association of antigenic peptides with the binding site of class I molecules may be required for correct folding of the heavy chain, association with β_2-microglobulin, and transport of the antigen-MHC complex to the cell surface.

ACKNOWLEDGMENTS

We thank George Klein for acting as catalyst to our collaboration; Jonathan Rothbard and G. Hammerling for supplying peptides and antibodies B22.249 and K10-56, respectively; Nigel Rust and the Nuffield Department of Surgery for time on the Orthocytofluoro-graf; Richard Klausner, Peter Cresswell, and Hidde Ploegh for helpful discussion; the editors of Nature for permission to reproduce Figures 1 A and B, 4–6, and 8; and the Medical Research Council, the National Cancer Institute, and the Swedish Cancer Society for support.

REFERENCES

Allen, H., J. Fraser, D. Flyer, S. Calvin, and R. Flavell. 1986. β-2 microglobulin is not required for cell surface expression of the murine class I histocompatibility antigen H-2b or of a truncated Db. *Proc. Natl. Acad. Sci.* **83:** 7447.

Allen, H., D. Wraith, P. Pala, B. Askonas, and R.A. Flavell. 1984. Domain interactions of H-2 class I antigens alter cytotoxic T-cell recognition sites. *Nature* **309:** 279.

Bastin, J., J. Rothbard, J. Davey, I. Jones, and A. Townsend. 1987. Use of synthetic peptides of influenza nucleoprotein to define epitopes recognized by class I restricted cytotoxic T lymphocytes. *J. Exp. Med.* **165:** 1508.

Bernabeu, C., M. Van de Rijn, P. Lerch, and C. Terhorst. 1984. β-2 microglobulin from serum associated with class I antigens on the surface of cultured cells. *Nature* **308:** 642.

Bjorkman, P.J., M.A. Saper, B. Samraoui, W.S. Bennett, J.L. Strominger, and D.C. Wiley. 1987a. Structure of the human class I histocompatibility antigen, HLA-A2. *Nature* **329:** 506.

———. 1987b. The foreign antigen binding site and T cell recognition regions of class I histocompatibility antigens. *Nature* **329:** 512.

Bodmer, H., J. Bastin, B. Askonas, and A. Townsend. 1989. Influenza specific cytotoxic T cell recognition is inhibited by peptides unrelated in both sequence and MHC restriction. *Immunology* **66:** 163.

Chen, B.P. and P. Parham. 1989. Direct binding of influenza peptides to class I HLA molecules. *Nature* **337:** 743.

DeMars, R., R. Rudersdorf, C. Chang, J. Strandtmann, N. Korn, B. Sidwell, and H.T. Orr. 1985. Mutations that impair a posttranscriptional step in expression of HLA-A and -B antigens. *Proc. Natl. Acad. Sci.* **82:** 8183.

Ey, P.L., S.J. Prowse, and C.R. Jenkin. 1978. Isolation of pure IgG1, IgG2a and IgG2b immunoglobulin from mouse serum using protein A-sepharose. *Immunochemistry* **15:** 429.

Gould, K., J. Cossins, J. Bastin, G.G. Brownlee, and A. Townsend. 1989. A fifteen amino acid fragment of influenza nucleoprotein synthesized in the cytoplasm is presented in class I restricted T lymphocytes. *J. Exp. Med.* **170:** 1051.

Hammerling, G.J., U. Hammerling, and H. Lemke. 1979. Isolation of twelve monoclonal antibodies against Ia and H-2 antigens. Serological characterisation and reactivity with B and T lymphocytes. *Immunogenetics* **8:** 433.

Hammerling, G.J., E. Rusch, N. Tada, S. Kimura, and U. Hammerling. 1982. Localization of allodeterminants on H-2Kb antigens determined with monoclonal antibodies and H-2 mutant mice. *Proc. Natl. Acad. Sci.* **79:** 4737.

Hildreth, J.E.K. 1982. N-D-gluco-N-methyl alkyl carboxyamide compounds: A new class of non-ionic detergents for membrane biochemistry. *Biochem. J.* **207:** 363.

Hochman, J.H., Y. Shimizu, R. DeMars, and M. Edidin. 1988. Specific associations of fluorescent β-2-microglobulin with cell surfaces. *J. Immunol.* **140:** 2322.

Hosken, N.A., M.J. Bevan, and F.R. Carbone. 1989. Class I restricted presentation occurs without internalization or processing of exogenous antigenic peptides. *J. Immunol.* **142:** 1079.

Kärre, K., H.G. Ljunggren, G. Piontek, and R. Kiessling. 1986. Selective rejection of H-2-deficient lymphoma variants suggests alternative immune defence strategy. *Nature* **319:** 675.

Klar, D. and G.J. Hammerling. 1989. Induction of assembly of MHC class I heavy chains with β-2 microglobulin by interferon-γ. *EMBO J.* **8**: 475.

Krangel, M.S., H.T. Orr, and J.L. Strominger. 1979. Assembly and maturation of HLA-A and HLA-B antigens in vivo. *Cell* **18**: 979.

Krangel, M.S., D. Pious, and J.L. Strominger. 1982. Human histocompatibility antigen mutants immunoselected in vitro. *J. Biol. Chem.* **257**: 5296.

Ljunggren, H.G. and K. Kärre. 1985. Host resistance directed selectively against H-2-deficient lymphoma variants. Analysis of the mechanism. *J. Exp. Med.* **162**: 1745.

Ljunggren, H.G., S. Paabo, M. Cochet, G. Kling, P. Kourilsky, and K. Kärre. 1989. Molecular analysis of H-2 deficient lymphoma lines; distinct defects in biosynthesis and association of MHC class I/β-2 microglobulin observed in cells with increased sensitivity to NK cell lysis. *J. Immunol.* **142**: 2911.

Maryanski, J.L., P. Pala, J. Cerrotini, and G. Corradin. 1988. Synthetic peptides as antigens and competitors in recognition by H-2 restricted cytolytic T cells specific for HLA. *J. Exp. Med.* **167**: 1391.

Nuchtern, J.G., J.S. Bonifacino, W.E. Biddison, and R.D. Klausner. 1989. Brefeldin A implicates egress from the endoplasmic reticulum in class I restricted antigen presentation. *Nature* **339**: 223.

Owen, M.J., A.M. Kissonerghis, and H.F. Lodish. 1980. Biosynthesis of HLA-A and HLA-B antigens in vivo. *J. Biol. Chem.* **255**: 9678.

Ozato, K. and D.H. Sachs. 1980. Monoclonal antibodies to mouse MHC antigens. III. Hybridoma antibodies reacting to antigens of the H-2b haplotype reveal genetic control of isotype expression. *J. Immunol.* **126**: 317.

Ploegh, H.L., L.E. Cannon, and J.L. Strominger. 1979. Cell free translation of the mRNAs for the heavy and light chains of HLA-A and HLA-B antigens. *Proc. Natl. Acad. Sci.* **76**: 2273.

Salter, R.D. and P. Cresswell. 1986. Impaired assembly and transport of HLA-A and -B antigens in a mutant T × B cell hybrid. *EMBO J.* **5**: 943.

Santos-Aguado, J., P.A. Biro, U. Fuhrmann, J.L. Strominger, and J.A. Barbosa. 1987. Amino acid sequences in the α1 domain and not glycosylation are important in the HLA-A2/βR2-microglobulin association and cell surface expression. *Mol. Cell. Biochem.* **7**: 982.

Tarentino, A.L. and F. Maley. 1974. Purification and properties of an Endo-β-N-acetylglucose aminidase from Streptomyces griseus. *J. Biol. Chem.* **249**: 811.

Taylor, P.M., J. Davey, K. Howland, J. Rothbard, and B.A. Askonas. 1987. Class I MHC molecules, rather than other mouse genes dictate influenza epitope recognition by cytotoxic T cells. *Immunogenetics* **26**: 267.

Townsend, A and H. Bodmer. 1989. Antigen recognition by class I-restricted T lymphocytes. *Annu. Rev. Biochem.* **7**: 601.

Townsend, A.R.M., F.M. Gotch, and J. Davey. 1985. Cytotoxic T cells recognize fragments of influenza nucleoprotein. *Cell* **42**: 457.

Townsend, A.R.M., J. Bastin, K. Gould, and G.G. Brownlee. 1986a. Cytotoxic T lymphocytes recognise influenza haemagglutinin that lacks a signal sequence. *Nature* **234**: 575.

Townsend, A., C. Öhlén, J. Bastin, H.-J. Ljunggren, L. Foster, and K. Kärre. 1989. Association of class I major histocompatibility heavy and light chains induced by viral peptides. *Nature* **340**: 443.

Townsend, A.R.M., J. Rothbard, F.M. Gotch, G. Bahadur, D. Wraith, and A.J. McMichael. 1986b. The epitopes of influenza nucleoprotein recognized by cytotoxic T lymphocytes can be defined with short synthetic peptides. *Cell* **44**: 959.

Townsend, A., J. Bastin, K. Gould, G. Brownlee, M. Andrew, B. Coupar, D. Boyle, S. Chan, and G. Smith. 1988. Defective presentation to class I-restricted cytotoxic T lymphocytes in vaccinia-infected cells is overcome by enhanced degradation of antigen. *J. Exp. Med.* **168**: 1211.

Warren, G. 1987. Signals and salvage sequences. *Nature* **327**: 17.

Yewdell, J.W. and J.R. Bennink. 1989. Brefeldin A specifically inhibits presentation of protein antigens to cytotoxic T lymphocytes. *Science* **244**: 1072.

Zinkernagel, R.M. and P.C. Doherty. 1979. MHC-restricted cytotoxic T cells: Studies on the biological role of polymorphic major transplantation antigens determining T cell restriction-specificity, function, and responsiveness. *Adv. Immunol.* **27**: 51.

Structural and Functional Aspects of HLA Class II Glycoproteins and the Associated Invariant Chain

P. CRESSWELL, J.S. BLUM,* M.S. MARKS, AND P.A. ROCHE
Department of Microbiology and Immunology, Duke University Medical Center, Durham, North Carolina 27710

A proliferative response by helper T cells requires that foreign antigens be presented in the context of syngeneic class II antigens by, for example, a macrophage (Unanue 1984). B cells can also function as antigen-presenting cells, and they exhibit a dramatically enhanced ability to present antigens for which their surface immunoglobulin is specific (Rock et al. 1984; Lanzavecchia 1985). The antigen must be "processed" by the presenting cell for optimal responses. A large body of data suggests that antigen-presenting cells incorporate bound antigens, proteolytically cleave or otherwise process them, and re-express them on the cell surface.

T-cell recognition of re-expressed processed antigens depends on the direct binding of such antigens by the class II molecules of the antigen-presenting cell. Experiments by Babbitt et al. (1985), confirmed and extended by others (Guillet et al. 1986; Sette et al. 1989), have shown that peptides presented "in the context of Ia" will physically associate with the appropriate Ia allelic products in vitro. Our own studies of the intracellular transport of class II antigens led to the hypothesis that such interactions in vivo might normally occur in an intracellular compartment rather than at the cell surface.

Our current view of HLA class II antigen biosynthesis is indicated schematically in Figure 1. When synthesized in the endoplasmic reticulum (ER), HLA-DR α and β subunits are cotranslationally core glycosylated to generate a single N-linked glycan on the β subunit and two on the α subunit. In the ER, the α and β subunits rapidly associate with a 31-kD third subunit, known as the invariant (I) chain (Machamer and Cresswell 1982). The I chain is not encoded by the major histocompatibility complex (MHC) (Claesson-Welsh et al. 1984) and exhibits no sequence homology with the α or β subunits, nor with any other known member of the immunoglobulin "superfamily" (Strubin et al. 1984). It contains two N-linked glycans and is one of a number of transmembrane glycoproteins that are inverted in the membrane, with the amino terminus of the major form of the I chain forming a cytoplasmic domain consisting of 30 amino acids (Strubin et al. 1986).

Within 30 minutes of their association in the ER, the three chains of the class II MHC are transported through the Golgi apparatus, where the N-linked glycans are processed into the complex, endoglycosidase H (endo H)-resistant form. O-linked glycans are also added to the I chain (Machamer and Cresswell 1984). After an additional 1–3 hours, proteolysis of the I chain occurs (Blum and Cresswell 1988), it dissociates from the class II MHC, and mature $\alpha\beta$ dimers are expressed on the cell surface (Cresswell and Blum 1988). Because the I chain remains associated throughout this period and does not appear to be significantly expressed on the cell surface (Accolla et al. 1985), we believe that for the entire 1–3-hour post-Golgi period, prior to cell-surface expression of mature class II glycoproteins, the class II/I chain complexes remain in an intracellular compartment. This compartment remains undefined but obviously has the potential of being the site where interactions with foreign antigens occur. We have demonstrated that $\alpha\beta$I complexes are accessible to the endocytotic route followed by the transferrin receptor during this period of intracellular residence (Cresswell 1985). The prolonged post-Golgi hiatus prior to cell-surface expression is unusual and may reflect a post-Golgi sorting event that routes class II/I chain complexes differently from other membrane glycoproteins. Such sorting functions are thought to be a property of the *trans*-Golgi network or *trans*-Golgi reticulum (TGR; Griffiths and Simons 1986), and the potential association of the TGR with endocytotic structures may be important in antigen presentation.

In the work reported here, we focus on three main areas of the cell biology of class II MHC antigens. First, we examine the behavior of the I chain in the absence of association with class II molecules, showing that it remains in the ER in a predominantly trimeric form, as indicated in Figure 1. Second, we focus on the nature of the intracellular $\alpha\beta$I complex. Finally, we present evidence indicating that peptides, known to be presented to T helper cells via class II molecules, can bind directly to HLA-DR molecules in vivo.

METHODS

Cells. Cell lines were maintained at 37°C in Iscove's modified Dulbecco's minimal essential medium (IDMEM, GIBCO), containing 5% fetal bovine serum (FBS). The B-LCL cells used were EHM (DR1), TRa1 (DR2), QBL (DR3), WT51 (DR4), Swei (DR5), HU301 (DRw6), BER (DR7), and BM9 (DR8). The

---

*Present address: Department of Cell Biology and Physiology, Box 8101, Washington University School of Medicine, 660 S. Euclid Avenue, St. Louis, Missouri 63110.

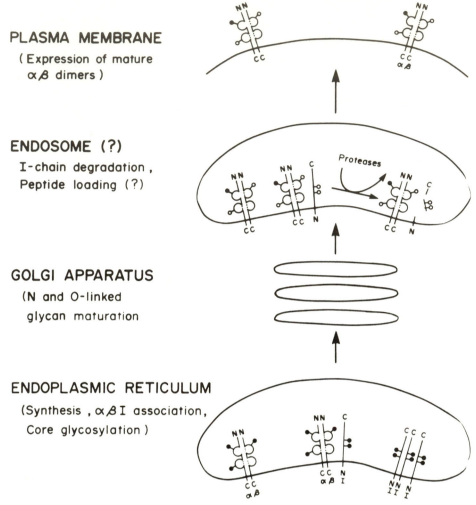

PLASMA MEMBRANE

(Expression of mature
αβ dimers)

ENDOSOME (?)

I-chain degradation,
Peptide loading (?)

GOLGI APPARATUS

(N and O-linked
glycan maturation

ENDOPLASMIC RETICULUM

(Synthesis, αβI association,
Core glycosylation)

Figure 1. Schematic representation of the assembly and transport of class II HLA glycoproteins to the cell surface. Dashed lines in the class II α and β subunits represent intrachain disulfide bonds. The "lollipops" on the α, β, and I chains represent N-linked glycans, either immature and endo-H-sensitive (●) or mature and endo-H-resistant (○).

class-II-negative T × B hybrid line 174 × CEM.T2 (T2) was also used (Salter et al. 1985).

Antisera and monoclonal antibodies. The monoclonal antibodies L243, DA6.147, XD5.A11, and VIC Y1 have been described previously (Blum and Cresswell 1988). The monoclonal anti-I chain antibody POP.I4.3 was prepared in this laboratory by immunizing a mouse with a preparation of whole cellular membranes from the T2 cell line. Immunoprecipitation and solid-phase radioimmunoassay indicated that it is specific for the human I chain. Rabbit antiserum MATILDA was prepared by injecting a female NZB rabbit with material that was first affinity-purified from T2 on a POP.I4.3 affinity column and further purified by gel filtration. The anti-I-chain amino-terminal (EQLP, N350) and carboxy-terminal (KESL, C351) peptide antisera were generous gifts from V. Quaranta (Scripps Clinic, La Jolla, CA).

Radiolabeling of B-LCL cells. For pulse-chase studies, B-LCL cells were labeled biosynthetically at 37°C for 10 minutes with [^{35}S]methionine, as described previously (Machamer and Cresswell 1982), in methionine-free medium containing 0.5 mCi/ml of Tran^{35}S label (>1000 Ci/mmole; ICN Radiochemicals). Chase conditions, Triton X-100 solubilization, and immunoprecipitations with monoclonal antibodies were carried out as described previously (Machamer and Cresswell 1982; Blum and Cresswell 1988).

Peptides and iodination. The synthetic peptide corresponding to influenza hemagglutinin 306-320 (C15G) was synthesized by Peninsula Laboratories (Belmont, CA). The peptide corresponding to the sequence encoded by exon 6 of HLA-A3 (A3E6, DRKGGSYT-QAA) was synthesized by Multiple Peptide Systems (San Diego, CA). The influenza hemagglutinin peptide was radiolabeled with ^{125}I using the chloramine-T method and possessed a specific activity of approximately 15,000 cpm/pmole.

Peptide binding to intact B-LCL cells. B-LCL cells (3×10^6) were incubated at 37°C for 18 hours in 2 ml IDMEM containing 2% FCS with ^{125}I-labeled C15G peptide (2×10^7 to 3×10^7 cpm). The cells were washed three times in serum-free IDMEM and extracted in 1 ml of 1% Triton X-100 in 0.15 M NaCl and 0.01 M Tris at pH 7.4 (TS) at 0°C for 30 minutes, as for conventional extractions and immunoprecipitation techniques (Machamer and Cresswell 1982). The extract was divided into four aliquots, and duplicates were precipitated using the monoclonal antibody L243 (anti HLA-DR), or a control antibody, and protein A–Sepharose (Sigma). Anti-H-2K^b (28-8-6S) or anti-HLA class I (w6/32) antibodies were used as controls. The protein A beads were washed three times with TS containing 0.05% Triton X-100 and then counted for ^{125}I, using an LKB CliniGamma 1272 gamma counter.

Affinity chromatography. Class II MHC molecules were purified from EHM (HLA-DR1), Swei (HLA-DR5), and BM9 (HLA-DR8) B-LCL cells by immunoaffinity chromatography in $C_{12}E_9$ detergent (Sigma), as described previously (Kelner and Cresswell 1986). For peptide-binding studies following elution from the affinity column, the material was purified further by high-performance liquid chromatography (HPLC), using a TSK-G4000 (7.5×600 mm) gel-filtration column equilibrated in a buffer of 50 mM sodium phosphate, and 1% octylglucoside (Sigma) at pH 7.0 (HPLC buffer). Class II molecules were detected by absorption at 214 nm and SDS-PAGE/Western blotting with anti-α- (DA6.147) and anti-β-subunit (XD5.A11) antibodies. The class II molecule concentration was calculated on the basis of the area of the pooled class II peak, relative to the area of a known amount of bovine serum albumin. I chain, for cross-linking studies, was purified from a POP.I4.3 affinity column and subjected to gel filtration on Sephacryl S-300 in 0.1 $C_{12}E_9$ detergent in 0.14 M NaCl and 0.02 M bicine (pH 8.5) prior to cross-linking.

Peptide binding to class II molecules. Approximately 2 pmoles of class II molecules was incubated with 20 pmoles of ^{125}I-labeled C15G in HPLC buffer alone, in the presence of 400 pmoles of unlabeled A3E6 or in the presence of 400 pmoles of unlabeled C15G. Following incubation for 15 hours at room temperature, a 1:5 dilution of 50% glycerol/5% octylglucoside was added to each sample, and the material was subjected to nondenaturing pore-limit polyacrylamide gel electrophoresis.

Electrophoresis. One-dimensional discontinuous polyacrylamide (10%) gel electrophoresis in SDS was performed as described previously (Laemmli 1970). For cross-linking experiments, 7% acrylamide separating gels were employed. Samples were eluted from beads or dissolved directly from ethanol precipitates by heating to 100°C for 5 minutes in 50–65 μl of SDS-

PAGE sample buffer. Various molecular-weight markers were used. For cross-linking experiments, α_2-macroglobulin was used under nonreducing (M_r 360,000) and reducing conditions (M_r 180,000) and stained with Coomassie blue. In some experiments, ^{14}C-labeled standards (Amersham) were used. These consisted of bovine cytochrome c (M_r 12,300), bovine erythrocyte carbonic anhydrase (M_r 31,000), chicken ovalbumin (M_r 44,500), bovine serum albumin (M_r 68,000), mouse IgG (M_r 55,000 heavy chain and M_r 22,500 light chain), and rabbit muscle phosphorylase b (M_r 92,500). In other experiments, prestained molecular-weight standards were purchased from Sigma and consisted of rabbit muscle triosephosphate isomerase (M_r 28,000), rabbit muscle lactic dehydrogenase (M_r 34,000), porcine heart fumarase (M_r 53,000), chicken muscle pyruvate kinase (M_r 66,000), rabbit muscle fructose-6-phosphate kinase (M_r 86,000), and *Escherichia coli* β-galactosidase (M_r 112,000).

Pore-limit PAGE was performed under nondenaturing conditions using a buffer of 90 mM Tris, 90 mM boric acid, and 2 mM EDTA at pH 8.6 (TBE), or in a discontinuous gel system, essentially as described by Laemmli (1970), without the addition of SDS. In each gel system, 1% octylglucoside was added to the gel buffers to prevent denaturation and precipitation of integral membrane proteins. The separating gels were formed using a linear gradient of 5–15% acrylamide, and the spacer gel contained 4% acrylamide. Following addition of the samples, the gel was run for 15 hours at 150 V, and the proteins were electrophoretically blotted to nitrocellulose. The relative molecular weight of class II molecules was estimated from a plot of log M_r versus R_f using bovine serum albumin monomer (M_r 68,000), dimer (M_r 136,000), and trimer (M_r 204,000) as standards.

Gels of [^{35}S]methionine-labeled material were treated with Enlightning (New England Nuclear-du Pont), prior to vacuum drying and autoradiography. Western blotting was carried out as described previously (Radka et al. 1984). For blots probed with monoclonal antibodies, ^{125}I-labeled Ox-20 (anti-mouse K chain; Cresswell 1985) was used as a secondary reagent. For rabbit antisera, ^{125}I-labeled *Staphylococcus aureus*–protein A was used.

Cross-linking. Pooled fractions from gel-filtration peaks were divided into 6–10 aliquots of equal volume. Each aliquot was treated for 30 minutes at 4°C with 3,3'-dithio*bis*(propionic acid *N*-hydroxysuccinimide ester) (DSP; Sigma) at concentrations ranging from 1.5 to 100 μg/ml. DSP was added to samples as $100 \times$ stocks in dimethylsulfoxide. Control samples were treated with dimethylsulfoxide alone. Cross-linking reactions were stopped by adding glycine or ammonium chloride to 10 mM, and samples were precipitated with ethanol. Cross-linked products were analyzed by one-dimensional SDS-PAGE under nonreducing conditions with 7% acrylamide separating gels. A control sample was analyzed by reducing SDS-PAGE to examine the polypeptide products prior to cross-linking. Gels of radiolabeled samples were analyzed by autoradiography, and gels of unlabeled samples were analyzed by Western blotting.

RESULTS

Invariant Chain Behavior in the Absence of Associated Class II Molecules

Variable sialic acid addition to the N- and O-linked glycans of the I chain results in a complicated pattern when HLA-DR/I chain complexes are subjected to two-dimensional gel electrophoresis. In pulse-chase analyses, this complexity develops with time as the class II molecules are transported through the Golgi apparatus (Machamer and Cresswell 1982). Figure 2 shows the contrasting simplicity of the pattern observed during a similar pulse-chase analysis of the I chain in a class-II-negative T × B hybrid cell line, T2. Only a trace amount of the I chain is processed to a sialic-acid-containing form (Ip), visible at 2–4 hours of chase, and the vast majority persists in an immature form even through 24 hours. The I chain in T2 remains endo-H-sensitive, consistent with retention in the ER or cis-Golgi (data not shown). On the basis of immuno-

fluorescence data, the I chain in T2 appears to be in the ER (M.S. Marks and P. Cresswell, in prep.). Thus, in the absence of class II association, the I chain appears to behave as a resident ER protein.

To determine whether the I chain in the absence of class II association is multimeric or monomeric, we have subjected the I chain from T2 to gel-filtration analysis and to chemical cross-linking, either following purification using a monoclonal antibody affinity column or in membranes solubilized in detergent with no further purification. In the latter case, cross-linked I chain multimers were detected by SDS-PAGE and Western blotting, using a rabbit antibody to the I chain. Figure 3A shows the results of such a cross-linking experiment, which indicate that the major form of the I chain in T2 is a trimer with an $M_r \sim 90,000$. Even in the absence of cross-linker, a substantial amount of the I chain runs as a dimer in nonreducing SDS-PAGE. This is so, even though membranes were prepared for extraction in the presence of iodoacetamide, which should prevent postisolation disulfide bond formation, indicating that interchain disulfide bonds between I chain subunits are likely to occur in vivo. Gel-filtration analysis of I chain using Sephacryl S-300 columns is also consistent with the I chain existing in a multimeric form. In sodium deoxycholate, the I chain has an $M_r \sim$

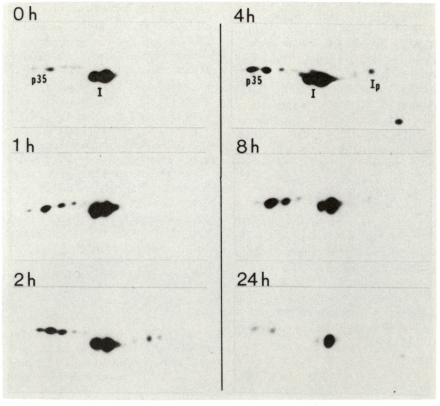

Figure 2. Pulse-chase analysis of I chain in the class-II-negative T × B hybrid cell line T2. The cells were pulsed for 10 min with [³⁵S]methionine and chased at 37°C for the times indicated. I chain was precipitated using the VIC Y1 monoclonal antibody and analyzed by two-dimensional gel electrophoresis and fluorography. A small amount of processed I chain (Ip) is visible at 2–4 hr of chase, but the majority of the I chain remains in an immature form throughout the chase period. p35 is a form of the I chain with an extended amino-terminal cytoplasmic region (Strubin et al. 1986).

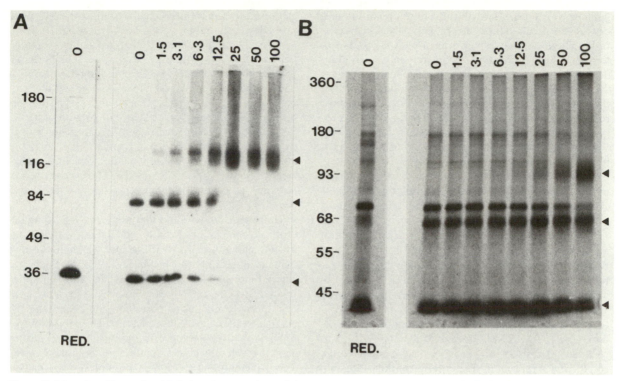

Figure 3. Non-class-II-associated I chain exists as a trimer. (*A*) Unlabeled T2 cells were extracted in $C_{12}E_9$ detergent, and extracts were applied directly to Sephacryl S-300 in $C_{12}E_9$ to partially purify the I chain and remove Tris from the extract. Peak fractions (predominantly in the excluded volume), identified by Western blotting, were pooled and treated with 0–100 µg/ml DSP. Cross-linked products were precipitated with ethanol, fractionated on one-dimensional SDS-PAGE, and analyzed by Western blotting with MATILDA anti-I-chain serum. An autoradiograph of the blot is shown, with positions of molecular-weight markers (*left*) and arrowheads indicating the positions of monomeric, dimeric, and trimeric I chains (*right*). (*B*) Detergent extracts of Swei cells, continuously labeled with [^{35}S]methionine for 8 hr, were applied to sequential affinity columns of L243-Bio-Gel (to remove mature HLA-DR complexes), DA6.147-Bio-Gel (to remove remaining immature HLA-DR complexes), and XD5.A11-Bio-Gel (to remove remaining class II complexes). Remaining excess I chain was purified on POP.I4.3-Bio-Gel. POP.I4.3 eluate was partially purified and desalted by gel filtration in $C_{12}E_9$, and peak fractions (identified by scintillation counting) were pooled and treated with 0–100 µg/ml DSP. Cross-linked products were precipitated with ethanol and analyzed by one-dimensional SDS-PAGE, fluorography, and autoradiography. (*Left*) Positions of molecular-weight markers run in parallel; (*right*) arrowheads indicate I-chain monomer, dimer, and trimer.

220,000. Affinity purification in CHAPS detergent appears to induce the formation of higher multimers. Affinity-purified I chain from T2 by gel-filtration chromatography in CHAPS has an $M_r \sim 500,000$, and cross-linking analyses using DSP indicate up to nine I chains per multimer (data not shown). On the basis of the minimal perturbation involved in the Western blotting experiments, we believe that the majority of the I chain in the T2 cell line is likely to be in the trimeric state.

The above result was obtained in a class-II-negative hybrid and has been confirmed in an additional class-II-negative B-LCL cell, a variant of P3HR-1 (Spiro et al. 1984; data not shown). Previous experiments have suggested that the I chain in human B-LCL cells is synthesized in excess of class II molecules and that it resides in the ER prior to its association with class II glycoproteins. We were therefore interested in whether the excess I chain in class-II-positive B-LCL cells also existed in a trimeric form. Figure 3B shows cross-linking of [^{35}S]methionine-labeled free I chain affinity purified from B-LCL Swei cells. All class II glycoproteins (DR, DQ, and DP), together with associated I chain, were

first removed by passing the detergent extract through a succession of anti-class-II monoclonal antibody affinity columns. Again, a fundamental trimer appears to form the core free I chain in these cells. The contaminating 70-kD band visible on the gel is not likely to be involved in any of the I-chain multimeric bands, because gel-filtration experiments indicate that it is not associated with the I chain. In sodium deoxycholate, gel-filtration analysis indicates that the I chain recovered from Swei cells by this procedure has a Stoke's radius equal to that of a globular protein of 220 kD, similar to I chain from T2 (data not shown). This is somewhat larger than expected for an I-chain trimer with an associated deoxycholate micelle, which might indicate either unexpectedly high detergent binding or asymmetry in the I-chain trimer.

Accumulation of High-molecular-weight Class II Complexes with Monensin and Leupeptin

In an earlier publication (Machamer and Cresswell 1984), we described the inhibition of class II antigen transport by the ionophore monensin. This compound induces vesicularization of the Golgi apparatus and causes the accumulation of $\alpha\beta$I complexes in B-LCL cells. These complexes have an $M_r \sim 270{,}000$ as determined by gel-filtration chromatography in sodium deoxycholate, a property initially ascribed to their association with a chondroitin-sulfate-containing form of the I chain (Kelner and Cresswell 1986). Our most recent experiments indicate that although a minor proportion of these high-molecular-weight complexes do contain the I chain-derived chondroitin sulfate proteoglycan, most do not. Preliminary cross-linking experiments similar to those described above for analysis of free I chain indicate that these complexes are higher-order multimers containing more than one α, β, and I subunit.

In additional studies, we have found that the proteinase inhibitor leupeptin also has profound effects on class II MHC antigen transport, causing the accumulation of HLA-DR $\alpha\beta$ dimers associated with a proteolytic fragment of the I chain (Blum and Cresswell 1988). Similar results were obtained by Nguyen et al. (1989). This fragment, termed leupeptin-induced protein (LIP), is a 21-kD species that retains the two N-linked glycans of the I chain. Figure 4 shows the results of a Western blotting experiment indicating that the LIP fragment contains the amino-terminal cytoplasmic domain of the I chain. HLA-DR molecules from Swei B-LCL cells, untreated or incubated for 18 hours with 0.5 mM leupeptin, were affinity-purified, using the antibody DA6.147 coupled to Bio-Gel A15m agarose. The eluted material was precipitated by ethanol, separated by SDS-PAGE, and electrophoreti-cally transferred to nitrocellulose, and the blots were probed with the rabbit antibodies 247 (anti-HLA-DR), MATILDA (anti-I chain), EQLP (anti-amino-terminal peptide of the I chain), or KESL (anti-carboxy-terminal peptide of the I chain). The 247 antibody detects DR α and β subunits, whereas MATILDA and both the anti-peptide sera detect the I chain. Only the anti-amino-terminal peptide antibody reacts with a band of 21 kD detectable in DR molecules purified from leupeptin-treated cells. From this experiment, the LIP fragment must result from the proteolytic cleavage of a significant portion (~ 100 amino acids) of the carboxy-terminal region of the I chain by a leupeptin-insensitive proteinase.

We have recently found that the HLA-DR complexes that accumulate in B-LCL cells treated with leupeptin are similar in size to those that accumulate upon monensin treatment. This is indicated in Figure 5, where detergent extracts of monensin- and leupeptin-treated B-LCL cells have been separated by nondenaturing PAGE, using pore-limit gels containing 1% octylglucoside, electrophoretically transferred to nitrocellulose and probed with a monoclonal antibody to class II β subunits and a rabbit antibody to the I chain. The accumulation of class II glycoproteins from the monensin- and leupeptin-treated B-LCL cells in a high-molecular-weight band ($\sim 300{,}000$) can clearly be seen. There is a corresponding accumulation of high-molecular-weight I chain for monensin-treated cells. The rabbit antiserum does not react with the LIP fragment (see Fig. 4) and was not informative for the leupeptin-treated B-LCL cells. Corroborating data

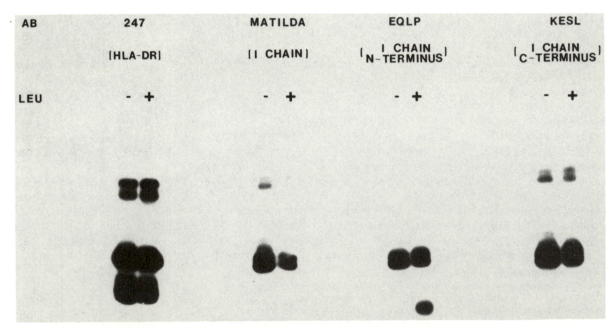

Figure 4. The I-chain fragment (LIP) that accumulates in leupeptin-treated cells contains the amino-terminal cytoplasmic domain. HLA-DR molecules were purified on a DA6.147-Bio-Gel affinity column either from Sweig B-LCL cells cultured for 18 hr in 0.5 mM leupeptin (+) or without added leupeptin (−). After ethanol precipitation, the samples were separated by SDS-PAGE and analyzed by Western blotting with the indicated antibodies. Only class II molecules from leupeptin-treated cells are associated with the LIP fragment, detectable by the anti-amino-terminal I-chain peptide serum.

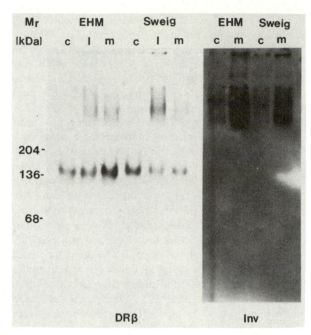

Figure 5. Leupeptin and monensin induce the accumulation of high-molecular-weight class II antigen-containing complexes. EHM or Sweig B-LCL cells were cultured with 0.5 mM leupeptin (l), 10 μM monensin (m), or with no additive (c). Triton X-100 extracts of the cells were separated by pore-limit PAGE in 1% octylglucoside in Tris-borate (5×10^5 cell equivalents per lane), and analyzed by Western blotting with XD5.A11 (anti-class-II β subunit) or MATILDA (anti-I chain). The accumulation of β subunits in a high-molecular-weight band can be seen in both leupeptin- and monensin-treated cells. A corresponding increase in the intensity of I chain in a similar band can be seen in monensin-treated cells.

showing the accumulation of large class II complexes containing LIP in leupeptin-treated cells have been obtained by gel filtration (data not shown).

On the basis of these results, our current picture of the αβI complex is that it exists as some form of a higher multimer, rather than as the simple trimeric structure indicated in Figure 1. Possibly, because the free I chain in the ER is a trimer, as shown in T2 as well as class-II-positive B-LCL cells, the αβI complex has a I-chain trimer as a core. Resolution of this problem awaits further experimentation. It also appears that complexes of class II glycoproteins with the LIP fragment have a higher multimeric structure. This structure presumably breaks down only after the I chain is completely degraded prior to cell-surface expression of the mature αβ dimer.

Peptide Binding to HLA-DR Antigens In Vivo

Peptides derived from protein antigens presented in a class-II-restricted manner to the T-helper cells have been shown to bind to the relevant class II allelic products in vitro. To examine specificity of peptide binding to a range of class II alleles, a simple assay that does not rely on the purification of significant amounts of class II glycoproteins, e.g., using intact cells, would

clearly be advantageous. An assay involving intact class II antigen-positive cells would also facilitate an analysis of in vivo binding mechanisms. With this in mind, we set out to determine whether we could directly demonstrate the binding of an influenza hemagglutinin-derived peptide (306-320, C15G) to HLA-DR molecules in vivo. This peptide has been shown to be presented in an HLA-DR1-restricted fashion to a T-helper cell clone (Rothbard et al. 1988). The principle of the assay was to simply incubate ^{125}I-labeled peptide at 37°C with HLA homozygous B-LCL cells carrying different HLA-DR alleles, wash the cells, extract them in a conventional manner with detergent, and precipitate the HLA-DR molecules with a specific monoclonal antibody, L243. Figure 6 shows the results of such an experiment. Clearly, six of the HLA-DR allelic products tested (DR1–DR6) are capable of binding ^{125}I-labeled peptide. No significant binding is detected for the DR7 and DR8 homozygous cells. No significant precipitation of counts per minute was obtained when the class II antigen-negative cell line T2 was used. The control antibody in the experiment shown is an isotype-matched anti-H-2K^b antibody, but a similar negative result is seen with the anti-HLA class I antibody, w6/32 (data not shown), confirming that the association is

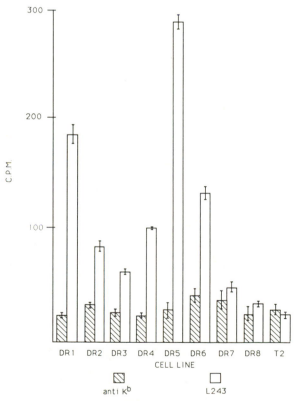

Figure 6. Specific binding of an influenza hemagglutinin peptide (306-320, C15G) to HLA-DR molecules in vivo. Conditions for incubation of ^{125}I-labeled peptide with B-LCL cells, detergent extractions, and immunoprecipitation with the anti-HLA-DR antibody L243 (open bars) or the anti-K^b antibody 28-8-6S (hatched bars) are described in the text. The error bars represent the range of duplicates.

specific for HLA-DR molecules. On the basis of the specific activity of the ^{125}I-labeled peptide, and assuming 10^6 HLA-DR molecules per cell, approximately 1–5% of the HLA-DR glycoproteins are binding peptide specifically.

To corroborate the in vivo peptide-binding studies, peptide-binding experiments were performed in vitro, using HLA-DR1, DR5, and DR8 antigens affinity-purified from DR homozygous B-LCL cells. The affinity-purified material was purified further using HPLC gel filtration in 1% octylglucoside. The HLA-DR glycoprotein was incubated with ^{125}I-labeled C15G peptide with or without a 20-fold excess of unlabeled C15G peptide or a 20-fold excess of unlabeled irrelevant peptide as a control. The class II peptide complexes were then separated from free ^{125}I-labeled peptide by nondenaturing pore-limit PAGE in 1% octylglucoside, electrophoretically transferred to nitrocellulose, and analyzed by autoradiography. Electrophoretic transfer was found preferable to conventional vacuum-drying techniques because of the tendency of the 5–15% gradient gels to crack upon drying.

The results of this analysis are shown in Figure 7. A clear band with bound ^{125}I-labeled peptide is visible with purified DR1 and DR5 glycoprotein. Generation of this band is inhibited by the presence of the specific competitor peptide. A band in the HLA-DR8 lane is visible but significantly weaker. Whether this is because the HLA-DR8 molecule has an intrinsically lower affinity for the peptide or whether the binding is lower because a greater proportion of HLA-DR8 molecules are occupied by high-affinity endogenous peptides is currently under investigation.

DISCUSSION

The biosynthesis and transport of class II MHC antigens are complex and still poorly understood. The unusual aspects of transport, i.e., the I chain association in the ER and dissociation in a post-Golgi compartment, are of unknown significance but seem likely to be functionally important. Clearly, the I chain itself, in the absence of class II association, behaves as a resident ER protein in the B-LCL cells studied here. Only minor amounts escape from the ER, determined by acquisition of sialic acid (Fig. 2) and resistance to endo H. Trimerization need not be a specific requirement for retention in the ER. Indeed, trimerization occurs prior to transport of certain glycoproteins out of the ER, including influenza virus hemagglutinin and vesicular stomatitis virus glycoprotein (Copeland et al. 1986; Kreis and Lodish 1986). One might speculate that the I chain contains a specific signal mediating retention in the ER, equivalent to the KDEL sequence characteristic of other resident ER proteins (Munro and Pelham 1987). Alternatively, a specific transport signal may be lacking.

When the I chain trimer associates with class II glycoproteins, transport of the complex out of the ER ensues. This may result from the masking of an ER retention signal in the I chain, or, alternatively, from the provision of a transport signal by the class II α and/or β subunits. The multimeric $\alpha\beta$I complex moves through the Golgi apparatus, as judged from the maturation of N-linked and O-linked glycans, but is not transported directly to the cell surface, as is the case for other membrane glycoproteins that follow the constitu-

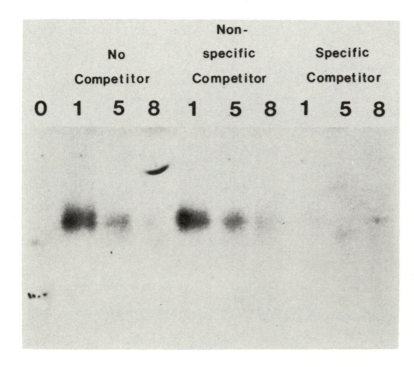

Figure 7. Analysis of ^{125}I-labeled C15G peptide binding to purified HLA-DR glycoproteins by discontinuous pore-limit PAGE in 1% octylglucoside. (Lane *0*) Free ^{125}I-labeled peptide was electrophoresed; (lanes *1*) HLA-DR1-peptide complexes; (lanes *5*) DR5-peptide complexes; (lanes *8*) DR8-peptide complexes. The specific competing peptide was unlabeled C15G; the nonspecific control peptide corresponded to the sequence encoded by exon 6 of HLA-A3. The band visibly migrated identically to purified HLA-DR glycoproteins visualized by Western blotting.

tive secretory pathway. The delay in cell-surface expression that occurs for class II molecules may also be a function of the I chain, because expression of mature $\alpha\beta$ dimers on the cell surface does not occur until the I chain is degraded.

The degradative dissociation of the I chain from class II MHCs is probably a consequence of the action of at least two proteinases. This is based on the results of the leupeptin experiments, because addition of this particular proteinase inhibitor blocks degradation of the I chain but allows the accumulation of the amino-terminal LIP fragment (Fig. 4). Presumably, in the absence of leupeptin, the LIP fragment is further degraded by a leupeptin-sensitive proteinase, possibly cathepsin B. The involvement of a leupeptin-sensitive proteinase in I chain degradation is especially intriguing in light of experiments by Berzofsky and co-workers, indicating that leupeptin and other cathepsin-B inhibitors (antipain and E64) block the in vivo generation of three distinct T-cell epitopes of myoglobin by antigen-presenting cells (Takahashi et al. 1989). These inhibitors were unable to block the response of T cells to myoglobin digested with cathepsin B in vitro. Thus, there is an interesting parallel between antigen processing and I chain degradation in that both may involve the same proteinase. An obvious hypothesis is that the two events may occur in the same intracellular compartment. Antigen processing, peptide binding to class II molecules, and I chain degradation might therefore form individual steps in a concerted mechanism, the end result of which is a class II–peptide complex, devoid of I chain, which is now free to be transported to the cell surface. Once there, it can be recognized by antigen-specific, class-II-restricted T-helper cells. The precise organelle where class II–peptide interactions occur remains undefined. An endosomal compartment seems a likely possibility, because cathepsins B and D have both been localized to macrophage endosomes (Diment and Stahl 1985). Clearly, however, understanding the detailed mechanisms involved in antigen processing will require considerably more investigation.

Whether any of the processes described above are involved in the binding of peptides to HLA-DR antigens in vivo, as shown in Figure 6, is unclear. Recently, other investigators have shown binding of a labeled influenza matrix peptide to intact cells and found a correlation with HLA-DR expression (Ceppellini et al. 1989). The speed of binding observed in these experiments (maximal binding in 45 min) suggests that simple cell-surface binding may account for their results. Preliminary kinetic experiments using the assay described here suggest somewhat slower binding, and specific binding was not demonstrable by simply washing the cells and counting them for ^{125}I. Precipitation of HLA-DR, with associated labeled peptide, was essential to demonstrate specificity and simultaneously proved that the peptide was indeed binding to HLA-DR molecules and not some other cellular protein. On the basis of the relatively broad specificity of binding observed, with six

of the eight tested HLA-DR allelic products showing binding, a definitive demonstration that DR molecules are responsible is critical. Clearly, the additional evidence (shown in Fig. 7) that HLA-DR5 glycoproteins are capable of binding the influenza hemagglutinin peptide in vitro validates the in vivo assay further. Additional experiments are in progress to determine whether the peptide binding in vivo involves simple surface exchange or internalization and interaction with newly synthesized class II glycoproteins.

ACKNOWLEDGMENTS

We thank Ms. Brenda Tapp for preparing the manuscript, Mr. Alan Payne for photography, and the other members of the laboratory for valuable discussions. This work was supported by grants AI-23081 and AI-23282 from the National Institutes of Health.

REFERENCES

Accolla, R.S., G. Carra, F. Buchegger, S. Carrel, and J.-P. Mach. 1985. The human Ia-associated invariant chain is synthesized in Ia-negative B-cell variants and is not expressed on the cell surface of both Ia-negative and Ia-positive parental cells. *J. Immunol.* **134:** 3265.

Babbitt, B.P., P.M. Allen, G. Matsueda, E. Mober, and E.R. Unanue. 1985. Binding of immunogenic peptides to Ia histocompatibility molecules. *Nature* **317:** 359.

Blum, J.S. and P. Cresswell. 1988. Role for intracellular proteases in the processing and transport of class II HLA antigens. *Proc. Natl. Acad. Sci.* **85:** 3975.

Ceppellini, R., G. Frumento, G.B. Ferrara, R. Tosi, A. Chersi, and B. Pernis. 1989. Binding of labeled influenza matrix peptide to HLA-DR in living B lymphoid cells. *Nature* **339:** 392.

Claesson-Welsh, L., P.E. Barker, D. Larhammer, L. Rask, F.H. Ruddle, and P.A. Peterson. 1984. The gene encoding the human class II γ chain is located on chromosome 5. *Immunogenetics* **20:** 89.

Copeland, C., R.W. Doms, E.M. Bolzain, R.G. Webster, and A. Helenius. 1986. Assembly of influenza hemagglutinin trimers and its role in intracellular transport. *J. Cell. Biol.* **103:** 1179.

Cresswell, P. 1985. Intracellular class II HLA antigens are accessible to transferrin-neuraminidase conjugates internalized by receptor-mediated endocytosis. *Proc. Natl. Acad. Sci.* **82:** 8188.

Cresswell, P. and J.S. Blum. 1988. Intracellular transport of class II HLA antigens. In *Processing and presentation of antigens* (ed. B. Pernis et al.), p. 43. Academic Press, New York.

Diment, S. and P. Stahl. 1985. Macrophage endosomes contain proteases which degrade endocytosed protein ligands. *J. Biol. Chem.* **260:** 15311.

Griffiths, G. and K. Simons. 1986. The Trans Golgi Network: Sorting at the exit site of the Golgi complex. *Science* **234:** 438.

Guillet, J.-G., M.-Z. Lai, T.J. Briner, J.A. Smith, and M.L. Gefter. 1986. Interaction of peptide antigens and class II major histocompatibility complex antigens. *Nature* **324:** 260.

Kelner, D.N. and P. Cresswell. 1986. Biosynthetic intermediates of HLA class II antigen from B lymphoblastoid cell lines. *J. Immunol.* **137:** 2632.

Kreis, T.E. and H.F. Lodish. 1986. Oligomerization is essential for transport of VSV viral glycoprotein to the cell surface. *Cell* **46:** 929.

Laemmli, U.K. 1970. Cleavage of structural proteins during assembly of the head of bacteriophage T4. *Nature* **227**: 680.

Lanzavecchia, A. 1985. Antigen-specific interaction between T and B cells. *Nature* **314**: 537.

Machamer, C.E. and P. Cresswell. 1982. Biosynthesis and glycosylation of the invariant chain associated with HLA-DR antigens. *J. Immunol.* **120**: 2564.

———. 1984. Monensin prevents terminal glycosylation of the N- and O-linked oligosaccharides of the HLA-DR-associated invariant chain and inhibits its dissociation from the $\alpha\beta$ chain complex. *Proc. Natl. Acad. Sci.* **81**: 1287.

Munro, S. and H.R.B. Pelham. 1987. C-terminal signal prevents secretion of lumenal ER proteins. *Cell* **48**: 899.

Nguyen, Q.V., W. Knapp, and R.E. Humphreys. 1989. Inhibition by leupeptin and antipain of the intracellular proteolysis of I_i. *Human Immunol.* **24**: 153.

Radka, S.F., C.E. Machamer, and P. Cresswell. 1984. Analysis of monoclonal antibodies reactive with human class II β chains by two-dimensional electrophoresis and Western blotting. *Human Immunol.* **10**: 177.

Rock, K.C., B. Benacerraf, and A.K. Abbas. 1984. Antigen presentation by hapten specific B-lymphocytes. 1. Role of surface immunoglobulin receptors. *J. Exp. Med.* **160**: 1102.

Rothbard, J.B., R.I. Lechler, K. Howland, V. Bal, D.D. Eckels, R. Sekaly, E.O. Long, W.R. Taylor, and J.R.

Lamb. 1988. Structural model of HLA-DR1 restricted T-cell antigen recognition. *Cell* **52**: 515.

Salter, R.D., D.N. Howell, and P. Cresswell. 1985. Genes regulating HLA class I antigen expression in T-B lymphoblast hybrids. *Immunogenetics* **21**: 235.

Sette, A., S. Buus, S. Colon, L. Miles, and H.M. Grey. 1989. Structural analysis of peptides binding to more than one Ia antigen. *J. Immunol.* **142**: 35.

Spiro, R.C., T. Sairenji, and R.E. Humphreys. 1984. Enhanced I_i expression after n-butyrate treatment of a P3HR-1 Burkitt's lymphoma subline which does not express HLA-D. *Hematol. Oncol.* **2**: 239.

Strubin, M., C. Berte, and B. Mach. 1986. Alternative splicing and alternative initiation of translation explain the four forms of the Ia-antigen associated invariant chain. *EMBO J.* **5**: 3483.

Strubin, M., B. Mach, and E.O. Long. 1984. The complete sequence of the mRNA for the HLA-DR-associated invariant chain reveals a polypeptide with an unusual transmembrane polarity. *EMBO J.* **3**: 869

Takahashi, H., K.B. Cease, and J.A. Berzofsky. 1989. Identification of proteases that process distinct epitopes on the same protein. *J. Immunol.* **142**: 2221.

Unanue, E.R. 1984. Antigen presenting function of the macrophage. *Annu. Rev. Immunol.* **2**: 324.

Intracellular Colocalization of Molecules Involved in Antigen Processing and Presentation by B Cells

F.M. Brodsky,* B. Koppelman,* J.S. Blum,† M.S. Marks,‡
P. Cresswell,‡ and L. Guagliardi*

*Department of Pharmacy, University of California, San Francisco, California 94143;
†Department of Cell Biology and Physiology, Washington University School of Medicine, St. Louis, Missouri 63110;
‡Department of Microbiology and Immunology, Duke University Medical Center, Durham, North Carolina 27710

The fact that T cells and B cells recognize different features of foreign antigen was first illustrated by the hapten-carrier effect (Mitchison 1971). Subsequently, the explanation for this phenomenon has become clear. Surface immunoglobulin (Ig) on B cells binds directly to foreign antigen, whereas T cells generally recognize antigen fragments bound to histocompatibility molecules (Unanue 1984; Allen 1987). The physical basis for antigen binding to histocompatibility molecules has been demonstrated by the resolution of the crystal structure of HLA-A2, which shows a characteristic peptide-binding site (Bjorkman et al. 1987). The generation of antigen fragments that can interact with histocompatibility molecules is called antigen processing, whereas the binding of antigen fragments to histocompatibility molecules and their export to the cell surface for recognition by a T-cell receptor is called antigen presentation. The studies described in this paper use immunoelectron microscopy to address the question of where antigen processing and presentation occur within the B cell.

Class I and class II histocompatibility molecules both present processed antigen to α/β T-cell receptors (Germain 1986). In general, class I molecules present antigen derived from endogenously synthesized proteins, whereas class II molecules most commonly present antigens internalized by the endocytotic pathway (Braciale et al. 1987; Wraith 1987). For class-I-mediated presentation, antigen can be produced either in the endoplasmic reticulum (ER), as in the case of viral surface glycoproteins, or in the cytosol, as in the case of viral nuclear or matrix proteins (Townsend and Bodmer 1989). It has been suggested that the assembly of the α chain with the β_2-microglobulin subunit of the class I molecule may actually require the presence of a peptide (Parham 1988b). If this is the case, then peptide binding by class I molecules probably occurs in the ER. Townsend presented data suggesting that peptide can influence association of β_2-microglobulin with class I α chain, thereby increasing surface expression of the peptide–class I complex (Townsend et al., this volume). On the basis of studies of T-cell receptor assembly and export, it is clear that degradation of newly synthesized surface glycoproteins can occur in a pre-Golgi intracellular compartment (possibly the ER itself) (Lippincott-Schwartz et al. 1988). Newly synthesized class I subunits may interact with the products of this degradative pathway and thereby export them to the surface for presentation. Class I molecules can present antigen fragments derived from antigens delivered artificially into the cytosol (Moore et al. 1988), as well as fragments of proteins synthesized in the cytosol. It is still a mystery how proteolytic fragments from cytoplasmic proteins can be presented by class I molecules. The interaction between cytosolic proteolytic processes and membrane-bound organelles is not yet understood, although mechanisms for translocation of cytosolic proteins into lysosomal compartments have been identified (Dice 1987). Additional mechanisms for transport of degraded peptides into the lumen of the ER may also exist, dependent on or independent from known protein translocation processes (Walter and Lingappa 1986). Most data suggest that processed antigen must interact with class I molecules early during their biosynthesis and transport to the cell surface. This is supported by the inhibition of class-I-mediated antigen presentation by emetine (Braciale et al. 1987) and Brefeldin-A (Nuchtern et al. 1989; Yewdell and Bennink 1989). Emetine prevents protein synthesis, and Brefeldin-A blocks export of newly synthesized proteins from the ER (Lippincott-Schwartz et al. 1989).

In contrast to class I histocompatibility molecules, class II molecules apparently bind processed antigen at a later stage in their transit through the cell (Germain 1986). In addition, the presented antigen is usually acquired by endocytosis from exogenous sources. Modeling the structure of class II molecules based on the class I crystal structure has indicated that class II molecules probably also have a peptide-binding site and an overall structure very similar to that of class I molecules (Brown et al. 1988). Thus, two similar molecules bind peptides from different sources and at different intracellular locations. One possible explanation is that class II molecules undergo a process of biosynthesis and export to the cell surface that differs from that of class I molecules. In the ER, class II α and β chains assemble with a third chain called γ chain, or invariant chain (I_i), which accompanies the class II α/β complex through the ER, Golgi, and trans-Golgi region (Cresswell et al. 1987). Most of the I_i dissociates from α/β prior to expression on the cell surface, although some surface I_i can be detected, as demonstrated by N. Koch (pers. comm.). This dissociation of α/β and I_i has been shown to require low pH and proteolytic activity (Nowell and Quaranta 1985; Blum and Cresswell 1988; Nguyen and Humphreys 1989). These conditions also cause fragmentation of internalized proteins. This coincidence suggests the possibility that dissociation of α/β and I_i is coordinate with binding of peptide by the α/β class II complex. In this scheme, I_i could be obscuring the peptide-binding site or changing the conformation of α/β such that peptides do not associate during the early transit of class II molecules through the cell. A second alternative is that I_i changes the intracellular trafficking of class II molecules so that they only encounter antigenic peptides at a late stage in their export to the surface. A third possibility is that the presence of I_i promotes exchange of peptides bound to α/β and its removal "fixes" a particular peptide in place. Stockinger et al. (1989) have recently demonstrated by transfection experiments that the presence of I_i in a cell is a prerequisite for the class-II-mediated presentation of processed, internalized antigen to T cells. In contrast, in the unusual case of measles virus infection, where endogenously synthesized antigen is presented by class II molecules, I_i is not required (Sekaly et al. 1988). Together, these data support the idea that I_i association influences the intracellular location where the α/β complex binds antigenic peptides.

Light microscopy and biochemical and functional studies have indicated that class II histocompatibility molecules encounter internalized proteins inside the cell. Pletscher and Pernis (1983) have shown intracellular colocalization of internalized Ig and class II molecules by two-color immunofluorescence. Cresswell (1985) has demonstrated that neuraminidase, internalized by coupling it to transferrin, is capable of cleaving sialic acids from processed I_i-α/β class II complexes (after their transit through the Golgi). Lanzavecchia (1985) has demonstrated that tetanus toxoid internalized via antigen-specific surface Ig can be presented by class II molecules to responding T cells. The electron microscopy studies described below were designed to determine the physical basis for these observations by mapping the intracellular routes accessed by class II histocompatibility molecules, I_i, and internalized surface Ig. These studies also investigate whether the pathways of class II molecules and internalized Ig intersect in compartments that contain the necessary proteinases and conditions for antigen processing. To mimic the uptake of multivalent antigen by surface Ig, anti-Ig coupled to 15-nm colloidal gold beads was used to cross-link surface Ig and induce its internalization at 37°C. At various time points following internalization, cells were fixed, embedded, and thin-sectioned for electron microscopy. The sections themselves were then labeled with antibodies to class II histocompatibility molecules, proteinases, and trafficking markers, iden-

tified by gold beads of different sizes (2, 5, and 10 nm). Physical evidence for the presence of class II histocompatibility molecules and I_i in the Ig uptake pathway was demonstrated. Furthermore, cathepsin B, a proteinase that is active at neutral as well as low pH (Barrett 1980), colocalized with internalized Ig, class II histocompatibility molecules, and I_i as early as 2 minutes following Ig internalization. The intracellular pathway containing internalized Ig with class II molecules and I_i was analyzed over a 30-minute period, with respect to the relative pH of the compartments entered and their proteinase content. The physical data obtained are highly consistent with functional data, suggesting that I_i is involved in antigen presentation, and demonstrate a rapid interaction between class II histocompatibility molecules and internalized Ig in the presence of proteinases.

EXPERIMENTAL PROCEDURES

Internalization of Ig and processing for electron microscopy. Human B-lymphoblastoid cells IM-9 (5×10^6) (Fahey et al. 1971) were washed twice with cold RPMI 1640 medium containing 1% fetal calf serum and incubated with polyclonal goat anti-human Ig (Tago) at 600 μg/ml for 60 minutes on ice. Cells were washed in cold medium and resuspended in rabbit anti-goat IgG conjugated to 15-nm gold beads (EY Labs), diluted 1:4, for 60 minutes on ice. Following a wash with cold medium, the cells were resuspended in prewarmed medium and allowed to internalize surface Ig for 2–30 minutes in a 37°C water bath. Cells were then chilled, pelleted, and fixed in 100 mM cacodylate buffer containing 0.2 mM $CaCl_2$, 4% sucrose, and 2% paraformaldehyde for 45 minutes at room temperature. Glutaraldehyde was added to a final concentration of 0.5%, and the cells were fixed for an additional 15 minutes. Washed cells were then osmicated (1% osmium, 1.5% ferricyanide) for 20 minutes (Coggeshall 1979) and stained with 2% aqueous uranyl acetate for 20 minutes. Fixed cell pellets were dehydrated in 50% and 70% ethanol for 5 minutes each and infiltrated with LR White resin (medium hardness, Polysciences) (Newman et al. 1983; Newman and Hobot 1987), using increasing ratios of resin to ethanol up to 100% resin. Dehydration and infiltration were performed at room temperature with gentle agitation. The cell pellets were transferred to gelatin capsules (Pelco) for polymerization. The LR White was hardened at 50°C for 24 hours without the addition of either hardener or accelerator. Ultrathin sections (700Å) were cut on a Reichert Ultracut "E" and mounted on unsupported 150-mesh nickel grids (Pelco).

Postembedment labeling. To label tissue sections with two different antibodies, one antibody (usually anti-I_i) was applied to one side of the ultrathin section, followed by the appropriate gold–anti-Ig conjugate, and the second antibody was applied to the opposite face and detected using a different size gold probe. All gold-conjugated anti-Ig was obtained from EY Labs. Antibodies and dilutions used are listed in Table 1. Before antibody labeling, sections on unsupported grids were floated on a drop of phosphate-buffered saline (PBS) containing 0.8% bovine serum albumin (BSA) and 0.1% gelatin (Janssen Pharmaceuticals, Inc.) for 10 minutes to prevent nonspecific sticking of proteins. The PBS/BSA/gelatin was also used for dilution of antibodies and for washing grids. In a typical double-labeling experiment, grids were placed on a drop of diluted MATILDA rabbit antiserum (anti-I_i) for 90 minutes, rinsed with five changes of PBS/BSA/gelatin, and then placed on a drop of mouse anti-rabbit Ig (34 μg/ml) (Accurate Chemicals) for 45 minutes. After washing, grids were incubated on a drop of goat anti-mouse Ig conjugated to either 2- or 5-nm gold beads and washed again. Following this first staining step, the labeled face of the section was coated with a thin film of Formvar (silver interference color). This step permits a second staining on the other side of the section without leakage of reagents from one side of the grid to the other (Deschepper et al. 1986). The remaining exposed surface of the section was then labeled with a second primary antibody and the appropriate antibody-gold probe. Monoclonal antibodies (MAbs) L243 and AP.6 were visualized with 5- or 10-nm gold, coupled to goat anti-mouse IgG. Anti-cathepsin D serum was followed by staining with mouse anti-rabbit Ig and goat anti-mouse Ig conjugated to 5- or 10-nm gold. Anti-cathepsin B was localized using 5-nm gold, coupled to rabbit anti-sheep Ig. Grids were then washed in distilled H_2O and dried. Sections were observed on a JEOL 100C electron microscope at 60 kV.

Labeling acidic vesicles with DAMP reagent. Surface Ig was first labeled at 4°C, using the two-step immunogold-binding procedure described above. Cells were then incubated for 30 minutes at 37°C with medium containing 50 μM 3-(2,4-dinitroanilino)-3'-amino-N-methyldipropylamine (DAMP; Molecular Probes) (Anderson et al. 1984). The DAMP reagent concentrated in acidic compartments was visualized on sections after reaction with the monoclonal anti-2,4-dinitrophenol (DNP) antibody 29B5 (1 μg/ml) and goat anti-mouse Ig coupled to 5-nm gold.

Scoring the labeled sections. Intracellular vesicles containing cross-linked, internalized Ig (labeled with

15-nm gold probes) were examined for the presence of the markers listed in Table 1. The 15-, 10-, 5-, and 2-nm immunogold complexes used to map three molecules on the same cell are readily distinguished by transmission electron microscopy. Vesicles containing internalized Ig were scored as having (1) no other labels, (2) I_i chain staining alone, (3) proteinase, DAMP, HLA-DR, or AP.6 labeling alone, or (4) both I_i and an additional marker. The percentage of Ig-containing vesicles with a given staining pattern is shown in Figure 5. A minimum of 50 Ig-containing vesicles were counted for each labeling combination. The specificity of the staining procedure was determined by quantitating the number of endocytotic vesicles (containing Ig) labeled when grids were incubated with an irrelevant, isotypically matched monoclonal antibody, normal mouse serum, normal rabbit serum, or in the absence of a primary antibody followed by the appropriate gold conjugate (and amplification step, if used). For example, to determine the background staining with rabbit antiserum, normal rabbit serum was used in place of the primary antiserum, amplified with mouse anti-rabbit Ig and visualized with goat anti-mouse IgG conjugated to gold. In single-labeling experiments, the percentage of endocytotic vesicles stained with an irrelevant antibody/antiserum ranged from 4% to 10%. In double-labeling procedures on opposite grid surfaces, the percentage of endocytotic vesicles labeled with both irrelevant antibodies was 4%.

Internalization assay. Internalization of cell-surface HLA-DR was measured using a modification of the procedure described by Watts and Davidson (1988). Briefly, cells were incubated at 5×10^6/ml in PBS and 0.5% BSA (PBS/BSA) containing iodinated L243 Fab fragments at 5×10^6 cpm/10^6 cells for 1 hour at 4°C. Following incubation, cells were spun down, resuspended in PBS/BSA at 1.3×10^7 cells/ml, and seeded at 2×10^5 cells/well in a 96-well V-bottom plate (Flow Labs). Cells were washed once, and pellets were resuspended in either 4°C PBS/BSA or 37°C PBS/BSA for varying periods of time to prevent or allow internalization of bound ligand. Plates were then spun, and remaining cell-surface-bound antibody was removed by resuspending pellets in either 150 μl 20 mM HCl, 150 mM NaCl (pH 1.7), or control PBS/BSA for 3 minutes prior to centrifugation. Finally, the cells were washed

Table 1. Antibodies Used to Characterize Intracellular Compartments

Target antigen	Antibody	Form	Concentration used	Source/reference
HLA-DR	L243	mouse MAb IgG2a	10 μg/ml	Lampson and Levy (1980)
I_i	MATILDA	rabbit antiserum	1/20	Cresswell et al. (this volume)
Cathepsin B (human)	anti-cathepsin B	sheep antiserum	1/20	The Binding Site, Ltd.
Cathepsin D (human)[b]	anti-cathepsin D	rabbit antiserum	1/20	Blum et al. (this volume)[a]
Endocytotic clathrin-coated vesicles	AP.6	mouse MAb IgG	10 μg/ml	Brodsky (1988)
DAMP (acidic vesicles)	anti-DNP (29B5)	mouse MAb IgG1	1 μg/ml	L. Herzenberg (Stanford University)

[a]Reference gives immunization protocol.
[b]Antigen was human placental cathepsin D, purified as described by Diment et al. (1988) and Takahashi and Tang (1981).

three consecutive times in PBS/BSA before being counted in a gamma counter. L243 Fab fragments were produced using pepsin, as described by Parham (1988a). L243 Fab fragments and purified B3/25 anti-transferrin receptor monoclonal antibody (Omary et al. 1980) were iodinated using Iodobeads (Pierce Chemicals) and 25 μg of protein with 1 mCi [^{125}I]sodium iodide for 5 minutes.

Percent internalization indicates the number of cell-associated counts after acid stripping, divided by the number of counts associated with unstripped cells. Background counts remaining associated with cells incubated at 4°C and acid-stripped were subtracted before calculating percent internalization. A typical sample analyzed after acid-stripping showed loss of 10% of the labeled cells.

RESULTS

Route of Ig Uptake

Electron microscopy studies of routes of surface Ig internalization were carried out using the IM-9 B-cell line. These Epstein-Barr virus (EBV)-transformed human B cells have been shown to secrete IgG (Fahey et al. 1971), and the experiments described below demonstrate their expression of surface Ig. Similar EBV-transformed B cells with surface anti-tetanus toxin Ig have been shown to present antigen efficiently to tetanus-toxin-specific T-cell clones (Lanzavecchia 1985). To induce internalization of surface Ig, a two-step cross-linking procedure was used, as outlined in Figure 1. At 4°C, goat anti-human Ig was bound to cells, followed by rabbit anti-goat Ig coupled to 15-nm colloidal gold. Cells were then warmed to 37°C, inducing endocytosis. At various times following induction of internalization, cells were fixed, processed for electron microscopy, and sectioned. Within 2 minutes, internalized surface Ig was visible in large pinocytotic vesicles (Fig. 2A) close to the plasma membrane. By 30 minutes (Fig. 2B), these vesicles doubled in size, accumulating more gold particles, and some were observed closer to the nucleus. The pinocytotic vesicles observed at 2 minutes averaged 200–500 nm, which is larger than clathrin-coated vesicles (50–100 nm) (Pearse and Bretscher 1981). These are formed either by extremely rapid uncoating and fusion of clathrin-coated vesicles or by direct invagination of larger areas of membrane. Observation of gold particles in highly invaginated areas of plasma membrane surrounded by finger-like extensions of membrane suggests that the Ig-containing pinosomes may form directly, without passing through a smaller clathrin-coated intermediate. Internalization by direct invagination would be nonselective, in contrast to the clathrin-mediated route, which concentrates and excludes particular cell-surface molecules (Brodsky 1988). Labeling of patches of the pinosome membrane with anticlathrin antibodies suggests further that the pinosomes result from direct invagination, cointernalizing any coated pits that might be forming.

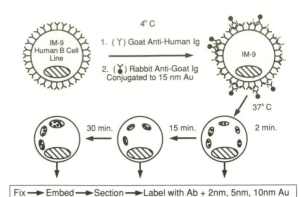

Figure 1. Procedure for cross-linking and internalization of cell-surface Ig. Cells were incubated with two layers of cross-linking anti-Ig antibodies. The second antibody was coupled to 15-nm colloidal gold. Cells were then warmed to induce internalization and processed for electron microscopy at the indicated times.

Markers Used to Characterize Intracellular Compartments

To determine whether the Ig-containing pinosomes are potential sites for antigen processing and presentation, sections of cells that had internalized Ig were labeled with the panel of antibodies listed in Table 1. Binding of these antibodies was detected with appropriate anti-Ig reagents coupled to 2-, 5-, and 10-nm colloidal gold. HLA-DR was localized using MAb L243. Biosynthetic studies have demonstrated that L243 recognizes only mature HLA-DR molecules composed of α and β chains that have already dissociated from I_i (Shackelford et al. 1981). However, staining of cell sections with L243 showed a low level of binding throughout the biosynthetic pathway (ER, Golgi, and trans-Golgi) with increased binding in the cell periphery and on the surface. This suggests that the fixation procedure used to prepare the cells for microscopy may reveal the L243-binding site on some immature HLA-DR molecules. Alternatively, there may be some dissociation of α/β and I_i throughout the biosynthetic pathway (Nguyen and Humphreys 1989). I_i was localized with a rabbit antiserum (MATILDA) produced against purified I_i (Cresswell et al., this volume). Staining was observed through the biosynthetic pathway and very occasionally on the cell surface.

The enzymes cathepsin B and cathepsin D have both been implicated in proteolytic cleavage of I_i, an event that correlates with its dissociation from the α/β class II chains (Blum and Cresswell 1988; Nguyen et al. 1989). Both enzymes have also been implicated in proteolysis of antigen by using inhibitors (Berzofsky et al. 1988; Watts et al., this volume), and cathepsin B was shown to be effective for artificial processing of myoglobin in vitro, rendering it presentable to T-cell clones (Takahashi et al. 1989). Cathepsins B and D were localized to Ig-containing vesicles using specific polyclonal antisera.

Ig-containing vesicles were also characterized with respect to their lumenal pH and the presence of mark-

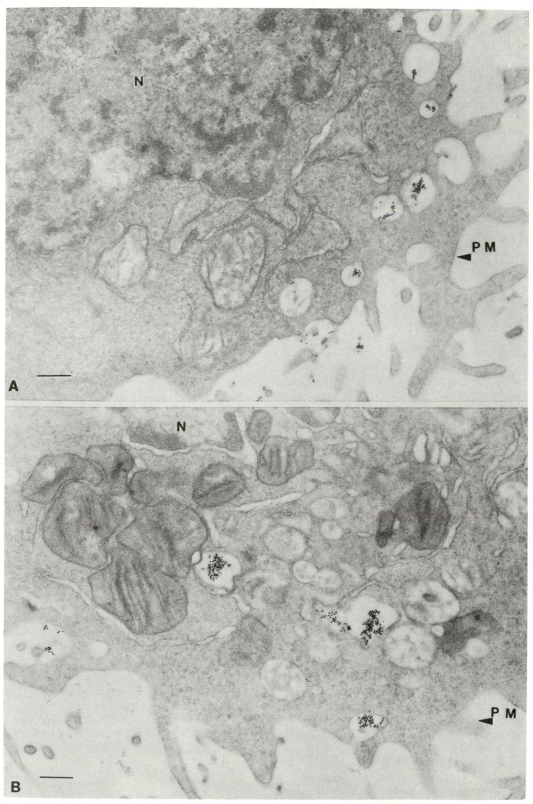

Figure 2. Intracellular compartments with internalized surface Ig. Surface Ig was cross-linked and internalized, as outlined in Fig. 1. Internalized 15-nm gold bound to surface Ig is shown in intracellular compartments formed after 2 min (*A*) and 30 min (*B*) of endocytosis. (PM) Plasma membrane; (N) nucleus. Bar, 0.33 μm.

ers for the endocytotic pathway. The DNP-derivatized amine, DAMP, passes freely across vesicular membranes until it is protonated, consequently accumulating in acidic, intracellular compartments (Anderson et al. 1984). Cells internalizing Ig were incubated simultaneously with DAMP. After processing for electron microscopy, DAMP was localized with the DNP-specific MAb 29B5 and colloidal gold coupled to anti-mouse Ig. Recently, it has been demonstrated that the adaptor components of clathrin-coated vesicles have a restricted intracellular distribution (Robinson 1987; Ahle et al. 1988). MAb AP.6, against the 100-kD α-adaptin, reacts only with vesicles in the cell periphery (Brodsky 1988) and inhibits endocytosis if microinjected into the cytoplasm (Chin et al. 1989). This antibody was used to identify vesicles derived from the endocytotic pathway. Interestingly, the Ig-containing vesicles present in cells after 30 minutes of Ig uptake were frequently labeled (57% of Ig-positive vesicles) with this antibody in small patches of the vesicular membrane. Such vesicles were less frequently labeled with anti-clathrin antibody (30% of Ig-positive vesicles). This suggests that these adaptor proteins remain bound to membrane that had undergone endocytosis, even after dissociation of the clathrin coat. Alternatively, the presence of these adaptor proteins might indicate the budding of recycling vesicles. As discussed below, the presence of I_i in compartments labeled with MAb AP.6 suggests intersection of the biosynthetic pathway with the endocytotic pathway.

Colocalization of Internalized Ig, Class II Molecules, I_i, and Cathepsin B

The distribution of the markers listed in Table 1 within compartments containing internalized Ig was analyzed by labeling tissue sections prepared from samples embedded after 2, 15, and 30 minutes of Ig uptake. Internalized Ig was marked by 15-nm gold particles, and other markers were identified using smaller (2-, 5-, or 10-nm) gold particles, coupled to anti-Ig reagents. Two minutes following induction of Ig internalization, I_i was observed in 50% of compartments with Ig that had undergone endocytosis. Figure 3 illustrates several compartments observed at 2 minutes containing both internalized surface Ig and I_i. These compartments are close to the plasma membrane. In Figure 3, A and B, I_i colocalized with Ig appears to be clustered, as though it were being delivered from a small intracellular vesicle. In Figure 3B, a single gold particle labeling I_i at the top of the vesicle may have entered the compartment from the cell surface. It is possible that I_i colocalizes with internalized surface Ig via both a surface and a secretory route. The small proportion of I_i detectable on the cell surface, however, suggests that the primary source of I_i is likely to be from an internal pool. Because I_i, which is not associated with class II α/β chains, does not leave the ER (Cresswell et al., this volume), the I_i observed in these peripheral endocytotic vesicles must be either still associated with class II α/β chains or

recently dissociated. In a separate experiment, 58% of the Ig-containing vesicles formed after 2 minutes of uptake also labeled with anti-HLA-DR, confirming the presence of class II α/β chains in these peripheral vesicles. The same percentage of Ig-containing vesicles formed at 2 minutes also label with anticlathrin and AP.6, recognizing endocytotic adaptor proteins. In a double-labeling experiment, it was observed that 80% of Ig-containing vesicles with I_i also contained cathepsin B. An additional 32% of Ig-containing vesicles labeled with cathepsin B alone. Cathepsin B staining was clustered, similar to that observed for I_i, again suggesting delivery from small transport vesicles. Thus, within 2 minutes of uptake, internalized surface Ig encounters HLA-DR, I_i, and cathepsin B.

Properties of the Endocytotic Pathway for Ig

Peripheral endocytotic compartments containing Ig formed over a period of 15–30 minutes after initiation of Ig internalization were characterized by double labeling with all of the markers listed in Table 1. Figure 4 shows two examples of double-labeling experiments. At 15 minutes, 50% Ig-containing compartments labeled with anti-HLA-DR, 52% labeled with AP.6, and 46% labeled with anti-cathepsin D. Figure 4A shows that some compartments had both HLA-DR and the AP.6 endocytotic marker. Of HLA-DR-positive Ig-containing compartments, 21% also labeled with cathepsin B. In a separate experiment labeling compartments present after 15 minutes of Ig uptake, 44% contained colocalized cathepsin D and I_i. This pattern of colocalization was also observed in samples prepared after 30 minutes of Ig uptake. Figure 4B shows I_i and cathepsin D colocalized with Ig, representing 28% of Ig-containing compartments after 30 minutes internalization.

Figure 5 summarizes the results of scoring double-labeled sections similar to those shown in Figure 4. The bars on the right-hand side of the figure indicate the percentage of Ig-containing vesicles with I_i and the percentage with an additional marker. The majority of Ig-positive I_i-positive vesicles (80–100%) are acidic, have the endocytotic adaptor protein, and contain cathepsin B, cathepsin D, and HLA-DR. These results indicate that from 2 to 30 minutes following endocytosis, Ig can be found with all the components required for antigen processing and presentation. The level of colocalization observed is a minimum estimate because the efficiency of antibody binding to proteins treated for electron microscopy is reduced to a variable degree, depending on the nature of individual antibody-antigen recognition sites.

Origin of HLA-DR and Proteinases Observed in Endocytotic Compartments

Previous studies of the distribution of lysosomal enzymes and I_i suggest that the most likely source of these

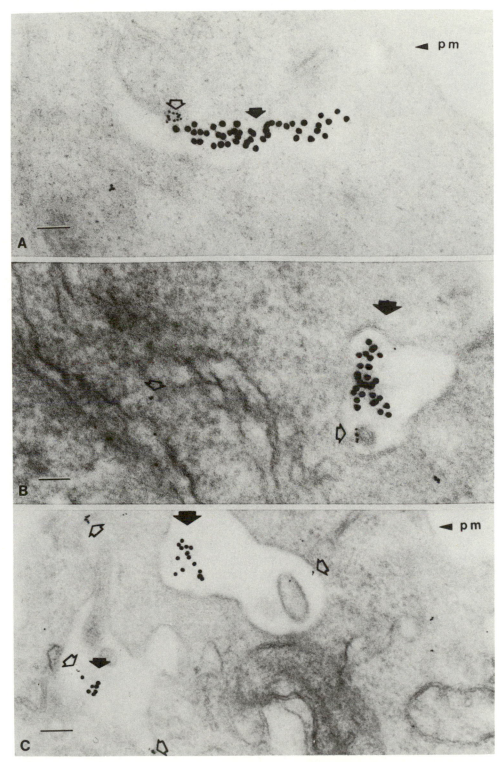

Figure 3. Colocalization of I_i with internalized surface Ig following 2 min of endocytosis. Surface Ig was labeled with 15-nm gold, cross-linked, and internalized for 2 min. Cells were embedded for electron microscopy, and sections were labeled with anti-I_i serum (MATILDA), detected with 5-nm colloidal gold. Three different views of peripheral intracellular compartments found on the same section are shown. Solid arrows indicate 15-nm gold (Ig), open arrows show 5-nm gold (I_i). (pm) Plasma membrane. In *B*, the plasma membrane is to the right of the vesicle shown, which seems to be connected to the cell surface by a thin neck of invaginated membrane. Bars: (*A*) 0.08 μm ; (*B*) 0.07 μm; (*C*) 0.11μm.

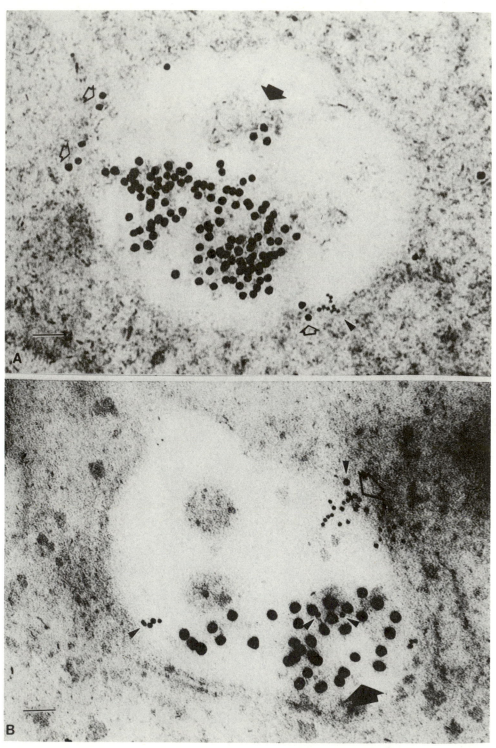

Figure 4. Example of double labeling of intracellular vesicles containing internalized Ig. (*A*) Surface Ig (15-nm gold; solid arrow) was internalized for 15 min; sections were labeled with AP.6 (10-nm gold; open arrows) and L243 (5 nm gold; arrowhead) to detect endocytotic adaptor proteins and HLA-DR, respectively. Bar, 0.05 μm. Note the characteristic staining of the vesicle surface by AP.6. (*B*) Surface Ig (15-nm gold; solid arrow) was internalized 30 min; sections were labeled with anti-I$_i$ (MATILDA, 10-nm gold; arrowheads) and anti-cathepsin D (5-nm gold; open arrow). Bar, 0.038 μm. Note the clustering of both I$_i$ and cathepsin D.

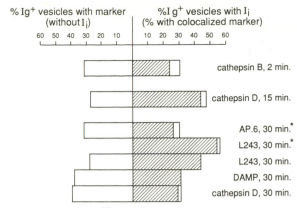

% Ig⁺ vesicles with marker (without I_i)

%I g⁺ vesicles with I_i (% with colocalized marker)

cathepsin B, 2 min.

cathepsin D, 15 min.

AP.6, 30 min.*

L243, 30 min.*

L243, 30 min.

DAMP, 30 min.

cathepsin D, 30 min.

Figure 5. Summary of double labeling of intracellular vesicles containing internalized Ig. Surface Ig labeled with 15-nm gold was internalized for 2, 15, or 30 min, and tissue sections were prepared and labeled with the markers indicated (specificity listed in Table 1). (*Right*) Ig-containing vesicles were scored for the presence of I_i and the percent positive plotted to the right of the center. The percentage of Ig-positive (Ig⁺) vesicles containing both I_i and the labeled marker is indicated by the shaded portion of the bar. (*Left*) The percentage of Ig-positive (Ig⁺) vesicles with the marker and without I_i. To determine the total percentage of Ig-positive vesicles with a particular marker, add the percent indicated at left plus the percent indicated by the shaded portion of the bar at right. All samples were double labeled as described in Experimental Procedures, except the samples indicated by an asterisk (*), where the two labeling antibodies were applied to the same side of the section. As seen for the L243 sample at 30 min, the two procedures give the same result. The times indicate the period allowed for Ig endocytosis prior to section preparation.

molecules is intracellular. Cathepsins B and D have both been identified in endosomes (Wiley et al. 1985; Roederer et al. 1987; Diment et al. 1988), whereas no evidence for surface cathepsin D has been found (Rodman et al. 1987). Cathepsin B has been demonstrated in plasma-membrane-enriched cell fractions (Sloane et al. 1987). However, the latter preparation might also contain early endosomes. P. Stahl showed data suggesting the existence of small transport vesicles that deliver cathepsin D from the Golgi to endosomal compartments (Blum et al., this volume). It is possible that cathepsin D, cathepsin B, and I_i localize to the Ig-containing endocytotic compartments by a similar mechanism. Knapp et al. (1989) demonstrated detection of I_i molecules on the cell surface, indicating the possibility of I_i colocalization with Ig by cointernalization. However, the number of intracellular gold particles labeling I_i far exceeds the rarely observed surface gold particle labeling I_i, suggesting a primarily internal source for these molecules.

To study the spontaneous internalization of HLA-DR, IM-9 cells were labeled with iodinated L243 Fab fragments at 4°C. After warming for various times to allow endocytosis, cells were chilled, and remaining surface Fab fragments were stripped off by an acid wash. Counts remaining associated with the cells indicate internalized HLA-DR molecules (Fig. 6). Very little internalized HLA-DR was detected. Similar

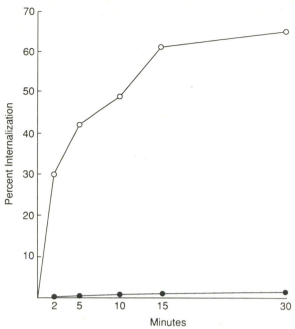

Figure 6. Internalization of class II molecules compared to transferrin receptor. Cells were incubated at 4°C with ¹²⁵I-labeled L243 Fab fragments to label HLA-DR (●) or with ¹²⁵I-labeled B3/25 IgG to label transferrin receptor (○). After warming to 37°C for indicated times, surface-bound Fab or IgG was removed by acid-stripping, and cells were counted for remaining associated radioactivity derived from internalized molecules. The percent internalization indicates the number of cell-associated counts after acid-stripping divided by the number of counts associated with unstripped cells. The maximum amount of internalized class II molecules in three separate experiments varied from 1.5% to 3.5%. This could be a slightly low estimate if the low viability after acid-stripping causes some loss of cell-associated internal counts. However, compared to the transferrin control, which would be subject to the same loss after acid-stripping, the class II molecules are internalized to a considerably lesser extent.

studies have confirmed that the internalization of cross-linked Ig does not significantly increase the internalization of HLA-DR. In contrast, a control experiment using bivalent, iodinated MAb B3/25 to induce internalization of transferrin receptor showed high levels of internalized monoclonal antibody after acid stripping. These results suggest that most HLA-DR observed in intracellular compartments in IM-9 cells is in transit to the cell surface. Biosynthetic studies have indicated that HLA-DR export is a slow process in comparison to export of class I molecules (Ploegh and Fuhrmann 1985; Cresswell et al. 1987; Harding and Unanue 1989; Nguyen and Humphreys 1989). It may be sequestered en route to the cell surface in compartments derived from the endocytotic pathway such as the Ig-containing vesicles analyzed in this work.

DISCUSSION

The studies described above characterize the intracellular pathway followed by internalized, cross-linked surface Ig. Induction of internalization by cross-linking was used to mimic uptake of multivalent antigen. Nonselective pinocytosis of cross-linked receptors seems to be the endocytotic mechanism utilized for internalization, in contrast to the clathrin-mediated uptake of Ig receptors bound by the monovalent antigen tetanus toxoid, coupled to colloidal gold (Watts et al., this volume). These results indicate that the degree of receptor cross-linking may influence the uptake mechanism. Studies by Tran et al. (1987) have indicated that following either selective (clathrin-mediated) or nonselective endocytosis, internalized ligands are delivered to the same endosomes, albeit with different efficiencies. Thus, the observations described above, which apply to uptake of multivalent antigen, may also be relevant to the pathway encountered by monovalent antigen. Studies investigating this possibility are in progress.

The immunoelectron microscopy studies presented here provide physical evidence for intracellular colocalization of internalized surface Ig, class II molecules, and I_i. Data on constitutive class II molecule internalization indicate that the biosynthetic pathway is the most likely source for the class II molecules observed in the Ig uptake pathway. The presence of I_i in this pathway further supports a biosynthetic origin for the class II molecules observed. These data suggest the existence of a pathway that delivers class II molecules from the trans-Golgi to early endosomes. Lysosomal enzymes cathepsin B and cathepsin D observed in Ig-containing endosomes might also be delivered from this pathway (Blum et al., this volume).

Antigen internalized by the Ig uptake pathway characterized above would be rapidly (within 2 min) exposed to cathepsin B, a proteolytic enzyme that has an optimum at pH 6 (Barrett 1980), well within endosomal pH (Mellman et al. 1986). Cathepsin B has also been implicated in cleavage of I_i and its dissociation from the α/β chains, because leupeptin, a cathepsin B inhibitor, prevents this process (Blum and Cresswell 1988). Labeling with DAMP after 30 minutes of Ig internalization indicates favorable acidic conditions for cathepsin D function, which has no activity at or above pH 7 (Barrett 1980). The acidic compartments observed are located in the cell periphery and contain I_i, again suggesting potential for I_i and antigen cleavage followed by surface export of class II α/β-peptide complexes. These colocalization studies demonstrate the feasibility of the proposal that dissociation of I_i from α/β is coordinate with binding of processed antigen and suggest that this primarily occurs prior to surface expression of class II molecules. This model is also compatible with the proposal that some antigen fragments may be generated by serum or cell-surface proteinases and internalized by nonselective pinocytosis into early endosomes, where they would encounter $\alpha/\beta-I_i$ complexes (Delovitch et al. 1988).

If the role of I_i is to prevent effective binding of antigen by α/β complexes until they reach a peripheral endocytotic compartment, then some apparent anomalies must be explained. In the cases where endogenously synthesized measles and hepatitis antigens are presented by class II molecules (Jin et al. 1988; Long and Jacobson 1989), these molecules must be delivered during biosynthesis or by recycling to the peripheral endosome. Alternatively, their proteolytic fragments might effectively compete with I_i for binding α/β in the ER. The presentation of such measles virus antigens by cells that lack I_i (Sekaly et al. 1988) would be expected because without I_i, the α/β complexes would presumably behave like class I molecules, binding antigenic fragments generated early in the biosynthetic pathway.

If peptide association with both class I and class II molecules occurs by the intracellular pathways discussed here, it would be expected that all surface class I and class II molecules should have bound peptide except for those class II molecules that retain I_i. In this context, the binding and presentation of exogenously added peptide to class II molecules by fixed cells (Shimonkevits et al. 1983; Unanue 1984; Ceppellini et al. 1989) and the demonstration of peptide binding by purified class I and class II molecules (Babbitt et al. 1985; Buus et al. 1986; Watts and McConnell 1986; Bouillot et al. 1989; Chen and Parham 1989) must be explained. The high concentration of peptides required and the low levels of binding detected suggest that most surface class I and class II molecules are occupied with peptide. The processes of fixation and extensive dialysis used in these experiments may actually contribute to replacement of a bound peptide by added peptide through mild denaturation processes. Although peptide dissociation from class II is slow (Buus et al. 1986), there is always a potential for a few unoccupied molecules to be generated at the cell surface or for class I molecules to escape the requirement for peptide during biosynthetic assembly, making these molecules available for binding by exogenously added peptide. The sensitive T-cell response assays, which require relatively few peptide-histocompatibility molecule complexes for triggering (Watts and McConnell 1986), most likely detect these rare binding events.

Although different interpretations have been proposed, the observed effects of chloroquine, emetine (Unanue 1984; Braciale et al. 1987), cycloheximide (Harding and Unanue 1989), and Brefeldin-A (Nuchtern et al. 1989) on class II-mediated antigen presentation are certainly compatible with the idea that I_i dissociation is required for effective binding of antigenic peptide. Pulse-chase and drug inhibition studies have indicated that the I_i-α/β class II complex accumulates in an intracellular pool following processing in the trans-Golgi (Machamer and Cresswell 1984; Nowell and Quaranta 1985). As discussed here, peptide association with class II molecules, resulting in an antigenic complex, could occur during or after this accumulation. The presence of a large intracellular pool of α/β-I_i complexes in B cells would explain why class-II-mediated presentation is not affected by Brefeldin-A inhibiting export from the ER (Lippincott-Schwartz et al. 1989) and is only affected by cycloheximide in macrophages that have a reduced intracellular pool of class

II molecules (Harding and Unanue 1989). Chloroquine has multiple effects on processes relevant to class-II-mediated presentation. It raises the pH of intracellular compartments affecting acid-dependent proteolysis of internalized proteins (Ohkuma and Poole 1978), inhibits recycling of internalized receptors back to the cell surface (Steinman et al. 1983), and prevents export of class II α/β chains to the cell surface by inhibiting dissociation from I_i (Nowell and Quaranta 1985). Thus, the effects of chloroquine do not distinguish whether peptide associates with class II molecules from a biosynthetic pool or following recycling.

Ceppellini et al. (1989) have demonstrated that complexes between exogenous peptide and class II molecules can be detected within 30 minutes when peptide is added to live cells. In contrast, detectable peptide binding to fixed cells is achieved only after an 18-hour incubation. This implies that peptide binding by class II major histocompatibility complex is a dynamic process and may require internalization of peptide to enhance association with class II molecules en route to the cell surface. Evidence presented by E. Unanue (Harding et al. 1989) indicated that on live cells, membrane-bound class II–peptide complexes have half-lives measurable in hours rather than days, as found for soluble biochemically generated class II–peptide complexes (Buus et al. 1986). The shorter half-life in cells could be the result of peptide exchange following class II molecule internalization, because it does not correlate with class II degradation rates. The mouse lymphoma cells and mouse macrophage cells studied by Harding and Unanue (1989) internalize their class II molecules to a greater extent than the human B-cell lines described here. Correspondingly, class II–peptide complexes on the human B-cell lines that show minimal class II internalization have longer half-lives of about 72 hours, as reported by A. Lanzavecchia (pers. comm.). It is possible that for cell lines internalizing a significant percentage of their surface class II molecules, peptide exchange might be a mechanism for binding peptides generated in the peripheral endocytotic pathway. However, it has yet to be demonstrated directly that internalized class II molecules recycle to the cell surface and could present exchanged antigenic peptides. The work described here characterizes a potential pathway for antigen processing and presentation by class II molecules in cells that internalize only a small percentage of surface class II molecules. The presence of I_i in peripheral endocytotic compartments that contain proteinases indicates the possibility that fragments of internalized antigen could be generated in the same compartment where I_i dissociates from class II α/β chains on their way to the cell surface.

ACKNOWLEDGMENTS

We thank D. Crumrine for technical assistance, I. Trowbridge for the B3/25 antibody, L. Herzenberg for the 29B5 antibody, A. Livingstone for comments on the manuscript, and G. Dela Cruz for manuscript preparation. This work was supported by grants from the National Institutes of Health, the National Science Foundation, and the Pew Charitable Trusts. L.G. was supported by a postdoctoral fellowship from the California Chapter of the American Heart Association. J.B. was supported by a postdoctoral fellowship from the Leukemia Society of America, Inc.

REFERENCES

Ahle, S., A. Mann, U. Eichelsbacher, and E. Ungewickell. 1988. Structural relationships between clathrin assembly proteins from Golgi and the plasma membrane. *EMBO J.* 7: 919.

Allen, P.M. 1987. Antigen processing at the molecular level. *Immunol. Today* 8: 270.

Anderson, R.G., J.R. Falck, J.L. Goldstein, and M.S. Brown. 1984. Visualization of acidic organelles in intact cells by electron microscopy. *Proc. Natl. Acad. Sci.* 81: 4838.

Babbitt, B.P., P.M. Allen, G. Matsueda, E. Haber, and E.R. Unanue. 1985. Binding of immunogenic peptides to Ia histocompatibility molecules. *Nature* 317: 359.

Barrett, A.J. 1980. The many forms and functions of cellular proteinases. *Fed. Proc.* 39: 9.

Berzofsky, J.A., S.J. Brett, H.Z. Streicher, and H. Takahashi. 1988. Antigen processing for presentation to T lymphocytes: Function, mechanism and implications for the T cell repertoire. *Immunol. Rev.* 106: 5.

Bjorkman, P.J., M.A. Saper, B. Samraoui, W.S. Bennett, J.L. Strominger, and D.C. Wiley. 1987. Structure of human Class I histocompatibility antigen, HLA-A2. *Nature* 329: 506.

Blum, J.S. and P. Cresswell. 1988. Role for intracellular proteases in the processing and transport of class II HLA antigens. *Proc. Natl. Acad. Sci.* 85: 3975.

Bouillot, M., J. Choppin, F. Cornille, M. Martinon, T. Papo, E. Gomard, M.-C. Fournie-Zaluski, and J.P. Levy. 1989. Physical association between MHC class I molecules and immunogenic peptides. *Nature* 339: 473.

Braciale, T.J., L.A. Morrison, M.T. Sweetser, J. Sambrook, M.-J. Gething, and V.J. Braciale. 1987. Antigen presentation pathways to class I and class II MHC-restricted T lymphocytes. *Immunol. Rev.* 98: 95.

Brodsky, F.M. 1988. Living with clathrin: Its role in intracellular membrane traffic. *Science* 242: 1396.

Brown, J.H., T. Jardetzky, M.A. Saper, B. Samraoui, P.J. Bjorkman, and D.C. Wiley. 1988. A hypothetical model of the foreign antigen binding site of class II histocompatibility molecules. *Nature* 332: 845.

Buus, S., A. Sette, S.M. Colon, D.M. Jenis, and H.M. Grey. 1986. Isolation and characterization of antigen-Ia complexes involved in T cell recognition. *Cell* 47: 1071.

Ceppellini, R., G. Frumento, G.B. Ferrara, R. Tosi, A. Chersi, and B. Pernis. 1989. Binding of labelled influenza matrix peptide to HLA-DR in living B lymphoid cells. *Nature* 339: 392.

Chen, B.P. and P. Parham. 1989. Direct binding of influenza peptides to class I HLA molecules. *Nature* 337: 743.

Chin, D.J., R.M. Straubinger, S. Acton, I. Näthke, and F.M. Brodsky. 1989. Adaptor proteins in peripheral clathrin-coated vesicles are required for receptor-mediated endocytosis. *Proc. Natl. Acad. Sci.* (in press).

Coggeshall, R.E. 1979. A fine structural analysis of the myelin sheath in rat spinal roots. *Anat. Rec.* 194: 201.

Cresswell, P. 1985. Intracellular Class II HLA antigens are accessible to transferrin-neuraminidase conjugates internalized by receptor-mediated endocytosis. *Proc. Natl. Acad. Sci.* 82: 8188.

Cresswell, P., J.S. Blum, D.N. Kelner, and M.S. Marks. 1987.

Biosynthesis and processing of class II histocompatibility antigens. *CRC Crit. Rev. Immunol.* **7**: 31.

Delovitch, T.L., J.W. Semple, P. Naquet, N.F. Bernard, J. Ellis, P. Champagne, and M.L. Phillips. 1988. Pathways of processing of insulin by antigen-presenting cells. *Immunol. Rev.* **106**: 195.

Deschepper, C.F., D.A. Crumrine, and W.F. Ganong. 1986. Evidence that the gonadotrophs are the likely site of production of angiotensin II in the anterior pituitary of the rat. *Endocrinology* **119**: 36.

Dice, J.F. 1987. Molecular determinants of protein half-lives in eukaryotic cells. *FASEB J.* **1**: 349.

Diment, S., M.S. Leech, and P.D. Stahl. 1988. Cathepsin D is membrane-associated in macrophage endosomes. *J. Biol. Chem.* **263**: 6901.

Fahey, J.L., D.N. Buell, and H.C. Sox. 1971. Proliferation and differentiation of human lymphoid cell lines and immunoglobulin synthesis. *Ann. N.Y. Acad. Sci.* **19**: 221.

Germain, R.N. 1986. The ins and outs of antigen processing and presentation. *Nature* **322**: 687.

Harding, C.V. and E.R. Unanue. 1989. Antigen processing and intracellular Ia: Possible roles of endocytosis and protein synthesis in Ia function. *J. Immunol.* **142**: 12.

Harding, C.V., R.W. Roof, and E.R. Unanue. 1989. Turnover of Ia-peptide complexes is facilitated in viable antigen-presenting cells: Biosynthetic turnover of Ia vs. peptide exchange. *Proc. Natl. Acad. Sci.* **86**: 4230.

Jin, Y., J.W.-K. Shih, and I. Berkower. 1988. Human T cell response to the surface antigen of hepatitis B virus (HBsAg). Endosomal and non-endosomal processing pathways are accessible to both endogenous and exogenous antigen. *J. Exp. Med.* **168**: 293.

Lampson, L.A. and R. Levy. 1980. Two populations of Ia-like molecules on a human B cell line. *J. Immunol.* **125**: 293.

Lanzavecchia, A. 1985. Antigen-specific interaction between T and B cells. *Nature* **314**: 537.

Lippincott-Schwartz, J., J.S. Bonifacino, L.C. Yuan, and R.D. Klausner. 1988. Degradation from the endoplasmic reticulum: Disposing of newly synthesized proteins. *Cell* **54**: 209.

Lippincott-Schwartz, J., L.C. Yuan, J.S. Bonifacino, and R.D. Klausner. 1989. Rapid redistribution of Golgi proteins into the ER in cells treated with Brefeldin A: Evidence for membrane cycling from Golgi to ER. *Cell* **56**: 801.

Long, E.O. and S. Jacobson. 1989. Pathways of viral antigen processing and presentation to CTL: Defined by the mode of viral entry. *Immunol. Today* **10**: 45.

Machamer, C.E. and P. Cresswell. 1984. Monensin prevents terminal glycosylation of the N- and O-linked oligosaccharides of the HLA-DR-associated invariant chain and inhibits its dissociation from the α-β chain complex. *Proc. Natl. Acad. Sci.* **81**: 1287.

Mellman, I., R. Fuchs, and A. Helenius. 1986. Acidification of the endocytic and exocytic pathways. *Annu. Rev. Biochem.* **55**: 663.

Mitchison, N.A. 1971. The carrier effect in the secondary response to hapten-protein conjugates. II. Cellular cooperation. *Eur. J. Immunol.* **1**: 18.

Moore, M.W., F.R. Carbone, and M.J. Bevan. 1988. Introduction of soluble protein into the class I pathway of antigen processing and presentation. *Cell* **54**: 777.

Newman, G.R. and J.A. Hobot. 1987. Modern acrylics for post-embedding immunostaining techniques. *J. Histochem. Cytochem.* **35**: 971.

Newman, G.R., B. Jasani, and E.D. Williams. 1983. A simple post-embedding system for the rapid demonstration of tissue antigens under the electron microscope. *Histochem. J.* **15**: 543.

Nguyen, Q.V. and R.E. Humphreys. 1989. Time course of intracellular associations, processing, and cleavages of I_i forms and class II major histocompatibility complex molecules. *J. Biol. Chem.* **164**: 1631.

Nguyen, Q.V., W. Knapp, and R.E. Humphreys. 1989. Inhibition by leupeptin and antipain of the intracellular proteolysis of I_i. *Hum. Immunol.* **24**: 153.

Nowell, J. and V. Quaranta. 1985. Chloroquine affects biosynthesis of Ia molecules by inhibiting dissociation of invariant (γ) chains from α-β dimers in B cells. *J. Exp. Med.* **162**: 1371.

Nuchtern, J.G., J.S. Bonifacino, W.E. Biddison, and R.D. Klausner. 1989. Brefeldin A implicates egress from endoplasmic reticulum in class I restricted antigen presentation. *Nature* **339**: 223.

Ohkuma, S. and B. Poole. 1978. Fluorescence probe measurement of the intralysosomal pH in living cells and the perturbation of pH by various agents. *Proc. Natl. Acad. Sci.* **75**: 3327.

Omary, M.B., I.S. Trowbridge, and J. Minowada. 1980. Human cell-surface glycoprotein with unusual properties. *Nature* **286**: 888.

Parham, P. 1988a. Preparation and purification of active fragments from mouse monoclonal antibodies. In *Handbook of experimental immunology* (ed. D.M. Weir et al.), vol. 1, p. 14.1. Blackwell Scientific Publications, Oxford.

——. 1988b. Presentation and processing of antigens in Paris. *Immunol. Today* **9**: 65.

Pearse, B.M.F. and M.S. Bretscher. 1981. Membrane recycling by coated vesicles. *Annu. Rev. Biochem.* **50**: 85.

Pletscher, M. and B. Pernis. 1983. Internalized membrane immunoglobulin meets intracytoplasmic DR antigen in human B lymphoblastoid cells. *Eur. J. Immunol.* **13**: 581.

Ploegh, H. and U. Fuhrmann. 1985. Manipulation of glycans on antigens of the major histocompatibility complex. In *Cell biology of the major histocompatibility complex* (ed. B. Pernis and H.J. Vogel), p. 133. Academic Press, Orlando, Florida.

Robinson, M.S. 1987. 100-KD coated vesicle proteins: Molecular heterogeneity and intracellular distribution studied with monoclonal antibodies. *J. Cell Biol.* **104**: 887.

Rodman, J.S., M.A. Levy, S. Diment, and P.D. Stahl. 1987. Immunolocalization of cathepsin D in macrophage endosomes. *J. Cell Biol.* **105**: 248a.

Roederer, M., R. Bowser, and R.F. Murphy. 1987. Kinetics and temperature dependence of exposure of endocytosed material of proteolytic enzymes and low pH: Evidence for a maturation model for the formation of lysosomes. *J. Cell. Physiol.* **131**: 200.

Sekaly, R., S. Jacobson, J.R. Richert, C. Tonnelle, H.F. McFarland, and E.O. Long. 1988. Antigen presentation to HLA class II-restricted measles virus-specific T-cell clones can occur in the absence of the invariant chain. *Proc. Natl. Acad. Sci.* **85**: 1209.

Shackelford, D.A., L.A. Lampson, and J.L. Strominger. 1981. Analysis of HLA-DR antigens by using monoclonal antibodies: Recognition of conformational differences in biosynthetic intermediates. *J. Immunol.* **127**: 1403.

Shimonkevitz, R., J. Kappler, P. Marrack, and H.M. Grey. 1983. Antigen recognition by H-2 restricted T cells. I. Cell-free antigen processing. *J. Exp. Med.* **158**: 303.

Sloane, B.F., J. Rozhin, J.S. Hatfield, J.D. Crissman, and K.V. Honn. 1987. Plasma membrane-associated cysteine protease in human and animal tumors. *Exp. Cell. Biol.* **55**: 209.

Steinman, R.M., I.S. Mellman, W.A. Muller, and Z.A. Cohn. 1983. Endocytosis and the recycling of plasma membrane. *J. Cell Biol.* **96**: 1.

Stockinger, B., U. Pessara, R.H. Lin, J. Habicht, M. Grez, and N. Koch. 1989. A role of Ia-associated invariant chains in antigen processing and presentation. *Cell* **56**: 683.

Takahashi, H., K.B. Cease, and J.A. Berzofsky. 1989. Identification of proteases that process distinct epitopes on the same protein. *J. Immunol.* **142**: 2221.

Takahashi, T. and J. Tang. 1981. Cathepsin D from porcine and bovine spleen. *Methods Enzymol.* **80**: 565.

Townsend, A. and H. Bodmer. 1989. Antigen recognition by

class I-restricted T lymphocytes. *Annu. Rev. Immunol.* **7**: 601.

Tran, D., J.L. Carpentier, F. Sawano, P. Gorden, and L. Orci. 1987. Ligands internalized through coated or non-coated invaginations follow a common intracellular pathway. *Proc. Natl. Acad. Sci.* **84**: 7957.

Unanue, E.R. 1984. Antigen-presenting functioning of the macrophage. *Annu. Rev. Immunol.* **2**: 395.

Walter, P. and V.R. Lingappa. 1986. Mechanism of protein translocation across the endoplasmic reticulum membrane. *Annu. Rev. Cell. Biol.* **2**: 499.

Watts, C. and H.W. Davidson. 1988. Endocytosis and recycling of specific antigen by human B cell lines. *EMBO J.* **7**: 1937.

Watts, T.H. and H.M. McConnell. 1986. High-affinity fluorescent peptide binding to I-A^d in lipid membranes. *Proc. Natl. Acad. Sci.* **83**: 9660.

Wiley, S.H., W. Van Nostrand, D.N. McKinley, and D.D. Cunningham. 1985. Intracellular processing of epidermal growth factor and its effect on ligand-receptor interactions. *J. Biol. Chem.* **260**: 5290.

Wraith, D.C. 1987. The recognition of influenza A virus-infected cells by cytotoxic T lymphocytes. *Immunol. Today* **8**: 239.

Yewdell, J.W. and J.R. Bennink. 1989. Brefeldin A specifically inhibits presentation of protein antigens to cytotoxic T lymphocytes. *Science* **244**: 1072.

Antigen Binding and Processing by B-cell Antigen-presenting Cells: Influence on T- and B-cell Activation

T.L. DELOVITCH, A.H. LAZARUS, M.L. PHILLIPS, AND J.W. SEMPLE

Banting and Best Department of Medical Research and Department of Immunology, University of Toronto, Toronto, Ontario, Canada M5G 1L6

The antigen specificity of an immune response is determined by the activation of relevant clones of lymphocytes via the recognition of an antigen by their surface antigen receptors. Whereas a surface immunoglobulin (sIg) on a B lymphocyte recognizes a determinant in the native conformation of a thymus-dependent soluble protein antigen, a T-cell antigen receptor (TCR) generally recognizes an epitope formed by the association of a processed antigenic peptide with a self major histocompatibility complex (MHC) molecule on the plasma membrane of an antigen-presenting cell (APC). The expression of antigen-specific sIg and surface MHC class II molecules enables B cells to present a self or foreign antigen at low concentration and function efficiently as antigen-specific APCs. B cells can also take up protein antigens by fluid-phase pinocytosis and function at higher antigen concentrations as antigen-nonspecific APCs in a manner similar to that of other types of sIg-negative APCs.

Despite these interesting differences in the mode of antigen recognition by B cells and T cells, much remains to be learned about the molecular basis of antigen-dependent B- and T-cell activation. For example, it is accepted that an antigen must first bind either specifically (sIg) or nonspecifically to a component(s) on the surface membrane of a B cell to be processed and presented to a T cell. However, the signals transduced by this antigen-binding step, which lead to either B-cell activation or inactivation, are not well defined. Multiple events have been proposed to occur in an APC subsequent to antigen binding. Evidence suggests that most protein antigens need to be processed by a proteinase(s) into peptides, some of which become destined for an interaction with an MHC class II molecule for presentation to a T cell. It is conceivable that this proteolysis is mediated by plasma-membrane-bound proteinases and/or intracellular proteinases, depending on the antigen. Antigen peptides formed at the plasma membrane may associate directly with cell-surface MHC class II molecules. Internalization of an antigen by endocytosis and/or pinocytosis is presumably required for it to be processed by an intracellular proteinase. Antigen peptides formed intracellularly may either be transported (in endosomes?) to the plasma membrane in association with MHC class II molecules or be transported independently to the plasma membrane,

where they can then interact with MHC class II. Recognition of such a peptide/MHC class II complex by an appropriate TCR is thought to mediate the antigen-specific activation of the host T cell.

The above sequence of events thus raises the possibility that the development of the T-cell repertoire and antibody response of an individual to a given antigen is influenced by the ability of APCs to bind antigen and to generate immunogenic peptides that can interact in a productive fashion with MHC class II molecules. Different APCs may process an antigen differently and produce a variety of immunodominant peptides. It is therefore essential that we examine how immunodominant peptides are generated in situ by an APC. In this paper, we describe experiments designed to delineate the role and specificity of antigen binding, antigen processing, antigen/MHC interaction, and antigen presentation by a B-cell APC on T-cell repertoire development and immune responsiveness.

MATERIALS AND METHODS

Antigens. 2,4,6-Trinitrobenzene sulfonic acid (TNBS) was used to couple the 2,4,6-trinitrophenyl (TNP) hapten to ovalbumin (OVA) in 200 mM H_3BO_3, 150 mM NaCl (pH 9.0) for 2 hours at 25°C.

Antibodies. The murine monoclonal antibody (MAb) 9B12 (IgG2b, κ) specific for insulin-degrading enzyme (IDE) was generously supplied by R. Roth (Stanford University). VC6 (IgG1, κ), a murine monoclonal antibody specific for an idiotope on 11-5.2.1.9 (11-5, mouse anti-I-A^k; Phillips et al. 1984), was used as a control antibody.

Calcium measurements. Cells (10^7/ml) were incubated with 2.5 μg/ml of the acetoxymethylester derivative of indo-1 in complete medium for 25 minutes at 37°C in 5% CO_2. The cells were then washed and resuspended in complete medium at 10^6/ml and held at 25°C until used. Cells were further washed and resuspended in 140 mM NaCl, 3 mM KCl, 1 mM $MgCl_2$, 10 mM glucose, 1.8 mM $CaCl_2$, and 20 mM HEPES (pH 7.2) immediately prior to use. The fluorescence emission of TA3 cells was measured in a thermostatically controlled cuvette at 37°C in a Hitachi F 4000 spectrofluorometer, using an excitation wavelength of 331 nm and an emission wavelength of 410 nm. The effect of the addition of antigen or antibody on the intracellular free calcium concentration ($[Ca^{++}]_i$) in these cells was assessed by adding the reagent "on line" to cells that maintained a stable $[Ca^{++}]_i$. Each analysis was calibrated by the addition of 5 μM ionomycin, followed by 1 mM MnCl (Grynkiewics et al. 1985).

IDE purification. CNBr-activated protein A–Sepharose was swelled and incubated with rabbit anti-mouse IgG for 18 hours at 4°C. The beads were washed in phosphate-buffered saline (PBS) and incubated with either the 9B12 or VC6 MAb for 3 hours at 4°C. The beads were then washed three times in ice-cold PBS before use. A 5-ml human erythrocyte pellet was washed three times in ice-cold PBS, and the cells were lysed by the addition of an equal volume of ice-cold milli-Q H_2O and ice. The erythrocyte homogenate was centrifuged at 12,000 rpm for 1 hour at 4°C. The supernatant was then immunoprecipitated with CNBr-activated protein A–Sepharose conjugated with anti-IDE (9B12) or VC6 (control) for 3 hours at 4°C. The Sepharose beads were washed six times in ice-cold PBS and mixed with 0.5 mg/ml of human insulin (HI) in 2 ml. The mixture was rotated for 18 hours at 37°C in a dry incubator, and the beads were removed by centrifugation. The supernatant was then applied to an Altex reversed-phase C18 column (4.6 × 150 mm) attached to a Beckman model 334 high-performance-liquid chromatography (HPLC) system.

Cellular processing. The processing of antigen by B-cell APCs was analyzed as described previously (Semple et al. 1989). Antibody inhibition of processing was performed by incubating 2×10^6 TA3 cells with a 1/20 dilution of either 9B12 or VC6 for 1 hour at 37°C and then cooling the cells on ice for 0.5 hour. The cells were incubated with ^{125}I-labeled HI for 1 hour on ice and then warmed to 37°C for 1 hour. The mixture was layered above 20% Percoll and centrifuged, and the supernatant above the Percoll was precipitated in 10% trichloroacetic acid (TCA). The TCA-soluble material was then applied to an Altex reversed-phase analytical C18 HPLC column and analyzed as described previously (Semple et al. 1989).

RESULTS AND DISCUSSION

Antigen Binding: Role in B-cell Activation and Desensitization

B cells can function efficiently as antigen-specific APCs at low antigen concentration (Lanzavecchia 1987; Pierce et al. 1988); however, they are also subject to antigen-induced tolerance for antibody formation in vivo at both low and high antigen dose. To further understand how the binding of an antigen at different concentrations ultimately controls the activation of a B cell to antibody formation, we developed an in vitro antigen-specific B-cell model to measure both low- and high-dose antigen-induced B-cell activation and de-

sensitization. We tested the effect of a thymus-dependent antigen on calcium signaling by utilizing TNP-specific transfected B cells (Bernard et al. 1988a,b; A.H. Lazarus et al., in prep.). The B-hybridoma cell line TA3.14.D5.1 (D5.1) was transfected previously with plasmid pR-HL$_{TNP}$ DNA to yield the 7.9 subclone, which expresses an anti-TNP-specific sIgM of the Sp6 idiotype (Bernard et al. 1988b). These cells present TNP-OVA about 1000-fold more efficiently than OVA to OVA/I-A^d-specific T cells, demonstrating that they utilize this TNP-specific sIgM to internalize, process, and present antigen to an appropriate T cell (Bernard et al. 1988a).

We have determined previously that 7.9 cells can be stimulated to undergo Ca^{++} signaling by anti-IgM, the anti-Sp603 anti-idiotype antibody, or the thymus-dependent antigen TNP-OVA. $[Ca^{++}]_i$ was measured as described previously (Grynkiewics et al. 1985), using the acetoxymethylester derivative of indo-1. The net fourfold increase in $[Ca^{++}]_i$ in response to TNP-OVA was dependent on both the antigen dose and the TNP/OVA molar ratio (A.H. Lazarus et al., in prep.). Both the multivalent antigen TNP$_6$-OVA (molar ratio of TNP/OVA is 6:1) and anti-Sp603 reciprocally inhibit each other's induced $[Ca^{++}]_i$ response (homologous desensitization). Anti-IgM also blocks the TNP$_6$-OVA-stimulated $[Ca^{++}]_i$ signal.

We then determined the effect of antigen concentration on homologous desensitization. Exposure to TNP$_6$-OVA at concentrations of ≤ 100 μg/ml desensitized 7.9 cells to stimulation with anti-IgM (Fig. 1a–c). However, when high concentrations of TNP$_6$-OVA were used, a different result was obtained. Following incubation of 7.9 cells with TNP$_6$-OVA at concentrations above 180 μg/ml, anti-IgM induced a virtually normal increase in $[Ca^{++}]_i$ (Fig. 1d). Although the relative increase in $[Ca^{++}]_i$ stimulated by either 100 or 180 μg/ml TNP$_6$-OVA was similar (Fig. 1c,d), the latter antigen concentration clearly did not desensitize 7.9 cells to subsequent signaling by anti-IgM.

Monovalent TNP-OVA conjugates with TNP/OVA molar ratio of $\leq 1:1$ did not elicit an increase in $[Ca^{++}]_i$ at low concentrations (A.H. Lazarus et al., in prep.). We therefore determined whether cross-linking of this monovalent antigen by an anti-carrier antibody would elicit a rise in $[Ca^{++}]_i$. The 7.9 cells were incubated first with 2.5 μg of TNP$_1$-OVA (molar ratio < 1:1) and then with either a rabbit anti-OVA antibody or normal rabbit serum (NRS). This treatment did not lead to a rise in $[Ca^{++}]_i$ (Fig. 2). However, when the cells were tested for stimulation of $[Ca^{++}]_i$ by anti-IgM, we observed that the TNP$_1$-OVA plus anti-OVA-pretreated cells were desensitized to stimulation by anti-IgM (Fig. 2a). Control cells that received TNP$_1$-OVA plus NRS were not desensitized to further stimulation by anti-IgM (Fig. 2b). These data indicate that cross-linking of cell-bound antigen is sufficient to induce desensitization in the absence of a change in $[Ca^{++}]_i$. Furthermore, because a low dose of antigen was used, it is possible that cross-linking of only a portion of sIgM molecules is

**Antigen
concentration**

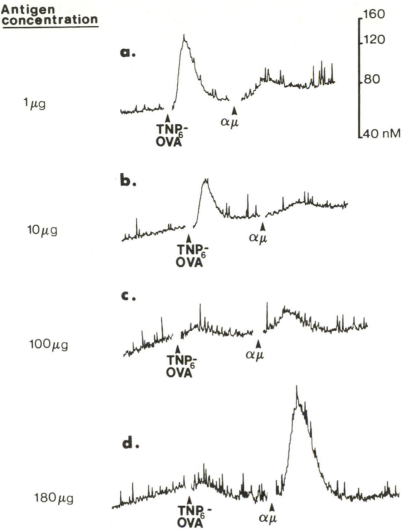

Figure 1. Homologous desensitization by antigen only occurs at low concentration. Transfected 7.9 cells were reacted with 1–180 μg/ml of TNP$_6$-OVA, followed by 15 μg/ml of purified goat anti-mouse IgM ($\alpha\mu$). The high (180 μg/ml) dose of TNP$_6$-OVA was ineffective at inducing desensitization in 7.9 cells (d).

required for desensitization. When high doses of antigen were tested, it was found that ≥ 180 μg/ml TNP$_6$-OVA did not lead to significant changes in [Ca^{++}]$_i$. In addition, we could find no evidence for desensitization (A.L. Lazarus et al., in prep.). The simplest conclusion is that although antigen probably bound to the cell, the conformation of the bound antigen was unable to stimulate a [Ca^{++}]$_i$ response or the process required for desensitization. We propose that in this TNP-specific B-cell system, productive antigen-sIgM interaction closely resembles a "precipitin reaction." Both low and high doses of antigen lie beyond the equivalence zone, do not cross-link sIgM, and do not give rise to a change in [Ca^{++}]$_i$. For this reason, low and high doses of antigen may not be effective in B-cell activation and could lead to B-cell unresponsiveness. Thus, our findings on the relationship between antigen concentration and antigen-induced B-cell sIg-mediated desensitization may have important implications toward under-

standing low- and high-dose antigen-induced B-cell tolerance.

Sites of Antigen Processing in a B-cell APC

Apart from the binding of an antigen to its specific sIg receptor on a B cell, it has been suggested that the binding of an antigen to other B-cell membrane components may enhance its processing prior to internalization and further processing in an intracellular compartment (Chain et al. 1988); i.e., an antigen may be processed both at the plasma membrane and intracellularly (Chain et al. 1988; Werdelin et al. 1988). However, the issue of whether multiple sites of processing of an antigen by a B-cell APC exist has still not been clearly resolved. We will review three sets of experiments conducted to test this possibility and to obtain further information on the cell biology of antigen processing by a B-cell APC.

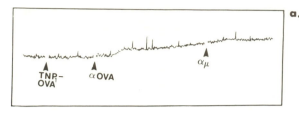

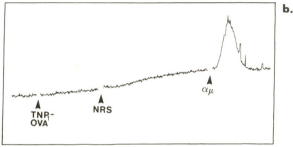

Figure 2. Cross-linking of membrane-bound antigen results in desensitization in 7.9 cells. Transfected 7.9 cells were reacted with 2.5 μg/ml of TNP-OVA containing <1 mole TNP/mole OVA (TNP$_1$-OVA), followed by a 1/100 dilution of either rabbit anti-OVA (αOVA) (a) or NRS (b). Both sets of cells were then reacted with 15 μg/ml of purified goat anti-mouse IgM (αμ). Although cross-linking of the TNP$_1$-OVA did not result in a [Ca^{++}]$_i$ signal, desensitization was achieved in these cells (a).

First, to determine if an antigen is internalized, processed, and recycled to the cell surface of an APC for presentation to T cells, we carried out an ultrastructural analysis of this pathway by following the kinetics and route of internalization and recycling of gold-labeled antigens in the TA3 mouse B-cell lymphoma APC (Lin et al. 1987). The antigens used were pork insulin (PI), a desoctyl peptide of PI that does not bind to the insulin receptor, myoglobin and apomyoglobin. Gold particles of 17 mM in diameter were used. The antigen/gold conjugates retained much of their T-cell immunogenicity. Our transmission electron micrographs demonstrated that each conjugate binds to the cell surface and is then internalized by 1 hour into several different types of endosomes, including pinocytic, phagocytic, and clear vesicles. The antigens are then transported in succession from these vesicles to the Golgi and post-Golgi membrane-associated vesicles and, finally, to the cell surface. Whereas about 50% of the insulin conjugates reappeared on the cell surface by 4 hours, it was apparent that more time was required for the return of the myoglobin conjugates to the cell surface. Because free gold particles did not follow this route, the pathway observed appeared to be antigen dependent and may represent a pathway by which antigen is internalized, processed, and recycled to the cell surface. However, we were unable to prove formally that the pathway we observed by electron microscopy is the functional pathway for processing and presentation.

Second, to attempt to identify such a functional pathway, we adopted a biochemical approach to study the kinetics, cellular sites of production, structure, and immunogenicity of insulin peptides formed in situ by B cells. A protocol was devised to examine the appearance of immunogenic insulin peptides in different compartments of TA3 B-cell APCs. TA3 cells were cultured for 1 hour at 4°C and then at various times ranging from 0 to 4 hours at 37°C with a physiological concentration (10^{-9} M) of HI ^{125}I-labeled at either A14 Tyr or B26 Tyr. Fractionation of TA3 cells into their intracellular, plasma-membrane-associated, and intracellular compartments, coupled with the use of HPLC, amino acid composition, and amino-terminal amino acid sequencing, enabled us to analyze several peptides derived from each compartment, as described previously (Delovitch et al. 1988; Semple et al. 1989). One HI peptide found in all three compartments is composed of residues A1-A14 disulfide-linked to B7-B26 (A1-A14/B7-B26). The presence of this peptide in the extracellular compartment likely resulted from digestion of HI by an enzyme(s) released from the APC. Extracellular processing of ^{125}I-labeled HI was inhibited completely by unlabeled HI and N-ethylmaleimide, an inhibitor of a previously described insulin-specific proteinase (Duckworth and Kitabchi 1981), partially by lysozyme but not by bovine serum albumin (BSA) or OVA. The processing of HI at both the plasma membrane and intracellularly was inhibited by chloroquine, monensin, and NH$_4$Cl, suggesting that both intracellular pH changes and endocytic and exocytic events may be required for these compartments to process insulin. Kinetic analyses revealed that the processing of insulin into the A1-A14/B7-B26 peptide is first detected by 15 minutes at the plasma membrane, by 30 minutes intracellularly, and, finally, by 60 minutes in the extracellular compartment. This peptide, when purified in an unlabeled form and in a sufficient quantity from the extracellular compartment, was immunogenic for PI/I-A^d-specific T cells; PI and HI A1-A14/B7-B26 peptides are identical in amino acid sequence and can be used interchangeably to assay their capacity to stimulate interleukin 2 (IL-2) secretion by PI/I-A^d-specific T cells. However, this peptide could not be presented efficiently to PI/I-A^d-reactive T cells by either glutaraldehyde-fixed TA3 APCs or planar membranes containing I-A^d molecules (Semple et al. 1989), suggesting that the A1-A14/B7-B26 peptide requires further processing to bind to an MHC class II molecule. Nonetheless, this set of data indicates that the processing of a soluble protein antigen such as insulin by a B-cell APC into an immunogenic peptide can occur at several cellular sites and that processing of insulin at the plasma membrane precedes that which takes place both intracellularly and extracellularly.

To determine the relevance of these sites of antigen processing to antigen presentation, we reasoned that it was necessary to assay whether insulin peptides formed at these cellular sites can associate with MHC class II molecules. In a third series of experiments, we used photoaffinity labeling and subcellular fractionation to identify the sites of formation of insulin peptide/MHC class II complexes in B-cell APCs. TA3 cells were incubated for various times from 1 minute to 1 hour, with radioiodinated photoreactive antigen prepared by derivatization of B29 Lys of beef insulin with N-[4-(4'-azido-3'-[^{125}I]iodophenylazo) benzoyl]-3-aminopropyl-N'-oxy-succinimide (Phillips et al. 1986), photocross-linked, washed, disrupted, and separated into subcellular fractions by discontinuous sucrose gradient centrifugation, as reported previously (Delovitch et al. 1988). MHC class II/insulin peptide formation in each subcellular membrane fraction was analyzed by SDS-PAGE. We found that insulin had to be processed to bind to MHC class II molecules under these conditions (observations of M.L. Phillips; see Delovitch et al. 1988). Binding of insulin to MHC class II molecules occurred within 1 minute of exposure of the cells to the antigen. Both at this time and at subsequent times (5 and 25 min), these MHC class II/insulin peptide complexes were located in fractions enriched in plasma membrane and in endosomes that could not be well resolved from plasma membrane. No such complexes were found in fractions containing Golgi or lysosomes.

On the basis of the above three sets of data that describe the kinetics, sites of internalization, recycling, processing into immunogenic peptides, and peptide/MHC complex formation of insulin in TA3 B cells, we have proposed a model for the pathway of processing and presentation of insulin by an antigen-nonspecific

B-cell APC (Fig. 3). Because insulin peptides can be found in the plasma membrane compartment and can associate with MHC class II at this cellular site rather soon after the exposure of TA3 cells to insulin, we propose that insulin can be processed by a membrane-bound proteinase(s) (antigen-degrading enzyme) into peptides that bind cell-surface-associated MHC class II molecules (Fig. 3, steps 1–3). Such peptide/MHC complexes may be internalized by pinocytosis (Fig. 3, steps 4 and 5). Alternatively, at step 5, antigen that was not degraded at the plasma membrane may be cointernalized with the antigen-degrading enzyme into an endosome, which may or may not require acidification to promote enzyme activity. Once activated, this enzyme degrades the antigen into fragments, some of which may be transported to other cellular sites to assume a particular function or otherwise be routed to a lysosome for complete degradation into amino acids. The endosomes formed at step 5 might fuse to give rise to another endosome (step 6), where preexisting peptide/MHC and antigen enzyme complexes may be dissociated and new complexes formed after additional processing of the antigen. Endosomes containing such complexes might then return to and fuse with the plasma membrane, ultimately allowing for the expression of various peptide/MHC class II (Ia) complexes at the cell surface (steps 7–9).

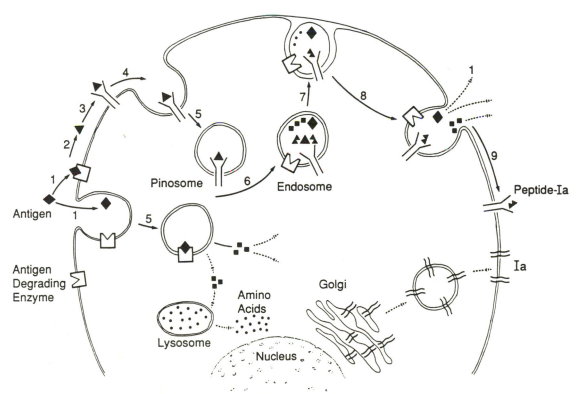

Figure 3. Model for the pathway of processing and presentation of an antigen by an antigen-nonspecific B-cell APC. Steps 1–4 demonstrate that the binding and processing of an antigen and the formation of peptide/MHC complexes can occur at the plasma membrane. Steps 5–9 illustrate those events of antigen processing that occur intracellularly in endosomes and ultimately lead to the surface expression of peptide/Ia complexes. Our studies suggest that insulin is processed both at the plasma membrane and in early endosomes by an IDE and that insulin peptide/MHC class II complexes are formed at both of these sites and not in the Golgi compartment.

It should be emphasized that this is a minimal model that may exclude some important and controversial features. First, note that in the case of a hormonal antigen such as insulin, an interaction between insulin and its surface receptor may be expected to have a role in the internalization and processing of insulin (Duckworth 1988). However, our photoaffinity labeling studies have failed to detect the binding of insulin to insulin receptors on TA3 cells under the conditions used (Phillips et al. 1986; Delovitch et al. 1988), perhaps due to the finding that TA3 cells express about 100-fold fewer insulin receptors than do adipocytes (M. Moule and M.L. Phillips, unpubl.). In addition, we and others have found that many insulin peptides that lack the insulin receptor binding site but require further processing for presentation to T cells stimulate IL-2 secretion by insulin-specific T cells. Thus, insulin-insulin receptor interactions may not play a major role in the proposed endocytic pathway that generates immunogenic insulin peptides. Consequently, we have omitted the insulin receptor from this model. Note also that despite the facts that there is a reservoir of newly synthesized Ia molecules that appear in the Golgi owing to the 3 hours required for the transport of these molecules from the Golgi to the cell surface (Blum and Cresswell 1988) and that this reservoir of Ia would be expected to provide an excellent site to capture antigen peptides for cotransport back to the cell surface, our results have not provided any evidence for the formation of complexes between insulin peptides and Golgi-associated MHC class II molecules. Although this result is consistent with the finding that intracellular Ia in TA3 cells is largely in a recycling pool derived from the plasma membrane by endocytosis (Harding et al. 1988), and this would disfavor the association of peptides with newly synthesized MHC class II molecules, we cannot eliminate the possibility that some peptides of antigens other than insulin do bind to MHC class II molecules (either recycled or synthesized de novo) located in the Golgi. It is also possible that some endosomes usually found in the *trans*-Golgi network exchange compartments after cell disruption and cosediment with fractions enriched in plasma membrane. However, the relative absence of any galactosyl transferase Golgi enzyme marker activity in our isolated fraction of TA3 plasma membrane (Delovitch et al. 1988) renders this possibility unlikely.

Proteolysis of Insulin by the IDE into Immunogenic Peptides

One of the main aims in the study of antigen processing is the identification of an enzyme(s) in an APC that digests a given antigen into immunogenic peptides that bind to MHC class II molecules and are presented to T cells. This is a challenging task, as it is estimated that $\leq 1\%$ of native antigen molecules are converted into immunogenic peptides, and thus the bulk of internalized antigen is normally degraded into nonstimulatory fragments (Unanue 1984).

In the case of insulin, however, considerable evidence obtained with nonlymphoid cells suggests that it is degraded predominantly by a relatively insulin-specific proteinase, termed IDE (Shii and Roth 1986; Duckworth 1988). IDE cleaves glucagon and insulin growth factor (IGF)-II at one-tenth the rate of insulin and does not cleave IGF-I or proinsulin (Misbin and Almira 1989). The monomer of IDE is a protein of M_r 110,000 that binds avidly to insulin ($K_d = 100$ nM) and functions as a neutral thiol metalloproteinase with a pH optimum ranging from about 6 to 7, depending on the cell type. Sulfhydryl inhibitors such as N-ethylmaleimide, which inhibit insulin degradation, also inhibit IDE activity. IDE activity is not inhibitable by leupeptin, pepstatin, and antipain. Interestingly, a portion ($\leq 10\%$) of IDE activity is associated with the plasma membrane of various cell types, including B lymphocytes (Yaso et al. 1987), whereas the bulk of IDE activity in B cells is found intracellularly (Shii and Roth 1986). Recent studies of insulin degradation in hepatocytes provide strong support for an endosomal location of IDE in these cells (Hamel et al. 1988).

It is thus of interest to investigate whether IDE represents the antigen-degrading enzyme proposed in Figure 3 that is responsible for the processing of insulin by a B-cell APC into peptides that bind to MHC class II molecules. TA3 B cells (2×10^6) were incubated with 2 μCi of ^{125}I-labeled HI (1 μCi each of HI ^{125}I-labeled at either A14 Tyr or B26 Tyr) for 1 hour at 4°C and then for either 0 or 1 hour at 37°C. The extracellular cell supernatants obtained after Percoll gradient centrifugation were precipitated with 10% TCA, cleared by ultracentrifugation, and applied to an Altex reversed-phase analytical C18 HPLC column equilibrated with 5 mM sodium phosphate. Peptides were eluted with an acetonitrile/phosphate (80:20 v/v) gradient (0–90% in 45 min), 1-ml fractions were collected, and their radioactivity was determined. Four main radioactive peptides were found to be released after 60 minutes into the extracellular compartment (Fig. 4a; for details, see Delovitch et al. 1988; Semple et al. 1989). Peptide 1 is the A1-A14/B7-B26 peptide referred to earlier in this paper, and peptide 2 consists of A7-A11 disulfide-linked to B7-B26 (A7-A11/B7-B26). The compositions of peptides 3 and 4 are unknown, but they contain residue B26. Preincubation of 2×10^6 TA3 cells for 1 hour at 37°C with the 9B12 anti-IDE monoclonal antibody prior to exposure of the cells to ^{125}I-labeled HI, as in Figure 4a, resulted in virtually complete inhibition of insulin processing, as evidenced by the relative absence of ^{125}I-labeled HI peptides 1–4 (Fig. 4b). Because 9B12 does not bind to the catalytic site of IDE and does not interfere with insulin binding of IDE (Shii and Roth 1986), it is possible that the inhibition of insulin processing by 9B12 is due to an alteration of normal enzyme trafficking that reduces the net amount of IDE available for the processing of insulin. Little, if any, reduction in insulin processing was obtained using VC6, a control monoclonal antibody specific for an idiotype of the 11-5 anti-I-A^k monoclonal antibody.

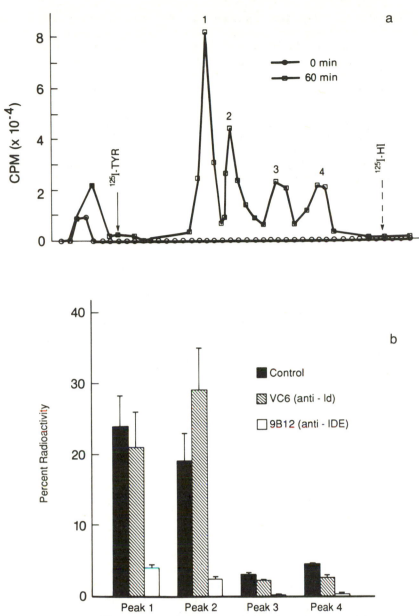

Figure 4. (*a*) HPLC chromatogram of ^{125}I-labeled HI peptides 1–4, derived from the extracellular compartment of TA3 B cells. TCA-soluble ^{125}I-labeled HI peptides obtained from the extracellular compartment after incubation of ^{125}I-labeled HI with TA3 APC for 1 hr at 4°C and then either 0 min (open circle) or 60 min (open box) at 37°C were resolved on a C18 reversed-phase HPLC column, as described previously (Semple et al. 1989). The positions of elution of ^{125}I-labeled tyrosine and ^{125}I-labeled HI are shown. (*b*) Inhibition of processing of insulin by anti-IDE. TA3 B cells were incubated as above with ^{125}I-labeled HI for 60 min at 37°C in the absence (solid bar) or presence of the VC6 anti-idiotype (hatched box) or 9B12 anti-IDE (open bar) MAbs. TCA-soluble ^{125}I-labeled HI peptides were separated by HPLC as above. Data from two independent experiments are expressed as the percent ± s.e.m. of total ^{125}I-radioactivity (cpm) loaded onto the C18 column. The detection of peptides 1–4 was inhibited by treatment of TA3 APC with anti-IDE.

Preliminary experiments also indicate that reactivity of TA3 cells with the 9B12 MAb and a fluoresceinated goat anti-mouse IgG resulted in the specific immunofluorescent staining of these B cells (J.W. Semple, unpubl.). These data suggest that IDE is present on the plasma membrane of TA3 B cells.

We reported previously that the processing of insulin by IDE generates insulin peptides that are capable of binding to MHC class II molecules on TA3 plasma

membranes (Delovitch et al. 1988), but we were unable to prove whether IDE alone or in conjunction with another TA3 cell enzyme(s) was responsible for the generation of these peptides. Thus, we compared the insulin peptides generated by the treatment of insulin with IDE alone in vitro to those insulin peptides derived by the proteolysis of insulin by TA3 APC in situ. Very similar HPLC profiles were obtained by incubation for 18 hours at 37°C of unlabeled HI with either

IDE (Fig. 5b) or TA3 APC (Fig. 5d). The peptides shown in Figure 5d are those derived from the extracellular compartment of TA3 cells. Only relatively few (≤20%) peptides (shaded peaks) differ between these two profiles, indicating that IDE is probably a major enzyme that processes insulin in TA3 cells.

The 20 unlabeled insulin peptides produced by IDE digestion were purified extensively by HPLC and characterized by amino acid analyses. These analyses enabled us to deduce the sites of cleavage of insulin by IDE (Fig. 6). IDE was reported previously to cleave ^{125}I-labeled insulin on the carboxyl side of residues A13 and A14 of the A chain and residues B9, B10, B14, B24, and B25 of the B chain (Duckworth et al. 1987, 1988). We have confirmed these sites using unlabeled HI and have identified several additional sites located after residues A11 and A17 of the A chain and residues B4, B12, B13, B15, B18, B20, B26, and B27 of the B chain. A number of interesting points emerge from these analyses. First, most of the major sites of cleavage of insulin by IDE are located in the hydrophobic core of insulin. Thus, processing of insulin by IDE might enable hydrophobic regions of insulin, which are normally buried within the native conformation of the water-soluble molecule to maximize its stability in water, to now be exposed and interact with MHC class II molecules and perhaps other membrane components

on the surface of an APC. The notion that an essential feature of antigen processing is the exposure of critical hydrophobic sites was discussed in previous reviews (Allen et al. 1987; Berzofsky et al. 1988). Second, the majority of the A- and B-chain IDE cleavage sites are in close physical proximity according to the three-dimensional structure of insulin, suggesting that the enzyme may recognize a specific conformational region (e.g., hydrophobic) in the intact molecule. The action of IDE therefore differs from that of many other types of proteinases that hydrolyze their substrates at bonds between defined residues located in hydrophobic, as well as more accessible hydrophilic, regions. For example, insulin can be cleaved at multiple sites by elastase, pepsin, and chymotrypsin, but none of these enzymes possess a high affinity or specificity for insulin and they are not restricted in their activity to a hydrophobic region of insulin. Presumably, the folding of the insulin molecule dictates its apparent preference and specificity for cleavage by IDE. Third, although IDE also cleaves insulin at many sites, most of these sites are located on the B chain. Unlike the other enzymes mentioned above, IDE generally leaves the A1-A14 peptide containing the A-loop region (A6-A11) intact. The A-loop region constitutes an immunodominant epitope that is recognized by an insulin-specific TCR (Delovitch et al. 1988). Moreover, as a result of IDE

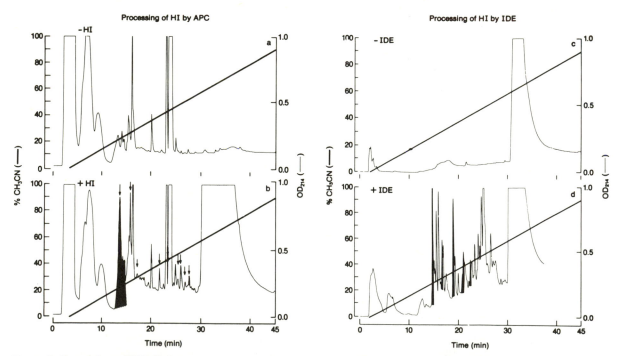

Figure 5. Comparison of HPLC chromatograms of insulin peptides processed either in situ by TA3 APC or in vitro by IDE. TA3 cells (3×10^6/ml) were incubated for 18 hr at 37°C in serum-free medium in the absence (a) or presence (b) of 0.5 mg/ml unlabeled HI. The TCA-soluble extracellular supernatants of these mixtures were chromatographed on a C18 HPLC column, as described in Fig. 4. Arrows in b indicate HI-derived peptides not observed in the control chromatogram shown in a. HI (0.5 mg/ml) was digested in vitro for 18 hr at 37°C with protein A–Sepharose beads conjugated with either the control VC6 MAb (−IDE) (c) or the anti-IDE 9B12 MAb (+IDE) (d), and the HI peptides were separated by HPLC, as outlined above. An erythrocyte lysate, used as a source of IDE, was previously passed through both sets of beads, and IDE was retained in an active form only by the 9B12-containing beads. Shaded peaks in b and d represent those peptides that differ between the two chromatograms. About 80% of the peptides in b co-elute with those seen in d. Peptides eluting at 26 min in b and at 17 min in d are the A1-A14/B1-B9 and A1-A14/B7-B26 peptides, respectively.

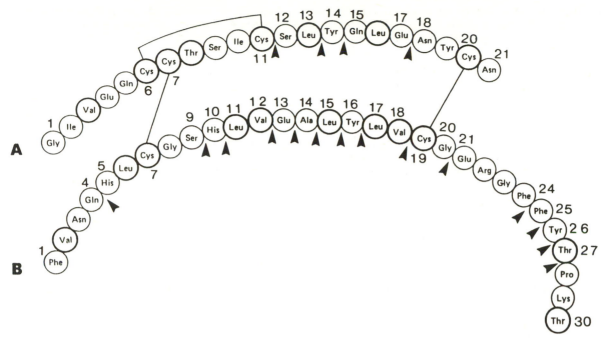

Figure 6. Deduced sites of cleavage of HI by human IDE. The IDE cleavage sites on the carboxyl side of various HI A- and B-chain residues are indicated by arrowheads.

cleavage, the A-loop region and the A1-A14 peptide, in particular, more often than not tend to be disulfide-linked to various B-chain residues (e.g., B1-B9, B5-B9, etc.) in heterodimeric insulin peptides. The formation of such heterodimeric peptides might result from the proposed sequence of sequential stages of processing of insulin (Duckworth 1988). A-chain residues seem to be more resistant to IDE cleavage than B-chain residues. B-chain residues located in the insulin receptor-binding site (B24-B27) are removed first upon digestion of insulin with IDE. The remainder of the molecule can act as an intermediate substrate of IDE action. Several such intermediates containing the A-loop region disulfide-linked to different B-chain residues may exist. This could potentially give rise to many A-loop-containing heterodimeric disulfide-linked insulin peptides that are similar but nonidentical in structure.

If heterodimeric insulin peptides generated by IDE digestion are able to bind to MHC class II molecules with different avidity and specificity, they could play a role in the development of the insulin-specific T-cell repertoire of an individual. This then raises the question of whether IDE actually digests insulin into peptides that bind to MHC class II molecules and are presented to T cells. We have accumulated considerable evidence that supports, but does not yet formally prove, this conclusion (Delovitch et al. 1988). The known sites of processing of insulin by IDE after residues B15, B16, and B26 coincide with the sites of enzymatic cleavage identified in the immunogenic A1-A14/B7-B15, A1-A14/B1-B16, and A1-A14/B7-B26 peptides that we have characterized. Processing of insulin by IDE is required to generate insulin peptides that are capable of binding to MHC class II antigens.

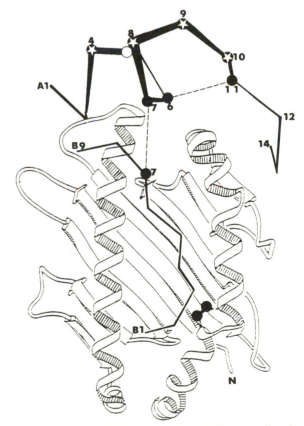

Figure 7. Proposed model of binding of the heterodimeric disulfide-linked insulin peptide A1-A14/B1-B9 to an MHC class II molecule. This model indicates that B-chain residues B1-B9 fit in the MHC class II groove and that A-chain residues A1-A14 extend beyond the groove. This may permit residues A4, A8, A9, and A10 (star) to bind to the TCR. Closed circle indicates Cys residue.

The photocross-linking of insulin to MHC class II molecules is inhibitable by intact B chain and various peptides containing amino-terminal, but not carboxy-terminal, B-chain residues. Neither intact A chain and peptide A1-A14 nor peptides containing A-chain carboxy-terminal residues inhibit this binding. This suggests that B-chain residues of disulfide-linked heterodimeric insulin peptides bind in the groove of an MHC class II molecule and the A-chain residues bind to the TCR. Because we found that A1-A14/B1-B9 is an insulin peptide that is produced with maximum yield upon IDE digestion of insulin (see Fig. 6b, fraction at 26 min), and if our current studies reveal that this peptide is a minimal processed insulin peptide that does not require further processing for presentation to T cells, we speculate that A1-A14/B1-B9 could bind to an MHC class II molecule and TCR as shown in Figure 7. Residues B1-B9 may fit into the MHC class II groove. Residues A4, A8, A9, and A10, which are variable between different mammalian insulins, may bind to the TCR. This configuration is compatible with a computer-generated three-dimensional model (P. Bjorkman, pers. comm.), which suggests that if the B-chain residues are accommodated in the groove of the MHC molecule, then the A-chain residues and the A-loop, in particular, would have to extend beyond the groove.

Our future studies will be devoted to further testing this model and to determining the nature of a minimal insulin T-cell determinant produced in vivo. This may be more easily achieved by determining which peptides of a metabolically labeled recombinant HI (Semple et al. 1988) are produced in various APCs in vivo. Of particular interest will be the study of insulin processing by APCs present in the thymus, since these results will have important bearing on the shaping of the T-cell repertoire during T-cell ontogeny.

ACKNOWLEDGMENTS

We thank Rosa Jara and Fernanda Teodoro for their excellent assistance with the preparation of this manuscript. We also extend special thanks to Andrew Crow, Pat Champagne, Janet Ellis, and Edwin Speck for their superb technical assistance. A.H.L. was the recipient of a postdoctoral fellowship from Les Fonds de la Recherche en Santé du Québec. J.W.S. was the recipient of a postdoctoral fellowship from Diabetes Canada. M.L.P. was supported by the University of Toronto, Banting and Best Diabetes Center. This work was supported, in part, by grants from the Medical Research Council of Canada, National Cancer Institute of Canada, and Canadian Diabetes Association.

REFERENCES

Allen, P.M., B.P. Babbitt, and E.R. Unanue. 1987. T cell recognition of lysozyme: The biochemical basis of presentation. *Immunol. Rev.* **98:** 71.

Bernard, N.F., P.C. Reid, M.L. Phillips, and T.L. Delovitch. 1988a. Correlation of presentation of insulin with surface I-A^d and Aα and Aβ mRNA expression by cloned B lymphoma hybridoma variants. *Immunol. Lett.* **19:** 143.

Bernard, N.F., P. Naquet, M. Watanabe, N. Hozumi, and T.L. Delovitch. 1988b. Possible role for specific surface immunoglobulin in antigen presentation. In *Antigen presenting cells: Diversity, differentiation, and regulation* (ed. L. Schook and J. Tew), p. 291. Alan R. Liss, New York.

Berzofsky, J.A., S.J. Brett, H.Z. Streicher, and H. Takahashi. 1988. Antigen processing for presentation to T lymphocytes: Function, mechanisms, and implications for the T cell repertoire. *Immunol. Rev.* **106:** 5.

Blum, J.S. and P. Cresswell. 1988. Role for intracellular proteases in the processing and transport of class II HLA antigens. *Proc. Natl. Acad. Sci.* **85:** 3975.

Chain, B.M., P.M. Kaye, and M.A. Shaw. 1988. The biochemistry and cell biology of antigen processing. *Immunol. Rev.* **106:** 33.

Delovitch, T.L., J.W. Semple, P. Naquet, N.F. Bernard, J. Ellis, P. Champagne, and M.L. Phillips. 1988. Pathways of processing of insulin by antigen-presenting cells. *Immunol. Rev.* **106:** 195.

Duckworth, W.C. 1988. Insulin degradation: Mechanisms, products and significance. *Endocrine Rev.* **9:** 319.

Duckworth, W.C. and A.E. Kitabchi. 1981. Insulin metabolism and degradation. *Endocrine Rev.* **2:** 210.

Duckworth, W.C., F.G. Hamel, J.J. Liepnicks, D.E. Peavy, M.P. Ryan, M.A. Hermodson, and B.H. Frank. 1987. Identification of A chain cleavage sites in intact insulin produced by insulin protease and isolated hepatocytes. *Biochem. Biophys. Res. Commun.* **147:** 615.

Duckworth, W.C., F.G. Hamel, D.E. Peavy, J.J. Liepnicks, M.P. Ryan, M.A. Hermodson, and B.H. Frank. 1988. Degradation products of insulin generated by hepatocytes and by insulin protease. *J. Biol. Chem.* **263:** 1826.

Grynkiewics, G., M. Poenie, and R.Y. Tsien. 1985. A new generation of Ca^{2+} indicators with greatly improved fluorescence properties. *J. Biol. Chem.* **260:** 3440.

Hamel, F.G., B. Posner, J.J.M. Bergeron, B.H. Frank, and W.C. Duckworth. 1988. Isolation of insulin degradation products from endosomes derived from intact rat liver. *J. Biol. Chem.* **263:** 6703.

Harding, C.V., F. Leyva-Cobian, and E.R. Unanue. 1988. Mechanisms of antigen processing. *Immunol. Rev.* **106:** 77.

Lanzavecchia, A. 1987. Antigen uptake and accumulation in antigen-specific B cells. *Immunol. Rev.* **99:** 39.

Lin, J., J.A. Berzofsky, and T.L. Delovitch. 1987. Ultrastructural study of internalization and recycling of antigen by antigen presenting cells. *J. Mol. Cell. Immunol.* **3:** 321.

Misbin, R.I. and E. Almira. 1989. Degradation of insulin and insulin-like growth factors by enzyme purified from human erythrocytes. Comparison of degradation products observed with A14 and B26-[^{125}I]monoiodo insulin. *Diabetes* **38:** 152.

Phillips, M.L., J.F. Harris, and T.L. Delovitch. 1984. Idiotypic analysis of anti-I-A^k monoclonal antibodies. I. Production and characterization of syngeneic anti-idiotypic mAb against an anti-I-A^k mAb. *J. Immunol.* **135:** 2587.

Phillips, M.L., C.C. Yip, E.M. Shevach, and T.L. Delovitch. 1986. Photoaffinity labeling demonstrates binding between Ia molecules and nominal antigen or antigen presenting cells. *Proc. Natl. Acad. Sci.* **83:** 5634.

Pierce, S.K., J.F. Morris, M.J. Grusby, P. Kaumaya, A. Van Buskirk, M. Srinivasan, B. Crump, and L.A. Smolenski. 1988. Antigen-presenting function of B lymphocytes. *Immunol. Rev.* **106:** 149.

Semple, J.W., S.A. Cockle, and T.L. Delovitch. 1988. Purification and characterization of radiolabeled human insulin from *E. coli*. Kinetics of processing by antigen presenting cells. *Mol. Immunol.* **25:** 1291.

Semple, J.W., J. Ellis, and T.L. Delovitch. 1989. Processing and presentation of insulin. II. Evidence for intracellular, plasma membrane-associated and extracellular degradation of human insulin by antigen-presenting B cells. *J. Immunol.* **142:** 4184.

Shii, K. and R.A. Roth. 1986. Inhibition of insulin degradation by hepatoma cells after microinjections of monoclonal antibodies to a specific cytosolic protease. *Proc. Natl. Acad. Sci.* **83:** 4147.

Unanue, E.R. 1984. Antigen-presenting function of the macrophages. *Annu. Rev. Immunol.* **2:** 395.

Werdelin, O., S. Mouritsen, B. Laub-Petersen, A. Sette, and S. Buus. 1988. Facts on the fragmentation of antigens in presenting cells, on the association of antigen fragments with MHC molecules in cell-free systems, and speculation on the cell biology of antigen processing. *Immunol. Rev.* **106:** 181.

Yaso, S., K. Yokono, J. Hari, K. Yonezawa, K. Shii, and S. Baba. 1987. Possible role of cell surface insulin degrading enzyme in cultured human lymphocytes. *Diabetologia* **30:** 27.

Processing of Immunoglobulin-associated Antigen in B Lymphocytes

C. Watts, M.A. West, P.A. Reid, and H.W. Davidson
Department of Biochemistry, Medical Sciences Institute, University of Dundee, DD1 4HN, United Kingdom

For most antigens presented in association with class II major histocompatibility complex (MHC) molecules, an intracellular processing step is required to produce a suitable ligand for binding to the class II MHC glycoproteins and, as a complex, to the T-cell receptor. The available evidence strongly suggests that following endocytosis, processing and unfolding take place in intracellular compartments and that suitable MHC/peptide complexes are then returned to the cell surface. Using T cells to assay for the appearance of processed determinants, it has been established that these antigen-processing events take approximately 1 hour and are sensitive to chloroquine and fixation of the antigen-presenting cells (APCs) and to inhibitors of endosomal/lysosomal proteinases (Ziegler and Unanue 1982; Lanzavecchia 1985; Buus and Werdelin 1986).

Analysis of MHC glycoproteins at the structural level (Bjorkman et al. 1987) and at the biochemical level (Buus et al. 1988) reveals the presumptive peptide products of antigen processing, whereas other work demonstrates that fragmented antigen or appropriate synthetic peptides can interact directly with MHC glycoproteins in vitro (Babbitt et al. 1985; Buus et al. 1986; Chen and Parham 1989) and in vivo (Shimonkevitz et al. 1983; Townsend et al. 1986), thereby bypassing the requirement for processing. These discoveries are powerfully suggestive of a sequence of events called "antigen processing" but MHC-bound peptides constitute the end point of the process and, in fact, we have little information on what actually happens to protein antigens during processing.

Several striking observations underline how important these processing steps are for class-II-restricted antigen presentation. For example, the T-cell response to a native protein antigen is often dominated by several determinants. However, T cells able to recognize other determinants are present in the repertoire because they can be readily elicited by peptide immunogens (see, e.g, Brett et al. 1988). It seems that the processing of the native antigen or the context in which a particular T-cell epitope is found, or the presence or absence of allelic forms of MHC other than that directly involved in presentation, can, individually or in combination, affect the efficiency of presentation of particular determinants (for review, see Gammon et al. 1987). Other work suggests that when APCs are engaged in processing antigen/immunoglobulin complex-

es, the range of T-cell determinants presented appears to be influenced by the immunoglobulin specificities involved. From the standpoint of the B-cell repertoire, it seems that "help" for the production of particular antibody specificities is more readily provided by some T-cell specificities than others (Manca et al. 1985, 1988; Ozaki and Berzovsky 1987).

Taken together, these findings suggest that factors influencing the course of antigen processing play a major role in determining which specificities in the repertoire become established and amplified. These factors may be particularly important in the context of vaccine design where, to be effective, primary immunogens must induce T-cell specificities that will be recalled following processing of the natural infectious agent.

We have made the assumption that an analysis of the processing of exogenous antigen will be facilitated when the input of native antigen consists of a single population of molecules bound to a defined cell-surface receptor, e.g., the immunoglobulin receptor on B lymphocytes. These conditions make it possible to follow the fate of antigen much as the fate of, for example, transferrin, low-density lipoproteins, or virus particles was followed in studies that first defined the receptor-mediated endocytotic pathway (for reviews, see Helenius et al. 1983; Goldstein et al. 1985; Wileman et al. 1985). Here, we review recent experiments on the endocytosis and processing of monovalent antigen by antigen-specific Epstein-Barr virus (EBV)-transformed B-cell clones (Lanzavecchia 1985; Watts and Davidson 1988; Davidson and Watts 1989).

METHODS

Methods relevant to the experiments described in this paper are outlined in the figure legends or can be found in Watts and Davidson (1988) and Davidson and Watts (1989).

RESULTS

Receptor-mediated Endocytosis of Antigen

In all of the experiments described here, cell-surface immunoglobulin (mIgG) receptors for the specific antigen under investigation (tetanus toxin) were saturated by incubating the various B-lymphoblastoid cell lines with 2–5 μg/ml ^{125}I-labeled tetanus toxin for 60–120 minutes at 0°C. The cells were washed free of unbound antigen and then incubated, generally at 37°C, for various time periods. At these times, two kinds of analyses were performed: (1) assessment of the redistribution of total radiolabel from its initial location on the cell surface to other cellular compartments and the external media, and (2) assessment of the fragmentation of specific antigen by SDS-gel electrophoresis.

Upon warming the cells to 37°C, antigen redistributed from the cell surface to an intracellular compartment, as judged by the fact that it could not be removed either by washing at low pH or by proteolysis. These treatments removed 90–95% of cell-surface antigen. Endocytosis of antigen proceeded without a lag, although the initial rates varied between 3% and 9% per minute of the initial antigen load, depending on the

particular B-cell clone (Fig. 1). The kinetics of endocytosis were independent of the number of receptors occupied (Fig. 2) and were observed for monovalent antigen, demonstrating that receptor cross-linking was not required. In Figure 3, tetanus toxoid–gold conjugates reveal that cell-surface-coated pits and vesicles appear to be responsible for the efficient endocytosis of antigen, which suggests that the membrane IgG expressed by these cells interacts either directly or indirectly with the assembly polypeptides (adaptins) which, together with clathrin, build up a coated pit (Pearse 1988). Moreover, the capacity to undergo endocytosis appears to be an intrinsic property of mIgG and not just of mIgG/antigen complexes because unoccupied receptors also undergo endocytosis (data not shown).

Recycling of Antigen

The kinetics of loss of labeled antigen from the cell surface were biphasic, resulting in a maximum of 40–60% (depending on the clone) of the initial antigen load becoming sequestered within the cells at the end of the phase of rapid redistribution (Fig. 1). After this point, antigen continued to be lost from the cell surface, but some 20–40 times slower than the initial rapid rate (Fig. 1). This can be explained, to a large extent, by the fact that antigen undergoing endocytosis recycles to the cell surface so that a steady state of endocytosis and recycling is established within 10–30 minutes (again depending on the clone) of endocytosis commencing. Evidence for such a steady state comes from experiments that either measure the rate of endocytosis of antigen still on the cell surface at time points after the

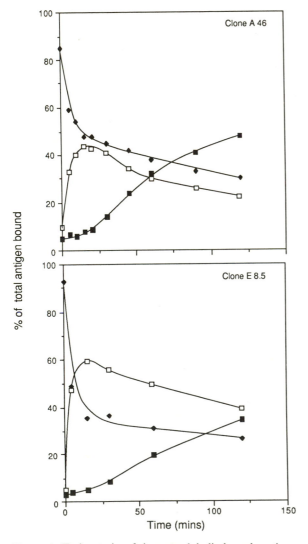

Figure 1. Endocytosis of immunoglobulin-bound antigen. Cells to which radiolabeled antigen had been bound at 0°C were incubated at 37°C for the indicated times. Radiolabel returned to the incubation medium (■), sequestered within the cells (□), and remaining on the cell surface (◆) was then assayed. (Reprinted, with permission, from Watts and Davidson 1988.)

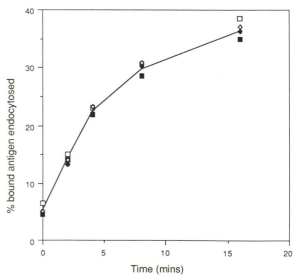

Figure 2. Kinetics of endocytosis of subsaturating monovalent antigen loads. Cells (clone A46) were preincubated with antigen concentrations (1×10^{-10} to 26×10^{-10} M) to achieve 7% (◇), 21% (■), 57% (◆), and 100% (□) occupancy of available receptors. The initial rates of antigen endocytosis were then assayed at 37°C. (Reprinted, with permission, from Watts and Davidson 1988.)

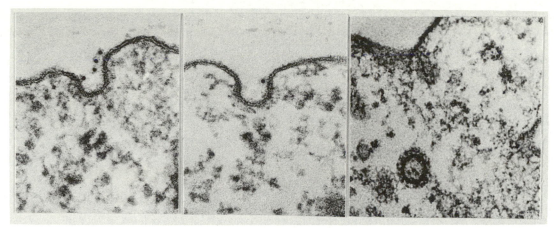

Figure 3. Antigen endocytosis through the coated pit/coated vesicle pathway. Monovalent tetanus toxoid was conjugated to 7 nm colloidal gold and incubated with clone 8.5 cells for 75 min at 0°C. After removing unbound antigen/gold complexes, the cells were incubated for 3 min at 37°C prior to fixation, embedding in Epon, and sectioning. Note that most gold particles (80–90%) were bound to uncoated regions of the plasma membrane.

initial rapid redistribution or measure directly the return to the surface of antigen having undergone endocytosis previously (Watts and Davidson 1988). It should be stressed that these experiments measure the cycling of intact antigen bound to mIg and not of MHC-bound processed antigen. The fact that a substantial proportion of the antigen that has undergone endocytosis is involved in a recycling process that appears to begin within minutes of endocytosis commencing, i.e., at a time when no degradation can be detected, argues against a significant contribution from processed MHC-associated antigen.

The B-cell receptor for specific antigen (mIgG) resembles other receptors (e.g., those for transferrin;

Watts 1985) in that it cycles constitutively, i.e., with or without ligand bound, and can return occupied to the cell surface. However, whereas apotransferrin dissociates at the cell surface when it encounters neutral pH (Dautry-Varsat et al. 1983; Klausner et al. 1983), antigen remains bound and subsequently undergoes re-endocytosis. Therefore, in contrast to, for example, the low-density lipoprotein receptor that returns unoccupied to the cell surface to be reused perhaps hundreds of times (Goldstein et al. 1985), mIgG may only be involved in the uptake of one or two molecules of antigen. Reuse of mIg is probably unnecessary in any case. The purpose of the B-cell immunoglobulin receptor for antigen is not to mediate wholesale antigen

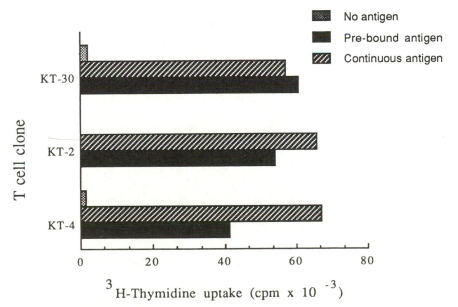

Figure 4. T-cell stimulation by a single receptor-bound pulse of antigen. B cells (clone 11.3) were incubated with 5 μg/ml tetanus toxoid of 0°C for 100 min. The cells were irradiated (4200 rads), washed to remove unbound antigen, and incubated with 2×10^4 tetanus-specific T cells in the presence or absence of 1 μg/ml tetanus toxin, as indicated. After 48 hr, [^{3}H]thymidine incorporation was measured, following a 16-hr pulse.

degradation but to permit the generation of processed determinants in sufficient number to recruit specific T-helper cells. In vitro T-cell stimulation assays using specific B cells as APCs demonstrate that B cells having antigen bound only to cell-surface immunoglobulin receptors can, following processing of this population, induce as effective a T-cell proliferation as can the same B cells cocultured with saturating amounts of antigen (Fig. 4). This holds true for many, although not all, B-cell/T-cell combinations when equal numbers of B and T cells are used (see also Lanzavecchia 1986; Roosnek et al. 1988). When antigen concentrations are well below those necessary to saturate cell-surface mIg receptors, it takes longer to capture sufficient antigen to achieve the same T-cell activation/recruitment (Lanzavecchia 1987).

The experiments described so far establish that B cells cause specific monovalent antigen to undergo endocytosis efficiently and that a considerable proportion of it is returned intact to the cell surface and then presumably undergoes re-endocytosis. The significance of this recycling pathway is not clear and may simply be a reflection of the fact that unoccupied receptors appear to follow a similar pathway and there is no easy means of diverting occupied receptors. However, an antibody/antigen complex of lower affinity might dissociate on being returned to the cell surface so there might be an element of selection imposed by this recycling process for those B cells expressing a higher affinity antibody whose interaction with antigen will withstand repeated recycling events.

Proteolytic Fragmentation of Antigen in B Cells

There is clearly an alternative to the recycling of intact antigen to the cell surface. After a lag of about 30 minutes, radiolabel begins to appear in the incubation medium and increases steadily over extended time courses (Fig. 1). At least 50% of this material cannot be precipitated with trichloroacetic acid (TCA), demonstrating that proteolysis of antigen is occurring in B cells. This release of TCA-soluble material into the medium can be blocked by chloroquine, by reducing the incubation temperature to 20°C (endocytosis still occurs, albeit more slowly), and is substantially inhibited by inhibitors of thiol proteinases such as leupeptin (Davidson and Watts 1989). Thus, the kinetics of antigen degradation and its susceptibility to inhibitors

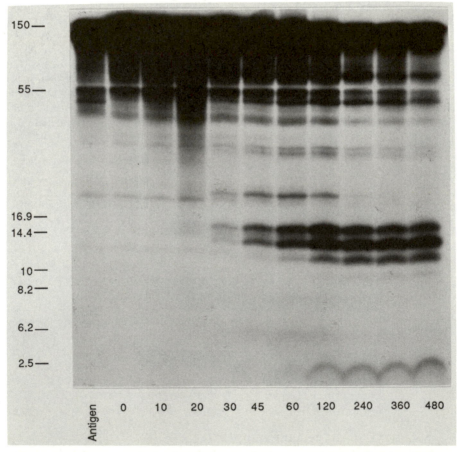

Figure 5. Fragmentation of antigen in specific B cells. Cells (clone 11.3) were preincubated with radioiodinated antigen for 2 hr at 0°C, washed, and incubated at 37°C for the indicated times (minutes). Aliquots (2×10^6 cells) were analyzed by SDS-gel electrophoresis and autoradiography. (*Left*) Molecular-weight standards. (Reprinted, with permission, from Davidson and Watts 1989.)

suggest (1) that it is occurring at some point along the endosome/lysosome pathway and (2) that it is likely to be part and parcel of the proteolytic process that gives rise to processed MHC-restricted antigen.

When B cells engaged in processing radioiodinated tetanus toxin were analyzed by SDS-gel electrophoresis, a clear pattern of fragmentation was observed. A typical experiment of this type is shown in Figure 5, where the fate of antigen bound to cell-surface mIgG on B-cell clone 11.3 has been followed. There was no detectable fragmentation of the 150-kD antigen during the first 30 minutes of incubation at 37°C, but distinct antigen fragments could be resolved on the gels thereafter. Some were rather short-lived, but others appeared either to accumulate or at least to reach a more or less steady-state level. After a 4-hour incubation period, approximately 75% of the starting antigen load had been returned to the medium, of which only one-third was TCA-precipitable. Of the antigen associated with the cells, about 10% was found on the cell surface and 15% within the cells. These antigen fragments were not observed in cells incubated at 20°C or in cells treated with chloroquine, whereas the thiol proteinase inhibitor leupeptin changed the fragmentation profile observed (Davidson and Watts 1989).

The antigen degraded by these cells might correspond to material dissociated from the immunoglobulin receptor and therefore not recycled but, instead, transported onward to a proteinase-containing compartment. Alternatively, antigen might be degraded still bound to its receptor. We obtained clear evidence for the latter possibility when we immunoprecipitated the mIg receptor from clone 11.3 cells engaged in antigen processing and found, somewhat to our surprise, that the observed antigen fragments were also precipitated (Davidson and Watts 1989). This finding demonstrated that the initial substrate for processing was the antigen/mIgG complex and suggested that the bound antigen fragments formed all or part of the epitope recognized by this antibody.

Epitope-directed Processing of Antigen

If the substrate offered to the processing system is the antigen/mIg complex, B cells with different epitope specificity might generate distinct fragmentation patterns. Two further experiments demonstrate that the nature of the antigen/immunoglobulin substrate undergoing endocytosis can influence the course of antigen processing dramatically.

We first examined the products of antigen processing in B-cell clones that had earlier been shown to have different epitope specificities (Lanzavecchia 1987; Watts and Davidson 1988; Demotz et al. 1989). The results shown in Figure 6 (left) reveal that a distinct set of iodinated products was generated in the three clones tested, two of which (11.3 and 8.5) were derived from the same donor (Lanzavecchia 1985). In each case, most of the fragments could be precipitated with an anti-immunoglobulin antibody, which strongly suggested that the distinct epitope specificity of each B-cell immunoglobulin gave rise to these patterns. A further experiment emphasized this point and excluded the possibility that other clonal differences, e.g., in proteinase expression, were responsible for these variations in processing. We reasoned that if an additional epitope on the antigen molecule was complexed with a Fab, a distinct processing pattern might arise following endocytosis of this Fab/antigen/mIg complex. Because each of the tetanus-specific B-cell clones secretes soluble immunoglobulin, we were able to make Fab fragments corresponding to each clone's specificity and test their effect on processing in the other clones. The result of such an experiment is shown in Figure 6 (right) and clearly demonstrates that processing within a single B-cell clone depends on the nature of the antigen substrate undergoing endocytosis. When epitopes other than that involved in receptor binding are occupied with Fabs, new fragments arise characteristic of the clone from which they derived. For example, in A46 and 8.5 cells, the 11.3 Fab gives rise to many, although not all, of the fragments observed in 11.3 cells (Fig. 6, lanes 4, 6, and 12). In reciprocal fashion, the A46 Fab induces a fragment characteristic of the processing pattern in A46 cells but not normally seen in 11.3 cells (lanes 2 and 7). In other cases, an added Fab blocks or strongly inhibits the accumulation of fragments that would otherwise be observed; for example, two fragments (~8 and 6 kD) characteristic of 8.5 cells were not observed when the 11.3 epitope was occupied (lanes 10 and 12). Taken together, these results reveal the importance of immunoglobulin specificity in B-cell antigen processing and also suggest that processing is likely to be perturbed by preexisting antibody specificities.

Processing of Membrane Immunoglobulin

What is the fate of the mIg receptor for antigen? When the abilities of anti-Fab (light chain or Cγ1) or anti-Fc region monoclonal antibodies to precipitate receptor-bound antigen are compared, they are nearly equally effective when all of the radiolabeled antigen is bound to cell-surface immunoglobulin receptors; however, as antigen processing proceeds, the anti-Fc region reagents become much less effective than anti-Fab reagents at precipitating antigen (see Fig. 7). SDS-gel analysis of the radiolabeled antigen precipitated at these later times reveals that the anti-Fc reagents only precipitate intact antigen and not the antigen fragments (data not shown). The most likely explanation is that the receptor itself has been cleaved and that the antigen fragments are bound to what may well resemble a Fab or (Fab')₂ fragment of the receptor. We are presently investigating whether there is any preferential order for processing of the antigen or receptor by identifying intermediates that may give rise to these species, i.e., processed antigen bound to an intact receptor or intact antigen bound to a cleaved receptor.

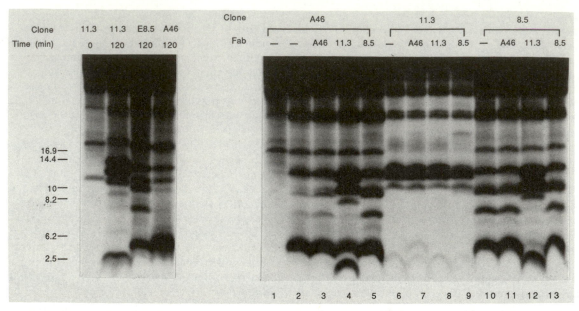

Figure 6. Epitope-directed antigen processing. B-cell clones were incubated with ^{125}I-labeled antigen at 0°C for 2 hr and then washed to remove unbound antigen. The cells either were resuspended in growth medium and incubated for 2 hr at 37°C (*left*) or were first incubated for 90 min at 0°C in growth medium containing 25 μg/ml unlabeled anti-tetanus toxin Fab fragments (prepared from antibodies secreted from each of the three clones) and then incubated for 2 hr at 37°C (*right*). Cell-associated antigen fragments were detected after electrophoresis and autoradiography. (Modified, with permission, from Davidson and Watts 1989.)

DISCUSSION

The studies outlined here show that membrane IgG allows the efficient receptor-mediated endocytosis of low levels of monovalent antigen, a property likely to be important in memory B-cell activation. Its high affinity for antigen over a wide range of pH, including that found in acidic intracellular compartments (Mell-

man et al. 1986), precludes the repeated reuse of receptors characteristic of receptor-mediated endocytosis of other ligands. Instead, tightly bound antigen is either recycled to the cell surface or, with a lower probability, delivered to a proteinase-containing environment. Exactly what determines whether an occupied receptor will be recycled or transported to an environment where proteinases are active is unclear and suggests a number of more general questions concerning transport of material through the endosome/lysosome system and the possible existence of distinct endosome populations active in receptor recycling or proteolytic degradation, but not both.

Reuse of receptors is apparently unnecessary because a single cohort of monovalent antigen molecules bound to surface mIgG receptors can generate sufficient processed determinants to drive effective collaborations with T cells, at least in vitro (Fig. 4; Lanzavecchia 1986). How and where in the cell these MHC/antigen complexes are generated and how the additional dimension of B-cell epitope specificity affects their formation are major unresolved questions. The influence of immunoglobulin specificity on antigen processing, hypothesized by others on the basis of preferred T-cell/immunoglobulin pairings (Berzofsky 1983; Manca et al. 1985), is clearly revealed by these studies on tetanus toxin processing.

A Possible Antigen Bridge between mIg and Class II MHC

What is the relationship between the longest-lived fragments, identifiable on SDS gels, most of which are

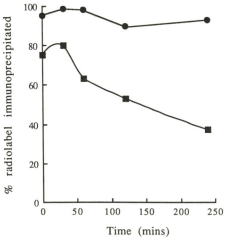

Figure 7. Processing of the mIg receptor for antigen. Cells (clone 11.3) were preincubated with radioiodinated antigen for 90 min at 0°C, washed, and incubated at 37°C. At the indicated times, cell lysates were prepared (Davidson and Watts 1989), and aliquots were subjected to immunoprecipitation with monoclonal antibodies QE 11 (●) or MK146 (■) specific for Fab (light chain) or Fc region, respectively, of human IgG. Precipitated radiolabel is expressed as a percentage of that in the cell lysates.

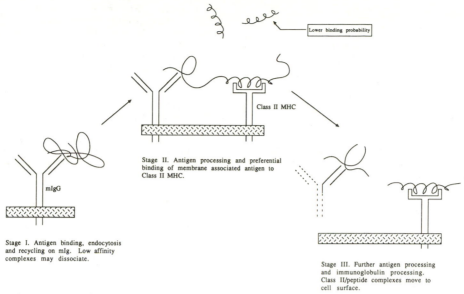

Figure 8. A possible antigen bridge between mIg and class II MHC. Endocytosis of mIg-bound antigen leads to processing of the immunoglobulin/antigen complex, as demonstrated in Fig. 6. Partially processed and unfolded forms may associate with class II MHC (with a vacant peptide-binding site) prior to release from the membrane surface. Further processing may cleave the bridge and the mIg and trim the MHC-bound peptide prior to transport to the cell surface. (For details, see text.)

immunoglobulin bound, and those parts of the antigen presented to T cells? Their longevity might favor their eventual association with a class II MHC site over those parts of the antigen that are more rapidly degraded, particularly if rates of association with the MHC are slow (Buus et al. 1986; but see also Ceppellini et al. 1989). On the other hand, these fragments may represent the end point of digestion and may not correspond to the most readily presented parts of the antigen. Nevertheless, the precursors of such distinct fragments are themselves likely to be distinct in each B-cell clone.

Such transient intermediates generated during processing may be difficult to visualize on SDS gels but may be immunologically relevant, particularly if still bound to an intact mIg receptor. An encounter or collision between MHC and partially processed antigen bound to the membrane, e.g., via immunoglobulin, may be a more frequent event than one between MHC and antigen dissociated from the plane of the membrane and freely distributed in the lumen of endosomal compartments. That is, those parts of the antigen that can be loaded onto the MHC in the two-dimensional membrane plane might be eventually expressed at a higher density than those parts released by cleavage into the bulk phase which might have to compete with many other peptides, including those derived from processed self proteins, for rebinding to the MHC on the membrane surface. This speculative model is outlined in Figure 8 and is, in a sense, a redrawing of the antigen bridge envisaged by Mitchison (1971) for B- and T-cell epitopes. We suggest that partially processed antigen might link a membrane immunoglobulin (immuno-globulin/Fc receptor in other APC types) and a class II MHC molecule, thus bridging a B-cell epitope and a potential T-cell epitope. Preferential immunoglobulin/T-cell pairings (Berzofsky 1983; Manca et al. 1985) might be explained by such a model, preferred T-cell epitopes being those that remain linked during processing, via such a bridge, to the immunoglobulin epitope responsible for antigen uptake. The formation of such a bridge would need to take place before the cleavage of the immunoglobulin receptor, which would presumably release it and any bound antigen into the bulk phase.

Whatever the precise details of the association of processed antigen with the MHC, the capacity to manipulate the pattern of processing within a single B-cell clone will allow us to investigate how the clear differences in processing evident at the biochemical level are reflected in differential presentation at the level detected by T cells. The perturbations induced by Fabs may be expected to block or enhance the presentation of particular T-cell epitopes. Blocking might arise as a result of coincidence of B- and T-cell determinants (Ozaki and Berzofsky 1987), whereas blockade by a Fab of a deleterious cleavage site might result in the enhanced presentation of particular regions of the antigen.

ACKNOWLEDGMENTS

We thank A. Lanzavecchia for cell clones and for valuable discussions. We are also grateful to Drs. S. van Heyningen and N. Fairweather and Mr. A. Sheppard (Wellcome Biotech) for gifts of tetanus toxin and toxoid. This work was supported by a Medical Research Council project grant, by the Nuffield Foundation, and by an EMBO short-term fellowship to C.W.

REFERENCES

Babbitt, B., P.M. Allen, G. Matsueda, E. Haber, and E.R. Unanue. 1985. Binding of immunogenic peptides to Ia histocompatibility molecules. *Nature* 317: 359.

Berzofsky, J.A. 1983. T-B reciprocity. An Ia-restricted epitope-specific circuit regulating T cell-B cell interaction and antibody specificity. *Surv. Immunol. Res.* 2: 223.

Bjorkman, P.J., M.A. Saper, B. Samraoui, W.S. Bennett, J.L. Strominger, and D.C. Wiley. 1987. Structure of the human class I histocompatibility antigen, HLA-A2. *Nature* 329: 506.

Brett, S.J., K.B. Cease, and J.A. Berzofsky. 1988. Influences of antigen processing on the expression of the T cell repertoire. *J. Exp. Med.* 168: 357.

Buus, S. and O. Werdelin. 1986. A group-specific inhibitor of both proteolytic degradation and presentation of the antigen dinitrophenyl-poly-L-lysine by guinea pig accessory cells to T cells. *J. Immunol.* 136: 452.

Buus, S., A. Sette, S.M. Colon, and H.M. Grey. 1988. Autologous peptides constitutively occupy the antigen binding site on Ia. *Science* 242: 1045.

Buus, S., A. Sette, S.M. Colon, D.M. Jenis, and H.M. Grey. 1986. Isolation and characterization of antigen-Ia complexes involved in T cell recognition. *Cell* 47: 1071.

Ceppellini, R., G. Frumento, G.B. Ferrara, R. Tosi, A. Chersi, and B. Pernis. 1989. Binding of labeled influenza matrix peptide to HLA DR in living B lymphoid cells. *Nature* 339: 392.

Chen, B.P. and P. Parham. 1989. Direct binding of influenza peptides to Class I HLA molecules. *Nature* 337: 743.

Dautry-Varsat, A., A. Ciechanover, and H. Lodish. 1983. pH and the recycling of transferrin during receptor-mediated endocytosis. *Proc. Natl. Acad. Sci.* 80: 2258.

Davidson, H.W. and C. Watts. 1989. Epitope-directed processing of specific antigen by B-lymphocytes. *J. Cell Biol.* 109: 85.

Demotz, S., A. Lanzavecchia, U. Eisel, H. Niemann, C. Widmann, and G. Corradin. 1989. Delineation of several DR-restricted tetanus toxoid T cell epitopes. *J. Immunol.* 142: 394.

Gammon, G., N. Shastri, J. Cogswell, S. Wilbur, S. Sadegh-Nasseri, U. Krzych, A. Miller, and E. Sercarz. 1987. The choice of T-cell epitopes utilized on a protein antigen depends on multiple factors distant from, as well as at, the determinant site. *Immunol. Rev.* 98: 53.

Goldstein, J.L., M.S. Brown, R.G.W. Anderson, D.W. Russell, and W. Schneider. 1985. Receptor mediated endocytosis: Concepts emerging from the LDL receptor system. *Annu. Rev. Cell Biol.* 1: 1.

Helenius, A., I. Mellman, D. Wall, and A.L. Hubbard. 1983. Endosomes. *Trends Biochem. Sci.* 8: 245.

Klausner, R.D., G. Ashwell, J. van Renswoude, J.B. Harford, and K.R. Bridges. 1983. Binding of apotransferrin to K562 cells: Explanation of the transferrin cycle. *Proc. Natl. Acad. Sci.* 80: 2263.

Lanzavecchia, A. 1985. Antigen-specific interaction between T and B cells. *Nature* 314: 537.

————. 1986. Antigen presentation by B lymphocytes: A critical step in T-B collaboration. *Curr. Top. Microbiol. Immunol.* 130: 65.

————.1987. Antigen uptake and accumulation in antigen-specific B-cells. *Immunol. Rev.* 99: 39.

Manca, F., D. Fenoglio, A. Kunkl, C. Cambiaggi, M. Sasso, and F. Celada. 1988. Differential activation of T cell clones stimulated by macrophages exposed to antigen complexed with monoclonal antibodies. A possible influence of paratope specificity on the mode of antigen processing. *J. Immunol.* 140: 2893.

Manca, F., A. Kunkl, D. Fenoglio, A. Fowler, E. Sercarz, and F. Celada. 1985. Constraints in T-B cooperation related to epitope topology on *E. coli* β-galactosidase. I. The fine specificity of T cells dictates the fine specificity of antibodies directed to conformation-dependent determinants. *Eur. J. Immunol.* 15: 345.

Mellman, I., R. Fuchs, and A. Helenius. 1986. Acidification of the endocytotic and exocytic pathways. *Annu. Rev. Biochem.* 55: 663.

Mitchison, N.A. 1971. The carrier effect in the secondary response to hapten-protein conjugates. II. Cell cooperation. *Eur. J. Immunol.* 1: 18.

Ozaki, S. and J.A. Berzofsky. 1987. Antibody conjugates mimic specific B cell presentation of antigen: Relationship between T and B cell specificity. *J. Immunol.* 138: 4133.

Pearse, B.M.F. 1988. Receptors compete for adaptors found in plasma membrane coated pits. *EMBO J.* 7: 3331.

Roosnek, E., S. Demotz, G. Corradin, and A. Lanzavecchia. 1988. Kinetics of MHC-antigen complex formation on antigen-presenting cells. *J. Immunol.* 140: 4079.

Shimonkevitz, R., J. Kappler, P. Marrack, and H.M. Grey. 1983. Antigen recognition by H-2 restricted T cells. II. Cell-free antigen-processing. *J. Exp. Med.* 158: 303.

Townsend, A.R.M., J. Rothbard, F.M. Gotch, B. Bahadur, D. Wraith, and A.J. McMichael. 1986. The epitopes of influenza nucleoprotein recognized by cytotoxic T lymphocytes can be defined with short synthetic peptides. *Cell* 44: 959.

Watts, C. 1985. Rapid endocytosis of the transferrin receptor in the absence of bound transferrin. *J. Cell Biol.* 100: 633.

Watts, C. and H.W. Davidson. 1988. Endocytosis and recycling of specific antigen by human B cell lines. *EMBO J.* 7: 1937.

Wileman, T., C. Harding, and P. Stahl. 1985. Receptor-mediated endocytosis. *Biochem. J.* 232: 1.

Ziegler, H.K. and E. Unanue. 1982. Decrease in macrophage antigen catabolism caused by ammonia and chloroquine with inhibition of antigen presentation to T cells. *Proc. Natl. Acad. Sci.* 79: 175.

Comparison of Orthorhombic and Monoclinic Crystal Structures of HLA-A2

D.R. Madden,* M.A. Saper,*† T.P.J. Garrett,*† P.J. Bjorkman,*‡
J.L. Strominger,* and D.C. Wiley*†
*Department of Biochemistry and Molecular Biology, †Howard Hughes Medical Institute,
Harvard University, Cambridge, Massachusetts 02138

The structure of the orthorhombic crystal form of the histocompatibility antigen HLA-A2 has been refined to 2.5 Å resolution. The structure of HLA-A2 had previously been determined to 3.5 Å using data from both orthorhombic and monoclinic crystals (Bjorkman et al. 1987a) and has now been refined to 2.7 Å resolution using the monoclinic data (M.A. Saper et al., in prep.). A comparison of the two structures, which have been independently refined on data from different crystal forms, shows that the structures are very similar. Differences are found only in areas where the electron density is weak (some surface side chains and amino- or carboxy-terminal residues), in those parts of the molecule subject to different packing contacts in the crystals, and in the orientation of a few side chains within the same envelope of electron density. The electron density found in the putative peptide-binding cleft of both HLA-A2 structures is similar in shape and can clearly be seen to reach into several "pockets" around the perimeter of the site.

The determination of the structure of the same molecule twice serves as a control for the level of noise in crystallographic structures, and thus acts as a measure of the significance of structural differences found between different histocompatibility antigens. HLA-Aw68, a second polymorphic class I molecule, crystallizes isomorphously with the orthorhombic form of HLA-A2 (Bjorkman et al. 1985). A comparison of these two alleles permits an assessment of the contribution of amino acid substitutions to the binding specificity of the cleft (T.P.J. Garrett et al., in prep.).

METHODS

Crystallization and data collection on orthorhombic crystals. Crystals formed in hanging drops of 14% polyethylene glycol and 25 mM MES (pH 6.5) as described previously (Bjorkman et al. 1985). They generally measured 150 μm $\times$ 150 μm $\times$ 60 μm. Data were collected from orthorhombic crystals of HLA-A2 ($P2_12_12_1$, $a = 60.36$ Å, $b = 80.81$ Å, $c = 111.9$ Å) at 4°C, using a Xentronics area detector (Durbin et al.

1986). Data were processed to 2.5 Å using the BUD-DHA software package (Blum et al. 1987) together with the CCP4 scaling programs (P. Evans, pers. comm.). The R-factor on intensities was 7.4% to 2.5 Å and 19.1% in the shell from 2.67 Å to 2.5 Å. Data were 93% complete to 2.5 Å and 88% complete (61% > 3σ) in the shell from 2.67 Å to 2.5 Å.

Refinement of a molecular model against orthorhombic data. A molecular model based on the monoclinic data had been partially refined to 2.7 Å using least-squares refinement (M.A. Saper et al., in prep.). A rotation and translation search at 3.5 Å yielded a preliminary transformation from monoclonic to orthorhombic coordinates (Saper et al. 1989). The model was then refined at 2.5 Å using orthorhombic data and a combination of simulated molecular dynamics, least-squares refinement, and manual rebuilding. During an initial round of refinement, data from 5.0 Å to 2.7 Å were used. The program X-PLOR (Brünger 1988) was used to perform energy minimization, overall B-factor refinement, a simulated heating to 1000° K for 0.5 psec, a simulated quenching at 300° K for 0.25 psec, and another round of energy minimization and B-factor refinement. In the second round, the procedure was essentially the same, except that data from 5.5 Å to 2.5 Å were used, B-factors were refined individually, and the simulated heating was modeled at 2500° K. The third round was identical to the second. At this point, simulated heating no longer brought a significant improvement in the R-factor, and subsequent refinement proceeded without it. The final round of refinement therefore involved several stages of manual rebuilding according to difference and $2F_o$-F_c maps, regularization of geometry using FRODO (Jones 1982; Pflugrath et al. 1984), together with X-PLOR energy minimization and individual B-factor refinement to convergence (Brünger 1988). At the end of the process, the resolution range was extended to 6.0 Å to 2.5 Å.

Monoclinic data collection and structure refinement. Data had been collected from monoclinic crystals ($P2_1$, $a = 60.35$ Å, $b = 80.40$ Å, $c = 56.49$ Å, $\beta = 120.42°$) and interpreted at 3.5 Å (Bjorkman et al. 1987a). The model used for comparisons was refined from 6 to 2.7 Å resolution (R-factors = 16.4%) by both geometry- and

‡Present address: Department of Biology, California Institute of Technology, Pasadena, California 91125.

energy-restrained least squares methods (M.A. Saper et al., in prep.).

Comparing the structures. A least-squares fitting algorithm was used to superimpose the α-carbons of the orthorhombic and monoclinic models (Kabsch 1978). The transformation obtained was also used to skew electron density difference maps from the monoclinic to the orthorhombic cell for comparison. A scale factor for comparing the orthorhombic and monoclinic maps was computed by least-squares fitting the electron density values at grid points within 2 Å of atoms in the α_1 and α_2 domains.

In all coordinate comparisons, carboxy-terminal residues 267–270 have been omitted, since there is very little density to support their positions (as is reflected in B-factors above 50 Å^2). Also, during round 3 of refinement, these residues were rebuilt up to 14 Å from their original positions, and these differences dominated the rms statistics.

RESULTS

Orthorhombic Crystal Structure of A2

The structure was refined from an initial R-factor of 37.0% to the current R-factor of 23.0% from 6.0 Å to 2.5 Å. The rms bond length deviation in the current structure is 0.019 Å, and the average deviation of angles is 3.27° (Table 1).

Comparison of the Orthorhombic and Monoclinic A2 Structures

Following a least-squares fit of the α-carbons, the rms difference between all atoms is 0.83 Å. For α-carbons, the rms difference is 0.34 Å. The net C$_\alpha$ rms change during the refinement was similar for domains α_1/α_2 (0.42 Å) and for domains α_3/β_2 (0.37 Å). Also, in the final comparison between the orthorhombic and monoclinic structures, the domains showed a similar overall C$_\alpha$ rms difference of 0.35 Å (α_1/α_2) and 0.31 Å (α_3/β_2).

A list of the 25 α-carbons with differences greater than 1.5*rms includes 14 residues involved in or adjacent to crystal contacts, five of them in the conserved contacts I and II (see below). Four involve amino- or carboxy-terminal residues with B-factors in at least one model of more than 45 Å^2, indicating that they are in areas of the map without good electron density. Six of the seven remaining residues have been affected by different choices in fitting side-chain χ angles to ambiguous density. The final difference, residue 163, appears to be affected by a nearby positive difference electron density peak in the cleft of the orthorhombic structure.

Crystal Contacts

The crystal contacts have been enumerated in Table 2. In the monoclinic crystal, there are four contacts

Table 1. Course of HLA-A2 Orthorhombic Refinement

Round:	start	1	2	3	4
R-factor (6.0–2.5 Å)	0.370	0.277	0.236	0.234	0.230
Geometry (rms deviation from equilibrium):					
bonds (Å)	0.024	0.018	0.019	0.019	0.020
angles (°)	3.0	3.6	3.7	3.3	3.3
peptide bond (°)	1.3	5.8	6.1	5.8	5.7
Average B-factor (Å^2):	16	17	16	24	16
Refinement method[a]:		MD/min	MD/min	build/ MD/min	build/ min
Refinement resolution (Å):		5.0–2.7	5.5–2.5	5.5–2.5	5.5–2.5/ 6.0–2.5
rms change from previous round, following superposition (Å):					
whole molecule (excluding residues 267–270):					
all atoms:		0.73	0.49	0.42	0.21
backbone:		0.40	0.22	0.13	0.072
side chain:		0.92	0.63	0.57	0.29
α_1/α_2:					
all atoms:		0.75	0.46	0.36	0.21
backbone:		0.39	0.22	0.13	0.077
side chain:		0.95	0.58	0.48	0.28
α_3/β_2 m (excluding residues 267–270):					
all atoms:		0.70	0.52	0.48	0.22
backbone:		0.39	0.22	0.14	0.066
side chain:		0.88	0.69	0.65	0.30

[a]Refinement techniques (see text for full details): (MD) simulated molecular dynamics; (min) least-squares energy minimization and B-factor refinement; (build) manual rebuilding or use of the FRODO regularization facility.

Table 2. Crystal Contact Patches, Orthorhombic and Monoclinic

Patch	Form found in	Residues involved	Δ rms backbone (Å)	Δ rms all atoms (Å)	Average B-factor (Å^2)[a]
I	ort, mon	17, 18[a], 19, 69, 72, 73[b], 75	0.29	0.83	16
I′	ort, mon	178, 181, 183, 186, 207[a], 209, 238[a], B13, B16, B19, B20	0.31	0.48	13
II	ort, mon	85[a], 121, 122, 135, 136, 137, 138[b]	0.22	0.69	10
II′	ort, mon	219, 222, 226, 249[b], 250[b], 253, 256, 257	0.41	0.73	17
III	mon	84, 142, 149	0.30	0.40	15
III′	mon	105, 106, 108	0.81	1.6	38
IV	mon	176	0.25	1.7	27
IV′	mon	196	0.46	0.91	38
V	ort	127, 131, 154, 155, extra density	0.44	1.5	19
V′	ort	192, 193, 195, 196[c], B74, B96, B98	0.41	0.72	24

Residues preceded by B indicate β_2-microglobulin.
[a]Orthorhombic structure only.
[b]Monoclinic structure only.
[c]Contacts the extra density in HLA-A2 cleft.

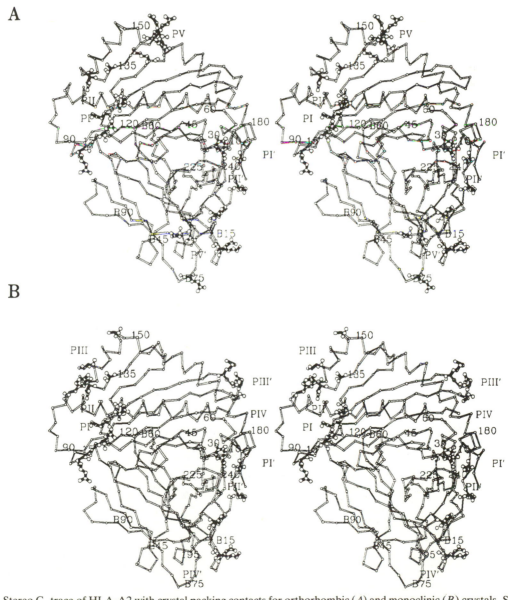

Figure 1. Stereo C$_\alpha$ trace of HLA-A2 with crystal packing contacts for orthorhombic (*A*) and monoclinic (*B*) crystals. Side chains involved in crystal contacts are shown with bold-faced bonds. Residue labels beginning with B indicate β_2-microglobulin. Roman numerals designate contact patches as listed in Table 2.

(eight patches) between symmetry-related molecules within the crystal, which have been labeled so that the two patches forming a contact share the same Roman numeral and are distinguished by being primed or unprimed. There are 39 residues in contacts in the orthorhombic structure and 38 in the monoclinic structure, out of a total of 359 residues in the HLA-A2 heavy chain and β_2-microglobulin. The monoclinic crystal has four contacts (I–IV). The orthorhombic packing shares only contacts I and II with the monoclinic crystal and has one additional contact (V) at the kink in the main α_2 helix.

The relatively conserved contact patch I involves a loop between strands of the $\alpha_1 \alpha_2 \beta$-sheet together with the outside and upper edge of the α_1 helix. Its contact partner, the I' patch, is a surface spanning the α_3- and β_2-microglobulin domains (Fig. 1). In the two crystal forms, the α-carbon paths of these contact residues are

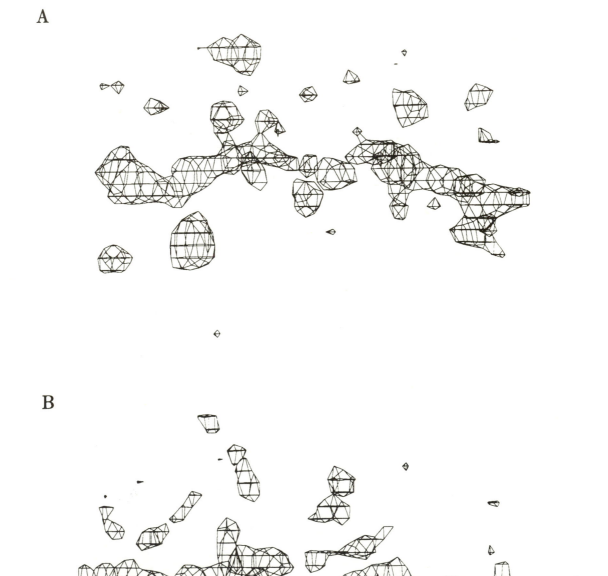

A

B

Figure 2. Electron density found in the HLA-A2 cleft. $2F_o$-F_c, calculated phases. (A) Orthorhombic data, contoured at 1 σ. (B) Monoclinic data, contoured as described in the text.

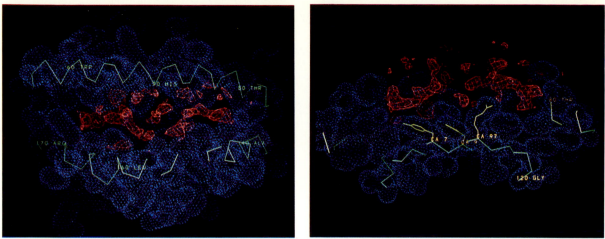

Figure 3. Orthorhombic extra electron density (red) shown in the context of a van der Waals dot surface (blue) of the HLA-A2 site. (*Left*) Top view and (*right*) side view, looking perpendicular to the axes of the α-helices.

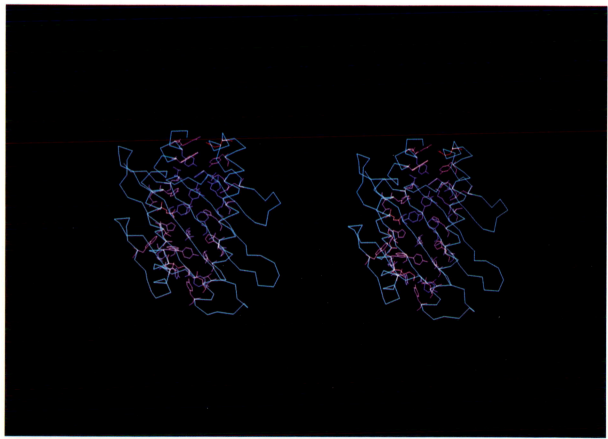

Figure 4. Stereo C$_\alpha$ trace of HLA-A2 α_1 and α_2 domains (blue) with the site residue side chains color-coded by temperature factor. The α_1 helix is to the right, with its amino terminus toward the top of the figure. Blue reflects a low temperature factor (minimum is 2.1 Å^2), and red reflects a high temperature factor (maximum is 30 Å^2).

identical, but there are some differences in the positions of patch I side chains, especially on the loop (residues 17–19) (Table 2).

Patch II is a surface under the end of the two helices and the edge of the β-sheet (near residue 121). It contacts (patch II′) β-turn and strand-terminal residues of the α_3 domain (Fig. 1). In this contact, the main-chain structure is again conserved, but there is some difference in the side-chain positions of the orthorhombic and monoclinic structures in both patches. Contacts I and II both involve residues for which the electron density is clear, as indicated by low values of the refined B-factors (Table 2).

Monoclinic contact III involves residues 84,142, and 149 contacting residues 105, 106, and 108 (Fig. 1B). These latter residues are located on an exterior loop, whose average temperature factor is 10 Å^2 higher than the remaining residues in the α_2 domain, and whose backbone rms difference between the two structures is 0.81 Å. Residue 84, conserved in many class I sequences, is at the end of helix H2 in α_1, whereas residues 142 and 149 are in helix H1 in α_2. Their main-chain rms deviations relative to the orthorhombic structure are slight (0.30 Å), whereas side chains move only 0.40 Å.

The single-residue contacts IV (176) and IV′ (196) in the monoclinic crystals have backbone rms differences with respect to the orthorhombic structure of 0.25 and 0.46 Å, respectively.

Contact V is found only in orthorhombic crystals and is formed by residues 154 and 155 of the H2a helix in α_2 and residues 127–131 on a β turn (S3 to S4 in α_2) of the sheet (Fig. 1A). The contact extends from the sheet to the helix and over the cleft so that residue 196 of the symmetry-related molecule comes within approximately 3.5 Å of the 1σ contour of the extra density (see below). It approaches the extra density near to the central break between the two major sections (Fig. 2), and thus may be contacting a relatively disordered element.

The backbone rms difference for these residues is 0.44 Å for patch V and 0.41 Å for patch V′. Most of this difference is accounted for by a rotation of the 127–131 loop relative to the rest of the molecule. Residues 126–132 have a backbone rms difference of 0.54 Å when the whole molecules are superimposed, but can be independently superimposed with a backbone rms difference of only 0.26 Å. The reorientation of the β-turn residues upward toward the H2a α_2 helix does not appear to alter the helix itself, since the nearest helical residues are essentially superimposable. The side chains of residues 154 and 155 differ in the two structures, although in the monoclinic structure they are characterized by high temperature factors (45 and 36 Å^2, respectively). In the orthorhombic structure an omit map of residue 154 shows a break in the side-chain density near the β-carbon. These two side-chain placements, therefore, must still be considered preliminary.

Extra Density

In the original report of the HLA-A2 structure, extra electron density was observed within the putative pep-

tide-binding cleft (Bjorkman et al. 1987a). This extra density has remained throughout the refinement of the HLA-A2 monoclinic and orthorhombic structures. The extra density found in the two crystals is remarkably similar both in the path traced and in the location of protrusions. The extra electron density reaches deeply into several of the pockets that are found in the van der Waals surface of the cleft (Fig. 3).

Temperature Factor of Residues within the Cleft

The residues in the site appear to be relatively immobile in the refined molecular structure. This is reflected in the temperature factors of the site residues, a crystallographic indication of atomic disorder. In Figure 4, the residues of the site have been color-coded to reflect their temperature factors and hence mobilities. Those residues that point into the site are well-fixed, as indicated by the preponderance of side chains colored blue through salmon in the cleft (Fig. 4). To give a sense of the color scale, tyrosine 59, whose side chain is the second along the α_1 helix from the amino terminus, has an average temperature factor of 18 Å^2 and is thus well-fixed. In the site, only residue 55, the amino-terminal side chain shown on the α_1 helix, has a higher average temperature factor (30 Å^2). The average temperature factor of all the site residues is only 12 Å^2 ($\sigma = 6.5$ Å^2), compared to 16 Å^2 ($\sigma = 11$ Å^2) for the molecule as a whole.

DISCUSSION

An analysis of two independent HLA-A2 crystals allows us to assess the independence of the protein structure from the crystal environment. The fundamental elements of tertiary structure are found to be identical. Significant differences are found only in some crystal-contact residues on loops or in the side-chain positions of some contact residues and their neighbors. The extra electron density is conserved in the different crystal forms, strongly suggesting that it represents some genuine feature associated with the HLA-A2 molecule, most likely some as yet unidentified peptide(s) bound in the cleft.

The results presented here appear to indicate specific recognition in the binding of the extra electron density. The extra density is most clearly defined where it reaches down into pockets on the periphery of the HLA-A2 cleft. Also, the side chains that define these pockets seem to be relatively well fixed, despite the fact that a heterogeneous population of peptides is probably bound. Thus, it seems likely that the cleft residues primarily adopt single conformations for the recognition of antigenic peptides.

Surface residues involved in a crystal contact in one of the two structures and exposed to an aqueous environment in the other generally adopt the same backbone conformation in both structures. Specifically, the differences in α-carbon positions found between non-conserved contacts in the two crystals, for the most part, are at or below the level found when comparing the entire molecular structure or residues involved in conserved contacts. This suggests that the crystallized structure is largely independent of the crystal environment and therefore likely to be closely related to that found in solution. There are, however, differences involving the backbone trace of relatively loosely constrained loops (contact III') and the positions of side chains, as seen in several contacts. It is thus fairly clear that the crystal environment can have a localized effect on surface residues.

Some residues on the top of the helices, thought to be likely candidates for T-cell receptor recognition (Bjorkman et al. 1987b), are involved in contacts in each crystal form. Also, residues 227 and 245, implicated in class I/CD8 interactions (Potter et al. 1989; Salter et al. 1989), are quite near to the contact patch II', which is found in both crystals. Although the molecule is unlikely to be affected at the level of gross structure by these crystal contacts, any detailed attempts to model the molecular interactions between HLA, CD8, and the T-cell receptor should take account of the possible influence of the crystal environment on specific side chains in these crystal contacts.

ACKNOWLEDGMENTS

The authors thank Anastasia Haykov for excellent technical assistance. This material is based on work supported in part under a National Science Foundation Graduate Fellowship (D.R.M.). We also thank Drs. Dean Mann (N.I.H.), D. Michael Strong and James Woody (U.S. Naval Research Unit), and Don Giard (M.I.T. Cell Culture Facility) for provision of cells which made this work possible.

REFERENCES

Bjorkman, P.J., J.L. Strominger, and D.C. Wiley. 1985. Crystallization and X-ray diffraction studies on the histocompatibility antigens HLA-A2 and HLA-A28 from human cell membranes. *J. Mol. Biol.* **186:** 205.

Bjorkman, P.J., M.A. Saper, B. Samraoui, W. Bennett, J.L. Strominger, and D.C. Wiley. 1987a. Structure of the human Class I histocompatibility antigen, HLA-A2. *Nature* **329:** 506.

———. 1987b. The foreign antigen binding site and T cell recognition regions of Class I histocompatibility antigens. *Nature* **329:** 512.

Blum, M., P. Metcalf, S.C. Harrison, and D.C. Wiley. 1987. A system for collection and on-line integration of X-ray diffraction data from a multiwire area detector. *J. Appl. Crystallogr.* **20:** 235.

Brünger, A. 1988. *X-PLOR manual (Version 1.5).* Yale University, New Haven.

Durbin, R., R. Burns, J. Moulai, P. Metcalf, D. Freymann, M. Blum, J. Anderson, S.C. Harrison, and D.C. Wiley. 1986. Protein, DNA, and virus crystallography with a focused imaging proportional counter. *Science* **232:** 1127.

Jones, T.A. 1982. FRODO: A graphics fitting program for macromolecules. In *Computational crystallography* (ed. D. Sayre), p. 303. Clarendon Press, Oxford.

Kabsch, W. 1978. A discussion of the solution for the best rotation to relate two sets of vectors. *Acta Crystallogr.* **A34:** 827.

Pflugrath, J.W., M.A. Saper, and F.A. Quiocho. 1984. New generation graphics system for molecular modeling. In *Methods and applications in crystallographic computing* (ed. S. Hall and T. Ashiaka), p. 407. Clarendon Press, Oxford.

Potter, T.A., T.V. Rajan, R.F. Dick II, and J.A. Bluestone. 1989. Substitution at residue 227 of H-2 class I molecules abrogrates recognition by CD8-dependent, but not CD8-independent, cytotoxic T lymphocytes. *Nature* **337:** 73.

Salter, R.D., A.M. Norment, B.P. Chen, C. Clayberger, A.M. Krensky, D.R. Littman, and P. Parham. 1989. Polymorphism in the α3 domain of HLA-A molecules affects binding to CD8. *Nature* **338:** 345.

Saper, M.A., P.J. Bjorkman, and D.C. Wiley. 1989. Iterative molecular averaging and phase refinement of two HLA-A2 crystal forms. In *Improving protein phases: Proceedings of the study weekend held at Daresbury Laboratory, 1988* (ed. S. Bailey et al). Science and Engineering Research Council, Daresbury.

Mutants of HLA-A2 in the Analysis of Its Structure and Function

J.L. Strominger, J. Santos-Aguado, S.J. Burakoff, M.A. Vega,
F.M. Gotch, P.A. Robbins, and A.J. McMichael

Department of Biochemistry and Molecular Biology, Harvard University, Cambridge, Massachusetts 02138;
Dana-Farber Cancer Institute, Harvard Medical School, Boston, Massachusetts 02115;
Institute for Molecular Medicine, John Radcliffe Hospital, Oxford, England OX3 9DU

A relatively large number of mutants of HLA-A2 have been constructed either (1) by site-directed mutagenesis of residues in the peptide-binding cleft or (2) by deletions of mini-exons 6 and/or 7 encoding portions of the intracytoplasmic region and have been used to analyze the structure and function of this molecule in the light of the structure revealed by X-ray crystallography (Madden et al., this volume).

Mutations in the Foreign Antigen-binding Cleft

Four immunological phenomena in which these molecules participate have been examined.

1. Recognition by monoclonal antibodies (Santos-Aguado et al. 1988). The localization of the amino acid residues involved in the serologic specificity of the HLA-A2 molecule has been investigated. At least three nonoverlapping serologic epitopes were identified. Mutations in the highly polymorphic region at amino acids 62–66 completely eliminated binding of monoclonal antibody MA2.1 (A2/B17 cross-reactive). Mutation at position 107 resulted in complete loss of monoclonal antibody BB7.2 binding (A2 allospecific). The recognition of other allotypic monoclonal antibodies was not affected by these mutations, and they therefore represent at least a third serologic epitope. Mutations at positions 152 and 156, known to be important for T-cell recognition, did not affect serologic recognition. Introduction of residues of HLA-B7 origin in the polymorphic segment spanning amino acids 70–80 created a molecule carrying the -Bw6 supertypic determinant as demonstrated by monoclonal antibody SFR8-B6 binding, but no determinant recognized by B7 allospecific monoclonal antibodies was detected.

2. Recognition by alloantisera (Santos-Aguado et al. 1989b). A small number of pregnancy alloantisera are allospecific and recognize the same epitopes detected by monoclonal antibodies at residues 62–66 and at residue 107 (which earlier data had indicated was a nonlinear epitope also involving residue 161).

3. Recognition by influenza virus-directed HLA-A2-restricted CTL.

   Epitope in matrix protein of a type A strain (McMichael et al. 1988). Cytotoxic T lymphocytes (CTL) specific for influenza A virus were prepared from 15 donors. Those with HLA-A2 recognized autologous or HLA-A2-matched B-lymphoblastoid cells in the presence of synthetic peptide representing residues 55–73 or 56–68 of the virus matrix protein sequence. Influenza A virus-specific CTL from donors without HLA-A2 or with an HLA-A2 variant type failed to respond to this peptide. CTL lines specific for HLA-A2 plus peptide did not lyse peptide-treated target cells from HLA-A2 variant donors. They also failed to lyse peptide-treated cells with point mutations that had been inserted into HLA-A2 at positions 62–63, 66, 152, and 156, and in some instances, mutations at positions 9 and 70. CTL lysed peptide-treated target cells with mutations in HLA-A2 at positions 43, 74, and 107. The results imply that this defined peptide epitope therefore interacts with HLA-A2 in the binding groove so that the long α helices of HLA-A2 make important contacts with the peptide at positions 66, 152, and 156. Different amino acids at position 9, which is in the floor of the peptide-binding groove of HLA-A2, and the closely related position 70, modulate the peptide interaction so that some T-cell clones react and some do not. These data raise the possibility that the same peptide may bind in the groove in two different ways.

   Epitope in nucleoprotein of a type B strain (Robbins et al. 1989). An influenza B virus nucleoprotein (BNP) peptide, residues 82–94, identified by very limited sequence homology with the influenza A matrix protein epitope, was recognized by HLA-A2-restricted CTL. Reciprocal inhibition of T-cell recognition by the two peptides suggests that the BNP peptide may have lower avidity for HLA-A2 molecules than the matrix peptide. The weak competitor activity of the BNP peptide for the matrix peptide may be explained by its location within the HLA-A2-binding cleft, which has been mapped using T-cell recognition of target cells expressing natural variants and site-specific mutants of HLA-A2. Mutations at residues 9, 99, 70, 74, 152, and 156 were found to abolish T-cell recognition of the BNP peptide. These results taken together with results obtained with the influenza A matrix peptide suggest that the two peptides bind differently in the peptide-binding site and, in particular, that binding of the

BNP peptide may involve residues 9, 99, 70, and 74 in a way that they are not involved in the binding of the matrix peptide (Fig. 1).

4. Recognition by a panel of allogeneic CTL (Santos-Aguado et al. 1989a). The complexity and fine specificity of the allospecific T-cell response generated against the human HLA-A2.1 molecule and the characterization of the antigenic determinants that anti-HLA-A2 alloreactive CTLs recognize in the molecule have been analyzed using as targets cell lines expressing HLA-A2 CTL-variants and the human rhabdomyosarcoma cell line (RD) transfected and expressing HLA-A2 mutants obtained by site-directed mutagenesis. Correlation of the specific reactivity pattern of the CTL clones with the three-dimensional structure of the HLA-A2.1 molecule allowed delineation of some molecular characteristics of the alloantigenic determinants seen in this molecule by human allospecific T-cell clones and led to the following conclusions: (1) Every clone displayed a different recognition pattern, illustrating the enormous epitope-diversity of this allogeneic T-cell response. The heterogeneity of the CTL clones was also demonstrated when monoclonal antibodies against monomorphic or polymorphic determinants in HLA molecules were used in cytotoxicity inhibition assays. (2) Residues shown to be important for allogeneic CTL recognition were located either in the α_1 or α_2 helix pointing into the site or in the bottom of the putative antigen-binding recognition site, just as they are for virus peptide-directed HLA-A2.1-restricted CTL recognition. Thus, allogeneic recognition must also involve recognition of some material in the foreign antigen-binding site of HLA-A2.1, most likely a self-peptide. The multiplicity of recognition patterns of the mutants seen with different CTL clones is compatible with a model in which a large number of different self-peptides are bound in different ways in the peptide-binding cleft of HLA-A2 (just as virus-derived peptides may be bound in distinct ways) and serve as the ligands for allogeneic recognition.

All of the data obtained are compatible with the proposed structure of HLA-A2. Antibodies recognize only residues that are exposed in the structure. Recognition of two different flu virus peptide epitopes (one from a type A strain and one from a type B strain) indicate that these two quite different peptides that are presented by HLA-A2 interact with different residues in the peptide-binding cleft and may be located in slightly different positions. The repertoire of allogeneic CTL is extremely large. The data are compatible with a model in which allogeneic CTLs recognize a variety of self-peptides bound in different ways in the cleft.

A. B NUCLEOPROTEIN PEPTIDE

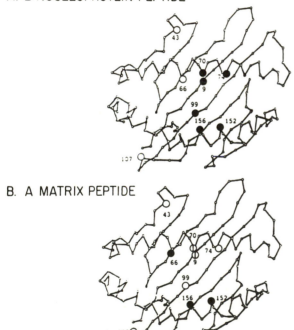

B. A MATRIX PEPTIDE

Figure 1. Definition of the binding sites for influenza B nucleoprotein peptide (*A*) and for influenza A matrix peptide (*B*) in HLA-A2. The figure is based on the crystal structure of HLA-A2 (see elsewhere in this volume) and shows the α-carbon backbone structure of the α_1 and α_2 domains looking down on the peptide-binding cleft. (Solid circles) Mutations that affect recognition of CTL lines; (lined circles) mutations that affect some clones; (open circles) mutations with no effect.

Deletions of Portions of the Intracytoplasmic Region

Finally, the deletion of mini-exons encoding portions of the 32 intracytoplasmic amino acids of HLA-A2 have been employed in a study of the constitutive endocytosis of HLA-A2 in a human T-cell line. First, HLA class I antigens present in the human leukemia T-cell line HPB-ALL were shown to be endocytosed in the absence of specific antibodies (constitutive endocytosis). In 1 hour, ~10% of class I molecules initially present at the cell surface were found intracellularly. Genetically engineered mutants of the HLA-A2 gene lacking exon 6 or 7 or both were used to analyze whether the cytoplasmic region contributes to the internalization. The results indicate that amino acids encoded by exon 7 (spanning amino acid residues 323–340) are required for internalization, whereas deletion of exon 6 had no effect. In addition, a comparison of the cytoplasmic sequences of receptors that are known to be internalized via coated pits and the present data revealed that they share a structural feature that could constitute a specific signal required for endocytosis (Vega and Strominger 1989) (Table 1). The biological significance of endocytosis and its possible relevance to antigen presentation remain to be explored.

Table 1. Cytoplasmic Domains of Molecules Endocytosed Via Coated Pits Share a Common Structural Feature

Molecule		Sequence	
		1 2 3 4 5	
HA[a]	538	N G S L Q Y – R I C L	547 (538–547)
LDLr (h)	802	F D N P V Y Q K T T E D E V H I	817 (790–839)
TRr (h, m)	15	G E P L S Y T R F S L A R Q V D	30 (1–65)
VSV G	496	K K R Q I Y T D I E M N R L G K	511 (483–511)
HLA-A2 (h)	326	S D S A Q G S D V S L T A C K V	341 (309–341)
M6Pr (b)	204	P H L A F W Q D L G N L V A D G	219 (191–257)
AsGr (r)	1	T K D Y Q D F Q H L D N E N	14 (1–38)
Pol lgr (rb)[b]	663	V S I G S Y – R T D I S M S D L	677 (653–755)
CD4 (h)	423	Q C P H R F Q K T C S P I	435 (396–435)

Data from Vega and Strominger (1989).

[a]Hemagglutinin sequence from a mutant that is endocytosed. It has tyrosine at position 543 instead of cysteine.

[b]The change of a single tyrosine (position in the sequence not indicated) within the cytoplasmic domain of the polyimmunoglobulin receptor impairs efficient endocytosis of this receptor. Two tyrosine residues occur within the cytoplasmic portion. Only the one here shows homology with the other receptors within the region numbered 1–5.

ACKNOWLEDGMENTS

This work was supported by National Institutes of Health grants AI-15669, AI-20182, and CA-47554. P.A.R. is a Fellow of the Leukemia Society of America. M.A.V. acknowledges postdoctoral support from the Consejo Superior de Investigaciones Científicas of Spain. The material presented is, in part, abstracted from the references cited. Only work carried out in the authors' laboratories has been referenced. Full documentation to the work of others can be found in the papers cited.

REFERENCES

McMichael, A.J., F.M. Gotch, J. Santos-Aguado, and J.L. Strominger. 1988. Effects of mutations and variations of HLA-A2 on recognition of a virus peptide epitope by cytotoxic T lymphocytes. *Proc. Natl. Acad. Sci.* **85:** 9194.

Robbins, P.A., L.A. Lettice, P. Rota, J. Santos-Aguado, J. Rothbard, A.J. McMichael, and J.L. Strominger. 1989. Comparison between two peptide epitopes presented to cytotoxic T lymphocytes by HLA-A2; evidence for discrete locations within HLA-A2. *J. Immunol.* **143:** (in press).

Santos-Aguado, J., J.A. Barbosa, P.A. Biro, and J.L. Strominger. 1988. Molecular characterization of serologic determinants in the human HLA-A2 molecule. *J. Immunol.* **141:** 2811.

Santos-Aguado, J., M.A.V. Crimmins, S.J. Mentzer, J.L. Strominger, and S.J. Burakoff. 1989a. Molecular characterization of allospecific cytotoxic T lymphocytes recognition sites in the HLA-A2 molecule using oligonucleotide-generated site specific mutants. In *Immunobiology of HLA* (ed. B. Dupont), vol. 2, p. 97. Springer-Verlag, New York and *Proc. Natl. Acad. Sci.* **86:** (in press).

Santos-Aguado, J., J.J. Yunis, E. Mildford, E.J. Yunis, and J.L. Strominger. 1989b. Molecular characterization of serological recognition sites in the HLA-A2 molecule using oligonucleotide-generated site specific mutants. In *Immunobiology of HLA* (ed. B. Dupont), vol. 2, p. 93. Springer-Verlag, New York.

Vega, M.A. and J.L. Strominger. 1989. Constitutive endocytosis of HLA class I antigens requires a specific portion of the intracytoplasmic tail that shares structural features with other endocytosed molecules. *Proc. Natl. Acad. Sci.* **86:** 2688.

Model for the Interaction of T-cell Receptors with Peptide/MHC Complexes

P.J. BJORKMAN* AND M.M. DAVIS†

*Division of Biology, California Institute of Technology, Pasadena, California 91125;
†Howard Hughes Medical Institute and Department of Microbiology and Immunology,
Stanford University, Stanford, California 94305

The immune response against a viral infection is mediated by two different types of cells known as B and T lymphocytes. The receptor on the B cell is the well-characterized antibody molecule, which exists in a membrane-bound form and in a secreted form involved in the initiation of complement-mediated killing and the inactivation of viral particles by direct binding. The recognition molecule on T cells is the membrane-bound T-cell antigen receptor, which has specificity for a combination of foreign antigen with a molecule of the major histocompatibility complex (MHC), as first demonstrated by Zinkernagel and Doherty (1974). MHC proteins exist in two closely related forms called class I and class II MHC molecules, both of which are cell-surface glycoproteins that are highly polymorphic in the human population. In general, class II MHC molecules are involved in interactions with T-helper cells, which cooperate with B cells to make antibody. Class I MHC molecules are recognized by T-killer cells, or cytotoxic T lymphocytes, that lyse virally infected cells. In both cases, T-cell recognition of antigen together with a "self" MHC molecule is termed MHC "restricted" recognition (for review, see Davis 1985; Kronenberg et al. 1986).

It has now been established that MHC-restricted T-cell receptors (TCRs) recognize peptide fragments of antigens (presumably derived from intracellular processing) bound to an MHC molecule at what appears to be a single site. Two major lines of evidence point to the involvement of peptides in T-cell recognition: Peptide fragments of an antigen added to the outside of fixed class II MHC-bearing target cells can be recognized by T-helper cells specific for the appropriate combination of antigen and MHC type (Shimonkevitz et al. 1983). Subsequently, short synthetic peptides (8–30 residues long) were shown to bind to purified class II proteins (Babbitt et al. 1985). In some cases, the binding of a particular peptide by an MHC molecule correlated with the ability of an animal of that MHC type to mount an immune response against the antigen from which the peptide was derived (Buus et al. 1987), suggesting a reason for the observation that there is a correlation between immunological response to an antigen and certain specificities of histocompatibility molecules (McDevitt et al. 1972). It has been much more difficult to demonstrate peptide binding to purified class I MHC molecules, although class I and class II MHC molecules are similar in domain organization, sequence, and presumably three-dimensional structure (Brown et al. 1988). However, virus-specific T-killer cells have been shown to lyse an uninfected target cell of appropriate class I specificity to which peptide fragments of a viral protein have been added (Townsend et al. 1986). By analogy with the work described for class II MHC molecules, it is assumed that the class I molecules on the target cell bind peptides, and that it is a peptide/MHC complex that is recognized by TCRs on the cytotoxic killer cells. Some T cells recognize foreign or "non-self" MHC molecules in the apparent absence of antigen, although in these cases, it is possible that the peptide-binding site is occupied by an endogenous peptide. The reactivity of T cells and antibodies against foreign MHC molecules leads to host rejection of transplanted tissue.

The discovery that MHC molecules bind antigenic peptides and present them to T cells has allowed the correlation of susceptibility to autoimmune disease with certain MHC alleles to be understood on a more molecular basis. Any given MHC molecule binds only a subset of peptides tested, and as discussed above, the ability to bind a peptide can determine the immune response to an antigen. Increased susceptibility to autoimmune diseases such as ankylosing spondylitis and insulin-dependent diabetes mellitus are found in individuals of certain MHC types, and such diseases arise when the body's immune system attacks its own proteins (for review, see Todd et al. 1988). It is thought that the MHC molecules correlated with autoimmune disease bind peptides from self proteins, leading to tissue damage by self-reactive T-cell clones.

One hopes that an increased understanding of the physical nature of antigenic peptide interactions with MHC molecules will allow the design of peptides to stimulate the immune response against a viral infection, or the design of high-affinity ligands that block the self-reactive recognition of MHC molecules involved in autoimmune diseases. Before this can be accomplished, we will need to understand not only the forces comprising the peptide/MHC complex, but also how TCRs bind to it. In this paper, we briefly discuss what the crystal structure of a human class I MHC molecule reveals about how histocompatibility molecules might interact with TCRs, and we present a hypothetical model for how MHC-restricted TCRs bind to the peptide/MHC complex. The three-dimensional structure of a TCR has not yet been determined, but because of the similarity between TCRs and antibodies, we can use the known structure of an Fab to serve as a first-order TCR model structure, in order to make an educated guess about how T-cell recognition of the peptide/MHC complex occurs.

TCR Structure and Potential Diversity

TCRs are membrane-bound disulfide-linked heterodimers that resemble the Fab fragments of immunoglobulins in sequence and domain organization (for review, see Kronenberg et al. 1986). Each polypeptide chain contains a domain with sequence similarity to antibody variable (V) domains, followed by a domain similar to an antibody constant (C) domain. Following the constant-like domain in each chain, there is a hinge region containing a cysteine residue involved in the formation of an interchain disulfide bond, and then a hydrophobic membrane-spanning sequence and short cytoplasmic tail. Figure 1 shows a schematic representation of the primary sequence organization of the four TCR polypeptide chains that make up the two different types of receptor heterodimers (α/β and γ/δ). As in immunoglobulins, both the α/β and γ/δ TCRs are assembled by the relatively random joining of different coding segments to C-region genes (V and J join to C in the case of α and γ chains; V, D, and J join to C in the case of β and δ chains). Although variability in TCR V regions is less localized than in immunoglobulin V regions, hypervariability is found in the locations corresponding to the three classic immunoglobulin hypervariable regions or complementarity-determining regions (CDRs) (Patten et al. 1984; Barth et al. 1985), which are known in antibodies to form the principal points of contact with antigen (Wu and Kabat 1970; Kabat et al. 1987). In both antibodies and TCRs, the first and second CDR are encoded within the V gene segment itself, and the third CDR is formed by the junction of the V gene segment with D and J gene segments (in the case of immunoglobulin heavy chains

and TCR β and δ chains) or with J gene segments alone (immunoglobulin light chains and TCR α and γ).

Although TCRs and immunoglobulins share a similar organization of diversity and mechanisms for its generation, a closer look at TCR diversity shows a striking concentration of sequence polymorphism in the CDR3-equivalent region as compared to this region in antibodies (discussed in more detail in Davis and Bjorkman 1988). In contrast, TCR diversity within the CDR1- and CDR2-equivalent regions is far less pronounced than in immunoglobulins. The primary cause of decreased TCR diversity in the first and second CDR regions is that there are far fewer TCR V gene segments than immunoglobulin V gene segments. Assuming that the V domains of TCRs pair to form a combining site (as is the case for antibody V regions), the combinatorial diversity resulting from a random pairing of TCR V domains shows even greater disparity from the amount of diversity resulting from antibody V region pairing. Estimates for the amounts of sequence diversity possible for immunoglobulins and TCRs are compared in Table 1. As a result of the many mechanisms generating diversity within the CDR3-equivalent or junctional region in TCRs, the potential diversity is estimated to be between 4 and 7 orders of magnitude higher in TCRs as compared to immunoglobulins. On the other hand, the amount of potential TCR nonjunctional diversity (within the CDR1- and CDR2-equivalent regions) is estimated to be between 10 and 1000 times less than that possible for antibodies.

To rationalize the striking concentration of TCR diversity within the junctional region and relative lack of diversity elsewhere, it should be relevant to consider what TCRs are known to do; namely, to recognize a large number of small molecules (i.e., peptides) embedded in physically larger and much less diverse MHC molecules. The simplest interpretation of the skewing of diversity in the TCR case toward the CDR3-equivalent region is that the amino acids in this region are mainly interacting with peptide determinants, and that residues within the much less diverse CDR1- and CDR2-equivalent regions are primarily involved in contacts to MHC determinants.

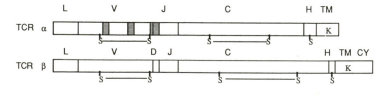

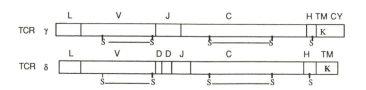

Figure 1. Schematic representation of primary structure of TCR polypeptides. Leader (L), variable (V), diversity (D), and joining (J) gene segment contributions are indicated for the variable domains. The constant portion of each TCR polypeptide is divided into the immunoglobulin-like constant (C) region, a hinge (H), transmembrane (TM) region, and cytoplasmic (CY) domain. The approximate locations of cysteine residues involved in disulfide bonds are indicated by an external "S" connected to another cysteine indicated by an external "S". The cysteine in the hinge region is presumed to form an interchain disulfide bond. The approximate location of CDR1-, CDR2-, and CDR3-equivalent regions are indicated by shading in the primary structure of the TCR α-chain.

Table 1. Sequence Diversity in T-cell Receptor and Immunoglobulin Genes

	Immunoglobulin		TCR α/β		TCR γ/δ	
	H	κ	α	β	γ	δ
Variable segments	250–1000	250	100	25	7	10
Diversity segments	10	0	0	2	0	2
Ds read in all frames	rarely	—	—	often	—	often
N-region addition	V-D, D-J	none	V-J	V-D, D-J	V-J	V-D1, D1-D2, D1-J
Joining segments	4	4	50	12	2	2
Variable region combinations	62,500–250,000		–	2500		70
Junctional combinations	$\sim 10^{11}$			$\sim 10^{15}$		$\sim 10^{18}$

Calculated potential amino acid sequence diversity in TCR and immunoglobulin genes without allowance for somatic mutation. The approximate number of V gene segments are listed for the four TCR polypeptides and contrasted with immunoglobulin heavy and light chains. CDR1 and CDR2 are encoded within the V gene segments. The pairing of random V regions generates the combinatorial diversity listed as "variable region combinations." Because there are fewer TCR V gene segments than immunoglobulin V gene segments, the combinatorial diversity is lower in TCRs than in immunoglobulins. Estimates for the number of unique sequences possible within the junctional region are contrasted for TCRs and immunoglobulins. Amino acids within CDR3 are encoded almost entirely within the D and/or J region gene segments. (The last few amino acids encoded by a TCR V gene segment can contribute to diversity within the TCR CDR3-equivalent region, but the effects of these residues on junctional diversity are not included in these calculations.) The mechanisms for generation of diversity within the junctional region that are used for this calculation include usage of different D and J gene segments, N region addition up to six nucleotides at each junction, variability in the 3′ joining position in V and J gene segments, and translation of D regions in different reading frames. Numbers are corrected for out-of-frame joining codon redundancy and N-region mimicry of germ-line sequences as described by Elliott et al. (1988).

At this point, it would be useful to compare the three-dimensional structure of a TCR to the structure of HLA-A2 to see if there is any structural reason to hypothesize the alignment of CDR1 and 2 with MHC residues, and CDR3 with residues on a bound peptide. Although the crystal structure of a TCR is unknown, sequence data suggest that TCR V regions are folded into β-sandwich structures resembling immunoglobulin V regions (Chien et al. 1984; Hedrick et al. 1984; Yanagi et al. 1984). In antibodies, the hypervariable or CDR regions are located on loops that connect β-strands, and the V regions from the heavy and light chains (V_H and V_L) are paired such that CDR1,2, and 3 from each domain are clustered at the ends of the Fab arms of the molecule, forming the antigen-binding site (for review, see Davies and Metzger 1983). In all of the three-dimensional structures of antibodies that are known, V_H and V_L domains have a conserved mode of interaction in which they are paired about an approximate twofold symmetry axis (i.e., one domain is related to the other by a 180° rotation). Thus, in different Fabs, the CDR loops are found in the same relative positions with respect to each other (Chothia et al. 1985). A study of immunoglobulin sequences and structures has identified conserved amino acids that are critical for maintaining the V_H–V_L contact surface, and most of these amino acids are found in homologous positions in TCR V region sequences (Novotny et al. 1986; Chothia et al. 1988). It is therefore likely that TCR V domains will not only fold into tertiary structures similar to antibody V regions, but that the chain pairing and resulting combining sites of TCRs will also be similar to those described for antibodies. This conclusion has been recently reached after a systematic study of immunoglobulin structures and a comparison of TCR and immunoglobulin sequences by Chothia et al. (1988). These authors conclude that TCR and anti-body V domains will share a similar β-sheet framework, as well as a similar domain interface. Strongly conserved residues are also found in TCR β sequences at sites homologous to those that form the conserved contact between the framework of the V and C domains of the immunoglobulin heavy chain, implying that V_β and C_β will associate in the same way as V_H and C_H1. We can therefore use what is known about antigen binding from crystal structures of Fab and of Fab/antigen complexes to serve as a guideline for understanding how TCRs bind to their ligand.

In antibodies, the first and second CDRs on V_L are separate from their counterparts on V_H, and the space between them is occupied by the CDR3 regions from each chain (Davies and Metzger 1983). In Figure 2A, the relative locations of the six CDR regions in an immunoglobulin combining site are shown (for our purposes to represent the approximate structure of a TCR combining site). In this view of the V_H–V_L pair, the pseudo twofold axis is perpendicular to the plane of the paper and located between the two CDR3 loops. Structural studies of antibodies complexed with protein antigens have shown that side chains from all six CDRs can contact the antigen, and that the entire antigen/antibody interface is a rather flat surface with protrusions and depressions in the antibody being complementary to the antigen surface (Amit et al. 1986; Colman et al. 1987; Sheriff et al. 1987). Assuming these details are also true for the combining site for a TCR, we now turn to a discussion of the structure of the TCR ligand, i.e., the peptide/MHC complex.

MHC Structure

The three-dimensional structure of HLA-A2, a human class I MHC molecule, has been determined (Bjorkman et al. 1987a,b), and it is likely that other

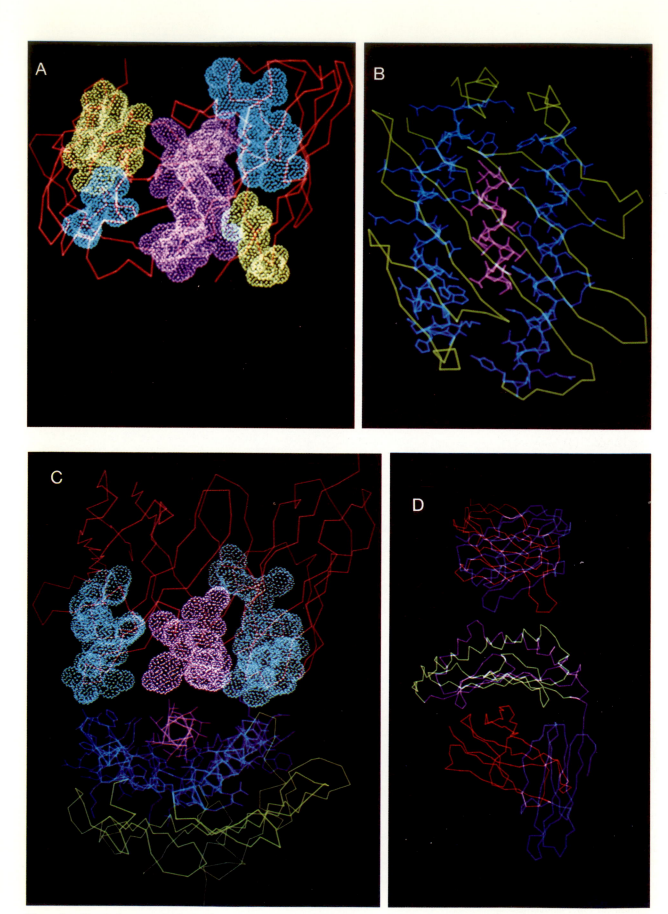

Figure 2. (*See facing page for legend.*)

class I as well as class II MHC molecules (Brown et al. 1988) will fold into similar tertiary structures. The HLA-A2 molecule is composed of two structural motifs: The membrane proximal α_3 and β_2 microglobulin domains are folded like immunoglobulin C domains, and the membrane-distal α_1 and α_2 domains consist of a platform of eight β-strands topped by two α-helices. The α_1 and α_2 domains have similar tertiary structures, each consisting of four β-strands and a long helical region. As is also the case for immunoglobulin and presumably TCR V domains, the α_1 and α_2 domains are related by an approximate twofold symmetry axis when they are paired in the HLA structure. Since these are the domains that show most of the polymorphism between different alleles, one would expect that the peptide-binding site and TCR recognition regions would be located on this part of the molecule. Several lines of evidence suggest the peptide-binding site on MHC molecules is the deep groove that separates the two α-helices on its top surface, and that this surface is therefore the part of the MHC molecule that the TCR recognizes: (1) The groove is located on the top of the molecule, and is thus in a likely position to interact with a molecule on the surface of another cell. (2) The groove is ~25 Å long and ~10 Å wide and deep, dimensions consistent with the expectation that MHC molecules bind a processed (i.e., peptide) form of an antigen. (3) Many of the residues that form the sides and the bottom of the site are highly polymorphic or have been identified to be critical for T-cell recognition of class I molecules, fitting with the expectation that MHC polymorphisms affect the peptide binding and T-cell reactivity. (4) The crystal structure of HLA-A2 shows that the site appears to be occupied by a molecule or mixture of molecules that evidently copurified and cocrystallized with HLA-A2. Although other interpretations are possible, it seems most likely that these molecules represent a heterogeneous mixture of endogenous peptides perhaps added during synthesis of HLA. If the peptide-binding site is occupied, the top surface of the peptide/MHC complex is relatively flat, as can be shown by model-building short peptides into the HLA-A2 structure. (In fact, in the original electron density maps of HLA-A2, the top surface of the molecule appears fairly level because of the presence of the unknown occupant[s] in this site.) A view of the top surface of HLA-A2 combined with a 12-residue peptide model-built (as an α-helix) into the presumed peptide-binding site is shown in Figure 2B (to scale with respect to the V regions combining site, Fig. 2A). The HLA-A2 structure is discussed in more detail by Bjorkman et al. (1987a,b).

A Model for TCR Recognition of the Peptide/MHC Complex

When the (hypothetical) TCR combining site is compared to the top surface of the peptide/MHC complex that is its ligand, it is interesting to note that the α-helices that make up the sides of the MHC peptide-binding site are separated by about the same distance as separates the CDR1 and 2 regions of one V domain from another (18 Å). Thus, the relatively flat surface of a peptide/MHC complex could interact with the combining site of an immunoglobulin-like TCR such that the limited diversity in the CDR1- and CDR2-equivalent regions on TCR V_α and V_β contacts the side chains of the MHC α-helices, leaving the centrally located and very diverse CDR3-equivalent regions to interact with the peptide. Using immunoglobulin V regions as a model for a TCR and HLA-A2 with a hypothetical peptide as the MHC molecule, this type of interaction is shown in Figure 2C. A more extensive discussion of this model for TCR recognition of peptide/MHC com-

Figure 2. Representation of the structures of (A) the immunoglobulin antigen-binding site, (B) the peptide-binding site of an MHC molecule, and (C) the alignment of CDRs in a hypothetical TCR over a peptide/MHC complex. (A) View from the top (the direction of antigen) of an immunoglobulin combining site (Fab J539; Suh et al. 1986) with the three CDRs on each chain highlighted with van der Waals surfaces (CDR1: yellow, CDR2: blue, CDR3: pink, carbon-α backbone of V_H and V_L shown in red). Similarities between TCRs and immunoglobulins suggest that TCR combining sites will preserve the same general features, having CDR1 and CDR2 from one domain separate from their counterparts on the partner domain and the space between them occupied by CDR3 from each domain (see text for details). (B) Top surface of an MHC molecule with the side chains of the amino acids located in two helices on either side of the peptide-binding site highlighted in blue. A hypothetical peptide (a 12-mer polyvaline) has been model-built into the peptide-binding site as an α-helix (shown in pink). Carbon-α backbone of HLA-A2 (Bjorkman et al. 1987a,b) is shown in green. Note that the distance between the MHC α-helices is approximately the same as the distance the first and second CDRs on one V domain are separated from their counterparts on the partner V domain (see part A). (C) Model for TCR interaction with a peptide/MHC complex. The molecules in this figure are rotated ~90° with respect to their orientation in parts A and B on this figure. The antibody V domains (top of figure) here represent a TCR bound to a peptide/MHC complex (bottom of figure). The carbon-α backbone of the V domains (red) is shown with the amino acids within CDR1 and CDR2 highlighted with blue van der Waals surfaces, and amino acids within CDR3 highlighted in pink van der Waals surfaces. The MHC carbon-α backbone is shown in green with side chains located on the α-helices highlighted in blue. A (hypothetical) peptide model built into the binding site as an α-helix is shown in pink. The relatively flat surface of the V region combining site is complementary to the peptide/MHC complex, with the first and second CDR from each V domain "fitting" over an MHC α-helix, leaving the centrally located CDR3 regions aligned over the peptide (see text for details). (D) Side view of model for TCR interacting with an MHC molecule. The V domains and MHC molecule have been rotated to show that there is sufficient space on the top surface of the MHC molecule for TCR V regions (here depicted as immunoglobulin V regions) to bind in several different registers along the MHC α-helices. The carbon-α backbone of V_H and V_L (here representing TCR V_α and V_β) are shown in red and blue (top of figure). At the bottom of the figure are the four domains of a class I MHC molecule (α_1: green, α_2: pink, α_3: blue, β_2-microglobulin: red).

plexes has been published (Davis and Bjorkman 1988), and a similar model has been suggested by Claverie and co-workers (Claverie et al. 1989).

This model for TCR and MHC/peptide interactions is consistent with some recent work correlating TCR α/β sequences with known antigen-MHC specificities. For example, in some cytochrome-c-specific T-cell clones, changes in the junctional region alter the specificity for peptide without altering MHC specificity (Fink et al. 1986; Winoto et al. 1986). Also, some of the TCRs from these clones show a selection for certain amino acids within the CDR3-equivalent region, suggesting that junctional residues are important for peptide recognition (Hedrick et al. 1988). This idea was tested by changing one of the conserved junctional residues by site-directed mutagenesis, with the result that the mutated TCR displayed a different fine specificity for antigen (Engel and Hedrick 1988).

Even within the confines of our model for TCR interaction with peptide/MHC complexes, however, one would not always expect a direct correlation of TCR junctional residues with specificity for a particular peptide, for the simple reason that changes in MHC residues could alter the conformation or orientation of a bound peptide, thus requiring a compensatory change in the TCR residues contacting the peptide. Also, we would not expect that the V_α and V_β gene segments used by T cells restricted to the same MHC molecule would always be the same, because the surface of a peptide/MHC complex is large enough to allow a TCR (assuming an immunoglobulin-like binding site) to bind in different registers along the MHC α-helices. In Figure 2D, the V-regions/MHC complex has been rotated by 90° so that the MHC α-helices are approximately in the plane of the paper to demonstrate that there is room on the top surface of the MHC molecule for a TCR molecule to bind in several different regions. In addition, because antibody (and presumably TCR) V regions pair with approximate dyad symmetry and because the MHC α_1–α_2 domains are approximately dyad symmetric, the interaction of CDR1 and CDR2 residues with MHC determinants and CDR3 with peptide determinants can be accomplished in either of two orientations related to each other by 180°. (In other words, the interaction depicted in Figure 2C would look the same if the V regions dimer were rotated by 180° about its pseudo-dyad axis, which is vertical in this figure).

It is likely that an exact correlation between TCR hypervariable region sequences and MHC and peptide specificities will never be possible, due to the spatial proximity of CDR residues in the combining site. Also, it is a bit of an oversimplification to assume that TCR interactions with ligand will exclusively involve residues in the CDR loops, because crystal structures of Fabs complexed to protein antigens have shown that framework residues adjacent to the CDR loops can contact the antigen (Amit et al. 1986; Sheriff et al. 1987). However, the structural complementarity between the MHC peptide-binding site and the (hypothetical) TCR

combining site depicted in Figure 2C may provide an explanation for the original suggestion by Jerne (1971) that T-cell antigen receptors and MHC molecules coevolved to have some affinity for each other and gives us some idea of what MHC-restricted TCR recognition means at the molecular level. This model also provides a rationale for the decreased number of TCR V gene segments as compared to immunoglobulin V gene segments, because the variability within the portion of the protein they encode is primarily predicted to interact with a limited number of MHC molecules within any given individual (on the order of 6 class I and 20 class II MHC molecules in a heterozygous individual). Finally, the model may serve as a useful framework for the design of experiments to alter TCR residues and test the effect on MHC or peptide recognition.

Thymic Selection

In a way that is not fully understood, the T cells that leave the thymus have receptors that can recognize foreign antigen plus self-MHC, but not self-MHC alone (or self-MHC plus a self-peptide) when they are in the periphery (for review, see Marrack and Kappler 1987). It is difficult to understand how this selection can occur, since the huge number of foreign peptides that the TCR must recognize are not present in the thymus. The selection of receptors is thought to operate on two levels: There is a "positive" selection for TCRs that recognize antigen in the context of their own MHC, and a "negative" selection against self-reactive receptors to ensure that individuals are tolerant to their own proteins. It has been suggested that all TCRs with some affinity for self-MHC are selected, but only thymocytes with a low affinity for self are allowed to mature because the process of tolerance deletes cells with TCRs that have a moderate to high affinity for self-MHC (Marrack and Kappler 1987). The TCRs with low affinity for self-MHC are assumed to have an increased affinity for some combination of self-MHC plus foreign peptide that they will encounter in the periphery.

It is difficult to understand, however, how a positively selected TCR could bind tightly enough to distinguish residues on a self-MHC molecule from a non-self molecule, yet apparently disregard interactions with any self-peptides that are present on MHC molecules in the thymus during selection. As can be seen by examination of the HLA-A2 structure, a TCR binding to the top surface of the peptide/MHC complex would, by necessity, interact with a bound peptide. In fact, because of the physical proximity of side chains contributed by the MHC molecule and side chains from the peptide, almost any shape of molecule recognizing the top of the MHC molecule could not help but interact with parts of a bound peptide. As a way around the dilemma of the absence of foreign peptides during positive selection, it has been postulated that the foreign peptides to which the TCR responds in the periphery resemble self-peptides that are bound to

MHC molecules in the thymus. As has been suggested by Marrack and Kappler (1987), the MHC molecules on the thymus cortical epithelial cells might bind a different spectrum of peptides than is found elsewhere in the animal. In this scenario, these peptides would not be found on bone-marrow-derived cells, hence the process of tolerance would not delete cells with TCRs specific for self-MHC plus a thymic cortical epithelial-specific peptide. These cells would then go on to join the peripheral T-cell pool, where they would respond to foreign peptides that resemble the peptide upon which they were selected. A variant of this idea suggests that spontaneous mutation of self-proteins could generate enough variants to self-peptides to allow TCRs to be selected to recognize a self-MHC plus a mutated self-peptide that resembles a foreign peptide to be encountered later in the periphery (Kourilsky and Claverie 1989). However, it is hard to imagine that enough variability in self-peptides would be generated to account for a T-cell response against a universe of foreign antigens.

Another way to reconcile the existence of positive selection with the absence of foreign antigens in the thymus would be to assume that the MHC molecules in the thymic cortical epithelium have empty peptide-binding sites, which is not unreasonable from a purely structural point of view. Since the residues lining the site in HLA-A2 are not exclusively hydrophobic (Bjorkman et al. 1987b), one could imagine that the peptide-binding site could be filled with water molecules, resulting in an empty MHC molecule with a structure similar to that of HLA-A2 (in which the site was found to be occupied by an unknown molecule or mixture of molecules). An empty class II MHC molecule is also a structural possibility, since an examination of the class II MHC sequences shows that the residues predicted to be in the peptide-binding site are also not particularly hydrophobic. If TCRs are positively selected by binding to MHC molecules with empty peptide-binding sites, they could recognize the MHC α-helices using residues within their CDR1 and CDR2 loops, leaving the selection of residues within the CDR3 junctional region to be almost completely unconstrained. Following a selection of TCRs with affinity for self-MHC, those TCRs with an affinity for self-MHC plus a self-peptide could be eliminated by whatever mechanism controls negative selection, leaving a number of TCRs capable of recognizing a self-MHC plus foreign peptide complex.

The idea that positive selection occurs on empty MHC molecules assumes that at least some MHC molecules in the thymic cortical epithelium are capable of reaching the cell surface without a bound peptide. However, recent results from Townsend's laboratory suggest that the intracellular assembly and cell-surface expression of class I MHC molecules are dependent on peptide binding (Townsend et al., this volume). It is still possible, though, that some small percentage of MHC molecules manage to reach the cell surface of the thymic cortical epithelium without a bound peptide.

TCRs that are positively selected by binding to these empty molecules could survive a subsequent negative selection step, whereas the majority of TCRs that are positively selected on MHC molecules occupied with a self-peptide would be eliminated during negative selection.

TCR Recognition of Superantigens

Recently, several self-antigens in combination with murine class II MHC molecules have been shown to form ligands that are recognized by virtually all T cells whose receptors bear certain V_β elements, without apparent regard to V_α, J_α, D_β, or J_β gene usage (Kappler et al. 1987, 1988; McDonald et al. 1988; Pullen et al. 1988). The best-studied such antigen is encoded within the Mls locus, and mice combining particular Mls and MHC haplotypes are found to have deleted T cells bearing certain V_β TCRs during the establishment of self-tolerance. Assuming that Mls products are processed and presented as peptides bound to MHC molecules, one interpretation of the correlation of TCR V_β sequences with reactivity to Mls is that specific germ-line V_β-encoded residues are in direct contact with antigen. Since this interpretation is in direct conflict with our model for TCR interaction with the peptide/MHC complex, we will discuss an alternative explanation for these data originally suggested by Janeway and colleagues (Janeway et al. 1989).

The molecular nature of the Mls product is not known, but it has been suggested to be many things, including a unique peptide bound to an MHC molecule (Kappler et al. 1988). However, the T-cell response to Mls differs in several ways from a response to conventional antigens that are recognized as peptides embedded in MHC molecules: The response is very strong, stimulating about 20% of all T cells, and is not strictly MHC restricted (Janeway et al. 1989). Recently, the T-cell response to certain bacterial enterotoxins has been found to closely resemble the response to Mls, both in its strength and in the correlation of certain V_β TCR chains with T-cell reactivity, and the Mls product and the enterotoxins are now being called "superantigens" (White et al. 1989). In the case of T-cell recognition of the bacterial enterotoxins, antigen processing (i.e., degradation into peptides) is not required, and furthermore, the intact protein has been shown to bind to purified class II MHC molecules (Fraser 1989). It is therefore likely that the T-cell response to the superantigens may represent a special mode of recognition in which the intact antigen has some intrinsic affinity for TCR V_β subunits. The model proposed by Janeway and colleagues (Janeway et al. 1989) suggests that a superantigen (the Mls product or an enterotoxin) binds as an intact protein to the sides of the class II MHC molecule and the V_β TCR subunit, effectively forming a bridge between the T cell and antigen-presenting cell. The interaction between the TCR and peptide/MHC complex is thus undisturbed by the superantigen and could be as we have proposed (Davis and Bjorkman

1988 and this paper). The MHC peptide-binding site could even be occupied by an endogenous peptide, since the superantigen is proposed to bind in a region distinct from this site. Recent data from the laboratory of Mathis and Benoist support the contention that superantigens do not interact with MHC molecules like conventional peptides, in that mutations within the peptide-binding site of a class II molecule that abrogated peptide presentation had no effect on the recognition of the enterotoxin SEB (Dellabona et al., this volume). The idea that superantigens are presented to T cells in a fundamentally different way from processed peptides bound in the MHC peptide-binding site is attractive, because it is difficult to envision how the V_β portion of the TCR could exclusively contact a peptide bound in the binding site of an MHC molecule as we understand the architecture of this site from the crystal structure of HLA-A2 (Bjorkman et al. 1987a,b).

REFERENCES

Amit, A.G., R.A. Mariuzza, S.E.V. Phillips, and R.J. Poljak. 1986. Three-dimensional structure of an antigen-antibody complex at 2.8 Å resolution. *Science* 233: 747.

Barth, R.K., B.S. Kim, B.S. Lan, N.C. Lan, T. Hunkapiller, N. Sobieck, A. Winoto, H. Gershenfeld, C. Okada, D. Hansburg, I.L. Weissman, and L. Hood. 1985. The murine T cell receptor uses a limited repertoire of expressed Vβ gene segments. *Nature* 316: 517.

Babbitt, B.P., P.M. Allen, G. Matsueda, E. Haber, and E.R. Unanue. 1985. Binding of immunogenetic peptides to immunoglobulin histocompatibility molecules. *Nature* 324: 317.

Bjorkman, P.J., M.A. Saper, B. Samraoui, W.S. Bennett, J.L. Strominger, and D.C. Wiley. 1987a. Structure of the human class I histocompatibility antigen, HLA-A2. *Nature* 329: 506.

———. 1987b. The foreign antigen binding site and T cell recognition regions of class I histocompatibility antigens. *Nature* 329: 512.

Brown, J.H., T. Jardetzky, M.A. Saper, B. Samraoui, P.J. Bjorkman, and D.C. Wiley. 1988. A hypothetical model of the foreign antigen binding site of class II histocompatibility molecules. *Nature* 332: 845.

Buus, S., A. Sette, S.M. Colon, C. Miles, and H.M. Grey. 1987. The relation between major histocompatibility complex (MHC) restriction and the capacity of Ia to bind immunogenic peptides. *Science* 235: 1353.

Chien, Y.-H., D. Becker, T. Lindsten, M. Okamura, D. Cohen, and M.M. Davis. 1984. A third type of murine T cell receptor gene. *Nature* 312: 31.

Chothia, C., D.R. Boswell, and A.M. Lesk. 1988. The outline structure of the T-cell αβ receptor. *EMBO J.* 7: 3745.

Chothia, C., J. Novotny, R. Bruccoleri, and M. Karplus. 1985. Domain association in immunoglobulin molecules. The packing of variable domains. *J. Mol. Biol.* 186: 651.

Claverie, J.-M., A. Prochnicka-Chalufour, and L. Bouguel-eret. 1989. Implications of a Fab-like structure for the T-cell receptor. *Immunol. Today* 10: 10.

Colman, P.M., W.G. Laver, J.N. Varghese, A.T. Baker, P.A. Tulloch, G.M. Air, and R.G. Webster. 1987. Three-dimensional structure of a complex of antibody with influenza virus neuraminidase. *Nature* 326: 358.

Davies, D.R. and H. Metzger. 1983. Structural basis of antibody function. *Annu. Rev. Immunol.* 1: 87.

Davis, M.M. 1985. Molecular genetics of the T cell receptor β chain. *Annu. Rev. Immunol.* 3: 537.

Davis, M.M. and P.J. Bjorkman. 1988. T-cell antigen receptor genes and T-cell recognition. *Nature* 334: 395.

Elliott, J.R., E.P. Rock, M.M. Davis, and Y.-H. Chien. 1988. The adult T cell receptor δ chain is diverse and distinct from that of fetal thymocytes. *Nature* 331: 627.

Engel, I. and S.M. Hedrick. 1988. Site-directed mutations in the VDJ junctional region of a T cell receptor β chain cause changes in antigenic peptide recognition. *Cell* 54: 473.

Fink, P.J., L.A. Matis, D.L. McElligott, M. Bookman, and S.M. Hedrick. 1986. Correlations between T-cell specificity and the structure of the antigen receptor. *Nature* 321: 219.

Fraser, J.D. 1989. High affinity binding of staphylococcal enterotoxins A and B to HLA-DR. *Nature* 339: 221.

Hedrick, S.M., E.A. Nielsen, J. Kavaler, D.I. Cohen, and M.M. Davis. 1984. Sequence relationships between putative T cell receptor polypeptides and immunoglobulins. *Nature* 308: 153.

Hedrick, S.M., I. Engel, D.L. McElligott, P.J. Fink, M.-L. Hsu, D. Hansburg, and L.A. Matis. 1988. Selection of amino acid sequences in the beta chain of the T cell antigen receptor. *Science* 239: 1541.

Janeway, C.A., J. Yagi, P.J. Conrad, M.E. Katz, B. Jones, S. Vroegop, and S. Buxser. 1989. T-cell responses to Mls and to bacterial proteins that mimic its behavior. *Immunol. Rev.* 107: 61.

Jerne, N.K. 1971. The somatic generation of immune recognition. *Eur. J. Immunol.* 1: 1.

Kabat, E.A., T.T. Wu, M. Reid-Miller, H.M Perry, and K.S. Gottesman. 1987. *Sequences of proteins of immunological interest*, 4th edition. Public Health Service, National Institutes of Health, Washington, D.C.

Kappler, J.W., N. Roehm, and P. Marrack. 1987. T cell tolerance by clonal elimination in the thymus. *Cell* 49: 273.

Kappler, J.W., U. Staerz, J. White, and P. Marrack. 1988. Self-tolerance eliminates T cells specific for Mls-modified products of the major histocompatibility complex. *Nature* 332: 35.

Kourilsky, P. and J.-M. Claverie. 1989. MHC restriction, alloreactivity, and thymic education: A common link? *Cell* 56: 327.

Kronenberg, M., G. Siu, L.E. Hood, and N. Shastri. 1986. The molecular genetics of the T-cell antigen receptor and T-cell antigen recognition. *Annu. Rev. Immunol.* 4: 529.

MacDonald, H.R., R. Schneider, R.K. Lees, R.C. Howe, H. Acha-Orbea, H. Festenstein, R.M. Zinkernagel, and H. Hengartner. 1988. T cell receptor Vβ use predicts reactivity and tolerance to Mls-encoded antigens. *Nature* 332: 40.

Marrack, P. and J. Kappler. 1987. The T cell receptor. *Science* 238: 1073.

McDevitt, H.O., B.D. Deak, D.G. Shreffler, J. Klein, J.H. Stimpfling, and G.D. Snell. 1972. Genetic control of the immune response. Mapping of the Ir-1 locus. *J. Exp. Med.* 128: 1.

Novotny, J., S. Tonegawa, H. Saito, D.M. Kranz, and H.N Eisen. 1986. Secondary, tertiary, and quaternary structure of the T-cell specific immunoglobulin-like polypeptide chains. *Proc. Natl. Acad. Sci.* 83: 742.

Patten, P., T. Yokota, J. Rothbard, Y.-H. Chien, K.-I. Arai, and M.M. Davis. 1984. Structure, expression and divergence of T cell receptor β-chain variable regions. *Nature* 312: 40.

Pullen, A.M., P. Marrack, and J.W. Kappler. 1988. The T-cell repertoire is heavily influenced by tolerance to polymorphic self-antigens. *Nature* 335: 796.

Sheriff, S., E.W. Silverton, E.A. Padlan, G.H. Cohen, S.J. Smith-Gill, B.C. Finzel, and D.R. Davies. 1987. Three-dimensional structure of an antibody-antigen complex. *Proc. Natl. Acad. Sci.* 84: 8075.

Shimonkevitz, R., J.W. Kappler, P. Marrack, and H.M. Grey. 1983. Antigen recognition by H-2 restricted T cells. Cell-free antigen processing. *J. Exp. Med.* 158: 303.

Todd, J.A., H. Acha-Orbea, J.I. Bell, N. Chao, Z. Fronek, C.O. Jacob, M. McDermott, A.A. Sinha, L. Timmerman, L. Steinman, and H.O. McDevitt. 1988. A molecular basis for MHC class II-associated autoimmunity. *Science* **240:** 1003.

Suh, S.W., T.N. Bhat, M.A. Navia, G.H. Cohen, D.N. Rao, S. Rudikoff, and D.R. Davies. 1986. The galactan-binding immunoglobulin Fab J539: An X-ray diffraction study at 2.6 Å resolution. *Proteins* **1:** 74.

Townsend, A.R.M., J. Rothbard, F.M. Gotch, G. Behador, D. Wraith, and A.J. McMichael. 1986. The epitopes of influenza nucleoprotein recognized by cytotoxic T lymphocytes can be defined with short synthetic peptides. *Cell* **44:** 959.

White, J., A. Herman, A.M. Pullen, R. Kubo, J.W. Kappler, and P. Marrack. 1989. The Vβ-specific superantigen staphylococcal enterotoxin B: Stimulation of mature T cells and clonal deletion in neonatal mice. *Cell* **56:** 27.

Winoto, A., J.L. Urban, N.C. Lan, J. Goverman, L. Hood, and D. Hansburg. 1986. Predominant use of a Vα gene segment in mouse T-cell receptors for cytochrome c. *Nature* **324:** 679.

Wu, T.T. and E.A. Kabat. 1970. An analysis of the sequences of the variable regions of Bence-Jones and myeloma light chains and the implications for antibody complementarity. *J. Exp. Med.* **132:** 211.

Yanagai, Y., Y. Yoshikai, K. Leggett, S.P. Clark, I. Aleksander, and T.W. Mak. 1984. A human T cell-specific cDNA clone encodes a protein having extensive homology to immunoglobulin chains. *Nature* **308:** 145.

Zinkernagel, R.M. and P.C. Doherty. 1974. Restriction of in vitro T-cell mediated cytotoxicity in lymphocytic choriomeningitis within a syngeneic or semi-allogeneic system. *Nature* **248:** 701.

T-cell Recognition of Superantigens: Inside or Outside the Groove?

P. DELLABONA,* J. PECCOUD, C. BENOIST, AND D. MATHIS

Laboratoire de Génétique Moléculaire des Eucaryotes du CNRS, Unité 184 de Biologie Moléculaire et de Génie Génétique de l'INSERM, Institut de Chimie Biologique, Faculté de Médecine, 67085 Strasbourg CEDEX, France

Conventional antigens usually stimulate only about one in 10^4 T cells, and alloantigens provoke a response from approximately 1% of the T-cell repertoire. Both types of antigen are surpassed by a newly recognized class of molecules capable of stimulating as many as one in five T lymphocytes. Included in this class are the staphylococcal enterotoxins (SEA-SEE), other bacterial toxins (toxic shock syndrome toxin, exfoliating toxin), the minor lymphocyte stimulatory antigens (Mls-1[a], Mls-2[a]), and the uncharacterized substances recognized by $V_\beta 17^+$, $V_\beta 11^+$, $V_\beta 5^+$, and $V_\beta 12^+$ T-cell receptors (TCRs) (for recent reviews, see Janeway et al. 1988, 1989b; Fleischer 1989; White et al. 1989). These molecules have recently been termed "superantigens" to connote their immunological potency (White et al. 1989). In the following discussion, we will focus on bacterial toxins as representative superantigens, since they, unlike the others listed, have been identified in molecular terms.

That superantigens are recognized by the TCR is now well established. T-cell responses to these molecules are clonally distributed (Fleischer and Schrezenmeier 1988; Janeway et al. 1989b; White et al. 1989) and can be blocked by anti-TCR, anti-CD3, and anti-CD4 monoclonal antibodies (MAbs) (Mollick et al. 1989; Yagi et al. 1989). Perhaps more convincing, these molecules do not stimulate all T cells—as do anti-CD3 MAbs and mitogens like concanavalin A—but only those bearing TCRs with a particular V_β region (or regions) (Kappler et al. 1989b; White et al. 1989; Yagi et al. 1989). If they are encountered by a mature T cell, activation and eventually proliferation ensue; if, on the other hand, they are encountered by a nonmature T cell during intrathymic differentiation, clonal deletion is the result (White et al. 1989; C. Janeway, pers. comm.). Although superantigens are almost certainly recognized by the TCR, it remains controversial whether they can bind directly to T cells (Fraser 1989; Mollick et al. 1989; Fischer et al. 1989 vs. Janeway et al. 1989a; and perhaps Fleischer and Schrezenmeier 1988).

That superantigens are recognized in association with major histocompatibility complex (MHC) molecules has also become increasingly evident. Several studies demonstrated a need for accessory cells and noted a correlation between efficiency as an accessory cell and level of MHC class II gene expression (Carlsson et al. 1988; Fleischer and Schrezenmeier 1988; Fischer et al. 1989; Fraser 1989; Scholl et al. 1989). This correlative argument has been rendered more convincing by the use of class-II-negative cell mutants (Fleischer and Schrezenmeier 1988) or class II gene transfectants (Mollick et al. 1989; Scholl et al. 1989; White et al. 1989). In addition, monoclonal antibodies specific for MHC class II molecules were able to block T-cell stimulation by bacterial toxins. (Fleischer and Schrezenmeier 1988; Fischer et al. 1989; Yagi et al. 1989). Finally, and most convincingly, a number of approaches have recently demonstrated direct binding of these molecules to class II complexes (Fischer et al. 1989; Fraser 1989; Janeway et al. 1989a; Mollick et al. 1989; Scholl et al. 1989).

Because recognition of superantigens demonstrably involves both the TCR and MHC class II molecules, they have excited much interest of late. The hope has been that T-cell recognition of bacterial toxins (or of mls) might serve as a paradigm for more conventional T-cell recognition events, in particular, during repertoire selection in the thymus. Unfortunately, it has remained controversial whether these substances are recognized just like conventional antigens, as peptides in the groove of the MHC complex, or whether they bind outside the groove and serve as TCR co-ligands (White et al. 1989 vs. Janeway et al. 1989b). We have attempted to resolve this controversy using varied approaches.

EXPERIMENTAL PROCEDURES

Cell lines. The T-cell hybridoma 3A9 was selected after screening a panel of hybridomas because it recognizes both a conventional antigen (hen egg white lysozyme [HEL]46-61) and several superantigens (SEB, exfoliating toxin, SEC1). This hybridoma has been described previously (Allen and Unanue 1984) and was a gift from P. Allen, Washington University, St. Louis, Missouri. The T hybridoma QO23-26.6 (26.6 for short) was provided by J. Kappler and P. Marrack, National Jewish Center for Immunology and Respiratory Diseases, Denver, Colorado.

The E_α:E_β (CA36.2.1) and E_α:E_β/Ii (CA36.2.1.Ii) transfectants have also been described previously

* Permanent address: Centro C.N.R. di Immunogenetica ed Istocompatibilità, Torino, Italy.

(Shastri et al. 1985; Stockinger et al. 1989) and were gifts from B. Malissen, Centre d'Immunologie de Marseille-Luminy, Marseilles, France, and B. Stockinger, Basel Institute for Immunology, Basel, Switzerland.

The A_α^k mutants have an alanine substitution at a single position along the putative α helix, except at positions 53 and 68, where alanine has been replaced by valine. A detailed description of the creation of the 30 mutant A_α^k cDNAs, carried in the expression vector pKCR7, will be presented elsewhere (J. Peccoud et al., in prep.). They were individually transfected into LMTK$^-$ cells together with a wild-type A_β^k cDNA in pKCR3 and the herpes simplex virus *tk* gene. HAT-resistant transfectants were selected for high A^k expression by staining with the pan-Ia reagent 40B followed by sorting. At the time of each antigen presentation assay, an aliquot of each of the antigen-presenting cell (APC) lines was reanalyzed by cytofluorimetry to ensure a consistent level of A^k expression; lines expressing aberrant levels were ignored.

Fixation experiments. APCs were fixed with either 0.05% glutaraldehyde or 0.5% paraformaldehyde in phosphate-buffered saline (PBS) for the indicated times. Lysine (0.2 M), glycine (0.2 M), or nothing was added to stop the reaction, and the cells were pelleted by centrifugation. They were washed and resuspended in tissue culture medium and used in a typical antigen presentation assay.

Antigen presentation assays. Each antigen presentation assay was conducted by adding 5×10^4 T-hybridoma cells to 5×10^4 APCs. Antigens were added to duplicate wells in five doses diluted in fivefold steps, or were not added (as a negative control). The highest concentrations were 3 μg/ml for HEL(46-61), 85 μg/ml for SEB, 23 μg/ml for exfoliating toxin, and 16

μg/ml for SEC1. After 24 hours, 50 μl of supernatant was harvested and tested for IL-2 content, using the IL-2-dependent cytotoxic T-lymphocyte line (CTLL), as described by van Ewijk et al. (1988). From the dose response curve derived for each APC line, it was possible to estimate the antigen presentation efficiency: W = the antigen concentration required by the KK line to provoke a half-maximum IL-2 response by the 3A9 cells; M = the antigen concentration required by the mutant to provoke the same level of IL-2 production; antigen presentation efficiency = W/M.

Competition assays. Competition experiments were set up in 96-well flat-bottomed microtiter plates by mixing 1.5×10^4 A_α^k:A_β^k wild-type transfected L cells with 5×10^4 3A9 cells. Nonsaturating concentrations of the target antigen (either SEB or HEL[46-61]) were added together with increasing concentrations of competitor antigen (either HEL[34-45] or A_α^k[6-20], ranging from 80 μg/ml down to 0 with twofold dilutions). After 24 hours, supernatant was collected and tested for IL-2 by the CTL assay.

RESULTS AND DISCUSSION

Fixation Experiments Indicate That SEB Is "Presented" Differently from a Conventional Antigen

Several groups have reported that fixed cells can serve as accessory cells for the stimulation of T lymphocytes by bacterial toxins (Carlsson et al. 1988; Fleischer and Schrezenmeier 1988; Yagi et al. 1989). This result has been taken as evidence that conventional antigens and superantigens are "presented" by MHC molecules in a fundamentally different fashion: The former, but not the latter, must first be processed to peptides. Unfortunately, some difficulties have been encoun-

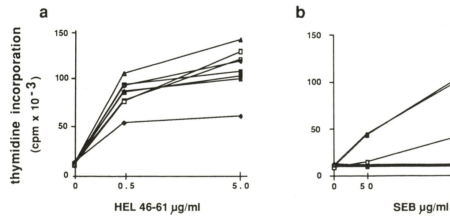

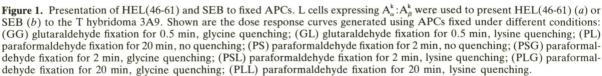

Figure 1. Presentation of HEL(46-61) and SEB to fixed APCs. L cells expressing A_α^k:A_β^k were used to present HEL(46-61) (*a*) or SEB (*b*) to the T hybridoma 3A9. Shown are the dose response curves generated using APCs fixed under different conditions: (GG) glutaraldehyde fixation for 0.5 min, glycine quenching; (GL) glutaraldehyde fixation for 0.5 min, lysine quenching; (PL) paraformaldehyde fixation for 20 min, no quenching; (PS) paraformaldehyde fixation for 2 min, no quenching; (PSG) paraformaldehyde fixation for 2 min, glycine quenching; (PSL) paraformaldehyde fixation for 2 min, lysine quenching; (PLG) paraformaldehyde fixation for 20 min, glycine quenching; (PLL) paraformaldehyde fixation for 20 min, lysine quenching.

tered in attempts to repeat these experiments in other systems (Carlsson et al. 1988; J.W. Kappler and P.C. Marrack, pers. comm.; our own unpublished results), so we decided to explore this issue systematically.

The T-cell hybridoma 3A9 recognizes HEL(46-61) and SEB in the context of the A^k class II complex. Hence, we could compare presentation of a superantigen and a conventional antigen to the same T-cell hybridoma by the same fixed APCs.

L cells expressing on A^k complex were chosen as APCs and were fixed with either glutaraldehyde or formaldehyde using various protocols. Consistent with previous reports, SEB presentation could be observed after APCs were fixed in conditions that abrogate presentation of intact proteins, but this was true of only certain conditions; namely, short fixation with paraformaldehyde (Fig. 1b). In contrast, presentation of HEL(46-61) proceeded to at least some degree after all protocols of APC fixation (Fig. 1a).

These results confirm that superantigens can be presented by fixed cells, implying that they can stimulate T cells in the absence of processing events and that they probably do not bind to MHC molecules as a peptide. This has been interpreted to indicate that superantigens bind outside the antigen groove, but it should be remembered that some conventional antigens like fibrinogen are also presented as large molecules that do not require processing and seem to have flexible segments that insert into the groove (for review, see Allen 1987). Interestingly, though, SEB stimulation of T cells is not completely resistant to fixation of APCs, unlike what was observed with a peptide antigen.

A second indication that stimulation of T cells by SEB does not require processing came from evaluating the role of Ii. Stockinger et al. (1989) have provided evidence that the class II invariant chain, Ii, is required for the presentation of intact protein but not of peptide antigens. Thus, we compared the ability of an $E_\alpha:E_\beta$ transfectant and an $E_\alpha:E_\beta/Ii$ transfectant to present SEB to the T-cell hybridoma 26-6. No difference was observed (Fig. 2), again suggesting that SEB does not need to be processed in order to stimulate a T cell.

Presentation Experiments with a Panel of Mutant APC Lines Indicate That SEB Binds Outside the Class II Molecule Antigen Groove

Brown et al. (1988) have derived a model for the structure of MHC class II complexes based on their crystallographic structure of a class I molecule. This model is consistent with the little physical information that is available (Gorga et al. 1989), is supported by the fact that identical peptides can be recognized by class I and class II restricted T cells (Perkins et al. 1989), and is consistent with data from a number of mutagenesis experiments (Ronchese et al. 1987a,b; Braunstein and Germain 1987; Buerstedde et al. 1989; Pierres et al. 1989). It predicts that antigens bind to class II complexes in a groove: one side formed by an α helix from the α chain, the other side by an α helix from the β chain, and the floor by β sheets from both chains.

To experimentally evaluate the Brown/Wiley model, we have created a set of 30 APC lines, each expressing a mutant A_α^k chain in association with a wild-type A_β^k chain. The mutants carry alanine substitutions at each residue from positions 50 to 79—i.e., each residue of the putative α chain α helix. A detailed description of the derivation and characterization of this panel of APC lines and an evaluation of their recognition by sets of monoclonal antibodies and T-cell hybridomas will be presented elsewhere (J. Peccoud et al., in prep.). Here, we have used the lines in an attempt to establish how superantigens bind to MHC class II molecules.

Since the hybridoma 3A9 recognizes HEL(46-61) and SEB in the context of the A^k class II complex, we could compare in a well-controlled fashion the ability of our mutant APC lines to present a conventional antigen and a superantigen. The T hybridoma was incubated with a wild-type, positive-control APC line (KK) and with each of the 30 mutant lines in the presence of five different antigen concentrations (0–3 μg/ml for HEL[46-61]; 0–85 μg/ml for SEB). The amount of IL-2 produced by 3A9 was measured by the CTLL assay, thus generating an antigen dose response curve for the wild-type and each mutant line. From these curves, the presentation efficiency of the mutants was quantitated on the basis of the amount of antigen required by the wild-type line to provoke the half-maximum IL-2 response versus the amount of antigen required by the mutant lines to provoke the same level of IL-2 production. Each line was evaluated in four independent experiments; the average values are listed in Table 1.

Presentation of HEL(46-61) to 3A9 cells was very sensitive to mutations within the A_α chain α helix. Alanine substitutions at seven positions had a > 100-fold effect on presentation, and alterations at a further seven positions had an effect that was between 10- and 100-fold. Four of the seven mutations that drastically altered HEL(46-61) presentation occur in a series: 59, 62, 66, 69, and when these are situated on the model class II structure, their side chains all point into the antigen groove (see Fig. 3). This picture is very

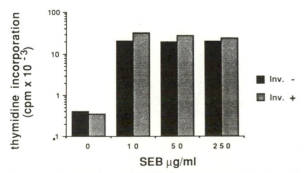

Figure 2. Presentation of SEB in the presence and absence of the invariant chain, Ii. Unfixed L cells expressing $E_\alpha^k:E_\beta^k$ (CA 36.2.1; Inv$^-$, solid bars) or $E_\alpha^k:E_\beta^k$ and Ii (CA36.2.1.Ii, Inv$^+$, hatched bars) were used to present SEB to the T hybridoma 26-6.

Table 1. Presentation by Mutant APCs

KK	HEL 46–61 1.0	SEB 1.0
50	0.3	0.5
51	0.6	0.7
52	0.04	0.2
53	n.d.	0.2
54	0.35	0.6
55	0.03	0.5
56	0.04	1.1
57	0.4	1.6
58	0.5	0.8
59	0.004	0.6
60	n.d.	n.d.
61	0.04	14.2
62	<0.001	1.0
63	0.8	2.5
64	0.03	0.2
65	<0.001	0.8
66	<0.001	0.4
67	0.05	0.2
68	<0.001	0.3
69	<0.001	1.1
70	0.3	0.6
71	0.002	100
72	0.5	3.3
73	0.3	1.0
74	0.06	0.3
75	1.1	2.5
76	0.6	0.3
77	0.3	0.8
78	0.8	2.5
79	0.4	0.6

Listed at the left are L-cell transfectants expressing the wild-type A_α^k chain (KK) or one of thirty mutant A_α^k chains (50–79), together with wild-type A_β^k. The mutants have an alanine substitution at a single position along the putative α helix, except at positions 53 and 68, where alanine has been replaced by valine. The values are the average of four determinations of antigen presentation efficiency (calculated as described in Experimental Procedures). n.d. indicates not determined.

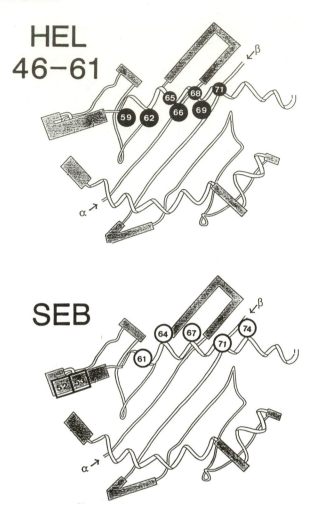

Figure 3. A_α^k residues for presentation of HEL(46-61) and SEB. Numbers in the upper panel indicate those residues whose alteration leads to >100-fold reduction in efficiency of HEL(46-61) presentation to the T hybridoma 3A9; numbers in the lower panel indicate those whose alteration leads to a >4-fold increase or decrease in SEB presentation.

similar to those we have produced with seven different T-cell hybridomas that recognize three different conventional antigens (J. Peccoud et al., in prep.).

3A9 recognition of SEB was clearly very different. Presentation of this molecule was not very sensitive to mutations within the A_α chain α helix: No alanine substitution reduced presentation as much as 10-fold, although two alterations did enhance presentation 10- to 100-fold. Moreover, the mutations that had the greatest effect on presentation (52, 53, 61, 64, 71) would be predicted to have side chains pointing away from the antigen groove (see Brown et al. 1988, legend to Fig. 3, for 52 and 53). A similar picture was produced when the panel of mutants was tested with 3A9 and two other superantigens—exfoliating toxin and SEC1 (not shown). A second T-cell hybridoma (with a different TCR V_β region) that recognizes SEB in the context of A^k showed a similar pattern of response: relatively minor influences by the alanine substitutions

and the most important effects by residues pointing away from the groove (not shown).

These results demonstrate quite clearly that HEL(46-61) and SEB bind differently to the A^k molecule. They also suggest that SEB does not bind in the antigen groove, but one must be aware of two caveats. First, it is possible that a portion of SEB binds in the groove but makes critical contacts only with the A_β chain. However, the fact that APCs expressing $A_\alpha^d:A_\beta^k$ and $A_\alpha^b:A_\beta^k$ complexes cannot present SEB to certain hybridomas even though $A_\alpha^k:A_\beta^k$, $A_\alpha^d:A_\beta^d$, and $A_\alpha^b:A_\beta^b$ complexes all can do so argues for both chains being contacted (our unpublished data). Second, it could have been that SEB residues contact multiple groove-pointing amino acids along the A_α α helix, but that no single interaction is absolutely essential for binding. However, the relatively low affinity of SEB for A^k (see below) would seem to argue against this interpretation. Nonetheless, we considered it important to provide independent evidence that SEB binds outside the antigen pocket, and we did this by performing a set of competition experiments.

Competition Experiments Confirm That SEB Binds Outside the Groove

Another means to determine whether superantigens bind in the antigen groove was to compare the ability of high-affinity groove-binding peptides to compete for HEL(46-61) versus SEB presentation to 3A9 cells. Two such competitors were employed: HEL(34-45) and A_α^k (6-20); both were known to be efficient competitors for A^k-restricted presentation of conventional peptides (E. Rosloniec, pers. comm.). The competitors were added in increasing concentrations to antigen presentation assays consisting of 3A9 cells, wild-type $A_\alpha^k:A_\beta^k$ APCs (B lymphoma or L cells, fixed or unfixed), and either HEL(46-61) or SEB. All of the experiments showed effective competition by the groove-binding peptides for HEL(46-61) but not SEB presentation. Data from a representative experiment are plotted in Figure 4.

It is highly unlikely that the results can be attributed to a higher affinity of SEB for the A^k molecule. To elicit an equivalent response in 3A9, 25 times more SEB than HEL(46-61) (on a molar basis) was required. In fact, the class II E molecule is probably the preferred target of SEB (Yagi et al. 1989).

CONCLUSION

There have been several hints that superantigens and conventional antigens interact differently with MHC class II molecules. First, fixation experiments suggested that SEs of molecular weight 20,000–30,000 could stimulate T cells without prior processing (Carlsson et al. 1988; Fleischer and Schrezenmeier 1988; Yagi et al. 1989). We have confirmed this result by employing a variety of fixation protocols and by demonstrating that

presentation of SEB is Ii-independent. Second, proteinase digestion experiments showed that SEs must remain intact for effective T-cell recognition to take place (Fraser 1989; J.W. Kappler and P.C. Marrack, pers. comm.). Third, effective stimulation by superantigens proceeds after "pulsing" either the APC or the responder T cell (Yagi et al. 1989), and there is at least some evidence that SEs can interact directly with the TCR (Fleischer and Schrezenmeier 1988; Janeway et al. 1989a). Fourth, the association and dissociation rates appear to differ greatly for binding of a bacterial toxin and a conventional peptide to MHC class II molecules (compare Scholl et al. 1989 with Buus et al. 1986). Although these arguments add up to a reasonably strong case, they are all rather indirect, and none is irrefutable.

In the experiments described herein, we have directly compared where a superantigen (SEB) and a conventional antigen (HEL[46-61]) bind on the class II A^k molecule. By two different approaches, we have demonstrated that SEB does not bind within the antigen groove, as do HEL(46-61) and all other peptide antigens tested to date.

If not inside the groove, where do superantigens bind? SEB and other toxins were presented less effectively by some of the APC lines that carry mutations along the back face of the proposed α chain α helix (e.g., positions 64, 67, 74). These molecules could lie across this face, interacting weakly at several sites along it. Alternatively, they could bind to regions of the A_α or A_β chain remote from the α helix, and the affected residues might exert only an indirect effect. Resolution of this issue will require extensive further investigation.

Our conclusion that conventional antigens and superantigens bind to MHC class II molecules in a very different fashion argues against the view that selection of T cells recognizing superantigens is a paradigm for selection events involving self-peptide antigens. Yet, it is undeniable that superantigens—in particular mls—exert a strong influence on the repertoire of T cells

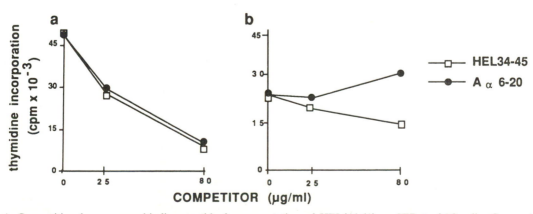

Figure 4. Competition by a groove-binding peptide for presentation of HEL(46-61) or SEB to 3A9 cells. Groove-binding peptides (HEL[34-45] and A_α[6-20]) were independently used to compete for the presentation of (*a*) HEL(46-61) or (*b*) SEB to the T hybridoma 3A9.

emerging in the periphery (Kappler et al. 1987, 1988, 1989a; Abe et al. 1988; Fry and Matis 1988; Hengartner et al. 1988; MacDonald et al. 1988; Pullen et al. 1988; Okada and Weissman 1989; White et al. 1989). Many questions arise about the evolution and normal function of these molecules.

ACKNOWLEDGMENTS

We thank Drs. Paul Allen, John Kappler, Philippa Marrack, David McKean, Brigitta Stockinger, and Bernard Malissen for the gift of cells; Dr. Ed Rosloniec for providing peptides; Caroline Waltzinger for helping with the cytofluorimetric analysis; and Philippe Gerber for innumerable harvestings. This work was supported by institutional grants from the INSERM and the CNRS; and by grants to D.M. and C.B. from the National Multiple Sclerosis Society and the National Institutes of Health (AI-26636-01). P.D. is supported by a fellowship from the Association pour la Recherche contre le Cancer and J.P. by a bursary from the CNRS and Roussel/UCLAF.

REFERENCES

Abe, R., M.S. Vacchio, B. Fox, and R.J. Hodes. 1988. Preferential expression of the T-cell receptor V$_\beta$3 gene by Mls^c reactive T cells. *Nature* 335: 827.

Allen, P.M. 1987. Antigen processing at the molecular level. *Immunol. Today* 8: 270.

Allen, P.M. and E.R. Unanue. 1984. Differential requirements for antigen processing by macrophages for lyzozyme-specific T cell hybridomas. *J. Immunol.* 132: 1077.

Braunstein, N.S. and R.N. Germain. 1987. Allele-specific control of Ia molecule surface expression and conformation: Implications for a general model of Ia structure-function relationships. *Proc. Natl. Acad. Sci.* 84: 2921.

Brown, J.H., T. Jardetzky, M.A. Saper, B. Samraoui, P.J. Bjorkman, and D.C. Wiley. 1988. A hypothetical model of the foreign antigen binding site of class II histocompatibility molecules. *Nature* 332: 845.

Buerstedde, J.M., A.E. Nilson, C.G. Chase, M.P. Bell, B.N. Beck, L.R. Pease, and D.J. McKean. 1989. Aβ polymorphic residues responsible for class II molecule recognition by alloreactive T cells. *J. Exp. Med.* 169: 1645.

Buus, S., A. Sette, S.M. Colon, D.M. Jenis, and H.M. Grey. 1986. Isolation and characterization of antigen-Ia complexes involved in T cell recognition. *Cell* 47: 1071.

Carlsson, R., H. Fischer, and H.-O. Sjögren. 1988. Binding of staphylococcal enterotoxin A to accessory cells is a requirement for its ability to activate human T cells. *J. Immunol.* 140: 2484.

Fischer, H., M. Dohlsten, M. Lindvall, H.-O. Sjögren, and R. Carlsson. 1989. Binding of staphylococcal enterotoxin A to HLA-DR on B cell lines. *J. Immunol.* 142: 3151.

Fleischer, B. 1989. Bacterial toxins as probes for the T-cell antigen receptor. *Immunol. Today* 10: 262.

Fleischer, B. and H. Schrezenmeier. 1988. T cell stimulation by staphylococcal enterotoxins. *J. Exp. Med.* 167: 1697.

Fraser, J.D. 1989. High-affinity binding of staphylococcal enterotoxins A and B to HLA-DR. *Nature* 339: 221.

Fry, A.M. and L.A. Matis. 1988. Self-tolerance alters T-cell receptor expression in an antigen-specific MHC restricted immune response. *Nature* 335: 830.

Gorga, J.C., A. Dong, M.C. Manning, R.W. Woody, W.S. Cauchey, and J.L. Strominger. 1989. Comparison of the secondary structures of human class I and class II major histocompatibility complex antigens by Fourier transform infrared and circular dichroism spectroscopy. *Proc. Natl. Acad. Sci.* 86: 2321.

Hengartner, H., B. Odermatt, R. Schneider, M. Schreyer, G. Wälle, H.R. MacDonald, and R.M. Zinkernagel. 1988. Deletion of self-reactive T cells before entry into the thymus medulla. *Nature* 336: 388.

Janeway, C.A., J. Chalupny, P.J. Conrad, and S. Buxser. 1988. An external stimulus that mimics Mls locus responses. *J. Immunogenet.* 15: 161.

Janeway, C.A., Jr., P. Portoles, J. Rojo, U. Dianzani, J. Yagi, S. Rath, and S. Buxser. 1989a. The interaction between the T cell receptor: CD4 complex and its class II MHC ligand. *UCLA Symp. Mol. Cell. Biol. New Ser.* (in press).

Janeway, C.A., Jr., J. Yagi, P.J. Conrad, M.E. Katz, B. Jones, S. Vroegop, and S. Buxser. 1989b. T-cell responses to Mls and to bacterial proteins that mimic its behavior. *Immunol. Rev.* 107: 61.

Kappler, J.W., E. Kushnir, and P. Marrack. 1989a. Analysis of Vβ17a expression in new mouse strains bearing the Vβh^a haplotype. *J. Exp. Med.* 169: 1533.

Kappler, J.W., N. Roehm, and P. Marrack. 1987. T cell tolerance by clonal elimination in the thymus. *Cell* 49: 273.

Kappler, J.W., U. Staerz, J. White, and P.C. Marrack. 1988. Self-tolerance eliminates T cells specific for Mls-modified products of the major histocompatibility complex. *Nature* 332: 35.

Kappler, J., B. Kotzin, L. Herron, E.W. Gelfand, R.D. Bigler, A. Boylston, S. Carrel, D.N. Posnett, Y. Choi, and P. Marrack. 1989b. V$_\beta$-specific stimulation of human T cells by staphylococcal toxins. *Science* 244: 811.

MacDonald, H.R., R. Schneider, R.L. Lees, R.C. Howe, H. Acha-Orbea, H. Festenstein, R.M. Zinkernagel, and H. Hengartner. 1988. T-cell receptor Vβ use predicts reactivity and tolerance to Mls^a-encoded antigens. *Nature* 332: 40.

Mollick, J.A., R.G. Cook, and R.R. Rich. 1989. Class II MHC molecules are specific receptors for staphylococcus enterotoxin A. *Science* 244: 817.

Okada, G.Y. and I.L. Weissman. 1989. Relative Vβ transcript levels in thymus and peripheral lymphoid tissues from various mouse strains. *J. Exp. Med.* 169: 1703.

Perkins, D.L., M.-Z. Lai, J.A. Smith, and M.L. Gefter. 1989. Identical peptides recognized by MHC class I- and II-restricted T cells. *J. Exp. Med.* 170: 279.

Pierres, M., S. Marchetto, P. Naquet, D. Landais, J. Peccoud, C. Benoist, and D. Mathis. 1989. I-Aα polymorphic residues that determine alloreactive T cell recognition. *J. Exp. Med.* 169: 1655.

Pullen, A.M., P. Marrack, and J.W. Kappler. 1988. The T-cell repertoire is heavily influenced by tolerance to polymorphic self-antigens. *Nature* 335: 796.

Ronchese, F., M.A. Brown, and R.N. Germain. 1987a. Structure-function analysis of the A$_\beta^{bm12}$ mutation using site-directed mutagenesis and DNA-mediated gene transfer. *J. Immunol.* 139: 629.

Ronchese, F., R.H. Schwartz, and R.N. Germain. 1987b. Functionally distinct subsites on a class II major histocompatibility complex molecule. *Nature* 329: 254.

Scholl, P., A. Diez, W. Mourad, J. Parsonnet, R.S. Geha, and T. Chatila. 1989. Toxic shock syndrome toxin 1 binds to major histocompatibility complex class II molecules. *Proc. Natl. Acad. Sci.* 86: 4210.

Shastri, N., B. Malissen, and L. Hood. 1985. Ia-transfected L-cell fibroblasts present a lysozyme peptide but not the native protein to lysozyme-specific T cells. *Proc. Natl. Acad. Sci.* 82: 5885.

Stockinger, B., U. Pessara, R.H. Lin, J. Habicht, M. Grez, and N. Koch. 1989. A role of Ia-associated invariant chains in antigen processing and presentation. *Cell* 56: 683.

van Ewijk, W., Y. Ron, J. Monaco, J. Kappler, P. Marrack, M. Le Meur, P. Gerlinger, B. Durand, C. Benoist, and D. Mathis. 1988. Compartmentalization of MHC class II gene expression in transgenic mice. *Cell* **53:** 357.

White, J., A. Herman, A.M. Pullen, R. Kubo, and J.W. Kappler. 1989. The V_β-specific superantigen staphylococcal enterotoxin B: Stimulation of mature T cells and clonal deletion in neonatal mice. *Cell* **56:** 27.

Yagi, J., J. Baron, S. Buxser, and C.A. Janeway, Jr. 1989. Bacterial proteins that mediate the association of a defined subset of T cell receptor: CD4 complexes with class II MHC. *J. Immunol.* (in press).

Antigen-binding Function
of Class II MHC Molecules

E.R. Unanue, C.V. Harding, I.F. Luescher, and R.W. Roof
Department of Pathology, Washington University School of Medicine, St. Louis, Missouri 63110

We view the histocompatibility molecules as a special transport system in antigen-presenting cells (APCs) that functions to rescue denatured or processed peptides from extensive intracellular digestion (Unanue and Allen 1987). This transport system operates by virtue of the property of the molecules of the major histocompatibility complex (MHC) to interact with peptides and unfolded proteins. At the same time, the peptide/MHC bimolecular complex constitutes the antigenic determinant that engages the $\alpha\beta$ T-cell receptor. Here, we briefly summarize salient earlier contributions and then describe our recent studies on the functions of class II MHC molecules (MHC-II).

Our initial studies indicated that protein antigens required a processing event in APCs before they could be recognized by T cells (Ziegler and Unanue 1981, 1982; Allen and Unanue 1984). This processing took place in acid intracellular vesicles and consisted of either the unfolding of the molecule or its fragmentation to small peptides. We concentrated our efforts on the examination of hen egg white lysozyme (HEL), a well-defined protein, immunogenic in various strains of mice. HEL recognition by T-cell hybridomas required its internalization by APCs in a process sensitive to chloroquine. However, peptides derived from HEL were presented by live macrophages in the presence of chloroquine. Macrophages lightly fixed in paraformaldehyde presented peptides but not the native HEL molecule. In contrast, macrophages that internalized and processed HEL presented it to T cells only if fixed after 30–60 minutes, indicating that the peptide/MHC-II complex became available and was resistant to the fixatives. Results similar to ours were also obtained in other laboratories using globular proteins as antigen (Chesnut et al. 1982; Shimonkevitz et al. 1983; Streicher et al. 1984; Kovac and Schwartz 1985).

The molecular explanation of this processing became apparent when it was found that the processed fragments could interact with purified MHC-II molecules (Babbitt et al. 1985, 1986). Using equilibrium dialysis, immunogenic peptides of HEL bound in detergent solution to affinity-purified I-A^k molecules. The binding was saturable with a K_d of 2–4 μM. Although HEL(46-61) could bind to I-A^k, it did not bind to I-A^d, corresponding to the restriction of its presentation by I-A^k. Thus, there was agreement between the binding pattern of a peptide and its immune gene response. This observation first implied that peptide binding was one

essential function of MHC molecules. It was later confirmed and extended by others, primarily by the laboratory of H. Grey (Buus et al. 1986a,b, 1987). In general, these observations supported the ideas of MHC function and the determinant selection hypothesis discussed in the 1970s (Rosenthal et al. 1977; Benacerraf 1978). (Rosenthal's laboratory first hypothesized that the selection of an antigenic determinant from a natural protein depended on the MHC haplotype of the APC.) Of key importance, too, are the more recent studies indicating that presentation of viral antigens by class I MHC molecules (MHC-I) also involves presentation of small peptide sequences (Townsend et al. 1985). The differences in presentation between MHC-I and MHC-II are most likely explained on the basis of their intracellular physiology (Morrison et al. 1986).

MHC-II molecules show a single binding site as gathered from data based on competition experiments with a range of unlabeled peptides (Babbitt et al. 1986; Buus et al. 1987; Guillet et al. 1987). The site, although unique, can interact with a variety of peptides. The binding site of MHC-II molecules apparently will include peptides of at least 8–12 amino acids. This estimate has been reached by examining the responses of peptide antigens of various sizes. The tertiary structure of a human class I MHC molecule, the HLA-A2 molecule (Bjorkman et al. 1987a,b), has revealed the combining site of the molecule. A similar structure has been proposed for class II molecules (Brown et al. 1988). The existence of a single combining site that accommodates only one peptide immediately explains the phenomenon of competition among protein antigens noted both in vivo and in vitro (Babbitt et al. 1986). In "antigenic competition," simultaneous immunization with two proteins results in a decrease in the response to one of them. This competition may take place at the level of uptake of the protein by the APC as well as at the level of binding of processed peptides to MHC-II molecules. In the latter case, antigenic competition probably takes place in the milieu of the endosome (see below). Furthermore, it is likely that the peptides that derive from one single protein may compete with each other for the combining site of the MHC-II molecules. Finally, a single binding site implies that many peptides must share the property of interacting with the same binding site of a given class II allele. Several peptide sequence motifs have now been proposed to explain the pattern of peptide binding to particular MHC alleles

Table 1. Binding Properties of HEL

Protein	Binding to MHC-II	MHC haplotype	Comment[a]
Native HEL	no binding	—	needs processing (1)
Peptide HEL(46–61)	2–4 μM	k	immunodominant peptide
Peptide HEL(52–61)	2–4μM	k	minimal size of immunodominant peptide
Murine(52–61)	competes with HEL peptide	n.d.[b]	self-peptides bind to MHC-II(2)
HEL(34–45)	2 μM	k	a second epitope in HEL (3)
Murine(34–45)	no binding	—	an Arg in murine peptide instead of Gln at residue 41 affects binding (4)

[a]References: (1) Allen and Unanue (1984); (2) Babbitt et al. (1986); (3) Allen et al. (1987a); (4) Lambert and Unanue (1989).

[b]Competes with HEL(46–61) on binding to I-A^k. n.d. indicates not determined.

(Berzofsky et al. 1987; Sette et al. 1987, 1989; Rothbard and Taylor 1988).

Our experience with lysozyme peptides is summarized in Table 1. There are key important points to note briefly:

1. The immunodominant sequence for H-2^k mice was found in the tryptic peptide HEL(46-61). (Immunodominance—the phenomenon whereby one of many possible peptides is presented—has yet to be entirely explained in molecular terms [Gammon et al. 1987]. The affinity of peptides for MHC-II must play a role, but it is certainly not the single factor. This underscores the need to detail the chemical profiles of protein degradation.)

2. The minimal-size functional peptide in the tryptic fragment HEL(46-61) was from residues 52–61. We made an "Ala map" by making peptides that had alanine substitutions at each position, which then enabled us to identify residues that contacted I-A^k and those that contacted the T-cell receptor (Allen et al. 1987b). Three MHC-II contact residues were identified, Asp-52, Ile-58, and Arg-61, as well as three T-cell receptor residues, Tyr-53, Leu-56, and Gln-57. These residues were intermingled in the molecule (Table 2). We have proposed that peptides mold and adopt particular conformations as they bind into the MHC-II combining site. For example, folding the peptide in an α-helix results in a segregation of each set of residues in the two planes of the helix.

3. It is of key importance to note that MHC molecules did not discriminate between self- and nonself-peptides (Babbitt et al. 1986). Thus, the murine lysozyme sequence 52–61 that differs from HEL(52–

61) by a Phe$\rightarrow$Leu change at residue 56 was not immunogenic, yet was able to bind to I-A^k. This observation is obviously important in the context of autoreactivity to self-protein antigens. Note that not all self-peptides bind to I-A^k (Lorenz et al. 1988). For example, the murine lysozyme peptide (34–45) will not bind to I-A^k because of an Arg$\rightarrow$Gln change at residue 41 (Lambert and Unanue 1989). Thus, foreign and self-peptides behave similarly; some bind, but others do not, depending on their structure and the MHC haplotype.

MATERIALS AND METHODS

The binding studies used affinity-purified I-A^k molecules (Babbitt et al. 1985) and peptide derivatives of HEL(52-61) (Allen et al. 1987b; Luescher et al. 1988). Fixed macrophages or B-lymphoma cell lines were used for presentation of peptides (Allen and Unanue 1984). The 3A9 T-cell hybridoma secretes interleukin 2 (IL-2) in response to stimulation with I-A^k/HEL(46-61) complexes and was used to assay the expression of these complexes in APCs.

RESULTS

Cellular Studies on Antigen Presentation

It is important to place the interaction of peptide with MHC-II molecules in the context of the live APCs. The site of catabolism of the antigen, the site of coupling of the antigen with MHC-II, and the turnover rate of MHC-II, either free or complexed with peptides, are all issues that need critical evaluation. Recent experiments studying the kinetics of the interaction of MHC-

Table 2. MHC-II and T-cell Contact Residues in HEL(52–61)

	52 Asp	53 Tyr	54 Gly	55 Ile	56 Leu	57 Gln	58 Ile	59 Asn	60 Ser	61 Arg
MHC-II contact	+						+			+
T-cell contact		+			+	+				
Spacer residue			+	+				+	+	

Data from Allen et al. (1987b).

II proteins and HEL peptides in live APCs, which have recently been published, are reviewed here.

Recent experiments compared the behavior of MHC-II molecules in macrophages and the B-cell lymphoma TA3 (H-2^{kxd}) (Harding and Unanue 1989; Harding et al. 1989). In one series of experiments, the turnover rate of the peptide/MHC-II complex was compared in these cells. Figure 1 shows that the complex was very long lived on the membranes of fixed TA3 cells but, in great contrast, exhibited a short life in live cells. The experiment was done by pulsing fixed cells with HEL(46-61) peptide, washing, and incubating for various periods at 37°C and then assaying for the amounts of I-A^k/HEL(46-61) remaining on the surface, using a T-cell hybridoma as our readout system. Alternatively, live cells were pulsed, washed, and then fixed at later times. After 72 hours, there was no major reduction in the amount of immunogenic complex displayed by the fixed B-lymphoma cells; in contrast, the half-life in live cells varied from 15 to 50 minutes in different experiments. In similar experiments with macrophages, there was no significant loss in the amount of peptide/MHC-II complex in fixed macrophages after 60 hours, whereas the half-life in viable macrophages was approximately 5 hours. Importantly, the turnover rate of radiolabeled MHC-II molecules (Fig. 2) indicated a half-life of 11 hours in the macrophage and 14 hours in TA3 cells.

The dissociation of isolated complexes of peptides and MHC-II molecules was also studied (Fig. 3). Purified I-A^k molecules were incubated with HEL(52-61); the bimolecular complex was isolated by Sephadex G-50 chromatography and concentrated; a 10,000-fold excess of unlabeled HEL(52-61) was added: The solution was fractionated at different times to determine the amounts of free and complexed peptides. As in the fixed cell, there was minimal dissociation of the pep-

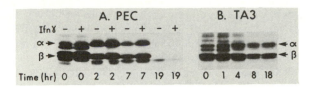

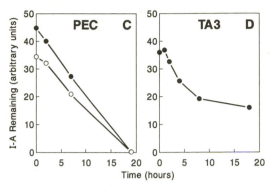

Figure 2. Half-life of I-A^k in macrophages (*A*, *C*) and B-lymphoma cells (*B*, *D*). The cells were labeled with [^{3}H]leucine for 1 hr, washed, and cultured for the indicated times. The amount of radioactivity associated with I-A^k was determined by immunoprecipitation, SDS-PAGE, and densitometry. The half-life of I-A^k is much longer than that of the I-A^k–HEL(46-61) complex (Fig. 1).

tide, in accordance with the results published with an ovalbumin peptide by the laboratory of H. Grey (Buus et al. 1986b).

In the studies mentioned above, the turnover of MHC-II/peptide complexes in viable cells was much

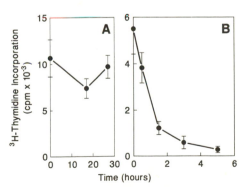

Figure 1. Turnover of the peptide/MHC-II complex is enhanced in live B-lymphoma cells (TA3). (*A*) TA3 cells were pulsed with peptide, fixed, and incubated for various periods before the addition of the T-cell hybridoma. (*B*) TA3 cells were pulsed with peptide HEL(46-61) (10 μM; 20 min at 37°C), washed, incubated for the indicated times, and fixed. The HEL(46-61)-specific T-cell hybridoma was then added, and the amounts of IL-2 were measured 24 hr later. I-A^k/HEL(46-61) complex was stably expressed in the fixed cells (*A*) but decreased with time in the live TA3 cells (*B*) (Harding et al. 1989).

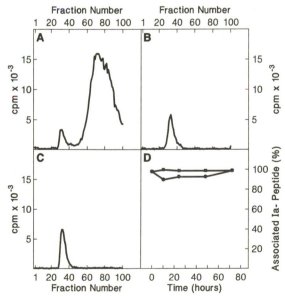

Figure 3. Dissociation of peptides from isolated peptide/MHC-II complexes. Purified I-A^k was incubated with ^{125}I-labeled HEL(52-61). The solution was passed through Sephadex G-50 to isolate the peptide/MHC-II complex (fractions 20–40). The isolated complex was then incubated in 10,000-fold excess of unlabeled peptide for 72 hr. After 0–72 hr, the complex was again passed over G-50 (*B*, 0 hr; *C*, 72 hr). The amount of peptide released is minimal (computed in *D*).

more rapid than that observed with fixed cells or with isolated peptide/MHC-II complexes. Thus, an active mechanism must exist to mediate the turnover of these complexes. The disappearance of I-A^k peptide complexes was very rapid in B-lymphoma cells, relative to the turnover of the I-A^k molecule. This suggests that the active turnover of the complexes was mediated by their dissociation to free peptide and I-A^k, which could then be recycled to present new peptides. In macrophages, the half-life of the complexes was somewhat longer (one-third to one-half the half-life of the I-A^k molecule); this suggests that recycling of I-A^k was less prevalent in macrophages and that turnover of the complexes largely reflected the turnover of the MHC-II molecule. These conclusions support other studies using cycloheximide and Brefeldin-A, which imply a greater degree of "recycling" of MHC-II molecules in B-lymphoma cells than in macrophages (see below, Table 3).

Dissociation of peptide/MHC-II complexes and recycling of MHC-II could be accomplished by internalization of MHC-II into a specialized intracellular organelle or endosome. We have also provided experimental evidence in support of internalization of MHC-II molecules. Both B-lymphoma cells and macrophages contained MHC-II in an intracellular compartment that remained in the cell for long periods after cessation of protein synthesis (Fig. 4) (Harding and Unanue 1989). This compartment was revealed by the binding of anti-MHC-II monoclonal antibodies to cells in the presence of saponin; saponin permeabilized the cells to allow the antibody to enter and bind intracellular MHC-II, causing an increment in antibody binding. The intracellular compartment was stable in both the B-lymphoma cells and macrophages kept in suspension but was markedly reduced when the macrophages adhered to plastic dishes. We directly observed endocytosis of MHC-II molecules in both B cells and macrophages in other experiments. Figure 5 shows that 25–30% of I-A^k molecules were internalized as measured by the uptake of monoclonal antibodies or their monovalent fragments. The internalized I-A^k molecule could be identified by Percoll density gradient fractionation in a light endosomal vesicle that sedimented in identical position as vesicles containing transferrin (cf. Creswell 1985). These vesicles were much lighter than lysosomes. In essence, these experiments indicate that

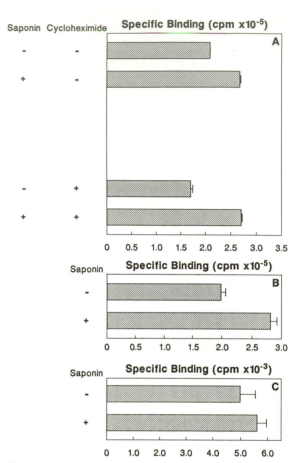

Figure 4. Intracellular MHC-II molecules revealed in B-lymphoma cells (TA3) (*A*) and macrophages (*B, C*) by the use of saponin. The binding of ^{125}I-labeled anti-I-A^k monoclonal antibody to cells was measured in the presence and absence of 0.02% saponin. Saponin increased the antibody binding to B cells, reflecting an intracellular pool of I-A^k. Cycloheximide exposure for 2 hr had no effect on the intracellular pool of MHC-II. Similar studies with macrophages are shown in *B* and *C*. (*B*) Macrophages were incubated in suspension; (*C*) macrophages were first plated on a culture dish, a manipulation that decreases intracellular MHC-II (Harding and Unanue 1989).

although the majority of I-A^k molecules are on the plasma membrane, there are a significant number (20–30%) found in a light endosomal organelle. We define endosomes as those intermediate organelles that harbor internalized proteins in their sojourn through the cell and prior to their fusion with lysosomes. In our view, it is likely that endosomes have key roles in protein processing and in the coupling of peptides to I-A^k, as well as in the peptide interchange suggested from the turnover studies described above.

Effects of Inhibitors of Protein Synthesis

Treatment of B-lymphoma cells and macrophages with cycloheximide produced strikingly different results. Both cell types were exposed to the drug first for 3 hours and then during a subsequent 90-minute incubation period with HEL; the cells were then fixed at

Table 3. Comparison between Macrophages and B-lymphoma Cells

	Macrophages	B-lymphoma cells
Cycloheximide	inhibits	does not inhibit
Brefeldin-A	inhibits	does not inhibit
Dextran	inhibits	does not inhibit
Peptide MHC-II half-life	4–5 hr	15–55 min
MHC-II recycling	slight	predominant

The degree of recycling of MHC-II is different in macrophages and B-lymphoma cells. The macrophages depend more on newly synthesized MHC-II.

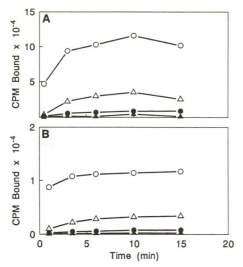

Figure 5. Uptake and endocytosis of ^{125}I-labeled monoclonal anti-I-A^k antibodies in macrophages (*A*) or B-lymphoma cells (TA3) (*B*). The graph shows the uptake after incubation with time at 37°C (0), the amounts internalized with time (△) (as determined by the amount of antibody resistant to treatment of the cells at acid pH, which removes surface-bound antibody). (●) Nonspecific uptake; (▲) nonspecific internalization. (Reprinted, with permission, from Harding and Unanue 1989.)

various intervals and the amount of peptide/MHC-II complex was assayed using T-cell hybridomas. Doses of cycloheximide that entirely inhibited protein synthesis did not affect the presentation of HEL by B cells but markedly inhibited that of the macrophage. The dramatic reduction in presentation in macrophages fol-

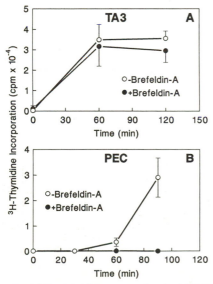

Figure 6. Brefeldin-A inhibits processing for MHC-II-restricted presentation in macrophages but not TA3 B-lymphoma cells. Both cell types were incubated in 0.5 μg/ml Brefeldin-A, beginning 3 hr before addition of HEL. HEL was then added for various periods at 37°C; the APCs were then fixed, and 3A9 T-hybridoma cells were added to assay the degree of HEL processing (Fig. 1). (*A*) B-lymphoma (TA3) cells (1 mg/ml HEL); (*B*) macrophages (0.5 mg/ml HEL).

lowing inhibition of protein synthesis was first reported by Jensen (1988).

These differences in antigen presentation between both B cells and macrophages have now been found in other situations. In recent experiments, we tested the effect of antigen processing of the fungal product Brefeldin-A, which inhibits the egress of molecules from endoplasmic reticulum (ER)–Golgi to plasma membranes (Lippincott-Schwartz et al. 1989). The cells were incubated with 0.5 μg/ml of Brefeldin-A beginning 3 hours before the addition of HEL. Similar to cycloheximide, Brefeldin-A inhibited the presentation of HEL by macrophages but not by TA3 cells (Fig. 6). Other differences between macrophages and B-lymphoma cells are found with regard to the inhibitory effects of some polysaccharides (see below). Incubation with several polysaccharides such as dextran inhibited presentation of HEL by macrophages and not by B-lymphoma cells (C.V. Harding and E.R. Unanue, unpubl.). Table 3 is a comparison of the various results using both cells. Again, it suggests to us that B-lymphoma cells may use a recycling pathway of MHC-II much more than macrophages do. The latter would depend more on nascent MHC-II molecules.

Some Biochemical Aspects of Peptide/MHC Interaction

Table 1 summarizes our experience with lysozyme peptides. We are currently examining conditions that can affect the primary interaction between ligand and MHC-II protein. Our hypothesis is that the endosomes where peptide/MHC-II interaction may take place contain components that can modulate this primary interaction. Using photoaffinity lysozyme peptide conjugates, we have been able to show that some phospholipids play an important role in this modulation. The data also suggest that the combining site of I-A^k, which holds HEL(52-61), is conformationally not fixed, but is pliable, resulting in variable interactions with peptides.

In our experiments, cell membranes from TA3 cells were exposed to HEL(46-61) conjugated to a photoaffinity moiety either at its amino terminus or at its carboxyl terminus. After UV irradiation, the I-A^k was detergent-solubilized and isolated using monoclonal antibodies to generate a covalent bond of the peptide to I-A^k; its component chains were then separated by SDS-PAGE. All the label was found associated with the α-chain (Luescher et al. 1988). The same results were obtained when the cell membranes were first solubilized, followed by incubation of the crude material with the probe and subsequent analysis. In contrast, handling of the I-A^k molecule during its purification (using affinity chromatography) led to decreased labeling, as well as labeling of the β-chain. Simple dialysis of the crude membrane preparation resulted in a decreased labeling, suggesting that a small soluble component was critical for the binding properties of the MHC-II molecule. Addition of certain lysophospholipids resulted in the reacquisition of strong labeling or labeling predominantly of either of the two chains (I.F. Luescher and E.R. Unanue, unpubl.). The binding kinetics of radiolabeled peptide and I-A^k was also studied in the presence of the lysophospholipids (in detergents). For example, the affinity constant for HEL(52-61) binding to I-A^k was 1×10^{-7} M to 3×10^{-7} M in the presence of lysophosphatidylserine, as compared to 2×10^{-6} to 4×10^{-6} in their absence. The increase was the result of a higher rate of association. The rate of dissociation was similarly slow with or without phospholipids (I.E. Luescher et al., in prep.).

We interpret these results to indicate that class II molecules, particularly in detergent, have a certain conformational flexibility, which affects their interaction with antigens. Conformational changes in the antigen-binding site conceivably originate in different mutual orientations in which the subunit chains assemble. These orientations may be affected by particular lipid/detergent interactions of the spanning domains of their subunits.

Studies from B. Benacerraf's (Falo et al. 1986) laboratory using phospholipases showed that these enzymes inhibited antigen presentation. These workers believed that the antigenic peptides could associate with phospholipids prior to their interaction with MHC-II molecules. An alternative explanation based on our own results is that enzymes affected the lipid surrounding the MHC-II molecule.

It is noteworthy that a single peptide bound to MHC-II gives rise to more than one antigenic site (Allen et al. 1985a,b; Cease et al. 1986; Baumhuter et al. 1987; Mills et al. 1988). We have obtained very striking results to support this point when examining the HEL(34-45) peptide (Table 1). HEL(34-45) is a second immunogenic peptide to which T-cell hybridomas have been developed. Its sequence is indicated in the legend to Figure 7. We synthesized peptides having alanine substitutions at each position and then tested each peptide for its binding to I-A^k, as well as for stimulation of two T-cell hybridomas. The striking results are depicted in Figures 7 and 8. The key point can be shown by the results with alanine substitution in the amino and carboxyl termini. Peptides with alanine substitutions at residues 43, 44, or 45 bound to I-A^k and so did peptides with substitution at residues 34, 35, or 36. Indeed, binding assay showed that the alanine-substituted peptides competed for the binding of radiolabeled HEL(52-61) to I-A^k. However, the alanine substitutions at the carboxyl terminus stimulated only one of the two hybridomas, whereas the peptides with alanine at the amino terminus stimulated the other. Thus, although the substituted peptides were able to bind to I-A^k, each had different stimulatory capacity for each T-cell hybridoma.

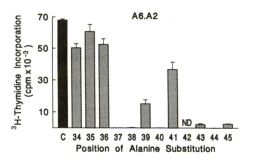

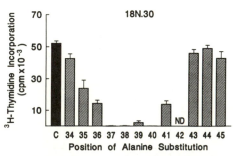

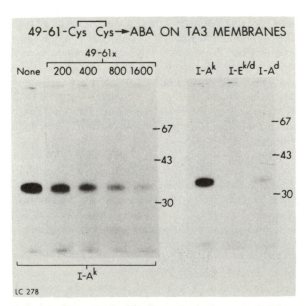

Figure 7. Photoaffinity labeling of membranes of B-lymphoma line TA3 (H-2^{kxd}) by a photoreactive conjugate of HEL(46-61). The photoreactive conjugate consisted of (4-axidobenzoyl) cystine, carboxy-terminally coupled to HEL(49-61). The membranes were incubated with the photoconjugate, UV-irradiated, and lysed in detergent; the I-A^k was precipitated and subjected to SDS-PAGE. (*Right*) Labeling of the α-chain of I-A^k with minimal labeling of I-A^d and none of I-E^k. (*Left*) Binding was inhibited by an excess of unlabeled peptide (Luescher et al. 1988).

Figure 8. Response of two T-cell hybridomas specific for HEL(34-45) to alanine-substituted peptides. The sequence of HEL(34-45) is Phe-Glu-Ser-Asn-Phe-Asn-Thr-Gln-Ala-Thr-Asn-Arg. (The murine counterpart has Tyr at residue 38, Arg at 41,and Tyr at 45.) Peptides were prepared with alanine substitutions at each residue and tested for binding and presentation to A6.A2 and 18N.30. Indicated is the production of IL-2 by the hybridomas upon interaction with the peptides (at 100 μM) presented by fixed macrophages (Lambert and Unanue 1989).

HEL(34-45) could be binding to I-A^k in different conformations or at different places in the combining site of MHC-II. The binding of different T-cell receptors, specific for each particular situation, would be affected differently by the alanine substitutions. Another alternative explanation is that the differences are explained by the T-cell receptor itself—the peptide could be located in the combining site in a single configuration, but T cells may show higher specificity for either the amino- or carboxy-terminal portion of the peptide.

The conclusion, regardless of the final explanation, is that small peptides do generate more than one antigenic specificity when bound to I-A^k. This point may be critical in the generation of diversity for T-cell systems. If the T cells recognize two or three amino acids within a peptide (Allen et al. 1987b), it implies that there should be other factors aside from the random sequence of amino acid to generate the antigenic diversity of peptides. After all, T-cell epitopes in proteins are no more cross-reactive than are the epitopes recognized by the antibody molecule. Conceivably, not only the sequence of T-cell contact residues, but also their spatial position within the MHC-II combining site—as a result of the way in which the MHC-II binding residues contact the MHC—will influence how the antigenic determinant is created.

Polysaccharides Do Not Bind to MHC-II Molecules but Interfere with Antigen Presentation

We have been interested in examining whether carbohydrate antigens interact with MHC-II molecules and/or affect antigen presentation. Carbohydrate antigens do not stimulate CD4 T cells and thus cannot induce the cellular and inflammatory manifestations of T-cell immunity (i.e., B-cell memory, macrophage activation, delayed hypersensitivity). Prodded by the late John Humphrey—who always maintained an interest in the response to polysaccharides—we recently examined whether these "thymus-independent antigens" could interact with MHC-II molecules. A variety of polysaccharides did not bind to the combining site of I-A^k, I-E^k, or I-A^d. The binding was tested either by competition on direct binding of radiolabeled HEL(52-61) to detergent-solubilized, affinity-purified I-A^k or by competition for binding of immunogenic peptides to fixed APCs (for antigen presentation to T-cell hybridomas). Tested compounds included dextrans of various sizes, dextran sulfate, Ficoll, lipopolysaccharides, the capsular polysaccharides of *Haemophilus influenzae*, *Neisseria meningitidis*, and *Diplococcus pneumoniae*, heparin, and a variety of di- and trisaccharides (R.M. Roof and E.R. Unanue, in prep.). Clearly, the hydrophilic nature of the carbohydrate moieties was not conducive to their interactions with the MHC-II combining site. The lack of association of carbohydrate antigens with MHC-II molecules explains their incapacity to stimulate CD4 T cells. Polysaccharides are believed to stimulate B cells, albeit in a limited way,

perhaps by virtue of their repeating epitope, which leads to extensive cross-linking of membrane Ig, and/or because they are intrinsically mitogenic (as is endotoxin from gram-negative bacteria).

A surprising observation was that many of the same polysaccharides that did not bind to MHC-II proteins inhibited the presentation of proteins, like HEL, which need a processing event (Leyva-Cobian and Unanue 1988) (Fig. 9). The experiments were done as follows: Peritoneal macrophages were isolated and incubated with the polysaccharides for periods of 1–3 hours, and the cells were washed, exposed to HEL for 30–60 minutes, fixed, and tested for the presence of the processed epitope found in HEL(46-61), using the T-cell hybridomas. Exposure to the carbohydrates decreased the amount of peptide associated with I-A^k, as evidenced by a reduction in the response of the specific T-cell hybridomas. However, the uptake and gross catabolism of HEL was not impaired in the cells given polysaccharides. The amounts of I-A^k on the macrophage surface and the presentation of HEL(46-61) were not affected. Because polysaccharides did not interfere with the binding of peptide to MHC-II, we are left with the possibility that they must influence cellular events that involve the association of vesicles containing HEL with those that bear MHC-II molecules. Perhaps the polysaccharides are concentrated in the same vesicles that bear MHC-II molecules and these molecules are impaired in their fusion with antigen-bearing vesicles, or vice versa.

The interference by polysaccharides must be of importance in infections with microorganisms that contain a high level of them. In this regard, we also obtained excellent inhibition of HEL administered after uptake of *Listeria monocytogenes* (Leyva-Cobian and Unanue 1988), and *Myobacterium leprae* or one of its products (phenolic glycolypid I) (F. Leyva-Cobian, unpubl.).

Some Views on Antigen Presentation

It is peculiar that the cellular immune system evolved to recognize antigenic determinants formed by linear sequences of amino acids. This development may have been the result of the need to develop a recognition system that not only required a vast diversity, but, at the same time, the capacity to recognize self-proteins versus nonself-proteins. One critical issue in antigen presentation is the balance between presentation of self- and nonself-peptides. Because the MHC-II molecules do not make such differentiation at the level of their binding sites, some other system must operate to ensure favorable presentation of foreign determinants during antigenic challenge. It is noteworthy that the presentation of self-peptides is important in certain tissues. The recent experiments of Lorenz and Allen (1988), indicating that thymus stromal cells naturally process a peptide from the self-protein hemoglobin, establish that some autologous proteins reach the thymus where a negative (or positive) selection of T cells can then take place.

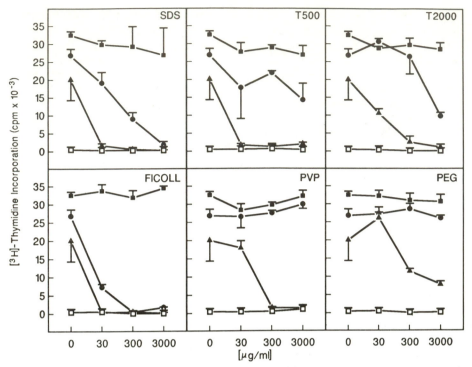

Figure 9. Inhibition of HEL presentation by polysaccharides and polyanionic molecules. Macrophages were incubated for 2 hr with the indicated concentrations of sodium dextran sulfate (SDS), dextrans of molecular weight 500,000 (T500) or 2×10^6 (T2000), Ficoll, polyvinylpyrrolidone (PVP), and polyethylene glycol (PEG); the cells were then washed and incubated with or without HEL ([□] without HEL; [▲] HEL at 10 μg/ml; [●] at 100 μg/ml; [■] at 500 μg/ml) for 1 hr, washed, and fixed. T-cell hybridomas specific for HEL(46-61) were then added, and their production of IL-2 was determined after 24 hr of incubation.

We believe that the intracellular processing events are critical for the APC to effectively present foreign proteins and override the antigenic competition by self-proteins. The plasma membrane contains MHC-II molecules that are free and unoccupied, but the exact number is uncertain. With binding affinities of HEL peptides of approximately 10^{-6} M and using B-lymphoma cells and our T-cell hybridomas, we have estimated that about 600–1000 peptide/MHC-II complexes per APC are required to stimulate T cells. This indicates that about 1% of the available MHC-II sites on an APC surface need to be occupied by an antigenic epitope to stimulate an immune response.

Self-proteins that compete with foreign peptides will derive from two sources: (1) *exogenous*—either proteins that are internalized and processed in endosomes (in a process akin to HEL) or peptides that are in the circulation and bind directly to surface MHC-II molecules and (2) *endogenous*—i.e., proteins that are synthesized and assembled in the ER and then handled in the Golgi. At this time, we have little appraisal of the extent to which any of these sources provides peptides for binding to MHC molecules. The degree of internalization of plasma proteins and generation of self-peptides is also unclear; we believe that this is a significant but limited process. There is also little evidence for significant amounts of circulating peptides in blood that bind to MHC.

The internally made proteins could be a major component in the competition with foreign peptides. Here

is where we see the major differences between the MHC-I and MHC-II systems. Although the work with immunoglobulins suggests that some endogenous peptides can be presented by MCH-II (Weiss and Bogen 1989), it is likely that the MHC-I system is the one that functions mainly to rescue the proteins from the ER-Golgi. The experiments from Braciale's laboratory (Morrison et al. 1986) and the recent experiments using Brefeldin-A (Yewdell and Bennick 1989) indicate that the pathway for presentation via MHC-I molecules is different from that of MHC-II. Endogenous proteins appear to be presented by MHC-I. If both MHC-I and MHC-II molecules are in ER-Golgi, then why does the MHC-II not become saturated with peptides that result from partial proteolysis of some of the endogenous protein? One very tentative speculation is (1) the MHC-II proteins do actually get loaded with self-peptides, but they unload as they reach the endosome in a manner similar to the turnover of foreign peptide/MHC-II complexes (Harding et al. 1989); (2) in ER-Golgi the MHC-II proteins do not bind peptides because their binding sites are not open, perhaps because of their interaction with other components. One possibility is that the invariant chains may bind and protect the MHC-II and prevent the binding of peptides until the endosome is reached; there, the invariant chain dissociates from the MHC-II molecules, which are free to bind peptide. Therefore, in endosomes, MHC-II proteins become available for peptide binding; these derive from a nascent pool or by way of the plasma

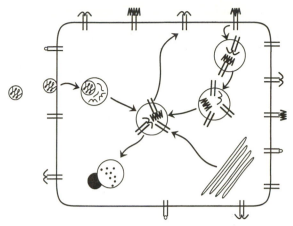

Figure 10. Our view of intracellular processing. A protein antigen is internalized in vesicles; the vesicles eventually reach endosomes that bear MHC-II (*center*). These contain nascent MHC-II and/or recycled MHC-II molecules.

membrane (either free or occupied by peptides that are subsequently released [Fig. 10]). Their binding to foreign antigens will depend on the relative amounts of foreign and self-proteins. The manipulations that result in effective immunization typically involve altering the antigen molecules to increase their uptake by the APC system. Further experimentation on the in vivo processing events should give valuable information as to how the presentation of self/nonself is balanced at the level of the APC.

ACKNOWLEDGMENTS

The research discussed in this paper was supported by grants from the National Institutes of Health and the Monsanto-Searle-Washington University agreement.

REFERENCES

Allen, P.M. and E.R. Unanue. 1984. Differential requirements for antigen processing by macrophages for lysozyme-specific T cell hybridoma. *J. Immunol.* **132:** 1077.

Allen, P.M., B.P. Babbitt, and E.R. Unanue. 1987a. T-cell recognition of lysozyme: The biochemical basis of presentation. *Immunol. Rev.* **98:** 171.

Allen, P.M., G.R. Matsueda, E. Haber, and E.R. Unanue. 1985a. Specificity of the T cell receptor: Two different determinants are generated by the same peptide and the I-A^k molecule. *J. Immunol.* **135:** 368.

Allen, P.M., D.J. McKean, B.N. Beck, J. Sheffield, and L.H. Glimcher. 1985b. Direct evidence that a class II molecule and a single globular protein generate multiple determinants. *J. Exp. Med.* **162:** 1264.

Allen, P.M., G.R. Matsueda, R.J. Evans, J.B. Dunbar, Jr., G. Marshall, and E.R. Unanue. 1987b. Identification of the T-cell and Ia contact residues of a T-cell antigen epitope. *Nature* **327:** 713.

Babbitt, B.P., P.M. Allen, G. Matsueda, and E.R. Unanue. 1985. Binding of immunogenic peptides to Ia histocompatibility molecules. *Nature* **317:** 359.

Babbitt, B.P., G. Matsueda, E. Haber, E.R. Unanue, and P.M. Allen. 1986. Antigenic competition at the level of peptide-Ia binding. *Proc. Natl. Acad. Sci.* **83:** 4509.

Baumhuter, S., C.J.A. Wallace, A.E.I. Proudfoot, C. Bron, and G. Corradin. 1987. Multiple T cell antigen determinant identified within a limited region of the horse cytochrome c molecule. *Eur. J. Immunol.* **17:** 651.

Benacerraf, B. 1978. A hypothesis to relate the specificity of T lymphocytes and the activity of I region specific Ir genes in macrophages and B lymphocytes. *J. Immunol.* **128:** 1809.

Berzofsky, J.A., K.B. Cease, J.L. Cornette, J.L. Spouge, H. Margalit, I.J. Berkower, M.F. Good, L.H. Miller, and C. DeLisi. 1987. Protein antigenic structures recognized by T cells: Potential applications to vaccine design. *Immunol. Rev.* **98:** 9.

Bjorkman, P.J., M.A. Saper, B. Samraoui, W.S. Bennett, J.L. Strominger, and D.C. Wiley. 1987a. Structure of the human class I histocompatibility antigen, HLA-A2. *Nature* **329:** 506.

———. 1987b. The foreign antigen binding site and T cell recognition regions of class I histocompatibility antigens. *Nature* **329:** 512.

Brown, J.H., T. Jardetzsky, M.A. Saper, B. Samraoui, P. Bjorkman, and D.C. Wiley. 1988. A hypothetical model of the foreign antigen binding site of class II histocompatibility antigens. *Nature* **332:** 845.

Buus, S., A. Sette, S.M. Colon, D.M. Jenis, and H.M. Grey. 1986a. Isolation and characterization of antigen-Ia complexes involved in T cell recognition. *Cell* **47:** 1071.

Buus, S., A. Sette, S.M. Colon, C. Miles, and H.M. Grey. 1987. The relation between major histocompatibility complex (MHC) restriction and the capacity of Ia to bind immunogenic peptides. *Science* **235:** 1353.

Buus, S., S. Colon, C. Smith, J.H. Freed, C. Miles, and H.M. Grey. 1986b. Interaction between a "processed" ovalbumin peptide and Ia molecules. *Proc. Natl. Acad. Sci.* **83:** 3968.

Cease, K.B., I. Berkower, J. York-Jolley, and J.A. Berzofsky. 1986. T cell clones specific for an amphipathic α-helical region of sperm whale myoglobin show differing fine specificities for synthetic peptides. A multiview/single structure interpretation of immunodominance. *J. Exp. Med.* **164:** 1779.

Chesnut, R., S. Colon, and H.M. Grey. 1982. Requirements for the processing of antigen by antigen presenting B cells. I. Functional comparison of B cell tumors and macrophages. *J. Immunol.* **129:** 2382.

Creswell, P. 1985. Intracellular class II HLA antigens are accessible to transferin-neuraminidase congregates internalized by receptor-mediated endocytosis. *Proc. Natl. Acad. Sci.* **82:** 8188.

Falo, L.P., B. Benacerraf, and K.L. Rock. 1986. Phospholipase treatment of accessory cells that have been exposed to antigen selectively inhibits antigen-specific Ia-restricted, but not allospecific stimulation of T lymphocytes. *Proc. Natl. Acad. Sci.* **83:** 6994.

Gammon, G., N. Shastri, J. Cogswell, S. Wilbur, S. Sadegh-Nassier, U. Krzych, A. Miller, and E. Sercarz. 1987. The choice of T-cell epitopes utilized on a protein antigen depends on multiple factors distant from, as well as at, the determinant site. *Immunol. Rev.* **98:** 53.

Guillet, J.G., M.Z. Lai, and T.J. Briner. 1987. Immunological self, non-self discrimination. *Science* **235:** 865.

Harding, C.V. and E.R. Unanue. 1989. Antigen processing and intracellular Ia. Possible role of endocytosis and protein synthesis in Ia function. *J. Immunol.* **142:** 12.

Harding, C.V., F. Leyva-Cobian, and E.R. Unanue. 1988. Mechanisms of antigen processing. *Immunol. Rev.* **106:** 77.

Harding, C.V., R.M. Roof, and E.R. Unanue. 1989. Turnover of Ia-peptide complexes is facilitated in viable antigen presenting cells: Biosynthetic turnover of Ia vs. peptide exchange. *Proc. Natl. Acad. Sci.* **86:** 4230.

Jensen, P.E. 1988. Protein synthesis in antigen processing. *J. Immunol.* **141:** 2545.

Kovac, Z. and R.H. Schwartz. 1985. The molecular basis of the requirement for antigen processing of pigeon cytochrome c prior to T cell activation. *J. Immunol.* **134:** 3233.

Lambert, L.E. and E.R. Unanue. 1989. Analysis of the interaction of the lysozyme peptide HEL(34045) with the I-A^k molecule. *J. Immunol.* **143**: 802.

Leyva-Cobian, F. and E.R. Unanue. 1988. Intracellular interference with antigen presentation. *J. Immunol.* **141**: 1445.

Lippincott-Schwartz, J., L.C. Yuan, J.S. Bonifacino, and R.D. Klausner. 1989. Rapid redistribution of Golgi proteins into the ER in cells treated with Brefeldin A: Evidence for membrane cycling from Golgi to ER. *Cell* **56**: 801.

Lorenz, R.G. and P.M. Allen. 1988. Direct evidence for functional self-protein/Ia-molecule complexes in vivo. *Proc. Natl. Acad. Sci.* **85**: 5220.

Lorenz, R.G., A.N. Tyler, and P.M. Allen. 1988. T cell recognition of bovine ribonuclease: Self/non-self discrimination at the level of binding to the I-A^k molecule. *J. Immunol.* **141**: 4124.

Luescher, I.F., P.M. Allen, and E.R. Unanue. 1988. Binding of photoreactive lysozyme peptides to murine histocompatibility class II molecules. *Proc. Natl. Acad. Sci.* **85**: 871.

Mills, K.H.G., D.S. Burt, J.J. Skeehel, and D.B. Thomas. 1988. Fine specificity of murine Class II-restricted T cell clones for synthetic peptides of influenza virus hemagglutinin. Heterogeneity of antigen interaction with the T cell and the Ia molecule. *J. Immunol.* **140**: 4083.

Morrison, L.A., A.E. Lukacher, V.L. Braciale, D. Fan, and T.J. Braciale. 1986. Differences in antigen presentation to MHC Class I- and Class II-restricted influenza virus specific T lymphocyte clones. *J. Exp. Med.* **163**: 903.

Rosenthal, A.S., M.A. Barcinski, and J.T. Blake. 1977. Determinant selection is a macrophage dependent immune response gene function. *Nature* **267**: 156.

Rothbard, J.B. and W.R. Taylor. 1988. A common sequence to T cell epitopes. *EMBO J.* **7**: 93.

Sette, A., S. Buus, S. Colon, J.A. Smith, C. Miles, and H.M. Grey. 1987. Structural characteristics of an antigen required for its interaction with Ia and recognition by T cells. *Nature* **328**: 395.

Sette, A., S. Buus, E. Appella, J.A. Smith, R. Chesnut, C. Miles, S.M. Colon, and H.M. Grey. 1989. Prediction of major histocompatibility complex binding regions of protein antigens by sequence pattern analysis. *Proc. Natl. Acad. Sci.* **86**: 3296.

Shimonkevitz, R., J. Kappler, P. Marrack, and H. Grey. 1983. Antigen recognition by H-2 restricted cells: I. Cell-free antigen processing. *J. Exp. Med.* **158**: 303.

Streicher, H.Z., I.J. Berkower, M. Busch, F.R.N. Gurd, and J.A. Berzofsky. 1984. Antigen conformation determines processing requirements for T cell activation. *Proc. Natl. Acad. Sci.* **81**: 6831.

Townsend, A.R.M., F.M. Gotch, and J. Davey. 1985. Cytotoxic T cells recognize fragments of influenza nucleoprotein. *Cell* **42**: 457.

Unanue, E.R. and P.M. Allen. 1987. The basis for the immunoregulatory role of macrophages and other accessory cells. *Science* **236**: 551.

Weiss, S. and B. Bogen. 1989. B lymphoma cells process and present their endogenous immunoglobulin to major histocompatibility complex-restricted T cells. *Proc. Natl. Acad. Sci.* **86**: 282.

Yewdell, J.A. and J.R. Bennink. 1989. Brefeldin A specifically inhibits presentation of protein antigens to cytotoxic T lymphocytes. *Science* **244**: 1072.

Ziegler, K. and E.R. Unanue. 1981. Identification of a macrophage antigen-processing event required for I-region-restricted antigen presentation to lymphocytes. *J. Immunol.* **127**: 1869.

———. 1982. Decrease in macrophage antigen catabolism by ammonia and chloroquine is associated with inhibition of antigen presentation to T cells. *Proc. Natl. Acad. Sci.* **78**: 175.

Studies on the Nature of Physiologically Processed Antigen and on the Conformation of Peptides Required for Interaction with MHC

H.M. Grey,* S. Demotz,* S. Buus,† and A. Sette*

*Cytel, La Jolla, California 92037; †Institute for Experimental Immunology, DK-2100, Copenhagen Ø, Denmark

Activation of class-II-restricted T cells requires the formation of a trimolecular complex between antigenic peptide fragments, class II major histocompatibility complex (MHC) molecules, and the T-cell receptor (Buus et al. 1987; Ogasawara et al. 1989). Much debate has been devoted to the conformational requirements for antigen molecules to bind MHC molecules and activate T cells. Different groups, mostly on the basis of indirect data, either functional or biochemical, have argued for or against regular secondary structures (mainly α helix) as the main conformational requirement. Using spectroscopy techniques, different groups have detected either positive or negative correlations between antigenicity and α-helical or β-sheet conformational propensity (Pincus et al. 1983; Heber-Katz et al. 1985; Carbone et al. 1987). Independent computer analysis suggested that regions with amphipathic (De Lisi and Berzofsky 1985; Margalit et al. 1987) and/or α-helical or β-sheet (Spouge et al. 1987) propensities may be frequently found within T-cell epitopes. Finally, two groups of investigators have argued in favor of α-helical requirements on the basis of segregation of residues apparently involved in contacting MHC molecules and T-cell receptors (Allen et al. 1987; Rothbard et al. 1988). However, when similar approaches were applied to other MHC/antigen combinations, we (Sette et al. 1987 and in prep.) and other investigators (Guillet et al. 1986; Fox et al. 1987; Ogasawara et al. 1989) failed to detect similar segregations.

In contrast to the substantial body of evidence characterizing the interaction between synthetic peptides and class II molecules, essentially no data are available on the nature of the antigen resulting from in vivo processing of protein molecules. Fragments are thought to arise from limited proteolytic degradation of native antigens inside acidic compartments of the antigen-presenting cells; however, up to now, no direct chemical characterization of physiologically processed peptides has been presented.

In this paper, we review experiments that we have performed to address the question of the conformation of peptides required for interaction with MHC, and we provide the first partial characterization of a physiologically processed antigen.

METHODS

Affinity purification of Ia^d. The B-cell lymphoma A20-1.11 was used as a source of I-A^d and I-E^d (Sette et al. 1989b). Class II molecules were purified using the monoclonal antibody MKD6 (I-A^d) or 14.4.4 (I-E^d), coupled to Sepharose 4B beads. Lysates were filtered and then purified, as described previously (Sette et al. 1987).

Binding of radiolabeled peptides to I-A^d molecules. Purified I-A^d (2–20 μM) was incubated with 0.1 μM ^{125}I-radiolabeled OVA (323–339) for I-A^d or λ rep 12-26 for I-E^d for 48 hours in the presence of detergent and a proteinase inhibitor cocktail (Sette et al. 1989b). The Ia/peptide complexes were separated from free peptide by gel filtration on a Sephadex G50 (Buus et al. 1986).

Peptide synthesis. Peptides were synthesized on an Applied Biosystems (Foster, California) 430A peptide synthesizer and radiolabeled as described previously (Sette et al. 1988). The synthesis of groups of analogous or overlapping peptides was simplified by combining automated synthesis with the manual method described by Houghten (1985). After the synthesis was completed, the peptide was cleaved from the resin, and the protecting groups were removed by treatment with 90% hydrogen fluoride in the presence of the appropriate scavengers. The peptides were then purified by reversed-phase HPLC.

Acid-eluted I-E^d peptides. I-E^d (350 μg), purified from 1.5×10^{10} hen egg lysozyme (HEL)-pulsed A20 cells (HEL-I-E^d), was acetonitrile-precipitated, treated for 30 minutes at 37°C with 2.5 M acetic acid, and then loaded on a Sephadex G10 column equilibrated with acetate buffer (Buus et al. 1988). The peptide material eluted in the void volume was collected and lyophilized twice.

Preparation and analysis of I-E^d/peptide complexes. To decrease the amount of antigenic material required to trigger IL-2 release by T hybridoma cells and thereby increase the sensitivity of our analysis, we developed a protocol whose incubation step mimics the conditions already established as optimal for in vitro

I-E^d/peptide complex formation (Sette et al. 1989b). The lyophilized peptides were dissolved in 10 μl of phosphate-buffered saline (PBS)/100 mM Tris (pH 7.2), supplemented with 1 mg/ml sodium azide and a cocktail of proteinase inhibitors (8 mM EDTA, 1.3 mM 1,10-phenanthroline, 73 μM pepstatin A, and 1 mM phenylmethylsulfonyl fluoride. To this, 10 μl of I-E^d at 1–2 mg/ml was added. After 1 day of incubation at room temperature, the samples were diluted to 250 μl with PBS containing 1 mg/ml sodium azide, 1% n-octyl-β-D-glucopyranoside (Sigma), 175 μg/ml L-α-phosphatidylcholine (Sigma), and 25 μg/ml cholesterol (Sigma). Planar membranes (PM) were prepared and tested in a T-cell stimulation assay as described previously (Buus et al. 1986; Coeshott et al. 1986).

Acid-eluted I-E^d peptides were analyzed on a μ-Bondapak C-18 reversed-phase HPLC column (Waters System, Milford, Massachusetts) by forming a linear gradient of 0.08% trifluoroacetic acid in water and 0.08% trifluoroacetic acid in acetonitrile (1%/minute). Fractions (1 ml) were collected and lyophilized.

Acid-eluted I-E^d peptides were also analyzed on a Sephadex G50 column (1.5 × 90 cm) equilibrated with 40 mM ammonium acetate and 20 mM acetic acid (Buus et al. 1988). Fractions (8 ml) were collected and lyophilized twice.

RESULTS

Effect of Proline Substitutions of OVA (323-336) on its I-A^d-binding Capacity

Proline is known to profoundly affect secondary structure of protein molecules (Chou and Fasman 1974; Nemethy and Scheraga 1977). It destabilizes both α helices and β-sheet structures and is often referred to as a "helix-breaker" and "β-sheet-breaker" (Chou and Fasman 1974, 1978; Nemethy and Scheraga 1977; Richardson 1981). Because of these effects, we systematically introduced proline substitutions within the

peptide, OVA (323-336), whose structural requirements for I-A^d binding have been previously analyzed in detail (Sette et al. 1987). Nine single amino acid substituted analogs, each carrying a proline substitution at one of the residues within 326–334 of OVA (323-336), were synthesized and tested for their capacity to bind to purified I-A^d (Table 1). Previous studies indicated that a core region encompassing residues 327–332 is crucial in determining the I-A^d-binding capacity of this peptide. It was therefore predicted that if the peptide was recognized in either an α-helix or β-sheet conformation, proline substitutions within or near this core would have a generalized detrimental effect on I-A^d-binding capacity.

The results indicated, however, that proline substitutions did not have a generalized detrimental effect; only two of the analogs (H$_{328}$ → P and A$_{329}$ → P) resulted in an appreciable (> fivefold) decrease in binding capacity. These data failed to document, therefore, either α helices or β sheets as relevant peptide conformations in their interaction with the I-A^d molecules. The localized effects of proline at positions 328 and 329 may be due to conformational restrictions in this particular portion of the peptide, or alternatively, may be due to H$_{328}$ and A$_{329}$ being contact residues that directly interact with I-A^d.

I-A^d-binding Capacity of a Panel of Synthetic Analogs of OVA (323-336) of Different Conformational Propensities

In previous studies, using amino- and carboxy-terminal truncation analysis, we had localized the region of OVA (323-339) that was critical for determining the I-A^d-binding capacity to the region 327–332. However, when this hexapeptide was synthesized, it did not bind I-A^d. That the failure to bind is related to the size of the peptide was indicated by the fact that good binding could be restored by adding 2–4 amino acids unrelated to the natural OVA sequence to the amino and carboxyl

Table 1. Effect of Proline Substitutions on the I-A^d-binding Capacity of OVA (323-336)

Substituted amino acid	Peptide sequence	Relative capacity to bind I-A^d
—	I S Q A V H A A H A E I N E	1.00
A 326	- - - P - - - - - - - - - -	0.83
V 327	- - - - P - - - - - - - - -	0.50
H 328	- - - - - P - - - - - - - -	0.03
A 329	- - - - - - P - - - - - - -	0.19
A 330	- - - - - - - P - - - - - -	0.83
H 331	- - - - - - - - P - - - - -	0.28
A 332	- - - - - - - - - P - - - -	0.48
E 333	- - - - - - - - - - P - - -	0.53
I 334	- - - - - - - - - - - P - -	0.77

The amount of each peptide necessary to inhibit by 50% the binding of ^{125}I-labeled OVA (323-339) to I-A^d was measured and was normalized to the capacity of unlabeled OVA (323-336) to inhibit binding. The 50% inhibitory concentration for OVA (323-336) before normalization was 19 μM. Data represent the average of 2–4 experiments.

Table 2. Effect of Different Synthetic Extensions of OVA (327-332) on its I-A^d-binding Capacity

Peptide sequence	Relative I-A^d binding $\pm$ S.E.M.	
I S Q A V H A A H A E I N E	1.00	—
E A E A – – – – – – E A E A	0.71	±0.10
Y T Y T – – – – – – Y T Y T	10.00	±4.41
G P G P – – – – – – G P G P	0.09	±0.02
Y T A – – – – – – A Y T	7.14	±3.22
Y T P – – – – – – P Y T	3.70	±1.50
A M A M – – – – – A M A M	6.30	±1.55
L E L E – – – – – – L E L E	0.44	±0.04
K M K M – – – – – K M K M	1.16	±0.33
A K A K – – – – – – A K A K	4.55	±1.90
E S E S – – – – – – E S E S	0.07	±0.002
K Q K Q – – – – – – K Q K Q	0.36	±0.03
P A P A – – – – – – P A P A	0.09	±0.02
D H D H – – – – – D H D H	0.02	±0.01
I Y I Y – – – – – – I Y I Y	0.07	±0.02
N V N V – – – – – N V N V	2.78	±2.06
T N T N – – – – – – T N T N	0.07	±0.04
P T P T – – – – – – P T P T	0.03	±0.02
Y N Y N – – – – – – Y N Y N	0.90	±0.09
N G N G – – – – – – N G N G	0.10	±0.10
V I V I – – – – – – V I V I	0.01	±0.01
N F N F – – – – – N F N F	0.76	±0.19
M H M H – – – – – M H M H	1.76	±0.22
D E D E – – – – – – D E D E	<0.01	—

Relative binding capacity was calculated as described in Table 1. The 50% inhibitory concentration for OVA (323-336) before normalization was 11 μM. Data represent the average of 2–3 experiments.

termini of this core region. This finding provided us with the opportunity to determine the relationship between the binding capacity of such core-extended peptides and the nature of the amino acids used to construct the extensions with respect to their predicted propensities to be associated with particular secondary conformations. Table 2 shows a panel of 23 such core-extended peptides, their sequences, and their relative I-A^d-binding capacities. Of the 23 analogs, 22 yielded significant binding. Of these, 8 had more than a tenfold reduction in binding capacity; 3 had a two- to tenfold reduction in binding capacity; 5 had an equivalent binding capacity to OVA (323-336); and 6 bound appreciably better than the native peptide. These data were then analyzed to determine the correlation, if any, between the MHC-binding capacity of a peptide and its conformational propensity, as determined by the Chou and Fasman (1978) algorithm. A plot of the calculated α-helical, β-sheet, and β-turn propensities versus the binding capacity of the corresponding analogs is shown in Figure 1. It is apparent from this analysis that no significant correlation exists. These data support, therefore, the conclusions derived from the analysis of the proline substitutions, that the formation of regular α-helical, β-sheet, or β-turn structures is not critical to the binding of the OVA peptide to I-A^d.

Characterization of Physiologically Processed Antigen

Taking advantage of the high stability of the complexes between MHC molecules and antigenic pep-tides, we decided to attempt the isolation and characterization of a naturally processed antigenic determinant from antigen (HEL)-pulsed A20-1.11 B-lymphoma cells (A20 cells). First, I-E^d molecules were purified by affinity chromatography from a lysate of HEL-pulsed A20 cells (HEL/I-E^d), and an aliquot of this I-E^d preparation was inserted into lipid PM. These complexes strongly stimulated IL-2 production by the I-E^d-restricted T-cell hybridoma 1H-11.3, for which the sequence HEL (107-116) had previously been identified as the minimal antigenic determinant (Adorini et al. 1988). Thus, this I-E^d preparation contained naturally processed material that included the HEL (107-116) determinant (Table 3, first row).

The naturally processed antigen contained in such I-E^d preparations was isolated by acid treatment of acetonitrile-precipitated HEL/I-E^d material, followed by Sephadex G10 chromatography (Buus et al. 1988). As assessed by SDS-PAGE, this step completely depleted the acid-eluted HEL/I-E^d peptide preparation of I-E^d (data not shown). The acid-eluted HEL-I-E^d peptides were then incubated with I-E^d molecules purified from A20 cells grown in the absence of HEL. The putative complexes were then inserted into PM as described in Methods. These antigen-presenting structures stimulated IL-2 release from 1 H-11.3 T cells, indicating that peptidic material containing the HEL (107-116) sequence was eluted from the I-E^d isolated from cells incubated with HEL, and these peptides could be rebound to I-E^d molecules and detected by their capacity to stimulate T cells (Table 1, last row).

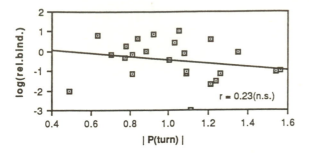

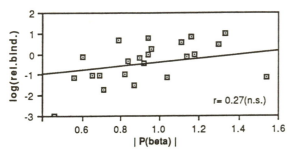

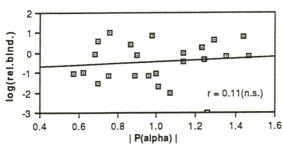

Figure 1. Correlation between relative I-A^d-binding capacity of the OVA (323-336) analogs (from Table 1) and their β-turn, β-sheet, and α-helix conformational parameters, calculated according to Chou and Fasman (1978) rules. (n.s.) Not significant at the 0.05 probability level.

Table 3. Isolation of Naturally Processed Antigenic Material from Antigen-pulsed B-lymphoma Cells

Addition of 1 mg/ml HEL to A20 cells[a]	Antigen incubated with I-E[b]	Units/ml IL-2 produced by 1 H-11.3T cells[c]
yes	—	1280
no	20 ng synthetic HEL(107-116)	20
no	200 ng synthetic HEL(107-116)	640
no	acid-eluted peptides from HEL/I-E[d]	80

[a]A20 cells were grown for 24 hr in the presence of 1 mg/ml HEL.
[b]I-E^d/peptide complexes were prepared by incubating I-E^d molecules with various peptide preparations, as described in the Methods section.
[c]I-E^d/peptide-bearing PM were tested in a T-cell hybridoma stimulation assay, as described previously (Buus et al. 1986; Coeshott et al. 1986).

to form T-cell stimulatory complexes. Material antigenic for 1 H-11.3 T cells was eluted within a restricted portion of the solvent gradient, between 34% and 40% acetonitrile. The activity profile suggested that at least three peptide species were produced by A20 cells during processing of HEL molecules (Fig. 2). The synthetic peptides HEL (107-116) and HEL (105-120), respectively, eluted at 34% and 40% acetonitrile, suggesting that the HEL fragments generated by A20 cells were structurally related to these peptides.

Next, the molecular weights of acid-eluted HEL/I-E^d peptides were estimated by Sephadex G50 chromatography. Each fraction was tested for its capacity to produce, when combined to I-E^d molecules, complexes antigenically active for 1 H-11.3 T cells. Stimulatory material was found in a single homogeneous peak, with apparent molecular weights of 1200 to 3500 (Fig. 3).

As a control, a radioiodinated synthetic peptide corresponding to ^{125}I-labeled-Y-HEL (105-120) was subjected to the purification procedures described above to evaluate the possibility that limited degradation of the antigenic material occurred during the isolation proce-

This, then, provided an assay with which naturally processed antigen could be characterized. To this end, an acid-eluted peptide preparation was subjected to reversed-phase HPLC, and each fraction was tested for its capacity, following incubation with I-E^d molecules,

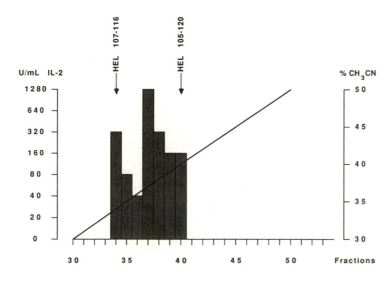

Figure 2. Reversed-phase HPLC analysis of a naturally processed MHC class-II-restricted determinant of lysozyme. Acid-eluted material obtained from 350 μg of HEL/I-E^d complexes was separated by reversed-phase HPLC. Fractions (1 ml) were collected, lyophilized, and tested as described in the Methods section. The elution positions of synthetic HEL (107-116) and HEL (105-120) peptides are indicated.

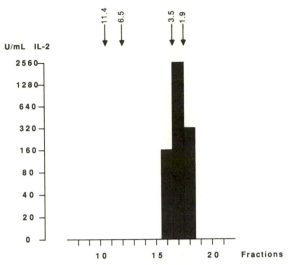

Figure 3. Gel filtration analysis of a naturally processed MHC class-II-restricted determinant of lysozyme. Acid-eluted material obtained from 350 μg of HEL/I-E^d complexes was chromatographed on a Sephadex G50 column. Fractions (8 ml) were collected and were lyophilized twice. One-fifth of each fraction was tested as described in the Methods section. The positions of molecular-weight markers are indicated (11.4 kD: cytochrome c; 6.5 kD: aprotinin; 3.5 kD: protamine A; 1.9 kD: Y-HEL [105-120]). In this experiment, I-E^d complexes prepared with 20 ng and 200 ng synthetic HEL (107-116) peptide stimulated the production of 1280 units/ml IL-2 and >2560 units/ml IL-2 by 1 H-11.3 T cells, respectively.

dure. As assessed by reversed-phase HPLC, no significant degradation could be detected, indicating that the antigenic HEL peptides characterized above were representative of those produced by processing within A20 cells (data not shown).

Proportion of I-E^d Occupied by HEL(107-116)-containing Peptides

To estimate the proportion of I-E^d molecules on HEL-pulsed A20 cells that were occupied by peptides containing the HEL (108-116) determinant detected by 1 H-11.3, we compared the antigenicity of an I-E^d preparation from HEL-pulsed A20 (HEL/I-E^d) with synthetic HEL (107-116)/I-E^d complexes prepared in vitro. The amount of synthetic HEL (107-116) peptide bound to I-E^d molecules was first determined by Scatchard analysis, as described previously (Buus et al. 1986). Thus, it was calculated that under saturating concentrations of HEL (107-116) peptide (>10 μg/ml), 7.5% of I-E^d molecules were occupied by this peptide. Then, various amounts of HEL (107-116)/I-E^d complexes were inserted into PM, and for each of them, the corresponding 1 H-11.3 T-cell stimulation was measured. The total amount of I-E^d inserted into each PM sample was kept constant by adding I-E^d purified from unpulsed A20 cells to obtain a direct correlation between the T-cell response and the density of antigenic complexes present in the PM (Fig. 4). It was found that naturally processed HEL/I-E^d complexes inserted at 16 nM into PM stimulated 1 H-11.3 T cells

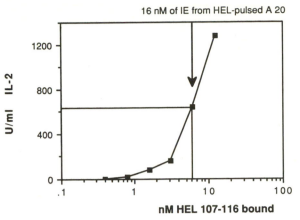

Figure 4. Occupancy of MHC class II molecules purified from lysozyme-pulsed B-lymphoma cells by lysozyme (107-116) determinants. Various concentrations of synthetic HEL (107-116) peptide bound to I-E^d molecules and inserted into PM were tested for their ability to trigger 1 H-11.3 T-cell stimulation. A known concentration of I-E^d molecules purified from HEL-pulsed A20 cells (16 nM) was inserted into PM and used to stimulate 1 H-11.3 T cells.

to produce 640 units/ml IL-2. As indicated in Figure 4, a similar T-cell activation was reached with 6 nM HEL (107-116) peptide bound to I-E^d molecules. Assuming that HEL (107-116)/I-E^d complexes were as stimulatory as HEL/I-E^d complexes, these data would indicate that 38% of the I-E^d molecules expressed by HEL-pulsed A20 cells were occupied by HEL (107-116) determinants. An independent method of estimating the degree of occupancy was based on the amount of antigenic peptides eluted from an HEL/I-E^d preparation after its separation on G50 gel filtration. In this experiment, antigenic material obtained from 2 nmoles of I-E^d yielded T-cell stimulatory activity corresponding to 2000–3000 units/ml IL-2. Similar levels of IL-2 production were reached using approximately 0.2 nmoles of synthetic HEL (107-116) peptide. Thus, by this calculation, it would appear that approximately 10% of the I-E^d molecules purified from HEL-pulsed A20 cells carried HEL (107-116) determinants. This figure is a minimal estimate, since the G50 fractions probably also contained non-HEL-derived I-E^d-binding peptides that would tend to compete with, and lower the efficiency of, binding of the HEL peptides to I-E^d.

DISCUSSION AND CONCLUSIONS

We have described herein the data obtained with two distinct sets of analogs of the peptide, OVA (323-336). The purpose of these experiments was to examine whether a correlation could be discerned between the capacity of these analogs to bind I-A^d molecules and their predicted propensity to form certain regulatory secondary structures, such as α helices and β sheets. First, we found that proline substitutions, despite their strong tendency to disrupt both α helices and β sheets, did not affect, in most cases, the capacity of the peptide analogs to bind I-A^d molecules. Second, we synthesized a number of peptide analogs in which the crucial I-A^d-binding region of the OVA peptide (OVA [327-332]) was extended in both directions with artificial sequences of differing conformational propensities. No correlation between the I-A^d-binding capacity of these analogs and their propensity to form α helices, β sheets, or β turns, as measured by the Chou and Fasman (1978) algorithm, was detected. Thus, a role for any regular secondary structure in peptide binding to I-A^d could not be documented. This conclusion is in accord with the experiments of Paterson and associates (Bhayani et al. 1988), who, using a similar approach but a different MHC/antigen combination (I-E^k/p cyt$_c$), also found a lack of correlation between T-cell immunogenicity and propensity of the peptides to form α helices.

The apparent contradiction with the previously reported (Rothbard et al. 1988) correlation between secondary structure propensity and capacity to serve as a T-cell epitope can be resolved, considering that immunogenicity and class II binding may be, in fact, two distinct, although overlapping, properties. It is conceivable, for example, that conformational propensities may play a role in some processing event distinct from MHC binding, such as directing where in a molecule proteolytic cleavage occurs. Furthermore, it should be noted that interpretation of all the data correlating MHC binding and antigen conformation should be considered with caution, since little is known about the applicability of conformational parameters derived from the study of three-dimensional structures of isolated proteins (Chou and Fasman 1974, 1978; Nemethy and Scheraga 1977; Richardson 1981) to the study of peptide/MHC interactions.

With the caveats mentioned above, on the basis of the data presented in this study, it is hypothesized that OVA peptide antigen is bound to class II molecules in an extended conformation similar to the "extended coil" of denatured proteins (which can, in fact, bind to Ia [Sette et al. 1989a] and serve, in some instances, as bona fide T-cell-activating antigens [Allen and Unanue 1984; Striecher et al. 1984]). This type of recognition would also be consistent with the repeated observation that some residues in the antigen molecule appear to be recognized jointly by both MHC and T-cell receptor, and with previously proposed models in which the antigen molecule is "sandwiched" between class II and T-cell receptor molecules (Fox et al. 1987; Sette et al. 1987). It should be stressed, however, that these conclusions are based on experiments with only a few peptide antigens. The distinct possibility exists that class II MHC molecules may bind different antigens in different conformations, or even that the same antigen may be bound in different conformations, depending on the MHC (Heber-Katz et al. 1985; F. Ronchese and R. Germain, pers. comm.).

In this paper, we have described techniques for the preparation of complexes between MHC molecules and naturally processed antigenic peptides that allowed us to initiate characterization of a naturally processed determinant of HEL. The microheterogeneity obtained upon HPLC analysis of the antigenic peptides produced by A20 cells indicates that processing does not lead to single unique peptide fragments, but rather to a series of related peptides ranging from approximately 10 to 30 residues in length. The observed heterogeneity may be due to cleavages at different positions within the HEL sequence, reflecting the usage of either different proteinases or proteinases displaying a broad substrate specificity.

Attempts to quantitate the proportion of HEL/I-E^d complexes bearing HEL (107-116) determinants yielded surprisingly high estimates (10–40%). These data can be rationalized at least in part, considering that HEL represented under the experimental conditions used about one-third of the total extracellular proteins (1 mg/ml HEL in 5% total calf serum). Furthermore, the HEL (107-116) peptide region is the major I-E^d-binding site of HEL (Adorini et al. 1988). Nevertheless, the efficiency of in vivo binding of HEL-processed fragments by I-E^d molecules appears to be quite high. If, however, naturally processed antigen had, for some unknown reason, an increased antigenic potency compared to the synthetic peptide, this could also contribute to the high biologic activity observed (Falo et al. 1986). Direct sequencing of naturally processed antigenic peptides should allow us to solve these issues.

ACKNOWLEDGMENTS

The expert secretarial assistance of Joyce Joseph and the skillful technical help of Virginia Ord and Doris Johnson are gratefully acknowledged.

REFERENCES

Adorini, L., A. Sette, H.M. Grey, M. Darsley, P.V. Lehmann, G. Doria, Z.A. Nagy, and E. Appella. 1988. Interaction of an immunodominant epitope with Ia molecules in T-cell activation. *Proc. Natl. Acad. Sci.* **85:** 5181.

Allen, P.M. and E.R. Unanue. 1984. Differential requirements for antigen processing by macrophages for lysozyme-specific T cell hybridomas. *J. Immunol.* **132:** 1077.

Allen, P.M., G.R. Matsueda, R.J. Evans, J.B. Dunbar, Jr., G.R. Marshall, and E. Unanue. 1987. Identification of the T cell and Ia contact residues of a T cell antigenic epitope. *Nature* **327:** 713.

Bhayani, H., F.R. Carbone, and Y. Paterson. 1988. The activation of pigeon cytochrome *c*-specific T cell hybridomas by antigenic peptides is influenced by non-native sequences at the amino terminus of the determinant. *J. Immunol.* **141:** 377.

Buus, S., A. Sette, and H.M. Grey. 1987. The interaction between protein-derived immunogenic peptides and Ia. *Immunol. Rev.* **98:** 115.

Buus, S., A. Sette, S.M. Colon, and H.M. Grey. 1988. Autologous peptides constitutively occupy the antigen binding site on Ia. *Science* **242:** 1045.

Buus, S., A. Sette, S.M. Colon, D.M. Jenis, and H.M. Grey. 1986. Isolation and characterization of antigen-Ia complexes involved in T cell recognition. *Cell* **47:** 1071.

Carbone, F.R., B.S. Fox, R.H. Schwartz, and Y. Paterson. 1987. The use of hydrophobic α-helix-defined peptides in delineating the T cell determinant for pigeon cytochrome c. *J. Immunol.* **138:** 1838.

Chou, P.Y. and G.D. Fasman. 1974. Prediction of protein conformation. *Biochemistry* **13:** 222.

———. 1978. Empirical predictions on protein conformation. *Annu. Rev. Biochem.* **47:** 251.

Coeshott, C.M., R.W. Chesnut, R.T. Kubo, S.F. Grammer, D.M. Jenis, and H.M. Grey. 1986. Ia-specific mixed leukocyte reactive T cell hybridomas: Analysis of their specificity by using purified class II MHC molecules in a synthetic membrane system. *J. Immunol.* **136:** 2832.

DeLisi, C. and J.A. Berzofsky. 1985. T cell antigenic sites tend to be amphipathic structures. *Proc. Natl. Acad. Sci.* **82:** 7048.

Falo, L.D., Jr., B. Benacerraf, and K.L. Rock. 1986. Phospholipase treatment of accessory cells that have been exposed to antigen selectively inhibits antigen-specific Ia-restricted, but not allospecific, stimulation of T lymphocytes. *Proc. Natl. Acad. Sci.* **83:** 6994.

Fox, B.S., C. Chen, E. Fraga, C.A. French, B. Singh, and R.H. Schwartz. 1987. Functionally distinct agretopic and epitopic sites: Analysis of the dominant T cell determinant of moth and pigeon cytochromes c with the use of synthetic peptide antigens. *J. Immunol.* **139:** 1578.

Guillet, J., M. Lai, T. Briner, J. Smith, and M. Gefter. 1986. Interaction of peptide antigens and class II major histocompatibility antigens. *Nature* **324:** 260.

Heber-Katz, E., M. Hollosi, B. Dietzschold, F. Hudecz, and G.D. Fasman. 1985. The T cell response to the glycoprotein D of the herpes simplex virus: The significance of antigen conformation. *J. Immunol.* **135:** 1385.

Houghten, R. 1985. General method for the rapid solid phase synthesis of large numbers of peptides: Specificity of antigen-antibody interaction at the level of individual amino acids. *Proc. Natl. Acad. Sci.* **82:** 5131.

Margalit, H., J.L. Spouge, J.L. Cornette, K.B. Cease, C. DeLisi, and J.A. Berzofsky. 1987. Prediction of immunodominant helper T cell antigenic sites from the primary sequence. *J. Immunol.* **138:** 2213.

Nemethy, G. and H.A. Scheraga. 1977. Protein folding. *Q. Rev. Biophys.* **10:** 239.

Ogasawara, K., W.L. Maloy, B. Beverly, and R.H. Schwartz. 1989. Functional analysis of the antigenic structure of a minor T cell determinant from pigeon cytochrome c. *J. Immunol.* **142:** 1448.

Pincus, M.R., F. Gerewitz, R.H. Schwartz, and H.A. Scheraga. 1983. Correlation between the conformation of cytochrome c peptides and their stimulatory activity in a T-lymphocyte proliferation assay. *Proc. Natl. Acad. Sci.* **80:** 3297.

Richardson, J.S. 1981. The anatomy and taxonomy of protein structure. *Adv. Protein Chem.* **34:** 167.

Rothbard, J.B., I. Lechler, K. Howland, V. Bal, D.D. Eckels, R. Sekaly, E.O. Long, W.R. Taylor, and J.R. Lamb. 1988. Structural model of HLA-DR1 restricted T cell antigen recognition. *Cell* **52:** 515.

Sette, A., L. Adorini, S.M. Colon, S. Buus, and H.M. Grey. 1989a. Capacity of intact proteins to bind to MHC class II molecules. *J. Immunol.* **143:** 1265.

Sette, A., S. Buus, S. Colon, C. Miles, and H.M. Grey. 1988. I-A^d-binding peptides derived from unrelated protein antigens share a common structural motif. *J. Immunol.* **141:** 45.

———. 1989b. Structural analysis of peptides capable of binding to more than one Ia antigen. *J. Immunol.* **142:** 35.

Sette, A., S. Buus, S. Colon, J.A. Smith, C. Miles, and H.M. Grey. 1987. Structural characteristics of an antigen required for its interaction with Ia and recognition by T cells. *Nature* **328:** 395.

Spouge, J.L., H.R. Guy, J.L. Cornette, H. Margalit, K. Cease, J.A. Berzofsky, and C. DeLisi. 1987. Strong conformational propensities enhance T cell antigenicity. *J. Immunol.* **138:** 204.

Streicher, H.Z., I.J. Berkower, M. Busch, F.R.N. Gurd, and J.A. Berzofsky. 1984. Antigen conformation determines processing requirements for T-cell activation. *Proc. Natl. Acad. Sci.* **81:** 6831.

Consequences of Self and Foreign Superantigen Interaction with Specific V_β Elements of the Murine TCR$\alpha\beta$

J.W. KAPPLER,[†‡] A. PULLEN,[*] J. CALLAHAN,[§] Y. CHOI,[*] A. HERMAN,[*]
J. WHITE,[*] W. POTTS,[‖] E. WAKELAND,[‖] AND P. MARRACK[*†‡§]

*Howard Hughes Medical Institute, Division of Basic Immunology, Department of Medicine, National
Jewish Center for Immunology and Respiratory Medicine, Denver, Colorado 80206; Departments of
†Medicine, ‡Microbiology and Immunology, and §Biophysics, Biochemistry, and Genetics, University
of Colorado Medical School, Denver, Colorado 80220; ‖Department of Pathology, University of
Florida College of Medicine, Gainesville, Florida 32610

The $\alpha\beta$ T-cell receptor (TCR$\alpha\beta$) recognizes a ligand composed of an antigen fragment complexed with a product of the major histocompatibility complex (MHC). The repertoire of receptors is limited both by the germ line of receptor variable elements and by selective events that take place during T-cell development. The current view is that the germ-line repertoire is expressed in the thymus randomly but that only those T cells bearing receptors that successfully interact with MHC molecules expressed on thymic cortical epithelial cells are allowed to mature (Bevan and Fink 1978; Zinkernagel et al. 1978; Kisielow et al. 1988; Sha et al. 1988). Furthermore, during the process of establishing tolerance to self-antigens, this positively selected population is further reduced by the deletion or inactivation of clones whose receptors continue to interact with self-antigen/MHC ligands (Kappler et al. 1987a, 1988; MacDonald et al. 1988; Pullen et al. 1988). Thus, positive and negative selections reduce expressed receptor repertoire in the periphery to a fraction of the germ-line repertoire.

Five variable elements contribute to the specificity of the TCR$\alpha\beta$: V_α (variable), J_α (joining), V_β, D_β (diversity), and J_β. Despite the fact that in most circumstances all five components together determine receptor specificity, a study of the variation of expression of individual V_β elements in different mouse strains has produced a wealth of information on genetic factors effecting the TCR$\alpha\beta$ repertoire. Several studies have shown the influence of thymic-positive selection on expression of particular V_β elements (Blackman et al. 1989; Palmer et al., this volume). More striking are the many mechanisms in mice that prevent the expression of particular V_β elements in individual mice. Some of these are genetic defects within the V_β complex (Chou et al. 1987a; Kappler et al. 1987b; Wade et al. 1988). However, the most surprising mechanism limiting V_β expression involves the induction of tolerance to a set of unusual self-antigens, which we have termed "superantigens" (White et al. 1989). Superantigens combine with MHC molecules to generate ligands that are recognized by all TCR$\alpha\beta$s bearing one or a few V_β elements with little input from the other receptor variable elements (Kappler et al. 1987a, 1988; MacDonald et al. 1988; Pullen et al. 1988). The consequence is that mice carrying these antigens delete nearly all T cells bearing the relevant V_β elements while establishing self-tolerance. Since there are only a total of 22 different V_β elements in the mouse, these self-superantigens drastically alter the repertoire of the mice in which they occur.

Superantigens have also been identified as products of microorganisms. Particularly striking examples are the toxins of *Staphylococcus aureus*, which cause a number of diseases in humans and other animals (Bergdoll 1983). These toxins have been recognized as powerful T-cell stimulants for many years, but the role of T cells in their mode of action has not been pursued. Recently, we and other investigators have shown that these toxins are superantigens in that each stimulates a set of human or mouse T cells bearing particular V_β elements (Choi et al. 1989; Janeway et al. 1989; Kappler et al. 1989b; White et al. 1989).

In this paper, we review some of the properties of the bacterial and the polymorphic murine superantigens and attempt to tackle the question of their possible function in bacteria and mice. We present evidence that T-cell stimulation by bacterial superantigens is critical to their toxic properties. In addition, we demonstrate that in mice widespread polymorphisms in superantigens as well as in V_β structural genes results in a state where the mouse population as a whole expresses all V_β elements but that the number of V_β elements expressed in an individual mouse is generally quite limited. We propose that this state may be an evolutionary equilibrium balancing the advantage of a large, diverse T-cell repertoire against the disadvantage of possessing too many potential targets for the microbial superantigen toxins.

RESULTS

Germ-line Limitations on V_β Expression

So far, 22 functional murine V_β elements have been described (Fig. 1). However, no mouse has been found

```
-2--4-16-10-1---5²-8³-5¹-8²-8¹-13-12-11-9--6--15---19-17-3---7--18--DJCβ1-DJCβ2--14- BALB/c,B6
                        x  x                                                          DBA,C3H,etc.

-2--4-16-10-1-···                      ···-6--15---19-17-3---7--18--DJCβ1-DJCβ2--14- SJL,SWR,
                                                                                     C57L,C57BR

-2--4-16-10-1-···                              ···-3---7--18--DJCβ1-DJCβ2--14- RIII

-2--4-16-10-1---5²-8³-5¹-8²-8¹-13-12-11-9--6--15---19-17-3---7--18--DJCβ1-DJCβ2--14- Florida
                        ?  x                                                          Wild Mice

-2--4-16-10-1-···                         ···----19-17-3---7--18--DJCβ1-DJCβ2--14- Florida
                                           ?  x                                       Wild Mice
```

Figure 1. Deletions and mutations within the mouse V_β complex. The genomic organization of the mouse V_β complex is shown for various laboratory strains and for wild mice from central Florida. Approximate position of deletions is shown. (X) V_β elements known to carry point mutations that inactivate the gene. Data are from this paper and Behlke et al. (1986), Malissen et al. (1986), Kappler et al. (1987b), Chou et al. (1987a,b), Lai et al. (1987, 1988), Wade et al. (1988), and Haqqi et al. (1989). Data from $V_\beta 19$ was from D. Loh (pers. comm.).

that carries all 22 functional V_β genes because various deletions and mutations eliminate at least some V_β elements in all mice examined thus far. Three V_β haplotypes have been identified in laboratory mice. The haplotype carried by most strains has a full complement of V_β genes; however, the $V_\beta 17$ gene carries a single-base mutation generating a termination codon near the 3' end of the coding region (Wade et al. 1988), and the $V_\beta 19$ gene is inactivated by a frameshift caused by a single-base deletion in the leader (D. Loh, pers. comm.). Loh and colleagues have described a large deletion in SJL and a few other strains of mice in the middle of the V_β complex, that eliminates nine functional V_β elements (Chou et al. 1987a). These strains have a functional $V_\beta 17$ and $V_\beta 19$ gene. Recently, a similar but more extensive deletion has been found in another laboratory strain, RIII (Haqqi et al. 1989).

Such massive elimination of functional V_β elements should be disadvantageous to mice since the mice carrying these deletions should have a substantially reduced TCR$\alpha\beta$ repertoire. Therefore, one could expect that in the wild the pressure of dealing with environmental pathogens might select against mice carrying the mutations and deletions. On the contrary, Huppi et al. (1988) have found that a deletion similar to that of SJL mice is common in mice from Hebrides. We have examined the V_β complex of a series of 39 wild mice from central Florida. Southern blot analysis of the $V_\beta 17$ gene in these mice showed a restriction-fragment-length polymorphism pattern identical to the inactive $V_\beta 17$ allele (Kappler et al. 1987b; Wade et al. 1988), and no T cells were detected in these mice reactive with an antibody specific for $V_\beta 17$. In addition, a deletion was found in the V_β complex in many of these mice. This deletion was intermediate in length between the two previously described deletions, involving 11 V_β elements (Fig. 1), and was frequent enough in these populations so that 10 of the 39 mice examined were homozygous for the deletion and therefore lacked any

T cells bearing the deleted V_β elements (Table 2). Thus, for some reason, mice in the wild tolerate at high-frequency genetic mutations and deletions that limit the TCR$\alpha\beta$ repertoire in some mice.

Deletion of T Cells by Polymorphic V_β-specific Self-superantigens

A similar picture of limited V_β expression has emerged during examination of the V_β-specific self-superantigens. We identified the first antigen of this type as a B-cell product that combined with the MHC class II molecule, IE, to form a ligand for virtually all T cells whose TCR$\alpha\beta$ contained $V_\beta 17a$ (Kappler et al. 1987b; Marrack and Kappler 1988). IE$^+$ mice carrying the functional $V_\beta 17a$ gene delete virtually all $V_\beta 17a^+$ T cells while establishing self-tolerance (Kappler et al. 1987a, 1989a). Since then, we and other investigators have identified the V_β specificity of a number of other self-superantigens. For example, mice carrying the minor lymphocyte-stimulating (Mls-1^a) antigen, long known as a powerful alloantigen, have been shown to eliminate virtually all T cells bearing $V_\beta 6$ (MacDonald et al. 1988), $V_\beta 8.1$ (Kappler et al. 1988), and $V_\beta 9$ (Happ et al. 1989). Likewise, mice carrying the Mls-2^a or Mls-3^a antigen eliminate T cells bearing $V_\beta 3$ (Pullen et al. 1988, 1989). Examples of these phenomena are shown in Figure 2 and 3, and the properties of the V_β-specific self-superantigens reported so far are summarized in Table 1.

Some of the most striking features of these antigens are the extensive polymorphisms controlling their expression. Thus, in every case, the superantigen and/or the MHC-restricting elements that present it are polymorphic, so that a functional ligand appears in only some strains of mice. For example, the superantigens that delete T cells bearing $V_\beta 17a$, $V_\beta 5$, or $V_\beta 11$ all require an IE molecule for presentation. Therefore, even in the presence of the superantigen, IE$^-$ strains of

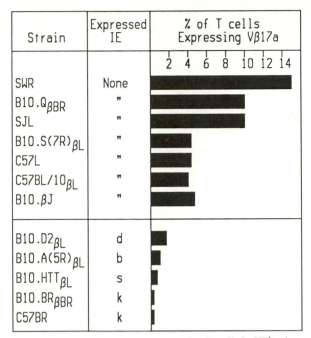

Strain	Expressed IE	% of T cells Expressing Vβ17a

Figure 2. Elimination of $V_\beta 17a$-bearing T cells in IE$^+$ mice. Peripheral T cells, prepared from a series of mice carrying a functional gene for $V_\beta 17$, were stained with a monoclonal antibody specific for $V_\beta 17$ and analyzed by flow cytometry (Kappler et al. 1987b). For each strain, the percentage of T cells bearing $V_\beta 17$ is shown along with the MHC class II molecules expressed in that strain. Each value shown is an average for those obtained in three or more mice. Standard errors were 10% or less.

mice do not present the antigen, and T cells bearing the relevant V_β elements are not deleted. In the case of Mls-1, Mls-2, and Mls-3, only the *a* allele of these loci encodes a superantigen. The relevant V_β elements are expressed normally in mice carrying the *b* allele. Furthermore, the class II molecule of H-2^q, IA^q, is unable

to present these Mls superantigens, so that an H-2^q strain, such as DBA/1 carrying the *a* allele at all three Mls loci, nevertheless expresses normal levels of the relevant V_β elements.

Again, one might suppose that in the wild the antigen and MHC alleles creating superantigen ligands would be selected against because they dramatically limit the TCRαβ repertoire. To test this idea, we used the available monoclonal antibodies to V_β elements to examine peripheral T cells from the 39 wild mice from Florida mentioned above. We were surprised to find that the pattern of V_β expression in these mice was consistent with the frequent expression of a number of the superantigens listed in Table 1. Figure 4 shows some relevant data from a few of the mice, and the data are summarized in Table 2. In each case, the presence of a functional V_β gene was established by good V_β expression on immature thymocytes (prior to induction of self-tolerance). T cells bearing each of the relevant V_β elements were severely depleted among mature T cells in some of the mice. For example, $V_\beta 3$-bearing T cells were deleted in most mice, indicating widespread distribution of an Mls-2/3^a-like antigen. Nearly all of these mice expressed an IE molecule, and deletion of $V_\beta 5$ T cells was very common. The evidence in laboratory mice suggests that the IE-dependent superantigens specific for $V_\beta 5$ and $V_\beta 11$ are polymorphic (Bill et al. 1989; Palmer et al., this volume). The results with these wild mice strengthen this conclusion, indicating that different antigens control interactions with these V_β elements and that at least one nonfunctional allele exists for each since the presence of an IE molecule is not sufficient for deletion of T cells bearing these V_β elements and the pattern of deletion for each is different.

The deletion of $V_\beta 6$- and $V_\beta 8.1$-bearing T cells in some of these mice indicated the presence of an Mls-1^a-like antigen. Interestingly, the pattern of reactivity with

Table 1. Self-superantigens in the Mouse That Delete T Cells Bearing Particular V_β Elements

Self-superantigen (gene location)	MHC-class-II-presenting elements	V_β elements	References[a]
Nonpolymorphic? B-cell product (unknown locus)	IE	17a	1
Mls-1^a (chromosome 1)	most IE some IA	6, 8.1, 9	2
Mls-2^a (single locus)	most IE some IA	3	3
Mls-3^a (linked to Ly-7)	most IE some IA	3	4
Polymorphic (unknown locus)	IE	5	5
Polymorphic (unknown locus)	IE	11	6
Polymorphic (unknown locus)	most IE some IA?	7	7

[a] (1) Kappler et al. (1987a, b, 1989a); Marrack and Kappler (1988); (2) Kappler et al. (1988); MacDonald et al. (1988); Happ et al. (1989); (3) Pullen et al. (1988, 1989); (4) Palmer et al. (this volume); (5) Bill et al. (1989); and (6) M. Happ et al. (pers. comm.).

H-2^k Strain	Mls 1	Mls 2/3	% T cells Expressing V$_\beta$8.1	% T cells Expressing V$_\beta$3
B10.BR	b	b	(bar to ~7)	(bar to ~3)
CBA/CaJ	b	b	(bar to ~6)	(bar to ~3)
C3H/HeJ	b	a	(bar to ~3)	(bar to ~3)
AKR/J	a	b	(bar to ~1)	(bar to ~7)

Figure 3. The *a* alleles of the Mls antigens eliminate T cells bearing V$_\beta$8.1 or V$_\beta$3. Peripheral T cells from the strains shown are analyzed as in Fig. 2 for expression of V$_\beta$8.1 or V$_\beta$3. V$_\beta$8.1 was analyzed using two monoclonal antibodies, one specific for V$_\beta$8.1 plus V$_\beta$8.2 and the other specific for V$_\beta$8.2 (Kappler et al. 1988). V$_\beta$3 was analyzed with a specific monoclonal antibody (Pullen et al. 1988).

a series of monoclonal antibodies specific for different combinations of the three members of the V$_\beta$8 family indicated both that the V$_\beta$8.2 element in these mice had lost reactivity with one of the antibodies and that T cells bearing this altered V$_\beta$8.2 were also deleted in Mls-1^a mice (Fig. 4). Consequently, we sequenced this variant V$_\beta$8.2 and produced a series of T-cell hybridomas from Mls-1^b wild mice bearing the variant V$_\beta$8.2. The hybridomas indeed showed a very high frequency of reactivity to spleen cells from Mls-1^a-bearing laboratory mice (data not shown), and the sequence showed five amino acid differences from the V$_\beta$8.2 of laboratory mice, two of which were changes to the corresponding amino acid in the known Mls-1^a reactive V$_\beta$8.1 gene (Table 3). Therefore, we conclude that the T-cell-deleting alleles of superantigens and the MHC molecules that present them are not selected against in wild mice but rather coexist stably with nondeleting allelic

forms. Furthermore, the conversion of the V$_\beta$8.2 gene to superantigen reactivity suggests that V$_\beta$ elements may be under selection pressure to be able to recognize superantigens.

Staphylococcus aureus Toxins Are Superantigens in Mice

The data on the distribution of V$_\beta$ expression in mice suggest that, despite the obvious advantage of a large T-cell repertoire for dealing with a wide variety of pathogens, mice for some reason purposely exist in a state where individuals generally express only a subset of the V$_\beta$ elements available to the species as a whole. Therefore, one can suppose that there is some offsetting disadvantage to having too many V$_\beta$ elements expressed in an individual mouse. We have been exploring the possibility that this phenomena is related to

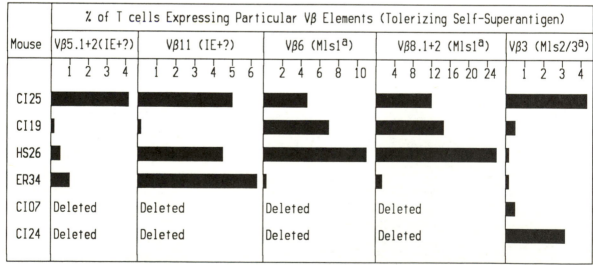

Figure 4. V$_\beta$ expression in six representative wild mice. Peripheral T cells from six mice taken from three different sites in central Florida were analyzed for V$_\beta$ expression, as in Fig. 2, using monoclonal antibodies specific for the V$_\beta$ elements shown. The self-superantigen capable of eliminating T cells bearing these V$_\beta$ elements are shown in parentheses. In those cases where a value is given, staining of immature cells in the thymus established the presence of a functional V$_\beta$ structural gene. Those cases marked as "deleted" indicate no staining in the thymus or periphery, indicating the absence of a functional structural gene. In many cases, the deletion of the gene was confirmed by Southern blot analysis.

Table 2. High Frequency of V_β Elimination in Wild Mice

			Mechanism of V_β elimination			
	homozygous gene deletion	homozygous gene mutation	tolerance to self-superantigens			
			Mls-1[a]	Mls-2/3[a]	IE[+]?	IE[+]?
V_βs eliminated	5.1 + 2 8.1 + 2 + 3 13, 12, 11 9, 6, 15	17	6, 8.1 9 8.2	3	5.1 + 2	11
Portion of wild mice with this elimination	10/39	39/39	8/29	32/39	21/29	2/29

toxic microbial products that are themselves V_β-specific superantigens and use this property in their mode of action.

A number of microbial products have been identified as potent T-cell stimulators in vitro in mouse and man. The related exotoxins of *S. aureus* are particularly good examples (Bergdoll 1983; Couch et al. 1988). In humans, these toxins are responsible for a large portion of food poisoning cases (staphylococcal enterotoxins A to E [SEA to SEE]), as well as other diseases such as scalded skin syndrome (exfoliating toxin) and toxic shock syndrome (toxic shock syndrome toxin [TSST-1]). Originally considered nonspecific mitogens, recent work has shown that these toxins must bind MHC molecules in order to stimulate T cells (Fischer et al. 1989; Fraser 1989) and that for each toxin only T cells bearing particular V_β elements respond (Choi et al. 1989; Janeway et al. 1989; Kappler et al. 1989b; White et al. 1989). Table 4 summarizes our results in mice using some of the *S. aureus* toxins. We found that each toxin stimulates a different set of V_β-bearing T cells. Even very closely related toxins (Couch et al. 1988), such as SEB and SEC1 or SEA and SEE, stimulate different T cells. Since most of the toxins stimulate T cells bearing any of several V_β elements, the proportion of total T cells stimulated is in some cases very high. For example, in the mouse SEB stimulates T cells bearing $V_\beta 3$, $V_\beta 8$, $V_\beta 7$, or $V_\beta 17a$. Depending on the strain of mouse, this can account for over 30% of all T cells. Similarly, in humans, we have found that these toxins stimulate T cells bearing particular V_β elements and that particular toxins often stimulate T cells bearing homologous V_β elements in mice and humans (Choi et al. 1989).

T Cells Bearing Specific V_βs Required in the Mode of Action of SEB

Despite the considerable variability of the primary sequences of these toxins, their ability to act as superantigens appears to be a conserved property. Furthermore, since each has a different V_β specificity, their superantigen function appears not to be an accidental consequence of the conservation of some common structural element required for some other function. Therefore, it is reasonable to suppose that the pathology associated with these toxins (e.g., vomiting, diarrhea, skin rashes, and shock) may be an indirect consequence of the massive in vivo activation of T cells and release of powerful lymphokine mediators rather than a direct effect of the toxins on the target tissue. This idea is difficult to test directly in humans where most of the pathology associated with these toxins has been identified so we have begun to study the effects of these toxins in mice in vivo.

We have begun our experiments with SEB. Mice given a single injection of SEB develop a shock-like syndrome within 24 hours. Usually, high doses are required ($> 50 \mu g$/mouse), correlating with the observation that this toxin, which was isolated from a strain of Staphylococcus that infects humans, must be used at a higher concentration in vitro to stimulate murine T cells than human T cells. The most obvious in vivo symptom in mice from this toxin is extremely rapid weight loss with wasting and in some cases death within 2–3 days. Those mice that survive for 3 days usually recover completely over the next few days. We have used this simple assay to assess the importance of the superantigen properties of SEB for its in vivo toxicity.

Table 3. Amino Acid Substitutions in the $V_\beta 8.2$ Gene of Wild Mice

Mouse	V_β	Mls-1[a] reactive	Binds MAb F23.2	Amino Acid				
				8	22	51	70	71
C57BL/6	8.2	−	+	N	N	G	E	N
Wild	8.2	+	−	S	D	D	K	E
C57BL/6	8.1	+	−	S	H	D	E	N

C57BL/6 sequences from Chou et al. (1987b). Amino acid numbering starts at the alanine at the amino termi of the mature proteins.

Table 4. *S. aureus* Toxins Are Superantigens in the Mouse

S. aureus toxin	Response of T cells bearing V_β				5				8									
	1	2	3	4	1	2	6	7	1	2	3	10	11	12	14	15	16	17
SEA	+	−	+	−	−	−	−	−	−	−	−	−	+	−	−	−	−	+
SEE	−	−	−	−	−	−	−	−	−	−	−	−	+	−	−	+	−	n.d.
SEB	−	−	+	−	−	−	−	+	+	+	+	−	−	−	−	−	−	+
SEC1	−	−	+	−	−	−	−	−	−	+	−	−	−	−	−	−	−	+
TSST	−	−	+	−	−	−	−	−	−	−	−	−	−	−	−	+	−	+

V_β usage was analyzed in T-cell blasts after stimulation with each of the toxins shown. Most data are from B10.BR mice (H-2^k). To analyze V_β elements that recognize IE-dependent superantigens IE$^-$ mice were used: B10.Q$_{\beta BR}$ mice for $V_\beta 17$ and B10.Q mice for $V_\beta 5$ and $V_\beta 11$. Staining with V_β-specific monoclonal antibodies was used where possible, otherwise RNA was prepared from each of the blast populations and V_β expression established using a quantitative dot blot. Either unstimulated (staining) or concanavalin-A-stimulated T-cell blasts (RNA dot blots) were used as control cells. Pluses indicate an enrichment in V_β expression in the toxin-stimulated T-cell blasts compared with the control cells of twofold or better. n.d. indicates not determined.

Nude mice and neonatal mice, both of which lack mature functional T cells, are extremely resistant to SEB (data not shown), implicating T cells in the mode of action of SEB. However, the hypothesis we wished to test was that the various mechanisms that mice use to limit V_β expression may be a protective mechanism to limit the possible targets for these toxins in vivo. Therefore, we devised an experiment to test this idea more directly. We bred mice that combined a genetic deletion with the appropriate tolerizing V_β-specific self-superantigens to lower drastically the levels of the T cells bearing the V_β elements recognizing SEB. One strain, B10.BR(βBR) contributed a genetic deletion involving all members of the $V_\beta 8$ family. The other (CBA/J) contributed the self-superantigens deleting $V_\beta 3^+$ (Mls-2^a or Mls-3^a) and $V_\beta 7^+$ (unknown locus) T cells. (B10.BR[βBR] × CBA/J)F$_1$ mice were bred with B10.BR(βBR) mice and the progeny screened for the homozygous gene deletion and heterozygous but dominant superantigens. These mice occurred approximately with the predicted 1 in 8 frequency. On average, the sum of $V_\beta(3 + 7 + 8)$ T cells in these mice was less than 6% compared with 32% in control B10.BR mice, which lack both the genetic deletion and the tolerizing self-superantigens. All mice in these experiments lacked $V_\beta 17^+$ T cells both because they expressed the IE-molecule of H-2^k and in some cases because they bore the inactive $V_\beta 17$ gene. The experimental and control mice were injected with SEB, and their weight was followed over the next several days (Table 5). Whereas the control mice with a high level of SEB-reactive T cells showed a typical response with rapid weight loss, the mice specifically low in SEB-reactive T cells were protected against the toxin.

These results demonstrate that V_β-specific T-cell stimulation is important in the mode of action of these toxins in mice. The advantage to the bacteria of massive T-cell activation is not immediately apparent; however, our preliminary experiments have shown that after SEB administration mice temporarily produce a poor T-cell response to other antigens, which may be of some advantage to the bacteria producing these toxins.

IMPLICATIONS

Our experiments establish that in mice the selective advantage of a large, diverse TCR$\alpha\beta$ repertoire is not strong enough to weed out any of the many polymorphisms that limit V_β expression in laboratory and wild mice. Rather, they suggest an equilibrium in which mice exist in a state where all V_β elements are available to the species as a whole, but individuals express only a subset of the total. This implies some selective disadvantage to the expression of too many V_β elements in one individual. We suggest that this disadvantage lies in the susceptibility of mice to microbial toxins that rely on the massive stimulation of T cells bearing particular V_β elements for their toxicity. Our finding that mice constructed to have the right combination of V_β gene deletions and tolerizing V_β-specific self-superantigens are resistant to the appropriate toxin is consistent with this view.

Our results imply that the V_β repertoire of the mouse population is very flexible, capable of changing rapidly to accommodate the threat either from a new pathogen, the immune response to which may require a particular V_β element, or from a new microbial toxin in which case elimination of particular V_β elements may

Table 5. Deletion of T Cells Bearing Approximate V_β Elements Protects Mice from SEB

Mouse	T cells bearing $V_\beta 3$, 8, or 7 (%)	Weight loss following SEB (%)		
		day 1	day 2	day 3
B10.BR	32	10.9 ±0.7	9.7 ±1.0	5.3 ±1.6
(B10.Q[βBR] × CBA/J)F$_1$ × B10.Q(βBR)	6	2.6 ±1.4	−0.2 ±1.1	2.6 ±1.1

Mice were given 50 μg of SEB intraperitoneally on day 0.

be protective. The self-superantigens are a particularly efficient way of limiting expression of particular V_β elements although keeping them in reserve for rapid reexpression should the need arise. Suppression of a particular V_β is achieved without altering the V_β structural gene in mice heterozygous for the relevant superantigen. Mice expressing V_β appear in every mating between superantigen heterozygous mice. For example, to maintain the lack of $V_\beta 6$ expression in 90% of mice, a V_β haplotype with a $V_\beta 6$ gene deletion must occur at a frequency of 95% in the gene pool, and the reemergence of $V_\beta 6$ can only come from matings involving the 10% of mice already expressing $V_\beta 6$. On the other hand, lack of $V_\beta 6$ expression can be maintained at the 90% level with a frequency of only 68% of the Mls-1[a] gene, and approximately 30% of matings, including those between two Mls-1[a] heterozygous mice each of which lacks $V_\beta 6$ expression, will yield at least some $V_\beta 6$-expressing progeny.

ACKNOWLEDGMENTS

We thank Mike Bevan, Uwe Staerz, Jerry Bill, Osami Kanagawa, Ed Palmer, and Craig Okada for providing anti-V_β monoclonal antibodies. We thank also Ella Kushnir, Terri Wade, and Rhonda Richards for their excellent technical assistance. This work was supported in part by U.S. Public Health Service grants AI-17134, AI-18785, and AI-22295.

REFERENCES

Behlke, M., H. Chou, K. Huppi, and D. Loh. 1986. Murine T cell receptor mutants with deletions of β-chain variable region genes. Proc. Natl. Acad. Sci. 83: 767.

Bergdoll, M. 1983. Enterotoxins. In Staphylococci and staphylococcal infections (eds. C.S.F. Easman and C. Adlam), p. 559. Academic Press, New York.

Bevan, M. and P. Fink. 1978. The influence of thymus H-2 antigens on the specificity of maturing killer and helper cells. Immunol. Rev. 42: 3.

Bill, J., V. Appel, and E. Palmer. 1989. The MHC molecule I-E is necessary, but not sufficient for the clonal deletion of Vβ11 bearing T cells. J. Exp. Med. 169: 1405.

Blackman, M.A., P. Marrack, and J. Kappler. 1989. Influence of the MHC on positive thymic selection of $V_\beta 17a^+$ T cells. Science 244: 214.

Choi, Y., B. Kotzin, L. Herron, J. Callahan, P. Marrack, and J. Kappler. 1989. Interaction of S. aureus toxin superantigens with human T cells. Proc. Natl. Acad. Sci. 86: 8941.

Chou, H., C. Nelson, S. Godambe, D. Chaplin, and D. Loh. 1987a. Germline organization of the murine T cell receptor β-chain genes. Science 238: 545.

Chou, H., S. Anderson, M. Louie, S. Godambe, M. Pozzi, M. Behlke, K. Huppi, and D. Loh. 1987b. Tandem linkage and unusual RNA splicing of the T cell receptor β-chain variable-region genes. Proc. Natl. Acad. Sci. 84: 1992.

Couch, J., M. Soltis, and M. Betley. 1988. Cloning and nucleotide sequence of the type E staphylococcal enterotoxin gene. J. Bacteriol. 170: 2954.

Fischer, H., M. Dohlsten, M. Lindvall, H. Sjögren, and R. Carlsson. 1989. Binding of staphylococcal enterotoxin A to HLA-DR on B cell lines. J. Immunol. 142: 3151.

Fraser, J.D. 1989. High-affinity binding of staphylococcal enterotoxins A and B to HLA-DR. Nature 339: 221.

Happ, M.P., D. Woodland, and E. Palmer. 1989. A third T cell receptor V_β gene encodes reactivity to Mls-1[a] gene products. Proc. Natl. Acad. Sci. (in press).

Haqqi, T., S. Banerjee, G. Anderson, and C. David. 1989. RIII S/J (H-2[r]). An inbred mouse strain with a massive deletion on T cell receptor V_β genes. J. Exp. Med. 169: 1903.

Huppi, K., B. D'Hoostelaere, B. Mock, E. Jouvin-Marche, M. Behlke, H. Chou, R. Berry, and D. Loh. 1988. T-cell receptor VTβ genes in natural populations of mice. Immunogenetics 27: 51.

Janeway, C.A., Jr., J. Yagi, P. Conrad, M. Katz, S. Vroegop, and S. Buxser. 1989. T cell responses to Mls and to bacterial proteins that mimic its behavior. Immunol. Rev. 107: 61.

Kappler, J.W., E. Kushnir, and P. Marrack. 1989a. Analysis of Vβ17a expression in new mouse strains bearing the Vβ[a] haplotype. J. Exp. Med. 169: 1533.

Kappler, J., N. Roehm, and P. Marrack. 1987a. T cell tolerance by clonal elimination in the thymus. Cell 49: 273.

Kappler, J.W., U. Staerz, J. White, and P.C. Marrack. 1988. Self-tolerance eliminates T cells specific for Mls-modified products of the major histocompatibility complex. Nature 332: 35.

Kappler, J., T. Wade, J. White, E. Kushnir, M. Blackman, J. Bill, R. Roehm, and P. Marrack. 1987b. A T cell receptor Vβ segment that imparts reactivity to a class II major histocompatibility complex product. Cell 49: 263.

Kappler, J., B. Kotzin, L. Herron, E. Gelfand, R. Bigler, A. Boylston, S. Carrel, D. Posnett, Y. Choi, and P. Marrack. 1989b. V_β-specific stimulation of human T cells by staphylococcal toxins. Science 244: 811.

Kisielow, P., H. Teh, H. Blüthmann, and H. von Boehmer. 1988. Positive selection of antigen-specific T cells in thymus by restricting MHC molecules. Nature 335: 730.

Lai, E., R. Barth, and L. Hood. 1987. Genomic organization of the mouse T-cell receptor β-chain gene family. Proc. Natl. Acad. Sci. 84: 3846.

Lai, E., P. Concannon, and L. Hood. 1988. Conserved organization of the human and murine T cell receptor β-gene families. Nature 331: 543.

MacDonald, H.R., R. Schneider, R.K. Lees, R.C. Howe, H. Acha-Orbea, H. Festenstein, R.M. Zinkernagel, and H. Hengartner. 1988. T-cell receptor V_β use predicts reactivity and tolerance to Mls[a]-encoded antigens. Nature 332: 40.

Malissen, M., C. McCoy, D. Blanc, J. Trucy, C. Devaux, A. Schmitt-Verhulst, F. Fitch, L. Hood, and B. Malissen. 1986. Direct evidence for chromosomal inversion during T-cell receptor β-gene rearrangements. Nature 319: 28.

Marrack, P. and J. Kappler. 1988. T cells can distinguish between allogeneic major histocompatibility complex products on different cell types. Nature 332: 6167.

Pullen, A.M., P. Marrack, and J.W. Kappler. 1988. The T cell repertoire is heavily influenced by tolerance to polymorphic self antigens. Nature 335: 796.

———. 1989. Evidence that Mls-2 antigens which delete $V_\beta 3^+$ T cells are controlled by multiple genes. J. Immunol. 142: 3033.

Sha, W., C. Nelson, R. Newberry, D. Kranz, J. Russell, and D. Loh. 1988. Positive and negative selection of an antigen receptor on T cells in transgenic mice. Nature 336: 73.

Wade, T., J. Bill, P.C. Marrack, E. Palmer, and J.W. Kappler. 1988. Molecular basis for the nonexpression of Vβ17 in some strains of mice. J. Immunol. 141: 2165.

White, J., A. Herman, A.M. Pullen, R. Kubo, J. Kappler, and P. Marrack. 1989. The Vβ-specific superantigen staphylococcal enterotoxin B: Stimulation of mature T cells and clonal deletion in neonatal mice. Cell 56: 27.

Zinkernagel, R., G. Callahan, A. Althage, S. Cooper, P. Klein, and J. Klein. 1978. On the thymus in the differentiation of H-2 self-recognition by T cells: Evidence for dual recognition? J. Exp. Med. 147: 882.

Structural Intermediates in the Reactions of Antigenic Peptides with MHC Molecules

K. DORNMAIR, B. ROTHENHÄUSLER, AND H.M. McCONNELL

Stauffer Laboratory for Physical Chemistry, Stanford University, Stanford, California 94305

Molecular complexes of class I and class II major histocompatibility complex (MHC) molecules and antigenic peptides are recognized by specific cytotoxic and helper lymphocytes (Schwartz 1985; Townsend and Bodmer 1989). Class II MHC/peptide complexes reconstituted in planar lipid bilayers are recognized by specific T-helper cells (Watts et al. 1984,1985). That is, specific antigenic peptides bind to affinity-purified class II MHC molecules in lipid membranes, the resulting MHC/peptide complexes have long lifetimes (Watts and McConnell 1986), and even after extensive washing, such MHC/peptide complexes trigger specific T-helper cells to release interleukin-2. However, there are major questions as to the mechanism by which exogenous peptides bind to MHC molecules in bilayer membranes. Such questions are raised by the difficulty of preparing MHC/peptide complexes of defined stoichiometry, with many preparations only showing 5–10% binding of added peptide (Watts and McConnell 1986; Sadegh-Nasseri and McConnell 1989). This raises the issue of the possible role of unidentified additional peptides, multiple conformational states of the MHC protein, the role of lipids, and so forth. To the extent that they are comparable, results obtained with solubilized MHC/peptide complexes in detergent micelles are similar to those obtained in the bilayer membranes (Babbitt et al. 1985; Buus et al. 1986; Guillet et al. 1987). Thus, peptide/MHC binding does not appear to be strongly affected by peptide/lipid or protein/lipid interaction. Kinetic studies of FpCytc and I-E^k in planar bilayer membranes provide evidence for sequential steps in both the association and dissociation reactions, with peptide/MHC specificity being already shown in the more rapid binding step (Sadegh-Nasseri and McConnell 1989). These kinetic data thus provide evidence for significant structural intermediates. The present work was undertaken to explore further the possibility that peptide binding and dissociation involves a protein-folding intermediate or even disassembly of the class II molecules.

METHODS

Cell lines and materials. As a source of I-E^k and I-A^d, we used the cell lines CH27 (Haughton et al. 1986) or A 20.1.11 (Kim et al. 1979), respectively. For the purification of I-E^k and I-A^d, we used the monoclonal antibodies 14-4-4 S (anti-I-E^k) (Ozata et al. 1980) or MKD6 (anti-I-A^d) (Kappler et al. 1981). The synthetic peptides pCytc(88-104) (representing amino acids 88–104 of pigeon cytochrome *c*) and FOva(323-339) (representing amino acids 323–339 of ovalbumin labeled at its amino terminus with fluorescein isothiocyanate [FITC]) were purchased from Peninsula Labs. The purity of pCytc(88-104) was >90%. CFpCytc (88-104) was kindly provided by G.K. Schoolnik (Stanford). The peptide was labeled at the amino terminus with carboxyfluorescein succinimidyl ester and purified to homogeneity.

Purification of I-E^k. The CH27 cells were maintained as described for A20-1.11 cells (Watts et al. 1984). They were washed in 10 mM Tris-HCl buffer (pH 8.3), 150 mM NaCl, 0.02% NaN$_3$, 10 μM phenylmethylsulfonyl fluoride (PMSF), 10 μg/ml aprotinin (Sigma). A whole-cell lysate was prepared in Nonidet-P40 (Turkewitz et al. 1983). A pool of glycoproteins was obtained by chromatography on lentil lectin-Sepharose 4B (Pharmacia) (Watts et al. 1984). I-E^k was purified by affinity chromatography: The antibody 14-4-4 S was coupled to CNBr-Sepharose (Pharmacia) at 2 mg/ml gel volume. The eluate from the lentil lectin column was applied to the antibody column. Nonidet-P40 was replaced by *n*-octyl β-D-glucopyranoside (OG) by washing the column with the tenfold column-volume of 30 mM OG. This buffer was used throughout all following procedures with I-E^k unless indicated otherwise and will be referred to as incubation buffer. I-E^k was eluted with 100 mM Na$_2$CO$_3$ buffer (pH 11.5), 500 mM NaCl, 0.02% NaN$_3$, 30 mM OG. The fractions were brought to pH 8.5 by letting the column eluate drop into 2 M Tris-HCl buffer (pH 7.0), 30 mM OG. The protein-containing fractions were pooled, dialyzed against incubation buffer, and stored at 4°C. For some experiments, I-E^k was reconstituted into lipid vesicles by dialysis (Watts et al. 1984). We used a mixture of dipalmitoylphosphatidylcholine, dilinoleoylphosphatidylcholine, and cholesterol at a molar ratio of 9:1:2.7 (Quill et al. 1987). Protein concentrations were determined according to the method of Lowry (1951).

Purification of I-A^d. A20.1.11 cells were grown in RPMI 1640 medium (GIBCO), supplemented with 10% NU Serum IV (Collaborative Research), 2 mM glutamine, 1 mM sodium pyruvate, 100 μg penicillin per ml, and 100 μg streptomycin per ml of medium. No 2-mercaptoethanol was added to the medium. Viability of the cells was >97%. Prior to lysis, cells were washed twice in cold phosphate-buffered saline (PBS). Cells were lysed in lysis buffer (0.5% Nonidet-P40 in 10 mM Tris, 140 mM NaCl, 1 mM PMSF, 0.02% merthiolate [pH 8.2]) for 20 minutes. The whole-cell lysate was clarified by centrifugation (2500 rpm for 10 min followed by 25,000 rpm for 90 min) and applied to a lentil lectin column. Elution of glycoproteins was in lysis buffer containing 10% methyl-α-D-mannopyranoside directly onto a MKD6 affinity column. After washing with 15 volumes PBS (1% OG [pH 7.4]), fractions containing I-A^d were eluted in 1% OG, 50 mM NaHCO$_3$, 0.5 M NaCl, 1 mM PMSF, 0.02% merthiolate (pH 11), and immediately brought to pH 9.2 with 10% acetic acid. This buffer will be referred to as elution buffer. All purification steps were performed in the cold. No proteinase inhibitors other than PMSF were added, to avoid contamination of I-A^d with low molecular weight polypeptide chains.

Sample incubation and SDS gel electrophoresis.

To study the stability of I-E^k, we incubated the protein in OG micelles or reconstituted into lipid vesicles at elevated temperatures or at low pH values. Three types of experiments were performed: The incubation time was kept constant, but (1) the pH or (2) the temperature was varied. (3) The samples were incubated at a given temperature for varying times and analyzed on SDS gels. For one lane on the gel we used 0.5–1.0 μg I-E^k in 40 μl of incubation buffer.

For I-E^k, the pH dependence was investigated by adding concentrated buffer. We used for pH 7.0, sodium phosphate; for pH 6.0, sodium 2[N-morpholino]ethane sulfonate; for pH 5.0, sodium citrate; for pH 4.0, sodium formate; for pH 3.0, sodium citrate; and for pH 2.0, sodium phosphate. The incubation was stopped by adjusting the pH to 8.6 with 2 M Tris-HCl buffer (pH 8.6). The temperature stability at constant incubation time was studied by incubating the samples at 20, 37, 50, 65, 75, and 100°C for 30 minutes each. We measured the kinetics by incubating the samples for 1, 5, 15, and 30 minutes and 2, 6, 24, and 48 hours at 37, 45, 55, 65, and 100°C. Only in the case of the 55°C kinetics, we additionally incubated for 120 hours.

For I-A^d, we investigated the temperature stability for constant incubation times. The samples were incubated for 15 minutes at 20, 27, 37, 47, 56, 68, and 78°C in elution buffer and subsequently were applied to the gel.

SDS gel electrophoresis was performed essentially according to the method of Laemmli (1970) with the following modifications: (1) The samples were not boiled in SDS before applying them to the gel. (2) No mercaptoethanol was added. (3) Both the stacking and the bottom gel were adjusted to pH 8.6. (4) The gels were run at low voltage to prevent the temperature exceeding 30°C. We used 12.5% gels. The gels were stained with silver (Heukeshoven and Dernick 1985) and scanned on an LKB UltraScan XL Laser Scanner. The background of the gels was subtracted. With some gels, we observed considerable variation of the width of

different protein bands, possibly due to the presence of high concentrations of OG. To correct for this fact, for each lane, the intensities of all bands were added, and the sum was normalized to 100%.

Fluorescence scanning experiments.

For the fluorescence scanning experiments on SDS gels, I-A^d (10 μl, 1 μM in elution buffer containing 50 μM FOva [323-339]) was incubated for 2 hours at 20°C. I-E^k (40 μl, 0.5 μM in incubation buffer containing 100 μM CFpCytc[88-104]) was incubated for 24 hours at 37°C. The samples were applied to SDS gels after the incubation.

The gels were scanned on a fluorescence microscope, which has been described previously (Watts et al. 1986). In this microscope, the fluorescence is excited by an argon ion laser in epi-illumination. Excitation was at 488 nm, and fluorescence at 535 nm was detected by a photomultiplier. For continuous scanning, gels were mounted on a motor-driven translation stage. Data acquisition and processing was done with a multichannel analyzer (LeCroy 3500). Sampling time was 1 second at a scanning speed of 40 μm/sec. The data on I-E^k were corrected for background fluorescence.

Binding of fluorescent peptides to I-A^d for FD experiments.

For the steady-state fluorescence depolarization (FD) experiments on fluorescein-labeled peptides bound to I-A^d, a tryptic digest of ovalbumin was labeled with FITC, partially purified on Sephadex G25, and fed to A20.1.11 cells. The digest (FDOva) contained the fragment Ova([323-339]), which specifically binds to I-A^d. A20.1.11 cells were grown as described above. After two washes in PBS, the cells were resuspended in serum-free medium and grown for a period of 8 hours. The cells were then collected (1500 rpm for 10 min), washed in PBS, and incubated for 4 hours in serum-free medium containing FDOva (700 μM total peptide, approximately 30 μM Ova [323-339]. Subsequent purification of I-A^d was carried out as described above, but washing of the lentil lectin and MKD6 affinity column was done until fluorescence could no longer be detected in the eluate. The fractions containing I-A^d were tested for fluorescent peptides. The fluorescent peptide was bound to I-A^d as judged by gel filtration on Sephadex G25 where it was migrating together with I-A^d. Under reducing conditions in SDS gels containing 2-mercaptoethanol, the complex of fluorescent peptide and I-A^d could be disassembled after boiling for 90 seconds in 2% SDS sample buffer. Total protein was determined by the method of Lowry (1951) and by tryptophan fluorescence at 350 nm. Total amount of peptide was determined by FITC fluorescence at 535 nm.

FD measurements.

Measurements of the FD of I-A^d complexed with FDOva as described above, and on the tryptophans of I-A^d, were done on a Fluorolog 2000 spectrofluorometer (Spex) that was equipped with film linear polarizers (Oriel) on rotating mounts. The response function of the instrument for different polarizations was determined. FD data were corrected for nonlinearities of the monochromators and the photomultiplier. The calibration of the setup was tested with FITC-labeled bovine serum albumin (Sigma) and an FITC-labeled tryptic digest of ovalbumin at various concentrations. For excitation, the light was vertically polarized, and the emission was detected for light polarized parallel (lp) and perpendicular (ls) to the excitation polarization. The depolarization $1/G$ was determined as $1/G = (lp - ls)/(lp + ls) - 1/3$. Index p: parallel polarizers. Index s: crossed polarizers. The spectral bandwidth was 10 nm. The sample stage was connected to a thermostat. Temperature jumps of 5°C could be accomplished within 1 minute. Cuvettes (Starna Cells) were silanized with octadecyltrichlorosilane and sealed airtight with Teflon tape.

The tryptophan fluorescence at varying temperatures was excited at the absorption maximum, and emission was detected at 350 nm. The concentration of I-A^d was 1 μM in elution buffer. The data are averages from three measurements for each temperature. Temperature was increased in steps of 4°C and 5°C and was held constant for 10 minutes prior to measurement.

The fraction of fluorescent peptides complexed with I-A^d at different temperatures was determined at 490/535 nm. The concentration of I-A^d was 1 μM in elution buffer. Approximately 10% of all I-A^d molecules were complexed with a fluorescent peptide of the FDOva digest. As long as the fluorescent lifetime of the fluorescent label is constant, depolarization data are linear functions of the quotient of temperature and viscosity of the solvent and the inverse rotational relaxation coefficient of the macromolecules. Dissociation of the peptide from the complex will result in a decrease of the rotational relaxation time of the peptide according to the difference in molecular weight of complex and free peptide. Thus, the dissociation rate constant of the complex and the fraction of released peptide at different temperatures can be determined (Weber 1952a,b; Steiner and Edelhoch 1962). Data were analyzed in terms of a reversible chain reaction similar to the reaction scheme that was suggested previously for the association and dissociation of FpCytc and I-E^k (Sadegh-Nasseri and McConnell 1989).

RESULTS

To investigate the physical chemical stability of I-E^k and I-A^d, we incubated the proteins either in OG micelles or reconstituted in phospholipids at different temperatures or pH values. Our first point of interest was to study the conditions where the α/β heterodimer disassembles into separated α or β chains. We found that the dimers were stable for at least several hours in 2% SDS if the samples were kept at room temperature and no mercaptoethanol was added. Thus, simple SDS gels provide a suitable technique to investigate the dissociation of the α/β heterodimeric protein. Two examples of such gels are shown in Figures 1 and 2.

Figure 1 shows I-E^k reconstituted into lipid vesicles after incubation at different pH values. Samples of I-E^k

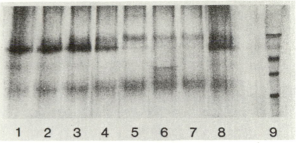

Figure 1. SDS gel of I-E^k reconstituted in lipid vesicles. The samples were incubated at room temperature for 30 min at the following pH values: (Lane 1) pH 8.3; (lane 2) pH 7.0; (lane 3) pH 6.0; (lane 4) pH 5.0; (lane 5) pH 4.0; (lane 6) pH 3.0; (lane 7) pH 2.0; (lane 8) pH 5.0 with 100 μM pCytc(88-104) added prior to incubation. The incubation was stopped by raising the pH to 8.3. The samples were applied to the gel without previous boiling. No mercaptoethanol was added. (Lane 9) Molecular-mass standards. The proteins used were bovine serum albumin (66 kD), egg albumin (45 kD), glycerinaldehyde-3-phosphate dehydrogenase (36 kD), and carbonic anhydrase (29 kD). Two facts may be responsible for the smearing of the bands: First, both the α and the β chains are glycosylated. It is a common observation that glycosylated proteins do migrate in smeared rather than in narrow bands on SDS gels. Second, the samples were not boiled in SDS before applying them to the gel, and no mercaptoethanol was added; thus, disulfide bridges are unreduced, and the proteins maintain a structure close to their folded structure. The proteins migrate as spheres rather than as a random coil. Minor parts may be unfolded, leading to a distribution of slightly different conformations and thus to a smeared band on the gel. This is also why the molecular masses for the disassembled α and β chains of I-E^k are 35 kD and 32 kD, respectively, and not 38.5 kD and 35 kD, as observed on reducing gels (Turkewitz et al. 1983).

were incubated at room temperature for 30 minutes each at different pH values, neutralized, and applied to the gel. At pH 8.3 (lane 1), about 90% of the proteins migrate with a molecular mass of 57 kD. This corresponds to the assembled complex of α and β chains. A weak band can be seen at 64 kD. About 10% of the proteins migrate in a broad band between 30 kD and 38 kD, corresponding to the disassembled α and β chains. By lowering the pH to 4.0 (lane 5), the intensity of both

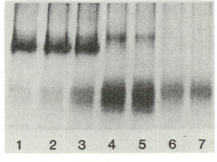

Figure 2. SDS gel of I-E^k. I-E^k in OG micelles was incubated for 30 min each at the temperatures given below and then cooled to room temperature. The incubation temperatures were: (Lane 1) 20°C; (lane 2) 37°C; (lane 3) 50°C; (lane 4) 65°C; (lane 5) 75°C; (lane 6) 100°C; (lane 7) 100°C with 100 μM pCytc(88-104) added prior to incubation.

the 64-kD band and the band between 30 kD and 38 kD increased, whereas, concomitantly, the intensity of the 57-kD band decreased. At pH 3.0 (lane 6), the 57-kD band has vanished almost completely. The intensity of the 64-kD band has slightly increased, but most of the proteins have disassembled into α and β chains, now migrating between 30 kD and 38 kD. At pH 2.0 (lane 7), all molecules are disassembled. Lane 8 is identical to lane 4, except that 100 μM of pCytc(88-104) was added to the sample prior to incubation. No difference between these samples can be seen on the gel. Thus, the presence of excess antigenic peptide did not stabilize the assembled protein against dissociation. For simplicity, we will refer to the conformation with molecular mass 57 kD as the compact (C) conformation, to the one with molecular mass 64 kD as the floppy (F) conformation, and to the disassembled chains as D.

Figure 2 shows a SDS gel where I-E^k was incubated at pH 8.3 in OG micelles at various temperatures for 30 minutes each. Lane 1 is identical to Lane 1 in Figure 1 (room temperature, pH 8.3). Elevated temperatures caused dissociation of the complex similar to the effects induced by lowering the pH. On raising the incubation temperature, the intensity of C decreased, and the intensity of D increased. Again F appeared at moderate temperatures and vanished at high temperatures. At 50°C (lane 3), the intensities of both the bands of F and D have increased, whereas the intensity of C has decreased. At 65°C (lane 4), C has vanished, the intensity of F is increased, but most of the proteins now have disassembled. At 75°C (lane 5), the intensity of F is slightly decreased, and at 100°C (lane 6), all the proteins have disassembled. Again the presence of 100 μM pCytc peptide during incubation at 100°C in lane 7 did not prevent I-E^k disassembly.

The same types of experiments were performed to study the pH stability of I-E^k in OG micelles and the temperature stability of I-E^k in lipids (data not shown). The pattern of the gels was similar to the patterns in Figures 1 and 2. I-E^k turned out to be more stable against low pH and temperature-induced dissociation when it was reconstituted into lipid membranes. To obtain the same effects on the intensity relations of the different bands on a particular lane, we had to lower the pH by about one unit, when I-E^k was in lipids compared to I-E^k in OG micelles, i.e., we observed the intensity C = F at pH 4.0 in lipids but already at pH 5.0 in OG micelles. The same holds for the temperature dependence: Here we had to raise the temperature about 10–15°C. Thus, the lipids stabilize the α/β heterodimer against temperature- and pH-induced dissociation. I-A^d in OG micelles showed behavior essentially similar to that of I-E^k. The compact structure migrated with molecular mass 60 kD and the floppy conformation with molecular mass 66 kD. I-A^d disassembled between 50 and 60°C, when incubated for 15 minutes in elution buffer.

To show that F is a structural intermediate in the consecutive reaction C → F → D, we investigated the

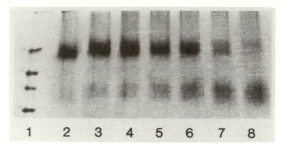

Figure 3. SDS gel of I-E^k in OG micelles. The samples were incubated at 55°C for 0 min (lane 2); 15 min (lane 3); 30 min (lane 4); 2 hr (lane 5); 6 hr (lane 6); 24 hr (lane 7); and 48 hr (lane 8). A sample incubated for 120 hr is not shown on this gel. Lane 1 shows molecular-mass standards (see Fig. 1).

kinetics of the disassembly of I-E^k. Figure 3 shows a gel where the I-E^k was incubated at 55°C in OG micelles for varying periods of time. This gel was scanned after it had been stained with silver. The relative intensities of C, F, and D are plotted versus time in Figure 4. The starting material (lane 1 in Fig. 3, $t = 0$ in Fig. 4) already showed a considerable dissociation of the C conformation into D. The extent of the dissociation was found to depend on the particular preparation used and on the age of the samples. However, it is evident from Figure 4 that C decreases with time and D increases, reaching nearly 100% for long incubation times. The most important point is the time course of F: It first increases, reaches a maximum, and decreases again. Such a time course is typical for intermediates of consecutive reactions. We have calculated the rate constant k_{CF} for the reaction C → F and found $k_{CF} = 1.9 \times 10^{-5}$ sec^{-1} for $T = 55$°C. For $T = 65$°C, we found $k_{CF} = 3.2 \times 10^{-5}$ sec^{-1} (data not shown). These rate constants

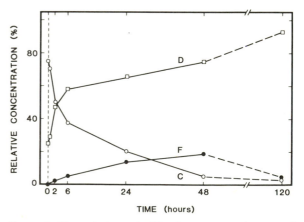

Figure 4. The gel shown in Fig. 3 was scanned on a gel scanner. After subtraction of the background, the intensities of the three bands at 64 kD (F), 57 kD (C), and 30–38 kD (D) were added and the sum was normalized to 100% for each lane separately (see Methods). With time, the intensity of C decreases, D increases, and F reaches a maximum and then decreases. This experiment thus demonstrates that the disassembly of C occurs as a consecutive reaction C → F → D. Judging the intensities of the bands by eye gives misleading results, not only because information gets lost during photography and printing, but also because the eye does not read the intensities linearly.

must be considered as apparent rate constants, since we did not allow for reversibility. Under the experimental conditions employed (incubation up to 48 hr), we were not able to resolve rate constants for the disassembly at 37, 45, and 100°C, because the disassembly was either too slow or too fast. To obtain order of magnitude estimates, we extrapolated the rate constants measured at 55°C and 65°C to 37°C by assuming an Arrhenius exponential change of k_{CF} with temperature. We found $k_{CF} = 7.3 \times 10^{-6} \ sec^{-1}$ for $T = 37°C$.

Independent evidence for a two-step reaction leading from C not directly to D but first to F and subsequently from F to D comes from FD measurements. The structural changes of I-A^d were monitored qualitatively as a function of temperature by FD of tryptophan (Fig. 5). For temperatures between 10°C and 53°C, the FD of tryptophan is linearly dependent on temperature. A small change in slope at about 33°C (corresponding to $T/\eta = 400$ K/cP) is observed. It is interpreted by the appearance of I-A^d in a state with slightly increased effective volume. It must be noted that this argument only holds by assuming that the lifetime of the trytophans is not altered when the protein undergoes its conformational change. However, an altered lifetime would also indicate a conformational change, since the probes are exposed to an environment with altered dielectric constant. Thus, a conformational change can be taken for granted. This is consistent with the data obtained from SDS gels that I-A^d undergoes the transition from the compact to the floppy conformation at about 37°C, i.e., at a slightly lower temperature than I-E^k. At temperatures higher than 53°C (corresponding to $T/\eta = 600$ K/cP), the FD data indicate a major structural transition that correlates with the dissociation of I-A^d into separated α and β chains. Thus, both

the transitions C → F and F → D may be observed by FD as well as by nonreducing SDS gels.

In the next experiments, we investigated the fate of a peptide bound to the MHC proteins. We wanted to determine during which transition of the protein the peptide is released. Buus et al. (1987) have reported an increase of the rate of dissociation of Ova(323-339) complexed with I-A^d in detergent micelles at elevated temperatures. In the experiments we report here, we followed the release of FOva that was bound to I-A^d in the temperature range between 10°C and 70°C. The release of peptide from the complex follows the same characteristic temperature dependence as found for FD of tryptophan. Figure 6 gives the temperature dependence of the depolarization $1/G$ of FDOva/I-A^d complex in elution buffer at pH 9.2. The two extreme cases, all this peptide bound in complex and all peptide dissociated from the complex, are represented by the straight lines a and d. Line d was determined in an experiment in which all bound peptide was released from the FDOva/I-A^d complex by boiling for 5 minutes prior to measurement. The solid line a was extrapolated from a calibration measurement with FITC-conjugated ovalbumin. A heating experiment is shown in curve b, with a stepwise heating as in Figure 5. On cooling, curve b was not reversible but followed line d for the free peptide. In c, a representative heating experiment is given, where temperature was held constant at 36°C and 41°C for extended times. Release of peptide leads to an exponential approach of the data points to the free peptide curve d.

Depending on the rate of heating, three characteristic temperature regimes can be distinguished: Regime I, where the release of the peptide from the complex occurs with half-lives of the order of days, is observed for temperatures lower than 33°C. At intermediate temperatures between 35°C and 53°C (regime II), the

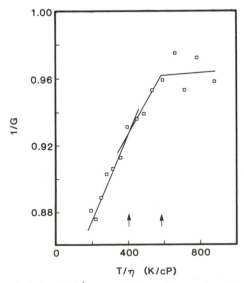

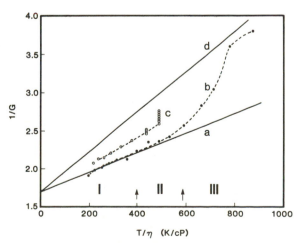

Figure 5. FD of I-A^d as a function of T/η, where T is the temperature and η is the viscosity of the solvent. Two breaks in the slope of the curve can be resolved: one at $T/\eta = 400$ K/cP (corresponding to 33°C) and one at $T/\eta = 600$ K/cP (corresponding to 53°C). These breaks indicate conformational changes of the protein.

Figure 6. FD of FDOva/I-A^d. (Line a) The fluorescent peptide was bound to I-A^d. (Line d) The fluorescent peptide was released from I-A^d by boiling. (Line b) FDOva/I-A^d was heated at a constant rate as described in the text. (Line c) FDOva/I-A^d was heated at temperatures increased to 36°C and 41°C and held constant for different times.

rate of dissociation increases rapidly. Halftimes for the dissociation of the complex are of the order of hours. At even higher temperatures (regime III), the peptide is released within minutes, at a rate that is comparable to the maximum heating rate of the instrument. At 41°C, the rate constant for the release of the peptide was determined as $k = 4 \times 10^{-5}$ sec^{-1}.

To address the question as to whether the observed characteristic changes with temperature are dominated by phase transitions in the detergent micelles, we recorded FD temperature scans with FDOva digest in elution buffer with 1% OG and with elution buffer containing 1% OG and 20 μg/ml N-7-nitro-2-1,3-benzoxadiazol 4-yl) dipalmitoyl phosphatidyl ethanolamine (NBD-DPPE). The results (data not shown) show that the measured changes of the dissociation of FDOva/I-A^d complex are not due to effects arising in the detergent micelles but are characteristic of the protein complex.

Another experiment was performed to investigate to which conformations of the MHC proteins a peptide may be bound. Thus, we incubated I-E^k and I-A^d with the fluorescent-labeled synthetic peptides CFpCytc(88-104) and FOva(323-339), respectively. The samples were applied to SDS gels, and these gels were scanned for peptide fluorescence before they were stained and scanned for proteins. Figure 7 shows the preliminary results of such an experiment. The fluorescence intensity is plotted versus the channel number, which is proportional to the migration length on the gel. Bars indicate where either the F, C, or D conformation has been detected on the silver-stained gel. It is evident that not

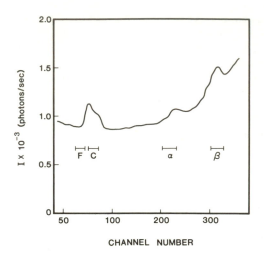

Figure 8. Fluorescence gel-scanning experiment on I-A^d. Essentially the same experiment as shown in Fig. 7 for I-E^k was performed on I-A^d. With this protein, the α and β chains are separated better on the gel. Here, three peaks were resolved: One again corresponds to the C conformation, and two correspond to the disassembled α and β chains.

only C is occupied with peptide, as one would expect, but also the disassembled chains have peptide bound. From this gel, we are not able to decide whether F is occupied with peptide and whether the α, the β, or both disassembled chains have peptide bound. The reason for this ambiguity is that the chains first migrate quite close to each other, and, second, the bands of the disassembled I-E^k are smeared (Turkewitz et al. 1983). To decide which of the chains do bind, we employed I-A^d, where the chains may be separated better on the gel. The preliminary result of this experiment is shown in Figure 8. Here, besides the C conformation, the fluorescent peptide is associated with the β chain of I-A^d. There might be association with the α chain too, but this peak is smaller than the β-chain peak. In conclusion, these experiments strongly suggest that immunogenic peptides may be bound to the disassembled chains.

DISCUSSION

It is evident from Figures 1 and 2 that the dissociation of I-E^k and I-A^d is not a simple one-step reaction leading from the α/β heterodimer to the dissociated α and β chains. When I-E^k is incubated at elevated temperature or at low pH, the heterodimer migrating with a molecular mass of 57 kD first adopts a structure migrating with molecular mass of 64 kD before it disassembles into the separated α and β chains. The same type of transition was observed for I-A^d. This suggests that it is common for class II MHC proteins to exist in at least two conformations, where the chains are assembled. Assuming that both conformations with assembled chains bind approximately the same number of SDS molecules, the change in the molecular mass is due to a change in the volume of the protein, which is

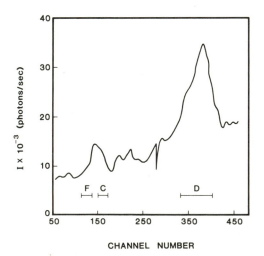

Figure 7. Fluorescence gel-scanning experiment on I-E^k. SDS gel was loaded with I-E^k previously incubated with the fluorescent peptide CFpCytc and scanned for fluorescence on a fluorescence microscope. Thereafter, it was stained and scanned for proteins. The curve gives the fluorescence intensity as a function of the channel number, which corresponds to the position on the gel. The bars indicate where I-E^k in its conformation C, F, or D has been identified on the stained gel. It is evident that two peaks may be identified that correspond to the C and D conformations.

consistent with FD data. We therefore refer to the structure with molecular mass of 57 kD as the compact (C) conformation and to the structure migrating with a molecular mass of 64 kD as the floppy (F) conformation.

To prove unambiguously that F is a structural intermediate of the α/β heterodimer I-E^k, we studied the kinetics of the disassembly at given temperatures. Figure 4 shows the typical pattern of a consecutive reaction C→F→D. At short times of incubation, the concentration of the starting conformation C is high, the concentration of the terminal conformation D is low, and within the limits of the detection sensitivity, no intermediate F is detected. With increasing incubation time, C decreases, D increases, and F first increases, reaches a maximum, and then decreases to almost zero. This is a typical time course of a consecutive reaction, where F is a reaction intermediate. Additionally, there is preliminary evidence that the reaction C→F is reversible. Recently, we succeeded in obtaining a pure preparation of the F conformation. This preparation could be transformed to the C conformation (K. Dornmair, unpubl.).

The possibility that F is identical to a β-chain trimer that has been observed for human MHC molecules (Gorga et al. 1987) can be excluded for the following reasons: First, a β-chain trimer or higher states of aggregation are unlikely to fit into a reaction scheme C→F→D as an intermediate. Second, an isolated β-chain trimer cannot refold to the α/β heterodimer. Thus, we conclude that the F conformation is a reaction intermediate during the disassembly of the compact α/β heterodimer.

This interpretation is consistent with the FD data on the tryptophan fluorescence and on FOva. The break in the slope at 33°C may be interpreted as reflecting the transition from the C to the F structure. Accordingly, the break at 53°C may be due to the transition F→D. The slope of the curve is flattened at 33°C and becomes nearly horizontal at 53°C. This slope depends on both the fluorescence lifetime of the probe and the volume of the protein. It is impossible to interpret these data in terms of alterations of the volume of I-A^d, since it is known that the fluorescence lifetime of tryptophan strongly depends on its environment and may vary significantly (Beecham and Brand 1985). Nevertheless, changes in the slope qualitatively indicate a conformational change of the protein.

The same holds for the FD data on the fluorescein-labeled peptide. However, the lifetime of fluorescein is known to vary only slightly on changes of its environment. Thus, it is possible in this case to interpret these data more quantitatively. A flat slope indicates the volume of the body undergoing rotational diffusion to be large; a steeper slope indicates a smaller volume. Therefore, the slopes of the lines a and d in Figure 6 are interpreted as being due to the I-A^d/peptide complex and the free peptide, respectively. The heating experiments (curves b and c) show two transitions at 33°C and 53°C. They are interpreted as being due to the transi-

tion C→F and F→D. Here the peptide is released from the disassembled chains. It should be noted that in regime II (33°C < T < 53°C), the steep slope of curve b results from the fact that depolarizations are additive. Therefore, in this regime, the three conformations C, F, and D coexist.

The fluorescence gel-scanning experiments provide preliminary evidence that the disassembled chains may bind peptides. Whereas we were unable to distinguish for I-E^k whether the peptide binds to the α or to the β chain, the experiments on I-A^d indicate that the peptide binds to the β chain and may also bind to the α chain. However, further experiments are necessary to establish the specificity of this binding. On the other hand, this finding is not too surprising. If the peptide is assumed to have extensive contact with both the α and β chain if they are assembled, then the disassembled chains should also be able to recognize the peptide. This holds under the proviso that partial binding sites do not undergo any significant conformational change during the disassembly. Since the number of amino acids participating in the peptide-chain interaction is smaller for disassembled chains, only the dissociation constant should increase.

This finding does not contradict the FD results discussed above, although the FD data show a peptide release during the disassembly of I-A^d, whereas the gel-scanning data indicate that the peptide may be bound to the separated chains. First, the experimental conditions were markedly distinct. Second, the FD data do not demonstrate complete dissociation under the conditions used to see the peptide association to the free chains. We thus hypothesize that the disassembled chains may exist in two states: one with bound peptide and another without.

We now consider three different intermediates of class II MHC proteins. The first is the kinetic intermediate C_i in the consecutive reaction from the initial complex to the terminal complex (C_t), found for I-E^k (Sadegh-Nasseri and McConnell 1989) and for I-A^d (B. Rothenhäusler et al., unpubl.). The second is a floppy conformation, which is a structural intermediate, and the third is the disassembled chains with bound peptide. Presently, it is not clear how these intermediates are related to each other. It is possible that either the floppy conformation or the disassembled chains are related to the kinetic intermediate, but at the moment we have no strong evidence either for or against this idea. The only hint that the kinetic intermediate and the floppy might be related comes from the comparison of rate constants measured in different experiments. From the FD data at 41°C, we calculated the rate constant for the release of the peptide from I-A^d as $k_r = 4 \times 10^{-5}$ sec^{-1}. From the kinetics of the disassembly of I-E^k, we judged the rate constant for the reaction C→F at 37°C as $k_{CF} = 7.3 \times 10^{-6}$ sec^{-1}. The rate constant for the formation of the dissociative kinetic intermediate has been found as $k = 6.3 \times 10^{-6}$ sec^{-1} (Sadegh-Nasseri and McConnell 1989). All these values are uncommonly small, and so they may be related.

ACKNOWLEDGMENTS

We thank Dr. R. Simoni for permission to use his gel scanner and Dr. G. Haughton for permission to use his CH27 cell line. This work was supported by the European Molecular Biology Organization under grant ALTF-113-1988 (K.D.), the Deutsche Forschungsgemeinschaft under grant Ro-721/1-1/2 (B.R.), and the National Insitutes of Health under grant 5R01 AI-13587-13.

REFERENCES

Babbitt, B.P., P.M. Allen, G. Matsueda, E. Haber, and E.M. Unanue. 1985. Binding of immunogenic peptides to Ia histocompatibility molecules. *Nature* **317**: 359.

Beecham, J.M. and L. Brand. 1985. Time resolved fluorescence of proteins. *Annu. Rev. Biochem.* **54**: 43.

Buus, S., A. Sette, and H.M. Grey. 1987. The interaction between protein-derived immunogenic peptides and Ia. *Immunol. Rev.* **98**: 115.

Buus, S., A. Sette, S.M. Colon, D.M. Jenis, and H.M. Grey. 1986. Isolation and characterization of antigen Ia complexes involved in T-cell recognition. *Cell* **47**: 1071.

Gorga, J.C., Y. Horejsi, D.R. Johnson, R. Raghupathy, and J.L. Strominger. 1987. Purification and characterisation of class II histocompatibility antigens from a homozygous human B cell line. *J. Biol. Chem.* **262**: 16087.

Guillett, J., M. Lai, T.J. Briner, S. Buus, A. Sette, H.M. Grey, J.A. Smith, and M.L. Gefter. 1987. Immunological self, non-self discrimination. *Science* **235**: 865.

Haughton, G., L.W. Arnold, G.A. Bishop, and T.J. Mercolino. 1986. The CH series of murine B-cell lymphomas. Neoplastic analogues of Ly-1$^+$ normal B-cells. *Immunol. Rev.* **93**: 35.

Heukeshoven, J. and R. Dernick. 1985. Simplified method for silver staining of proteins in polyacrylamide gels and the mechanism of silver staining. *Electrophoresis* **6**: 103.

Kappler, J.W., B. Skidmore, J. White, and P. Marrack. 1981. Antigen inducible, H-2 restricted Interleukin-2 producing T-cell hybridomas. Lack of independent antigen and H-2 recognition. *J. Exp. Med.* **153**: 1198.

Kim, K.J., C. Kanellopoulos-Langevin, R.M. Merwin, D.H. Sachs, and R. Asofsky. 1979. Establishment and characterization of Balb C lymphoma lines with B cell properties. *J. Immunol.* **122**: 549.

Laemmli, U.K. 1970. Cleavage of structural proteins during assembly of the head of bacteriophage T4. *Nature* **277**: 680.

Lowry, O.H., N.J. Rosebrough, A.L. Farr, and R.J. Randall. 1951. Protein measurement with the Folin phenol reagent. *J. Biol. Chem.* **193**: 255.

Ozata, K., N. Mayer, and D.H. Sachs. 1980. Hybridoma cell lines secreting monoclonal antibodies to mouse H-2 and IA antigens. *J. Immunol.* **124**: 533.

Quill, H., L. Carlson, B.S. Fox, J.N. Weinstein, and R.H. Schwartz. 1987. Optimization of antigen presentation to T cell hybridomas by purified Ia molecules in planar membranes. *J. Immunol. Methods* **98**: 29.

Sadegh-Nasseri, S. and H.M. McConnell. 1989. The kinetic intermediate in the reaction of an antigenic peptide and IE^k. *Nature* **338**: 274.

Schwartz, R.H. 1985. T-lymphocyte recognition of antigen in association with gene products of the major histocompatibility complex. *Annu. Rev. Immunol.* **3**: 237.

Steiner, R.F. and H. Edelhoch. 1962. Fluorescent protein conjugates. *Chem. Rev.* **62**: 457.

Townsend, A. and H. Bodmer. 1989. Antigen restriction by class I restricted T lymphocytes. *Annu. Rev. Immunol.* **7**: 601.

Turkewitz, A.P., C.P. Sullivan, and M.F. Mescher. 1983. Large-scale purification of murine IA^k and IE^k antigens and characterization of the purified proteins. *Mol. Immunol.* **20**: 1139.

Watts, T.H. and H.M. McConnell. 1986. High affinity fluorescent peptide binding to IA^d in lipid membranes. *Proc. Natl. Acad. Sci.* **83**: 9660.

Watts, T.H., H.E. Gaub, and H.M. McConnell. 1986. T-cell mediated association of peptide antigen and major histocompatibility complex protein detected by energy transfer in an evanescent wave-field. *Nature* **320**: 179.

Watts, T.H., J. Gariepy, G.K. Schoolnik, and H.M. McConnell. 1985. T cell activation by peptide antigen: Effect of peptide sequence and method of antigen presentation. *Proc. Natl. Acad. Sci.* **82**: 5480.

Watts, T.H., A.A. Brain, J.W. Kappler, P. Marrack, and H.M. McConnell. 1984. Antigen presentation by supported planar membranes containing affinity purified IA^d. *Proc. Natl. Acad. Sci.* **81**: 7564.

Weber, G. 1952a. Polarization of the fluorescence of macromolecules. I. Theory and experimental methods. *Biochemistry* **51**: 145.

———. 1952b. Polarization of the fluorescence of macromolecules. II. Fluorescent conjugates of ovalbumin and bovine serum albumin. *Biochemistry* **51**: 155.

Molecular Studies of Antigen Processing and Presentation to T Cells by Class II MHC Molecules

J.A. Berzofsky, A. Kurata, H. Takahashi, S.J. Brett, and D.J. McKean*

*Molecular Immunogenetics and Vaccine Research Section, Metabolism Branch, National Cancer Institute, National Institutes of Health, Bethesda, Maryland 20892; *Department of Immunology, Mayo Medical School, Rochester, Minnesota 55905*

In contrast to antibodies, which generally recognize native protein antigens free in solution, T cells require a much more complex mechanism for antigen recognition. In general, antigen receptors on both helper and cytotoxic T cells bind to antigen only on the surface of another cell (Unanue 1984; Unanue and Allen 1987), usually after some type of metabolic processing, resulting in fragmentation and/or unfolding of the native structure (Shimonkevitz et al. 1983; Allen and Unanue 1984; Streicher et al. 1984; Berzofsky et al. 1988), and then only when the resultant processed antigen is associated with a cell-surface molecule encoded by the major histocompatibility complex (MHC) of the target or antigen-presenting cell (APC) (Benacerraf 1978; Rosenthal 1978). Although processing has long been thought to involve proteolysis, the details of the chemistry and intracellular pathways involved are still not fully resolved. In the case of antigen seen with class II MHC molecules, inhibitors of endosomal function suggested that processing occurred in an intracellular endosomal compartment (Ziegler and Unanue 1982). In addition, antigen recognized with class II MHC molecules has been followed by electron microscopy through a pathway involving endosomes, Golgi, and return to the surface of the cell (Lin et al. 1988), although such studies cannot prove that this is the pathway relevant for immunologic processing. In the case of antigens recognized in association with class I MHC molecules, evidence is accumulating that processing is nonendosomal and occurs somewhere in the cytoplasm (Germain 1986; Morrison et al. 1986; Moore et al. 1988; Yewdell et al. 1988). The net result appears to be similar in both cases, except for the type of MHC molecule involved.

Using inhibitors of processing to compare the requirements for processing of native protein, unfolded protein, and short proteolytic fragments or synthetic peptides, early evidence indicated that small peptides generally do not require processing like the native protein (Shimonkevitz et al. 1983; Allen and Unanue 1984; Streicher et al. 1984). In addition, although some denatured forms of protein do require processing, unfolding of the protein frequently seems to be sufficient for bypassing the need for processing without the need for proteolysis (Allen and Unanue 1984; Streicher et al. 1984; Allen 1987a; Berzofsky et al. 1988; Lee et al. 1988; Régnier-Vigouroux et al. 1988). This led to the

hypothesis that the purpose of processing was to expose residues that are necessary for the antigenic determinant to interact simultaneously specifically with both the MHC molecule and the T-cell receptor. That two such subsites must exist for concurrent interaction with the MHC molecule and the T-cell receptor was postulated on the basis of functional data (Hansburg et al. 1983; Heber-Katz et al. 1983). These portions of the antigenic determinant were suggested to be called the agretope (for *antigen restriction tope*) and the epitope (a narrower use of a preexisting term that had been synonymous with antigenic determinant), respectively (Heber-Katz et al. 1983). Subsequent work with antigenic sites that appeared to fold as α-helices suggested that these subsites could be separated on different sides of a secondary structure, such as the cylinder of a helix, even though the residues involved were interspersed rather than separated linearly along the amino acid sequence (DeLisi and Berzofsky 1985; Berkower et al. 1986). A detailed analysis of the epitopic and agretopic residues of one such site indicated that such a separation was likely to be the case (Allen et al. 1987b). Other types of structures were also suggested on the basis of studies of peptides with amino acid substitutions (Sette et al. 1987). It has become clear that although T-cell receptor recognition of antigen is much more complex than antibody recognition, one simplifying feature is that the products of processing do not need to maintain the native tertiary structure, so that synthetic peptides can often be used to study T-cell determinants more readily than they can be used to study antibody determinants. We have taken advantage of this simplification to try to study the molecular mechanisms of antigen processing and presentation.

All studies of this sort have been greatly aided by the solution of the three-dimensional structure of a human class I MHC molecule by X-ray crystallography (Bjorkman et al. 1987a,b) and by the subsequent modeling of the structure of a class II MHC molecule on the basis of the class I structure (Brown et al. 1988). Exon-shuffling experiments indicated the functional roles of different domains of MHC molecules (Germain et al. 1985; Landais et al. 1986; Lechler et al. 1986), and finer mapping has involved the use of natural and chemically induced mutants (Hockman and Huber 1984; Kanamori et al. 1984; Allen et al. 1985; Brown et al. 1986), as well as site-directed point mutations (Cohn et al.

1986; Ronchese et al. 1987; McMichael et al. 1988; Buerstedde et al. 1989). Therefore, to complement our studies of functional residues in the antigenic determinant with mutant synthetic peptides, we have used a series of site-directed mutants of a class II MHC molecule (Buerstedde et al. 1988b) to study how individual amino acids in the active site of the MHC molecule participate in the activation of T-cell clones specific for defined antigenic determinants (Brett et al. 1989b). Thus, this paper addresses, with regard to T-cell recognition in association with class II MHC molecules, the role of antigen processing in determining which antigenic determinants are immunodominant, the molecular mechanisms of antigen processing, the role of MHC residues in presentation of antigen, and finally, the role of individual residues of an antigenic determinant in interaction with the MHC molecule and the T-cell receptor. The latter two studies both suggest that the same antigenic determinant can interact in more than one way with the same MHC molecule.

Role of Antigen Processing in Determinant Selection and Immunodominance

The repertoire of antigen determinants on a protein antigen that dominate the T-cell response is determined both by factors intrinsic to the structure of the antigenic determinant itself and by factors extrinsic to the antigenic determinant, such as the way the whole molecule is processed or the available MHC molecules in the individual or animal immunized (see Berzofsky 1986, 1988a,b), as well as other regulatory mechanisms in the host, such as suppression, idiotype networks, and competition among MHC molecules (Gammon et al. 1987). In a limiting-dilution T-cell frequency analysis, we have observed that a single immunodominant determinant can so dominate the T-cell response to a protein that the presence of T cells responding to this determinant–MHC molecule complex can lead to genetic high responsiveness. Conversely, in their absence, genetic low responsiveness to the whole protein can result, even though other antigenic sites of the protein may be

recognized equally in association with either high or low responder MHC molecules (Kojima et al. 1988). Therefore, one goal of our laboratory has been to understand the factors that determine immunodominance.

One approach we have taken in understanding the role of antigen processing in immunodominance has been to compare the responses to the same antigenic determinant when provided as the whole native antigen molecule or as a short synthetic peptide corresponding to nearly the minimal antigenic site (Brett et al. 1988). Both B10.BR (H-2^k) and B10.S (H-2^s) congenic strains of mice, which differ only in their MHC complex, are high responders to equine myoglobin, and in B10.S mice, the T-cell proliferative response is dominated by cells that recognize a determinant located to 102-118 (Berkower et al. 1982; Brett et al. 1988, 1989a). However, in B10.BR mice immunized with equine myoglobin, virtually no T-cell proliferative response can be detected to the 102-118 peptide (Fig. 1) (Brett et al. 1988). Indeed, in B10.BR mice, the response appears to be dominated by T cells that see a site unique to equine myoglobin among more than a dozen myoglobins studied (S.J. Brett and J.A. Berzofsky, unpubl.). The failure of B10.BR mice immune to equine myoglobin to respond to 102-118 could have been due to either of the two classic mechanisms of immune response (Ir) genetic low responsiveness: (1) a failure of this determinant to bind to the class II MHC molecules of that strain or (2) a hole in the T-cell repertoire (Berzofsky 1987). However, that neither of these mechanisms explained the results in this case is seen from the results in Figure 1 (right). When B10.BR mice were immunized with the synthetic peptide 102-118 itself, their T cells responded quite well to this peptide in vitro (Brett et al. 1988). Thus, the peptide 102-118 of equine myoglobin must be able to bind to a class II MHC molecule of these mice, and there must be T cells in their T-cell repertoire that can react with this determinant. What then is the mechanism that prevents animals immunized with the whole protein from manifesting this response? A clue comes from the

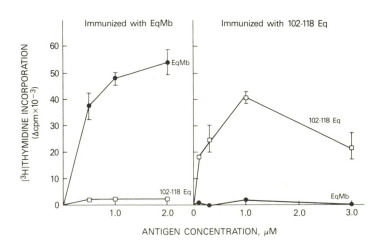

Figure 1. Reciprocal non-cross-reactivity of native equine myoglobin and peptide 102-118 in B10.BR mice. (*Left*) Mice were immunized subcutaneously in the tail with 100 μg native equine myoglobin in complete Freund's adjuvant (CFA); 8 days later, 10^4 lymph node T cells were cultured with 5×10^5 irradiated spleen cells and the indicated concentrations of antigens in 0.2 ml medium. The cultures were pulsed with 1 μCi [^{3}H]thymidine on the fourth day and harvested on the fifth day with a mash harvester; thymidine incorporation was measured by scintillation counting. (*Right*) Mice were immunized subcutaneously with 4 nmoles of synthetic equine myoglobin peptide 102-118 in CFA; 8 days later, 4×10^5 lymph node cells were cultured with the indicated concentrations of antigen and harvested as above. (Modified, with permission, from Brett et al. 1988.)

observation that the T cells from B10.BR mice immunized with peptide 102-118 fail to respond in vitro to the native equine myoglobin (Fig. 1, right). This suggests either that the whole molecule includes some structure that induces suppression of this response or that the difference lies in the way the native protein is processed to produce fragments. The response to 102-118 of equine myoglobin was mapped to the I-A^k class II MHC molecule, and individual T-cell clones were isolated (Brett et al. 1988). The fact that individual clones show the same response to peptide but not whole equine myoglobin excludes suppressor T cells from the list of possible mechanisms.

We are left with mechanisms that relate to the way the antigen is processed. Because T cells from congenic B10.S mice immunized with peptide 102-118 of equine myoglobin cross-reacted quite well in vitro with native equine myoglobin (Brett et al. 1988), destruction of the determinant during processing of the protein cannot explain the results in B10.BR mice unless there is an H-2-linked difference in processing between B10.S and B10.BR mice. Although there is no precedent for such H-2-linked differences in processing, we excluded such a mechanism by using F$_1$ hybrid-presenting cells. These F$_1$ cells processed the native protein and presented this epitope to B10.S T-cell clones, as well as B10.S APCs did. Thus, they did not destroy the determinant. Nevertheless, they did not present this determinant from the native protein to 102-118 peptide-specific B10.BR T-cell clones any better than homozygous B10.BR APCs did (Brett et al. 1988). We concluded that the problem was not a difference in processing between strains but rather a difference in presentation of the same determinant on the minimal length synthetic peptide and that of the products of natural processing of the native protein antigen. Probably the fragment containing this determinant produced by processing the native equine myoglobin was larger than the synthetic peptide and contained structures that hindered binding to the A^k molecule but did not hinder binding to the A^s molecule (Fig. 2). Support for this type of interpretation came from independent experiments with a T-cell clone specific for 102-118 of sperm whale myoglobin in association with A^d. This clone responded to native sperm whale myoblobin and cross-reacted with the corresponding 102-118 peptide of equine myoglobin but did not respond to native equine myoglobin (Brett et al. 1988). Artificial processing of equine myoglobin to a large cyanogen bromide fragment, 56-131, half the size of the whole protein, overcame this problem. Again, in this case, it appears that the problem is in hindering structures on the product of natural processing that prevent binding either to A^d or to the receptor of this clone. Similar results have been reported in the case of lysozyme (Shastri et al. 1986; Gammon et al. 1987), and such hindering interactions have been proposed as a reason that processing may be needed for cytochrome c (Kovac and Schwartz 1985). Recently, a similar interpretation has been suggested for a role of processing in presentation of an epitope of influenza virus in associa-

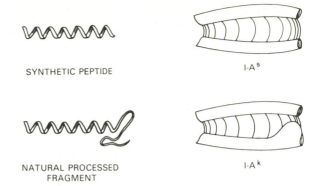

SYNTHETIC PEPTIDE

NATURAL PROCESSED FRAGMENT

I-A^s

I-A^k

Figure 2. Schematic diagram illustrating the difference between synthetic peptide and natural processed fragment of myoglobin in binding to two different allelic I-A molecules. Although the synthetic peptide can be presented by both I-A molecules, results suggest that the naturally processed fragment is presented only by I-A^s, not I-A^k, probably because additional peptide sequence in the natural fragment hinders interaction with the latter, as schematically represented by the bulge partially occluding the peptide-binding groove in I-A^k. Thus, hindering structures present after processing can prevent an otherwise potent determinant from being immunodominant. (Reprinted, with permission, from Berzofsky et al. 1988.)

tion with a class II MHC molecule (Bodmer et al. 1989). One case in which such a hindering structure has been localized very close to the antigenic determinant itself has been studied recently in the case of staphylococcal nuclease (Vacchio et al. 1989). The results are also consistent with a negative effect of increased peptide length sometimes seen in studying nested peptides covering an antigenic determinant (Cease et al. 1986; Sette et al. 1989). We conclude that antigen processing is very important in preventing or not preventing certain potentially dominant determinants from becoming immunodominant.

Proteinases That Process Distinct Epitopes on the Same Protein

For the reasons just stated, it will be important to be able to predict the sites of cleavage of a native protein during processing and the structures of the resultant fragments. As a first attempt in this endeavor, we have undertaken the identification of proteinases that are required for processing myoglobin to produce three different nonoverlapping epitopes, as defined with different T-cell clones and synthetic peptides (Takahashi et al. 1989). The approach was to test a series of inhibitors specific for intracellular endosomal trafficking in general or specific for each of the four classes of proteinases, thiol, serine, carboxyl, metalloproteinases, on the presentation of native myoglobin or the appropriate peptide to each of the T-cell clones. If production of fragments carrying each epitope depended on cleavages with a different set of proteinases, then one would expect different inhibitors to be effective with the different clones. On the other hand, if all of the processing of myoglobin depended primarily on a single proteinase, then the same inhibitors might inhibit presentation of all three epitopes. In each case, we used inhibitor concentrations that neither inhibited presentation of the synthetic peptide appropriate for that clone nor inhibited class II MHC expression by fluorescence flow cytometry, so the effects observed were not nonspecific toxicity or inhibition of steps other than processing that would be expected to affect presentation of both the peptide and the native molecule. Under these conditions, we found that monensin, as an inhibitor of intracellular trafficking, and inhibitors of thiol proteinases inhibited presentation of myoglobin to all three T-cell clones, whereas inhibitors of the other three classes of proteinases had no reproducible or significant effect on presentation of myoglobin to any of the clones (Table 1) (Takahashi et al. 1989). We concluded that an intracellular thiol proteinase was necessary for presentation of all three epitopes. The best candidate for such a proteinase would be cathepsin B. Therefore, we asked whether cathepsin B pretreatment of myoglobin was also sufficient for presentation to all three clones without further processing. We found that presentation of cathepsin-B-treated myoglobin, like that of the synthetic peptides, was not inhibited by monensin (or any of the inhibitors of thiol proteinases, as a control to ensure that digestion was adequate) (Fig. 3) (Takahashi et al. 1989). We conclude that an intracellular thiol proteinase, such as cathepsin B, is both necessary and sufficient for processing myoglobin to present all three nonadjacent epitopes and therefore

may be the only proteinase involved in most of the processing of myoglobin. As there is evidence that leupeptin and other inhibitors of thiol proteinases can inhibit processing of a number of antigens (Buus and Werdelin 1986; Puri et al. 1986; Puri and Factorovich 1988), this conclusion may not only pertain to myoglobin (Takahashi et al. 1989). To determine whether this observation would be of value in predicting cleavage sites, we examined retrospectively the fragments of myoglobin produced by APCs reported by McKean et al. (1983) and found that we could explain the molecular weights reported (Takahashi et al. 1989). Therefore, knowledge of the major proteinase involved in processing may be of value in prospectively predicting cleavage sites as well.

Lack of Cross Presentation by Allelic I-A Molecules That Present the Same Peptide Determinant

Because the same immunodominant determinant, 102-118, could be presented in association with three different allelic I-A class II MHC molecules and because we had T-cell clones specific for this site in association with each I-A molecule, we were in a position to ask whether cross-presentation could occur of the peptide by one I-A molecule to a T cell that normally recognized it with another I-A molecule. This question was raised by the suggestion (Claverie and Kourilsky 1986; Werdelin 1987) that T cells may recognize only the peptide epitope and that MHC restriction may result from the selection of different antigenic peptides,

Table 1. The Same Proteinase Inhibitors Inhibit Presentation of Three Different Epitopes of Myoglobin

T-cell clone		14.1	TK.G4	3.2
MHC restriction		I-E^d	I-A^d	I-E^k
Epitope in myoglobin		132-146	102-118	59-80
Category of inhibitor	Inhibitor[a]	Inhibition[b] (%)		
Intracellular transport	monensin	98.5	98.4	98.5
Thiol proteases (■)	■ E-64	99.0	90.3	98.8
	■□ leupeptin	94.5	77.4	96.6
	■□ antipain	97.0	81.3	82.5
Serine proteinases (□)	□ TLCK	0.0	2.5	17.0
	□ TPCK	0.0	0.0	0.0
	□ chymostatin	4.8	0.0	0.0
Acid proteinases (●)	● pepstatin	0.0	0.0	0.0
Metalloproteinases (○)	○ phosphoramidon	4.2	0.0	0.0
	○ 1,10-phenanthroline	0–19.4	0.0	0–47.3

Three distinct clones were used that see different portions of sperm whale myoglobin in association with different class II MHC molecules. Splenic APCs were pretreated with inhibitors for 30 min and then with antigen without removal of inhibitors for 2–3 hr. After three washes, they were irradiated and added to the indicated T-cell clone. Proliferation was measured after 4 days. Results show inhibition of presentation of native myoglobin in a range of inhibitor concentration that had no effect on peptide presentation.

[a]TLCK is N-p-tosyl-L-lysine chloromethyl ketone, and TPCK is N-p-tosylamino-2-phenylethyl chloromethyl ketone.

[b]Percentage of inhibition was calculated by the following formula based on means of quadruplicate cultures from maximum inhibition at nontoxic concentration of each proteinase or transport inhibitor.

% Inhibition = 100 × (1 − myoglobin with inhibitor/myoglobin without inhibitor).

All data shown above have been reproduced in three separate experiments. (Summarized from Takahashi et al. 1989.)

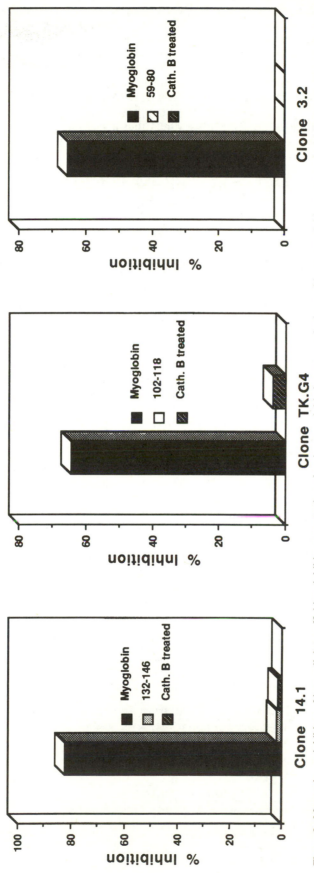

Figure 3. Monensin, an inhibitor of intracellular trafficking, inhibits presentation of native myoglobin but not synthetic peptide or myoglobin pretreated with cathepsin B, an indication that cathepsin B treatment is sufficient to bypass the need for endosomal processing. Myoglobin was treated with cathepsin B (1 unit/ml) at 37°C for 30 min in the presence of 0.07 M cysteine and 0.4 M citrate at pH 5.0. Splenic APCs were incubated with or without monensin (0.2 μM for clones 14.1 and 3.2 and 4 μM for clone TK.G4) for 30 min, and then, without removal of inhibitor, with the indicated antigen for 2–3 hr at 37°C; they were then washed, irradiated, and cultured with the indicated T-cell clone for 4 days in the absence of additional antigen. On the third day, the cultures were pulsed with 1 μCi [³H]thymidine, and on the fourth day they were harvested. The percentage of inhibition was calculated as in the footnote to Table 1. The peptide used for each clone corresponded to the epitope recognized by that clone. (Based on the data of Takahashi et al. 1989.)

or different conformations of these peptides, by different MHC molecules. Although we could not be sure that T cells specific for 102-118 of myoglobin with I-A^d, I-A^s, and I-A^k all recognized the peptide in the same conformation, this peptide appeared to be presented in an amphipathic α-helical conformation (DeLisi and Berzofsky 1985; Cease et al. 1986), and clones restricted to all three I-A molecules seemed to depend on the same three critical residues, Glu/Asp-109, His-113, and His-116 (Cease et al. 1986; Brett et al. 1989a). These three residues line up on the same side of the peptide, if it is folded as an α-helix. Furthermore, the minimal peptide lengths for the different T cells were closely overlapping: 106-118 for I-A^d- and I-A^k-restricted clones and 102-117 for I-A^s-restricted clones (Brett et al. 1989a). Using these clones, we asked whether each I-A molecule could cross-present the peptide to clones of the other type (Table 2). We found that no cross-presentation could be observed in any combination (Table 2). Failure to cross-present could be due to a requirement for each T cell to recognize not only the same epitope peptide, but also polymorphic amino acids residues characteristic of the particular I-A molecule. Alternatively, the T cells could be specific for the peptide only, but highly specific for subtle differences in conformation or orientation in the different MHC molecules not detected by specificity studies cited. For these reasons, we have studied further the role of individual amino acid residues of the I-A molecule involved in stimulation of peptide-specific T-cells and have examined the possibility that the same peptide may bind in more than one way to even the same MHC molecule.

Use of Site-directed MHC Mutants to Identify MHC Residues Involved in Antigen Presentation

Turning to the role of the MHC molecule in selecting which sites are immunodominant in a given individual or inbred strain of animals, we have asked which polymorphic amino acid residues in the β chain of the I-A^k class II MHC molecule contribute to presentation of

different determinants to defined T-cell clones. This was approached using a series of site-directed mutants of the A$_\beta$^{k} chain, each with a single substitution of a polymorphic residue from the sequence of the A$_\beta$^{d} chain, or with a cluster of several such substitutions (Buerstedde et al. 1988a). The use of such natural mutants assures that these allowed substitutions are less likely to disrupt the overall structure of the chain; because the T-cell clones studied recognize antigen with A^k but not A^d, we can ask which of the changes accounts for loss of activity. The mutant genes were transfected into M12.C3 (Glimcher et al. 1985), a mutant H-2^d B-lymphoma cell line that does not express its own class II MHC molecules. It can express endogenous A$_\alpha$^{d} chain if transfected with a β chain that can pair with it. Thus, when transfected with a β chain alone, it expresses A$_\beta$^{k} mutant/A$_\alpha$^{d} pairs, but when cotransfected with A$_\alpha$^{k} as well, the A$_\beta$^{k} mutant chains preferentially pair with the A$_\alpha$^{k}. None of the A^k-restricted T-cell clones responded to antigen with transfectants expressing either wild-type or mutant A$_\beta$^{k} chains paired with A$_\alpha$^{d} chains (Brett et al. 1989b). The A$_\alpha$^{k} chain appeared to be necessary in all cases, consistent with the exon-shuffle studies cited above (Lechler et al. 1986). Results with β-chain mutants at positions 12, 13, or 14 were difficult to interpret because of their possible effect on chain pairing and their lower expression. The three-for-one substitution at position 65 resulted in loss of presentation to all seven clones tested, specific for different epitopes. Because this substitution is thought to be in a kink between helices that may be accommodated without disrupting the helices but may be outside the peptide-binding groove (Brown et al. 1988), it is likely that these residues interact directly with the T-cell receptor (Fig. 4). Residues 85, 86, 88, on the α-helix of the β chain, seem to affect some clones and not others, even ones specific for the same epitope, 102-118. These residues are thought to be near one end of the α-helix of the β chain, where they might be able to interact with the antigenic peptide but might also interact directly with the T-cell receptor. Thus, the inability of the mutant carrying substitutions at 85, 86,

Table 2. Failure to Detect Cross-presentation of 102-118 to T-cell Clones Responsive to the Same Peptide on Three Different I-A Molecules

| T-cell clone | Restriction | Antigen-presenting cells | | |
| | | B10.BR I-A^k | B10.S I-A^s | B10.D2 I-A^d |
		([^{3}H]thymidine incorp, Δ cpm)		
10C9	1-A^k	22,816[a]	306[b]	350[b]
1-1C4	I-A^k	35,451	314[b]	500[b]
4-2D2	I-A^s	690	9,348	828
4-2D8	I-A^s	419	81,987	473
9.27	I-A^d	n.d.[c]	549	49,917

Modified, with permission, from Brett et al. (1989a).
[a] Underscore indicates positive response.
[b] In the presence of anti-I-A^k monoclonal antibody to block presentation by residual contaminating feeder cells carrying I-A^k.
[c] n.d. indicates not determined.

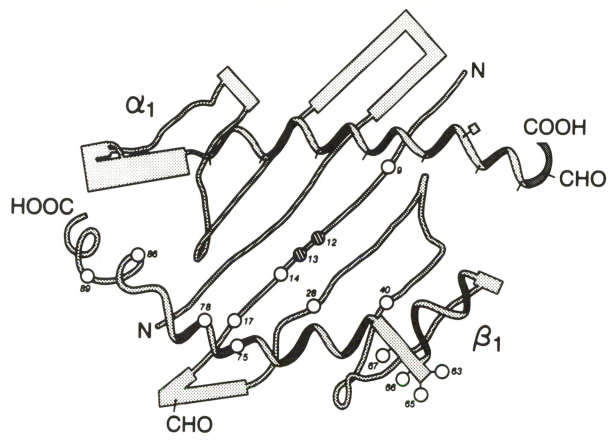

Figure 4. Schematic drawing of the predicted α-carbon structure of the class II MHC molecule based on the hypothetical model of Brown et al. (1988). The expected locations of residues at which site-directed mutations were made, as used in this study, are shown. (Modified from Brown et al. 1988; reprinted, with permission, from Brett et al. 1989b.)

and 88 to present myoglobin to one of the three clones specific for 102-118 could be due to a requirement for one of these residues as a contact residue with the T-cell receptor of that particular clone and not the others, or could be due to an affect of these substitutions on the way the peptide binds to the MHC molecule that alters its recognition by that clone and not the others. Because the mutant presents the same site to the other two clones, the problem is not simply interference with binding; therefore, direct measurements of peptide binding would not distinguish these alternatives. At present, we have no way to distinguish them.

A similar situation exists for the mutant at position 9, except that the residue in question in this case is assumed, from the class II MHC model (Brown et al. 1988), to be on the floor of the peptide-binding groove, pointing up toward the peptide but probably inaccessible to the T-cell receptor. Therefore, it is more likely that the effects of substitutions at this position are mediated by interaction with the peptide and not the T-cell receptor. The fact that this substitution completely abrogates the ability to stimulate clone 10A6, specific for 122-130, but not clones specific for 102-118 (Table 3), suggests that the agretopic residues of 122-130 interact with histidine residue 9, and the substitution with valine prevents binding (Brett et al. 1989b).

However, with only a single clone of this specificity, we cannot rule out the possibility from these data that the peptide still binds, but in an altered way that cannot be recognized by clone 10A6. Measurement of binding by competition studies is being carried out to test this possibility further.

Of perhaps even greater interest is the difference in presentation of the antigenic determinant 102-118 to different T cells by this mutant at position 9. All three T-cell clones specific for this site actually show about a twofold enhancement in response with the mutant compared with the wild-type A^k molecule (Table 3), when stimulated with whole equine myoglobin (Brett et al. 1989b). These clones had to be stimulated with the whole protein because they are so much more responsive to the synthetic peptide 102-118 that they respond to peptide with residual feeder cells in the presence of any allogeneic APC, despite attempts by multiple methods to eliminate carryover of feeder cells (Brett et al. 1989a). Therefore, studies with the synthetic peptide were not possible. An uncloned T-cell line specific for equine myoglobin 102-118 was also studied (Brett et al. 1989b). This line also responded better to the synthetic peptide and gave too low a response with the native protein to study easily. With the peptide, this clone gave a response only about 11% as high, using

Table 3. Effects of I-A^k Single or Regional Amino Acid Mutations on Antigen-specific T-cell Activation

Residue		Location on hypothetical class II structure[a]	Antigen-specific T cells[b]	102-118 equine[c]			122-130[c] (10A6)	Unique equine myoglobin[c,d]		
				10A10	10C9	1-IC4		4-5C4	1-3C8	10D9
9		S1', pointing up into helix	3/7	170	202	215	—	29	—	—
12		S1', pointing down	7/7	—	—	—	—	—	—	—
13	A	S1', pointing up into site	7/7	—	—	—	—	—	—	—
14		S1', pointing down	2/7	101	106	43	27	159	17	85
17		S1'-S2', connecting loop	3/7	118	155	24	13	75	19	46
19		S1'-S2', glycosylation site	3/7	32	51	8.4	—	91	—	38
63	B	H1'-H2', kink between helices	0/6	78	107	135	51	161	47	n.d.
65		H1'-H2', kink between helices	7/7	—	—	—	—	—	—	—
75	C									
78		H3', into site	2/6	174	117	136	2.9	240	20	n.d.
85	D									
86		H3'	1/7	60	91	9.8	225	163	425	105
88										

Reprinted, with permission, from Brett et al. (1989b).

[a]Based on Brown et al. (1988).

[b](x/y) More than 30% loss of reactivity with x antigen-restricted T cells out of a total of y T-cell clones examined.

[c]Mean percentage proliferative response compared with wild-type response over two to five individual experiments at the optimal antigen concentration of 2 μM equine myoglobin. (—) No response above background levels.

[d]n.d. indicates not determined.

424

the mutant at position 9 as it did with the wild-type A^k molecule (Brett et al. 1989b). Thus, the effect of the mutation at position 9 on the response of the 102-118-specific line was opposite that for the clones shown in Table 3. The difference in the form of the antigen used in culture complicates interpretation; but because the response was increased and not diminished when the whole protein was used, we cannot explain the results as a problem of the processed fragment of the protein interacting with the mutant MHC molecule. It remains possible that residue 9 in the wild-type A^k structure interferes with the binding of some part of the processed protein, but not the synthetic peptide, and that the substitution of valine for histidine actually relieves this hindrance. However, one would then have to explain independently how the same substitution interferes with recognition of the synthetic peptide, where such structures of the processed fragment would not be present. We believe that the simplest explanation of all the results with this mutant is that the agretope of 102-118 itself interacts with residue 9 in such a way that the antigenic determinant (on both the peptide and the processed fragment) binds differently to the mutant and that different T cells prefer either one configuration of bound peptide or the other. Again, direct binding measurements would not distinguish the alternatives. Therefore, we think the data suggest that even with the wild-type A^k molecule, different T cells prefer to see the same determinant in different configurations (orientations or conformations). The mutation at position 9 would stabilize the configuration preferred by some T-cell clones and enhance their response, and destabilize the configuration preferred by other T-cell clones and thus diminish their response. We use the term configuration because the difference in the way the determinant binds may not be a difference in conformation of the determinant itself, which could remain an α-helix in both cases (Cease et al. 1986), but rather in the orientation or positioning of the determinant in the groove. Thus, it is likely that a single determinant can be presented in more than one configuration by the same MHC molecule.

Parallel studies of peptide presentation by site-directed mutants of the human HLA-A2 molecule have recently led to similar conclusions for peptide binding to class I MHC molecules (McMichael et al. 1988). If different determinants bind to different contact residues in the groove of the MHC molecule, and even the same determinant can bind to the same MHC molecule in different ways, then it should be difficult to find consistent sequence motifs to explain all determinants that are presented by any given MHC molecule.

Effect of Amino Acid Substitutions in an Antigenic Peptide on Binding to and Presentation by a Class II MHC Molecule

Finally, we have explored this same question from the point of view of the residues in the antigenic peptide that are involved in binding to the MHC molecule and in recognition by the T-cell receptor. As indicated

below, this completely different approach leads to a very similar conclusion. In this case, we have used a different antigenic peptide of myoglobin, 133-146, which we believe is presented in helical form, by I-E^d class II MHC molecules (Berkower et al. 1985, 1986). A series of 36 peptides were synthesized in our laboratory, each with a single amino acid substitution at 1 of 12 positions (A. Kurata and J.A. Berzofsky, in prep.). For each position, three different peptides were made with different substitutions (Fig. 5). These peptides were studied for their ability to stimulate two distinct but very similar T-cell clones, 14.1 and 14.5, with previously indistinguishable fine specificity. Prior to this study, the only difference in specificity noted between these clones was the response to Mls[a] by 14.1, but not 14.5 (H. Kawamura and J.A. Berzofsky, unpubl.). The peptides that failed to stimulate were also studied for binding to E^d by their ability to inhibit competitively presentation of the wild-type peptide. The results are summarized in Table 4 and will be presented in detail elsewhere (A. Kurata and J.A. Berzofsky, in prep.).

Substitutions that affected antigenic potency (molar concentration required to stimulate the T-cell clones) were largely confined to residues 138-145. The strategy that has been developed recently for this type of analysis (Allen et al. 1987b; Sette et al. 1987) is to interpret substitutions that affect both stimulation of T cells and competition for binding to the MHC molecule as indicative of a residue that interacts with the MHC mole-

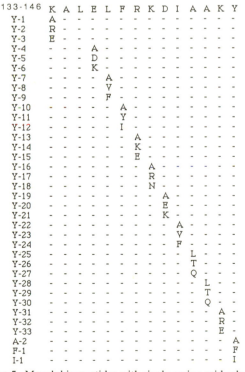

Figure 5. Myoglobin peptides with single amino acid substitutions used for analysis of residues interacting with I-E^d or with the receptor of T-cell clones specific for peptide 133-146 of sperm whale myoglobin. Amino acids are indicated in single-letter code. (Based on A. Kurata and J.A. Berzofsky, in prep.)

Table 4. Effect of Single Amino Acid Substitutions on Peptide Stimulation of T-cell Clones and Competition for Binding to I-E[d]

Substituted peptides		Stimulatory activity[a] T clone		Inhibitory activity[a] T clone		Interpretation[b] T clone	
		14.5	14.1	14.5	14.1	14.5	14.1
Y-1	133 K→A	++	++				
Y-2	133 K→R	++	++				
Y-3	133 K→E	++	++				
Y-4	136 E→A	+	++				
Y-5	136 E→D	+	++				
Y-6	136 E→K	++	++				
Y-7	137 L→A	+/−	++				
Y-8	137 L→V	++	++				
Y-9	137 L→F	++	++				
Y-10	**138 F→A**	−	−	++	+/−	T	**Ia**
Y-11	138 F→Y	++	++			N	N
Y-12	**138 F→I**	−	−	++	−	T	**Ia**
Y-13	139 R→A	−	−	−	−	Ia	Ia
Y-14	139 R→K	−	−	+	−	T?	Ia
Y-15	139 R→E	+/−	−		−		Ia
Y-16	140 K→A	−	+/−	−		Ia	
Y-17	**140 K→R**	−	++	++		T?	**N**
Y-18	140 K→N	+/−	−		−		Ia
Y-19	141 D→A	−	−	−	−	Ia	Ia
Y-20	141 D→E	−	−	−	−	Ia	Ia
Y-21	141 D→K	−	−	+	+	T?	T?
Y-22	**142 I→A**	++	−		+	**N**	**T?**
Y-23	142 I→V	++	++			N	N
Y-24	**142 I→F**	−	++	+/−		**Ia**	**N**
Y-25	143 A→L	−	−	+	−	T	Ia
Y-26	143 A→T	+/−	−		+		T?
Y-27	**143 A→Q**	−	−	++	−	T	**Ia**
Y-28	144 A→L	−	−	+	+	T?	T?
Y-29	144 A→T	+	++			N	N
Y-30	144 A→Q	++	++			N	N
Y-31	145 K→A	+/−	+				
Y-32	145 K→R	++	++				
Y-33	145 K→E	+/−	+/−				
A-2	146 Y→A	++	++				
F-1	146 Y→F	++	++				
I-1	146 Y→I	++	++				
Sw133–146		++	++				

[a](++, +, +/−, −) Relative potencies are based on the concentration required for half maximal stimulation of each clone or inhibition of presentation of wild-type peptide to a given clone. Each value represents a complete dose-response curve, done twice. (Modified from A. Kurata and I. A. Berzofsky, in prep.)

[b](Ia) substitution affects binding of peptide to Ia; (T) substitution affects recognition by T-cell receptor but not Ia; (N) substitution affects neither of the above.

cule and substitutions that affect stimulation of T cells, but not the ability to compete for presentation, as indicative of a residue that interacts with the T-cell receptor. In trying to apply this strategy, we noted several problems in interpreting the results in Table 4.

First, at position 140, two of the substitutions, K → A and K → N, affect stimulatory capacity for both T-cell clones and also abrogate the ability to compete for

presentation of wild-type peptide, indicative of interference with binding to I-E. However, the third substitution, K → R, affects the ability to stimulate one T cell and not the other, suggestive of a residue interacting with the T-cell receptor; this interpretation is supported by the finding that the substituted peptide competes quite well for presentation to the clone that it does not stimulate. Therefore, in the wild-type peptide in which residue 140 is a lysine, with which molecule does it interact? The most consistent explanation of all three substitutions is that residue 140 interacts with the Ia (class II MHC) molecule and that substitution of alanine or asparagine is sufficient to disrupt binding, whereas substitution of arginine allows binding but in a slightly different conformation or orientation that affects recognition by one T-cell clone and not the other.

Second, residue 142 behaves paradoxically. Substitution of alanine for isoleucine results in loss of activity for clone 14.1 without affecting clone 14.5, whereas substitution of phenylalanine for isoleucine has the reciprocal effect. Initially, then, these results suggest that isoleucine is part of the T-cell receptor-binding site and substitutions differentially affect binding to the receptors of different clones but not binding to MHC. However, when we examined competition for presentation of wild-type peptide to the clone that that substituted peptide could not stimulate, we found that binding to Ia appeared to be diminished, especially in the case of 142 I→F tested on clone 14.5 (Table 4). This result did not seem consistent with the result that the stimulatory potency, as measured by the molar concentration for half-maximal stimulation, for the other clone, 14.1, was not diminished at all. The only internally consistent explanation for these results seems to be that the peptide binds in more than one way to the same MHC molecule and that the two T-cell clones recognize it in different positions. As it is bound for presentation to clone 14.1, residue 142 interacts with the T-cell receptor, not the Ia molecule. The receptor of clone 14.1 seems to be able to accommodate the substitution of phenylalanine for isoleucine without loss of binding but does not bind when isoleucine is replaced by alanine. In contrast, as the peptide is bound for presentation to clone 14.5, residue 142 interacts with the Ia molecule (I-E^d) and this interaction cannot accommodate the substitution of phenylalanine for isoleucine but can accommodate the substitution of alanine for isoleucine.

Finally, in three cases, substitutions completely abrogated stimulation of both clones and yet had a differential effect on competition for presentation of wild-type peptide to the two clones (Table 4). The substituted peptides 138 F→I and 143 A→Q completely lost the capacity to compete for presentation to clone 14.1, and peptide 138 F→A was greatly diminished in this capacity; yet all three competed extremely well for presentation of wild-type peptide to clone 14.5. These results suggest again that the peptide can bind in more than one way to the I-E^d molecule and is seen in different conformations or orientations by the two clones. As the peptide is presented to clone 14.5, residues 138 and 143 appear to interact with the T-cell receptor and not the Ia molecule, and the substitutions interfere with T-cell recognition but not presentation by Ia. In contrast, as the peptide is presented to clone 14.1, the same residues appear to interact with the Ia molecule and the substitutions prevent or greatly diminish binding.

All of these results thus independently point to the same conclusion, that the same peptide can bind to the same MHC molecule in more than one way. Although the two T-cell clones see the same segment of the peptide, they see it in different conformations or orientations in the MHC groove. It is actually possible that the conformation of the peptide itself is nearly the same, but the orientation slightly shifted. For instance, if the peptide were an amphipathic α-helix (Fig. 6), as predicted (DeLisi and Berzofsky 1985; Berkower et al. 1986; Margalit et al. 1987), residues 138 and 142 would be approximately opposite residue 140, and residues 139 and 141 would be on either side of it. Thus, if residue 140 (lysine) interacted with a negatively charged amino acid on the floor of the groove, residues 139 and 141 could interact with the helical walls of the groove and residues 138 and 142 would be in a position that would allow interaction with either the T-cell receptor or the Ia molecule. Because these residues are offset on the circumference of the cylinder of the helix, and both have long side chains, a slight rotation of the cylinder of the helical peptide would favor 138 to interact with the T-cell receptor and 142 with the Ia, or vice versa. However, the two postulated configurations for peptide binding would have to be sufficiently different that a substitution that completely abrogated binding to Ia in one configuration would not affect binding at all to the same Ia molecule when binding occurred in the other configuration. Furthermore, cases of binding as measured by undiminished stimulation of one T-cell clone, in the absence of competition for presentation to the other clone, suggest binding of peptide to sites that overlap little, if at all, within the peptide-binding groove of the MHC molecule. Using additional substitutions and direct binding measurements, we hope to resolve these issues. However, we believe that regardless of the final details of the antigenic structures as

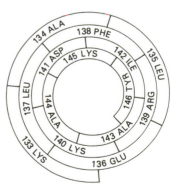

Figure 6. Spiral diagram showing a two-dimensional representation of an α-helix, viewed down the axis of the cylinder. The sequence of sperm whale myoglobin 133-146 is shown arrayed as such a helix, in which residues 139, 140, and 141 could interact with the I-E^d molecule, and residues 138 and 142 with either the I-E^d molecule or the T-cell receptor. Residues in different layers of the spiral are in different turns of helix, at different distances along the axis of the helix, and not farther out from the axis of the helix as it might appear in this two-dimensional representation. (Based on A. Kurata and J.A. Berzofsky, in prep.)

bound to I-E^d, the data imply that at least two modes of binding must exist for the same peptide presented by the same MHC molecule.

CONCLUSIONS

The results of these studies demonstrate that presentation of antigenic determinants by MHC molecules to T cells is more complex than had been envisaged. First, the natural products of processing may behave differently from the short synthetic peptides that correspond to little more than the minimal antigenic site. This emphasizes the need to better define and predict the products of processing, as we have tried to do by identifying the enzymes involved in processing. Second, even the same peptide may bind in multiple ways to the same MHC molecule, creating different complex structures for recognition by T-cell receptors. Data examining the effects of mutations in the MHC molecule and mutations in the antigenic peptide both support the same conclusions from opposite directions. This gives us more confidence that the conclusions will be generally valid. For these reasons, it will be more difficult to interpret the results of single substitutions in peptides, because a substitution that appears to affect T-cell receptor interaction and not MHC binding may not be a contact residue for the T-cell receptor. Rather, it may affect binding to MHC qualitatively instead of quantitatively, so that the peptide still binds with comparable affinity but in a different conformation or a different position or orientation within the groove. Even substitutions that affect binding quantitatively could do so by affecting the preferred conformation of the peptide rather than by being contact residues for the MHC molecule. In addition, if different peptides bind to different contact residues of the MHC molecule and possibly in different parts of the groove, and even the same peptide can bind in different ways in the same MHC molecule, then it may not be possible to find a sequence motif that explains all peptides that are presented by a given MHC molecule. Modeling studies are under way to try to better understand these structure-function relationships, but the ultimate answers may have to await the determination of a crystal structure for a class II MHC molecule with a peptide bound, or perhaps two distinct structures for the same peptide–MHC molecule complex.

ACKNOWLEDGMENTS

We thank Drs. Alfred Singer and Ronald N. Germain for helpful discussions.

REFERENCES

Allen, P.M. 1987a. Antigen processing at the molecular level. *Immunol. Today* **8**: 270.

Allen, P.M. and E.R. Unanue. 1984. Differential requirements for antigen processing by macrophages for lysozyme-specific T cell hybridomas. *J. Immunol.* **132**: 1077.

Allen, P.M., D.J. McKean, B.N. Beck, J. Sheffield, and L.H. Glimcher. 1985. Direct evidence that a class II molecule and a simple globular protein generate multiple determinants. *J. Exp. Med.* **162**: 1264.

Allen, P.M., G.R. Matsueda, R.J. Evans, J.B. Dunbar, Jr., G.R. Marshall, and E.R. Unanue. 1987b. Identification of the T-cell and Ia contact residues of a T-cell antigenic epitope. *Nature* **327**: 713.

Benacerraf, B. 1978. A hypothesis to relate the specificity of T lymphocytes and the activity of I region-specific Ir genes in macrophages and B lymphocytes. *J. Immunol.* **120**: 1809.

Berkower, I., G.K. Buckenmeyer, and J.A. Berzofsky. 1986. Molecular mapping of a histocompatibility-restricted immunodominant T cell epitope with synthetic and natural peptides: Implications for antigenic structure. *J. Immunol.* **136**: 2498.

Berkower, I., G.K. Buckenmeyer, F.R.N. Gurd, and J.A. Berzofsky. 1982. A possible immunodominant epitope recognized by murine T lymphocytes immune to different myoglobins. *Proc. Natl. Acad. Sci.* **79**: 4723.

Berkower, I., H. Kawamura, L.A. Matis, and J.A. Berzofsky. 1985. T cell clones to two major T cell epitopes of myoglobin: Effect of I-A/I-E restriction on epitope dominance. *J. Immunol.* **135**: 2628.

Berzofsky, J.A. 1986. Structural features of protein antigenic sites recognized by helper T cells: What makes a site immunodominant? In *The year in immunology 1985-1986* (ed. J.M. Cruse and R.E. Lewis, Jr.), p. 28. Karger, Basel.

———. 1987. Ir genes: Antigen-specific genetic regulation of the immune response. In *The antigens* (ed. M. Sela), p. 1. Academic Press, New York.

———. 1988a. Immunodominance in T lymphocyte recognition. *Immunol. Lett.* **18**: 83.

———. 1988b. The structural basis of antigen recognition by T lymphocytes: Implications for vaccines. *J. Clin. Invest.* **82**: 1811.

Berzofsky, J.A., S.J. Brett, H.Z. Streicher, and H. Takahashi. 1988. Antigen processing for presentation to T lymphocytes: Function, mechanisms, and implications for the T-cell repertoire. *Immunol. Rev.* **106**: 5.

Bjorkman, P.J., M.A. Saper, B. Samraoui, W.S. Bennett, J.L. Strominger, and D.C. Wiley. 1987a. Structure of the human class I histocompatibility antigen HLA-A2. *Nature* **329**: 506.

———. 1987b. The foreign antigen binding site and T cell recognition regions of class I histocompatibility antigens. *Nature* **329**: 512.

Bodmer, H.C., F.M. Gotch, and A.J. McMichael. 1989. Class I cross-restricted T cells reveal low responder allele due to processing of viral antigen. *Nature* **337**: 653.

Brett, S.J., K.B. Cease, and J.A. Berzofsky. 1988. Influences of antigen processing on the expression of the T cell repertoire: Evidence for MHC-specific hindering structures on the products of processing. *J. Exp. Med.* **168**: 357.

Brett, S.J., K.B. Cease, C.S. Ouyang, and J.A. Berzofsky. 1989a. Fine specificity of T cell recognition of the same peptide in association with different I-A molecules. *J. Immunol.* **143**: 771.

Brett, S.J., D. McKean, J. York-Jolley, and J.A. Berzofsky. 1989b. Antigen presentation to specific T cells by Ia molecules selectively altered by site-directed mutagenesis. *Int. Immunol.* **1**: 130.

Brown, J.H., T. Jardetzky, M.A. Saper, B. Samraoui, P.J. Bjorkman, and D.C. Wiley. 1988. A hypothetical model of the foreign antigen binding site of class II histocompatibility molecules. *Nature* **332**: 845.

Brown, M.A., L.A. Glimcher, E.A. Nielsen, W.E. Paul, and R.N. Germain. 1986. T-cell recognition of Ia molecules selectively altered by a single amino acid substitution. *Science* **231**: 255.

Buerstedde, J.M., L.R. Pease, M.P. Bell, A.E. Nilson, G. Buerstedde, D. Murphy, and D.J. McKean. 1988a. Identification of an immunodominant region on the I-A$_\beta$ chain using site-directed mutagenesis and DNA mediated gene transfer. *J. Exp. Med.* **167**: 473.

Buerstedde, J.M., L.R. Pease, A.E. Wilson, M.P. Bell, C. Chase, G. Buerstedde, and D.J. McKean. 1988b. Regulation of murine MHC Class II molecule expression. Identification of A$_\beta$ residues responsible for allele-specific cell surface expression. *J. Exp. Med.* **168**: 823.

Buerstedde, J.M., A.E. Wilson, C.G. Chase, M.P. Bell, B.N. Beck, L.R. Pease, and D.J. McKean. 1989. A$_\beta$ polymorphic residues responsible for Class II recognition by alloreactive T cells. *J. Exp. Med.* **169**: 1645.

Buus, S. and O. Werdelin. 1986. A group-specific inhibitor of lysosomal cysteine proteinases selectively inhibits both proteolytic degradation and presentation of the antigen dinitrophenyl-poly-L-lysine by guinea pig accessory cells to T cells. *J. Immunol.* **136**: 452.

Cease, K.B., I. Berkower, J. York-Jolley, and J.A. Berzofsky. 1986. T cell clones specific for an amphipathic alpha helical region of sperm whale myoglobin show differing fine specificities for synthetic peptides: A multi-view/single structure interpretation of immunodominance. *J. Exp. Med.* **164**: 1779.

Claverie, J.M. and P. Kourilsky. 1986. The peptidic self model: A reassessment of the role of the major histocompatibility complex molecules in the restriction of the T cell response. *Ann. Inst. Pasteur Immunol.* **137D**: 425.

Cohn, L.E., L.H. Glimcher, R.A. Waldmann, J.A. Smith, A. Ben-Nun, J.G. Seidman, and E. Choi. 1986. Identification of functional regions on the I-A$_\beta$ molecule by site-directed mutagenesis. *Proc. Natl. Acad. Sci.* **83**: 747.

DeLisi, C. and J.A. Berzofsky. 1985. T cell antigenic sites tend to be amphipathic structures. *Proc. Natl. Acad. Sci.* **82**: 7048.

Gammon, G., N. Shastri, J. Cogswell, S. Wilbur, S. Sadegh-Nasseri, U. Krzych, A. Miller, and E.E. Sercarz. 1987. The choice of T-cell epitopes utilized on a protein antigen depends on multiple factors distant from as well as at the determinant site. *Immunol. Rev.* **98**: 53.

Germain, R.N. 1986. The ins and outs of antigen processing and presentation. *Nature* **322**: 687.

Germain, R.N., J.D. Ashwell, R.I. Lechler, D.H. Margulies, K.M. Nickerson, G. Suzuki, and J.Y.L. Tou. 1985. "Exon-shuffling" maps control of antibody and T-cell-recognition sites to the NH$_2$ terminal domain of the class II major histocompatibility polypeptide A$_\beta$. *Proc. Natl. Acad. Sci.* **82**: 2940.

Glimcher, L.H., D.J. McKean, E. Choi, and J.G. Seidman. 1985. Complex regulation of class II gene expression: Analysis with class II mutant cell lines. *J. Immunol.* **135**: 3542.

Hansburg, D., T. Fairwell, R.H. Schwartz, and E. Appella. 1983. The T lymphocyte response to cytochrome c. IV. Distinguishable sites on a peptide antigen which affect antigenic strength and memory. *J. Immunol.* **131**: 319.

Heber-Katz, E., D. Hansburg, and R.H. Schwartz. 1983. The Ia molecule of the antigen-presenting cell plays a critical role in immune response gene regulation of T cell activation. *J. Mol. Cell. Immunol.* **1**: 3.

Hockman, P.S. and B.T. Huber. 1984. A Class II gene conversion event defines an antigen-specific Ir gene epitope. *J. Exp. Med.* **160**: 1925.

Kanamori, S., W.S. Walsh, T.H. Hansen, and H.Y. Tse. 1984. Assessment of antigen specific restriction sites on Ia molecules as defined by the bm12 mutation. *J. Immunol.* **133**: 2811.

Kojima, M., K.B. Cease, G.K. Buckenmeyer, and J.A. Berzofsky. 1988. Limiting dilution comparison of the repertoires of high and low responder MHC-restricted T cells. *J. Exp. Med.* **167**: 1100.

Kovac, Z. and R.H. Schwartz. 1985. The molecular basis of the requirement for antigen processing of pigeon cytochrome c prior to T cell activation. *J. Immunol.* **134**: 3233.

Landais, D., C. Waltzinger, B.N. Beck, A. Staub, D.J. Mc-

Kean, C. Benoist, and D. Mathis. 1986. Functional sites on Ia molecules: A molecular dissection of A$_\alpha$ immunogenicity. *Cell* **47**: 173.

Lechler, R.I., F. Ronchese, N.S. Braunstein, and R.N. Germain. 1986. I-A-restricted T cell antigen recognition. Analysis of the roles of A-α and A-β using DNA-mediated gene transfer. *J. Exp. Med.* **163**: 678.

Lee, P., G.R. Matsueda, and P.M. Allen. 1988. T cell recognition of fibrinogen. A determinant on the Aα-chain does not require processing. *J. Immunol.* **140**: 1063.

Lin, J., J.A. Berzofsky, and T.L. Delovitch. 1988. Ultrastructural study of internalization and recycling of antigen by antigen presenting cells. *J. Mol. Cell. Immunol.* **3**: 321.

Margalit, H., J.L. Spouge, J.L. Cornette, K. Cease, C. DeLisi, and J.A. Berzofsky. 1987. Prediction of immunodominant helper T-cell antigenic sites from the primary sequence. *J. Immunol.* **138**: 2213.

McKean, D.J., A. Nilson, A.J. Infante, and L. Kazim. 1983. Biochemical characterization of B lymphoma cell antigen processing and presentation to antigen-reactive T cells. *J. Immunol.* **131**: 2726.

McMichael, A.J., F.M. Gotch, J. Santos-Aguado, and J.L. Strominger. 1988. Effect of mutations and variations of HLA-A2 on recognition of a virus peptide epitope by cytotoxic T lymphocytes. *Proc. Natl. Acad. Sci.* **85**: 9194.

Moore, M.W., F.R. Carbone, and M.J. Bevan. 1988. Introduction of soluble protein into the class I pathway of antigen processing and presentation. *Cell* **54**: 777.

Morrison, L.A., A.E. Lukacher, V.L. Braciale, D.P. Fan, and T.J. Braciale. 1986. Differences in antigen presentation to MHC class I and class II-restricted influenza virus specific cytolytic T lymphocyte clones. *J. Exp. Med.* **163**: 903.

Puri, J. and Y. Factorovich. 1988. Selective inhibition of antigen presentation to cloned T cells by protease inhibitors. *J. Immunol.* **141**: 3313.

Puri, J., P. Lonai, and V. Friedman. 1986. Antigen-Ia interaction and the proteolytic processing of antigen: The structure of the antigen determines its restriction to the A or E molecule of major histocompatibility complex. *Eur. J. Immunol.* **16**: 1093.

Ronchese, F., M.A. Brown, and R.N. Germain. 1987. Structure-function analysis of the A-β-bm12 mutation using site-directed mutagenesis and DNA-mediated gene transfer. *J. Immunol.* **139**: 629.

Rosenthal, A.S. 1978. Determinant selection and macrophage function in genetic control of the immune response. *Immunol. Rev.* **40**: 136.

Régnier-Vigouroux, A., M.E. Ayeb, M.-L. Defendini, C. Granier, and M. Pierres. 1988. Processing by accessory cells for presentation to murine T cells of apamin, a disulfide-bonded 18 amino acid peptide. *J. Immunol.* **140**: 1069.

Sette, A., S. Buus, S. Colon, C. Miles, and H.M. Grey. 1989. Structural analysis of peptides capable of binding to more than one Ia antigen. *J. Immunol.* **142**: 35.

Sette, A., S. Buus, S. Colon, J.A. Smith, C. Miles, and H.M. Grey. 1987. Structural characteristics of an antigen required for its interaction with Ia and recognition by T cells. *Nature* **328**: 395.

Shastri, N., A. Miller, and E.E. Sercarz. 1986. Amino acid residues distinct from the determinant region can profoundly affect activation of T cell clones by related antigens. *J. Immunol.* **136**: 371.

Shimonkevitz, R., J. Kappler, P. Marrack, and H. Grey. 1983. Antigen recognition by H-2 restricted T cells. I. Cell free antigen processing. *J. Exp. Med.* **158**: 303.

Streicher, H.Z., I.J. Berkower, M. Busch, F.R.N. Gurd, and J.A. Berzofsky. 1984. Antigen conformation determines processing requirements for T-cell activation. *Proc. Natl. Acad. Sci.* **81**: 6831.

Takahashi, H., K.B. Cease, and J.A. Berzofsky. 1989. Identification of proteases that process distinct epitopes on the same protein. *J. Immunol.* **142**: 2221.

Unanue, E.R. 1984. Antigen-presenting function of the macrophage. *Annu. Rev. Immunol.* **2:** 395.

Unanue, E.R. and P.M. Allen. 1987. The basis for the immunoregulatory role of macrophages and other accessory cells. *Science* **236:** 551.

Vacchio, M.S., J.A. Berzofsky, U. Krzych, J.A. Smith, R.J. Hodes, and A. Finnegan. 1989. Sequences outside a minimal immunodominant site exert negative effects on recognition by staphylococcal nuclease-specific T-cell clones. *J. Immunol.* **143:** (in press).

Werdelin, O. 1987. T cells recognize antigen alone and not MHC molecules. *Immunol. Today* **8:** 80.

Yewdell, J.W., J.R. Bennink, and Y. Hosaka. 1988. Cells process exogenous proteins for recognition by cytotoxic T lymphocytes. *Science* **239:** 637.

Ziegler, H.K. and E.R. Unanue. 1982. Decrease in macrophage antigen catabolism caused by ammonia and chloroquine is associated with inhibition of antigen presentation to T cells. *Proc. Natl. Acad. Sci.* **79:** 175.

Structural Analysis of a Peptide-HLA Class II Complex

J.B. ROTHBARD, R. BUSCH, C.M. HILL, AND J.R. LAMB*

Laboratory of Molecular Immunology, Imperial Cancer Research Fund, Lincoln's Inn Fields, London, WC2A 3PX;
*Department of Immunology, Hammersmith Hospital, London, W12 0HS, United Kingdom

The identification and sequencing of the antigen receptor of T cells (Haskins et al. 1983; Hedrick et al. 1984; Yanagi et al. 1984), coupled with the demonstration that major histocompatibility complex (MHC) proteins specifically bind immunogenic peptides (Babbitt et al. 1985; Buus et al. 1986; Chen and Parham 1989) and the solution of the crystal structure of HLA-A2 (Bjorkman et al. 1987a,b), collectively have led to a working model of how T cells recognize protein antigens (Davis and Bjorkman 1988). This unique recognition mechanism apparently has evolved to allow receptors on two separate cells to contact a common peptide ligand. As valuable as these experimental results have been for increasing our understanding of T-cell recognition, they also have raised several different, but equally perplexing, questions. The principal issue our laboratory has concentrated on is how can a single, conserved MHC antigen combining site specifically recognize a very large number of diverse peptides? Although the MHC molecules are members of one of the most polymorphic families of proteins yet defined, the amino acids comprising the combining site of any one allele are constant. This is in stark contrast to the other proteins known to bind antigen, i.e., antibodies and the antigen receptors of T cells, which both create diverse binding sites by genetic rearrangement and, in the case of antibodies, additional somatic mutations (Honjo 1983; Moller 1987; Davis and Bjorkman 1988).

The interactions between ligand and receptor can be divided broadly into those contacts involving the amino acid side chains of the ligand as distinguished from those involving the atoms comprising its main-chain backbone. If the side chains of the ligand or substrate are essential for recognition, then identical or related amino acids should be present in the primary sequences of those compounds that bind, whereas if the majority of the critical contacts are with the atoms comprising the peptide bonds of the ligand, no structural similarity in the primary sequences of the ligands will be apparent. In addition, if many peptides bind with a preferential conformation in a similar location in the combining site and make many contacts via their side chains, then those peptides that bind should be able to be aligned to display structural similarities at homologous positions in their sequence.

Such similarities were identified when the T-cell determinants restricted by either MHC class I or class II proteins were analyzed (Rothbard and Taylor 1988).

Further similarities were seen when the number of defined determinants increased, which allowed them to be segregated by restriction element. The spacing of the homologous amino acids in these motifs also was quite consistent. A large number of sequences could be aligned to reveal structurally similar residues at relative positions 1, 4, 5, and 8—positions that would comprise a common facade if the peptides folded in a helical conformation when bound by the MHC molecules. A separate analysis of T-cell determinants also concluded that this conformation might be important in T-cell recognition (DeLisi and Berzofsky 1985).

If valid, the presence of these similarities within many T-cell determinants would be consistent with many peptides interacting with the MHC proteins via their amino acid side chains and occupying a common position in the antigen combining site. To test these ideas, we initially identified an alignment of two peptides recognized by HLA-DR1-restricted T cells based on structurally similar residues at relative positions 1, 4, 5, and 8. Using this alignment as a guide, residues of one sequence were substituted for the corresponding amino acid in the second to generate two sets of hybrid peptides. In each case, six amino acids, which constituted a face of the putative helical peptide, were the minimum residues necessary for stimulation of the T-cell clones. In addition to identifying residues critical for clonally specific recognition, this approach provided information on the structural requirements for binding and placed constraints on the potential conformations the peptides could adopt when part of the complex. However, this strategy had the inherent weakness that the putative MHC contact residues were identified on the basis of sequence homology between the two peptides and not with the use of direct binding assays.

Three groups have attempted to define the orientation of peptide determinants when part of the complex by correlating the inability of natural determinants containing point substitutions to stimulate the T-cell clone with their capacity to bind the restriction element. Substitution of every position in a lysozyme peptide with alanine generated a family of analogs whose ability to bind purified I-A^k and/or stimulate a T-cell clone provided sufficient information to allow a helical conformation of the bound peptide to be postulated (Allen et al. 1987). However, the results of a more extensive study using a similar strategy to dissect a helper determinant in ovalbumin failed to identify residues unequivocally interacting with either macromolecule

(Sette et al. 1987). Consequently, a regular conformation could not be identified, primarily because the majority of peptides containing single substitutions were still able to bind the class II protein. A separate analysis of T-cell recognition by clones specific for a cytochrome peptide also could not identify a regular conformation for a bound peptide (Ogasawara et al. 1989).

In our study, the ability to detect binding of biotinylated peptides to MHC class II proteins on cell surfaces was used to develop a model for the relative orientation and conformation of an influenza hemagglutinin peptide in the antigen combining site of HLA-DR1. Only when an unnaturally large amino acid was incorporated into each position of the peptide could important residues for binding clearly be identified. The peptide was placed in the binding site on the basis of the presence of potential complementary contact residues in the MHC molecule and the effects of a number of analogs on T-cell recognition and binding. The assay also allowed screening of a large number of HLA-DR alleles for their ability to bind the peptide. The ability of both a surprisingly large number of DR alleles to bind the peptide and any one MHC protein to bind a large variety of peptides is discussed in the context of the model.

MATERIALS AND METHODS

Peptides. The peptide representing residues 307–319 of influenza hemagglutinin (PKYVKQNTLK-LAT), which previously was shown to be recognized by DR1-restricted T cells (Rothbard et al. 1988), was the parent sequence for the analogs used in this study. Long-chain biotin (Hofmann et al. 1982) was placed unambiguously at each position by substituting lysine at the desired position, replacing lysines 308, 311, and 316 with arginine, and acetylating the α-amino group. The peptides were synthesized using standard solid-phase methods as described previously (Rothbard et al. 1988) on an Applied Biosystems 430 A synthesizer and were biotinylated with excess sulfosuccinimidyl 6-(biotinamido) hexanoate (Pierce). The biotinylated peptides were purified by reversed-phase HPLC and analyzed by amino acid analysis and fast atom bombardment mass spectrometry. Biotinylation was further confirmed by positive reaction with dimethylaminocinnamaldehyde (McCormick and Roth 1970).

Binding assay. This assay has been described in detail elsewhere (R. Busch et al., in prep.). Briefly, two Epstein-Barr virus (EBV)-transformed B-cell lines homozygous for HLA-DR1 Dw1, MAJA, and METTE, and the class II-deficient EBV-B-cell line, RJ 2.2.5 (Accolla 1983), were incubated at 3×10^5 cells per well with each biotinylated peptide (50 μM) in 96-well plates (200 μl) at 37°C for 4 hours, followed by fluorescein isothiocyanate (FITC)-streptavidin (4.22 μg/ml; Calbiochem). Cell-surface DR expression was quantified by staining with fluoresceinated L243 anti-DR monoclonal antibody (Shackelford et al. 1983) (Becton Dick-

inson; 30 min, 4°C). After each incubation, cells were washed with phosphate-buffered saline (PBS) containing 0.1% bovine serum albumin. Stained cells were analyzed by flow cytometry using a FACScan analyzer (Becton Dickinson). Only viable cells, identified on the analyzer by their ability to exclude propidium iodide, were included in the analysis. In inhibition studies, competing peptides or unlabeled L243 was included in the assay. To determine whether differential proteolysis was a factor, a mixture of proteinase inhibitors (TPCK, 10 μg/ml; PMSF, 50 μg/ml; leupeptin, 1 μg/ml; aprotinin, 1 μg/ml; soybean trypsin inhibitor, 10 μg/ml) were coincubated with cells and the biotinylated peptide.

Measurement of helicity. The helicity of the natural peptide (HA 307–319), or derivatives that either were acetylated, amidated, or both, was measured by the magnitude of the negative Cotton effect at 222 nm in a range of water/trifluoroethanol (TFE) mixtures. On the scale shown, 10 $\mathrm{M}^{-1}\mathrm{cm}^{-1}$ was taken to represent 100% helix. All peptides underwent simple helix-coil transitions as judged by the presence of isodichroic points around 203 nm and the minima in the circular dichroism (CD) spectrum at 222 and 207 nm for the helical conformation, and at 196 nm for the unordered conformation. CD spectra were recorded on a JASCO J-600 spectropolarimeter at approximately 0.15 mg/ml peptide in a 1-mm quartz cuvette. Absorption spectra of peptide stocks were recorded on a Hewlett-Packard diode array spectrophotometer. CD spectra of biotinylated peptides were measured in 50% PBS (pH 7.2)/TFE.

RESULTS AND DISCUSSION

Peptide Binding to HLA-DR on B-cell Surfaces

To determine whether immunogenic peptides could be shown to bind MHC class II molecules on the surface of intact cells, a T-cell determinant from influenza hemagglutinin (HA; residues 307–319) (Rothbard et al. 1988), which is recognized by a HLA-DR1-restricted T-cell clone, was assayed for its ability to bind EBV-transformed human B lymphocytes (B-LCL) homozygous for HLA-DR1. These cells were chosen because they were homozygous, well-characterized cell lines that express unusually high levels of HLA class II proteins. Because of concerns about high background fluorescence and a low specific signal, the peptide was not directly fluoresceinated. Instead, it was conjugated to a biotinyl group to take advantage of the amplification that can be obtained by using multiply fluoresceinated streptavidin.

When the DR1-homozygous B-LCL, MAJA, was incubated with the peptide, stained with fluoresceinated streptavidin, and analyzed for green fluorescence by flow cytometry, the cell-surface fluorescence was approximately five times higher than in the absence of peptide (Fig. 1A). The signal was two orders of magnitude less intense than that obtained by indirect immunofluorescence with a monoclonal antibody specific for a determinant present on many human class II molecules.

All detectable fluorescence with this peptide was shown to be specific by using RJ 2.2.5 cells (Accolla 1983). These cells, like MAJA line, are human B-lymphoblastoid cells transformed by EBV, except that they do not express class II proteins because of a mutation in a regulatory protein required for class II expres-

sion (Hume et al. 1987). Consequently, they provide an excellent control for the specificity of the fluorescent signal because they should display an identical cell surface except for the absence of MHC class II proteins and any allelic variation of surface proteins between the cell lines. When RJ 2.2.5 cells were used in the assay, the fluorescence in the presence of peptide was indistinguishable from background (Fig. 1B). This demonstrated that the large majority of the fluorescent signal on the cells expressing DR1 was specific and strongly

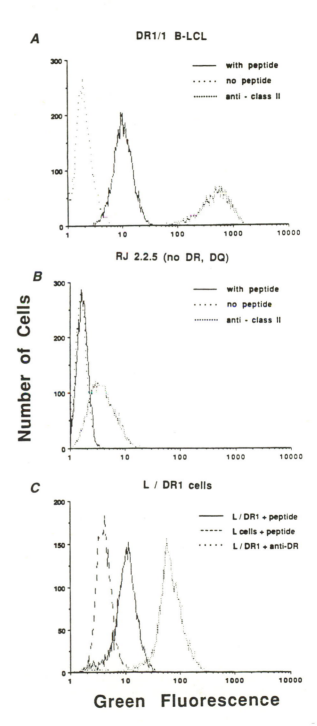

Figure 1. Binding of a biotinylated analog of HA 307-319 to surfaces of B cells transformed by EBV. (*A*) The DR-homozygous B-LCL, MAJA (HLA-A2,3, B35, C4, Bw6, DR1 Dw1, DQw1, DP4) was incubated with HA 307-319 containing long-chain biotin at the amino terminus and stained with FITC-streptavidin (——). Surface expression of class II MHC proteins was shown by indirect immunofluorescence using the anti HLA-D MAb, 31.1 (·······). Background fluorescence in the absence of biotinylated peptide was determined by incubation only with streptavidin (· · · ·). (*B*) Binding of the HA analog (——) and MAb 31.1 (·······) to the class II-deficient B-cell line, RJ 2.2.5 (HLA-A3, 19; B51, 35; C3,4; Bw4, 6; DR, DQ-negative; DP-low). Fluorescence in the absence of peptide (· · · ·) is indistinguishable from fluorescence with peptide. (*C*) Binding of the biotinylated HA peptide to L cells transfected with HLA-DR1. Transfectants (——) or untransfected L cells (----) were incubated with 100 μM peptide overnight. The levels of DR expression (·······) on the transfected L cells were measured by indirect immunofluorescence using the anti-DR monoclonal antibody, L243.

suggested that the peptide bound to class II MHC proteins or other proteins whose expression was coregulated.

L cells transfected with genes encoding α and β chains of human class II molecules (Lechler et al. 1988) were used to demonstrate that the peptide binds to HLA-DR. A distinct fluorescent signal was observed when the HA peptide was incubated with cells transfected with DR1, but was absent on normal L cells (Fig. 1C). In contrast, the fluorescence on L cells expressing DQw1 was indistinguishable from that of untransfected cells (data not shown). However, because the level of DQ expression on these transfectants was low, the possibility that the peptide can weakly interact with DQ cannot be ruled out.

Further evidence that the peptide directly interacted with HLA-DR on the surface of B-LCL was that the fluorescent signal could be modulated by coincubating the B-LCL with peptide and an anti-DR monoclonal antibody (Shackelford et al. 1983). Increasing amounts of antibody progressively reduced the fluorescent signal (Fig. 2A). However, complete inhibition of the signal by incubation with this antibody could not be obtained due to the difficulty of getting sufficiently high antibody concentrations to block the binding without cross-linking the cells and removing them from the gate of the FACS analyzer. Using Fab fragments of the antibody did not solve the problem. Nevertheless, the reduction of the fluorescent signal closely paralleled the saturation of cell-surface DR1 by the antibody (Fig. 2B), indicating that the majority of the fluorescent signal was due to the formation of a peptide/MHC class II complex and not to nonspecific binding on the cell surface.

The natural determinant also was shown to compete with the biotinylated peptide, demonstrating that both occupy the same site on DR1. Half inhibition could be obtained at relatively low (sevenfold) molar excess of the competitor over the biotinylated peptide (Fig. 2C). As the concentration of the competitor was increased, the fluorescence decreased, reaching 80% inhibition at a molar ratio of 110. A higher excess of competitor could not be obtained because of the limited solubility of the natural determinant and the need for relatively large amounts of biotinylated peptide in order to observe a distinct fluorescent signal.

Binding of the biotinylated peptide was detectable only after 30 minutes and continued to increase even after a 16-hour incubation (data not shown). Because binding to the class-II-deficient cells was not detectable, even at the longest incubation time, we can assume the increase in fluorescence with time reflects the kinetics of association of the peptide with HLA-DR. The low rate of cell-surface binding is consistent with the previously reported kinetics of association between peptides and purified class II molecules in detergent (Buus et al. 1986). When cells were incubated with peptide, stained with streptavidin, washed, and further incubated at 37°C, a gradual, slight reduction in cell-surface fluorescence was observed over several hours

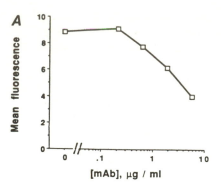

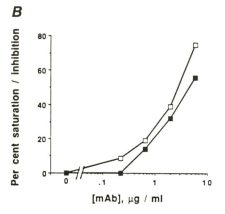

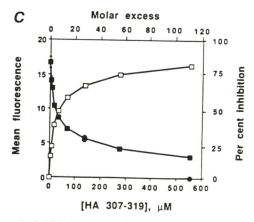

Figure 2. Inhibition of peptide binding by an anti-DR monoclonal antibody and the natural HA determinant. (*A*) MAJA cells were incubated with the peptide (50 μM) in the presence of varying amounts of protein-A-Sepharose-purified L243 anti-DR antibody (Shackelford et al. 1983), stained, and analyzed as in Fig. 1. Results are displayed as mean fluorescence per cell minus background. At concentrations above 10 μg/ml, the antibody agglutinated the cells. (*B*) Comparison of the reduction in fluorescent signal by L243 (■) and the fraction of DR molecules bound by antibody (□) as determined by indirect immunofluorescence using varying amounts of L243 as in *A*, followed by fluoresceinated rabbit anti-mouse Ig. (*C*) MAJA cells were coincubated with the biotinylated HA analog and varying amounts of HA 307-319. Both the fluorescence (■; scale on left) and the fractional reduction in fluorescent signal (□; scale on right) are shown. RJ 2.2.5 cells incubated with biotinylated peptide and competitor gave no signal (●).

(data not shown). The kinetic data demonstrated that binding does not approach a true equilibrium over the time of the assay and that dissociation is negligible on the time scale of the staining procedure.

The incubation temperature was a critical factor in the generation of the fluorescent signal. Peptide binding to DR1 was halved at 25°C and reduced by two thirds at 4°C relative to 37°C. However, a variety of inhibitors of antigen processing (sodium azide, colchicine, cytochalasin B, chloroquine, and ammonium chloride) had no effect, suggesting that internalization of the peptide was not required for binding.

The ease of the assay and the availability of the homozygous B-LCL allowed us to examine the ability of the biotinylated HA peptide to bind to 22 cell lines expressing different DR types (Fig. 3). Remarkably, even though the fluorescence signal (Fig. 3A) varied significantly between cell lines, detectable fluorescence distinct from background was present in each case with the exception of the class-II-deficient cell line. The variation in fluorescence could not be explained by

differences in DR expression between cell lines (shown in Fig. 3B). When peptide binding was corrected for these variations by dividing the fluorescence obtained with peptide by that obtained with the anti-DR monoclonal antibody (Fig. 3C), significant differences between cell lines remained, which allowed classification of the cells into groups having haplotypes with high (DR14a Dw16, DR13a Dw18, DR13b Dw19, DR16 Dw21), low (DR17 Dw3, DR9, DR4 Dw15), or intermediate (all others) capacity for associating with the HA peptide.

The broad range of binding exhibited by this peptide is surprising, particularly in the context of MHC-restricted recognition. However, two important features of this assay, which might contribute to the large degeneracy of binding, should be emphasized: (1) The assay requires a large amount of peptide (50 μM) relative to that necessary for stimulation of T cells and (2) the assay is performed in the absence of any competitive peptides. At physiologically relevant concentrations of peptide, the binding to the different cell lines

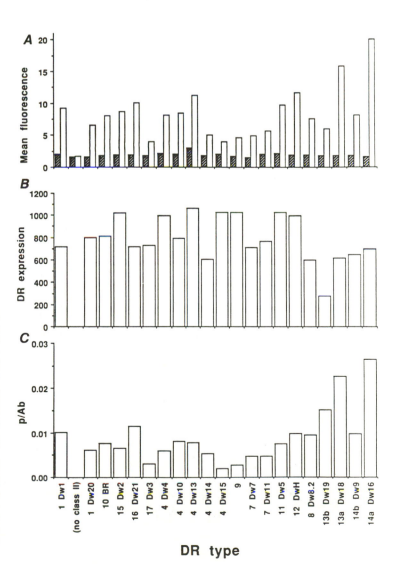

Figure 3. Binding of the HA peptide to B-LCL homozygous for different DR alleles. (A) Mean fluorescence on cell lines homozygous for the DR types indicated, when incubated with peptide (open bars) and without peptide (hatched bars). The cell lines used were MAJA (DR1 Dw1), LWAGS (DR1 Dw20), EFI-ND (10BR), PGF (DR15 Dw2), WT18 (DR16 Dw21), WT20 (DR17 Dw3), PRIESS (DR4 Dw4), AL10 (DR4 Dw10), JHF (DR4 Dw13), PE117 (DR4 Dw14), HIN-ND (DR4 Dw15), KOZ (DR9), MANN (DR7 Dw7), DBB (DR7 Dw11), IDF (DR11 Dw5), HERLUF (DR12 Dw H), OLL (DR8 Dw8.2), DAUDI (DR13b Dw19), ARNT (DR13a Dw18), WT52 (DR14b Dw9), and AZL (DR14a Dw16). (B) Mean fluorescence on the same cells stained with directly fluoresceinated L243 anti-DR monoclonal antibody (Becton Dickinson). (C) Relative peptide binding (from panel A) divided by relative antibody binding (from panel B).

might be quite different. In addition, when incubated with a variety of peptides, as in the case of a natural influenza infection, this particular peptide might not occupy the majority of sites on the class II molecules. However, the lowest levels of cell-surface fluorescence measured in this assay are relevant to T-cell responsiveness: DR4 Dw15-expressing cells, which bound the biotinylated HA analog most weakly, presented the natural HA determinant to a HA-specific T-lymphocyte clone equally well over a range of concentrations as the autologous restriction element, DR1 Dw1, which binds the biotinylated peptide at intermediate levels (J. Rothbard et al., in prep.). In addition, the broad range of binding reported here is unique to the HA peptide. Four other T-cell determinants also bind the 22 B-LCL, but the high-binding alleles are not identical for each peptide (J. Rothbard et al., in prep.). If generally true, these results indicate that a major factor in MHC restriction of T-cell recognition must arise from MHC/T-cell receptor interactions and not simply from different capacities to bind peptide.

Identification of Amino Acids Critical for Binding

Previous experiments exchanging amino acids between two DR1-restricted determinants suggested that both peptides adopted an α helix when bound (Rothbard et al. 1988). In this model, the side chains of the amino acids comprising the upper face of a helical peptide extend out of the antigen combining site, and the residues that form the opposite facade and the sides of the helix make important contacts with complementary residues of the HLA molecule. Consequently, substitution of individual residues of the peptide by a bulky amino acid should differentially affect the stability of the complex, depending on the steric requirements of each contact and the relative importance of each amino acid in binding. However, the structure of the antigen combining site of the MHC molecule has evolved to bind multiple, unrelated peptides and, therefore, is expected to tolerate many point substitutions in a peptide with only slight effects on the apparent affinity of binding. This might be why previous studies (Sette et al. 1987) examining binding of ovalbumin peptide analogs to murine class II molecules have failed to unambiguously define critical MHC contact residues. However, an unnaturally large side chain might cause greater steric interference with binding than substitution with any natural amino acid, thereby allowing us to observe a greater reduction in binding upon altering a critical residue.

To test this hypothesis, a set of peptides containing a derivative of biotinylated lysine with an additional hydrocarbon spacer, long-chain biotin (LCB) (Hofmann et al. 1982), substituted for each residue of the hemagglutinin peptide was synthesized. When peptides containing lysine-LCB at each position were incubated with the cells, marked differences were seen in the

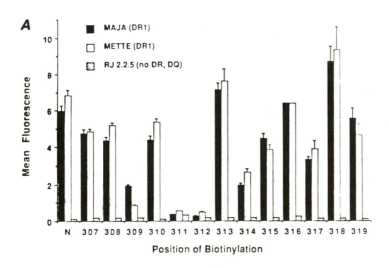

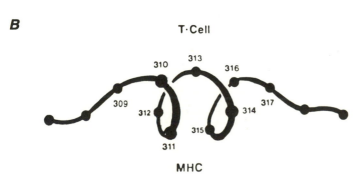

Figure 4. Differential binding of analogs of HA 307-319, biotinylated at each position, to DR1-homozygous, EBV-transformed B cells. (*A*) Each peptide (50 μM) was incubated with transformed B-cells homozygous for DR1 Dw1 (MAJA ■ and METTE □) or the DR-negative B-cell line, RJ2.2.5 (hatched), stained, and analyzed by flow cytometry. The relative amount of peptide bound to cells was judged by the intensity of green fluorescence per cell, averaged over all viable cells. Background as determined by control incubations in the absence of biotinylated peptide was subtracted. The results shown are the average of three assays with the standard deviation displayed with error bars. (*B*) Model of the conformation adopted by the peptide when bound to DR1, deduced from the binding results shown in *A*. Residues 309–317 are folded into an α helix, with an orientation that permits residues 310, 313, and 316 to point away from, while 309, 311, 312, 314, 315, and 317 would be directed toward the antigen combining site. The amino acids at both termini, which tolerate biotinylation, are not drawn as part of the helix because of their apparent conformational flexibility.

resultant fluorescent signal (Fig. 4A). Strong fluorescence was present when lysine-LCB was either placed at the amino terminus or substituted for Pro-307, Lys-308, Val-310, Asp-313, Lys-316, and Ala-318. In contrast, no detectable fluorescence was observed when peptides containing lysine-LCB at residues 311 and 312 were used, whereas substitution at 309, 314, 315, or 317 resulted in reduced fluorescence.

A loss of the fluorescent signal upon biotinylating any residue might occur because the ability of the peptide to bind to DR1 is reduced by the modification, or because the peptide still binds, but with the biotinyl group sterically unavailable to streptavidin. In the latter case, no fluorescent signal should be apparent at any concentration, because steric inaccessibility should not depend on the amount of peptide in the assay. The appearance of a fluorescent signal when analogs containing lysine-LCB at 309, 311, and 312 were used at concentrations well above 50 μM (data not shown) indicated that biotinylation affected the apparent affinity of the analogs for DR1.

The ability of the analogs to bind to the restriction element on cell surfaces could have been affected by the biotinylation in a number of different ways: (1) by interfering with a critical contact between the peptide and the class II proteins; (2) by altering the propensity of the peptide to adopt the conformation in which it bound to DR1; or (3) by changing the susceptibility of the analog to proteolytic degradation. The second possibility was unlikely because each of the 14 peptide analogs had indistinguishable circular dichroism spectra (data not shown) in TFE/water mixtures containing TFE concentrations at which the helical propensities of closely related, unbiotinylated HA analogs were significantly different (vide infra). The third possible explanation for the different fluorescent signals generated by each analog, differential proteolysis, was more difficult to disprove. However, none of the low fluorescent signals was increased in the presence of a cocktail of proteinase inhibitors (TPCK, PMSF, leupeptin, aprotinin, and soybean trypsin inhibitor). Therefore, the differences in fluorescence appear to arise from the varying capacity of the class II molecule to bind the analogs, reflecting the differential effect of biotinylation at each position on the affinity of the interaction.

If this interpretation is true, then the assay provides a quantitative measure of the involvement of each amino acid of the peptide in the formation of the complex: The lower the signal, the more important the amino acid is. Therefore, we can conclude that Tyr-309, Lys-311, Glu-312, and, to a lesser extent Thr-314, Leu-315, and Leu-317, contribute to the formation of the complex.

The peptide might bind to DR1 in a variety of ways. However, the distinct variations in fluorescence observed when the different analogs were assayed implied that the number of conformations and orientations of the bound peptide was limited. In all possible modes of binding, residues 311 and 312 form critical contacts with the restriction element, because biotinylation at

these positions eliminated the fluorescent signal at the peptide concentration used. A further constraint on the possible conformations of the bound peptide was that the fluorescent profile peaked at every third residue (310, 313, and 316) within the central portion of the peptide, with significantly less fluorescence in between. The periodicity suggested that the central core adopted a helical conformation. However, the results were not consistent with the peptide's being helical over its entire length, because analogs containing lysine-LCB at 308 and 318 resulted in a strong signal. If the peptide adopted a perfect helix with 310, 313, and 316 pointing up, these residues should point down. The ability to tolerate substitution with biotinylated lysine at both ends of the peptide might be explained by an increased accessibility of the termini of the helix or by deviations from an ideal α helix. A model based on this interpretation of the pattern of fluorescence is shown in Figure 4B, consisting of a helical core (residues 309–317), with the two amino acids at each end of the peptide exhibiting greater conformational freedom and not modeled as part of the repeating structure.

Stabilization of a Helical Conformation Results in Increased Antigenicity

If the hemagglutinin peptide binds the restriction element as an intact or partial α helix, then stabilization of this conformation should improve the potency of the peptide. Recent experiments have demonstrated that stabilization of the macrodipole of an α helix can result in a significant increase in the helical content of relatively short peptides (Shoemaker et al. 1987). One way to stabilize the macrodipole is to remove the charges at the amino and carboxyl termini of the peptide by acetylation and amidation.

The natural hemagglutinin peptide and several analogs were examined for secondary structure content by CD in a range of water/TFE mixtures. The unacetylated and unamidated hemagglutinin peptide exhibited only low helicity even at high TFE concentration (Fig. 5A), as judged by absorption of circularly polarized light at 222 nm. Amidation, acetylation, and, to a greater extent, combined acetylation and amidation, substantially increased the helicity of the hemagglutinin peptide. When tested in proliferation assays with the T-cell clone, HA1.7, the acetylated and amidated peptide stimulated the clone at approximately two orders of magnitude lower concentrations than the natural sequence (Fig. 5B).

Recognition and Competition by Analogs Containing Point Substitutions

To begin to understand the physical and chemical requirements at each position of the peptide for binding to DR1 and recognition by the T-cell receptor of HA 1.7, sets of peptides containing point substitutions at each position in the sequence were synthesized. Each peptide was assayed over a concentration range from

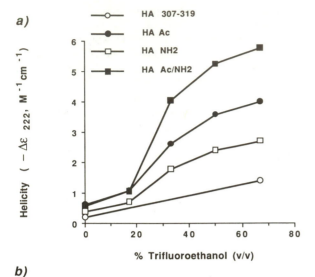

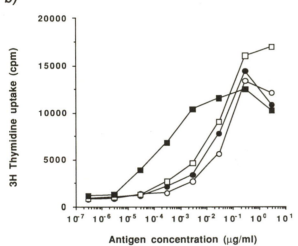

Figure 5. Chemical modification of HA 307-319 resulted in both greater helical propensity and increased antigenicity. (*a*) Helicity of the natural peptide (HA 307-319), or derivatives that were either acetylated (HA Ac), amidated (HA NH2), or both (HA Ac/NH2), measured in varying water/trifluoroethanol mixtures. (*b*) T-cell proliferation in response to acetylated and amidated analogs of HA 307-319. The response to the natural sequence is shown for comparison.

0.03 to 30 μg/ml for its ability to stimulate the hemagglutinin-specific clone. The proliferative responses relative to the natural sequence at 0.3 μg/ml are shown in Figure 6A. As in previous studies on both class I- and class II-restricted T-cell recognition (Allen et al. 1987; Sette et al. 1987; Gotch et al. 1988; Ogasawara et al. 1989; Rothbard et al. 1989), relatively few substitutions resulted in peptides that were recognized better than the natural sequence (R, K-307; Q-310; K-314).

Several peptides containing a point substitution, which resulted in complete loss of recognition by HA1.7, were tested for their ability to displace the natural sequence containing an amino-terminal LC-biotin from the antigen-combining site of DR1 on the surface of an EBV-transformed B-cell line (Fig. 6B). Interestingly, with the exception of a peptide contain-

ing serine at 309, they all successfully competed to varying extents. Some of the best competitors were analogs that contained substitutions at positions shown to tolerate long-chain biotin and that were postulated to point outward from the site (307, 308, 310, 313, and 316). Surprisingly, analogs containing substitutions at residues believed important for binding (311, 312, and 314) also bound sufficiently well to compete effectively.

Taken together with the earlier experiments on ovalbumin and cytochrome peptides (Sette et al. 1987; Ogasawara et al. 1989) and related studies on class-I-restricted determinants (Gotch et al. 1988; Rothbard et al. 1989), these findings indicate there is not an absolute requirement for a single amino acid in most positions in T-cell determinants. Monosubstitutions in the peptide may change the detailed interactions with the MHC protein or the surface of the peptide/MHC complex as seen by the T-cell receptor, but without significantly reducing the amount of peptide bound to the restriction element. Consequently, experiments using analogs containing point substitutions to determine relative orientation of the peptide can lead to results that are difficult to interpret. Only if, as shown above using long-chain biotinylated lysine, the substitutions are sufficiently drastic will distinct variations in binding be apparent. This high degree of tolerance to sequence variation in the peptide might be expected for a binding site containing several amino acids of different physical character in close proximity to each residue of the agretope. In addition, the flexibility of the side chains in the binding site might allow the MHC protein to accommodate the steric effects of monosubstitutions.

HA Peptide Does Not Bind All DR Alleles Equally

The results of earlier studies with allogenic presenting cell panels had indicated that the DR1-restricted T-cell clone HA1.7, isolated from a DR1,3 individual, responded to antigen presented by DR4- but not by DR7-expressing cells (Eckels et al. 1984). To confirm the results of the panel study, the restriction specificity of the T cells was examined, using murine L cells transfected with HLA-DR genes. Cells expressing either DR1 Dw1 or DR4 Dw15 were able to present HA 307-319 equally effectively to the cloned T cells. In contrast, cells expressing DR7 Dw7 failed to stimulate any response. Given that the *a* chains are conserved between DR molecules, the sequence of the β1 domain of DR1 Dw1 and DR4 Dw15, but not DR7 Dw7, must be sufficiently similar to allow equivalent interactions to occur between the peptide and the antigen receptor of HA1.7.

The amino acid sequences of the β1 domains of these class II molecules are compared in Table 1. DR1, DR4 Dw15, and DR7 differ in sequence in the central strands of the β-pleated sheet (positions 9, 11, 13, 28, 30, and 32), as well as in the positions corresponding to the helical section of the β chain. In contrast, DR1 Dw1 and DR4 Dw15 differ only in the strands and not the helix, with the exception of a single substitution at

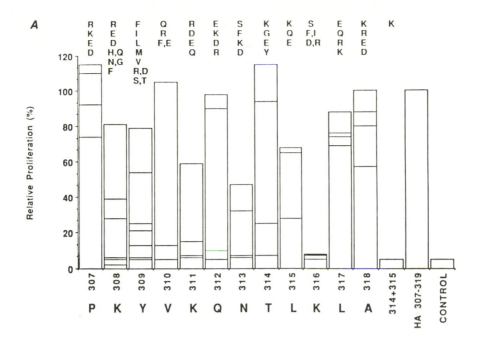

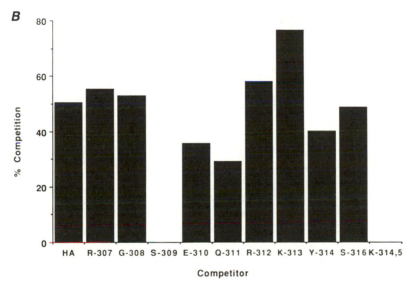

Figure 6. (*A*)The ability of peptide analogs of HA 307-319 containing substitutions to stimulate the HA-specific T-cell clone. The proliferation assays were performed as described in Methods. Proliferation to the substituted peptides is expressed as a percentage of the response observed to the natural sequence (HA 307-319) at the optimal concentration (0.3 μg/ml), although each peptide was tested over a dose range from 0.3 to 30 μg/ml. The horizontal axis represents the sequence of the natural determinant; monosubstitutions at each position are shown above the histogram in order of decreasing proliferation. Where the two peptides gave indistinguishable proliferation, they are shown on the same line. A disubstituted peptide containing two lysines at positions 314 and 315 also is included. The proliferative response of cloned T cells cultured with accessory cells in the absence of antigen is shown as a control. (*B*) Percent competition of monosubstituted HA peptides for binding of the amino-terminally biotinylated HA analog to the DR1 Dw1 homozygous B-cell line, MAJA. Cells were simultaneously incubated with 50 μM biotinylated peptide and 300 μM (sixfold molar excess) competitor peptide, stained, and analyzed as described in Methods.

residue 57. As shown earlier, the peptide binds each of the alleles. Because a single T-cell clone and peptide antigen were used in these experiments, differential responsiveness cannot have arisen from differences in the T-cell receptor or mechanisms of tolerance induction. Therefore, the inability of the clone to be stimulated by DR7 Dw7$^+$-presenting cells must be due to

either sequence variation in the β-chain helix interfering with the interaction with the T-cell receptor or the peptide binding differently to DR7 Dw7 than DR1 or DR4 Dw15.

To analyze the degeneracy further, EBV-transformed B cells representative of the different DR4 Dw subtypes were used to present HA 307-319 to the

Table 1. Primary Amino Acid Sequence of the β1 Domains of the HLA-DR1, DR4 DW, and DR7 DW7 Class II Proteins

```
                  10          20          30          40          50
DR1 DW1    G D T R P R F L W Q L K F E C H F F N G T E R V R L L E R C I Y N Q E E S V R F D S D V G E Y R A V
DR4 DW4    - - - - - - - E - V - H - - - - - - - - - - - - - - - F - D - Y F - H - - - Y - - - - - - - - - - -
DR4 DW10   - - - - - - - E - V - H - - - - - - - - - - - - - - - F - D - Y F - H - - - Y - - - - - - - - - - -
DR4 DW13   - - - - - - - E - V - H - - - - - - - - - - - - - - - F - D - Y F - H - - - Y - - - - - - - - - - -
DR4 DW14   - - - - - - - E - V - H - - - - - - - - - - - - - - - F - D - Y F - H - - - Y - - - - - - - - - - -
DR4 DW15   - - - - - - - E - V - H - - - - - - - - - - - - - - - F - D - Y F - H - - - Y - - - - - - - - - - -
DR7 DW7    - - - Q - - - - G - Y K - - - - - - - - - - - - - - - Q F - - - L F - - - - - - - - - - - F - - - - -

                                                                        90
                  60          70          80
DR1 DW1    T E L G R P D A E Y W N S Q K D L L E Q R R A A V D T Y C R H N Y G V G E S F T V Q R R
DR4 DW4    - - - - - - - - - - - - - - - - K - - - - - - - - - - - - - - - - - - - - - - - - -
DR4 DW10   - - - - - - - - - - - - - I - - D E - - - - - - - - - - V - - - - - - - - - - - - -
DR4 DW13   - - - - - - - - - - - - - - - - - E - - - - - - - - - - V - - - - - - - - - - - - -
DR4 DW14   - - - - - S - - - - - - - - - - - - - - - - - - - - - - V - - - - - - - - - - - - -
DR4 DW15   - - - - - S - - - - - - - I - - D - - G Q - - - V - - - - - - - - - - - - - - - - -
DR7 DW7    - - - - - V - - S - - - - - I - - D - - G Q - - - V - - - - - - - - - - - - - - - - -
```

cloned T cells. Marked variations in the efficiency of antigen presentation were observed when the subtypes were compared (Table 2). Accessory cells expressing DR4 Dw4 were capable of inducing only two thirds of the maximum stimulation observed with DR1. DR4 Dw13- and DR4 Dw14-positive EBV-transformed B-cell lines were even less effective, inducing only a marginal proliferative response, and DR4 Dw10 cells failed to present the peptide. These differences could not be accounted for by variation in the level of surface DR because, by flow cytometric analysis, the DR density on all of the EBV B-cell line was very similar. Furthermore, the identical pattern of responsiveness was observed when fixed cells were used (data not shown), suggesting that the inability of DR4 Dw10 EBV-B cells to present was not the result of differential processing (Fox et al. 1988). Interestingly, the relative ability of the alleles to present the natural sequence did not correlate with their capacity to bind the peptide. When normalized for DR expression, the peptide with glutamine at 312 and biotinylated at the amino terminus bound Dw13 > Dw4 > DR1 ~ Dw10 > Dw14 ~ Dw15.

In contrast with the sequence comparison of DR1 and DR4 Dw15, which differ in residues composing the β-pleated sheets, alignment of the DR4 subtypes revealed variations at six positions all present in the helical portion of the β chain (Table 2). The equal efficiency of DR1 and DR4 Dw15 to present antigen indicated that substitution of serine for aspartic acid at position 57 was not critical for recognition. However, a conservative replacement of lysine for arginine at position 71 significantly reduced the ability of DR4 Dw4 B cells to present antigen relative to DR4 Dw15. In addition, mutation of glycine to valine at position 86 also affected recognition, because DR4 Dw14 differs from DR1 only at this position. DR4 Dw13 has a valine at position 86 as well as a glutamic acid at 74 but, nevertheless, can present the peptide as well as DR4 Dw14. DR4 Dw10, the least effective allele, differs from DR1 at four positions, leucine to isoleucine at 67, glutamine to aspartic acid at 70, arginine to glutamic acid at 71, and glycine to valine at 86. In the proposed model for

MHC class II molecules (Brown et al. 1988), residues 67 and 71 point into the antigen combining site, whereas 70 and 74 are situated on the upper surface of the helix and potentially could interact with the T-cell receptor. Residues 57 and 86 are present at opposite ends of the site and are not centrally located.

If the differences in the ability of the alleles to present the peptide reflect their differential ability to bind HA 307-319, the variation might be apparent when screened using the set of biotinylated analogs. The set of peptides was assayed for their ability to bind each of the homozygous B-cell lines. The patterns of fluorescence observed with DR1 Dw1, DR4 Dw4, and Dw13 expressing B cell lines were similar (Fig. 7, A–C). In each case, the fluorescence varied significantly between analogs, with peaks of fluorescence present at every third residue (310, 313, 316) in the central portion of the peptide. This result was consistent with a previously postulated model for the HA peptide in the binding site of HLA-DR1 (Fig. 4B) in which the residues of the central core adopt an α-helical conformation with residues 310, 313, and 316 of the peptide pointing away from the MHC-binding site and residues 309, 311, 312, 314, 317, and perhaps 315 interacting with the class II molecule, whereas both amino and carboxyl termini have greater flexibility and tolerate biotinylation indiscriminately. The similarity between the binding patterns to DR1, DR4 Dw4, and DR4 Dw13 expressing cells indicated that the peptide adopted a similar conformation on these three restriction elements, even though residue 315 appeared to be more important for binding on the DR4 subtypes. In contrast, the pattern for DR4 Dw10 was different (Fig. 7D), with significant variations in fluorescence apparent over fewer amino acids, residues 310–315. Greater fluorescence was observed for the analogs with substitutions at residues 313 and 314 than at 310, 311, 312, and 315. The different fluorescent profiles indicated that the peptide bound DR4 Dw10 in a conformation dissimilar to that adopted on DR1, DR4 Dw4 and Dw13, and suggested that this could be the explanation for the nonresponsiveness of the T-cell clone observed when the peptide was presented in the context of DR4 Dw10.

Table 2. Differential Response of Cloned T Cells to HA 307–319 Presented by EBV-transformed B Cells Expressing the DRdw Subtypes (Gregerson et al. 1986)

| HLA-DR specificity | Amino acids at β-chain positions | | | | | | | Proliferative response (Δcpm) (3 μg/ml) |
	57	67	69	70	71	74	86	
DR1	D	L	E	Q	R	A	G	34288
DR4 dw4	D	L	E	Q	K	A	G	22793
dw10	D	I	E	D	E	A	V	2435
dw13	D	L	E	Q	R	E	V	17554
dw14	D	L	E	Q	R	A	V	14562
dw15	S	L	E	Q	R	A	G	38416

Culture conditions and proliferation were determined as described in Methods. Results are expressed as Δcpm with the background response of T cells cultured with EBV-transformed B cells (<3500 cpm) subtracted from proliferation observed when antigen is present.

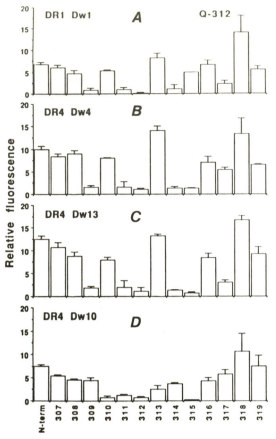

Figure 7. Binding of biotinylated HA analogs to EBV-transformed human B-lymphoblastoid cells homozygous for DR1 and DR4 Dw subtypes. Sets of HA analogs, long-chain biotinylated at either the terminal α amino group or via lysines substituted at the positions indicated, (*A–D*), were assayed for binding to EBV-B cells expressing DR1 Dw1 (*A*), DR4 Dw4 (*B*), DR4 Dw13 (*C*), or DR4 Dw10 (*D*). Results are expressed as mean fluorescence (arbitrary units) minus background, and with error bars indicating the standard deviations of the relative fluorescence pattern from three separate experiments. None of the analogs bound to the class-II-deficient EBV-B cell line, RJ 2.2.5.

To determine whether the variations in the fluorescence profiles generated on each allele could be interpreted in terms of simple changes in the preferred conformation of the bound peptide, the fluorescence profiles were normalized and subtracted from each other to quantify the differences. Comparison of the fluorescence profiles for DR4 Dw4 and Dw13 did not reveal significant differences for any of the residues comprising the central core (309–317), indicating that the peptide bound in manner sufficiently similar to both alleles that no differences can be detected using this method. However, when the pattern seen on DR4 Dw4 was compared to that on DR1 (Fig. 8A), significant changes in the fluorescence profile were apparent at several positions. The largest changes on DR4 Dw4 relative to DR1 were the increased fluorescence when lysine-LCB was substituted for residues 310, 313, and 317 and a decrease for the analog with lysine-LCB at

position 315. An increase in fluorescence indicates that the position becomes more tolerant of biotinylation and implies that the residue becomes less important in stabilizing the complex. The opposite is true for a decrease in fluorescence. When viewed in the context of a helical model for the central core of the peptide (Fig. 4B), the observed differences in the fluorescent pattern between DR4 Dw4 and DR1 can be explained by a small rotation of the helix about its axis, increasing the accessibility of residues 313, 317, and 310, while decreasing that of residue 315. Failure to observe significant differences at other positions emphasized that the rotation cannot be too great to perturb their contacts. In addition, the rotation must be sufficiently limited to allow the identical T-cell receptor to recognize the peptide bound to either DR1 or DR4 Dw4 and Dw13.

Comparing a normalized pattern for binding to DR4 Dw10 with that for DR1 results in a greater number of differences than seen when comparing DR4 Dw4 with DR1 (Fig. 8A). The fluorescent signals generated with peptides biotinylated at positions 309, 314, and 317 are increased, whereas biotinylation at 310, 313, and 315 decreased the fluorescence. These differences cannot be explained by a single rotation of the bound peptide about a helical axis. However, the changes are consistent with the amino-terminal half of the central core (residues 309–313) rotating clockwise as shown in Figure 8B, while the carboxy-terminal half (314–317) rotates counterclockwise. This could be due either to the central hydrogen bonds of the helix breaking, resulting in an opening of the helix by twisting either end, or to an increase in the pitch of the helix and the number of residues per turn on DR4 Dw10 compared to DR1. Again, the differences in the conformation of the peptide bound to DR1 and DR4 Dw10 must be quite small, because, in either case, the residues of the central core that best tolerate biotinylation segregate on the same face of the helical wheel shown in Figure 8B.

The experiments reported in this paper are consistent with the model of the antigen receptor of the T cell contacting the surface of the complex formed by the helices of the α and β chains of the class II molecule and those residues of the antigen that are sterically available (Davis and Bjorkman 1988). The ability of the receptor to cross-react with either other peptides bound by the same restriction element or the same peptide on different alleles will depend on the similarity of the contact surface of each peptide/MHC complex. Changes in this surface can arise either from (1) substitutions of residues in the β-chain helix of class II or in the bound peptide that point directly toward the T-cell receptor (e.g., residues 70 of the β chain or residue 313 of the HA peptide; Fig. 1B) or (2) the peptide binding the restriction element in slightly different conformations (e.g., binding to DR4 Dw10 compared to DR1; Fig. 8). Depending of the details of the contacts between the peptide and the class II molecule, the exact atoms that constitute the upper surface of the complex will differ. In general, how the residues comprising the

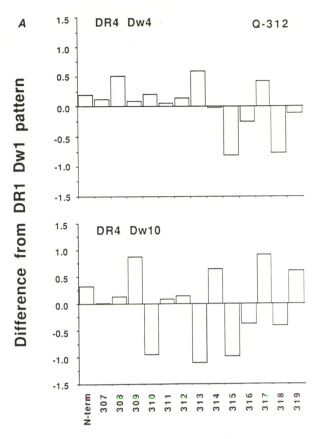

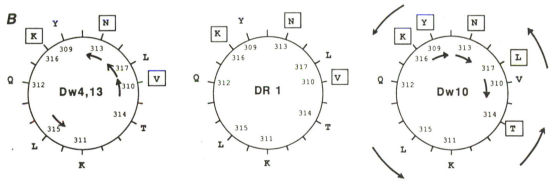

Figure 8. (*A*) Quantitation of the differences in the fluorescence found when the biotinylated HA analogs were tested on cells homozygous for DR1, DR4 Dw4, and DR4 Dw10. To eliminate the effects of variations in DR expression between cell lines and the apparent affinity of individual alleles for the HA peptide from the data shown in Figure 7*A*–*D*, the fluorescence generated by each analog on any cell line was divided by the mean fluorescent signal of all analogs for that cell line. The resultant normalized fluorescence profile generated for DR1 Dw1 was then subtracted from that for DR4 Dw4 or DR4 Dw10. (*B*) Interpretation of the differences in the fluorescence profiles between alleles in terms of minimal conformational adjustments in the peptide helix. Residues of the central core that gave peaks in the fluorescence profile (Fig. 7A) are boxed. Arrows indicate the sense of rotation of a residue that would be consistent with the differences between the fluorescent signals generated on different alleles by the analog biotinylated at that position. The rotations of the peptide main chain on DR4 Dw4 or Dw13 and DR4 Dw10 are shown relative to DR1. For DR4 Dw10, rotations for residues 309–313 have been shown inside and those for residues 314–317 outside the helical wheel to emphasize that the amino and carboxyl termini appear to twist in opposite directions. Differences in length between arrows do not imply quantitative differences in the degree of rotation.

sides of the helices of the antigen combining site and the antigenic peptide interact with each other might be an important factor in determining the detailed T-cell receptor contact surface of the peptide/class II complex. Clearly, experimental proof of such subtle

changes will require the crystallographic determination of the structure of the class II/peptide complex. However, the strategy of using a combination of functional assays and binding studies to model the class II/peptide complex can be extended by introducing single amino acid mutations in the restriction element as well as in the peptide. This will permit the dissection of the detailed contributions of individual residues in T-cell recognition and HLA restriction, which will both complement the crystallographic studies and be required to understand how the T-cell repertoire is established.

ACKNOWLEDGMENTS

We thank Kevin Howland and Caroline Fenton for excellent technical assistance; Drs. Steve Martin and Peter Bailey, National Institute for Medical Research, Mill Hill, for help with the circular dichroism measurements; Dr. Julia Bodmer and Steve Marsh for the anti-DR monoclonal antibodies and EBV-transformed B-cell lines; Dr. Roberto Accolla for the class-II-negative B-cell line, RJ 2.2.5; and Wendy Senior for help with preparation of the manuscript.

REFERENCES

Accolla, R. 1983. Human B cell variants immunoselected against a single Ia antigen subset have lost expression of several Ia antigen subsets. *J. Exp. Med.* **157:** 1053.

Allen, P., G. Matsueda, R. Evans, J. Dunbar, G. Marshall, and E. Unanue. 1987. Identification of the T cell and Ia contact residues of a T cell antigenic epitope. *Nature* **327:** 713.

Babbitt, B., P.M. Allen, G. Matsueda, E. Haber, and E. Unanue. 1985. The binding of immunogenic peptides to Ia histocompatibility molecules. *Nature* **317:** 359.

Bjorkman, P., M. Saper, B. Samraoui, W. Bennett, J. Strominger, and D. Wiley. 1987a. Structure of the human class I histocompatibility antigen, HLA-A2. *Nature* **329:** 506.

———. 1987b. The foreign antigen binding site and T cell recognition regions of class I histocompatibility antigens. *Nature* **329:** 512.

Brown, J., T. Jardetzky, M. Saper, B. Samraoui, P. Bjorkman, and D. Wiley. 1988. A hypothetical model of the foreign antigen combining site of class II histocompatibility molecules. *Nature* **332:** 845.

Buus, S., A. Sette, S. Colon, D. Jenis, and H. Grey. 1986. Isolation and characterisation of antigen-Ia complexes in T cell recognition. *Cell* **47:** 1071.

Chen, B. and P. Parham. 1989. Direct binding of influenza peptides to class I HLA molecules. *Nature* **337:** 743.

Davis, M. and P. Bjorkman. 1988. T cell antigen receptor genes and T cell recognition. *Nature* **334:** 395.

DeLisi, C. and J. Berzofsky. 1985. T cell antigenic sites tend to be amphipathic structures. *Proc. Natl. Acad. Sci.* **82:** 7048.

Eckels, D., T. Sell, S. Bronsen, A. Johnson, R. Hartzman, and J.R. Lamb. 1984. Human helper T cell clones that recognize different influenza hemagglutinin determinants are restricted by different HLA D region epitopes. *Immunogenetics* **19:** 409.

Fox, B., F. Carbone, R. Germain, Y. Patterson, and R. Schwartz. 1988. Processing of minimal antigenic peptide alters its interaction with MHC molecules. *Nature* **331:** 538.

Gotch, F., A. McMichael, and J. Rothbard. 1988. Recognition of influenza A matrix protein by HLA-A2 restricted cytotoxic T lymphocytes. Use of analogues to orientate the matrix peptide in the HLA-A2 binding site. *J. Exp. Med.* **168:** 2045.

Gregersen, P., M. Shen, Q. Song, P. Merryman, S. Degar, T. Seki, J. Maccari, D. Goldberg, H. Murphy, J. Schwenzer, C. Wang, R. Winchester, G. Nepom, and J. Silver. 1986. Molecular diversity of DR4 haplotypes. *Proc. Natl. Acad. Sci.* **83:** 2642.

Haskins, K., J. Kappler, and P. Marrack. 1983. The major histocompatibility complex-restricted antigen receptor on T cells. Isolation with a monoclonal antibody. *J. Exp. Med.* **157:** 1149.

Hedrick, S., E. Nielsen, J. Kavaler, D. Cohen, and M. Davis. 1984. Sequence relationships between putative T-cell receptor polypeptides and immunoglobulins. *Nature* **308:** 153.

Hofmann, K., G. Titus, J. Montibeller, and F. Finn. 1982. Avidin binding of carboxyl substituted biotin and analogues. *Biochemistry* **21:** 978.

Honjo, T. 1983. Immunoglobulin genes. *Annu. Rev. Immunol.* **1:** 499.

Hume, C., R. Accolla, and J. Lee. 1987. Defective HLA class II expression in a regulatory mutant is partially complemented by activated *ras* oncogenes. *Proc. Natl. Acad. Sci.* **84:** 8603.

Lechler, R., V. Bal, J. Rothbard, R. Germain, R. Sekaly, E. Long, and J. Lamb. 1988. HLA-DR restricted antigen induced activation of human helper T lymphocyte clone using transfected murine cell lines. *J. Immunol.* **141:** 3003.

McCormick, D. and J. Roth. 1970. Specificity, stereochemistry, and mechanism of the color reaction between p-dimethylaminocinnamaldehyde and biotin analogs. *Anal. Biochem.* **34:** 226.

Moller, O., ed. 1987. Role of somatic mutation in the generation of lymphocyte diversity. *Immunol. Rev.* **96:** 1.

Ogasawara, K., W. Maloy, B. Beverly, and R. Schwartz. 1989. Functional analysis of the antigenic structure of a minor T cell determinant from pigeon cytochrome C. *J. Immunol.* **142:** 1448.

Rothbard, J. and W. Taylor. 1988. A sequence pattern common to T cell epitopes. *EMBO J.* **7:** 93.

Rothbard, J., R. Pemberton, H. Bodmer, B.A. Askonas, and W.R. Taylor. 1989. Identification of residues necessary for clonally specific recognition of a cytotoxic T cell determinant. *EMBO J.* (in press).

Rothbard, J., R. Lechler, K. Howland, V. Bal, D. Eckels, R. Sekaly, E. Long, W. Taylor, and J. Lamb. 1988. Structural model of HLA-DR1 restricted T cell antigen recognition. *Cell* **52:** 515.

Sette, A., S. Buus, S. Colon, J. Smith, C. Miles, and H. Grey. 1987. Structural characteristics of an antigen required for its interaction with Ia and recognition by T cells. *Nature* **328:** 395.

Shackelford, D., L. Lampson, and J. Strominger. 1983. Separation of three class II antigens from a homozygous human B cell line. *J. Immunol.* **130:** 289.

Shoemaker, K., P. Kim, E. York, J. Stewart, and R. Baldwin. 1987. Test of the helix dipole model for stabilization of a helices. *Nature* **326:** 563.

Yanagi, Y., Y. Yoshikai, K. Leggett, S. Clark, I. Aleksander, and T. Mak. 1984. A human T cell specific cDNA clone encodes a protein having extensive homology to immunoglobulin chains. *Nature* **308:** 145.

Study on the Immunogenicity of Human Class-II-restricted T-cell Epitopes: Processing Constraints, Degenerate Binding, and Promiscuous Recognition

P. Panina-Bordignon,* S. Demotz,† G. Corradin,† and A. Lanzavecchia*
*Basel Institute for Immunology, Basel; †Institut de Biochemie, University of Lausanne, Epalinges, Switzerland

T lymphocytes recognize peptides derived from intracellular processing of antigens that have bound to major histocompatibility complex (MHC) molecules. Thus, the immunogenicity of a given epitope has three essential requirements: (1) The appropriate fragment must be generated by the processing machinery; (2) an MHC molecule must be present capable of binding this fragment; and (3) specific T cells must be available in the repertoire. Failure at any one of these steps results in failure to respond.

Data from experimental animal systems indicate that the capacity to respond to a given antigen is controlled by MHC gene products (Benacerraf 1978) and that the lack of an MHC molecule capable of binding antigen is the most frequent cause of unresponsiveness. Indeed, MHC molecules are highly polymorphic, and it has been shown that a given peptide can bind to only one or a few alleles, but never to all (Babbitt et al. 1985; Guillet et al. 1986; Buus et al. 1987). In addition, there are cases where the processing machinery fails to generate a given T-cell epitope (Buchmüller and Corradin 1982; Brett et al. 1988; Bodmer et al. 1989; Michalek et al. 1989). Finally, the response may fail because specific T cells have been deleted by self-tolerance (Vidovic and Matzinger 1989).

To understand what are the major constraints to a class-II-restricted response in humans, we studied the immunogenicity of three tetanus toxin (tt) epitopes in tetanus toxoid (TT)-immune donors. We found that two out of three epitopes are universally immunogenic, since they activate many different T-cell clones restricted by different class II molecules. Surprisingly, we found that processing patterns may vary from donor to donor, since the antigen-presenting cells (APCs) of some donors, although capable of presenting denatured TT, are unable to generate a given epitope when pulsed with native tt. Finally, we found that, whereas some T cells show the classic form of allele-specific MHC restriction, others have a promiscuous pattern of restriction, since they can recognize the peptide in the context of many MHC alleles. The finding of such promiscuous clones allows us to speculate about the basis of the MHC restriction specificity.

METHODS

Synthetic peptides. p2 (tt 830-844 QYIKANSKFIGITEL), p30 (tt 947-967 FNNFTVSFWLRVPKVSASHLE), and p4 (tt 1274-1283 GQIGNDPNRDIL) have been mapped and synthesized as described previously (Demotz et al. 1989a). Native tt was obtained from Calbiochem (La Jolla, California). TT was obtained from the Swiss Serum Institute, Bern. Reduced carboxymethylated TT (RCM-TT) was prepared as described previously (Demotz et al. 1989b).

Isolation of peptide-specific T-cell clones. The cloning and maintenance of human T cells have been described in detail elsewhere (Lanzavecchia et al. 1988). The medium was RPMI 1640 supplemented with 2 μM L-glutamine, 1% nonessential amino acids, 1% Na pyruvate, 50 μg/ml kanamycin, and either 5% human serum (HS) or 10% fetal calf serum (FCS). Peripheral blood mononuclear cells (PBMC) from HLA-typed, TT-primed donors were cultured at 7×10^5/ml in RPMI-HS with p2, p4, or p30 (10 μM) or medium alone in several 200-μl cultures in 96-well flat-bottom microplates. After 6 days, human recombinant IL-2 (Roche, Nutley, New Jersey) was added at 30 units/ml, and after 4 additional days, the cultures were inspected for cell growth. Cultures with growing cells occurred at higher frequency in peptide-stimulated cultures as compared to control cultures without peptide. The positive cultures were further expanded in IL-2 and tested for their capacity to recognize the peptide. As a rapid screening assay, an aliquot of T cells was transferred to a U-bottom plate, washed three times, and resuspended in 200 μl RPMI-FCS in the presence or absence of the peptide at 20 μM. Since human activated T cells express class II molecules, they are able to present the peptide to each other, resulting in a visible agglutination after 6 hours at 37°C. Positive cultures were cloned by limiting dilution, and peptide-specific clones were isolated and maintained using phytohemagglutinin and irradiated allogeneic PBMC as described previously (Lanzavecchia et al. 1988). Only one specific clone was kept from each positive well.

Proliferation assay. Cultures were set up in 200-μl RPMI-FCS in flat-bottom microplates. T cells (3×10^4) were cultured with 2×10^4 irradiated (6000 R) Epstein-Barr virus (EBV) transformed B cells or with 10^5 irradiated (3500 R) PBMC. TT, tt, or peptides were either added in culture or used to pulse the EBV B cells. After 2 days, the cultures were pulsed with 1 μCi [^{3}H]thymidine (Amersham, sp. act. 5 Ci/mM), and the radioactivity incorporated was measured after an additional 16 hours by liquid scintillation.

Determination of the T-cell restriction pattern. The isotype of class II molecules recognized by each T-cell clone was determined by antibody-blocking experiments. T cells were cultured with autologous EBV B cells, limiting concentrations of peptide and anti-DR (L243, ATCC, 1:4 culture supernatant), anti-DQ (SVPL3, provided by H. Spits), or anti-DP (B7.21, provided by J. Trowsdale), both as ascites diluted 1:1000. To identify the DR- or DP-restricting alleles, we used a panel of allogeneic HLA-homozygous EBV B cells as APCs. The cells were pulsed for 2 hours at 37°C with the peptide or medium alone, washed 4 times, and irradiated (6000 R). We found proliferation in response to unpulsed allogeneic cells in only very rare cases.

RESULTS

Two of Three Epitopes of Tetanus Toxin Are Universally Immunogenic

In mice, the affinity of certain peptides for certain MHC molecules seems to be the major factor determining whether an individual responds or not (Babbitt et al. 1985; Buus et al. 1987). To investigate whether this is also a major constraint for the immunogenicity of class-II-restricted epitopes in humans, we asked whether three tt peptides (p2, p30, and p4), previously identified as T-cell epitopes, are recognized by TT-immune donors bearing different MHC haplotypes.

PMBC from HLA-typed, TT-primed donors were restimulated in vitro with the three peptides under culture conditions that allow the expansion of one single precursor. This allowed us to easily identify the responder donors, quantify the response, and isolate

from each donor a number of independent peptide-specific T-cell clones.

The results are summarized in Table 1. Clones specific for p30 and p2 were isolated at the first attempt from all donors tested, irrespective of their DR type, indicating that these two peptides are universally immunogenic epitopes. On the contrary, p4-specific clones were isolated from only half of the donors tested. All the clones isolated proliferate in response to low concentrations of the specific peptide (0.02–1 μM), as well as to the complete TT molecule presented by autologous APCs, demonstrating that they are indeed TT-specific (data not shown).

For each clone, we determined the isotype of the restriction molecule by blocking experiments with anti-DR, -DP, and -DQ monoclonal antibodies and identified the restricting allele using a panel of HLA-homozygous EBV B cells as APCs. The results, summarized in Table 1, are shown in more detail in the following tables. p30-specific clones are either DR- or DP-restricted, and we have identified at least 4 DR (DRw11, w11JVM, 7, 9) and 2 DP alleles (DP2 and 4) as restriction molecules. p2-specific clones are all DR-restricted. Indeed, a large number of DR alleles can serve as restriction molecules for p2: DR1, w15, w18, 4Dw4, w11, w13, 7, 8, 9, w52b, and other DR alleles not yet well characterized.

We conclude that p30 and p2 are universally immunogenic, since all TT-immune donors carry high-affinity specific T cells. This property must in part be due to their ability to bind to several class II molecules. This is not true, however, for all tt peptides, since p4 can be recognized only in association with DRw52a and 52c molecules.

The availability of peptides with degenerate class II binding allowed us to ask whether or not T cells will be able to discriminate the same peptide bound to different class II molecules.

T Cells Can Always Distinguish p30 Bound to Different Class II Molecules

Table 2 shows the restriction pattern of six representative p30-specific clones. Although p30 binds to several class II molecules, T cells are always able to

Table 1. Two of Three tt Epitopes Are Universally Immunogenic

Epitope	Responders[a]	Clones characterized	Restriction molecules
p30 (tt 947–967) FNNFTVSFWLRVPKVSASHLE	18/18	60	DRw11, w11JVM, 7, 9, and others[b] DP2, 4, and others
p2 (tt 830–844) QYIKANSKFIGITEL	15/15	90	DR1, w15, w18, 4Dw4, w11, w13, 7, 8, 9, w52b, and others
P4 (tt 1273–1284) GQIGNDPNRDIL	5/10	54	DRw52a, 52c

[a]PBMC from DR-typed donors were stimulated with peptide. Specific clones were isolated and characterized for restriction specificities.

[b]The restriction element could not be identified using the available panel of typed APCs.

Table 2. p30 Can Be Recognized in Association with Several DR and DP Alleles

p30-pulsed APCs	Proliferative response (cpm × 10^{-3})[a]					
	5S3 DRw11JVM[b]	2GS5 DRw11	MS3 DR9	SS2 DR7	1BS1 DP2	5S5 DP4
QBL (DRw18, DP2)	0	0	0	0	72	0
JVM (DRw11JVM, DP2)	99	0	0	0	25	0
ATH (DRw11, DP2)	0	71	0	0	39	0
HHK (DRw13, DP4)	0	0	0	0	0	230
DKB (DR9, DP4)	0	0	12	0	0	78
PITOUT (DR7)	0	0	0	128	0	165

[a]Different clones were tested for their capacity to proliferate to p30-pulsed APCs. Proliferation to unpulsed APCs was always <1000 cpm. The proliferative response of DR-restricted clones was inhibited by anti-DR monoclonal antibody and that of DP-restricted clones by anti-DP monoclonal antibody.

[b]Indicates the restriction molecule utilized by the clone.

distinguish between complexes of p30 bound to each of them; i.e., they are always "monogamous" in their restriction specificity, each clone recognizing only one particular peptide/MHC combination.

This monogamous pattern of reactivity is expected if the different class II molecules present the peptide in different allele-specific conformations (Rosenthal and Schevach 1973; Kourilsky and Claverie 1986). When we tested truncated forms of p30 for their capacity to trigger T cells with different restriction patterns (Table 3), we found that indeed p30 contains three different epitopes: one (953-967) recognized by DRw11-restricted clones, one (947-960) recognized by clones restricted to DR7 and DR9, and one (949-960) recognized by DP2- and DP4-restricted clones. These data indicate that, in the case of p30, the restriction specificity is primarily determined at the level of the peptide/MHC interaction.

T Cells May or May Not Distinguish p2 Bound to Different DR Molecules

When we analyzed the restriction of p2-specific clones, we found two different patterns. Some clones are clearly monogamous, since they recognize p2 in association with only one DR allele, whereas other clones are "promiscuous," since they recognize p2 in association with two or more DR alleles.

Examples are shown in Figure 1. Clone GM2.11 recognizes, with the same high affinity, p2 bound to DR1, w15, 4Dw4, and 7, and, with lower affinity, p2 bound to DR8 and 9. In contrast, monogamous clones can discriminate between p2 bound to these alleles. Another promiscuous clone recognizes p2 bound to DRw11, w11JVM, and w13, whereas monogamous clones can discriminate among these three DR (data not shown). In all cases, the clonality of T cells has been proved by subcloning. These data indicate that, in the case of p2, the restriction specificity is not determined by the p2/DR complex, but is rather the property of the individual T cell.

These results can be most easily explained if we assume that some peptides can bind in a very similar conformation to a set of DR alleles. In this case, there will be the chance for a T cell to recognize the peptide in a monogamous or a promiscuous way, depending on which MHC residues (polymorphic, public, or monomorphic) contact the T-cell receptor (TCR) (Davis and Bjorkman 1988).

The analysis of truncated peptides (Table 4) indeed shows that p2 contains only one epitope (831-842) that is recognized in the context of every DR molecule tested (DR1–9, 52a, and 52b) by both monogamous and promiscuous clones.

It should be noted that monogamous and promiscuous patterns of restriction are also detectable for clones recognizing p4. p4-specific clones, in fact, are either monogamous, i.e., restricted to either 52a or 52c; or promiscuous, i.e., restricted to both 52a and 52c (see Fig. 1). In summary, for both p2 and p4, the restriction is determined not only by the allele-specific binding, but also by the TCR specificity.

Table 3. p30 Contains Three Epitopes Recognized in Association with Different Class II Molecules

	Proliferative response of T cells restricted to different class II molecules[a]				
	DRw11	DR7	DR9	DP2	DP4
947 967					
F N N F T V S F W L R V P K V S A S H L E	++	++	+	++	++
N - - - - - - - - - - - - - - - - - - E	n.d.	−	−	++	+
T - - - - - - - - - - - - - - - - - - E	n.d.	−	−	−	−
S - - - - - - - - - - - - - - - - - - E	++	−	−	−	−
W - - - - - - - - - - - - E	−	−	−	−	−
F - - - - - - - - - - - - K	−	+	+	++	++

[a]Clones with different restriction were tested for their capacity to proliferate to APCs pulsed with different concentrations of truncated peptides. (++) Response to <1 μM peptide; (+) response to 1–10 μM peptide; (−) no response to 10 μM peptide. n.d. indicates not determined.

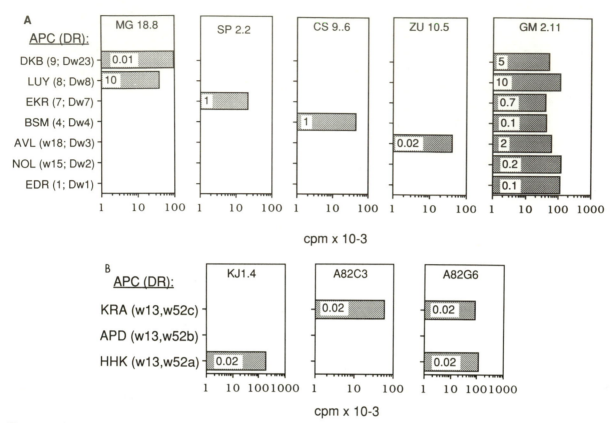

Figure 1. Monogamous and promiscuous recognition of peptides in association with DR molecules. (*A*) T-cell clones specific for p2; (*B*) clones specific for p4. The bars show the proliferative response of the T-cell clones to homozygous EBV B cells that had been pulsed with different concentrations of p2 or p4. Proliferation to unpulsed APCs was in all cases <1000 cpm. The proliferative response was in all cases inhibited by anti-DR and not by anti-DQ or anti-DP monoclonal antibodies. The number reported within each bar indicates the μM concentration of peptide required to induce 30% of the maximum response.

APCs from Some Donors Fail to Generate the p30 Epitope When Pulsed with Native tt

Since the donors used for this study have been immunized with alum-adsorbed TT, which is partially denatured, we were interested to determine whether all APCs would be able to process native tt and generate all three epitopes studied. Table 5 shows a representative experiment, where the APCs of four DR5$^+$ donors were pulsed with either RCM-TT or native tt and tested for their ability to trigger two DR5-restricted clones specific for p30 or p2. The APCs from two of the four donors fail to present native tt to a p30-specific clone.

This failure is not due to the lack of the appropriate restriction molecule, since the same cells can present RCM-TT to other p30-specific T cells. Neither is it due to a general processing defect, since the same cells can process and present native tt to a p2-specific T-cell clone. In addition, this defect is not limited to EBV B cells, since PBMC from the same donors also fail to present native tt. Finally, this defect cannot be overcome by increasing the antigen concentration over 30-fold (data not shown). Similar epitope-specific processing defects can also be found for the generation of the p4 epitope from native tt (S. Demotz et al., in prep.).

Table 4. p2 Contains Only One Epitope That Is Recognized in Association with Several DR Molecules

	Proliferative response of T-cell clones restricted to DR[a]								
	DR1	DRw15	DRw18	DR4Dw4	DRw11	DRw13	DR7	DR9	DRw52b
830 844									
Q Y I K A N S K F I G I T E	++	++	++	++	++	++	++	++	++
Y – – – – – – – – – – E L	++	++	+	+	+	+	++	+	+
I – – – – – – – – – – E	–	–	–	–	–	–	–	–	–
Q – – – – – – – – – – T	+	+	+	+	+	+	++	++	+
Q – – – – – – – – – I	–	–	–	–	–	–	–	–	–

[a]p2-specific clones restricted to different DR molecules with both monogamous and promiscuous patterns were tested for their capacity to proliferate to APCs pulsed with different concentrations of truncated p2 peptides. (++) Response to <1 μM peptide; (+) response to 1–10 μM peptide; (–) no response to 10 μM peptide.

Table 5. Delineation of an Epitope-specific Processing Defect

| DRw11[+] APCs (donor) | Proliferative response (cpm $\times 10^{-3}$)[a] | | | |
| | KT30 | | KT2 | |
	tt	RCM-TT	tt	RCM-TT
EBV B (KK)	73	39	54	32
PBMC (KK)	10	75	29	67
PBMC (GC)	74	58	60	75
EBV B (521)	2	67	21	20
EBV B (GG)	5	48	20	39
PBMC (GG)	1	103	n.d.	n.d.

[a]Two DRw11-restricted T-cell clones (KT30, p30-specific and KT2, p2-specific) were cultured with DRw11[+] APCs from various donors that had been pulsed (overnight at 37°C) with tt (40 μg/ml) or RCM-TT (60 μg/ml). The proliferative response to APCs alone was $<2 \times 10^3$ cpm. n.d. indicates not determined.

DISCUSSION

What Are the Major Constraints to the Immunogenicity in a Class-II-restricted Response in Humans?

The response to a foreign antigen has three essential requirements: (1) An appropriate antigen fragment must be generated; (2) this fragment must bind to an MHC molecule, and (3) specific T cells must be present. Data from experimental animal systems indicate that, although each of these three steps may be limiting, the most serious constraint usually comes from the level of peptide/MHC binding, which varies from allele to allele (Babbitt et al. 1985; Guillet 1986; Buus et al. 1987).

This study represents the first systematic analysis of the immunogenicity of class-II-restricted T-cell epitopes in humans. Our results indicate that two out of three tt epitopes fulfill all the criteria of immunogenicity in donors immunized with TT. The fact that all donors develop p2- and p30-specific T cells indicates that, in all individuals, these epitopes are generated by processing, bind to a class II molecule, and find specific T cells.

A key feature of these universally immunogenic peptides is their degenerate binding to class II molecules. The degeneracy shown here is still a minimum estimate, since the donor panel does not cover all the class II specificities and since we have isolated and characterized a relatively small number of specific clones.

One should note that such degenerate binding is not shared by all tt peptides, since p4 can be presented only by two very homologous DR alleles. Direct binding assays of these peptides to isolated DR molecules essentially confirm the data obtained with T-cell clones (A. Sette, pers. comm.).

Although, on one hand, the constraints imposed on MHC/peptide association are less severe than expected from the data obtained with mice, on the other hand, our study reveals unexpected constraints at the level of processing of native molecules that might greatly limit the availability of T-cell epitopes. In fact, the APCs of some donors, although capable of presenting RCM-TT to a p30-specific T-cell clone, are unable to present

native tt to the same clone. This defect is epitope-specific and is present in both EBV B cells and PBMC from the same donor and, in this respect, differs from the processing defect that Michalek et al. (1989) have recently described in different B-cell tumors from the same strain of mice.

Our data indicate that processing constraints are imposed primarily by the native structure of a protein and that, therefore, denaturation may enhance its immunogenicity. This is the case with TT, which is partially denatured and can therefore prime p30-specific T cells even in donors that are unable to generate the p30 epitope from the native molecule. For these reasons, one should consider that perhaps not all the T cells generated in response to a denatured antigen will be able to recognize the native molecules; it might be anticipated that T-cell immunity to a denatured protein may not always confer protection to a live pathogen. However, since our findings indicate that in humans MHC binding might not be such a severe constraint to immunogenicity, it is possible to exploit peptides such as p2 and p30 that bind to several class II molecules for the development of synthetic vaccines that will be active in a large proportion of the population.

Restriction Specificity Can Be Set at Three Different Levels

The availability of peptides that bind to several class II molecules and the analysis of the restriction specificity of more than 200 clones generate some speculations about the mechanisms that determine the T-cell restriction specificity. T cells are known to be exquisitely specific for both the antigen and the allelic form of MHC molecules (Katz et al. 1973; Zinkernagel and Doherty 1974). This restriction specificity may be set in three nonmutually exclusive ways.

First, some peptides bind only to some alleles. If a peptide binds to MHCa and does not bind to MHCb, there is obviously no chance for an a-restricted T cell to recognize the peptide on MHCb.

Second, the MHC molecules might shape the peptide in particular allele-specific conformations (Rosenthal and Schevach 1973; Kourilsky and Claverie 1986). A peptide *x* may bind to both MHCa and MHCb by interacting with different polymorphic residues. In this case, the two MHC molecules will present the peptide in different conformations or frames and, therefore, T cells that see *x* on MHCa will not be able to see *x* on MHCb.

Third, the TCR might contact the peptide and the MHC independently. If a peptide *x* binds to both MHCa and MHCb in the same conformation by interacting with monomorphic or public residues, there is the chance for the T cells to recognize the peptide on both alleles (if the TCR will contact MHC residues shared between the two) or with only one of them (if the TCR will contact allele-specific residues). Although in the first two cases the restriction specificity is primarily determined at the level of peptide binding, in the third case it is an intrinsic property of the TCR.

Although there is experimental evidence for the first point (Babbitt et al. 1985), there is still debate concerning the second and third possibilities, since it is difficult to distinguish between conformational effects and distinct contact sites (Matzinger 1981; Schwartz 1985; Kourilsky and Claverie 1986; Davis and Bjorkman 1988). Our data demonstrate that all three mechanisms contribute to determining the restriction specificity and that their relative contribution varies from case to case. In this respect p30, p2, and p4 provide three different examples.

p30 contains three distinct epitopes: 953-967, recognized in association with DR5w11; 947-960, recognized in association with DR7 and DR9; and 949-960, recognized in association with DP2 and DP4. Thus, different class II molecules will offer different epitopes to T cells that will consequently discriminate between the complexes of p30 and the different class II molecules. A similar finding has been recently reported for a malaria peptide (Sinigaglia et al. 1988). Thus, in this case, the restriction specificity is determined primarily by the way in which the peptide binds to the MHC.

In contrast, p2 provides a new case, since it contains only one epitope (831-842) that can be recognized by T cells in association with most DR molecules, suggesting that p2 may interact in the same way with all of these different DR alleles. This view is supported by the existence of promiscuous clones that recognize p2 in association with a number of DR alleles, implying that, on these DRs, p2 is displayed in a similar conformation.

The fact that the same p2/DR complex can be recognized by both monogamous and promiscuous clones can be most easily explained if we assume that the TCR of monogamous clones contacts the peptide and polymorphic MHC residues, whereas the TCR of promiscuous clones contacts the peptide and public or monomorphic MHC residues. Thus, in the case of p2, the restriction specificity is most likely to be determined at the level of the interaction of the TCR with the DR molecules.

Finally, p4 provides still a different example, since the restriction specificity is in this case determined first by its selective binding to only two DR alleles, and second by the specificity of the TCR.

It should be noted that promiscuous clones are most frequently found when the epitope is recognized in association with the DR molecules. It is thus tempting to speculate that the DR α chain might be a factor favoring promiscuous recognition because it provides monomorphic residues to contact the TCR.

Is There an Advantage in the Monomorphism of the DR α Chain?

MHC polymorphism has an obvious advantage for the species because it avoids the escape maneuvers made by pathogens, but it is, at the same time, a disadvantage for the individual, because it may result in a great variability in the capacity to bind peptides and generate an immune response. A good compromise would be that all the alleles of a given MHC molecule share the capacity to bind a large and common set of peptides and, at the same time, each of them possesses idiosyncratic binding specificities. We suggest that the DR α and β chains may serve these complementary functions, i.e., that DRα provides a common peptide-binding site able to bind a large set of universally immunogenic peptides, and DRβ provides each allele with idiosyncratic binding specificities.

There are two points in favor of this argument. The first is our finding that there are peptides, such as p4, that bind only to very few homologous alleles, whereas other peptides, such as p2, bind to most, if not all, DR molecules. It is tempting to speculate that p4 interacts primarily with the β chains of 52a and 52c, which are unique and very similar in the β sheets, and p2, which can bind and be recognized on many alleles, may bind to the monomorphic α chain. This is obviously an extreme view, since the binding of a peptide to the α or β chain only is neither proved nor likely. However, the recent finding that the minimal structure for peptide binding may be a small pocket on the MHC molecule (see Madden et al., this volume) indirectly supports the idea that α and β chains might contribute two partially distinct peptide-binding sites.

The second point comes from the conservation of the function of DR and I-E α chains in evolution. It has been recently shown that the DR α chain can substitute in transgenic mice for the mouse I-E α chain and the hybrid DRα/IEβ molecules can faithfully reconstitute I-E-dependent responses (Lawrance et al. 1989). Similarly, it has been reported that mouse I-E can present an influenza hemagglutinin peptide to a DR1-restricted human T-cell clone (Lechler et al. 1988). These findings suggest that, despite the divergence of DR and I-E α chains (25% amino acid difference), these two chains are quite similar as far as their function is concerned. Indeed, all the differences are accounted for by residues that do not participate in the peptide-binding groove, whereas the residues in the groove are remarkably conserved.

These considerations suggest to us an evolutionary speculation. The α chain might have been preserved in DR and I-E because it is a particularly good structure for peptide binding, whereas the β chain would have been allowed to diversify to provide each allele with idiosyncratic specificities.

ACKNOWLEDGMENTS

We thank Gerda Hügli for expert technical assistance, Drs. Gennaro De Libero, Jim Kaufmann, and Polly Matzinger for critical reading and constructive comments. G.C. is supported by a grant from the Swiss Science Foundation. The Basel Institute for Immunology was founded and is supported by F. Hoffman-La Roche and Co., Basel, Switzerland.

REFERENCES

Babbitt, B.P., G. Matsueda, E. Haber, E.R. Unanue, and P.M. Allen. 1985. Binding of immunogenic peptides to Ia histocompatibility molecules. *Nature* **317:** 359.

Benacerraf, B. 1978. A hypothesis to relate the specificity of T lymphocytes and the activity of I Region-specific Ir genes in macrophages and B lymphocytes. *J. Immunol.* **120:** 1809.

Bodmer, H.C., F.M. Gotch, and A.J. McMichael. 1989. Class I cross-restricted T cells reveal low responder allele due to processing of viral antigen. *Nature* **337:** 653.

Brett, S.J., K.B. Cease, and J.A. Berzofsky. 1988. Influences of antigen processing on the expression of the T cell repertoire. Evidence for MHC-specific hindering structures on the products of processing. *J. Exp. Med.* **168:** 357.

Buchmüller, Y. and G. Corradin. 1982. Lymphocyte specificity to protein antigens. V. Conformational dependence of activation of cytochrome c-specific T cells. *Eur. J. Immunol.* **12:** 412.

Buus, S., A. Sette, S.M. Colon, C. Miles, and H.M. Grey. 1987. The relation between major histocompatibility complex (MHC) restriction and the capacity of Ia to bind immunogenic peptides. *Science* **235:** 1353.

Davis, M.M. and P.J. Bjorkman. 1988. T-cell antigen receptor genes and T-cell recognition. *Nature* **334:** 395.

Demotz, S., P. Matricardi, A. Lanzavecchia, and G. Corradin. 1989a. A novel and simple procedure for determining T cell epitopes in protein antigens. *J. Immunol. Methods* (in press).

Demotz, S., A. Lanzavecchia, U. Eisel, H. Niemann, C. Widmann, and G. Corradin. 1989b. Delineation of several DR-restricted tetanus toxin T cell epitopes. *J. Immunol.* **142:** 394.

Guillet, J.G., M.Z. Lai, T.J. Briner, J.A. Smith, and M.L. Gefter. 1986. Interaction of peptide antigens and class II major histocompatibility antigens. *Nature* **324:** 260.

Katz, D.H., T. Hamaoka, and B. Benacerraf. 1973. Cell interactions between histoincompatible T and B lymphocytes II. Failure of physiological cooperative interactions between T and B lymphocytes from allogeneic donor strains in humoral responses to hapten-protein conjugates. *J. Exp. Med.* **137:** 1405.

Kourilsky, P. and J.-M. Claverie. 1986. The peptidic self model: A hypothesis on the molecular nature of the immunological self. *Ann. Inst. Pasteur Immunol.* **137D:** 3.

Lanzavecchia, A., E. Roosnek, T. Gregory, P. Berman, and S. Abrignani. 1988. T cells can present antigens such as HIV gp120 targeted to their own surface molecules. *Nature* **334:** 530.

Lawrance, S.K., R. Karlsson, J. Price, V. Quaranta, Y. Ron, J. Sprent, and P.A. Petron. 1989. Transgenic HLA DRa faithfully reconstitutes IE controlled immune functions and induces cross-tolerance to Ea in Ea mutant mice. *Cell* (in press).

Lechler, R.I., V. Bal, J.B. Rothbard, R.N. Germain, R. Sekaly, E.O. Long, and J. Lamb. 1988. Structural and functional studies of HLA-DR restricted antigen recognition by human helper T lymphocyte clones by using transfected murine cell lines. *J. Immunol.* **141:** 3003.

Matzinger, P. 1981. A one receptor view of T cell behaviour. *Nature* **292:** 497.

Michalek, M.T., B. Benacerraf, and K.L. Rock. 1989. Two genetically identical antigen-presenting T cell clones display heterogeneity in antigen processing. *Proc. Natl. Acad. Sci.* **86:** 3316.

Rosenthal, A.S. and E.M. Schevach. 1973. Function of macrophages in antigen recognition by guinea pig T lymphocytes I. Requirement for histocompatibility macrophages and lymphocytes. *J. Exp. Med.* **138:** 1194.

Schwartz, R.H. 1985. T lymphocyte recognition of antigen in association with gene products of the major histocompatibility complex. *Annu. Rev. Immunol.* **3:** 237.

Sinigaglia, F., M. Guttinger, J. Kilgus, D.M. Doran, H. Matile, H. Etlinger, A. Trzeciak, D. Gillessen, and R. Pink. 1988. A malaria T cell epitope recognized in association with most mouse and human MHC class II molecule. *Nature* **336:** 778.

Vidovic, D. and P. Matzinger. 1989. Unresponsiveness to a foreign antigen can be caused by self tolerance. *Nature* **336:** 222.

Zinkernagel, R.M. and P.C. Doherty. 1974. Immunological surveillance against altered self components by sensitized T lymphocytes in lymphocytic choriomeningitis. *Nature* **251:** 547.

Binding of Self-antigens to Ia Molecules

R.G. LORENZ, J.S. CHEN, S.G. WILLIAMS, AND P.M. ALLEN
Department of Pathology, Washington University School of Medicine, St. Louis, Missouri 63110

It is now clear that helper T cells recognize a bimolecular ligand composed of a foreign protein fragment bound to an Ia molecule on the surface of an antigen-presenting cell (APC) (for review, see Schwartz 1985; Unanue and Allen 1987). The demonstration of the direct binding of an immunogenic peptide to an Ia molecule has greatly simplified our thinking as to the nature of the ligand of the T-cell receptor (TCR) (Babbitt et al. 1985; Buus et al. 1986). However, it has also raised several other important questions, including the capacity of Ia molecules to distinguish self from foreign molecules. We and other investigators have in vitro evidence showing that major histocompatibility complex (MHC) molecules could not distinguish between foreign and self-peptides, but there was no direct proof that in vivo this was occurring (Babbitt et al. 1986; Lakey et al. 1986). The major difficulty in examining the processing and presentation of self-proteins was the lack of an experimental system by which one could directly examine in-vivo-processed self-proteins. We have recently developed a unique experimental system by which we were able to directly detect self-antigen/Ia complexes that were formed in vivo.

Generation and Characterization of Self-hemoglobin-reactive T Cells

During the course of investigating the ability of self-proteins to compete for the processing and presentation of foreign proteins, we examined the self-protein, murine hemoglobin (Hb). From this initial study, we developed a system by which we could generate T cells reactive against self-Hb (Lorenz and Allen 1988a). The basis of this system was the existence of alleles of the β chain of murine Hb (Hbb) that were independent of the H-2 haplotype. We used two mouse strains, CE/J and CBA/J, both of which possess the identical H-2^k complex, but which have different Hb β-chain alleles. We purified Hb from CBA/J animals (Hbb^d) and injected it into CE/J mice (Hbb^s). The CE/J mice gave a vigorous T-cell response against the allelic differences of the Hb molecules, and we were able to generate a panel of 57 T-cell hybridomas. We determined that 54 of the cell lines were restricted by the I-E^k molecule, whereas 3 were restricted by the I-A^k molecule. To confirm their antigen specificity, we initially used an antigen-presenting B-cell hybridoma, TA3. None of the hybridomas displayed any reactivity to the TA3 cells in the absence of antigen, but a vigorous response

was detected when Hb from CBA/J mice (Hbb^d) was added. The TA3 cells have previously been shown to be excellent stimulators of autologous mixed lymphocyte reaction. This lack of reactivity indicated that these T cells were not auto-Ia-reactive. As expected, no response was observed when Hb from CE/J mice (Hbb^s) was added. This panel of T-cell hybridomas appeared to have conventional reactivity, in that they did not recognize either I-A^k, I-E^k, or Hb alone but did recognize the allelic product of the murine Hbb^d locus when presented by an Ia-bearing APC.

It was next shown in two different assay systems that murine Hb had to be processed by an APC prior to recognition by a T-cell hybridoma (Lorenz and Allen 1988b). Chloroquine-treated or prefixed TA3 cells were unable to present the native Hb molecule, whereas untreated TA3 cells were able to present it. The determinant on the Hb β-chain protein Hb^{Bd} that was recognized by these T-cell hybridomas was then ascertained by identifying a tryptic fragment of Hb that was able to stimulate these T cells. Purified Hb^{Bd} (composed of 80% major and 20% minor Hb^{Bd} proteins) was digested with trypsin, and each fragment was separated using HPLC. Each fraction was then tested for its ability to stimulate the T cells using the TA3 cells as the APC. Surprisingly, all T cells responded to the same 10-amino-acid tryptic fragment Hb^{Bdmin}(67-76). There are potentially 13 amino acid differences between the Hb^{Bs} and the Hb$^{Bdmajor/minor}$ proteins, and 3 of these 13 differences were located in the Hb^{Bdmin}(67-76) sequence (Table 1). In our further studies, we have mainly used two of the T-cell hybrids, YO1.6, which is I-E^k-restricted, and WK5.1, which is I-A^k-restricted. We have obtained identical results with these two cell lines, and for simplicity only the results from the YO1.6 cells are usually shown.

Detection of Self-Hb/Ia Complexes In Vivo

The purpose in generating and characterizing these T-cell hybridomas was to use them as probes to detect the presence of self-Hb/Ia complexes in vivo. These T cells were exactly what we had desired, in that they specifically recognized an allelic fragment of murine Hb that required processing by an APC. The T cells should recognize self-Hb complexed to self-Ia molecules when CBA/J tissues are examined, if self-proteins are processed and presented in a manner similar to foreign antigens. We initially examined resident peritoneal macrophages (Mϕ) from CBA/J mice for the presence

Table 1. Summary of the Ability of Self-peptides to Bind to Ia Molecules

Peptide	Species	Sequence	Restriction element	Ability of mouse self-peptide to bind to the restriction element	Reference
HEL(52–61)	hen	D Y G I L Q I N S R	A^k		Babbitt et al. (1986)
	mouse	- - - - F - - - -		yes	Lambert and Unanue (1989)
HEL(34–45)	hen	F E S N F N T Q A T N R	A^k	no	Lorenz et al. (1988)
	mouse	- - - Y - - R - - - Y			
RNase(43–56)	cow	V N T F V H E S L A D V Q A	A^k	no	Lorenz et al. (1988)
	mouse	- - - - - P - - - - - -			
RNase(90–104)	cow	S K Y P N C A Y K T T Q A N K	E^k		J.S. Chen et al. (in prep.)
	mouse	- - - D - - - Y Q -		no	Lakey et al. (1986)
PCC(81–104)	pigeon	I F A G I K K K A E R A D L L A Y L K Q A T A K	E^k	yes	
	mouse	- - - - - - - G - - - - - - - - K - - N E		yes	Lorenz and Allen (1988a)
Hb^{Bdmin}(67–76)	mouse(CBA)	V I T A F N E G L K	E^k	yes	S.G. Williams et al. (in prep.)
Hb^s(67–76)	mouse(CE)	- - - - S D - - N		no	

The amino acid sequence for each peptide determinant is given using the standard one-letter codes. The corresponding murine sequence is given underneath the foreign sequence; only the amino acids that differ are shown. A "yes" indicates that the self-peptide can bind to the Ia molecule shown, as determined by either a direct binding assay (Babbitt et al. 1985) or a functional competition assay (Babbitt et al. 1986).

of these complexes. Mφ were purified by adherence and then tested for their ability to stimulate either the YO1.6 or WK5.1 cells without the addition of any exogenous antigen. These Mφ were able to stimulate the YO1.6 and WK5.1 cells in a dose-dependent manner. This was direct evidence that self-Hb/Ia complexes are expressed constitutively in vivo. To extend these findings, many controls were performed. As expected, CE/J Mφ did not stimulate the cells without the addition of exogenous antigen. We also proved that the complexes we were detecting were generated in vivo and not in vitro by treating the Mφ with chloroquine during their adherence step and then fixing. As with the live Mφ, good stimulation was observed when all the potential in vitro processing was inhibited by chloroquine. Similarly, when the Mφ were fixed prior to the addition of the T cells, they were fully able to stimulate the T cells. Thus, the Hb/Ia complexes we detected had to be formed in vivo.

After the initial examination of Mφ for the expression of these self-antigen/Ia complexes, we next tested a variety of tissues for their expression. We were able to detect these self-Hb/Ia complexes in a wide variety of organs as well as in purified cell populations. The complexes were detected in spleen, lymph nodes, liver, kidney, brain, heart, and thymus. This finding of ubiquitous expression of these self-Hb/Ia complexes indicates that these complexes are not restricted to cells of the lymphoid organs, and it appears that any tissue that contains Ia-bearing cells can process and potentially present self-Hb. In addition to these different organs, we also tested several different purified cell populations including alveolar macrophages, peripheral blood mononuclear cells, and splenic B cells. Again, all of these populations had detectable self-Hb/Ia complexes.

Despite our demonstration that the panel of T cells was specific for Hb^{Bdmin}(67-76), it was still possible that the reactivity we were detecting was not due to the recognition of Hb but of some other stimulating molecules. We have three lines of evidence that the observed reactivity was against the self-Hb/Ia molecule and not some cross-reactive molecule. Since the CBA/J and CE/J mice differ at many loci, it was possible that the CE/J T cells were detecting some allelic product on CBA/J cells besides Hb. We had found the Hb/Ia complexes in every tissue examined, and it was important to find a negative CBA/J tissue. We decided to test bone marrow macrophages (BMM) that were grown in vitro from bone marrow cells in the presence of colony-stimulating factor 1. These BMM were induced to express Ia antigens by treatment with IFN-γ and then tested for their ability to stimulate the YO1.6 cells. No reactivity was detected without the addition of any exogenous antigen. The BMM were able to stimulate the YO1.6 cells when exogenous Hb was added. Therefore, the YO1.6 cells do not appear to be recognizing some other allelic product on the CBA/J cells, since the BMM could not stimulate the cells without the addition of exogenous antigen.

A second possibility was that a Mls difference caused the observed reactivity. Since both the CE/J and CBA/J mice express the Mls-1^a and Mls-2^a alleles, the reactivity we observed could not be explained by an Mls difference (Table 2) (Lorenz and Allen 1988b). Supporting this conclusion is the observation that CBA/CaJ mice express the Mls-1^b and Mls-2^b alleles and were fully able to stimulate the YO1.6 cells. Conversely, C58/J mice express the Mls-1^a and Mls-2^a alleles but also express the Hbb^s allele, and they did not stimulate the YO1.6 cells. Thus, our observed reactivity does not correlate with either Mls-1 or Mls-2 reactivity.

The third line of evidence that the reactivity is due to the recognition of self-Hb/Ia complex involves the use of H-1 congenic mouse strains. The H-1 locus and the Hbb locus have both been localized to chromosome 7, and the two loci have never been separated by recombination. H-1 congenic mouse strains were used to prove that the observed reactivity was localized to the H-1/Hbb locus. Since these H-1 congenics were on a B10(H-2^b) background, we had to generate F$_1$ animals with B10.BR animals to introduce the YO1.6 restriction element, I-E^k. Spleen cells from (B10.BR × B10.129[5M])F$_1$ mice stimulated the YO1.6 cells, whereas cells from the (B10.BR × B10.D2)F$_1$ mice did not stimulate (Fig. 1). B10.129(5M) and B10.D2 mice only differ at the H-1 and H-2 loci. Since we already know that the H-2 complex does not code for the stimulating allele, the molecule must be encoded by the H-1/Hbb loci. Thus, the reactivity we detected in these mice maps to approximately a 180-kb fragment on chromosome 7 containing H-1 and Hbb. When all of these results are taken together, it seems without a doubt that the panel of Hb-reactive T-cell hybridomas

Table 2. YO1.6 Reactivity Does Not Correlate with Mls Phenotype of the Stimulating Cells

					YO1.6 Stimulation	
Mouse strain	H-2	Hbb	Mls-1	Mls-2	no exogenous antigen	hemoglobin
CBA/J	k	d	a	a	+	+
CBA/CaJ	k	d	b	b	+	+
C3H/HeJ	k	d	b	a	+	+
CE/J	k	s	a	a	−	+
C58/J	k	s	a	a	−	+

Resident peritoneal macrophages were tested for their ability to stimulate the YO1.6 cells as described previously (Lorenz and Allen 1988a). Macrophages were tested either without the addition of any exogenous antigen or with the addition of 100 μg/ml Hb^{Bd}. (+) The cells stimulated the YO1.6 cells; (−) no stimulation was observed.

YO1.6 Reactivity Maps to the Hbb/H-1 Locus

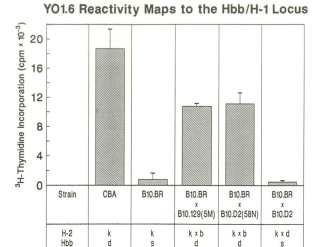

Strain	CBA	B10.BR	B10.BR x B10.129(5M)	B10.BR x B10.D2(58N)	B10.BR x B10.D2
H-2	k	k	k × b	k × b	k × d
Hbb	d	s	d	d	d
H-1	a	c	c × b	c × a	c × c

Figure 1. The ability to stimulate the YO1.6 cells maps to the Hbb/H-1 locus on chromosome 7. Spleen cells from each of the indicated strains were tested for their ability to stimulate the YO1.6 cells without the addition of exogenous antigen. The level of T-cell stimulation was determined by quantitating the amount of IL-2 released. The B10.BR and (B10.BR × B10.D2)F_1 cells were able to stimulate if exogenous Hb^{Bdmin}(67-76) was added.

are recognizing the Hb^{Bdmin}(67-76) determinant bound to an I-E^k molecule and not any other cross-reactive determinant. The reactivity we detected corresponds to the recognition of self-Hb/Ia complexes. From this set of experiments, we concluded that (1) self-Hb/Ia complexes are expressed constitutively in vivo, (2) in vivo Ia molecules do not discriminate between self and foreign antigens, and (3) these self-Hb/Ia complexes are expressed in a wide variety of tissues.

Thymic Cortical Epithelial Cells Express Self-antigen/Ia Complexes

In our initial experiments, we detected the constitutive expression of self-Hb/Ia complexes in the thymus. We then wanted to ascertain when and where in the thymus these complexes were being expressed. We had assumed that CBA/J mice were tolerant to their own Hb, and we confirmed this by immunizing CBA/J mice either with the Hb^{Bdmin}(67-76) peptide or intact Hb. In both cases, we did not observe any response (unpubl.). The Hb system provided us with a unique opportunity to examine the presence of self-antigen/Ia complexes in the thymus that were formed in vivo. We proposed that these self-Hb/Ia complexes that we detected in the thymus could be directly involved in the elimination of the self-Hb-reactive T cells. We then designed and implemented experiments that examined when during fetal life these complexes arose, and which cells in the thymus expressed these complexes. During neonatal life, γδ T-cell receptors start to rearrange around day 15, whereas the αβ T-cell receptors appear between days 16 and 17. If these Hb/Ia complexes were in-

volved in the process of eliminating these self-reactive T cells (negative selection), then we reasoned that they should occur prior to or at the same time that the TCRs are expressed. We isolated thymuses from day-14 to day-19 fetuses and tested them for their ability to stimulate the YO1.6 T-cell hybrid. We detected stimulation at all days tested, including day 14 (Lorenz and Allen 1989). These complexes were present in the thymus prior to the expression of the TCR, and, thus, they would be available for the process of negative selection.

We next determined which Ia-bearing cells in the thymus were expressing these self-Hb/Ia complexes. Three different Ia$^+$ thymic populations were purified: (1) thymic cortical epithelial cells (also referred to as nurse cells and abbreviated as TNC), (2) thymocyte rosettes (abbreviated as T-ROS) that are found in the cortico-medullary junction and contain Ia$^+$ dendritic cells and Ia$^-$ macrophages surrounded by thymocytes, and (3) medullary Ia$^+$ macrophages and dendritic cells (also referred to as low-density cells and abbreviated as Mφ/DC). Each of these cell populations was purified and tested for its ability to stimulate the YO1.6 cells. All three cell populations were able to stimulate approximately equally on a per-cell basis (Lorenz and Allen 1989). The surprising finding was that the cortical epithelial cells expressed these self-Hb/Ia complexes. It has been proposed that the cortical epithelial cells are involved in the process of positive selection and express a different set of self-proteins complexed to their Ia molecules. What our results showed is that, at least for the self-antigen Hb, the cortical epithelial cells expressed the same self-Hb/Ia complexes as the bone-marrow-derived dendritic cells and macrophages. Since cortical epithelial cells had previously been shown not to be able to present antigen to T-cell clones (Kyewski et al. 1984), we had to ensure that our nurse cells were not contaminated with other APCs. By fluorescence-activated cell sorting (FACS) analysis, we determined that the reactivity we observed could not be due to contaminating bone-marrow-derived cells. We also showed that the complexes that we were detecting were formed in vivo and were not generated during the isolation procedure. This was done by mixing thymuses from CE/J(H-2^k, Hbb^s) and BALB/c(H-2^d, Hbb^d) and then isolating the TNC. Since the YO1.6 cells are H-2^k-restricted and Hb^{Bd}-specific, the only way these complexes could form would be for Hb^{Bd} to be processed in vitro by the H-2^k cells. The TNC from this mixture did not stimulate the YO1.6 cells, indicating that the complexes we had detected in CBA/J thymuses were formed in vivo.

The main finding from this work was that the cortical epithelial cells expressed a self-antigen/Ia complex derived from an antigen that circulates in the blood. Earlier studies had shown the existence of a blood/thymus barrier, but our work and other studies have shown that self-proteins can enter the cortex of the thymus. Nieuwenhuis and his colleagues (1988) have shown that antibodies injected into the peritoneum can enter the thymus through a transcapsular route via the lymphatics, which is how we propose that the Hb got into the cortex. It would appear that the cortex may be accessible to many more self-proteins than originally thought, and that, at least for some antigens, the process of negative selection could actually occur in the cortex. Obviously, other self-antigens will have to be examined to determine the extent of self-antigens that the TNC can present. It has been proposed previously that the engagement of the TCR in the absence of a costimulatory molecule may result in the elimination of that T cell (Bretscher and Cohn 1970). There are many experiments that have convincingly shown that it is the bone-marrow-derived cells that are involved in negative selection (for review, see Sprent and Webb 1987). Other papers besides ours have indicated that thymic epithelium is involved in tolerance (Jordan et al. 1985; Ohki et al. 1987; Boguniewicz et al. 1989; Suzuki et al. 1989). As with most long-standing arguments in immunology, it seems likely that both sides end up being correct. We believe that for some self-proteins, the TNC may be involved in negative selection. For other self-antigens that may not be accessible to the TNC, negative selection may be occurring in the medulla on bone-marrow-derived cells. Our findings do not exclude epithelial cells from also being involved in the process of positive selection. Obviously, many more experiments will have to be performed before all of the critical and fascinating processes occurring in the thymus can be completely elucidated.

Ability of Self-peptides to Bind to Ia Molecules

It is now obvious that, in general, Ia molecules do not distinguish between self and foreign proteins. One of the first in vitro examples of this was obtained during the examination of the hen egg white lysozyme determinant, HEL(52-61). HEL(52-61) was shown to directly bind to the I-A^k molecule, which raised the question whether or not the corresponding self mouse lysozyme determinant, which only differs from the hen lysozyme determinant by a single amino acid, could also bind to I-A^k. It was ascertained using the direct binding assay that the mouse(52-61) peptide could bind to I-A^k in a manner indistinguishable from the HEL(52-61). Therefore, the I-A^k molecule could not distinguish between self and foreign determinants. Pierce and her colleagues obtained similar results with the pigeon cytochrome c determinant 81-104, in that the self-molecule was able to bind to the I-E^k molecule (Lakey et al. 1986).

To extend this analysis, we examined the I-A^k-restricted determinant of bovine ribonuclease, RNase(43-56). When this sequence was compared to the corresponding murine molecule, there was only a single amino acid difference. When the bovine and the mouse peptides were tested for their ability to bind to I-A^k, only the bovine molecule was able to bind. This indicated that the I-A^k molecule for this particular

determinant could distinguish between self and foreign antigens. This finding only pertains to this individual determinant and the I-A^k molecule. It is almost certain that there are other determinants on the murine RNase molecule that can bind to I-A^k, and the mouse RNase(43-56) determinant may bind to other alleles of Ia. All of these self-proteins are nonimmunogenic. If the self-determinant can bind to the Ia molecule, we propose that the self-reactive T cells are deleted. If the self-determinant cannot bind, there is no need to delete those reactive T cells, since the ligand cannot form. Thus, the overall tolerance to self-proteins is probably a collection of both clonal deletion and inability to bind to Ia.

We have now further extended this type of analysis to two I-E^k determinants, RNase(90-104) and Hb^{Bdmin}(67-76). For the RNase(90-104) determinant, the corresponding self-molecule, which differs by three residues, could not bind to I-E^k. The Hb system as described above is somewhat different from the lysozyme or ribonuclease systems, in that it involves allelic products of the Hbb locus. The Hb^{Bdmin}(67-76) and the Hb^{Bs}(67-76) peptides can be considered self-determinants in the two H-2^k strains we have examined (CBA/J and CE/J). From the results we have obtained through the use of YO1.6 cells, it is clear that the Hb^{Bdmin}(67-76) determinant must be able to bind to I-E^k molecules. This finding has also been confirmed in a functional competition assay. When the Hb^{Bs}(67-76) determinant was tested, it was unable to bind to the I-E^k molecule.

When all of the determinants and Ia molecules were analyzed, it appeared that approximately half of the corresponding self-determinants cannot bind to the restriction element (Table 1). We believe that this finding is due in part to our experimental systems, which have focused on immunodominant determinants and therefore may select for peptides that have corresponding self-sequences that cannot bind to Ia molecules. Many immunological systems have for obvious reasons used small well-defined proteins such as lysozyme, cytochrome c, and ribonuclease. All of these molecules have corresponding self-proteins, which limits the potential number of determinants that can be recognized because of the process of self-tolerance. A potential determinant would be more immunogenic (i.e., more T cells could respond) if the corresponding self-peptide could not bind to the Ia molecule. Obviously, this is not absolute, since the HEL(52-61) determinant is the immunodominant determinant of lysozyme in H-2^k strains, and the corresponding self-molecule binds to I-A^k. Since most physiological antigens, such as bacteria and viruses, will most likely not have corresponding self-molecules, the potential number of determinants that can be recognized by T cells is not affected by self-tolerance. Obviously, many more determinants will have to be examined before the relative effect of self-antigens binding to Ia molecules on the T-cell repertoire can be ascertained.

REFERENCES

Babbitt, B.P., P.M. Allen, G.R. Matsueda, E. Haber, and E.R. Unanue. 1985. Binding of immunogenic peptides to Ia histocompatibility molecules. *Nature* **317:** 359.

Babbitt, B.P., G.R. Matsueda, E. Haber, E.R. Unanue, and P.M. Allen. 1986. Antigenic competition at the level of the peptide-Ia binding. *Proc. Natl. Acad. Sci.* **83:** 4509.

Boguniewicz, M., G.H. Sunshine, and Y. Borel. 1989. Role of the thymus in natural tolerance to an autologous protein antigen. *J. Exp. Med.* **169:** 285.

Bretscher, P. and M. Cohn. 1970. A theory of self-nonself discrimination. *Science* **169:** 1042.

Buus, S., S. Colon, C. Smith, J.H. Freed, C. Miles, and H.M. Grey. 1986. Interaction between a "processed" ovalbumin peptide and Ia molecules. *Proc. Natl. Acad. Sci.* **83:** 3968.

Jordan, R.K., J.H. Robinson, N.A. Hopkinson, K.C. House, and A.L. Bentley. 1985. Thymic epithelium and the induction of transplantation tolerance in nude mice. *Nature* **314:** 454.

Kyewski, B.A., C.G. Fathman, and H.S. Kaplan. 1984. Intrathymic presentation of circulating non-major histocompatibility complex antigens. *Nature* **308:** 196.

Lakey, E.K., E. Margoliash, G. Flouret, and S.K. Pierce. 1986. Peptides related to the antigenic determinant block T cell recognition of the native protein as processed by antigen-presenting cells. *Eur. J. Immunol.* **16:** 721.

Lambert, L.E. and E.R. Unanue. 1989. Analysis of the interaction of the lysozyme peptide HEL(34-45) with the I-A^k molecule. *J. Immunol.* **143:** 802.

Lorenz, R.G. and P.M. Allen. 1988a. Direct evidence for functional self protein/Ia-molecule complexes in vivo. *Proc. Natl. Acad. Sci.* **85:** 5220.

———. 1988b. Processing and presentation of self proteins. *Immunol. Rev.* **106:** 115.

———. 1989. Thymic cortical epithelial cells can present self antigens in vivo. *Nature* **337:** 560.

Lorenz, R.G., A.N. Tyler, and P.M. Allen. 1988. T cell recognition of bovine ribonuclease: Self-non-self discrimination at the level of binding to the I-Ak molecule. *J. Immunol.* **141:** 4124.

Nieuwenhuis, P., R.J.M. Stet, J.P.A. Wagenaar, A.S. Wubbena, J. Kampinga, and A. Karrenbeld. 1988. The transcapsular route: A new way for (self-) antigens to by-pass the blood-thymus barrier. *Immunol. Today* **9:** 372.

Ohki, H., C. Martin, C. Corbel, M. Coltey, and N.M. Le Douarin. 1987. Tolerance induced by thymic epithelial grafts in birds. *Science* **237:** 1032.

Schwartz, R.H. 1985. T-Lymphocyte recognition of antigen in association with gene products of the major histocompatibility complex. *Annu. Rev. Immunol.* **3:** 237.

Sprent, J. and S.R. Webb. 1987. Function and specificity of T cell subsets in the mouse. *Adv. Immunol.* **41:** 39.

Suzuki, G., T. Moriyama, Y. Takeuchi, Y. Kawase, and S. Habu. 1989. Split tolerance in nude mice transplanted with 2'-deoxyguanosine-treated allogeneic thymus lobes. *J. Immunol.* **142:** 1463.

Unanue, E.R. and P.M. Allen. 1987. The basis for the immunoregulatory role of macrophages and other accessory cells. *Science* **236:** 551.

Molecular Studies of Human Response to Allergens

D.G. Marsh, P. Zwollo, S.K. Huang, B. Ghosh, and A.A. Ansari

Division of Clinical Immunology, Department of Medicine, Johns Hopkins University School of Medicine
Good Samaritan Hospital, Baltimore, Maryland 21239

Atopic allergy is a common disease that provides an appropriate model for studying the genetic and molecular basis of human immune responsiveness and its relationship to immunological disease (Marsh 1975; Marsh et al. 1981). In the case of allergy, unlike most other immunological diseases, a clear *causal* relationship has been established between specific immune responsiveness (detected by the presence of serum IgE antibodies) and the expression of a specific atopic disease. A large number of highly purified, well-characterized allergens are now available, and many more identified allergens await characterization (Marsh et al. 1986; Marsh and Norman 1988). Especially in the case of allergy to inhaled antigens, natural exposure is toward immunogenically limiting antigen doses (typically less than 1 μg/year [Marsh 1975]), which facilitates the study of *Ir* genes. Immunization with much higher doses of antigen than encountered by natural exposure forms the basis of conventional allergen immunotherapy (Rx) and is, therefore, ethically acceptable. Thus, one can "fingerprint" human immune responsiveness to a wide variety of allergenic macromolecules (and fragments thereof) under different conditions of antigen dosage and relate these immune response fingerprints to defined genetic markers such as those encoded by the HLA complex.

By analogy with data from animal studies (Allen et al. 1987; Buus et al. 1987; Guillet et al. 1987), the initiation of human immune responses to soluble antigens (i.e., most allergens) almost certainly involves the presentation of antigen fragments by class II major histocompatibility complex (MHC) (Ia) molecules to receptors on T_H cells. The following experimental findings support this hypothesis: (1) Striking associations have been observed between particular HLA-D phenotypes and specific immune responsiveness to certain highly purified pollen allergens in atopic subjects (Table 1); (2) studies using human T-cell clones demonstrate the role of HLA-D in the presentation of *Dermatophagoides* (house-dust mite) allergens to human T cells (O'Hehir et al. 1988; Lamb et al. 1989).

Significant HLA-D associations are usually observed with immune responsiveness to "minor" allergens, such as *Amb a* V (formerly Ra5) from *Ambrosia artemisiifolia* (short ragweed) pollen (Lapkoff and Goodfriend 1974; Mole et al. 1975), toward which only about 10% of ragweed-allergic subjects produce serum IgE

antibodies (Marsh et al. 1982a). The present studies focus on *Amb a* V (M_r 5000) and its homologs from two further *Ambrosia* species, namely, *Amb t* V (M_r 4400) and *Amb p* V ($M_r \sim 5000$) from *trifida* (giant) and *psilostachya* (western) ragweeds, respectively (Goodfriend et al. 1985; Marsh et al. 1987b). The sequences of *Amb a* V and *Amb t* V are compared in Figure 1; the sequence of *Amb p* V is not known, although its observed antigenic cross-reactivity with *Amb a* V and similar amino acid composition suggest a strong homology with *Amb a* V (Marsh et al. 1987b and unpubl.). Human immune responsiveness to these small, cystine-rich *Amb* V polypeptides is significantly associated with HLA-DR2 and Dw2 (Marsh et al. 1982a,b; Roebber et al. 1985; Marsh 1986; Marsh et al. 1987b and unpubl.). For the combination of two study groups (Table 1) (Marsh et al. 1982a), 95% of IgE antibody-positive and 85% of IgG antibody-positive "natural" responders to *Amb a* V (response resulting primarily from natural pollen exposure) were found to type as "DR2.2." In a companion study (Marsh et al. 1982b), *all* DR2.2$^+$ subjects, along with a small proportion of DR2.2$^-$ subjects, made IgG antibody to *Amb a* V following ragweed Rx. As discussed in this paper, we have subsequently observed a few rare DR2.2$^+$/*Amb a* V$^-$ subjects after Rx (by serum IgG and IgE antibody measurement). Other than the two subjects indicated in Table 1, we have never found any DR2.2$^-$/IgE antibody-positive subjects in a total of over 50 Caucasoid, 4 black, and 1 Oriental *Amb a* V IgE antibody-positive subjects studied.

Amb t V is virtually non-cross-reactive antigenically with *Amb a* V and *Amb p* V, although *Amb a* V and *Amb p* V are cross-reactive using antibodies from several subjects (Roebber et al. 1985; Marsh et al. 1987b and unpubl.). Thus, concordant responsiveness to *Amb a* V/*Amb p* V on the one hand and *Amb t* V on the other hand does not result simply from antigenic cross-reactivity; more probably, it reflects concordance of immune recognition of similar *Amb* V agretopes by the same Ia molecule. From the known linkage disequilibrium between HLA-DR2 and DQw1 (Baur et al. 1984), we would predict that this Ia molecule is one of the two Ia molecules encoded by DR2.2 or the single DQ1.2 Ia molecule. A DP molecule is unlikely to be involved, because of the weak linkage disequilibria between DP and DR alleles.

The molecular biological and cellular immunological studies presented here are designed to address the

Present address for all authors: Johns Hopkins Asthma and Allergy Center, 301 Bayview Boulevard, Baltimore, Maryland 21224.

Table 1. Significant Associations of HLA Phenotypes with Specific Antibody Responsiveness toward Highly Purified Pollen Allergens in Caucasoid Subjects

Allergen	M_r	Major HLA association	Westinghouse subjects		clinic patients		Overall p values[a]
			positive	negative	positive	negative	
Ambrosia artemisiifolia and *A. trifida* (short and giant ragweeds)							
Amb a V	5,000	DR2/Dw2	9/9 (100%)	20/83 (24%)	27/29 (93%)	10/56 (18%)	$<10^{-9}$
Amb a VI	11,500	DR5	11/13 (85%)	14/103 (14%)	6/15 (40%)	4/66 (6%)	$<10^{-6}$
Amb t V	4,400	DR2/Dw2	3/4 (75%)	0/13 (0%)	3/3 (100%)	1/7 (14%)	$<10^{-3}$
Lolium perenne (perennial rye)							
Lol p I	27,000	DR3	23/70 (33%)	9/65 (14%)	14/39 (36%)	2/28 (7%)	$<10^{-3}$
Lol p II	11,000	DR3	11/28 (39%)	21/107 (20%)	9/19 (47%)	7/48 (15%)	10^{-3}
Lol p III	11,000	DR3	13/30 (43%)	19/105 (18%)	13/23 (57%)	3/44 (7%)	$<10^{-5}$

No significant HLA-D associations were found for responsiveness to: *Amb a* I (M_r 37,800), *Amb a* III (M_r 12,300), *Phl p* V (M_r 15,000), *Der f* I (M_r 24,000), and *Der f* II (M_r 14,500). Data taken from Marsh et al. (1982a, 1987a); Roebber et al. (1985); Freidhoff et al. (1988); Ansari et al. (1989c); P.W. Heymann et al. (unpubl.); A.A. Ansari et al. (unpubl.).

[a] p values (Fisher's Exact Test) are given for analyses of IgE antibody data, except that IgG antibody data from immunized patients were used for *Amb t* V, since an insufficient number of IgE antibody-positive subjects were available.

predicted involvement of one of the DR2.2 Ia molecules, or the DQ1.2 Ia molecule. We have also investigated the possible molecular basis of the secondary associations of *Amb* V responsiveness with certain other HLA-D types (DR2.21, DR4, DR9, and DQw3), which mainly become evident following high-dose Rx with ragweed antigens.

We have studied the DRB and DQB1 genes of 67 selected Caucasoid atopic subjects by dot-blotting with sequence-specific oligonucleotides (SSOs) and sequencing of polymerase chain reaction (PCR)-amplified second exons (Zwollo et al. 1989a,b and in prep.). Three *Amb a* V-specific T-cell clones were isolated from a DR2.2$^+$ individual and used in antigen-presentation studies (Huang and Marsh 1989; S.K. Huang et al., in prep.). The combined data from these two experimental approaches strongly suggest that the DR$\alpha\beta_1$2.2 molecule is the major *Amb* V–*Ir* gene product. Further data indicate that HLA-DR2.21, and

either HLA-DR4 and DR9, or HLA-DQw3, may be secondary *Amb a* V–*Ir* gene products.

MATERIALS AND METHODS

Antigens. Highly purified ragweed allergens, *Amb a* V, *Amb t* V, and *Amb p* V, and highly purified rye grass allergen, *Lol p* III (control), were prepared as described previously (Roebber et al. 1982, 1985; Ansari et al. 1987; Marsh et al. 1987b and unpubl.).

Measurement of serum IgE and IgG antibodies to the Amb V allergens. Serum antibodies to the various highly purified ragweed or grass antigens were measured before, during, and after Rx with the respective antigens using double antibody radioimmunoassays that are capable of detecting ~ 0.6 ng/ml IgE antibody and 3 ng/ml serum IgG antibody (Marsh et al. 1982a; Ansari et al. 1987).

Study subjects. From a large group of ragweed-allergic Caucasoid subjects, 67 patients were chosen, most of whom had participated in previous genetic studies (Marsh et al. 1982a,b, 1987b; Zwollo et al. 1989a). It is important to note that these patients are *highly selected* to include all individuals we could find who had unusual combinations of HLA and *Amb a* V immune response phenotypes. Also, we made a special effort to sample all DR4$^+$ and DR9$^+$ subjects, whether they were responders or nonresponders. Thus, the typical DR2.2$^+$/*Amb a* V$^+$ subjects are very much underrepresented in the sample (P. Zwollo et al., in prep.).

All of these subjects were studied by SSO–dot-blot analysis; DNA sequencing of the second exons of DRB genes was performed in 17 subjects and, of these, DQB1 second exons were sequenced in 15 individuals. The subjects selected for sequencing included those having unusual combinations of HLA-D and *Amb a* V response phenotypes (P. Zwollo et al., in prep.). The majority of the subjects (including all of the *Amb a* V

```
        1        5         10        15
Amb a V:  L  V  P C  A  W  A G  N  V C  G  E  K  R
Amb t V:  D  D  G  L C  -  Y  E G  T  N C  G  K  V  G

        16       20        25        30
Amb a V:  A Y  C  C  S  D  P G  R  Y  C  P  W  Q  V
Amb t V:  K Y  C  C  S  P  I G  K  Y  C  -  -  -  -

        31       35        40        45
Amb a V:  V  C  Y  E S  S  E  I  C  S K  K C  G (K)
Amb t V:  V  C  Y  D S  K  A  I  C  N K  N C  T
```

Figure 1. Comparison of the amino acid sequences of *Amb a* V and *Amb t* V. Data were taken from Mole et al. (1975) and Goodfriend et al. (1985). Residues that are either identical or closely homologous are boxed; identical residues are shown in bold type. Using the Berzofsky algorithm (Margalit et al. 1987), we found segments 21–24 (*Amb a* V) and 19–24 (*Amb t* V) to be amphipathic using blocks of 7 amino acids, and segments 24–26 (*Amb a* V) and 9–23 (*Amb t* V) to be amphipathic using blocks of 11 amino acids. The corresponding sequence of *Amb p* V is presently unknown, but from the similarity of amino acid composition and the strong cross-reactivity between *Amb a* V and *Amb p* V, it is believed to be similar to that of *Amb a* V (Marsh 1986; Marsh et al. 1987b).

nonresponders by natural pollen exposure) were given high-dose ragweed Rx, as discussed elsewhere (Marsh et al. 1982b; P. Zwollo et al., in prep.).

HLA typing. The HLA serological and mixed lymphocyte reaction (MLR) typing was performed in the Immunogenetics Laboratory of W. Bias at the Johns Hopkins University School of Medicine (Marsh et al. 1982a). The typing data were confirmed and expanded by restriction fragment length polymorphism (RFLP) typing (Zwollo et al. 1989a and in prep.).

Nomenclature of HLA-D genes and encoded polypeptides. Our nomenclature for HLA-D alleles is based on that proposed by other investigators (Todd et al. 1987; IUIS HLA Nomenclature Subcommittee 1988). We will use the gene designation (e.g., DRB1, formerly named $DR\beta_1$), followed by an asterisk and the serological specificity associated with the encoded gene product (e.g., DRB1*2). DRB1 will be used to designate the more polymorphic and DRB3 the less polymorphic expressed DRB "loci" that map in the order: centromere-DQA1-DRB1-DRB2 (pseudogene)-DRB3 in most haplotypes. In addition, DRB4 will be used to designate the less polymorphic locus that encodes DRw53 specificities found in DR4, 7, and 9 haplotypes that contain two pseudogenes (cf. Gorski et al. 1987).

Where appropriate, the Dw type defined by the MLR will be used as a suffix to designate the DRB or DQB sequences more precisely. For example, DRB1*2.2, DRB3*2.2, and DQB1*1.2 will be used to designate, respectively, the unique DNA sequences of the expressed DRB1-, DRB3-, and DQB1-locus alleles found in almost all Caucasoid DR2/Dw2/DQw1 haplotypes. The polypeptides encoded by the A and B genes will be denoted by Greek letters α and β, respectively, followed by a Roman numeral subscript corresponding to the locus number, and by the specificity designation. For example, $DR\beta_1 2.2$ denotes the β polypeptide encoded by DRB1*2.2. According to recent studies, the more acidic and more polymorphic of the β polypeptides encoded by the DR2.2 and DR2.12 haplotypes, which were previously thought to be the products of DRB1 genes (Lee et al. 1987), are now almost certainly the products of the DRB3 genes (Kawai et al. 1989; J.L. Bidwell and J. Trowsdale, pers. comm.). Thus, $DR\beta_1 2$ will be used to designate the more basic and $DR\beta_{III} 2$ the more acidic β polypeptides, respectively, which is the converse of designations suggested previously (cf. Lee et al. 1987; Todd et al. 1987).

The term "allelic polymorphic regions (APRs)" will be used to denote the regions of HLA-D genes and their encoded polypeptide chains where two or more polymorphic amino acid residues are known to be clustered. The APRs for $DR\beta$ are as follows: *APR1*, amino acid residues 9-13; *APR2*, residues 25-38; *APR3*, residues 57-60; *APR4*, residues 67-74. The DQβ APRs are as follows: *APR1*, residues 9-13; *APR2*, residues 26-38; *APR3*, residues 55-57; *APR4*, residues 86 and 87. In and around most of these regions, one also finds

residues where two variants have been defined in different DRβ or DQβ polypeptides (Todd et al. 1987; Horn et al. 1988; Kappes and Strominger 1988).

DNA purification. Genomic DNA was purified from patients' peripheral blood lymphocytes or from homozygous typing cell (HTC) lines (controls), as described previously by Zwollo et al. (1989a).

RFLP analysis. Briefly, purified genomic DNA was digested with *Eco*RI and fractionated by agarose gel electrophoresis (Zwollo et al. 1989a). The DNA restriction fragments were transferred from the gel to a nylon filter (New England Nuclear) by Southern blotting and allowed to hybridize with ^{32}P-labeled DRB or DQB1 full-length cDNA probes (kindly supplied by T. Sasazuki, Japan, and E. Long, NIH, Bethesda, MD). After stringent washing, the filters were exposed to X-ray film.

PCR amplification of DRB and DQB1 second-exon gene segments. PCR amplification of the majority of the second exons of DRB genes (codons 6-88) and DQB genes (codons 14-88 or 90) from purified genomic DNA samples was performed as described elsewhere (P. Zwollo et al., in prep.), using the approach developed by Saiki et al. (1988). In brief, genomic DNA (0.5 μg) from an allergic patient or HTC was amplified for 28 cycles of denaturation, annealing, and chain extension using *Taq* polymerase, nucleotides, and appropriate oligonucleotide primers for the 5' ends of the "plus" and "minus" strands flanking the respective second exons of DRB or DQB1 genes. Restriction enzyme sites were included at the 5' ends of the primers to facilitate M13 cloning.

M13-cloning of DRB- and DQB1-amplified products and dideoxy sequencing. Ten percent of the DRB- or DQB1-amplified products was digested with appropriate restriction enzymes, ligated into an M13 vector, and transfected into the *Escherichia coli* strain JM103 (P. Zwollo et al., in prep.). Recombinants were screened for HLA-DRB or DQB inserts by hybridization with a DRB or a DQB1 full-length cDNA probe (Zwollo et al. 1989a). The single-stranded phage DNA was isolated and sequenced by the dideoxy procedure using the Sequenase enzyme. dITP was used in the place of dGTP, where necessary, to resolve ambiguous sequences in GC-rich regions.

Dot-blot analyses of PCR-amplified HLA-DRB and DQB1 segments. These analyses were performed as described by P. Zwollo et al. (in prep.) using 17 SSOs for DRB APR sequences and 14 SSOs for DQB1 APR sequences, using methodology similar to that of Erlich et al. (1986). DQA SSO–dot-blotting data were also available on some of these individuals through collaboration with H. Erlich, Cetus Corporation (P. Zwollo et al., in prep.).

For the analysis of DRB and DQB1 gene segments, 5% of each PCR-amplified DNA sample (2.5 μl) was denatured and applied to a nylon filter using a dot-blot apparatus; the filter was baked at 80°C for 2 hours. After prehybridization, a ^{32}P-labeled SSO (10 ng) was added and allowed to hybridize to the PCR-amplified DNA on the filters for 1 hour at $(T_d - 3)$°C (T_d is the theoretical temperature of dissociation of 50% of the SSO [see, e.g., Todd et al. 1987]). Where necessary, the filters were washed at increasingly higher temperature, followed by exposure to X-ray film at each step, in order to reveal the specific SSO hybridization patterns. The SSOs were subsequently stripped from the filters with 0.4 N NaOH for 30 minutes at 30°C, and the filters were reused several times with different SSOs. Additional control "framework" SSOs from conserved DRB or DQB regions were used with the filters to estimate the relative amounts of the respective amplified DNAs that had been applied.

Generation of Amb a *V-specific T-cell clones.* Isolation of *Amb a* V-specific T-cell clones was attempted from several DR2.2$^+$, highly *Amb a* V$^+$ subjects who had received short ragweed Rx and were known to have high levels of IgE and IgG antibodies to *Amb a* V (Huang and Marsh 1989; S.K. Huang et al., in prep.). Two black patients, who had very high levels of IgE antibody prior to Rx and IgG antibody levels in excess of 20 μg/ml during Rx, were included. The cloning procedure was a modification (S.K. Huang et al., in prep.) of that used by O'Hehir et al. (1987). Briefly, isolated peripheral blood mononuclear cells (PBMC) (1×10^6 cells/ml) from the patient were stimulated in vitro with 1 μg/ml purified *Amb a* V in culture medium (RPMI 1640 containing 1% penicillin, 1% streptomycin, 10% fetal calf serum, and 1% L-glutamine). T-cell blasts were isolated 7 days later, and blast cells (1×10^5 cells/ml) were restimulated with *Amb a* V (1 μg/ml) together with irradiated (5000 rads), autologous PBMC (1×10^6 cells/ml) as antigen-presenting cells (APCs) in culture medium. Two to three days after the antigen activation, recombinant IL-2 (10 units/ml) and fresh culture medium were added for the remaining 5 days of culture. Following an additional 2–3 culture cycles, T-cell blasts were cloned (0.3–1 cell/well) in 96-well round-bottomed plates in the presence of *Amb a* V (1 μg/ml) and autologous APCs (1×10^5 cells/well) in culture medium supplemented with recombinant IL-2 (20 units/ml). Subcloning was performed as described above.

Proliferation assays. A total of 1×10^4 cloned T cells per well were incubated with 1×10^5 autologous or allogeneic APCs, with or without *Amb a* V (0.5 μg/ml, unless otherwise indicated), for 3 days. The allogeneic APCs included 13 HTCs, DR2.2 (2 lines), 2.12 (2 lines), 2.21 (2 lines), 2.22, 4.4, 4.10, 4.14, w11, w8 and 9, as well as a number of selected patients' cells (see Results). All of the APCs were irradiated (5000 rads) before use. The cell cultures were then pulsed with 1 μCi of [^{3}H]thymidine, harvested 18 hours later onto glass fiber paper, and counted. The results from triplicate cultures are expressed as mean counts per minute (cpm) ± S.E.

Inhibition of Amb a *V-specific T-cell proliferation by monoclonal antibodies.* Purified anti-DR framework (L243), anti-DQ common polymorphic epitope (Leu-10), and anti-DP monomorphic epitope (B7/21) monoclonal antibodies (MAbs) were purchased from Becton Dickinson Inc. Ascites fluid containing MAb Hu30, which recognizes DR$\alpha\beta_I$2.2 (and DR$\alpha\beta_I$2.12), but at higher concentration also cross-reacts weakly with DR$\alpha\beta_{III}$2.2 and DR$\alpha\beta_I$1 (Sone et al. 1985; Kawai et al. 1989), was a gift from Drs. Wakisaka and Aizawa, Sapporo, Japan. Control ascites fluid containing MAb H5A4 (anti-CD11$_b$) was provided by B. Bochner, Johns Hopkins University.

Cultures were set up as described above for the proliferation assays, except that the concentration of *Amb a* V used was 0.5 μg/ml. At the start of each culture, 1.0 μg/ml each anti-DR, DQ, or DP purified monoclonal antibody was added. MAb Hu30 was similarly tested using 1:100 to 1:10,000 dilutions of ascites fluid. Control MAb H5A4 was used at 1:100 dilution of ascites fluid. A further set of cultures was run in parallel using the nonspecific T-cell mitogen, phytohemagglutinin (PHA) (2 μg/ml), in the place of *Amb a* V, to serve as an additional control.

Inhibition of Amb a *V presentation by* Amb t *V and* Amb p *V.* We assayed the inhibitory effect of *Amb t* V or *Amb p* V on the presentation of *Amb a* V to the cloned T cells by autologous APCs (Huang and Marsh 1989; S.K. Huang et al., in prep.). The APCs (5×10^5 cells/ml) were preincubated with or without each of the inhibitors (or *Lol p* III as a control antigen) at 0.1–10 μg/ml in culture medium for 10 hours at 37°C and washed three times. The prepulsed APCs (1×10^5 cells/well) were then cultured with cloned T cells (1×10^4 cells/well) in the presence or absence of *Amb a* V (0.1 μg/ml) for 60 hours. Again, PHA (2 μg/ml) in the place of *Amb a* V served as an additional control. Cultures were pulsed for an additional 18 hours with 1 μCi of [^{3}H]thymidine and counted. The results were expressed as described for the proliferation assays.

RESULTS

SSO–Dot-blot and DNA Sequencing Data for *Amb a* V Responders and Nonresponders

Our SSO–dot-blot studies of the APRs of the DRB and DQB1 alleles of 67 *highly selected* ragweed-allergic Caucasoid patients (see Materials and Methods), and sequencing of certain subjects, produced the following results (Zwollo et al. 1989b and in prep.). Of the patients, 25 were identified as being DR2.2$^+$ by serological, MLR, and/or RFLP typings. These subjects included 11 typical DR2.2$^+$/*Amb a* V$^+$ IgE/IgG antibody responders *before* ragweed Rx (of whom 7 who received Rx are shown in Fig. 2a), 11 IgG antibody responders after ragweed Rx (10 are shown in Fig. 2b and one [CSz] in Fig. 2c), and 3 quite atypical DR2.2$^+$/ *Amb a* V$^-$ subjects after Rx (non-responders MB and

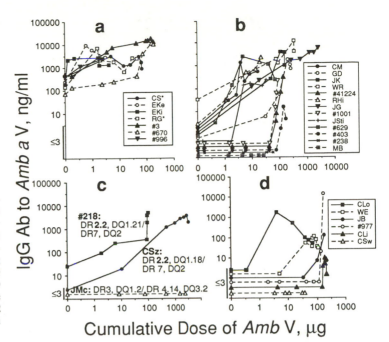

Figure 2. Immunoglobulin G antibody responses to *Amb a* V following ragweed Rx. (*a*) DR2.2+, DQ1.2+ subjects who possessed detectable IgE antibody in their sera prior to Rx. (*b*) DR2.2+, DQ1.2+ subjects who possessed no detectable IgE antibody in their sera prior to Rx (one subject possessed a small amount of IgG antibody). (*c*) People having atypical HLA-D phenotypes (see text). (*d*) Subjects who were found to possess DRB1*2.21 or DRB1*2.22 phenotypes from DNA studies. (Adapted, from P. Zwollo et al., in prep.)

#238, and very weak responder #403 [Fig. 2b]). All 25 of these subjects were shown to possess the DRB *Eco*RI 6.5-kb and DQB *Eco*RI 2.3-kb DNA fragments characteristic of the Dw2 phenotype. Also, all had SSO typings consistent with DRB1*2.2 and DRB3*2.2 sequences in their APRs 1, 2, and 4. For 8 subjects who were sequenced, the second-exon DNA sequences were identical to published DRB1*2.2 and DRB3*2.2 sequences (Todd et al. 1987; Kappes and Strominger 1988; Horn et al. 1988). One responder Dw2± subject (#218), who possessed the DRB *Eco*RI 6.5-kb but not the DQB *Eco*RI 2.3-kb fragment, was also found to possess the DRB1*2.2 and DRB3*2.2 second-exon sequences characteristic of Dw2.

All of the aforementioned individuals, except subject #218 and one of the DRB2.2+/*Amb a* V+ individuals (CSz), had typical Dw2-associated DQB1*1.2 sequences; the exceptional subjects #218 and CSz had different sequences, DQB1*1.21 and DQB1*1.18 (usually found in MLR types Dw21 and Dw18). The finding of these unusual sequence DRB–DQB combinations in responders implicates either a DR2.2 $\alpha\beta_I$ or $\alpha\beta_{III}$ molecule as the major *Amb a* V–*Ir* gene product. (Note that subject #218 responded to *Amb a* V as a result of natural pollen exposure. No typical DR2.21,DQ1.21 subject responded until ragweed Rx was performed [see below]). The conclusion that a DR2.2 molecule is involved is supported by our finding one *non*responder after prolonged Rx (JMc) who possessed the DQB1*1.2 sequence, but not the DRB1*2.2 and DRB3*2.2 sequences. Based on the known linkage disequilibria between specific DR and DQ alleles (Baur et al. 1984), the inferred haplotypes of these three atypical subjects are as shown in Figure 2c. Of further interest, the MLR and RFLP typings for the *Amb a* V

responder subject CSz are indistinguishable from those found for subjects having typical Dw2+ haplotypes, suggesting functional and genetic similarity between DR2.2,DQ1.18 and DR2.2,DQ1.2 haplotypes.

We investigated six DR2+/Dw2− subjects, none of whom showed any evidence of IgE or IgG antibodies before ragweed Rx. After ragweed Rx, four produced IgG antibody, one made a trace IgG antibody response, and one failed to respond (Fig. 2d). Five of these subjects were found to possess DRB1*2.21 sequences, and one subject (WE), an *Amb a* V responder after Rx, had a DRB1*2.22 sequence. We found the expected DNA sequences for DRB3*2.21, known to be identical for Dw21 and Dw22 haplotypes (Liu et al. 1988), in all six patients.

Besides the typical DR2.2+/*Amb a* V+ subjects, we have only found two unusual DR2.2−/*Amb a* V IgE antibody-positive individuals (before Rx), both of whom were included in this study. These subjects (JKo and ML) possessed DRB and DQB1 sequences and SSO typings consistent with DR8, 9, 53/DQ4, 3.3 and DR3, 4.14, 52a, 53/DQ2, 3.2 phenotypes, respectively. Several other DR4+ subjects (having all three common DR4 variants) and one DR9+ subject made IgG antibody to *Amb a* V either before (one case, patient MS) or after Rx. One subject (LL) had a questionable serological typing of "DR4," but no DRB1*4 sequence was found (Fig. 3). The common feature among these responder individuals is that they all have variants of DQw3 in association with DR4 (DQ3.1 and 3.2) and DR9 (DQ3.3). However, about 50% of DR4+/DQw3+ subjects were nonresponders to *Amb a* V after Rx. (Note that our sample included DR4+ and DR9+ subjects, irrespective of their *Amb a* V responder status; see Materials and Methods).

DR2⁻ SUBJECTS

Patient   DRB1   DQB1

IgE Ab⁺/IgG Ab⁺ before Rx:
JKo	9,	8	3.3, 4
ML	4.14, 17(3)	3.2, 2

IgE Ab⁻/IgG Ab⁺ before Rx;
IgG Ab⁺ after Rx:
MS	4.10, 7	3.2, 2

IgE Ab⁻/IgG Ab⁻ before Rx:
IgG Ab⁺ after Rx:
WL*	9,	11(5)	3.3, 3.1
SG*	4.10,	11(5)	3.2, 3.1
LFl*	4.10,	1.1	3.1, 1.1
LL	?	1.1	3.1, 1.1
DHa	4.4,	1.1	3.1, 1.1
JHo*	4.4,	1.1	3.1, 1.1
JSt	4.14,	7	3.2, 3.3
VH	4.4,	1.1	3.1, 1.1

Patient   DRB1   DQB1

IgE Ab⁻/IgG Ab⁻ before Rx;
IgG Ab⁻ after Rx:
1297	4.4,	1.1	3.2, 1.1
3017	4.4,	7	3.1, 2
3018	4.4,	11(5)	3.2, 1.1
LBo	4.14,	10	3.2, 1.1
MBa*	4.14,	17(3)	3.2, 1.1
JMc*	4.14, 17(3)	3.2, 1.2
LBe	4.14,	17(3)	3.2, 2
3002	4.14,	7	3.2, 2
3084	4.14,	11(5)	3.2, 3.1

Plus 15 DR4⁻, DR9⁻ non-responders

Specificities underlined were confirmed
by dideoxy sequencing

Figure 3. HLA phenotypes of HLA-DR2⁻ responders and nonresponders to *Amb a* V. Patient LL appears to be a DRB1*1.1 homozygote. (Data from P. Zwollo et al., in prep.)

Cellular Immunological Experiments Using *Amb a* V

Three *Amb a* V-specific T-cell clones (AP 1.2, AP 6, and AP 9), obtained from one of the allergic black patients, AP (SSO–dot-blot typing, DR2.2, 6a; DQ1.2, –), were established following extensive in vitro cloning and antigen stimulation. All three clones were found to be CD4⁺ by fluorescence-activated cell sorter (FACS) analysis. In addition, we obtained a polyclonal T-cell line from the other black subject (patient BE; SSO–dot-blot typing, DR2.2, 9, DQ1.2, 2) following repeated *Amb a* V and IL-2 stimulation, but have so far been unable to obtain clones from this line.

The MHC class II restriction specificity of the three clones was examined by testing the ability of various HTCs and patients' APCs to present *Amb a* V to the T cells, and of anti-HLA-D monoclonal antibodies to block *Amb a* V presentation by autologous APCs. (Only anti-HLA-DR, -DQ, and -DP experiments have been performed so far with the T-cell line.) For the first type of experiment, panels of HTCs and of PMBCs from patients were selected to include the different DR2 and DR4 variants, as well as DRw11, DRw8, and DR9, all of which are found in some *Amb a* V responders (Figs. 2 and 3). Regardless of the DQ phenotype and *Amb a* V responder status of the patient, all APCs bearing DR2.2 and DR2.12, and only these phenotypes, were able to present *Amb a* V to all of the cloned T cells (Figs. 4 and 5 show representative experiments). In particular, the cells of atypical *Amb a* V⁺ patients #218 and CSz, who have DR2.2, but not DQ1.2 (Fig. 2c), as well as one unusual DR2.2⁺/DQ1.2⁺/*Amb a* V⁻ subject (MB), were all able to present the antigen to all three clones. These results

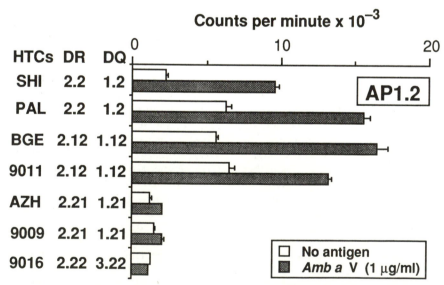

Figure 4. MHC restriction of *Amb a* V-specific T-cell proliferation of clone AP1.2 using HTCs as APCs. Cloned T cells (5 × 10⁴ cells/ml) were stimulated with (1 μg/ml) or without *Amb a* V antigen in the presence of irradiated HTCs (5 × 10⁵ cells/ml) having known DR, DQ phenotypes (indicated). The proliferative response of clone AP1.2 to *Amb a* V was measured as [³H]thymidine incorporation (mean cpm ± S.E. for triplicate cultures) as described in Materials and Methods. Results for further experiments using other HTCs were negative.

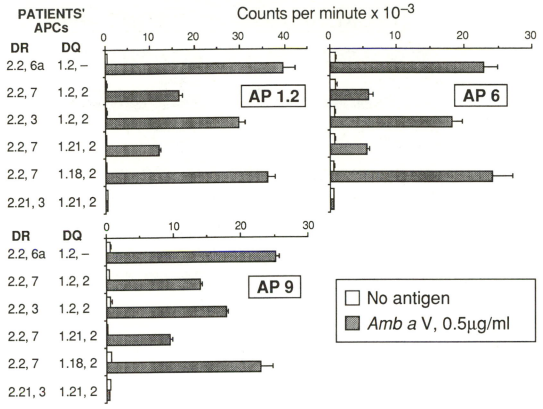

Figure 5. MHC restriction of *Amb a* V-specific T-cell proliferation of three clones using patients' cells as APCs. *Amb a* V (0.5 μg/ml) was presented to three T-cell clones (1 × 10⁴ cells/well) derived from patient AP by autologous APCs (top experiment in each set) or a panel of patients' APCs. The class II MHC phenotypes of patients' APCs are shown. [³H]thymidine incorporation (cpm ± S.E. for triplicate cultures) was measured as described in Materials and Methods. Results for other experiments using APCs from patient WE (DR2.22⁺) and several other patients (including DR4⁺ subjects) were negative, similar to those using APCs from DR2.21⁺ patient CLo. (Data from S.K. Huang et al., in prep.)

concur with the sequencing data and suggest that a DR gene product ($\alpha\beta_I$ or $\alpha\beta_{III}$) is important in *Amb a* V presentation.

To define further the restriction specificity of the *Amb a* V-specific T-cell response, the inhibitory effects of various anti-HLA-D monoclonal antibodies were examined on *Amb a* V-induced proliferation of two T-cell clones, AP1.2 and AP9, using autologous APCs (Fig. 6). First, of the three anti-HLA-D common-epitope monoclonal antibodies (anti-DR, anti-DQ, and anti-DP), only anti-DR was effective in blocking the proliferative responses of both clones to *Amb a* V. Inhibition was directly dependent on the dose of the anti-DR monoclonal antibody (data not shown). Similar evidence for DR restriction was also obtained using the T-cell line of patient BE (data not shown). Second, and most significantly, the anti-DR$\alpha\beta_I$2.2 monoclonal antibody (Hu30) blocked, in a dose-dependent manner, the responses of the cloned T cells to *Amb a* V (Fig. 6). The blocking effects of both anti-DR and Hu30 monoclonal antibodies were specific, since the control ascites at equivalent dilution was not inhibitory (Fig. 6); furthermore, stimulation of both clones with PHA was not inhibited by either monoclonal antibody

at the highest test concentrations used in the blocking experiments (data not shown).

We confirmed that Hu30 was much more specific for DR$\alpha\beta_I$2.2 than DR$\alpha\beta_{III}$2.2 by separate analyses using DR$\alpha\beta_I$2.2 and DR$\alpha\beta_{III}$2.2 transfectant mouse L-cell lines kindly provided by J. Trowsdale (Wilkinson et al. 1988). Staining with graded concentrations of MAb Hu30 (plus fluorescent anti-mouse IgG) showed that at 1:500 and 1:5000 dilutions of ascites fluid, the monoclonal antibody recognizes only the DR$\alpha\beta_I$2.2 transfectant (data not shown). Note that MAb Hu30 significantly inhibited T-cell responses to *Amb a* V even at a 1:10,000 dilution (Fig. 6). These results strongly suggest that the DR$\alpha\beta_I$2.2 heterodimer is the restriction element controlling *Amb a* V-specific T-cell response.

Inhibition of *Amb a* V-specific T-cell Activation by the *Amb a* V Homologs *Amb t* V and *Amb p* V

To test the hypothesis that T-cell responsiveness to both *Amb t* V and *Amb p* V is, like *Amb a* V, also restricted by a DR2.2 Ia molecule, we first examined whether either molecule was able to activate the cloned *Amb a* V-specific T cells. As shown in Figure 7, neither

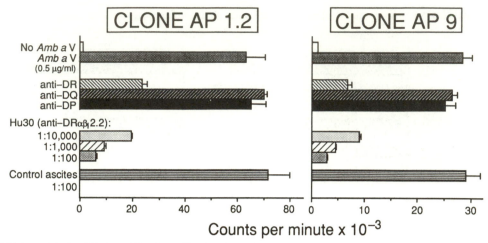

Figure 6. Inhibition of *Amb a* V-induced T-cell proliferation by anti-HLA-D monoclonal antibodies. T-cell clones, AP1.2 and AP 9 (1×10^4 cells/well), were incubated with or without 0.5 μg/ml *Amb a* V in the presence of autologous APCs and various anti-HLA-D monoclonal antibodies as indicated. Monoclonal antibody concentrations used: anti-DR, anti-DQ, and anti-DP, 1 μg/ml; Hu30, 1:100–1:10,000 dilutions of ascites fluid; control ascites (H5A4), 1:100 dilution. [^{3}H]Thymidine incorporation in mean cpm ± S.E. for triplicate cultures. (Adapted from S.K. Huang et al., in prep.)

Amb t V nor *Amb p* V was able to stimulate clones AP1.2 and AP9, in the presence of autologous APCs, at antigen concentrations ranging between 0.1 μg/ml and 10 μg/ml. We then determined whether either *Amb* V homolog could inhibit *Amb a* V antigen presentation in the same system (Fig. 7). Autologous APCs, when prepulsed for 10 hours at 37°C with *Amb t* V or *Amb p* V, followed by extensive washing, lost their ability to present *Amb a* V to clones AP1.2 and AP9 as the concentrations of the inhibitors were increased. The inhibitory function of both *Amb* V homologs was specific, since a control antigen, *Lol p* III, had no effect on cloned T-cell responses to *Amb a* V, even at a 100-fold higher concentration. Furthermore, neither *Amb* V homolog was cytotoxic, since no inhibition was observed in the mitogenic responses of either clone to

PHA (data not shown). These data strongly suggest that both *Amb t* V and *Amb p* V share similar or identical agretopes with *Amb a* V.

DISCUSSION

The results of our SSO–dot-blot (plus DNA-sequencing) studies of DRB and DQB1 second exons, and our studies using T-cell clones, strongly implicate the DR$\alpha\beta_1$2.2 molecule as the primary restriction element in human immune responsiveness to the *Amb a* V allergen. This class II MHC molecule contains the more basic of the two DRβ polypeptides associated with Dw2 (see Nomenclature). First, we found three unusual HLA-DRB/DQB sequence combinations, not previously reported in the literature—two *Amb a* V re-

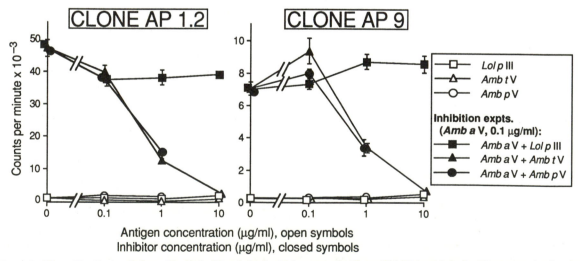

Figure 7. Direct T-cell stimulation with *Amb t* V and *Amb p* V (open symbols), and inhibition of *Amb a* V presentation by *Amb t* V and *Amb p* V (closed symbols). *Lol p* III was used as the control antigen. Results are expressed in terms of [^{3}H]thymidine incorporation (mean cpm ± S.E.) from triplicate cultures. (Adapted from S.K. Huang et al., in prep.)

sponders (#218 and CSz) who had DRB1*2.2 and DRB3*2.2, but not DQB1.2 (which is in strong linkage disequilibrium with DRB2.2 in Caucasoid populations), and one nonresponder who had DQB1.2 but not DRB1*2.2 and DRB3*2.2 (Fig. 2c). Taken together, these data implicate either the $DR\alpha\beta_I 2.2$ or the $DR\alpha\beta_{III} 2.2$ molecule as the major Amb a V–Ir gene product. Second, antigen-presentation studies (cf. Figs. 4 and 5), using three T-cell clones from a single individual, with various HTCs and allogeneic cells from selected patients (including #218 and CSz) as APCs, support this finding. This conclusion is further supported by the positive anti-DR blocking data in antigen-presentation studies using the T-cell clones (Fig. 6), as well as similar studies using a T-cell line from another patient. Finally, the positive blocking experiments using MAb Hu30 in antigen presentation to the T-cell clones (Fig. 6) strongly implicate $DR\alpha\beta_I 2.2$ as the principal restriction element. A more direct test would be of Amb a V presentation by a $DR\alpha\beta_I 2.2$ transfectant cell line; this has been attempted unsuccessfully using transfected L cells. Possibly, these cells are unable to process the disulfide-rich Amb a V molecule effectively.

As already noted, almost all subjects who respond to Amb a V following ultralow-dosage natural exposure to short ragweed pollen type as DR2/Dw2 (DR2.2); in such cases, $DR\alpha\beta_I 2.2$ appears to be a necessary requirement for Amb a V responsiveness. Most of the remaining DR2.2+ subjects respond to Amb a V after Rx with much higher Amb a V doses (Marsh et al. 1982a; P. Zwollo et al., in prep.). The presence of DR2.2 may be an *insufficient* requirement for responsiveness after ragweed Rx in only a few exceptional cases, such as those included in this study (patients MB and #238 [and weak responder #403]; Fig. 2b). These patients, who are highly atopic to several allergens other than Amb a V, may require higher cumulative Amb a V doses to produce IgG antibody responses, or they may be completely deficient with respect to class

II-restricted recognition of Amb a V (e.g., in their functional T-cell repertoires). Indeed, for some DR2.2+ patients, factors such as "holes" in the expressed T-cell repertoires, differential levels of expression of $DR\alpha\beta_I 2.2$, and absence of idiotype priming may contribute to nonresponsiveness to Amb a V under conditions of low-dose natural exposure or artificial immunization with small amounts of antigen (cf. Marsh 1986).

Besides the aforestated $DR\alpha\beta_I 2.2$ restriction, we also found evidence for restriction by other class II specificities, especially for patients who had received ragweed Rx with much higher doses of Amb a V. We found one atopic Oriental subject, who possesses a low level of IgG antibody (but no IgE antibody) to Amb a V, who types as DRB2.12 by SSO–dot-blot analysis (S.K. Huang et al., in prep.). This preliminary evidence, together with the observation that Dw12+ HTCs can present Amb a V to the cloned T cells of patient AP (Fig. 4), and a close similarity in the amino acid sequences of the β_I polypeptides of DR2.2 and DR2.12 (including residues that are believed to be involved in binding to antigen fragments; Fig. 8), suggests that $DR\alpha\beta_I 2.12$ is capable of substituting for $DR\alpha\beta_I 2.2$ in Amb a V presentation.

A proportion (3/5) of DR2.21+ subjects and one DR2.22+ atopic subject were able to produce adequate IgG antibody responses to Amb a V, but only after receiving ragweed Rx, usually at high antigen dosage (Fig. 2d). Furthermore, HTCs having specificities Dw21 or Dw22, and patients' APCs possessing DRB1*2.21 and DRB1*2.22 according to our DNA studies, were *not* able to present Amb a V to the T-cell clones derived from a DR2.2 subject (Figs. 4 and 5). The immunization data suggest that Dw21+ and Dw22+ APCs are less efficient in Amb a V presentation than Dw2 (resulting in a lower immune responsiveness); the antigen-presentation data show that the presentation of Amb a V peptide(s) is qualitatively different in the case of Dw21+ and Dw22+ cells than for Dw2+ or Dw12+

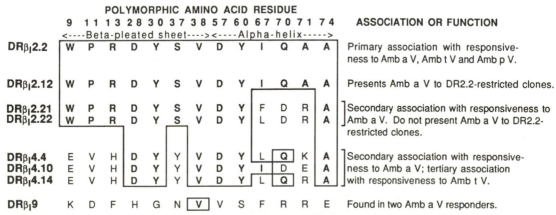

	POLYMORPHIC AMINO ACID RESIDUE													ASSOCIATION OR FUNCTION
	9	11	13	28	30	37	38	57	60	67	70	71	74	
	<----Beta-pleated sheet---->					<----Alpha-helix----->								
$DR\beta_I 2.2$	W	P	R	D	Y	S	V	D	Y	I	Q	A	A	Primary association with responsiveness to Amb a V, Amb t V and Amb p V.
$DR\beta_I 2.12$	W	P	R	D	Y	S	V	D	Y	I	Q	A	A	Presents Amb a V to DR2.2-restricted clones.
$DR\beta_I 2.21$	W	P	R	D	Y	S	V	D	Y	F	D	R	A	Secondary association with responsiveness to Amb a V. Do not present Amb a V to DR2.2-restricted clones.
$DR\beta_I 2.22$	W	P	R	D	Y	S	V	D	Y	L	D	R	A	
$DR\beta_I 4.4$	E	V	H	D	Y	Y	V	D	Y	L	Q	K	A	Secondary association with responsiveness to Amb a V; tertiary association with responsiveness to Amb t V.
$DR\beta_I 4.10$	E	V	H	D	Y	Y	V	D	Y	I	D	E	A	
$DR\beta_I 4.14$	E	V	H	D	Y	Y	V	D	Y	L	Q	R	A	
$DR\beta_I 9$	K	D	F	H	G	N	V	V	S	F	R	R	E	Found in two Amb a V responders.

Figure 8. Comparison of polymorphic amino acid residues of HLA-DRβ polypeptides that are postulated to point into the antigen-binding groove (Brown et al. 1988) and may be implicated in Amb a V binding. Only residues known to possess three or more amino acid variants in different β chains are shown. The DRβ polypeptides are designated as follows: position of locus that encodes the polypeptide (given as a Roman numeral subscript), DR serotype, period, Dw type determined by MLR (see Nomenclature section of Materials and Methods for further details).

cells. These differences may be a reflection of significant amino acid differences at positions 67, 70, and 71 in the β_I polypeptides (Fig. 8).

Other than patient LL, further Amb a V responders possess DR4.4, 4.10, or 4.14, or DR9 (Fig. 3). With three exceptions (JKo, ML, and MS), these subjects possess only moderate or low levels of serum IgG antibody to Amb a V only following Rx. The DRβ_I sequences of these DR4 subtypes, but not of DR9, show some similarity with DRβ_I2.2 in the hypothesized antigen-binding region (Fig. 8). (DRw53, which is associated with DR4 and DR9, has a DRβ_{IV} sequence very different from DRβ_I2.2; furthermore, DRw53 is unlikely to be involved in immune response to Amb a V, since it is also associated with the nonresponder phenotype, DR7.) Thus, it is possible that DR$\alpha\beta_I$4 molecules may bind the same or a similar Amb a V peptide as DR$\alpha\beta_I$2.2. As an alternative, perhaps more plausible hypothesis, class II molecules constituting three subtypes of DQw3, namely, DR4-associated DQ3.1 and 3.2 and the DR9-associated DQ3.3 molecule, which have identical DQα and very similar DQβ polypeptides, may form independent restriction elements for an Amb a V peptide. (The typing of patient LL as DQB1*3.1 would seem to support this hypothesis; however, his DQA typing was DQA1*4 [DR5-associated]. We found two nonresponders after ragweed Rx who possessed the DRB1*7,DQB1*3.3 phenotype. However, the associated DQA1 sequence [DQA1*2] was quite different from that associated with DR4 and DR9 [DQA1*3] [P. Zwollo et al., in prep.], as previously observed [Horn et al. 1988].) Cloning of T cells from DR4$^+$ and DR9$^+$ Amb a V responders will be necessary to investigate these hypotheses.

We have found that IgG antibody responsiveness to Amb t V and to Amb p V is associated with DR2.2 (Roebber et al. 1985; Marsh et al. 1987b and unpubl.), suggesting that major agretopes of these molecules may also be involved in binding to DR$\alpha\beta_I$2.2. To begin investigating this hypothesis, we used the Amb a V T-cell clones in antigen-presentation experiments. Amb t V and Amb p V did not directly stimulate these clones; however, they did block Amb a V-induced response in a dose-dependent manner (Fig. 7). These two observations indicate distinct T-cell epitopes but similar or identical agretopes on the Amb V molecules. Interestingly, Amb p V, but not Amb t V, cross-reacts with Amb a V at the B-cell level (Marsh et al. 1987b and unpubl.).

We have made preliminary investigations of the nature of the Amb a V agretope by use of synthetic peptides related to portions of the Amb a V molecule that show quite strong homology with Amb t V, specifically residues 12–26 and 31–44 (Fig. 1). (Note that there is evidence for amphipathicity within the regions 12–26 in the case of Amb a V and Amb t V; see legend to the figure.) To facilitate peptide synthesis, most of the cysteine residues were substituted by alanine. Experiments using these peptides for presentation to the T-cell clones, or in the blocking of Amb a V presenta-

tion, have so far not produced definitive data, although there is suggestive evidence that peptide 31–44 may bind to the class II molecule. Further experiments are in progress to examine this question, including the use of fragments of Amb a V produced by reduction and alkylation and/or proteolytic digestion.

As an alternative to the peptide-synthesis approach, we are in the process of isolating Amb a V and Amb t V cDNAs from cDNA libraries of short and giant ragweed pollens. These clones will be used in site-directed mutagenesis experiments to define the agretopes/T-cell epitopes on Amb a V and Amb t V and, hopefully, to circumvent the problem of the high proportions of S–S bonds in these molecules.

Besides the Amb V homologs, we have extended our studies to another set of allergens showing sequence homology, namely, the Lol p I, II, and III allergens from Lolium perenne (rye grass) pollen (Ansari et al. 1989a,b; Esch and Klapper 1989), for which we have data suggesting that responsiveness to all three allergens may be associated with the amino acid sequence EYSTS found in the first APR of the β_I polypeptide of DR3, DR5, and DR6 (Ansari et al. 1989c).

The complete elucidation of an HLA-A (class I MHC) structure by X-ray crystallography (Bjorkman et al. 1987), together with computer modeling of related HLA-D structures (Brown et al. 1988; Bjorkman and Davis, this volume), has allowed the prediction of which specific class II residues interact with the antigen fragment and the T-cell receptor (see other chapters in this volume). Using antigen-specific T-cell clones and direct class II–antigen peptide-binding studies, we believe that it will be possible to define more clearly the molecular basis of immune responsiveness to defined allergen molecules. Since there are so many different allergen molecules available for study, many of which have already been sequenced, or soon will be sequenced using recombinant DNA technology, allergy offers a unique model for studying the molecular basis of human immune responsiveness.

ACKNOWLEDGMENTS

We thank many colleagues and collaborators who contributed to these studies. Particularly, we thank Eva Ehrlich-Kautzky for excellent technical assistance in the DNA sequencing studies and Dr. Henry Erlich and Stephen Scharf of Cetus Corporation for help in our establishing the PCR technology. This work was supported by National Institutes of Health grants AI-19727 and AI-20059.

REFERENCES

Allen, P.M., B.P. Babbitt, and E.R. Unanue. 1987. T-cell recognition of lysozymes; the biochemical basis of presentation. Immunol. Rev. 98: 172.

Ansari, A.A., T.K. Kihara, and D.G. Marsh. 1987. Immunochemical studies of Lolium perenne (rye grass) allergens Lol p I, II, III. J. Immunol. 139: 4034.

Ansari, A.A., P. Shenbagamurthi, and D.G. Marsh. 1989a. Complete amino acid sequence of *Lolium perenne* (perennial rye grass) allergen, *Lol p* II. *J. Biol. Chem.* **264**: 11181.

———. 1989b. Complete primary structure of a *Lolium perenne* (perennial rye grass) allergen, *Lol p* III: Comparison with known *Lol p* I and II sequences. *Biochemistry* **28**: 8665.

Ansari, A.A., L.R. Freidhoff, D.A. Meyers, W.B. Bias, and D.G. Marsh. 1989c. Human immune responsiveness to *Lolium perenne* (rye) grass pollen allergen *Lol p* III (Rye III) is associated with HLA-DR3 and DR5. *Hum. Immunol.* **25**: 59.

Baur, M.P., N. Neugebauer, and E.D. Albert. 1984. Reference tables of two-locus haplotype frequencies for all MHC marker loci. In *Histocompatibility testing 1984* (ed. E.D. Albert et al.), p. 677. Springer-Verlag, Berlin.

Bjorkman, P.J., M.A. Saper, B. Samraoui, W.S. Bennett, J.L. Strominger, and D.C. Wiley. 1987. Structure of the human class I histocompatibility antigen, HLA-A2. *Nature* **329**: 506.

Brown, J.H., T. Jardetzky, M. Saper, B. Samraoui, P.J. Bjorkman, and D.C. Wiley. 1988. A hypothetical model for the foreign antigen binding site of Class II histocompatibility molecules. *Nature* **332**: 845.

Buus, S., A. Sette, and H. Grey. 1987. The interaction between protein derived immunogenic peptides and Ia. *Immunol. Rev.* **98**: 115.

Erlich, H.A., E.L. Sheldon, and G. Horn. 1986. HLA typing using DNA probes. *Biotechnology* **4**: 975.

Esch, R.E. and D.G. Klapper. 1989. Isolation and characterization of a major cross-reactive grass Group I allergenic determinant. *Mol. Immunol.* **26**: 557.

Freidhoff, L.R., E. Ehrlich-Kautzky, D.A. Meyers, S.H. Hsu, W.B. Bias, and D.G. Marsh. 1988. Association of HLA-DR3 and total serum immunoglobulin E level with human immune response to *Lol p* I and *Lol p* II allergens in allergic subjects. *Tissue Antigens* **31**: 211.

Goodfriend, L., A.M. Choudhury, D.G. Klapper, K.M. Coulter, G.D. Dorval, J. DeCarpio, and C.K. Osterland. 1985. Ra5G, a homologue of Ra5 in giant ragweed pollen: Isolation, HLA-DR-associated activity and amino acid sequence. *Mol. Immunol.* **22**: 899.

Gorski, J., P. Rollini, and B. Mach. 1987. Structural comparison of the genes of two HLA-DR supertypic groups: The loci encoding DRw52 and DRw53 are not truly allelic. *Immunogenetics* **25**: 397.

Guillet, J.-G., M.-Z. Lay, T.J. Briner, S. Buus, S. Alessandro, H.M. Grey, J.A. Smith, and M.L. Gefter. 1987. Immunological self, nonself discrimination. *Science* **235**: 866.

Horn, G., T. Bugawan, C.M. Long, and H.A. Erlich. 1988. Allelic variation of the HLA-DQ loci: Relationship to serology and to insulin-dependent diabetes susceptibility. *Proc. Natl. Acad. Sci.* **85**: 6012.

Huang, S.K. and D.G. Marsh. 1989. Genetic restriction of human T-cell clones to short ragweed allergen, *Amb a* V. *Am. J. Hum. Genet.* **55**: A196.

International Union of Immunological Studies (IUIS) HLA Nomenclature Subcommittee. 1988. Nomenclature for factors of the HLA system. 1987. *Immunogenetics* **28**: 391.

Kappes, D. and J.L. Strominger. 1988. Human class II major histocompatibility complex genes and proteins. *Annu. Rev. Biochem.* **57**: 991.

Kawai, J., A. Ando, T. Sato, T. Nakasatsuji, K. Tsuji, and H. Inoko. 1989. Analysis of gene structure and antigen determinants of DR2 antigens using DR gene transfer into mouse L cells. *J. Immunol.* **142**: 312.

Lamb, J.R., A.B. Kay, and R.E. O'Hehir. 1989. HLA Class II restriction specificity of *Dermatophagoides* spp. reactive T lymphocyte clones that support IgE synthesis. *Clin. Exp. Allergy* (in press).

Lapkoff, C.B. and L. Goodfriend. 1974. Isolation of a low molecular weight ragweed pollen allergen: Ra5. *Int. Arch. Allergy Appl. Immunol.* **46**: 215.

Lee, B.S.M., N.A. Rust, A.J. McMichael, and H.O. McDevitt. 1987. HLA-DR2 subtypes from an additional supertypic family of *DRβ* alleles. *Proc. Natl. Acad. Sci.* **84**: 4591.

Liu, C.-P., F.H. Bach, and S. Wu. 1988. Molecular studies of a rare DR2/LD-5a/DQw3 HLA Class II haplotype. *J. Immunol.* **140**: 3631.

Margalit, H., J.L. Spouge, J.L. Cornette, C. DeLisi, and J.A. Berzofsky. 1987. Prediction of immunodominant helper T-cell antigenic sites from the primary sequence. *J. Immunol.* **138**: 2213.

Marsh, D.G. 1975. Allergens and the genetics of allergy. In *The antigens*, Volume III. (ed. M. Sela), p. 271. Academic Press, New York.

———. 1986. Defining human immune response fingerprints toward ultra-pure allergens: Immunochemical and genetic aspects of responsiveness toward the *Amb* V (Ra5) homologues. *J. Allergy Clin. Immunol. (Suppl.)* **78**: 242.

Marsh, D.G. and P.S. Norman. 1988. Antigens that cause atopic disease. In *Immunological diseases*, 4th edition (ed. M. Samter et al.), p. 1027. Little, Brown and Company, Boston.

Marsh, D.G., D.A. Meyers, and W.B. Bias. 1981. The epidemiology and genetics of atopic allergy. *N. Engl. J. Med.* **305**: 1551.

Marsh, D.G., L.R. Freidhoff, E. Ehrlich-Kautzky, W.B. Bias, and M. Roebber. 1987a. Immune responsiveness to *Ambrosia artemisiifolia* (short ragweed) pollen allergen *Amb a* VI (Ra6) is associated with HLA-DR5 in allergic humans. *Immunogenetics* **26**: 230.

Marsh, D.G., L. Goodfriend, T.P. King, H. Løwenstein, and T.A.E. Platts-Mills. 1986. Allergen nomenclature. *Bull. WHO* **64**: 767.

Marsh, D.G., L.R. Freidhoff, D.B.K. Golden, E. Ehrlich-Kautzky, M. Roebber, D.A. Meyers, and C.L. Holland. 1987b. Genetic studies of immune response to the *Amb a* V homologues. *Fed. Proc.* **46**: 1047. (Abstr.)

Marsh, D.G., S.H. Hsu, M. Roebber, E. Ehrlich-Kautzky, L.R. Freidhoff, D.A. Meyers, M.K. Pollard, and W.B. Bias. 1982a. HLA-Dw2: A genetic marker for human immune response to short ragweed pollen allergen Ra5. I. Response resulting primarily from natural antigenic exposure. *J. Exp. Med.* **155**: 1439.

Marsh, D.G., D.A. Meyers, L.R. Freidhoff, E. Ehrlich-Kautzky, M. Roebber, P.S. Norman, S.H. Hsu, and W.B. Bias. 1982b. HLA-Dw2: A genetic marker for human immune response to short ragweed pollen allergen Ra5. II. Response after ragweed immunotherapy. *J. Exp. Med.* **155**: 1452.

Mole, L.E., L. Goodfriend, C.B. Lapkoff, J.M. Kehoe, and J.D. Capra. 1975. The amino-acid sequence of allergen Ra5. *Biochemistry* **14**: 1216.

O'Hehir, R.E., A.J. Frew, A.B. Kay, and J.R. Lamb. 1988. MHC class II restriction specificity of cloned human T lymphocytes reactive with *Dermatophagoides farinae* (house dust mite). *Immunology* **64**: 627.

O'Hehir, R.E., D.B. Young, A.B. Kay, and J.R. Lamb. 1987. Cloned human T lymphocytes reactive with *Dermatophagoides farinae* (house dust mite): A comparison of T- and B-cell antigen recognition. *Immunology* **62**: 635.

Roebber, M., D.G. Klapper, and D.G. Marsh. 1982. Two isoallergens of short ragweed component Ra5. *J. Immunol.* **129**: 120.

Roebber, M., D.G. Klapper, L. Goodfriend, W.B. Bias, S.H. Hsu, and D.G. Marsh. 1985. Immunochemical and genetic studies of *Amb t* V (Ra5G), an Ra5 homologue from giant ragweed pollen. *J. Immunol.* **134**: 3062.

Saiki, R.K., D.H. Gelfand, S. Stoffel, S.J. Scharf, R. Higuchi, T. Horn, K.B. Mullis, and H.A. Erlich. 1988. Primer-directed enzymatic amplification of DNA with a thermostable DNA polymerase. *Science* **239**: 487.

Sone, T.K., K. Tsukamoto, K. Hirayama, Y. Nishimura, T. Takenouchi, M. Aizawa, and T. Sasazuki. 1985. Two distinct class II molecules encoded by the genes within the HLA-DR subregion of HLA-Dw2 and Dw12 can act as stimulating and restriction molecules. *J. Immunol.* **135:** 1288.

Todd, J.A., J.I. Bell, and H.O. McDevitt. 1987. HLA-DQβ gene contributes to susceptibility and resistance to insulin-dependent diabetes mellitus. *Nature* **329:** 599.

Wilkinson, D., R.R.P. De Vries, J.A. Madrigal, C.B. Lock, J.A. Morgenstern, J. Trowsdale, and D.M. Altmann. 1988. Analysis of HLA-DR glycoproteins by DNA-mediated gene transfer. Definition of DR2β gene products and antigen presentation to T cell clones from leprosy patients. *J. Exp. Med.* **167:** 1442.

Zwollo, P., A.A. Ansari, and D.G. Marsh. 1989a. Association of class II DNA-restriction fragments with responsiveness to *Ambrosia artemisiifolia* (short ragweed) pollen allergen *Amb a* V. *J. Allergy Clin. Immunol.* **83:** 45.

Zwollo, P., E. Ehrlich-Kautzky, A.A. Ansari, H.A. Erlich, and D.G. Marsh. 1989b. HLA-D sequence polymorphism in responders and non-responders to short ragweed allergen, *Amb a* V. *FASEB J.* **3:** A1099.

Monoclonal Antibodies and the Epitope Distribution of HLA Class II Polymorphisms

J.G. BODMER, S.G.E. MARSH, AND J.M. HEYES
Tissue Antigen Laboratory, Imperial Cancer Research Fund, Lincoln's Inn Fields,
London WC2A 3PX, United Kingdom

Antisera produced by feto-maternal stimulation were originally used for the identification of HLA antigens. In 1964, through the use of such antisera, a two-allele polymorphism then called LA, now HLA-A (Payne et al. 1964), was identified. At the time, it was thought to be independent of van Rood's 4a, 4b polymorphism, now called HLA-Bw4 and HLA-Bw6 (van Rood and van Leeuwen 1963). The failure to see that the HLA-A locus products were closely linked to the HLA-B locus products was due partly to the complexity of some of the antisera and partly to the lack of reproducibility of the then available assays, which gave rise to apparent recombinants with too high a frequency to support close linkage.

Some years later, it was realized that many HLA typing sera showing extra reactions on B-lymphoblastoid cell lines contained antibodies to class II products (Bodmer et al. 1976a) and chronic lymphatic leukemia (CLL) cells (Bodmer et al. 1976b). These sera were used to identify an Ia-related group by their reactions on B-lymphocyte-derived cells that had been stripped of β_2-microglobulin to block their class I sites or simply had class I reactions blocked by antisera to β_2-microglobulin. Later, using antisera that were absorbed to remove HLA class I antibodies (Barnstable et al. 1977) to test peripheral B lymphocytes and B-lymphoblastoid lines, five groups of sera (OX1–5) that correlated with cellularly defined HLA-class II specificities were identified. Recent reanalysis of the data shows that OX1 identifies DQw3, OX2 is DQw2, OX3 is DQw1, and OX4 is "all but DQw2." In addition, mixed in these groups were sera identifying DR7 and DRw52. Although definition of both class I and class II antigens with such polyclonal antisera has improved, it still requires complex analysis and, for class II, extensive absorption of antibodies that then may be weak and are certainly in limited supply.

Early Monoclonal Antibodies

Development of the technique for producing monoclonal antibodies (Kohler and Milstein 1975) was welcomed as a possible replacement for typing with antisera. Early fusions of spleen cells from mice immunized with whole human cells (Barnstable et al. 1977) or purified HLA protein (Brodsky et al. 1979; Trucco et al. 1979), producing both monomorphic and polymorphic class I and class II antibodies, encouraged this possibility. However, it soon became apparent that some specificities were preferentially produced in many immunizations, whereas antibodies to a large number of class I and class II specificities were never produced.

Ten years later, the situation concerning the availability of monoclonal antibodies for HLA typing offered for the 11th International Histocompatibility Workshop is as follows. For HLA class I, there are 50 potentially useful antibodies for HLA-A, 27 for HLA-B, and only 2 for HLA-C, but since many of these are against the same specificity, e.g., HLA-A2, 28, there are not nearly enough for a comprehensive typing. For class II, there are 55 DR antibodies and 6 DP antibodies; again not covering the range of specificities. Interestingly, there are more than 30 HLA-DQ antibodies, covering the full range of DQ specificities so far identified.

Epitope Sequence Mapping of HLA-DR and DQ Monoclonal Antibodies

The difference between HLA-DQ and the other class II HLA loci in the apparent immunogenicity of their products was clearly worth studying. Class II sequences have been collected from many laboratories (Marsh and Bodmer 1989), and the positions of polymorphic residues that correlated with the specificities of HLA-DR and DQ antibodies have been mapped on to the sequences (Figs. 1 and 2). These sites are not necessarily the binding sites of the antibodies, since it is thought to be unlikely (M. Sternberg, pers. comm.) that antibodies could bind directly to some of the sites in the bottom of the groove of the three-dimensional class II structure (Fig. 3), which is based on the published class I structure (Bjorkman et al. 1987) and is similar to the published putative class II structure (Brown et al. 1988).

HLA-DR Specificities

Comparing the antibody-specific sites on DR and DQ shown in Figures 1 and 2, it is immediately clear that the sites of most of the DR antibodies, as indicated by the boxed areas in Figure 1, are much more complex than the DQ sites shown in Figure 2. That is, in DR sequences, a particular site or epitope appears to be shared between many of the DR alleles. Figure 1 shows the DR antibody-specific residues, or epitopes, and from the complex patterns indicated by arrows it is

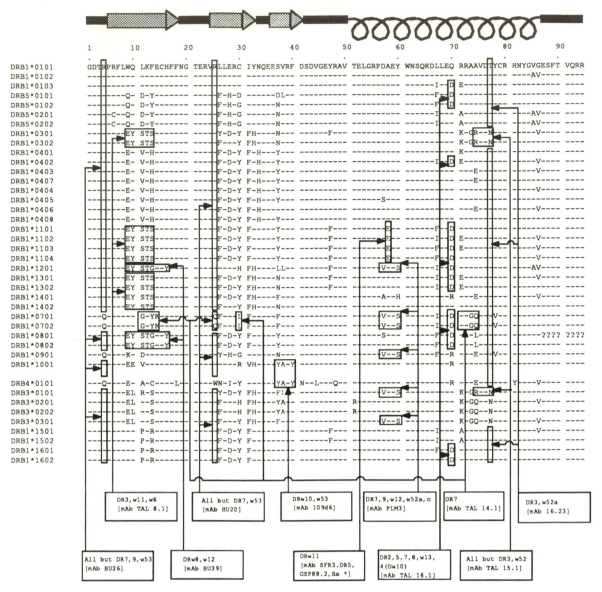

Figure 1. DRβ sequences indicating potential monoclonal antibody binding sites. The amino acid sequences of the first domains of 41 DRβ alleles. The standard one-letter amino acid code is used; a dash indicates identity to the DRB1*0101 sequence. Sites correlating with the reactivity of a monoclonal antibody are boxed. The monoclonal antibody specificity and the name of at least one antibody for this specificity are given at the bottom of the figure; arrows indicate which of these sites is implicated for each antibody. Above the sequences is a schematic of the proposed secondary structure: Arrows represent β strands, spirals represent α helices, and bars represent turns and bends. Official HLA nomenclature is used for naming the alleles. Human monoclonal antibodies are indicated by an asterisk.

clear that such specificities as "all but DR7, 9, w53" (residue 4) and "all but DR3 and DRw52" (residue 77) appear more often than simple specificities such as DRw11 at position 58, or DR7, which is not definitively mapped to a single site.

There are at least two monoclonal antibodies identifying DR7 alone: SFR16.DR7M (10W3050) (Kennedy et al. 1989; Marsh and Bodmer 1989),[1] a rat antibody; and TAL13.1, made in this laboratory

against a mouse L cell transfected with the DR7α and β genes. In addition, DR7 is one of the specificities for which there are a large number of reproducibly reacting pregnancy antisera. This suggests that whichever is the "binding" site of the antibodies, it is very immunogenic to rats, mice, and humans. It also seems that a number of apparently monomorphic antibodies, such as DA2 (Brodsky et al. 1979) and CA2 (Charron and McDevitt 1979), when tested on a large panel of L cells transfected with different class II genes, fail to react with the DR7 transfectant but react with DP transfectants, covering up the hole in their DR reactivity. Thus one, or perhaps more than one, of the possible DR7 sites

---

[1]Kennedy et al. (1989) is the relevant reference for all the 10th Workshop antibodies mentioned in this paper. Other antibodies are described by Marsh and Bodmer (1989).

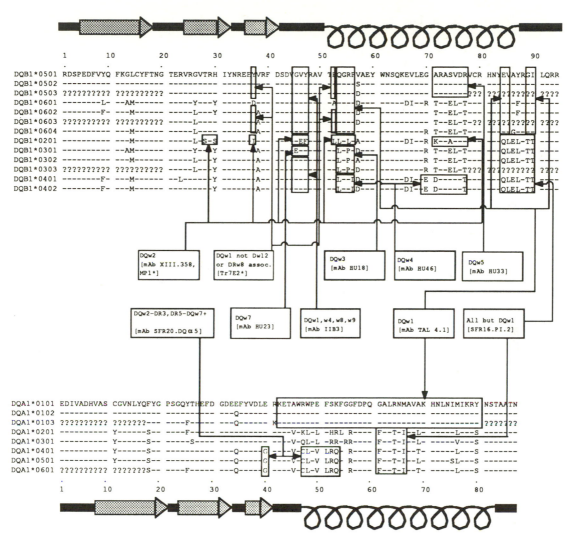

Figure 2. DQα and β sequences indicating potential monoclonal antibody binding sites. The amino acid sequences of the first domains of 13 DQβ and 8 DQα alleles. The standard one-letter amino acid code is used; a dash indicates identity to either the DQB1*0101 or DQA1*0101 sequence. Sites correlating with reactivity of a monoclonal antibody are boxed. The monoclonal antibody specificity and the name of at least one antibody for this specificity are given in the center of the figure; arrows indicate which of the sites is implicated for each antibody. Above and below the sequences is a schematic of the proposed secondary structure: Arrows represent β strands, spirals represent α helices, and bars represent turns and bends. Official HLA nomenclature is used for naming the alleles. Human monoclonal antibodies are indicated by an asterisk.

shown in Figure 1 is important enough, possibly by its effect on the conformation of the molecule, to affect reactivity of a large proportion of antibodies.

Specific sites for other antibodies mapped both to sites in the groove and on the α helix are shown in Figure 1. Tucked in the end of groove (37–40) is the site for 109d6, an antibody to DRw53 and DRw10 (Toguchi et al. 1984). Of particular interest is the region in the groove between residues 9 and 16. This region includes the allele-specific residues for a large number of the DR alleles. There are already antibodies against several of these: 9–13 for the DR3, w11, w6 specificity of TAL8.1; 9–12 for the wider specificity DR3, w11, w12, w6, w8 of EIII15/4 (site not shown) (Trucco et al. 1979); 9–16 DRw8, w12 seen by HU39

(Nakayama et al. 1987); and 11–14, one of the DR7-specific sites. In this region, there are also allele-specific sequences for DR1, DR2, DR4, and DR9, although no monoclonal antibodies have so far been raised against them. This region in the groove, therefore, appears to be especially important for DR specificity and, presumably, for its influence on antigen recognition.

HLA-DQ Specificities

DQβ chain. For DQβ, on the other hand, the situation seems simpler than for DRβ. There is a site on the DQβ chain between 52 and 56 that has a different sequence for each of DQw1, 2, 3, and 4, and that is the probable site for antibodies identifying each of these specificities. This is not clear, however, in the case of DQw2, for which there are at least five possible sites (Fig. 2). There are two other sites located in the region 52–56; the DQw1, w4 site recognized by KS11 (10W3091) at 54–55 and the site for DQw3, w4 recognized by TAL12.1 produced in this laboratory, at 52–53 (data not shown). Site 45–47 has four sequence variations: the DQw7 site, one of the DQw2 sites, the "all but DQw2 site" (not shown), and the DQw1, w4, w8, w9 site, all of which have antibodies directed against them.

DQα chain. We have mapped two possible sites on the DQα chain, somewhere in the region 42–80 for DQw1 and 61–66 for "all but DQw1" seen by SFR16-PI.2 (Radka et al. 1985), but neither of these is a unique site, and the antibody sites could also be mapped to the DQβ chain. There is one antibody, however, SFR20-DQα5 (Amar et al. 1987), which by its pattern of reactivity sees a site on the DQA1*0401, 0501, and 0601 sequences at position 40 or 47–53. A second (human) antibody TrC5 (Kolstad et al. 1989) recognizes only the DQA1*0501 sequence, thus implicating positions 75–76 as its reactive site (not shown).

The Three-dimensional Class II Structure

Taking the postulated three-dimensional class II structures for HLA-DR and DQ mentioned above, the polymorphic sites derived from Figures 1 and 2 were mapped on to them. On the structures, shown in Figure 3, the amount of polymorphism is indicated by the color of the different variable amino acid positions. Thus, blue indicates two alternative residues, green indicates three, and so on. Comparing the structures, two features are immediately noticeable. One is, apart from the obvious fact that the DRα chain is invariant, that the level of polymorphism is much greater on the DR structure than on the DQ structure. At some amino acid sites on DR, as many as five, seven, or even eight variants have been seen. On the DQ structure, the maximum number of variants at any site is four, with the majority of polymorphic sites having only two alternatives. The other difference lies in the distribution of the polymorphic sites. On DR, the majority of polymorphism is seen in the groove, whereas on DQ the majority of polymorphic sites are on the α helices, with very few variations in the groove. It is of interest to ask whether this difference is reflected in the antibodies made to DR or DQ. Comparison of Figure 1 and Figure 3 (top) shows that the polymorphic sites in the groove match the reactivity of six or seven antibodies, as has been discussed above. For DQ, on the other hand, as shown in Figure 2 and Figure 3 (bottom), there is just one region in the groove, at position 36, against which an antibody may have been made. However, since there is another unique site for this specificity at position 52 that is very exposed, position 36 is not necessarily the antibody-binding site. Thus, the inter-esting contrast is observed between DQ antibodies that appear to be directed mainly at the two very obvious and accessible sites, 42–46 and 52–57, and DR antibodies that are directed at sites in the groove and along the top of the α helix. The two regions that are most immunogenic and variable in DQ are highly conserved in DR.

Mouse, Rat, and Human Antibodies

There are not yet enough data to say whether the range of monoclonal antibodies raised so far is restricted by the fact that most of them have been made in mouse or rat. Because of the complexity of human antisera, it is difficult to make comparisons between monoclonal antibody and human polyclonal serum specificity. The recognition of the DR7 site by mouse, rat, and human has been mentioned above. The DRw11 site at residue 58 similarly has been recognized by a mouse monoclonal antibody, GSP 88.2 (10W3036), a rat antibody, SFR3.DR5 (10W3037), and a human monoclonal antibody, HA (Hancock et al. 1988). Against DR products there is also another human monoclonal antibody, TrB12 (Kolstad et al. 1987), which seems to be a simple DRw52 antibody, a specificity not so far seen by a mouse. It is of interest that the human antibodies so far made that correlate with the mouse antibodies are to the simple DR specificities, as was discussed earlier. This could be because any human will carry many of the non-allele-specific epitopes and will therefore see narrower differences.

In DQ, pregnancy antisera, mouse and human monoclonal antibodies have been made against both DQw2 and DQw1, w4. A human monoclonal antibody TrC5 (Kolstad et al. 1989) sees a subset of the DQα alleles seen by the rat antibody SFR20-DQα5 and so probably does not bind to the same site. There is also a human antibody Tr7E2 (Hansen et al. 1987), which sees a subset of DQw1 and which has no mouse counterpart. It will be interesting in the light of further data to analyze the contribution of mouse, or mouse strain, differences compared with human, or human ethnic and individual, differences to the repertoire of antibodies that can be raised against human HLA class II polymorphic epitopes.

It seems unlikely, however, even at this stage, that repertoire differences between human and mouse could be entirely responsible for the differences between DR and DQ in the distribution of the sites against which antibodies have been raised. What is certain is that the differences in distribution and level of polymorphism between DR and DQ must be factors in the evolution and function of the human class II region.

ACKNOWLEDGMENTS

We thank Amanda Sadler, Genevieve Rabiasz, Lorna Kennedy, and Peter Krausa for their help with production and screening of the monoclonal antibod-

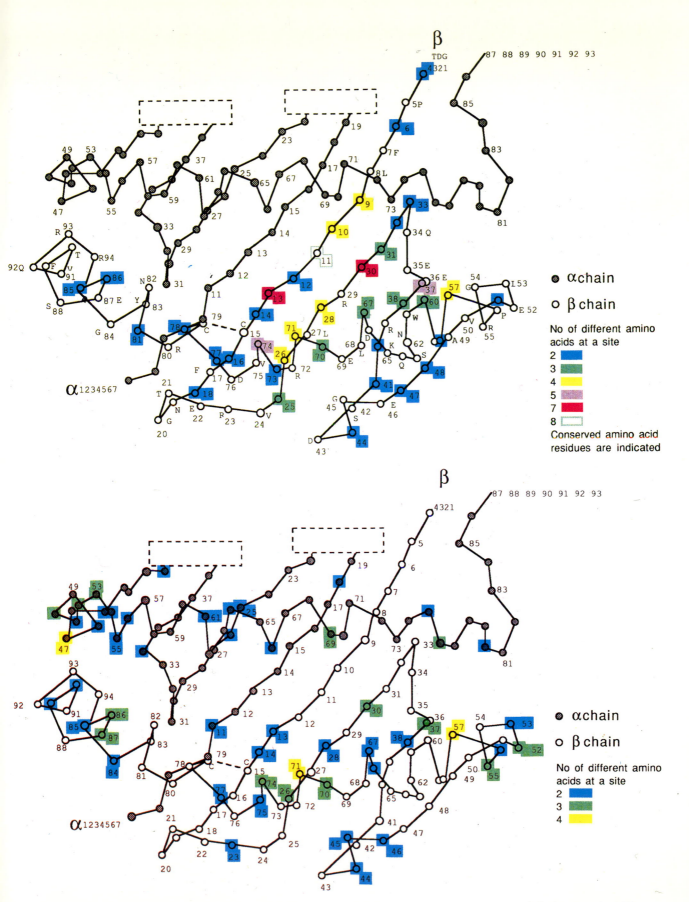

Figure 3. Postulated structures for DR (*top*) and DQ (*bottom*) based on the crystal structure of class I (Bjorkman et al. 1987). Colors indicate the degree of polymorphism at each residue. The structures between residues 19 and 22 and 38 and 48 (boxed) are omitted because of lack of homology at these sites with class I. (Reprinted, with permission, from Marsh and Bodmer 1989.)

475

ies; Jillian Maddox for help with the three-dimensional structure studies, and Walter Bodmer for his helpful comments.

REFERENCES

Amar, A., S.F. Radka, S.L. Holbeck, S.J. Kim, B.S. Nepom, K. Nelson,and G.T. Nepom. 1987. Characterization of specific HLA-DQα allospecificities by genomic, biochemical and serologic analysis. *J. Immunol.* **138:** 3986.

Barnstable, C.J., E.A. Jones, W.F. Bodmer, J.G. Bodmer, B. Arce-Gomez, D. Snary, and M.J. Crumpton. 1977. Genetics and serology of HLA-A-linked human Ia antigens. *Cold Spring Harbor Symp. Quant. Biol.* **41:** 443.

Bjorkman, P.J., M.A. Saper, B. Samraoui, W.S. Bennett, J.L. Strominger, and D.C. Wiley. 1987. Structure of the human class I histocompatibility antigen, HLA-A2. *Nature* **329:** 506.

Bodmer, W.F., E.A. Jones, D. Young, P.N. Goodfellow, J.G. Bodmer, H.M. Dick, and C.M. Steel. 1976a. Serology of human Ia type antigens detected on lymphoid lines: An analysis of the VI workshop sera. In *Histocompatibility testing 1975* (ed. F. Kissmeyer-Nielsen), p. 677. Munksgaard,Copenhagen.

Bodmer, W.F., J.G. Bodmer, P.R. Cullen, H.M. Dick, K. Gelsthorpe, R. Harris, S.D. Lawler, P. McKintosh, and P.J. Morris. 1976b. Ia antigens on chronic lymphocytic leukaemic lymphocytes? Associations between the reactions of VI workshop sera on CLL and lymphoid line cells. In *Histocompatibility Testing 1975* (ed. F. Kissmeyer-Nielsen), p. 685. Munksgaard, Copenhagen.

Brodsky, F.M., P. Parham, C.J. Barnstable, M.J. Crumpton, and W.F. Bodmer. 1979. Monoclonal antibodies for analysis of the HLA system. *Immunol. Rev.* **47:** 3.

Brown, J.H., T. Jardetzky, M.A. Saper, B. Samraoui, P.J. Bjorkman, and D. Wiley. 1988. A hypothetical model of the foreign antigen binding site of class II histocompatibility molecules. *Nature* **332:** 845.

Charron, D.J. and H.O. McDevitt. 1979. Analysis of HLA-D region associated molecules with monoclonal antibody. *Proc. Natl. Acad. Sci.* **76:** 6567.

Hancock, R.J.T., A. Martin, G.J. Laundy, J. Smythe, I. Roberts, H. Cooke, S. Pera, P. Bowerman, and B.A. Bradley. 1988. Production of monoclonal human antibody to HLA-DR5 (DRw11) by mouse/human heterohybridomas. *Hum. Immunol.* **22:** 135.

Hansen, T., A. Kolstad, G. Mathisen, and K. Hannestad. 1987. A human-human hybridoma (Tr7E2) producing cytotoxic antibody to HLA-DQw1. *Hum. Immunol.* **20:** 307.

Kennedy, L.J., S.G.E. Marsh, and J.G. Bodmer. 1989. Cytotoxic monoclonal antibodies. In *Immunobiology of HLA*, vol. I: *Histocompatibility testing 1987* (ed. B. Dupont), p. 301. Springer-Verlag, New York.

Kohler, G. and C. Milstein. 1975. Continuous culture of fused cells secreting antibody of predefined specificity. *Nature* **256:** 495.

Kolstad, A., T. Hansen, and K. Hannestad. 1987. A human-human hybridoma antibody (TrB12) defining subgroups of HLA-DQw1 and -DQw3. *Hum. Immunol.* **20:** 219.

Kolstad, A., B. Johansen, and K. Hannestad. 1989. Two HLA-DQ-specific human-human hybridoma antibodies (TrG6;Trc5) define epitopes also expressed by a transcomplementing hybrid DQ molecule (DQw7α/DQw4β). *Hum. Immunol.* **24:** 15.

Marsh, S.G.E. and J.G. Bodmer. 1989. HLA DR and DQ epitopes and monoclonal antibody specificity. *Immunol. Today* **10:** 305.

Nakayama, T., K. Ogasawara, H. Ikeda, H. Kunikane, M. Kasahara, N. Ishikawa, Y. Fukasawa, S. Hawkin, H. Kojima, A. Wakisaka, and M. Aizawa. 1987. A cytotoxic monoclonal antibody (HU-39) that detects DRw8+ DRw12. *Hum. Immunol.* **19:** 117.

Payne, R., M. Tripp, J. Weigle, W.F. Bodmer, and J. Bodmer. 1964. A new leukocyte isoantigen system in man. *Cold Spring Harbor Symp. Quant. Biol.* **29:** 285.

Radka, S.F., S.J. Stewart, and S.A. Smith. 1985. Analysis of HLA-DQ molecules with a monoclonal antibody detecting a DQ polymorphism absent from DQw1 homozygous cells. *Hum. Immunol.* **14:** 206.

Toguchi, T., G. Burmester, A. Nunez-Roldan, P. Gregersen, S. Seremetis, S. Lee, I. Szer, and R. Winchester. 1984. Evidence for the separate molecular expression of four distinct polymorphic Ia epitopes on cells of DR4 homozygous individuals. *Hum. Immunol.* **10:** 69.

Trucco, M.M., G. Garotta, J.W. Stocker, and R. Ceppellini. 1979. Murine monoclonal antibodies against HLA structure. *Immunol. Rev.* **47:** 219.

van Rood, J.J. and A. van Leeuwen. 1963. Leukocyte grouping: A method and its application. *J. Clin. Invest.* **42:** 1382.

T-lymphocyte Recognition of a Membrane Glycoprotein

T.J. BRACIALE, M.T. SWEETSER, L.R. BROWN, AND V.L. BRACIALE

Department of Pathology, Washington University School of Medicine, St. Louis, Missouri 63110

The vertebrate immune system is a complex of interacting cells and their soluble products. This system presumably evolved to deal with the threat of invasion by extracellular and intracellular microorganisms (see Mims 1982). The solution to this problem for vertebrates was to develop soluble and cell-associated effectors that can inhibit the replication of these organisms in the body. The thymus-derived (T) lymphocytes are critical cells involved both in the induction of the major specific soluble effector molecule, i.e., antibody, and in the direct expression of cell-associated effector activity, i.e., cytolysis of parasitized cells and the release of nonspecific mediators capable of orchestrating the inflammatory system.

In contrast to antibody molecules, T lymphocytes do not recognize foreign microorganisms and their products directly. Rather, they recognize antigens in association with products of the major histocompatibility gene complex (MHC) (Doherty et al. 1976). Two main classes of MHC products have been identified and characterized: Class I MHC products are displayed on the surfaces of most cell types in the vertebrate body; class II MHC products are, for the most part, constitutively displayed on cell types of lymphoreticular origin, although class II MHC expression can be induced on a variety of cell types through the action of cytokines. Two distinct subsets of T lymphocytes have been defined that recognize antigens in association with either class I or class II MHC products. Class I MHC-restricted T lymphocytes (henceforth referred to as class I T cells) are believed to function as direct cytolytic effectors, although they do secrete several cytokines upon exposure to antigen and class I MHC (Klein et al. 1982; Morris et al. 1982). Class II MHC-restricted T cells (henceforth referred to as class II T cells) primarily mediate their effector activity by cytokine release, although this T-cell subset can exhibit cytolytic activity in vitro (Feighery and Stastny 1979; Kaplan et al. 1984; Lukacher et al. 1985).

The antigen receptor on T lymphocytes does not recognize foreign antigens in their native form. Rather, this receptor recognizes nonnative "processed" fragments of protein antigens bound to MHC gene products (Unanue 1984). Strong evidence for this view initially came from studies of antigen recognition by class II T cells (Babbitt et al. 1985; Buus et al. 1986). More recently, evidence from the analysis of antigen recognition by class I T cells has also supported this concept (Townsend et al. 1985, 1986; Bjorkman et al. 1987).

A unifying feature of protein antigen recognition by T cells, then, is the preferential recognition of nonnative forms of these foreign moieties by both class I and class II T cells. Are there are any differences in antigen recognition between class I and class II T cells? Along with the obvious difference in restriction by class I and class II MHC molecules, there is evidence that the predominant pathway of antigen presentation to these two T-cell subsets is different (Morrison et al. 1986; Braciale et al. 1987).

We have examined the presentation and recognition of the influenza virus hemagglutinin glycoprotein (HA) by class I and class II T lymphocytes. This molecule is a constituent of the influenza virus virion (Lamb 1983) and, as such, can be presented to the immune system as a component of the virion particle or as an isolated polypeptide. Because the HA is synthesized de novo during infection of cells and is transported to the infected cell surface through the vesicular transport pathway (Copeland et al. 1986; Gething et al. 1986), the newly synthesized gene product in the infected cell is also available for recognition by the immune system. In this paper, we have used a series of mutant HA gene constructs to define the pathways through which the HA glycoprotein is processed and presented to T cells. Our data indicate that the pathways of HA presentation to class I and class II T cells are distinct. These results are discussed in terms of the intracellular compartments where antigen processing for class I and class II MHC presentation is localized.

RESULTS

Identification of an HA Site Recognized by Class I and Class II Cytolytic T Lymphocytes

We have recently identified and characterized two immunodominant sites on the A/Japan/305/57 (H2N2) HA recognized by class I (H-2K^d)-restricted murine T cells obtained from H-2^d haplotype donors (Braciale et al. 1989). These sites consist of an HA1 site corresponding to HA residues 202-221 and a carboxy-terminal site within the transmembrane anchor domain of the HA corresponding to residues 523-545. For studies on the generation of these two sites, we constructed a mutant HA gene (HAΔR1) that encodes a mutant HA lacking residues 248-409 of the primary HA translation product. This deletion mutant, which retains the HA 202-221 and HA 523-545 sites, is recognized by HA-specific class I cytolytic T lymphocytes (CTL) of the H-2^d, but not the H-2^k, haplotype (Braciale et al. 1989). The failure of HA-specific class I T cells from H-2^k mice to recognize the mutant lacking residues 248-409 raised the possibility that the HA sites(s) recognized by class I T cells of the H-2^k haplotype mapped within this deleted coding region (Braciale et al. 1989).

Using HA deletion mutants and a panel of synthetic peptides corresponding to portions of the 248-409 region of the A/Japan/305/57 HA, we identified a site within the deleted HA 248-409 region that is recognized by H-2K^k-restricted, HA-specific CTLs. This site could be mimicked by a synthetic peptide corresponding to HA residues 252-271. In separate studies, we examined the capacity of HA-specific class II T cells (Lukacher et al. 1985; Morrison et al. 1986) to recognize Ia$^+$ cells treated with the synthetic HA 252-271 peptide and other peptides corresponding to portions of the 248-409 region. Unexpectedly, we found that a subset of CD4$^+$, I-A^d-restricted, HA-specific T-cell clones recognize I-A^d target-expressing cells treated with the HA 252-721 synthetic peptide. These clones (U5, V4, N2.7) belong to the Th-1 T-cell subset and exhibit antigen-specific cytolytic activity on Ia$^+$ target cells (Lukacher et al. 1985). Figure 1 shows the peptide dose dependence of recognition and lysis by the three I-A^d-restricted clones. HA-specific clones U5, V4, and N2.7 and an HA-specific K^k-restricted T-cell line of CBA/J origin were tested for lytic activity on ^{51}Cr-labeled LK35.1 target cells treated with the HA 252-271 peptide. Both the class I and class II T cells efficiently recognize the K^k/I-A^d-expressing LK35.1 target cells over a range of peptide concentrations.

The results in Figure 1 indicate that a single peptide of the A/Jap/57 HA region encompassed by residues 252-271 contains sites recognized by class I and class II T cells. To define more accurately the boundaries of these epitopes and the critical residues for T-cell recog-

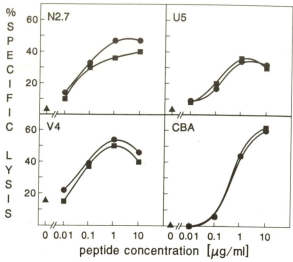

Figure 1. Dose dependence of peptide recognition by class I and class II MHC-restricted T cells. The CD4$^+$, H-2I-A^d-restricted murine clones U5, V4, and N2.7 were tested, along with a bulk line of CD8$^+$, H-2K^k-restricted T cells for recognition of LK35.1 target cells treated with the indicated concentrations of the synthetic A/Jap/57 HA 252-271 peptide (■), synthetic peptide HA MD252-271 (●), or untreated targets (▲). Lysis of peptide-treated target cells was determined in a standard 6-hr ^{51}Cr release assay.

nition, we synthesized a set of nested truncated peptides spanning the HA 252-271 region and screened target cells treated with these peptides for recognition by class I and class II CTLs. As shown in Table 1, amino-terminal deletions down to position 255 enhance recognition by H-2K^k-restricted T cells, with optimal lysis achieved with a peptide spanning residues 255-271. Deletion of residues 252-256 abolished recognition by class I T cells but had no effect on class II T cells. Deletion of residues 252-257, however, diminished recognition by both class I and class II T cells. At the

Table 1. Efficiency of Peptide Recognition by T Cells

Synthetic peptide	MHC class I (K^k restricted)[a]	MHC class II (I-A^d restricted)
252 255 260 265 271		
T I N F E S T G N L I A P E Y G F K I S	+	+++
M D T I N F E S T G N L I A P E Y G F K I S	+	+++
N L I A P E Y G F K I S	–	–
S T G N L I A P E Y G F K I S	–	+++
F E S T G N L I A P E Y G F K I S	+++	+++
T G N L I A P E Y G F K	–	++
E S T G N L I A P E Y G	–	++
N F E S T G N L I A P E	++	–
T I N F E S T G N L I A P E Y G F	++	++
T I N F E S T G N L I A	+	

Recognition of a nested set of synthetic peptides spanning the HA 252–271 site. LK35.1 target cells were treated with the indicated synthetic peptide and tested for lysis by the I-A^d-restricted class II clones U5, V4, and N2.7 or the K^k-restricted class I clones K8-3, K8-4, and K8-5, derived from the bulk CD8$^+$ line (see Fig. 1).

[a](–) No lysis of the peptide-treated targets by T-cell clones; (+) one-half maximal lysis of targets at a peptide concentration of >10 μg/ml; (++) one-half maximal lysis of targets at peptide concentrations of 0.1–1 μg/ml (+++) one-half maximal lysis of targets at peptide concentrations of <0.1 μg/ml.

carboxyl terminus, deletion of any residues diminished recognition by both T-cell subsets. The glycine at position 267 does, however, appear more critical for class II T-cell recognition because carboxy-terminal truncated peptides lacking positions 267-271 are no longer recognized by class II T cells. Class I T cells show diminished, but still significant, recognition of truncated peptides lacking carboxy-terminal residues from 264 to 271. Overall, these data suggest that an overlapping set of core residues are required for recognition of the HA 252-271 site by both class I and class II T cells.

Pathways of HA 252-271 Presentation to Class I and Class II T Cells

Because class I and class II T cells recognize an overlapping set of amino acids in the HA 252-271 site, it was of interest to ascertain whether HA protein, either introduced exogenously or synthesized de novo in infected cells, was processed for presentation to both class I and class II T cells. To examine the exogenous (endosomal) pathway, we pulsed LK35.1 cells with noninfectious (UV-inactivated) A/Jap/57 virions. This noninfectious form of antigen provides native HA protein in the virion particle but is unable to direct de novo HA expression in the antigen-presenting or target cells (Morrison et al. 1986; Braciale et al. 1987). To examine the endogenous presentation route, we infected target cells with a purified recombinant vaccinia virus preparation expressing the A/Jap/57 HA gene off the vaccinia p11 promoter. This expression vector lacks detectable HA in the recombinant virion preparation and can only provide HA expressed de novo in the antigen-presenting cells. As Figure 2 shows, both K^k-restricted and I-A^d-restricted T cells recognize target cells treated with the HA 252-271 peptide. Similarly, both class I and class II T cells recognize target cells infected with

A/Jap/57 virus, which provides both a source of virion-associated exogenous HA and HA expressed de novo as a result of infection of the target cells. However, only class II T cells recognized cells pulsed with noninfectious virions and only class I T cells recognized target cells infected with HA-encoding recombinant vaccinia virus. This finding is consistent with the view that processing and presentation of the HA 252-271 site through the exogenous (endosomal) pathway lead only to interaction of processed antigen with class II MHC molecules and recognition by class II T cells, whereas endogenous (cytosolic) processing of the HA 252-271 site leads only to charging of class I MHC molecules and recognition by class I T cells. These findings are in keeping with our previous observations that the pathways of antigen presentation to class I and class II T cells are distinctly different (Morrison et al. 1986).

T-cell Recognition of the HA 252-271 Site Expressed De Novo from a Synthetic Minigene

Because the "preprocessed" HA 252-271 site in the form of the synthetic peptide can be recognized by both class I and class II T cells when added exogenously to cells, it was of interest to determine whether preprocessed HA 252-271 expressed de novo in the cell is also recognized by both T-cell subsets. To express the HA 252-271 site de novo, we constructed a synthetic minigene (see Sweetser et al. 1988) consisting of oligonucleotides encoding a methionine translation start site and a coding triplet introducing a consensus Kozak's sequence (encoding an aspartate), followed by the nucleotide sequence encoding the HA 252-271 site and a termination codon (Fig. 3A). This HA MD252-271 minigene was expressed in a recombinant vaccinia vector. As shown in the Northern blot of Figure 3B, the mRNA transcribed off the HA MD252-271 minigene is primarily associated with free (cytoplasmic) ribosomes in cells infected with the vaccinia vector. The band of minigene RNA (HA MD252-271) in the lane corresponding to membrane-associated ribosomes is due to contamination in the fractionation of free and membrane-associated polysomes. Similar contamination was seen in the membrane-bound polysome fraction from cells expressing a signal minus mutant A/Jap/57 HA gene (HA-S$^-$) lacking the gene segment encoding the HA signal sequence (Gething and Sambrook 1982).

When we examined the capacity of the HA 252-271-specific class I and class II T-cell clones to recognize LK35.1 cells expressing the 22-amino-acid product of the minigene, we found that cells expressing the minigene product are recognized only by class I T cells (Fig. 4). The class II T cells fail to recognize this preprocessed endogenous antigen, although exogenous peptide is efficiently recognized. Thus, we were unable to bypass the block in class II T-cell recognition of HA processed and presented by the endogenous pathway by expressing the preprocessed site de novo in the cell. This finding suggests that the block in presentation to class II T cells by the endogenous pathway does not lie

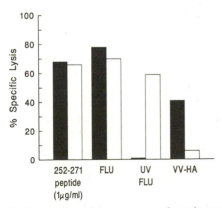

Figure 2. Recognition of exogenous and newly synthesized HA by HA 252-271-specific, class I and class II T-cell clones. LK35.1 target cells were infected with A/Jap/57 virus (FLU) or a recombinant vaccinia encoding the A/Jap/57 HA (VV-HA), or treated with a noninfectious influenza virion preparation (UV FLU) or the synthetic HA 252-271 peptide at a concentration of 1 μg/ml. The target cells were then tested for recognition by the K^k-restricted class I T-cell clone (solid bars) or the I-A^d-restricted class II T-cell clone (open bars).

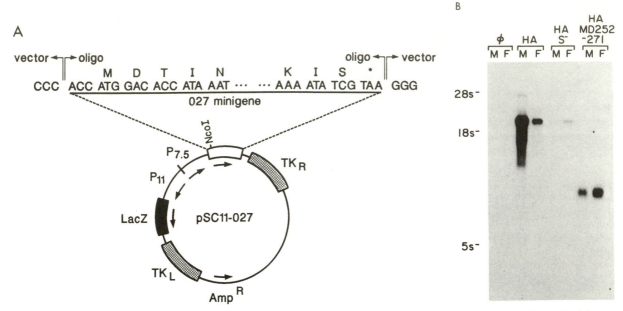

Figure 3. Construction and expression of the HA MD252-271 minigene. (*A*) A double-stranded synthetic oligonucleotide was synthesized, which contains an ATG initiator codon and bases encoding an aspartate residue and the amino acids of the HA 252-271 site. This synthetic oligonucleotide was introduced into the pSC11 insertion vector and inserted into vaccinia at the *tk* locus, as described previously (Sweetser et al. 1988). (*B*) Cells were infected with vaccinia virus vectors encoding the full-length HA, a signal minus form of the HA (HA-S⁻), or the HA MD252-271 minigene. Four hours after infection, cells were lysed and polysomes were separated into membrane-bound (M) and free (F) fractions. mRNA associated with these polysomes was extracted and subjected to Northern analysis, using a labeled 252-271 oligonucleotide probe. Each line contains 2.5 μg of RNA, which represents all membrane-bound RNA and approximately one-fiftieth of the free RNA from 3×10^7 to 5×10^7 cells.

at the level of intracellular processing but likely reflects a defect in the capacity of class II MHC molecules to be charged by processed endogenous antigen.

We have attempted to track the 22-amino-acid minigene product in the cell by biosynthetic labeling. To date, we have been unable to directly precipitate the product using a heterogeneous antisera against the HA 252-271 site. Our preliminary evidence indicates that

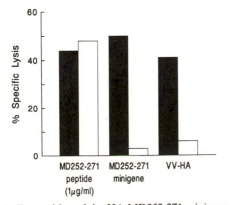

Figure 4. Recognition of the HA MD252-271 minigene product by HA 252-271-specific class I and class II T cells. LK35.1 target cells were infected with recombinant vaccinia vectors encoding the full-length HA or the HA MD252-271 minigene and tested for recognition, along with HA MD252-271 peptide-treated cells for recognition by the K^k-restricted class I clone K8-5 (■) or by the I-A^d-restricted class II clone V4 (□). (For other details, see Figs. 3 and 4.)

this translation product is unstable and rapidly degraded after synthesis.

HA Recognition by Human Class II T Cells

Our initial studies on T-cell recognition and the pathways of influenza HA glycoprotein presentation were carried out with murine T-cell clones. Because these studies suggested that the pathways of HA presentation to class I and class II T cells are different, it was of interest to extend this analysis to another species—the human. We previously isolated human class II T-cell clones with specific cytolytic activity in vitro, which are directed to the A/Jap/57 HA (Kaplan et al. 1984). For studies on HA presentation pathways, we utilized a $CD4^+$ cytolytic clone, V1. This clone is restricted by HLA-DRw11 in its recognition of a region of the HA defined by residues 126-145 (L. Brown, in prep.).

The first issue we examined was whether human $CD4^+$ cells, like class II MHC-restricted, HA-specific murine T cells, would fail to recognize HLA-DR⁺ cells expressing the HA de novo as a result of infection with the recombinant vaccinia virus encoding the HA gene. When this analysis was carried out (Fig. 5), the DRw11-restricted clone V1 gave a heretofore unexpected pattern of recognition. As anticipated, V1 recognizes autologous Epstein-Barr virus (EBV)-transformed lymphoblastoid target cells, either infected with A/Jap/57 virus or treated with noninfectious virions or purified HA. In each case, HA is available to enter the

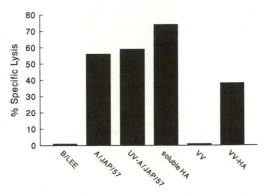

Figure 5. Recognition of exogenous and newly synthesized HA by the human CD4$^+$, HLA-DRw11-restricted T-cell clone. An HLA-DRw11-expressing human lymphoblastoid cell line was either infected or treated with the following: infectious type-B influenza strain B/Lee (B/LEE); infectious A/Jap/57 virus (A/JAP/57); noninfectious A/Jap/57 virions (UV-A/JAP/57); purified A/Jap/57 HA at a concentration of 1 μg/ml (soluble HA); wild-type vaccinia virus (VV); or the HA-encoding recombinant vaccinia vector (VV-HA). The target cells were tested for lysis by the HA-specific, CD4$^+$ clone V1 in a standard ^{51}Cr release assay.

exogenous (endosomal) pathway for processing and charging of class II MHC. Unexpectedly, this HA-specific clone could also recognize target cells expressing the HA de novo after infection with the vaccinia HA vector (Fig. 5).

One explanation for the capacity of the HA-expressing vaccinia to sensitize the lymphoblastoid cell targets for recognition by clone V1 was that the HA contaminating the vaccinia virion preparation entered the cell through the exogenous pathway in a fashion analogous to soluble HA glycoprotein (Braciale et al. 1987). If so, then target cell sensitization by the vaccinia HA vector for recognition by the class II clone V1 should be insensitive to inhibitors of protein synthesis, as had been reported previously in the murine system (Morrison et al. 1986). When human lymphoblastoid target cells were infected with the vaccinia HA vector

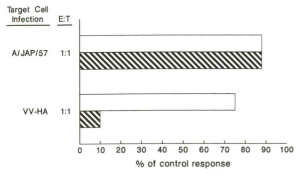

Figure 6. Effect of emetine on target cell sensitization by an infectious virus or an HA-encoding recombinant vaccinia vector. Human lymphoblastoid cells were infected with A/Jap/57 virus or vaccinia HA (VV-HA) in the absence (open bars) or presence (hatched bars) of 10^{-5} M emetine and tested for recognition by CD4$^+$, DRw11-restricted human T cells in a 6-hr ^{51}Cr release assay.

in the presence of the protein synthesis inhibitor emetine, emetine markedly inhibited target cell sensitization and recognition by V1 (Fig. 6). On the other hand, when target cells were infected with A/Jap/57 virus, where HA protein was present in the virion inoculum, emetine had no effect on target cell sensitization and recognition by V1 (Fig. 6). These data indicated that HA protein expressed and processed de novo in the infected cell is recognized by CD4$^+$ class II T cells in the human.

Hemagglutinin Mutants Define the Pathway of HA Processing and Presentation to Class II T Cells

The finding of class II T-cell recognition of lymphoblastoid target cells expressing only newly synthesized HA raised the possibility that in the human, antigen processed and presented through the endogenous pathway is recognized by class II T cells. An alternative explanation for the dichotomy between the findings with human and murine T cells would be that the human lymphoblastoid cells and murine B-lymphoma target cells differ in their transport and recycling of HA. In most cells types, newly synthesized HA at the surface of an infected (or transfected) cells recycles back in to the cell via coated pits and eventually into endosomes/lysosomes but does so very slowly (Lazarovits and Roth 1988). It was possible that in contrast to murine cells, HA expressed on the surface of human lymphoblastoid cells rapidly recycles into endosomes and hence into the exogenous processing pathway where charging of class II MHC molecules and target cell sensitization for class II T-cell recognition can occur. Consistent with this notion is our recent evidence that murine L cells transfected with the DRw11 molecule are recognized by clone V1 when infected with A/Jap/57 virus, where HA is available in the virion, but not when infected with the HA-encoding recombinant vaccinia vector where only newly synthesized HA is available (L. Brown, unpubl.).

Because HA synthesized de novo in the lymphoblastoid cells was recognized by V1, we could utilize a panel of mutant HA gene constructs that are defective in HA synthesis or transport through various intracellular compartments to study HA presentation. The products of each of these mutant HA genes are processed, presented, and recognized by class I T cells (T.J. Braciale, unpubl.), yet are blocked at different points in their transport to the cell surface. These mutants include (1) HA-S$^-$, a mutant gene encoding the signal minus form of the A/Jap/57 HA, which does not translocate into the endoplasmic reticulum (ER) (Gething and Sambrook 1982); (2) the HAΔR1 mutant (Braciale et al. 1989) and an HA mutant, HA67ER, which has a single cysteine-to-serine amino acid substitution at position 67 (M.-J. Gething, pers. comm.), both of which encode a signal sequence and enter the ER (both mutant gene products are improperly folded and are rapidly degraded within the ER); (3) a mutant HA gene, HA164, which contains a gene segment encoding a carboxy-

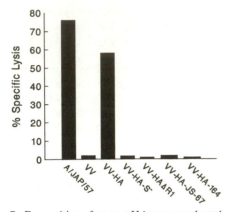

Figure 7. Recognition of mutant HA gene products by class II MHC-restricted CTL. (For details of mutant HA expression and transport, see Results.)

terminal 16-amino-acid extension to HA (Doyle et al. 1985). This mutant HA is properly synthesized, folded, and transported through the Golgi; however, it accumulates in a secretory vesicle in transit to the cell surface and never reaches the cell surface.

When target cells expressing mutant HA constructs were examined for recognition by V1, none of these constructs were recognized by the class II T-cell clone V1 (Fig. 7). Thus, these data suggest that the endogenous presentation pathway does not lead to class II T-cell recognition even in the human and that expression of the HA gene product through the vesicular transport pathway up to the level of the secretory vesicles is insufficient to allow presentation of HA to class II T cells.

DISCUSSION

We have examined the pathways of presentation of a membrane glycoprotein antigen—the influenza hemagglutinin—to both class I and class II T lymphocytes. We have observed that a minigene encoding a site recognized by both class I and class II T cells, when expressed in an antigen-presenting cell, is recognized only by class I T cells. In addition, we have gone on to examine the recognition of a series of mutant HA genes that are defective in synthesis and/or blocked in transport through the vesicular transport pathway. These analyses revealed that the transport of HA protein to the cell surface is required for processing and presentation of the polypeptide to class II T cells.

Our results with the HA MD252-271 minigene have several implications. First, they indicate that antigen presented through the endogenous (cytosolic) pathway does not charge class II MHC for recognition by class II T cells. By preprocessing the site, we were able to bypass any constraints on class II MHC charging and recognition imposed by processing enzymes or antigen fragmentation. As discussed below, interaction of antigen processed through the endogenous pathway with MHC probably occurs in the ER. Because both class I and class II MHCs are assembled and initially localized

in this compartment, antigen processed through the endogenous pathway should be available to both; yet only class I MHC is charged by the functional criterion of class I T-cell recognition. This fact strongly suggests that class II MHC in the ER and possibly in other intracellular compartments, e.g., Golgi stacks during its transit to the cell surface, is unable to interact with processed antigen fragments.

Because the minigene message is translated off free ribosomes, the 22-amino-acid product of this gene is most likely initially released into the cell cytoplasm after termination of translation. This minigene product must then transit through at least one membrane to reach class I MHC. Like the HA MD252-271 minigene product, the product of a minigene encoding the HA 523-545 class I T-cell site, which includes the transmembrane hydrophobic domain of the HA, has also been shown to be recognized by class I T cells (Sweetser et al. 1988) and must have access to the class I compartment as well. It is therefore unlikely that these peptides move from the cytoplasm to the class-I-containing compartment by simple diffusion, because a sequence like the HA anchor region contains a stop-transfer sequence and should remain lipid associated. As an alternative, we propose that there is a cytoplasmic-specific transporter that binds the minigene product (and presumably processed antigen fragments as well) and serves to target and translocate the peptide fragment into the compartment containing class I MHC. A likely candidate protein for this transporter is a heat-shock protein, because members of this family can bind to nonnative proteins and have an affinity for hydrophobic residues (Pelham 1986). This putative transporter may recognize sequences in processed antigen containing amino acid motifs (see, e.g., Rothbard and Taylor 1988) characteristic of sites capable of binding to MHC. Interestingly, in preliminary studies, the HA MD252-271 minigene product appears to be unstable and rapidly degraded in the cell cytoplasm. Thus, a transporter like a heat-shock protein could, by capturing antigenic fragments, serve a dual purpose of protecting processed antigen from further degradation, as well as targeting and translocating the processed antigenic fragment.

In marked contrast to our results with minigene expression in the murine system, we found that EBV-transformed lymphoblastoid cells could present newly synthesized HA to human class II T cells. Although newly synthesized HA recycles from the cell surface into endosomes/lysosomes very slowly in most cell types (Lazarovits and Roth 1988), it is possible that cell-surface HA is rapidly turning over into the endosomal processing pathway in human lymphoblastoid target cells, rather than using HA processed through the cytosolic pathway. Consistent with this notion is our preliminary evidence using transfected murine L cells expressing HLA-DRw11 as targets. When these murine cells are infected with a vaccinia virus encoding the full-length HA gene, the target cells are not recognized by human class II T cells. The HA may turn over rapidly into endosomes in certain human cells and slowly in most murine cells.

Because the human class II T cells could recognize lymphoblastoid cell targets expressing newly synthesized HA off a vaccinia vector, it was possible to use HA mutants to examine further the requirements for HA presentation to class II T cells. The results of these analyses were quite clear. HA mutants, whether blocked at the level of translocation from the cytoplasm into the ER (the HA signal minus mutant), rapidly degraded in the ER (HAΔR1, HA67ER), or blocked at the level of the post-Golgi transport vesicle (HA164), all failed to be recognized by class II T cells. The likeliest explanation for the efficient recognition of the full-length parental HA gene product in the face of no recognition of these mutants is that the HA protein must transit to the cell surface to be processed and presented to class II T cells.

Figure 8 summarizes our current view of the mechanism of presentation of a membrane glycoprotein like the HA to class I and class II T cells. In the simplest model, the glycoprotein is translated off ribosomes bound to the ER and cotranslationally translocated into the ER where the protein folds into its native form and where presumably a portion of the translocation product (perhaps misfolded or denatured during synthesis/translocation) must also be fragmented by ER-associated proteinases (see Lippincott-Schwartz et al. 1988). Although our results are consistent with this model, we do not favor this orthodox view, in part, because it is difficult to understand how the membrane-embedded HA 523-545 anchor site becomes accessible to class I MHC. An alternative hypothesis is that either a small but significant portion of the HA is synthesized off free ribosomes or a portion of the HA translocation product does not translocate into the ER. In either

instance, nonnative HA is in the cytoplasm. As noted above, certain hydrophobic residues on this denatured translocation product may be captured by a cytosolic transporter molecule that could serve to protect these regions from proteolytic degradation by cytoplasmic proteinases as well. The transporter would target the captured antigenic fragments to the ER, where translocation and interaction with class I MHC can occur.

Our data suggest that class II MHC in the ER is not able to bind processed antigen in a form capable of subsequent recognition by class II T cells. We suggest that the peptide-binding site of the class II MHC molecule is blocked or that the molecule is not sufficiently mature to accommodate peptide and requires further maturation during transit to the cell surface before it can bind processed antigen fragments. Class I MHC molecules, on the other hand, are charged with processed antigen, e.g., HA fragments, in the ER and transit to the cell surface fully charged and capable of stimulating class I T cells.

Our data on HA recognition strongly suggest that a newly synthesized membrane glycoprotein must travel to the cell surface and recycle into the endosomal compartment before proteolytic fragmentation and charging of class II MHC can occur. We would suggest that all protein antigens (or self-constituents serving as tolerogens) must enter the endosome (exogenous pathway) for processing and presentation to class II T cells. The failure of exogenous native protein to charge class I MHC molecules may reflect either the inaccessibility of newly synthesized class I MHC to enter the endosomal processing compartment on its way to the surface or the inability of cell-surface class I MHC to recycle into the endosomes. Alternatively, because newly synthesized class I MHC may transit to the cell surface already charged with processed antigen, it may be un-

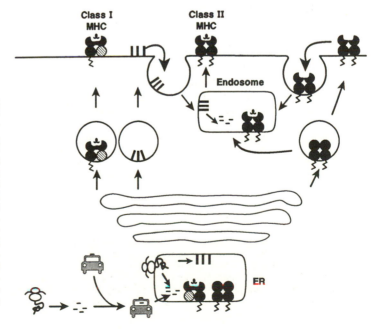

Figure 8. Pathways of membrane glycoprotein presentation to class I and class II MHC-restricted T cells. Class I pathway: Newly synthesized cytoplasmic protein is fragmented, transported (car), and translocated into the ER. Newly synthesized protein off membrane-bound polyribosomes is cotranslationally translocated to the ER, where it is fragmented. Class I MHC can bind antigenic fragments in the ER and is transported to the cell surface. Class II pathway: Newly synthesized class II MHC goes to an endosome enroute to cell-surface expression or undergoes endocytosis after cell-surface expression. Endogenously produced antigen, which is internalized subsequent to cell-surface expression, or exogenous antigen enters an endosome compartment and undergoes fragmentation. Class II MHC binds antigenic fragments in the endosome and undergoes exocytosis to the cell surface.

able to bind processed antigen derived from the endosomal processing pathway. Presumably, cell-surface class I MHC would not recycle at a rate rapid enough to be adequately charged with processed antigen in the endosome. Class II MHC, on the other hand, may not become competent to bind antigen fragments until it transits to the cell surface and recycles into an endosome or until newly synthesized class II MHC intersects with the endosomal compartment (Cresswell 1985).

This mechanism for presentation of antigen to class I and class II T cells has certain implications for self-tolerance in the thymus and periphery. Accordingly, cytosolic and nuclear protein would not be recognized by class-II-restricted T cells (or induce self-tolerance) unless these proteins can leave the cytoplasm and enter the endosome. One mechanism to achieve this is cell destruction, with release of these constituents into the extracellular space. The need to achieve self-tolerance against cytoplasmic and nuclear proteins could, in part, at least be an impetus for the extensive ongoing cell destruction in the thymus. Also because both cytosolic and membrane-associated proteins readily enter the endogenous presentation pathway, tolerance to self-constituents processed through the class I T-cell pathway may be more extensive than tolerance induced by processing through the endosomal pathway. If so, then the repertoire of class I T cells directed to foreign antigens may be more limited than that to class II T cells due to deletion of a larger fraction of potentially self-reactive T cells. These and other predictions of this hypothesis await experimental verification.

ACKNOWLEDGMENTS

The authors thank Drs. Mary-Jane and Joe Sambrook for providing the HA-JS67, the HA-S⁻, and the HA-164 hemagglutinin mutants; Drs. David Sweetser, Charles Rice, and Jeffrey Gordon for advice in the construction and expression of the hemagglutinin minigenes; Dr. Benjamin Schwartz for continuing collaboration and support in the study of human T lymphocyte responses to influenza; and Mr. John Gorka for production and HPLC analyses of synthetic peptides. The expert technical support of Mrs. Michelle Weber and Mrs. Belinda Counts is gratefully acknowledged as is the dedicated and expert secretarial services of Mrs. Jerri Smith.

REFERENCES

Babbitt, B., P.M. Allen, G. Matsueda, E. Haber, and E.R. Unanue. 1985. Binding of immunogenic peptides to Ia histocompatibility molecules. *Nature* **317:** 359.

Bjorkman, P.J., M.A. Saper, B. Samraoui, W.S. Bennett, J.L. Strominger, and D.C. Wiley. 1987. Structure of the human class I histocompatibility antigen, HLA-A2. *Nature* **329:** 506.

Braciale, T.J., M.T. Sweetser, L.A. Morrison, D.J. Kittlesen, and V.L. Braciale. 1989. Class I major histocompatibility complex restricted cytolytic T lymphocytes recognize a limited number of sites on the influenza hemagglutinin. *Proc. Natl. Acad. Sci.* **86:** 277.

Braciale, T.J., L.A. Morrison, M.T. Sweetser, J. Sambrook, M.-J. Gething, and V.L. Braciale. 1987. Antigen presentation pathways to class I and class II MHC-restricted T lymphocytes. *Immunol. Rev.* **98:** 95.

Buus, S., A. Sette, S.M. Conlon, D.M. Jenis, and H. Grey. 1986. Isolation and characterization of antigen-Ia complexes involved in T cell recognition. *Cell* **47:** 1071.

Copeland, C.S., R.W. Doms, E.M. Balzau, R.G. Webster, and A. Helenius. 1986. Assembly of influenza hemagglutinin trimers and its role in intracellular transport. *J. Cell. Biol.* **103:** 1179.

Cresswell, P. 1985. Intracellular class II HLA antigens are accessible to transferrin-neuraminidase conjugates internalized by receptor-mediated endocytosis. *Proc. Natl. Acad. Sci.* **82:** 8188.

Doherty, P.C., R.V. Blanden, and R.M. Zinkernagel. 1976. Specificity of virus-immune effector T cells for H-2K or H-2D compatible interactions: Implications for H-antigen diversity. *Transplant Rev.* **29:** 89.

Doyle, C., M.G. Roth, J. Sambrook, and M.-J. Gething. 1985. Mutations in the cytoplasmic domain of the influenza virus hemagglutinin affect different stages of intracellular transport. *J. Cell Biol.* **100:** 704.

Feighery, C. and P. Stastny. 1979. HLA-D region-associated determinants serve as targets for human cell-mediated lysis. *J. Exp. Med.* **149:** 485.

Gething, M.-J. and J. Sambrook. 1982. Construction of influenza hemagglutinin genes that code for intracellular and secreted forms of the protein. *Nature* **300:** 598.

Gething, M.-J., K. McCammon, and J. Sambrook. 1986. Expression of wild-type and mutant forms of influenza hemagglutinin: The role of folding in intracellular transport. *Cell* **46:** 939.

Kaplan, D.R., R. Griffith, V.L. Braciale, and T.J. Braciale. 1984. Influenza virus-specific human cytotoxic T cell clones: Heterogeneity in antigenic specificity and restriction by class II MHC products. *Cell. Immunol.* **88:** 193.

Klein, J.R., D.H. Raulet, M.S. Pasternack, and M.J. Bevan. 1982. Cytotoxic T lymphocytes produce immune interferon in response to antigen or mitogen. *J. Exp. Med.* **155:** 1198.

Lamb, R.A. 1983. The influenza virus RNA segments and their encoded proteins. In *Genetics of influenza viruses* (ed. P. Palese and D.W. Kingsbury), p. 21. Springer-Verlag, New York.

Lazarovits, J. and M. Roth. 1988. A single amino acid change in the cytoplasmic domain allows the influenza virus hemagglutinin to be endocytosed through coated pits. *Cell* **53:** 743.

Lippincott-Schwartz, J., J.S. Bonfacino, L.C. Yuan, and R.D. Klausner. 1988. Degradation from the endoplasmic reticulum: Disposing of newly synthesized proteins. *Cell* **54:** 209.

Lukacher, A.E., L.A. Morrison, V.L. Braciale, B. Malissen, and T.J. Braciale. 1985. Expression of specific cytolytic activity by H-2I region-restricted, influenza virus-specific T lymphocyte clones. *J. Exp. Med.* **162:** 171.

Mims, C.A. 1982. *The pathogenesis of infection disease*, 2nd edition. Academic Press, New York.

Morris, A.G., Y.-L. Lin, and B.A. Askonas. 1982. Immune interferon release when a cloned cytotoxic T cell line meets its correct influenza-infected target cell. *Nature* **295:** 150.

Morrison, L.A., A.E. Lukacher, V.L. Braciale, D.P. Fan, and T.J. Braciale. 1986. Differences in antigen presentation to MHC class I- and class II-restricted influenza virus-specific cytolytic T lymphocyte clones. *J. Exp. Med.* **163:** 903.

Pelham, H.R.B. 1986. Speculations on the functions of the major heat shock and glucose-regulated proteins. *Cell* **46:** 959.

Rothbard, J.B. and W.R. Taylor. 1988. A sequence pattern common to T cell epitopes. *EMBO J.* **7**: 93.

Sweetser, M.T., V.L. Braciale, and T.J. Braciale. 1988. Class I MHC-restricted recognition of cells expressing a gene encoding a 41 amino acid product of the influenza hemagglutinin. *J. Immunol.* **141**: 3324.

Townsend, A.R.M., F.M. Gotch, and J. Davey. 1985. Cytotoxic T cells recognize fragments of the influenza nucleoprotein. *Cell* **42**: 457.

Townsend, A.R.M., J. Rothbard, F.M. Gotch, G. Bahadur, D. Wraith, and A.J. McMichael. 1986. The epitopes of influenza nucleoprotein recognized by cytotoxic T lymphocytes can be defined with short synthetic peptides. *Cell* **44**: 959.

Unanue, E.R. 1984. Antigen-presenting function of the macrophage. *Annu. Rev. Immunol.* **2**: 395.

B- and T-cell Recognition of Influenza Hemagglutinin

D.B. Thomas, D.S. Burt, B.C. Barnett, C.M. Graham, and J.J. Skehel
National Institute for Medical Research, London NW7 1AA, United Kingdom

It has been frequently observed that antibodies or B cells recognize distinct regions of globular proteins from T cells: B cells recognize conformational epitopes at molecular surfaces, whereas T cells require proteins to be processed and presented as peptides in association with either class I or class II molecules of the major histocompatibility complex (MHC) (Benjamin et al. 1984; Schwartz 1985). Estimates of the specificity and diversity of class-II-restricted T cells have been derived from studies of the in vitro proliferative responses of T cells to antigens such as cytochrome *c* (Schwartz 1985), lysozyme (Allen et al. 1984; Shastri et al. 1985), and myoglobin (Berkower et al. 1986; Livingstone and Fathman 1987), which indicate that T cells recognize limited regions of a molecule in a haplotype-specific manner. Such limited diversity is consistent with current views of antigen processing (Babbit et al. 1985; Buus et al. 1986), as initially postulated in the determinant selection model (Benacerraf 1978; Rosenthal 1978). Moreover, the ability of antigenic peptides from unrelated proteins to compete for antigen presentation in association with the same MHC restriction element is consistent with their binding to a single receptor site (Guillet et al. 1987). In many instances, a common procedure has been used to establish antigen-specific T-cell clones, in vitro, from the lymph nodes of mice immunized 6–8 days previously with antigens in Freund's adjuvant (Kimoto and Fathman 1980), and there have been a few reports of analyses of the antigen-specific T-memory population resident in the spleen and elicited by natural infection.

The hemagglutinins (HAs) of influenza viruses are viral membrane components against which neutralizing antibodies are directed (Webster et al. 1982). Their antigenic properties have been extensively analyzed using natural and monoclonal-antibody-selected antigenic variants to determine the location of antibody-binding sites (Gerhard et al. 1981; Wiley et al. 1981; Caton et al. 1982; Both et al. 1983) on the surface of the membrane distal components of the molecule (Wilson et al. 1981). In a similar approach, we and other investigators have studied the recognition pattern of CD4[+] cells (Hurwitz et al. 1984; Mills et al. 1986; Thomas et al. 1987; Brown et al. 1988; Barnett et al. 1989; Burt et al. 1989; Graham et al. 1989) elicited by natural infection with influenza virus.

The majority of CD4[+] clones that we have analyzed recognize regions of the HA1 subunit that have previously been shown to be antibody-binding sites. Recognition is sensitive to amino acid substitutions that have occurred in these regions of natural variant viruses and monoclonal-antibody-selected variants, and synthetic peptides have allowed us to identify multiple and nonoverlapping T-cell epitopes that are recognized in the context of a single class II restriction element, either I-A[k] or I-A[d]. There are no evident structural similarities between individual peptides that we have used, and they fail to compete for antigen presentation to individual CD4[+] clones, indicating that the putative peptide-binding site of the class II molecule may accommodate a variety of antigenic peptides. The extensive commonality between B-cell and T-cell recognition specificities suggests that, in vivo, the B-memory cell may play a central role in the processing and selective presentation of peptide fragments to T cells. Since mice of different haplotypes appear to recognize different antigenic regions of HA, MHC polymorphism may be a significant factor in the selective pressure for antigenic drift within the population and may influence the neutralizing antibody response of an individual to virus infection.

METHODS

Mice and viruses. BALB/c and CBA/Ca mice were bred under specific pathogen-free conditions at the National Institute for Medical Research and used at 3 months of age. X31 is a recombinant virus between A/Aichi/68 (A/Aichi) and A/PR/8/34 (PR8) with A/Aichi glycoproteins (H3N2) and PR8 internal proteins (Kilbourne 1969). Natural variant viruses were all of the H3N2 subtype and were isolated from major influenza outbreaks between 1968 and 1984. Monoclonal-antibody-selected mutants were produced by growing X31 in eggs in the presence of neutralizing monoclonal antibodies. The amino acid sequence of HA from each virus was deduced from the nucleotide sequence of the RNA gene. All viruses were grown in embryonated hen eggs, and virus titers were determined in hemagglutination assays, using turkey erythrocytes, and are expressed as HA units (HAU)ml.

Viral fragments. The HA glycoprotein was obtained from purified X31 by bromelain digestion (BHA) and purified by sucrose density gradient centrifugation (Brand and Skehel 1972). Fragments of X31 were prepared by digestion with trypsin following pH 5 treatment of the virus (Skehel et al. 1982). The tryptic products were separated by sucrose density gradient centrifugation into a soluble glycopeptide fraction, residues 28–328 of HA1, and an insoluble aggregate containing the remainder of the virion.

Synthetic peptides. Peptides were synthesized according to the sequence of HA1 from X31 virus (Fig. 1) by a manual solid-phase procedure (Merrifield 1963) modified to allow simultaneous multiple synthesis (Houghten 1985) using fluorenylmethoxycarbonyl (Fmoc) amino acids. Alternatively, synthetic peptide HA1 186-200 and analogs thereof (HA1 186-200 S193N; HA1 186-200 A198E) were synthesized simultaneously using an LKB BIOLYNX 4170 peptide synthesizer, and all reagents were supplied by LKB Biochrom Ltd., Cambridge, United Kingdom. The purity of synthetic peptides was determined by HPLC and amino acid analysis.

T-cell clones and proliferation assays. CD4$^+$ T-cell clones, specific for the HA of X31 virus, were established from the spleens of individual CBA/Ca or BALB/c mice primed by intranasal infection (2–5 HAU). They were maintained in vitro by restimulation with ultraviolet-activated X31 virus (100 HAU/ml) and antigen-presenting cells (APC) (irradiated, syngeneic

spleen cells; 2×10^6/ml) every 10–12 days, with the addition of interleukin 2 (IL-2)-containing supernatant, from concanavalin A (Con A)-activated rat spleen cell culture medium, and APC after 3 days of stimulation. The antigen specificity of CD4$^+$ clones was determined in proliferation assays, 10–12 days after stimulation with X31 virus. T cells (2×10^4) were incubated with virus (50–500 HAU/ml) or peptide (0.005–5 μM) and APC in flat-bottom 96-well microtiter plates for 48 hours, and [^{3}H]thymidine (1 μCi/well) incorporation into acid-precipitable material was determined after a further 4-hour incubation.

RESULTS

Ia^k- and Ia^d-restricted T-cell Recognition of Influenza HA

Our approach to identify the T-cell recognition sites of HA has been to establish a large panel of CD4$^+$ T-cell clones, by limiting dilution, from individual CBA/Ca or BALB/c donor mice primed by intranasal infection with X31 virus, a recombinant virus between A/Aichi/2/68 and A/PR/8/34 that contains the H3N2 surface glycoproteins. All of the CD4$^+$ clones that

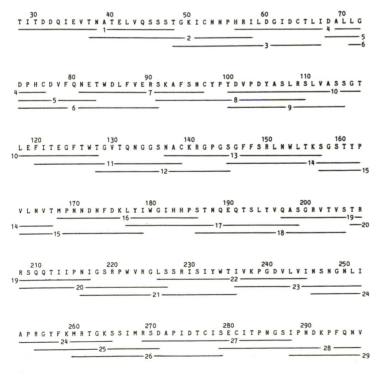

Figure 1. Amino acid sequence of the HA1 subunit of influenza HA (HA1 28-328) based on the H3N2 recombinant virus X31. Synthetic peptides and their code numbers are indicated.

responded in proliferation assays to PR8 virus but not to the purified HA of X31 were assumed to be specific for conserved internal proteins of the virion and were not studied further. A total of 67 CD4⁺ clones were characterized from nine individual BALB/c mice, and 55 CD4⁺ clones from seven CBA/Ca donors. All were found to be H3 subtype-specific and to recognize the tryptic cleavage fragment of X31, HA1 28-328.

Recognition of Synthetic Peptides of HA1 28-328

To determine the sequences within HA1 recognized by each of the above T-cell clones, their proliferative responses to synthetic peptides, corresponding to the sequence of HA1 residues 28-328 and overlapping by 10 amino acid residues, were determined (Fig. 1). Typical proliferative responses of CBA/Ca-derived T-cell clones are shown in Figure 2 and indicate recognition of four distinct and nonoverlapping epitopes contained within the HA1 sequences 68–83, 120–139, 226–245, and 246–265.

In Figure 3, we have represented all of the Ia^d- and Ia^k-restricted T-cell recognition sites defined so far on α-carbon traces of the HA. It is evident that a majority of the T-cell epitopes for both haplotypes are within surface regions of the HA1 polypeptide that are recognized by neutralizing antibodies (Wiley et al. 1981).

Diversity of the Ia^d-restricted Repertoire for Natural Variant Viruses

All of the I-A^d- and I-A^k-restricted T-cell clones so far characterized are sensitive in their recognition of natural variant viruses to the substitutions that have occurred in antigenic sites of the HA1 subunit and illustrate the extensive diversity of the class-II-restricted repertoire for a protective antigen. Figure 4 summarizes the complex pattern of recognition specificities exhibited by BALB/c T-cell clones for natural variant viruses isolated between 1969 and 1984, for laboratory mutant viruses, and for the corresponding synthetic peptides recognized by the relevant clones. A comparison of the response patterns of different donors to the panel of variant viruses fails to reveal any repeat antigenic specificities and illustrates the unique profile of clonotypic specificities expressed by individuals. Nevertheless, it is evident that a majority of I-A^d-restricted T cells recognize a common region of the HA1 subunit, corresponding to HA1 177-199, and are sensitive to amino acid substitutions in natural variants in that area.

Single Substitutions in Laboratory Mutants Abrogate CD4⁺ T-cell Recognition

Laboratory mutant viruses of X31, selected in ovo with neutralizing monoclonal antibodies to HA, differ

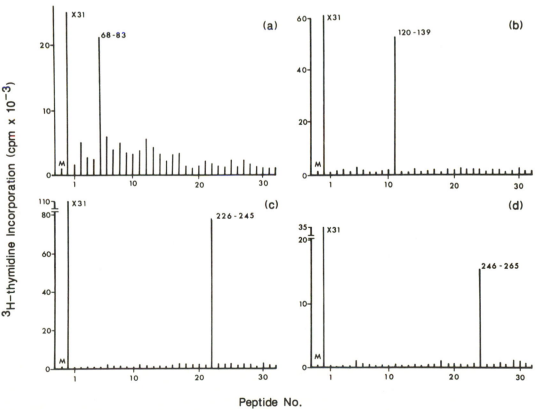

Figure 2. Proliferative responses to CD4⁺ clones from CBA/Ca mice to a panel of HA1 synthetic peptides (see Fig. 1) tested at a single concentration (1 μg/ml).

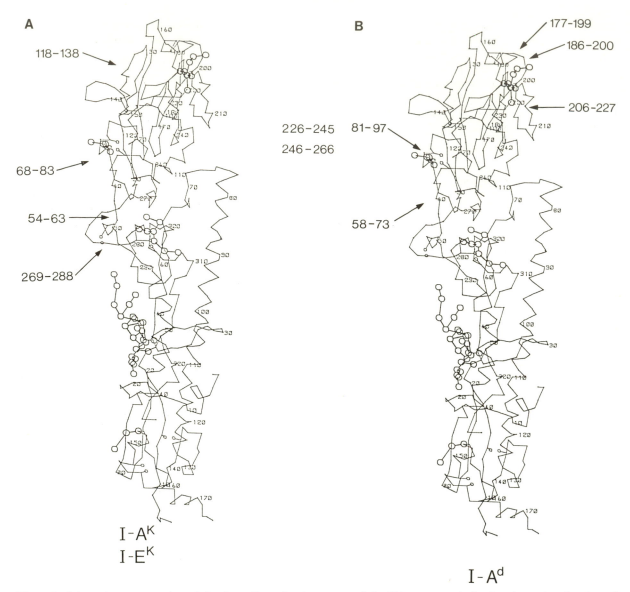

Figure 3. Schematic representation of the three-dimensional structure of the HA monomer indicating the surface location of I-A^k-restricted epitopes (*A*) and I-A^d-restricted epitopes (*B*). The I-E^k-restricted epitopes, HA1 226-245 and HA1 246-265, are within conserved and "buried" regions.

from the parental virus by one, or occasionally two, amino acid substitutions in the globular head region of the HA; responses to these mutants confirm the heterogeneity of CD4$^+$ T-cell recognition.

In BALB/c mice, a majority of I-A^d-restricted T cells recognize peptide HA1 177–199, corresponding to the amino acid sequence of antibody-binding site B (Wiley et al. 1981). Antigenic site B includes residues 186–199 of an α-helix and adjacent residues on the upper edge of the sialic acid receptor-binding site. This region has featured in antigenic drift of H3N2 subtype viruses and is an immunodominant region for BALB/c antibody responses (Staudt and Gerhard 1983). All of the HA1-specific T-cell clones from donors 1, 2, 4, 5, and 6 (Fig. 4) are sensitive to at least one residue

change within site B at residues 189, 193, 198, or 199. The fine specificity of individual CD4$^+$ T-cell clones is illustrated by their ability to discriminate between mutant viruses with different substitutions at position 193 (S→N, S→R, or S→I), whereas the substitution 198 A→E abrogates recognition by a majority of site-B-specific T-cell clones.

Antigenic site E is defined by the substitution 63 D→N that introduces an N-glycosylation site ($N_{63}C_{64}T_{65}$); oligosaccharide attachment prevents antibody recognition (Skehel et al. 1984). All of the T-cell clones from donors 7 and 8 are sensitive to this single substitution in a laboratory mutant virus but differ in their fine specificity for a further mutant virus with the substitution 63 D→Y.

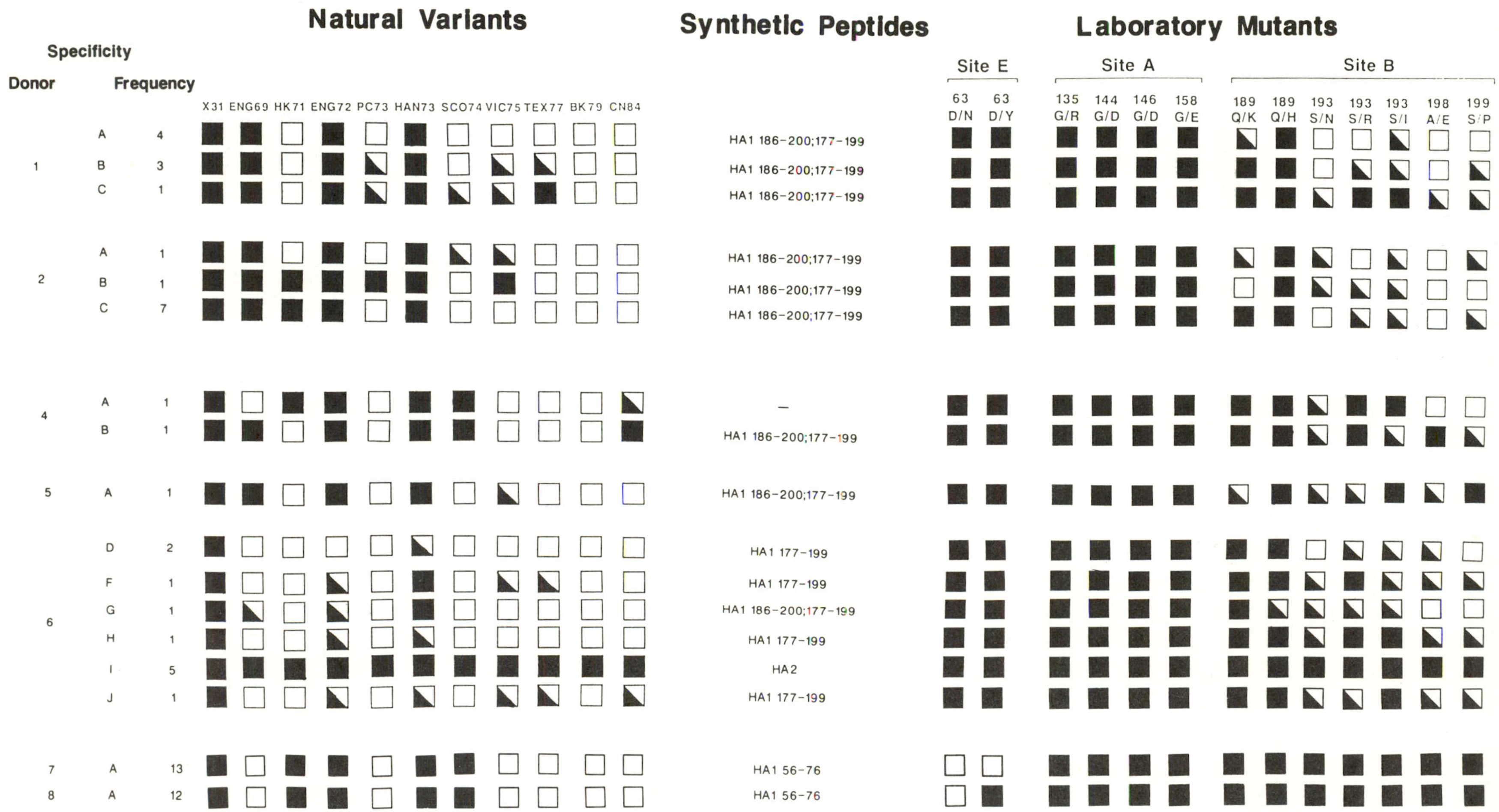

Figure 4. Diversity of I-A^d-restricted T-cell repertoire for influenza hemagglutinin (H3 subtype). The proliferative responses of CD4$^+$ T-cell clones from individual BALB/c mice, primed by natural infection, were determined against natural variant viruses isolated between 1969 and 1984, monoclonal-antibody-selected laboratory mutants, or HA1 synthetic peptides. T-cell responses were compared with the parental X31 response and considered as positive (>50% ■), weak (10–40% ◩), or negative (<10% □) after testing at a range of virus concentrations (50–500 HAU/ml).

Single Substitutions in Synthetic Peptides Mirror CD4[+] T-cell Recognition Specificity for Mutant Viruses

The sensitivity of the I-A[d]-restricted T-cell clones to the single residue changes in laboratory mutant viruses might be due to changes in the processing of HA or to effects on interactions of peptides with class II or the T-cell receptor (TCR). We therefore determined whether the same residue changes, at peptide level, would affect T-cell recognition.

Synthetic peptide analogs of HA1 186-200, differing at positions known to have changed in both natural variant and mutant viruses, at residues 189 (Q→K) or 193 (S→N) or 198 (A→E), were assayed for stimulation of HA1 186-200 specific clones (Fig. 5).

189 Q→K: Recognition was unaffected by this substitution, which was consistent with the specificities shown for mutant HAs with the equivalent change (Fig. 4).

193 S→N: Clones 1B, 4B, and 5A were sensitive to the S193N substitution in a mutant virus (Fig. 4) and exhibited a shift in the dose-response curves to recognition of the analog peptide HA1 186-200 (S 193N) only at high antigen concentrations, suggesting that the S193N substitution was affecting the association of peptide with the TCR and/or Ia molecule. Clone 2B, in contrast, recognized the synthetic peptide analog but discriminated between the corresponding mutant and the parental X31 virus, indicating that the S193N sub-

stitution might be affecting processing of the mutant virus.

198 A→E: The most consistent correlation between T-cell specificity for analog peptides and mutant HAs was seen for this residue; clones 1B, 2B, and 5A failed to recognize HA1 186-200 (A198E) at all peptide concentrations tested; this mirrored their specificities for a mutant HA with the same substitution. In contrast, clone 4B recognized the peptide analog, albeit at increased peptide concentrations, and was insensitive to the same A198E substitution in the mutant HA.

We have also found a similar correlation for I-A[k]-restricted T-cell clones that recognize synthetic peptide HA1 48-68 and are sensitive to substitutions in natural variants at residues 54 (N→S) or 63 (D→N). Introduction of the same residue changes in peptide analogs abrogates or severely reduces T-cell responses (Mills et al. 1988). It is remarkable, therefore, that the recognition specificity exhibited by CD4[+] T-cell clones for antibody-selected mutant viruses of X31 with single substitutions in the HA1 subunit should be mirrored in their specificity for synthetic peptide analogs containing the same amino acid substitutions.

Although a majority of CD4[+] clones from both haplotypes recognize antibody-binding regions of the HA1 subunit, we have found that the small number of I-E[k]-restricted epitopes identified map to conserved regions HA1 226-245 and HA1 246-265 and fail to discriminate between natural variant viruses.

Competition between HA1 Peptides for Antigen Presentation

Since CD4[+] clones specific for HA1 186-200 were sensitive to single amino acid substitutions in peptide analogs, it appears that the same residue changes in mutant viruses at 193 or 198 were affecting either TCR peptide or Ia-peptide interaction rather than the processing of the HA molecule. We undertook a series of competitive inhibition studies, therefore, in attempts to discriminate between these two possibilities. We reasoned that inhibition of T-cell recognition of the stimulatory peptide by an excess of nonstimulatory analog peptide would indicate a direct effect of the substituted residue on TCR interaction, whereas failure to inhibit could be interpreted as lack of association of the analog peptide with Ia or recognition by TCR.

The analog peptide HA1 186-200 (A198E) failed to inhibit proliferation of clone 2B, suggesting that the 198 A→E substitution prevents analog peptide-Ia interaction (Fig. 6); this contrasted with the marked inhibition seen for clone 5A, indicating that the nonstimulatory peptide did bind to Ia. Since the analog peptide HA1 186-200 (S193N) was recognized by clones 1B, 4B, and 5A (Fig. 4), but at greatly increased concentrations compared to the parent peptide (1.5 μM vs. 0.05 μM), competition studies were done at analog peptide concentrations (0.05-0.5 μM) that were insufficient to elicit a significant proliferative response. Addition of the peptide analog reduced the response of these clones

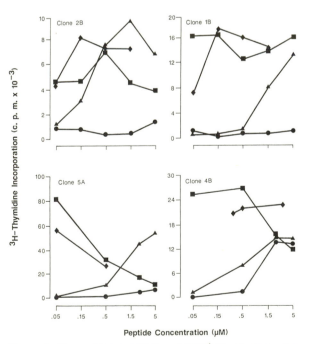

Figure 5. Recognition specificity of CD4[+] T-cell clones for HA1 synthetic peptide analogs containing single residue drift substitutions. The proliferative responses of clones 1B, 2B, 4B, and 5A (see Fig. 4) from individual BALB/c donors to synthetic peptide HA1 186-200 and analogs thereof: (◆) HA1 186-200, (■) HA1 186-200 Q189K, (▲) HA1 186-200S193N, and (●) HA1 186-200A198E.

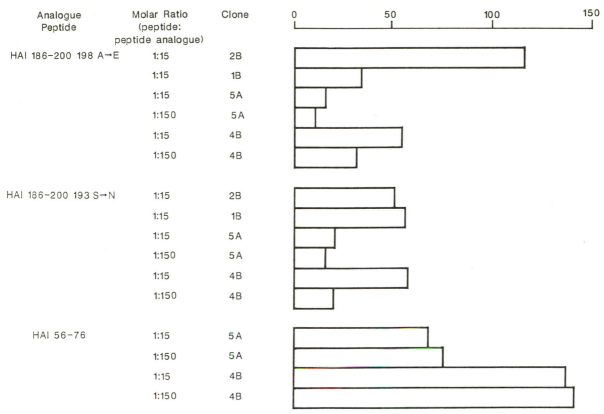

Figure 6. Competition for antigen presentation between synthetic peptides of HA1. Analog peptides, with single amino acid drift substitutions at residues 193 (S → N) or 198 (A → E), or the unrelated peptide HA1 56-76, were preincubated with irradiated, syngeneic BALB/c spleen cells for 1 hr before addition of the stimulatory peptide HA1 186-200 and an I-A^d-restricted clone, either 1B, 2B, 4B, or 5A.

to HA1 182-202, suggesting that the 193 S → N substitution was affecting the interaction of peptide with TCR.

Since antigenic peptides from unrelated proteins, but recognized in association with the same Ia restriction element, have been shown by other investigators (Guillet et al. 1986) to compete for antigen presentation, we included a further I-A^d-restricted peptide, HA1 56-76, in these competition studies. Although there was no obvious homology between HA1 56-76 and HA1 182-202 peptides, the requirements for the association of peptide with Ia might demand that both peptides interact with common residues in the receptor-binding site and therefore compete for antigen presentation. HA1 56-76 failed to inhibit proliferation to HA1 182-202, even when present at a 150-fold molar excess.

DISCUSSION

Extensive sequence analyses of the HAs of natural variant viruses of the H3N2 subtype, isolated between 1969 and 1984, and of monoclonal-antibody-selected mutant HAs have allowed the structural location of antigenically important regions of the HA1 polypeptide chain (Wiley et al. 1981; Webster et al. 1982; Both et

al. 1983). In the studies presented here, we have shown that I-A^k- or I-A^d-restricted CD4$^+$ T-cell clones recognize four of these regions, exhibit extensive diversity in their recognition of mutant viruses, and are able to discriminate between synthetic peptides containing amino acid substitutions identical to those in the mutant HA molecules. I-E^k-restricted T-cell clones, a minor proportion of the T-cell clones so far characterized, do not discriminate between natural variants and monoclonal-antibody-selected mutants and recognize residues within the sequences of HA1 226-245 and HA1 246-265. Both of these regions contain substantial sequences of amino acids that have been conserved during antigenic drift, which may account for the cross-reactivity of these T-cell clones.

Previous studies have also identified HA-specific class-II-restricted T cells that are sensitive to antigenically important amino acid substitutions. Thus, Hurwitz et al. (1984) have described H-2^d-restricted T-cell clones that recognize peptides equivalent to residues HA1 109-119 and HA1 126-138 of H1N1 subtype viruses but fail to respond to monoclonal-antibody-selected mutant viruses with single amino acid substitutions at positions HA1 115 E → K or HA1 136 S → P. Similarly, Brown et al. (1988) have described H-2^d-restricted clones that are sensitive to amino acid substitutions at residues HA1 60 and 63.

What is the basis and significance of this apparent commonality between antibody and T-cell recognition specificity? Reciprocity between B-cell and T-cell repertoires was postulated by Berzofsky (1983) to be the consequence of an "Ia-restricted epitope-specific circuit," although there has been little structural information to support this hypothesis. Furthermore, the role of surface Ig receptors of B cells in antigen presentation is well documented (Kappler et al. 1982; Lanzavecchia 1985; Abbas 1988), and antigen-specific B cells, which recognize conformational features of a protein, can, after intracellular processing, present peptides at their surface in association with Ia. From our results, it is possible that the interaction of surface receptors of B-memory cells with specific regions of the HA may result in the selective processing of these regions so that T-memory cells are focused on a common antigenic site. As a consequence, MHC restriction of the T-cell repertoire may, in turn, influence the neutralizing antibody response to viral infection so that the antibody response mounted by an individual is directed at a limited number of the available surface antigenic sites. Whatever the structural basis for the commonality of the class-II-restricted T-cell repertoire and the neutralizing antibody response to HA, the sensitivity of CD4$^+$ clones to substitutions that arise during antigenic drift may be an important factor in the ability of mutant influenza viruses to evade immune recognition. In the future, we plan to investigate the molecular basis for this commonality of the B-cell and T-cell repertoires both in vitro, by examining antigen processing and by antigen-specific B-cell populations, and in vivo, by an analysis of the T-cell repertoire of transgenic mice with B cells expressing HA-specific, surface immunoglobulins.

REFERENCES

Abbas, A.K. 1988. A reassessment of the mechanisms of antigen-specific T-cell-dependent B-cell activation. *Immunol. Today* 3: 89.

Allen, P.M., D.J. Strydom, and E.R. Unanue. 1984. Processing of lysozyme by macrophages: Identification of the determinant recognised by two T cell hybridomas. *Proc. Natl. Acad. Sci.* 81: 2489.

Babbitt, B.P., P.M. Allen, G. Matsueda, E. Haber, and E.R. Unanue. 1985. Binding of immunogenic peptides to Ia histocompatibility molecules. *Nature* 317: 359.

Barnett, B.C., C.M. Graham, D.S. Burt, J.J. Skehel, and D.B. Thomas. 1989. The immune response of BALB/c mice to influenza haemagglutinin: Commonality of the B cell and T cell repertoires and their relevance to antigenic drift. *Eur. J. Immunol.* 19: 515.

Benacerraf, B. 1978. A hypothesis to relate the specificity of T lymphocytes and the activity of I-region-specific Ir genes in macrophages and B lymphocytes. *J. Immunol.* 120: 1809.

Benjamin, D.C., J.A. Berzofsky, I.J. East, F.R.N. Gurd, C. Hannum, S.J. Leach, E. Margoliash, J.G. Michael, A. Miller, E.M. Prager, M. Reichlin, E.E. Sercarz, S.J.S. Gill, P.E. Todd, and A.C. Wilson. 1984. The antigenic

structure of proteins: A reappraisal. *Annu. Rev. Immunol.* 2: 67.

Berkower, I., G.K. Buckenmeyer, and J.A. Berzofsky. 1986. Molecular mapping of a histocompatibility-restricted immunodominant T cell epitope with synthetic and natural peptides: Implications for T cell antigenic structure. *J. Immunol.* 136: 2498.

Berzofsky, J.A. 1983. T-B reciprocity: An Ia-restricted epitope-specific circuit regulating T cell–B cell interaction and antibody specificity. *Surv. Immunol. Res.* 2: 223.

Both, G.W., C.H. Shi, and E.D. Kilbourne. 1983. Haemagglutinin of swine influenza virus: A single amino acid change pleiotropically affects viral antigenicity and replication. *Proc. Natl. Acad. Sci.* 80: 6996.

Brand, C.M. and J.J. Skehel. 1972. Crystalline antigen from the influenza virus envelope. *Nature* 238: 145.

Brown, L.E., R.A. French, J.M. Gawler, D.C. Jackson, M.L. Smith, E.M. Anders, G.W. Tregear, L. Duncan, P.A. Underwood, and D.O. White. 1988. Distinct epitopes recognised by I-A^d-restricted T cell clones within antigenic site E on influenza virus haemagglutinin. *J. Virol.* 62: 305.

Burt, D.S., K.H.G. Mills, J.J. Skehel, and D.B. Thomas. 1989. Diversity of the Class II (I-A^k/I-E^k)-restricted T cell repertoire for influenza haemagglutinin and antigenic drift: Six non-overlapping epitopes on the HA1 sub-unit are defined by synthetic peptides. *J. Exp. Med.* 170: 383.

Buus, S., S. Colon, C. Smith, J.H. Freed, C. Miles, and H.M. Grey. 1986. Interaction between a "processed" ovalbumin peptide and Ia molecules. *Proc. Natl. Acad. Sci.* 83: 3968.

Caton, A.J., G.G. Brownlee, J.W. Yewdell, and W. Gerhard. 1982. The antigenic structure of the influenza virus A/PR/8/34 haemagglutinin (H1 subtype). *Cell* 31: 417.

Gerhard, W., J. Yewdell, M.E. Frankel, and R. Webster. 1981. Antigenic structure of influenza virus haemagglutinin defined by hybridoma antibodies. *Nature* 290: 713.

Graham, C.M., B.C. Barnett, I. Hartlmayr, D.S. Burt, R. Faulkes, J.J. Skehel, and D.B. Thomas. 1989. The structural requirements for class II (I-A^d)-restricted T cell recognition of influenza haemagglutinin: B cell epitopes define T cell epitopes. *Eur. J. Immunol.* 19: 523.

Guillet, J.G., M.-Z. Lai, T.J. Briner, J.A. Smith, and M.L. Gefter. 1986. Interaction of peptide antigens and class II major histocompatibility complex antigens. *Nature* 324: 260.

Guillet, J.G., M.-Z. Lai, T.J. Briner, S. Buus, A. Sette, H.M. Grey, J.A. Smith, and M.L. Gefter. 1987. Immunological self, nonself discrimination. *Science* 235: 865.

Houghten, R.A. 1985. General method for the rapid solid-phase synthesis of large numbers of peptides: Specificity of antigen-antibody interaction at the level of individual amino acids. *Proc. Natl. Acad. Sci.* 82: 5131.

Hurwitz, J.L., E. Katz, C.J. Hackett, and W. Gerhard. 1984. Characterisation of the murine T$_H$ response to influenza virus haemagglutinin: Evidence for three major specificities. *J. Immunol.* 133: 3371.

Kappler, J., J. White, D. Wegmann, E. Mustain, and P. Marrack. 1982. Antigen presentation by Ia$^+$ B cell hybridomas to H-2 restricted T cell hybridomas. *Proc. Natl. Acad. Sci.* 79: 3604.

Kilbourne, E.D. 1969. Future influenza vaccines and the use of genetic recombinants. *Bull. WHO* 41: 643.

Kimoto, M. and C.G. Fathman. 1980. Antigen-reactive T cell clones. I. Transcomplementing hybrid I-A-region gene products function effectively in antigen presentation. *J. Exp. Med.* 152: 759.

Lanzavecchia, A. 1985. Antigen-specific interactions between T and B cells. *Nature* 314: 537.

Livingstone, A.M. and C.G. Fathman. 1987. The structure of T cell epitopes. *Annu. Rev. Immunol.* 5: 477.

Merrifield, R.B. 1963. Solid phase peptide synthesis. I. The synthesis of a tetrapeptide. *J. Am. Chem. Soc.* 85: 2149.

Mills, K.H.G., J.J. Skehel, and D.B. Thomas. 1986. Extensive diversity in the recognition of influenza virus haemagglutinin by murine T helper clones. *J. Exp. Med.* **163:** 1477.

Mills, K.H.G., D.S. Burt, J.J. Skehel, and D.B. Thomas. 1988. Fine specificity of murine Class II-restricted T cell clones for synthetic peptides of influenza virus haemagglutinin: Heterogeneity of antigen interaction with the T cell and the Ia molecule. *J. Immunol.* **140:** 4083.

Rosenthal, A.S. 1978. Determinant selection and macrophage function in genetic control of the immune response. *Immunol. Rev.* **40:** 136.

Schwartz, R.H. 1985. T lymphocyte recognition of antigen in association with gene-products of the major histocompatibility complex. *Annu. Rev. Immunol.* **3:** 237.

Shastri, N., A. Oki, A. Miller, and E.E. Sercarz. 1985. Distinct recognition phenotypes exist for T cell clones specific for small peptide regions of proteins. *J. Exp. Med.* **162:** 332.

Skehel, J.J., D.J. Stevens, R.S. Daniels, A.R. Douglas, M. Knossow, I.A. Wilson, and D.C. Wiley. 1984. A carbohydrate side-chain on haemagglutinins of Hong Kong influenza viruses inhibits recognition by a monoclonal antibody. *Proc. Natl. Acad. Sci.* **81:** 1779.

Skehel, J.J., P.M. Bayley, E.B. Brown, S.R. Martin, M.D.

Waterfield, J.M. White, I.A. Wilson, and D.C. Wiley. 1982. Changes in the conformation of influenza virus haemagglutinin at the pH optimum of virus-mediated membrane fusion. *Proc. Natl. Acad. Sci.* **79:** 968.

Staudt, L.M. and W. Gerhard. 1983. Generation of antibody diversity in the immune response of BALB/c mice to influenza virus haemagglutinin. *J. Exp. Med.* **157:** 687.

Thomas, D.B., J.J. Skehel, K.H.G. Mills, and C.M. Graham. 1987. A single amino acid substitution in influenza haemagglutinin abrogates recognition by monoclonal antibody and a spectrum of subtype-specific L3T4⁺ T cell clones. *Eur. J. Immunol.* **17:** 133.

Webster, R.G., W.G. Laver, G.M. Air, and G.C. Schild. 1982. Molecular mechanisms of variation in influenza viruses. *Nature* **296:** 115.

Wiley, D.C., I.A. Wilson, and J.J. Skehel. 1981. Structural identification of the antibody binding sites of Hong Kong influenza haemagglutinin and their involvement in antigenic variation. *Nature* **289:** 373.

Wilson, I.A., J.J. Skehel, and D.C. Wiley. 1981. Structure of the haemagglutinin membrane glycoprotein of influenza virus at 3Å resolution. *Nature* **289:** 366.

Control of Cellular and Humoral Immune Responses by Peptides Containing T-cell Epitopes

M.T. Scherer,* B.M.C. Chan,* F. Ria,* J.A. Smith,†
D.L. Perkins,* and M.L. Gefter*

*Department of Biology, Massachusetts Institute of Technology, Cambridge, Massachusetts 02139;
†Departments of Molecular Biology and Pathology, Massachusetts General Hospital,
and Department of Pathology, Harvard Medical School, Boston, Massachusetts 02114

T cells are known to recognize antigen in the form of peptides bound to major histocompatibility complex (MHC)-encoded class II molecules (Babbit et al. 1985; Schwartz et al. 1985; Buus et al. 1987; Guillet et al. 1987). Experiments with MHC-encoded class II molecules in planar membranes show that the binding of the T-cell receptor (TCR) to the peptide/MHC complex may not be sufficient for activation of the responding T cells (Quill and Schwartz 1987). One signal to the T cells is the binding of the TCR/CD3 complex to the antigen/MHC. As proposed by Bretscher and Cohn (1970), lymphocytes may be tolerized unless they see a second signal. This second signal for T cells can be provided in principle by the antigen-presenting cell (APC), either through the secretion of soluble cytokines or by the interaction of molecules on the APC and T-cell surface. To test this hypothesis, we exposed mice to peptides containing known T-cell epitopes without adjuvant in order to expose the T cells only to the first (TCR) signal.

The biological relevance of the existence of various APC types such as macrophages, B cells, and dendritic cells in vivo is still unclear. As mentioned above, the second signal necessary for the activation of T cells may be provided by APCs (Quill and Schwartz 1987). It is also possible that different types of APCs may provide different second signals and may thus affect the quantitative and qualitative outcome of immune responses. In this paper, the responding T cells from mice immunized with the amino-terminal fragment of λ repressor cI 1-102 using different immunization protocols are characterized with respect to the distribution of T-cell epitopes recognized, as well as their functional phenotypes upon presentation of T-cell epitopes by different APCs in vitro.

The protein context of a peptidic T-cell epitope also influences the T-cell response specific for that epitope (Shastri et al. 1986). Thus, the immune response to a T-cell epitope may be hidden when it is covalently linked to another T-cell epitope. This can be due, for example, to competition between epitopes for binding to the MHC peptide-binding site (Guillet et al. 1987). Antigen processing can also explain differential expression of epitopes, depending on the context. Thus, neighboring or distal residues could influence processing so that a particular T-cell epitope is unavailable to

bind MHC. We compare the activity of an ovalbumin-derived peptide epitope that is suppressed when covalently linked to an epitope of greater immunogenicity in an antigenic and tolerogenic system.

MATERIALS AND METHODS

Animals. Strains BALB/cByJ, C57BL/6 mice were obtained from Jackson Laboratories, Bar Harbor, Maine.

Cell cultures and assay conditions. All cultures and assays were performed according to established procedures (Lai et al. 1987).

Antigens. Bacteriophage λ repressor cI protein fragment p1-102 and synthetic peptides were prepared as described previously (Lai et al. 1987). p12-26^{N14} is residues 12–26 of cI with asparagine substituted for aspartic acid at position 14.

Cell lines. BW5147.G.4.Oau^R.1(α-,β-) was a gift from W. Borne. A20.2J (I-A^d, I-E^d) was a gift from J. Kappler and P. Marrack. CTLL.2 was a gift from D. Raulet. CT.4S (Hu-Li et al. 1989) and 11B11 (anti-IL-4) (Ohara and Paul 1985) were a gift from W. Paul. S4.B6 (anti-IL-2) was a gift from T. Mosmann. Class II MHC L-cell transfectants RT 2.3.3H (I-A^d) and RT 10.3H2 (I-E^d) were a gift from R. Germain.

Antibodies. Monoclonal antibodies were produced by harvesting cell supernatants from B-cell hybridomas. Supernatants were centrifuged and sterile filtered to remove any residual cells. 11B11 supernatant was used at 10%, and S4B6 supernatant was used at 50%.

Antisera. BALB/c mice were tolerized by injection of p12-26 i.v. in saline, or saline alone as a control. They were immunized 10 days after the first tolerization with p12-26 i.p. (50 μg emulsified in complete Freund's adjuvant [CFA]). Mice received a booster immunization 14 days after the primary injection of p12-26 i.p. (50 μg emulsified in incomplete Freund's adjuvant [IFA]). Mice were bled 7 days after the first immunization and 8 days after the booster immunization (data shown). Antibodies were measured by enzyme-linked immunosorbent assay (ELISA) (Good et al. 1988).

Isolation of T-cell hybridomas. Mice were immunized either s.c. at the base of the tail and in both thighs or i.p. with 100 μg of bacteriophage λ repressor p1-102 in either CFA, IFA, or alum. After 7 days, draining lymph nodes were removed from mice with s.c. immunizations, and spleen cells were removed from those with i.p. immunizations. Cells were stimulated in vitro with p1-102 at 50 μg/ml for 2 days before fusion with BW5147. Fusion hybrids were prepared according to established procedures (Gefter et al. 1977).

All the T-cell hybridomas reported here have been subcloned at least once by limiting dilution method (Walker et al. 1982). 9C127 and 1E1 are hybridomas made from BALB/c mice. 3D054.8 is a clone specific for OVA(325-336).

Tolerization of adult mice. Mice 4–8 weeks old were injected i.v. in the tail vein with 300 μg of deaggregated peptide dissolved in 100 μl of saline on day 0. After 5 days, another 300 μg of peptide was injected i.v. On day 10, the mice were immunized s.c. with peptide in CFA as described above.

Lymphokine assays. IL-2 assays were performed as described previously (Lai et al. 1987). Assay for IL-4 was performed using the IL-4-dependent cell line CT.4S according to the method of Hu-Li et al. (1989), with the slight modification that tritium incorporation in DNA was measured 6 hours after the addition of 1 mCi of tritiated thymidine.

Lymphocyte proliferation assays. T-lymphocyte proliferation assays were performed according to methods described by Lai et al. (1987).

RESULTS

We have previously shown that the T-cell response in BALB/c mice to the amino-terminal fragment of λ repressor (p1-102) is predominantly directed to a synthetic peptide (p12-26) containing residues 12–26 (Guillet et al. 1987; Roy et al. 1989). Proliferation of p1-102-immunized T cells is equivalent in response to either p1-102 or p12-26, and over 90% of BALB/c-derived T-cell hybrids made against p1-102 respond to p12-26. In addition, p12-26 can serve to recruit help, since immunization of mice with p12-26 produces anti-p12-26 antibodies (Roy et al. 1989). When BALB/c mice are exposed to p12-26 by intravenous injection, they become unresponsive to later immunization with p12-26 s.c. in CFA. The same is true for p12-26^{N14}, a related peptide that cross-reacts with p12-26 (Fig. 1). The tolerization procedure decreases lymphocyte proliferation (Fig. 1a) and almost eliminates IL-2 secretion (Fig. 1b) of draining lymph node cells. The effect is epitope-specific, since i.v. injection of saline alone or of unrelated peptides has no effect. In addition, C57BL/6 mice can be tolerized to their immunodominant epitope in p1-102, p73-88 (data not shown). This tolerization protocol also eliminates T-cell help, since treated mice can no longer produce antibodies to p12-26 (Table 1).

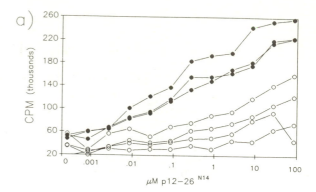

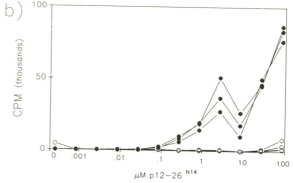

Figure 1. Response of lymphocytes from BALB/c mice immunized with p12-26^{N14} s.c. (○) Mice tolerized by two i.v. injections of p12-26^{N14}; (●) control mice. (*a*) Proliferation; (*b*) IL-2 secretion as measured by proliferation of CTLL cells.

The reduced response cannot be due to a sudden high concentration of soluble antigen inactivating T cells, since the same tolerization effect can be seen when antigen is injected i.p. in IFA 10 days before immunization (data not shown).

The tolerance effect lasts for at least 6 weeks (Table 2). The T-cell proliferation is initially reduced to only 20% of that of immunized mice, whereas the IL-2 secretion is reduced even more, to less than 5%. After 42 days, the IL-2 secretion of tolerized T cells seems to have increased to 15% of that of control T cells, whereas only one of two mice tested have reduced proliferation. Studies are continuing to investigate further the duration of the T-cell nonresponsiveness.

The T-cell tolerance could be due to the inactivation of antigen-specific T cells or the induction of suppressor

Table 1. Antibody Response to p12–26

Mouse	Pre-bleed (μg/ml)	Immunized (μg/ml)
Tolerized	<2	19
Tolerized	3	12
Tolerized	3	15
Tolerized	3	5
Control	2	528
Control	4	378
Control	2	99
Control	3	363

Table 2. Persistence of Tolerization Effects

Day immunized	% of Control	
	IL-2	proliferation
1	3, 2	19, 19
5	1, 2	28, 38
9	6, 20	14, 39
41	11, 17	17, 103

BALB/c mice were i.v. tolerized on day −5 and day 0 p12–26. Mice were immunized at various times thereafter and tested for specific proliferation and IL-2 secretion 7 days later.

T cells. To test the latter possibility, mixtures of lymphocytes from tolerized and nontolerized mice were compared with mixtures of lymphocytes from nonimmunized and nontolerized mice. It is expected that if tolerization were due to the induction of suppressor T cells, then the suppressor T cells present in tolerized mice should suppress the response of immunized T cells, whereas mixing with nonimmunized T cells should have no effect. As seen in Figure 2, the proliferation of immunized cells mixed with tolerized cells was the same as that of immunized cells mixed with nonimmune cells. If anything, the response was a bit higher, as could be expected, because tolerized cells still proliferate at 20% of the control level. Furthermore, the proliferation clearly rises as more immunized cells are added, until, with 99% control immunized cells and only 1% tolerized or nonimmunized cells, the response is normal. The same result was obtained with IL-2 secretion (data not shown).

We then investigated the immune response to a molecule in which two T-cell epitopes were combined. The two epitopes chosen were residues 12–26 (p12-26) of λ repressor and residues 325–336 (OVA-D) of egg ovalbumin, with valine residue 327 changed to aspartic acid to reduce binding to I-A^d (Sette et al. 1987). Both epitopes are I-A^d-restricted, and p12-26 and ova325-336 are immunodominant in their respective proteins when injected into BALB/c mice (Guillet et al. 1987; Shimonkevitz et al. 1987). We synthesized a long joint

peptide, 12-26-GPG-OVA-D, containing p12-26 linked to OVA-D by a glycine-proline-glycine bridge (see Table 3). T cells from BALB/c mice immunized with OVA-D proliferate and secrete IL-2 when stimulated in vitro with OVA-D. Similarly, T cells from mice immunized with p12-26 proliferate and secrete IL-2 in response to either p12-26 or the joint peptide (Fig. 3a). In contrast, lymphocytes from mice immunized with the long peptide respond in vitro to the long peptide and to p12-26, but not to OVA-D (Fig. 3e). Thus, the OVA-D epitope is hidden when present within the joint peptide. The basis for this result could be easily explained by competition between the two epitopes for binding to MHC-encoded class II molecules and perhaps also to a third epitope created at the junction of the two fused epitopes. This epitope suppression is not due to the inability of BALB/c-presenting cells to present OVA-D from within the long peptide, since the long peptide stimulates the ova325-336-restricted T-cell hybridoma 3DO54.8 when presented on I-A^d-transfected L cells (Fig. 4a). I-A^d-transfected L cells (Fig. 4b) and fixed or live H-2^d A20 cells (Fig. 4c) can also present the joint peptide to p12-26-specific hybridomas 9C127(I-A^d-restricted) and 1E1 (I-E^d-restricted). Thus, processing of the joint peptide is not required, at least for presentation of the p12-26 epitope in vitro.

Mice immunized with p12-26, which 10 days earlier had been tolerized by i.p. injection with either p12-26 (Fig. 3b) or the joint peptide (Fig. 3d) in IFA, have diminished responses, whereas mice given saline or OVA-D-tolerized mice proliferate normally in response to either p12-26 or the joint peptide (Fig. 3a,c). Similarly, mice immunized with the joint peptide that were previously tolerized with the joint peptide cannot respond to either p12-26 or the joint peptide (Fig. 3h), and those tolerized to p12-26 cannot respond to p12-26 (Fig. 3f) but can respond to a lesser extent to the joint peptide, possibly because T cells specific for the junction were not tolerized. Control mice tolerized to OVA-D (Fig. 3g) or not tolerized (Fig. 3e) respond to both p12-26 and the joint peptide. Mice immunized with OVA-D that were previously tolerized with OVA-D cannot respond to OVA-D or the joint peptide (Fig.

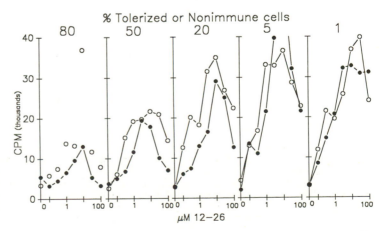

Figure 2. Proliferation of lymphocytes from mice immunized with p12-26. Lymphocytes from control mice were mixed with various percentages of lymphocytes from either tolerized mice (○) or nonimmunized mice (●).

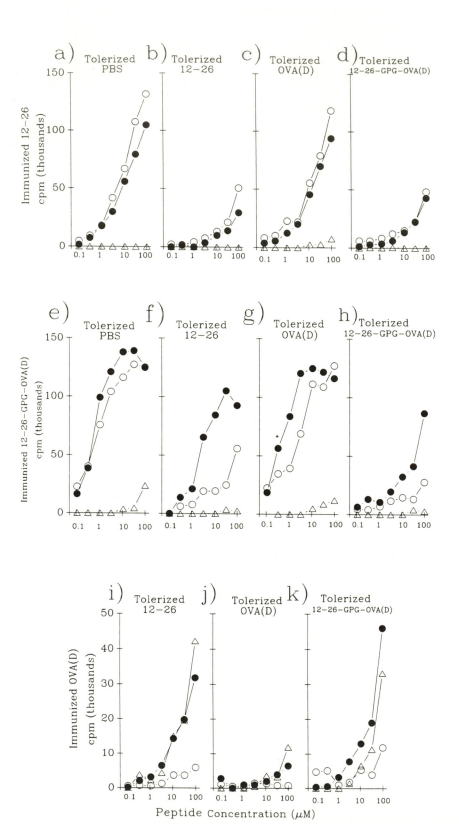

Figure 3. IL-2 secretion of lymphocytes from BALB/c mice. Lymphocyte response to in vitro stimulation with (●) joint peptide, (○) p12-26, (△) OVA-D. (*a*) Mice sham-tolerized and immunized with p12-26; (*b*) mice tolerized with p12-26 and immunized with p12-26; (*c*) mice tolerized with OVA-D and immunized with p12-26; (*d*) mice tolerized with joint peptide and immunized with p12-26; (*e*) mice sham-tolerized and immunized with joint peptide; (*f*) mice tolerized with p12-26 and immunized with joint peptide; (*g*) mice tolerized with OVA-D and immunized with joint peptide; (*h*) mice tolerized with joint peptide and immunized with joint peptide; (*i*) mice tolerized with p12-26 and immunized with OVA-D; (*j*) mice tolerized with OVA-D and immunized with OVA-D; (*k*) mice tolerized with joint peptide and immunized with OVA-D.

Table 3. Sequences of Peptides Used

P12–26	L E D A R R L K A I Y E K K K
P12–26[N14]	L E N A R R L K A I Y E K K K
OVA-D	Q A D H A A H A E I N E
Joint peptide	L E D A R R L K A I Y E K K K G P G Q A D H A A H A E I N E

3j), but mice that were tolerized with p12-26 do respond (Fig. 3i). However, mice tolerized with the joint peptide and immunized with OVA-D still respond to both OVA-D and the joint peptide (Fig. 3k). Thus, the OVA-D epitope is hidden within the joint peptide during tolerization as well as immunization. It appears that tolerization to T-cell epitopes occurs when such epitopes are presented by APCs but in the absence of a "second signal."

The mode of immunization is known to influence the immune response (Warren et al. 1986). For the purposes of this study, we may ask what types of second signals promote what types of immune responses. T-cell hybridomas were prepared from BALB/c mice immunized with p1-102 in CFA s.c., CFA i.p., IFA s.c., IFA i.p., and alum i.p. They were originally screened by measuring IL-2 secretion, as tested for by the ability to sustain growth of the IL-2-dependent cell line CTLL. Previous studies (Roy et al. 1989) have shown that p12-26 is the immunodominant epitope in BALB/c mice immunized with p1-102 in CFA s.c.. As shown in Table 4, p12-26 was also immunodominant in immunized mice using the five different protocols of immunization. About 90% of all p1-102-specific hybrids respond to p12-26. In addition, about half of the non-p12-26 hybrids were found to respond to a second p1-102 peptide, p46-62.

The p46-62- and p12-26-specific hybrids were further characterized with respect to their production of IL-4, using the IL-4-dependent clone CT.4S as indicator cells. Interestingly, over 50% of the p46-62-specific hybridomas produced IL-4 upon stimulation by B cells (A20) as APCs (Table 5). In contrast, less than 5% of the p12-26-specific hybridomas produced IL-4. A representative p12-26-specific hybridoma, 1PA12-1, produced IL-2 when given p12-26 presented on either the B cell A20 or I-A^d-transfected L cells (Fig. 5a,b). The CTLL response was inhibitable by anti-IL-2 antibody. In contrast, there was no response when the supernatants were tested on CT.4S cells (Fig. 5c,d). Thus, T

cells that recognize p46-62 often secrete IL-4, whereas those that recognize p12-26 rarely do. It is possible that this observation is due to presentation by distinct subsets of APCs that may direct responding T cells to express different functional phenotypes. We propose that APCs that can process p1-102 to give rise to p46-62 leading to IL-4 production are a subset of APCs distinct from those that process p1-102 primarily to p12-26. Evidence supportive of this possibility was obtained by comparing the ability of B cells (A20) and I-A^d-transfected L cells to stimulate IL-4 production from the identified hybridomas. A representative p46-62-specific hybridoma, 1SI46l-1.1, produces IL-2 when A20 cells are used as APCs, as shown by a CTLL response that is inhibitable by anti-IL-2 and not by anti-IL-4 (Fig. 6a). IL-4 production was also observed by stimulation of CT.4S, which is inhibited by anti-IL-4 and not by anti-IL-2 (Fig. 6c). The small decrease in the CT.4S response in the presence of anti-IL-2 may be due to a synergistic effect of IL-2 on IL-4 secretion on CT.4S stimulation (Hu-Li et al. 1989), as well as to the nonspecific toxicity of the antibody culture supernatant used. When I-A^d-transfected L cells are used to present p46-62, production of IL-2 but not IL-4 is observed (Fig. 6b,d). No hybrid tested has been able to secrete significant amounts of IL-4 when I-A^d-transfected L cells were used as APC. This is not due simply to a dose-response shift of the L cells as compared to A20 cells. The dose response of using L cells shifts 3-fold for the IL-2 response (Fig. 6a,b), whereas there is no IL-4 response while using L cells even at 32 μM of p46-62, 32-fold more antigen than required with A20 cells (Fig. 6c,d).

DISCUSSION

One known mechanism of thymic tolerance depends on the deletion of thymic T cells reactive to self-peptides bound to MHC-encoded molecules of thymic APCs (Kappler et al. 1987; Kisielow et al. 1988). This

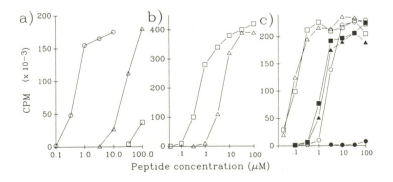

Figure 4. Hybridoma response to in vitro stimulation with peptides. Open symbols are live APCs, and filled symbols are fixed APCs. (*a*) 3D054.8 T-cell hybridoma and I-A^d-transfected L cells; (○) OVA, (△) joint peptide, (□) OVA-D. (*b*) 9C127 T-cell hybridoma and I-A^d-transfected L cells; (△) joint peptide, (□) p12-26. (*c*) 1E1 T-cell hybridoma and A20 cells; (○, ●) p1-102, (△, ▲) joint peptide, (□, ■) p12-26.

Table 4. Epitopes of BALB/c Hybridomas Immunized with cI p1–102

Immunization protocol	Number of hybrids			
	1–102 +	12–26 +	12–26⁻ tested with peptides	46–62 +
Alum i.p.	436	389	27	12
CFA i.p.	252	216	19	9
CFA s.c.	134	121	7	2
IFA i.p.	413	379	27	12
IFA s.c.	199	179	17	9
Total	1434	1284	97	44

mechanism can only delete those T cells that react to self-proteins that are expressed or travel to the fetal thymus. Expression in the fetal thymus of every self-T-cell epitope found in every protein in the organism would be extremely difficult. Even if tolerance is needed only for those proteins that are accessible to the immune system, and assuming efficient transport of all proteins to the fetal thymus, many proteins are only expressed after birth or later. T cells reactive to proteins expressed late in development would be able to leave the thymus and initiate autoimmune disease later in life. The fact that this does not occur argues for some sort of peripheral, continuing tolerance mechanism. We have found evidence for such a mechanism in that, by exposing a mouse to a T-cell epitope i.v. in saline or i.p. in IFA, the mouse later has a drastically diminished T-cell response to the same epitope when administered later using CFA as the adjuvant. This reduction or tolerance is epitope-specific, lasts for at least 6 weeks, and is not due to the induction of suppressor T cells. It also completely inhibits the antibody response to the epitope, presumably by blocking T-cell help.

We propose that the immune system in its resting state, i.e., unstimulated by an infectious agent or gross tissue damage, is normally in a tolerogenic state. All T cells that see antigen in that state are turned off either by clonal deletion or by clonal anergy. Only when the immune system is turned on by frank infection, by such

Table 5. IL-4-producing BALB/c Hybridomas from Mice Immunized with cI p1–102

Immunization protocol	Number of IL-4-producing clones/total clones	
	p12–26	p46–62
Alum i.p.	0/11	4/7
CFA i.p.	0/20	2/4
CFA s.c.	1/16	not recovered
IFA i.p.	2/30	4/11
IFA s.c.	1/15	5/5
Total	4/92 (4.3%)	15/27 (55.6%)

agents as the bacterial antigens and mitogens found in the mycobacteria, or by the presence of soluble cytokines, are T cells able to respond by proliferating, secreting IL-2, and helping B cells. Furthermore, all of the T-cell epitopes we have tested that are capable of eliciting an immune response are just those epitopes that can also serve to induce tolerance. Thus, it would appear that epitopes processed and presented in the absence of a second signal lead to tolerance. The observations presented here readily explain the classic low zone tolerance to soluble proteins.

Results from the present study clearly demonstrate a regulatory effect of competing epitopes present within the same peptide upon the immune response. Thus, a majority of the T-cell response to the joint peptide is

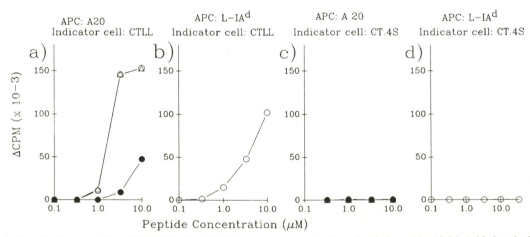

Figure 5. Lymphokine secretion of 1PA12-1 cells. Hybridoma response to in vitro stimulation with p12-26. Added to the indicator cells was (○) nothing, (●) anti-IL-2, (△) anti-IL-4. (a) IL-2 response with A20 cells; (b) IL-2 response with transfected L cells; (c) IL-4 response with A20 cells; (d) IL-4 response with transfected L cells.

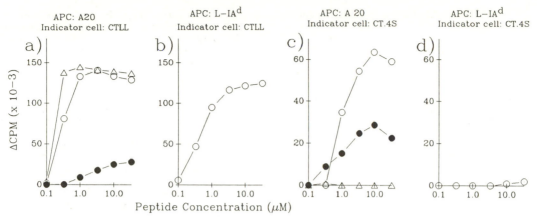

Figure 6. Lymphokine secretion of 1SI46-1.1 cells. Hybridoma response to in vitro stimulation with p46-62. Added to the indicator cells was (○) nothing, (●) anti-IL-2, (△) anti-IL-4. (*a*) IL-2 response with A20 cells; (*b*) IL-2 response with transfected L cells; (*c*) IL-4 response with A20 cells; (*d*) IL-4 response with transfected L cells.

directed toward the more immunogenic epitope (12-26), leading to an apparent suppression of the response to the less immunogenic epitope (OVA-D). It is also clear that competition occurs between T-cell epitopes during the induction of tolerance. Again, the more immunogenic epitope (12-26) is tolerized, and the less immunogenic epitope (OVA-D) is ignored. The T-cell response to the less immunogenic epitope can be elicited readily in mice tolerized with the joint peptide. Therefore, the processing mechanisms of APCs inducing immunity and those inducing tolerance seem to be the same, and the less immunogenic epitopes, such as OVA-D within the joint peptide 12-26-GPG-OVA-D, are hidden for both immunization and tolerization.

Many different cell types such as B cells, macrophages, and dendritic cells can serve in vitro as APCs (Chesnut and Grey 1981; Ziegler and Unanue 1981; Sunshine et al. 1983). The involvement of the different APCs used in an immune response in vivo are unknown. However, activation of T cells by the different APCs may vary because of differences in their endocytic and processing properties (Guidos et al. 1984). Thus, the immune response may be modulated by the involvement of different types of APCs during the activation of T cells. In addition, the type of adjuvant and the route of immunization may have selective effects on the APCs used in the immune response. In our study, we observed no significant difference in the T-cell response induced in BALB/c mice immunized with λ repressor p1-102 using different combinations of adjuvants and routes of immunization. However, over 50% of T-cell hybridomas specific for p46-62 secreted IL-4, whereas less than 5% of hybridomas specific for p12-26 did. The fact that all IL-4-producing hybrids also secrete IL-2 may be attributable to the fusion partner, BW5147, which has been shown to be capable of IL-2 production (Hagiwara et al. 1988) or, more likely, to the fact that the hybrids were initially screened for their abilities to secrete IL-2. We propose the existence of at least two different types of APCs that have different antigen-processing mechanisms to

explain these results. One type of APC processes p1-102 in such a way that both epitopes 12-26 and 46-62 are presented, with epitope 12-26 being dominant. T cells activated by these APCs produce only IL-2, phenotypically similar to T-helper type 1 (T_H1) cells. The other type of APC processes p1-102 in such a way that the 46-62 epitope predominates. T cells activated by this type of APC often secrete IL-4, phenotypically similar to T_H2 cells. An alternate explanation is that a single type of APC may be differentially activated to alter both its processing activity, i.e., to produce and present different epitopes, and its concomitant different second signals that alter the activation of responding T cells in such a way that their lymphokine production and thus their effect on the qualitative nature of the antibody response is altered. These possibilities are currently being explored.

REFERENCES

Babbit, B., P. Allen, G. Matsueda, E. Haber, and E. Unanue. 1985. Binding of immunogenic peptides to Ia histocompatibility molecules. *Nature* **317:** 359.

Bretscher, P. and M. Cohn. 1970. A theory of self-nonself discrimination. *Nature* **169:** 1042.

Buus, S., A. Sette, S. Colon, C. Miles, and H.M. Grey. 1987. The relation between major histocompatibility complex (MHC) restriction and the capacity of Ia to bind immunogenic peptides. *Science* **235:** 1353.

Chesnut, R.W. and H.M. Grey. 1981. Studies on the capacity of B cells to serve as antigen-presenting cells. *J. Immunol.* **126:** 1075.

Gefter, M.L., D.H. Margulies, and M.D. Scharff. 1977. A simple method for polyethylene glycol-promoted hybridization of mouse myeloma cells. *Somatic Cell Genet.* **3:** 231.

Good, M.F., D. Pombo, V.F. de la Cruz, L.H. Miller, and J.A. Berzofsky. 1988. Parasite polymorphism present within minimal T cell epitopes of *Plasmodium falciparum* circumsporozoite protein. *J. Immunol.* **235:** 1059.

Guidos, C., M. Wang, and K.-C. Lee. 1984. A comparison of the stimulatory activities of lymphoid dendritic cells and macrophages in T proliferative responses to various antigens. *J. Immunol.* **133:** 1179.

Guillet, J.-G., M.-Z. Lai, T. Briner, S. Buus, A. Sette, H.M.

Grey, J.A. Smith, and M.L. Gefter. 1987. Immunological self, nonself discrimination. *Science* **235:** 865.

Hagiwara, H., T. Yokota, J. Luh, F. Lee, K.-I. Arai, N. Arai, and A. Zlotnik. 1988. The AKR thymoma BW5147 is able to produce lymphokines when stimulated with calcium ionophore and phorbol ester. *J. Immunol.* **140:** 1561.

Hu-Li, J., J. Ohara, C. Watson, W. Tsang, and W.E. Paul. 1989. Derivation of a T cell line that is highly responsive to IL-4 and IL-2 (CT.4R) and of an IL-2 hyporesponsive mutant of that line (CT.4S). *J. Immunol.* **142:** 800.

Kappler, J.W., N. Roehm, and P. Marrack. 1987. T cell tolerance by clonal elimination in the thymus. *Cell* **49:** 273.

Kisielow, P., H. Bluthmann, U.D. Staerz, M. Steinmetz, and H. von Boehmer. 1988. Tolerance in T-cell-receptor transgenic mice involves deletion of nonmature CD4$^+$8$^+$ thymocytes. *Nature* **333:** 742.

Lai, M.-Z., D.T. Ross, J.-G. Guillet, T.J. Briner, M.L. Gefter, and J.A. Smith. 1987. T lymphocyte response to bacteriophage λ repressor cI protein. *J. Immunol.* **139:** 3973.

Ohara, J., and W.E. Paul. 1985. B cell stimulatory factor BSF-1: Production of monoclonal antibody and molecular characterization. *Nature* **315:** 333.

Quill, H. and R.H. Schwartz. 1987. Stimulation of normal inducer T cell clones with antigen presented by purified Ia molecules in planar lipid membranes: Specific induction of a long-lived state of proliferative nonresponsiveness. *J. Immunol.* **138:** 3704.

Roy, S., M.T. Scherer, T.J. Briner, J.A. Smith, and M.L. Gefter. 1989. Murine MHC polymorphism and T cell specificities. *Science* **244:** 572.

Schwartz, R.H., B.S. Fox, E. Fraga, C. Chen, and B. Singh. 1985. The T lymphocyte response to cytochrome c. *J. Immunol.* **135:** 2598.

Sette, A., S. Buus, S. Colon, J.A. Smith, C. Miles, and H.M. Grey. 1987. Structural characteristics of an antigen required for its interaction with Ia and recognition by T cells. *Nature* **328:** 395.

Shastri, N., A. Miller, and E.E. Sercarz. 1986. Amino acid residues distinct from the determinant region can profoundly affect activation of T cell clones by related antigens. *J. Immunol.* **136:** 371.

Shimonkevitz, R., J. Kappler, P. Marrack, and H.M. Grey. 1987. Antigen recognition by H-2 restricted T cells II. A tryptic ovalbumin peptide that substitutes for processed antigen. *J. Immunol.* **133:** 2067.

Sunshine, G.H., D.P. Gold, H.H. Wortis, P. Marrack, and J.W. Kappler. 1983. Mouse spleen dendritic cells present soluble antigens to antigen-specific T cell hybridomas. *J. Exp. Med.* **158:** 1745.

Walker, E., N.L. Warner, R. Chesnut, J. Kappler, and P. Marrack. 1982. Antigen-specific, I region restricted interactions *in vitro* between tumor cell lines and T cell hybridomas. *J. Immunol.* **128:** 2164.

Warren, H.S., F.R. Vogel, and L.A. Chedid. 1986. Current status of immunological adjuvants. *Annu. Rev. Immunol.* **4:** 369.

Ziegler, K. and E.R. Unanue. 1981. Identification of a macrophage antigen-processing event required for I-region-restricted antigen presentation to T lymphocytes. *J. Immunol.* **127:** 1869.

Examining the Crypticity of Antigenic Determinants

A. Ametani, R. Apple, V. Bhardwaj, G. Gammon,
A. Miller, and E. Sercarz

Department of Microbiology, University of California, Los Angeles, California 90024-1489

During the past decade, we have studied the T-cell response to a tightly folded protein antigen, hen egg white lysozyme (HEL), in an effort to understand why T cells become activated to only particular dominant determinants. In several recent reviews (Gammon et al. 1987; Apple et al. 1989; Sercarz 1989), these experiments and interpretations have been described in detail, and at the outset we will summarize them briefly, before we address the major focus of this report, the possible basis of crypticity.

MHC Dependence of T-cell Response

The CD4[+] T-cell response to HEL in the mouse is very much dependent on the nature of the major histocompatibility complex (MHC) and differs greatly in various haplotypes. The binding site on a particular class II molecule interacts with a motif found in a variety of peptides with a similar constellation of charged/polar and hydrophobic residues (Guillet et al. 1987; Sette et al. 1989). Almost the entire HEL molecule can be responded to, even in the small sample of three independent haplotypes we and others have studied—b,d, and k (Gammon et al. 1987; Adorini et al. 1988). It seems difficult to conclude that the secondary structure, e.g., helicity, of any particular determinant as it exists within the native molecule, has any relationship to immunogenicity.

Dominant and Cryptic Determinants

Certain immunodominant determinants will activate T cells after injection of the native antigen, whereas other minor and cryptic determinants fail to do so unless they are removed from the native molecule and used as peptides for immunization. Our studies indicate that some determinants are rarely revealed during natural processing of HEL: Such determinants can be termed *cryptic*. Even after priming with a cryptic peptide, the response to it cannot be elicited with the native protein except at very high concentrations (> 10 μM); this distinguishes cryptic determinants from *minor* determinants, which, although giving a poor response from the native immunogen, seem to be produced in large enough quantities in vitro to stimulate previously primed cells.

Distant Residues Can Affect Determinant Recognition

The molecular context determines which peptide will win out in the competition between different agretopes for the binding site on a class II molecule. As a highly compact antigen molecule is nicked and unfolded, certain determinants will be unearthed first, and those with a high affinity for a class-II-binding site will probably bind; the interaction between class II and the unfolding molecule will take place well before the molecule is catabolized into 10–15-amino-acid peptides. This early interaction can explain several interesting experimental situations, described in detail elsewhere (Shastri et al. 1986a,c), where amino acid residues at some distance from the site of T-cell-receptor engagement with the peptide/MHC ligand nevertheless affect the intensity and quality of responsiveness. This interaction and its sequelae could be considered Ia-guided processing (Sercarz et al. 1986) and suggest that the future course of processing could be strongly influenced by the initial, protective binding to the most favorable agretope. Our results are not in accord with the prevalent paradigm that the antigen is dissociated into small peptides before attachment to the MHC.

Dominance and Crypticity Are Not Absolute

There really is no such entity as an immunodominant, or a cryptic determinant, in an absolute sense. Dominance is strictly a characteristic of a particular antigen in a particular haplotype; as will be shown later, the same can be applied to crypticity. In earlier reports, we have described the hierarchies of determinant usage in several mouse strains and evidence supporting the belief that a major explanation for hierarchy is the availability of determinants. The existence of crypticity indicates that binding ability alone of a determinant within an antigen molecule cannot be the sole factor affecting its use, but that topology and geography of the molecule will be implicated. In this article, we will explore certain factors that especially play a role in determining crypticity of a peptide determinant.

RESULTS

Actually, some of these same factors influence the hierarchy of responses to individual determinants and can be described conveniently by examining the relationship between hierarchy and tolerance.

Hierarchy of Determinant Usage and the Induction of Tolerance

The induction of self-tolerance in the thymus by clonal deletion requires the presentation of antigen in association with MHC-encoded structures. Hence, tolerance is MHC-restricted (Groves and Singer 1983; Rammensee and Bevan 1984) and the *same* epitope recognized during stimulation of peripheral T cells to induce an immune response appears to cause tolerance (Gammon et al. 1986a,b). Although differences exist between these events in the thymus and in the periphery, the two processes must be similar in many ways. It would be expected that the features of antigen structure described above that affect antigen presentation will also be important in tolerance induction. The factors that adjust the level of responsiveness to each determinant on an antigen can be divided into three categories: those affecting the efficiency of presentation; those altering the pre-immune T-cell repertoire; and regulation by other cell types. A major determinant must do well in each of these three categories, whereas a minor determinant may not be able to withstand a single failure. We have proposed that during tolerance induction to certain antigens, only T cells recognizing well-presented determinants would be deleted and those responsive to poorly presented determinants would escape tolerization (Gammon and Sercarz 1989). The loss or preservation of responsiveness to individual determinants will not exactly match the hierarchy of determinants, because although efficiency of presentation is important in both situations, other factors regulate normal responses. For example, T cells specific for a self-molecule will be deleted regardless of their frequency. Since all major determinants need to be efficiently presented, the responses to them should be tolerized. Accordingly, the reactivities that are spared in tolerant animals will be to poorly presented determinants, which for this reason are minor.

The support for this model comes from a system of experimentally induced tolerance; i.e., tolerance induced by i.v. injection of 2 mg HEL. It had previously been shown that although HEL-tolerant B10.A mice did not respond to HEL immunization, they could respond to certain HEL fragments following direct immunization with them (Oki and Sercarz 1985). These latter responses were cross-reactive with whole HEL, raising a paradox, namely, the lack of response to HEL priming despite the presence of HEL-reactive T cells. To examine this in more detail, tolerant mice were challenged with several HEL peptides known to contain T-cell-inducing determinants. Two of these peptides, 20-35 and 46-61, contained major determinants, and the remaining three, 1-17, 30-53, and 74-96, contained minor or cryptic determinants only. The data (see Table 1) clearly showed that responsiveness to both major determinants was lost, as well as to 1-17, but responsiveness to one of the minor-determinant-bearing peptides, 30-53, and to cryptic 74-96, was preserved (Gammon and Sercarz 1989). This explains the above-mentioned paradox: The loss of reactivity to the major determinants diminished the overall response to HEL, whereas the preservation of reactivity to the minor determinants did not apparently affect the total response because these determinants only constitute a very minor part of it.

Why was the 1-17 specific response tolerized by HEL? We have argued that hierarchy and ease of tolerance induction will diverge when the response to a determinant is poor due to a deficient T-cell repertoire or immunoregulation.

1. *Deficient repertoire.* 1-17 may actually be well presented, hence the response to it lost. In fact, in C3H strain mice (Adorini et al. 1988), 1-17 contains a major determinant recognized in association with I-E^k. Additionally, it binds E^k relatively strongly (Adorini et al. 1988). This suggests that the much weaker response to 1-17 following HEL immunization in B10.A mice, which express E^k, is a repertoire/T$_s$ regulation problem.

2. *Immunoregulation.* It is possible that both a T$_s$-inducing determinant and a T$_H$-inducing determinant are present on 1-17. Some indirect evidence was presented earlier that a T$_s$-inducing determinant for B10.A occurred at the amino terminus (Oki and Sercarz 1985).

In the rest of this paper, we will examine crypticity, which is due in the main part to a failure of processing and presentation. Additionally, it may allow activation of proliferative T cells without any suppressor-cell activation. Thus for most minor determinants, e.g., 30-53 and 1-17, once the mice have been peptide-primed, the responses can be recalled with the whole molecule. However, there are some determinants, e.g., 74-96, where the recall of responsiveness is very much better with the peptide (100 ×) than with the whole molecule.

Table 1. Responsiveness to Peptides in Adult B10.A Mice Tolerant to HEL

Ag[a] (priming in CFA and challenge in vitro)	Dominance status	Response[b]
HEL	−	−
1–17	minor	−
20–35	major	−
30–53	minor	+
46–61	major	−
74–96	cryptic	+

[a]HEL tolerant mice were primed with antigen or peptide and challenged with the same material in vitro. (Ag) Antigen; (CFA) complete Freund's adjuvant.

[b]The proliferative response result is shown. The minus sign means no significant proliferation.

Crypticity of a Strong MHC-binding Determinant

The determinant found within peptide 85-96 is an excellent example of a cryptic determinant that nevertheless has a high-affinity interaction with the MHC. Buus et al. (1987) tested various peptides from HEL for their binding to different restriction elements, and 85-96 fell in the strongest interaction class (4^+) with E^k. Despite this demonstrated ability to interact with E^k, and despite the ready induction of a response to the isolated peptide, *no* 85-96-specific T-cell clones appear after footpad immunization with HEL in complete Freund's adjuvant. Thus, as observed from the popliteal lymph nodes of B10.A mice, this region in HEL molecules includes a cryptic determinant for T cells (Gammon et al. 1987).

Shastri et al. (1986b) established a T-cell hybridoma specific for 87-96 of HEL (A01T.13.1). All clones recognizing this part of HEL are restricted to E^k molecules (Shastri et al. 1986c). We tested the IL-2 response of this clone in response to HEL and synthetic peptides 74-96, 81-96, and 85-96 by using the CH27 B-cell lymphoma as antigen-presenting cells (APC), which display both A^k and E^k molecules. Figure 1 shows dose response curves in the IL-2 stimulation assay. A01T.13.1 cells were not stimulated significantly by native HEL (data not shown) or peptide 74-96, but responded to peptides 81-96 and 85-96. This response was stronger to peptide 85-96 than to peptide 81-96. One explanation for the difference in response between peptides 81-96 and 85-96 is that region 81-84 hinders the binding with E^k molecules or interferes with recognition by the T-cell receptor (TCR) of A01T.13.1. Berzofsky has referred to hindering structures (Brett et al. 1988) as "hinderotopes," which are distinct from T-cell epitopes or agretopes.

However, unresponsiveness of this T-cell hybridoma to peptide 74-96 cannot solely be caused by the hindering ability of region 74-84. Shastri et al. (1986b) showed that A01T.13.1 responded to peptide 74-96 presented by CA36.1.3 cells, which are L fibroblasts transfected with $E_\alpha{}^k$ and $E_\beta{}^k$ genes, but which lack A^k molecules. Actually, peptide 74-96 consists of two cryptic determinants juxtaposed on the peptide (Shastri et al. 1986c; Gammon et al. 1987). These are 74-86 (or 74-82) restricted to A^k, and 85-96 (or 87-96) restricted to E^k (Shastri et al. 1986b; Gammon et al. 1987). The A^k-restricted A01T.2.11 T-cell hybridoma is specific for the amino-terminal region of 74-96 and was also established by Shastri et al. (1986b). This hybrid recognizes the complex derived from 74-96 and A^k on the surface of peptide-pulsed CH27 cells. Accordingly, at least a portion of peptide 74-96 must be available for presentation by CH27 cells. It is possible that binding of the agretope within 74-82 to the A^k molecule could occur in CH27 cells, making it difficult for complexes of E^k to form with the agretope within region 87-96; at least, not enough of the latter complexes would form for detection by A0T.13.1 cells. This may be termed "competitive capture." We suggest that formation of complexes of region 87-96 and E^k might similarly be missed in CH27 cells pulsed with native HEL because of the competitive capture of region 74-96 by A^k, or by other regions binding more strongly at some distance from 74-96. It remains to test L-fibroblast transfectants with both E^k and A^k expression to see whether the existence of the extra A^k restriction element now prevents the activation of T cells specific for 87-96/E^k.

The competitive capture may occur through a simple interaction between peptide 74-96 and A^k, in which the A^k-reactive agretope is more available than the E^k-reactive agretope. Capture should be favored when the molar ratio of peptide to class II molecules is low. When the peptide is in excess, any peptide 74-96 still remaining after all A^k sites are filled might then bind to E^k. Another possibility is that L-fibroblast transfectants express a relatively large amount of E^k, whereas CH27 cells do not have enough E^k. We have no direct evidence that, in fact, peptide is limiting in the in vivo experiments, but surely in vitro, no matter how high the concentration of 74-96, A01T.13.1 does not respond. It should be remembered that the actual field of interaction occurs on the surface of APC and may be complicated; it may be difficult to apply physicochemical binding characteristics within a lipid membrane directly to the interaction in the cellular system (Ceppellini et al. 1989).

A third molecule (Nairn et al. 1984; Lakey et al. 1987) has been implicated in peptide antigen presentation. If this third molecule is able to assist peptides in interacting with Ia molecules, for example, from one end of the peptide, another pathway could be imagined for selective binding of peptide 74-96 to A^k rather than E^k.

Figure 2 shows dose response curves of A^k-restricted A01T.2.11 specific for 74-86, A^k-restricted A04H.H4.3 specific for 20-35, and A^k-restricted kLy4.3, kLy7.11, and h4Ly50.5 specific for 46-61. LK35.2, a B-cell-

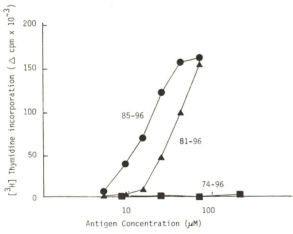

Figure 1. The response of T-cell hybridoma clone A01T.13.1 to HEL peptides 74-96, 81-96, and 85-96. CH27 cells were incubated with A01T.13.1 cells and various concentrations of the antigen peptides. [^{3}H]Thymidine incorporation of HT-2 cells was measured as an indication of the amount of IL-2 produced by the T-cell hybridoma.

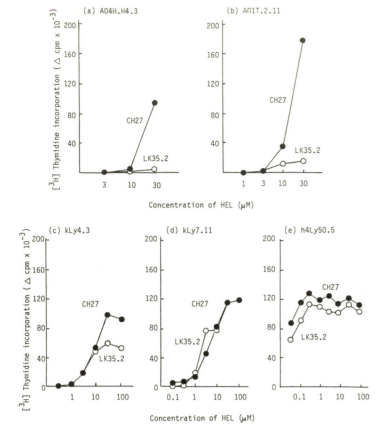

Figure 2. Comparison of the response to T-cell hybridomas A04H.H4.3, A01T.2.11, kLy4.3, kLy7.11, and h4Ly50.5. Each T-cell hybridoma clone was incubated with several concentrations of HEL, in the presence of CH27 or LK35.2 antigen-presenting cells. [^{3}H]Thymidine incorporation of HT-2 cells was measured.

lymphoma hybridoma used as an APC, displays A^k, E^k, A^d, and E^d; these cells were pulsed with HEL for presentation to the T-cell hybridomas. Examination of these curves indicates that, whereas LK35.2 functions about as well as CH27 in activating the three 46-61 hybrids, it is much worse with the 74-86- and 20-35-specific hybrids. Region 46-61 has strong binding ability to A^k and very poor binding to A^d/E^d (Buus et al. 1987). On the other hand, regions 20-35 and 74-86 can bind to A^d. Therefore, in the cases shown in Figure 2, other Ia molecules than A^k, namely A^d, may have been involved in competitive capture. Similar dose response curves to LK35.2 cells were obtained by using TA3 cells as APC (which is an H-$2^{a/d}$B cell/H-2^d B lymphoma hybridoma). This type of competitive capture may actually be quite commonplace.

The occurrence of competitive capture by Ia molecules is compatible with the model we have proposed earlier for Ia-guided processing (Sercarz et al. 1986). If processing or cleaving by proteinases were assumed to be *followed* by interaction with Ia molecules, different presentation patterns by CH27 (A^k,E^k) cells than by CA36.1.3 (only E^k) as compared to LK35.2 and TA3 cells (A^kE^k, A^dE^d) as APC could be explained by a difference in proteolysis. For example, specific cleavage within region 87-96 by proteinases present only in CH27 cells might prevent detectable formation of E^k/region 87-96 complexes.

We find it hard to imagine that individual APC from the same species have a unique set of protineases with independent specificities. More studies are needed about the various features of each APC related to antigen processing and presentation. Furthermore, more needs to be learned about in vitro and in vivo stimulation of the A01T.13.1 clone, which was originally established by immunization with peptide 74-96. The suggestions that there is heterogeneity in antigen processing by individual APC (Michalek et al. 1989) and that specific enzymes produce particular determinants (Puri and Factorovich 1988) do not necessarily indicate different cleavage points on the same antigen by unique protineases in each APC, even if different forms of antigen, such as a fragment vis-a-vis the whole native protein, could give a different pattern by proteinases. Rather, varying conditions in different APC may disclose certain antigenic cleavage sites differentially, so that the pattern of products would indeed be dissimilar in each APC, despite a similar panel of proteolytic enzymes in each.

Adjoining Dominant and Cryptic Determinants

Another example of MHC-specific crypticity is seen with peptide 116-129. Peptide 116-129 induces a strong I-A-restricted proliferative response in lymph node cells (LNC) following peptide immunization in both

H-2^k and H-2^d animals. However, the 116-129/A^k determinant is easily recalled with HEL, whereas the 116-129/A^d determinant is not. Similarly, 116-129/A^k responses can be readily demonstrated in LNC following HEL immunization of H-2^k mice, whereas 116-129/A^d responses are not elicited in H-2^d animals under identical conditions, illustrating the point that the MHC is directly implicated in crypticity.

To explore the availability of the 116-129 determinant, experiments have been conducted on the specificity of the T-cell proliferative response following immunization with the carboxy-terminal cyanogen bromide fragment of HEL (L3 = 106-129). Essentially, these experiments analyze the effect of an additional 10 amino-terminal amino acids on the elicitation of a 116-129 response. Furthermore, amino acids 108–116 constitute a dominant determinant, in the context of E^d.

Immunization of I-E^d-bearing mouse strains (BALB/c, B10.D2) with reduced, carboxymethylated-L3 results in a T-proliferative response that strongly favors the 108-120/E^d response over the 116-129/A^d response. Immunization of an I-E$^-$ mouse strain (B10.GD) results in a 116-129/A^d response, but not as strong as that following direct peptide 116-129 immunization. Immunization of A^{k}E^k mice (B10.A) with either L3 or peptide 116-129 results in equivalent proliferative responses to 116-129/A^k.

Through the addition of the amino-terminal 10 amino acids, a potent E^d determinant with its agretope is juxtaposed to the 116-129/A^d determinant, and it may not be surprising that predominant activation of T cells recognizing 108-120/E^d determinant ensues. In support, amino acids 112-116 form a basic-spacer-basic-spacer-basic (B X B X B) binding motif as defined by Sette et al. (1989). In the absence of I-E molecules, the removal of the strong competition from E^d allows a 116-129/A^d response to occur unimpeded. Whether this represents a case of competitive capture by the E^d restriction element, preventing the attached 116-129 residues from any chance of interacting with A^d, is still a moot question. The observation of lower 116-129 responses in I-E$^-$ mice following L3 immunization in comparison to direct peptide 116-129 immunization suggests that region 106-115 may also contain some hinderotope activity. Such a hinderotope could either impede peptide/MHC formation or block TCR interactions with critical triggering peptide/MHC residues, and these possibilities are currently under examination. Distinguishing hinderotopes from competing agretopes should be possible by altering crucial agretypic residues in the 10-amino-acid extension that can be shown in separate binding tests to obliterate the E^d-binding activity.

Chimeric Peptides

It has been demonstrated in the two previous examples that naturally occurring adjoining determinants affect each other. Preparation of a chimeric peptide, unnaturally juxtaposing a dominant determinant with a subdominant one, would also permit study of this type of interaction. In the myelin basic protein (MBP)/EAE system, it is known that the N-acetylated-1-9 peptide is dominant in H-2^u mice after injection of MBP, whereas 35-47 is subdominant. It is also known that the addition of nonsense amino acid residues at the carboxy-terminal side of 1-9 greatly increases the immunogenicity of the peptide. Attaching acetyl-1-9 amino-terminal to 35-47 has a most interesting effect, as illustrated in Table 2. Costimulation with 1-11 and 35-47 induces a rather small response to both peptides, clearly less than that induced to 1-11 after MBP immunization. However, the chimeric peptide induces an exceedingly strong response that is recalled very efficiently by the joined peptide, 1-11: 35-47, but not by its short components. It appears that a junctional determinant with high affinity for an H-2^u restriction element was created. This remains to be tested with minimal junctional peptides.

The natural product of processing MBP may very well be a peptide much longer than the minimal 1-9, perhaps resembling 1-20. The extra residues may stabilize the required determinant structure or enhance its interaction with the MHC with some quasi-specific binding to pockets in the cavernous site. Augmenting effects by addition of unrelated, but reactive residues has been seen with several other peptide determinants. However, in these experiments, a dominant determinant is subjugated by the addition of what is presumably a still more effective determinant. It is evident that neighboring residues can seriously affect the apparent specificity of a response. This response may be produced through the use of an independent agretope, but it is also conceivable that one of the two initial agretopes is used and the induced shape of the rest of the molecule constitutes a set of very immunogenic TCR-reactive epitopes.

In fact, the subjugated determinant on the chimeric peptide has been converted to a cryptic determinant. This result illustrates the complexity in dominance determination that may occur when potential determinants overlap. Given the rather broad specificity of Ia molecules, it seems reasonable to suppose that such overlapping determinants may often occur naturally.

Table 2. Subjugation of Dominant Determinant by Newly Created Chimeric Determinant

In vitro challenge	Immunization with[a]	
	1–11 + 35–47	1–11:35–47
	(cpm × 10^{-3})	
1–11	6.1	16.7
35–47	1.9	11.4
1–11:35–47	8.6	120.7

[a]Three mice in each group were immunized with the mixed peptides or the chimeric peptide in complete Freund's adjuvant, and their draining lymph nodes were cultured in vitro for 5 days and pulsed on the last day with [^{3}H]thymidine. The experiment shown is representative of three others.

Moreover, the potential dominance/crypticity of Ac-1-11 in MBP underlies another basic theme in our studies: Dominance and crypticity are not inherent qualities of determinants and very much relate to surrounding structures.

DISCUSSION

General Features of Crypticity

It is clear that a cryptic determinant in one haplotype is not necessarily cryptic in another: Crypticity is MHC-restricted and *not* a structural characteristic of the determinant, any more than dominance. We can attempt to categorize several reasons why potential determinants might not be expressed after immunization with a native molecule and would appear cryptic: (1) Their agretopes may never be revealed to their class II restriction element during normal processing (nondisclosure). (2) The natural end product of processing is so large that there are regions of the fragment that hide the determinant and hinder access to the MHC (agretypic hinderotope) or that (3) hinder access to the T-cell receptor on the large majority of T cells specific for the determinant (epitypic hinderotope). (4) Neighboring agretopes on the same antigenic molecule compete with the determinant in question for binding to the same restriction element (agretope competition). (5) Agretopes on other determinants have a higher affinity and availability for a *different* restriction element (determinant capture).

In this paper, we have attempted to explore the problem of dominance and crypticity by focusing on this last point of aggressive determinant capture by unrelated MHC restriction molecules. In particular, we studied three cases of physically associated determinants, restricted to different MHC elements. Such interaction between these determinants should not occur if antigen molecules were quickly processed to small 10–15-amino-acid minimal peptides before access to the class II restriction elements in the endosome.

In earlier work, we have enumerated several instances in which distant residues have an effect on the eventual outcome of a "determinant competition." Whether a particular determinant will ever be disclosed to class II molecules may very well be determined by the structure of the starting antigenic material presented to the organism (either the native molecule or some fragment or derivative of it). Because certain forms of the antigen may reveal or obscure favored residues for given proteolytic enzymes, the whole pathway of processing can differ owing to structural aspects of the immunogen. A related perspective to these effects, occurring at a distance from the site of determinant recognition, involves prediction of an early interaction between class II molecules and an unfolded, but only partially fragmented form of the antigen (Shastri et al. 1985). Attachment at an early point to class II would serve to protect the determinant in question and seriously influence the subsequent processing of the molecule in still unknown directions.

This type of view would predict that when known determinants adjoin each other on a long peptide, some competitive or hindering effect will be observed. In this rather preliminary experimental presentation, we have begun to examine such situations. In the three examples shown here, we have particularly chosen to study cases in which the two apposed determinants are restricted to *different* restriction elements, so that ordinarily there would be little reason for competition between the peptides for binding to class II. This approach should be able to dissociate competitive capture from hinderotope effects. In capture models, in the presence of limiting antigen concentrations as is presumed to occur in vivo, binding by one type of class II restriction element of the long peptide could preempt any binding by the other restriction element.

Alternatively, the long peptide bearing the two determinants can be considered a single determinant with a hindering (or enhancing) tail protruding in one direction or the other. As was pointed out above in the example of the amino-terminal peptide from MBP, an extension with 10 irrelevant amino acids in the carboxy direction greatly improved binding, as well as stimulation of responsiveness for clones directed to the 1–9 peptide. Entry into, or interaction with the cavernous, tortuous site on the floor of the MHC groove may be readily influenced by the addition or subtraction of small numbers of amino acids. However, if it is true that the MHC binds unfolded, but only partially fragmented molecules, it may not be all that difficult to make an initial contact with the binding site. Evidence from McConnell's laboratory (H.M. McConnell, pers. comm.) is consistent with the idea that the class II site may be slightly open and floppy at the outset, perhaps providing easier access for larger molecules. After the initial binding, readjustment within the site may lead to firm attachment of the optimal agretope. In such cases as the MBP chimeric peptide, it is conceivable that a multiplicity of agretopes within a defined region might enhance the overall antigenicity of a peptide. Advantage might be taken of this possibility by designing vaccine peptides with overlapping agretopes: The winning agretope would differ in each haplotype, but individuals with different haplotypes could each be effectively immunized with the same peptide preparation.

ACKNOWLEDGMENTS

This work was supported in part by National Institutes of Health grants CA-24442 and AI-11183, American Cancer Society grant IM-466, and a grant from the Multiple Sclerosis Society. A.A. is a Cancer Research Institute fellow; R.A. is supported by Tumor Immunology training grant CA-09120. Hybridomas kLy4.3, kLy7.11, and h4Ly50.5 were kindly provided by Dr. John Freed, National Jewish Hospital, Denver, Colorado; and hybridomas A01T.2.11 and A01T.13.1 were a gift from Dr. Nilabh Shastri, University of California, Berkeley, California. We thank Iris Sheldon for preparation of the manuscript, and Elaine Pickett and Denise Edger for technical assistance.

REFERENCES

Adorini, L., E. Appella, G. Doria, and Z.A. Nagy. 1988. Mechanisms influencing the immunodominance of T cell determinants. *J. Exp. Med.* **168:** 2091.

Apple, R., J. Clarke, J. Cogswell, G. Gammon, M.E. Katz, U. Krzych, R. Maizels, F. Manca, A. Miller, S. Nasseri, A. Oki, S. Wilbur, and E. Sercarz. 1989. The causes and consequences of immunodominance at the T cell level. In *The immune response to structurally defined proteins: The lysozyme model* (ed. S. Smith-Gill and E. Sercarz), p. 267. Adenine Press, New York.

Brett, S.J., K.B. Cease, and J.A. Berzofsky. 1988. Influences of antigen processing on the expression of T cell repertoire: Evidence for MHC-specific hindering structures on the products of processing. *J. Exp. Med.* **168:** 357.

Buus, S., A. Sette, S.M. Colon, C. Miles, and H.M. Grey. 1987. The relation between major histocompatibility complex (MHC) restriction and the capacity of Ia to bind immunogenic peptides. *Science* **235:** 1353.

Ceppellini, R., G. Frumento, G.B. Ferrara, R. Tosi, A. Chersi, and B. Pernis. 1989. Binding of labelled influenza matrix peptide to HLA DR in living B lymphoid cells. *Nature* **339:** 392.

Gammon, G. and E. Sercarz. 1989. How some T cells escape tolerance induction. *Nature* (in press).

Gammon, G., A. Oki, N. Shastri, and E.E. Sercarz. 1986a. Induction of tolerance to one determinant on a synthetic peptide does not affect the response to a second linked determinant. *J. Exp. Med.* **164:** 667.

Gammon, G., K. Dunn, N. Shastri, A. Oki, S. Wilbur, and E.E. Sercarz. 1986b. Neonatal T cell tolerance to minimal immunogenic peptides is caused by clonal inactivation. *Nature* **319:** 413.

Gammon, G., N. Shastri, J. Cogswell, S. Wilbur, S. Sadegh-Nasseri, U. Krzych, A. Miller, and E.E. Sercarz. 1987. The choice of T-cell epitopes utilized on a protein antigen depends on multiple factors distant from, as well as at the determinant site. *Immunol. Rev.* **98:** 53.

Groves, E.S. and A. Singer. 1983. Role of the H-2 complex in the induction of T cell tolerance to self minor histocompatibility antigens. *J. Exp. Med.* **158:** 1483.

Guillet, J.-G., M.-Z. Lai, T.J. Briner, S. Buus, A. Sette, H.M. Grey, J.A. Smith, and M.L. Gefter. 1987. Immunological self, nonself discrimination. *Science* **235:** 865.

Lakey, E.K., E. Margoliash, and S.K. Pierce. 1987. Identification of a peptide binding protein which plays a role in antigen presentation. *Proc. Natl. Acad. Sci.* **84:** 1659.

Michalek, M.T., B. Benacerraf, and K.L. Rock. 1989. Two genetically identical antigen-presenting cell clones display heterogeneity in antigen processing. *Proc. Natl. Acad. Sci.* **86:** 3316.

Nairn, R., M.L. Spengler, M.D. Hoffman, M.J. Solvay, and D.W. Thomas. 1984. Macrophage processing of peptide antigens: Identification of an antigenic complex. *J. Immunol.* **133:** 3225.

Oki, A. and E.E. Sercarz. 1985. T cell tolerance studied at the level of antigenic determinants. 1. Latent reactivity to lysozyme peptides that lack suppressogenic epitopes can be revealed in lysozyme tolerant mice. *J. Exp. Med.* **161:** 897.

Puri, J. and Y. Factorovich. 1988. Selective inhibition of antigen presentation to cloned T cells by protease inhibitors. *J. Immunol.* **141:** 3313.

Rammensee, H.G. and M.J. Bevan. 1984. Evidence from in vitro studies that tolerance to self-antigens is MHC restricted. *Nature* **308:** 741.

Sercarz, E., ed. 1989. The architectonics of immune dominance: The aleatory effects of molecular position on the choice of antigenic determinants. In *Chemical immunology,* vol. 46: *Antigenic determinants and immune regulation.* Karger, Basel. (In press.)

Sercarz, E., S. Wilbur, S. Sadegh-Nasseri, A. Miller, F. Manca, G. Gammon, and N. Shastri. 1986. The molecular context of a determinant influences its dominant expression in a T cell response hierarchy through "fine processing." In *Progress in immunology* (ed. B. Cinader and R.G. Miller), vol. 4, p. 227. Academic Press, Orlando, Florida.

Sette, A., S. Buus, E. Appella, J.A. Smith, R. Chesnut, C. Miles, S.M. Colon, and H.M. Grey. 1989. Prediction of major histocompatibility complex binding regions of protein antigens by sequence pattern analysis. *Proc. Natl. Acad. Sci.* **86:** 3296.

Shastri, N., A. Miller, and E.E. Sercarz. 1985. The expressed T cell repertoire is hierarchical: The precise focus of lysozyme-specific T cell clones is dependent upon the structure of the immunogen. *J. Mol. Cell. Immunol.* **1:** 369.

———. 1986a. Amino acid residues distinct from the determinant region can profoundly affect activation of T cell clones by related antigens. *J. Immunol.* **136:** 371.

Shastri, N., J. Kobori, D. Munt, and L. Hood. 1986b. Diversity of T-cell receptor structures specific for minimal peptide/Ia determinants: Implications for immune response gene defects. In *Regulation of immune gene expression* (ed. M. Teldmann and A. McMichael), p. 167. Humana Press, Clifton, New Jersey.

Shastri, N., G. Gammon, S. Horvath, A. Miller, and E.E. Sercarz. 1986c. The choice between two distinct T cell determinants within a 23 amino acid region of lysozyme depends upon structure of the immunogen. *J. Immunol.* **137:** 911.

Expression and Function of Human Major Histocompatibility Complex HLA-DQw6 Genes in the C57BL/6 Mouse

T. SASAZUKI,* T. IWANAGA,* T. INAMITSU,* Y. YANAGAWA,* M. YASUNAMI,*
A. KIMURA,* K. HIROKAWA,† AND Y. NISHIMURA*
*Department of Genetics, Medical Institute of Bioregulation, Kyushu University, Fukuoka 812;
†Department of Pathology, Tokyo Metropolitan Institute of Gerontology, Tokyo 173, Japan

Both human and murine major histocompatibility complex class II molecules control immune responses and susceptibility to disease (Ballet et al. 1983; Sasazuki et al. 1983; Schwarts 1984; Todd et al. 1988). HLA class II molecules are heterodimers of α and β chains, and HLA class II genes on a haploid encode at least one or two DR molecules, one DQ molecule, and one DP molecule (Todd et al. 1988). Among these HLA class II molecules, DR molecules act as major restriction molecules in antigen presentation and major stimulatory molecules in allogeneic mixed lymphocyte reaction (MLR) (Nishimura and Sasazuki 1983; Sone et al. 1985; Hirayama et al. 1986, 1987). On the other hand, little is known of the biological function of DQ and DP molecules. The murine DQ counterpart (Auffray et al. 1984; Long et al. 1984), I-A molecules, function as immune response (Ir) gene products and potently stimulate MLR (Schwarts 1984). An antigen-specific and DQ-restricted human T-cell clone was reported to have the ability of the DQ molecule to present antigen (Lamb and Feldman 1984).

Characteristic features of DQ molecules are as follows: (1) Both α and β chains are polymorphic and are homologous to murine I-A molecules (Auffray et al. 1984; Long et al. 1984); (2) the expression of DQ molecules is much less than that of DR molecules in B cells and monocytes (K. Fujisawa et al., in prep.); (3) most DQ β chains, except those from HLA-Dw9, Dw 12, and DB7 haplotypes, do not utilize exon 5 encoding cytoplasmic 8 amino acids due to the one-base substitution at the intron/exon junction right before exon 5 (Tsukamoto et al. 1987). We reported that HLA-linked immune suppression (Is) genes control antigen-specific low responsiveness as a dominant genetic trait (Sasazuki et al. 1978, 1980a,b; Nishimura and Sasazuki 1983). Because Is genes are in strong linkage disequilibrium with DQ alleles and because anti-DQ monoclonal antibodies (MAbs) can restore the strong immune response in low responders (Hirayama et al. 1987), we have directed much attention to the biological function of DQ molecules. We describe here the generation of a stable line of HLA-DQw6 transgenic C57BL/6 (DQw6-B6) mice to be used to elucidate the biological function of DQ molecules.

EXPERIMENTAL PROCEDURES

Transgenic mice. The HLA-DQw6A gene was isolated from a genomic DNA library constructed from an Epstein-Barr virus (EBV)-transformed B-lymphoblastoid cell line, EB-TOK, homozygous for HLA-DR2-DQw6-Dw12 haplotype, using λ charon 4A as a cloning vehicle. The isolated DQw6A gene was subcloned into pTZ19R at the EcoRI site and used for injection as a 13-kb EcoRI fragment. Isolation of the DQw6B gene was carried out as described previously (Tsukamoto et al. 1987). An 18-kb EcoRI fragment of the DQw6B gene from λDQβ Dw12 was connected to an EcoRI-PstI fragment containing a part of exon 6 and 3′ untranslated region from a cDNA clone (pDQβ101) to construct an intact DQw6B gene subcloned into pTZ 19R. pDQw6B DNA was linearized by partial digestion with EcoRI and used for injection. The DQw6A gene contained 0.8 kb of the 5′-flanking region and about 6 kb of the 3′-flanking region. The DQw6B gene contained 10 kb of the 5′-flanking region (Fig. 1a). A mixture of DQw6A and DQw6B DNA was injected into 40 fertilized eggs from C57BL/6 mice. Four neonate pups were obtained, and tail DNA from these mice was analyzed. One mouse harbored both DQw6A and DQw6B genes. The existence of DQw6 transgenes in the DQw6-B6 mice was investigated by Southern blot analyses, using pDQα107 and pDQβ101 as probes, as described by Maniatis et al. (1982).

S1 mapping. Various tissues were obtained from a DQw6-B6 mouse and total RNA was isolated by CsCl density gradient. Total RNAs (10 μg) from various tissues as well as from B6 spleen cells and 1 μg of total RNAs from EBV-transformed B-lymphoblastoid cell lines were analyzed by nuclease-S1 protection analysis, as described previously (Kimura et al. 1986). SacI-SacI fragment (720 bp) of pDQα107 and BamHI-EcoRI fragment (850 bp) of pDQβ101 were cloned into mp18 and mp19, respectively, and labeled homogeneously with ^{32}P as the probe, using [α-^{32}P]dCTP.

Immunohistology and flow cytometry. Tissue specificity of the expression of DQw6 molecules was investigated by the immunohistochemical method, using

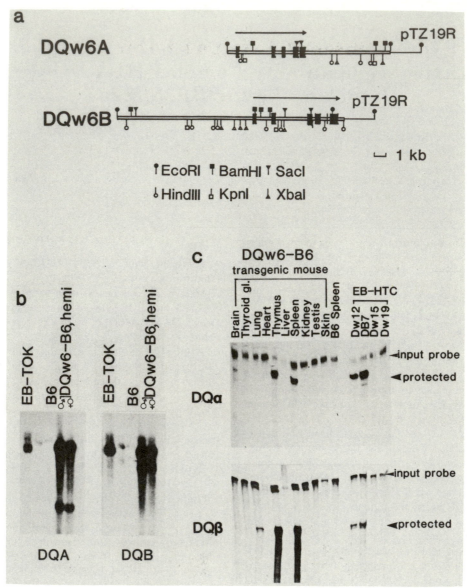

Figure 1. Restriction map and expression of HLA-DQw6A and DQw6B genes introduced into a HLA-DQw6 transgenic B6 mouse. (*a*) Restriction map of DQw6A (DQA1*0103) gene and DQw6B (DQB1*0104) gene introduced into a B6 mouse. (*b*) Southern blot analysis of tail DNA digested with *Bam*HI from the HLA-DQw6 transgenic mouse. (*c*) Nuclease-S1 analysis of DQw6A and DQw6B mRNA in the HLA-DQw6 transgenic mouse and EBV-transformed human B-lymphoblastoid cell lines established from HLA-D homozygous typing cells (EB-HTC). HLA-Dw12 and DB7 are positive for DQw6 genes.

frozen tissue sections, biotinylated anti-DQ MAb, HU-11[1] (Kasahara et al. 1983), and peroxidase-conjugated avidin. Immune-competent cells were stained directly with monoclonal antibodies conjugated with either fluorescein isothiocyanate (FITC) or phycoerythrin (PE), as described elsewhere (K. Fujisawa et al., in prep.). In some cases, cells were stained with biotinylated monoclonal antibodies followed by binding with avidin conjugated with either FITC or PE. Cells were then analyzed using a fluorescence-activated cell sorter (FACS).

Immunoprecipitation and two-dimensional polyacrylamide gel electrophoresis. Spleen cells from control B6 mice or transgenic DQw6-B6 mice were metabolically labeled by incubation in methionine-free RPMI 1640 medium containing 10% dialyzed fetal calf serum and 1 mCi of L-[35S]methionine (Amersham) for 6 hours and then were lysed with extraction buffer (10 mM Tris-HCl [pH 7.2], 0.15 M NaCl, 0.02% NaN_3, 0.5% Nonidet P-40). Radiolabeled cell lysates were precleared with formalin-fixed *Staphylococcus aureus* Cowan Strain 1 (SaC, Calbiochem) and purified anti-I-$A^b\beta$ MAb, 25-9-17, or the ascites containing the anti-HLA-DQ MAb, HU-11, was added, and immunoprecipitation was carried out with SaC. The precipitates

---

[1]HU-11 reacts to HLA-DQw4, DQw5, and DQw6 molecules.

were analyzed by two-dimensional polyacrylamide gel electrophoresis (PAGE), as described previously (Sone et al. 1985), in which nonequilibrium pH gradient electrofocusing was applied in the first dimension, followed by SDS-PAGE in the second dimension, then the precipitates were autoradiographed.

Analyses of immunological tolerance to the DQw6 molecules. Tolerance to DQw6 molecules in the DQw6-B6 mice was investigated in MLR and in antibody production directed against the DQw6 molecule. Lymph node cells (5×10^5) were cocultivated with mitomycin-c-treated spleen cells (5×10^5) for 4 days, and MLR was quantitated by measuring the incorporation of [^{3}H]thymidine into T lymphoblasts, as described previously (Sone et al. 1985). DQw6-B6 mice were crossed with C3H mice to obtain DQw6-positive F_1 (DQw6-B/C F_1) and DQw6 negative F_1 (B/C F_1), and then immunized intraperitoneally three times at 2-week intervals with the human cell line EB-TOK (10^7), homozygous for HLA-DR2-DQw6-Dw12. Antisera were obtained 2 weeks after the last immunization and were absorbed with the L cells. Subsequently, anti-DQw6 or anti-DR2 antibodies in these antisera were detected by indirect immunofluorescence staining of L cells, L-cell transfectants expressing DQw6 genes, or DR2 genes derived from EB-TOK. These target cells were treated with FITC-conjugated Fab′2 fragment of goat anti-mouse IgG + M (TAGO) as a negative control.

T-cell proliferation assays. DQw6-B6, B6, and C3H mice (8–12 weeks old) were immunized by giving 0.2 ml of soluble antigens (10–50 μg) emulsified with complete Freund's adjuvant in the hind foot pads and base of the tail. Popliteal, inguinal, and paraaortic lymph nodes were removed 7–12 days later, and a single-cell suspension was prepared by pressing lymph nodes between slide glasses. Cells were suspended in RPMI-1640 medium (GIBCO) supplemented with 10% heat-inactivated horse serum, 100 units/ml penicillin, 100 μg/ml streptomycin, 2 mM L-glutamine, 50 μM 2-mercaptoethanol, and 20 mM HEPES. The lymph node cells (5×10^5) were then cultivated in 0.2 ml of complete medium, with or without soluble antigens (20–100 μg/ml) or lectins (1–5 μg/ml). Culture was set up in triplicate in 96-well flat-bottom tissue culture plates (Falcon) at 37°C in a humidified atmosphere of 5% CO_2 and 95% air. Proliferative responses of T cells were assessed by the incorporation of [^{3}H]thymidine during a 24-hour pulse following an 84-hour incubation for soluble antigens and during a 12-hour pulse following a 48-hour incubation for lectins. In blocking experiments on the immune response with monoclonal antibodies, 1000-fold diluted ascites form of anti-HLA-DQ MAb, HU-11, or 8-fold diluted culture supernate containing anti-I-A$^b\alpha$,3JP (Janeway et al. 1984), or 6 μg/ml purified anti-I-A$^b\beta$ MAb, 25-9-17 (Ozato and Sachs 1981), or a 20-fold diluted culture supernate containing anti-CD4 (L3T4) MAb, GK1.5 (Dialynas et al. 1983), was added to the culture.

Antigen-specific T-cell line. A T-cell line specific to the streptococcal cell wall antigen (SCW) was established from lymph node cells of the DQw6-B6 mice preimmunized with SCW (20 μg), as described previously by other investigators (Kimoto and Fathman 1980). In brief, lymph node cells (5×10^6/ml) were stimulated with SCW (20 μg/ml) for 5–7 days, and T lymphoblasts were collected by density gradient centrifugation with Ficoll-Conray. T lymphoblasts (1×10^5/ml) were cultivated with irradiated (30 Gy from a cesium source) DQw6-B6 spleen cells (2×10^6/ml) for 14 days. Viable T cells (1×10^5/ml) were collected and stimulated with SCW (20 μg/ml) in the presence of irradiated DQw6-B6 spleen cells (2×10^6/ml) for 7 days. This cycle of stimulation and resting culture was repeated four or five times to establish a T-cell line specific to SCW. A T-cell line (5×10^4) was cocultivated with SCW (50 μg/ml) and mitomycin-c-treated murine L cells (3×10^4) transfected with both DQw6A and B genes for 72 hours; the proliferative response of the T-cell line was measured as described above.

RESULTS

Expression of the HLA-DQw6 Transgenes in DQw6-B6 Mice

A stable line of the HLA-DQw6 transgenic mouse (DQw6-B6) was established, and the DQw6-B6 mouse was integrated with 3–5 copies of DQw6 A and B genes linked together tandemly (Fig. 1b). Genetic analysis of the F_1 mice between the HLA-DQw6 transgenic founder mouse and B6 mouse revealed a 1 to 1 segregation ratio of the HLA-DQw6 genes. Analysis of F_1 and backcross progeny, using the transgenic and NOD mice, revealed that the HLA-DQw6 transgenes were not linked to the H-2 complex. Thereafter, DQw6-B6 mice hemizygous for DQw6 and their transgene-negative littermates were used for study.

Expression of DQw6 genes was first investigated at the mRNA level. Because DQw6 A and B cDNA probes cross-hybridized I-A$^b\alpha$ and β mRNA, respectively, and because sizes of the mature DQw6 A and B mRNA were similar to those of mature I-A$^b\alpha$ and β mRNA, respectively, the exonuclease-S1 protection assay was used. With this method, the 720-bp and 850-bp protected bands corresponding to DQw6 A and B mRNAs, respectively, were observed. As shown in Figure 1c, DQw6 mRNA was expressed in the thymus and spleen, and a trace amount of mRNA was expressed in brain and lungs; the liver, heart, kidneys, and all other tissues tested showed no evidence of DQw6 mRNA.

The tissue distribution of DQw6 molecules examined immunohistologically was exactly the same as that of I-A^b molecules; DQw6 molecules were expressed on both the cortex and medulla of the thymus, and in lymph nodes, spleen, bone marrow, skin, and lungs; they were negative in liver, kidneys, muscle, and uterus. Expression of DQw6 molecules in immune-competent cells was investigated, following immuno-fluorescence staining and analyses made using FACS. As shown in Figure 2a, DQw6-positive cells were included in the I-A^b-positive cells in the spleen, and about 30–40% of the I-A^b-positive cells were positive for DQw6. The majority of DQw6-positive spleen cells were positive for surface immunoglobulin M, and a small population of DQw6-positive cells were positive for CD11b (Mac-1), thereby indicating that both B cells and macrophages express DQw6 molecules (data not shown). Little or no expression of DQw6 was observed in activated lymph node T cells cultured with 5 μg/ml concanavalin A for 4 days (Fig. 2b). On the other hand, expression of DQw6 in spleen cells was markedly induced by cultivation of the cells with 50 units/ml murine recombinant interleukin-4 (rIL-4) for 24 hours (Fig. 2c).

As shown in Figure 3, anti-DQ MAb, HU-11, precipitated a pair of DQw6 α and β chains from spleen cells of a DQw6-B6 mouse, but not from B6 spleen cells. On the other hand, anti-I-A^bβ MAb, 25-9-17, precipitated a pair of I-A^b α and β chains from spleen cells of both DQw6-B6 and B6 mice. The charge of the DQw6 α chain was more basic than that of the I-A^bα chain, and the charge of the DQw6β chain was more acidic than that of I-A^b β chain, hence, we could readily differentiate the DQw6 from the I-A^b molecules on the two-dimensional PAGE profile. The two-dimensional PAGE profile of DQw6 molecules from DQw6-B6 was much the same as that from EB-TOK, homozygous for HLA-DR2-Dw12-DQw6 (Sone et al. 1985) (data not shown). There was no difference in the amount and profile of I-A^b molecules between the DQw6-B6 mouse

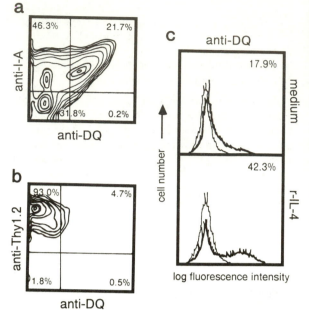

Figure 2. Cytofluorometric analyses of DQw6 molecules in the HLA-DQw6 transgenic mouse, DQw6-B6. Monoclonal antibodies used were HU-11, 040-10 (Meiji) or anti-mouse Thy 1.2 (Becton Dickinson) directed against HLA-DQ, I-A or Thy 1.2, respectively. The percentages of cells stained positively are indicated. (*a*) Expression of DQw6 and I-A^b molecules on spleen cells of the DQw6-B6 mouse. In panels *a* and *b*, log fluorescence intensity of PE and FITC are plotted on the x and y axis, respectively, and the lines separate the positive and negative staining defined by a control staining. (*b*) Little or no expression of DQw6 molecules on Thy 1.2-positive T cells activated by concanavalin A in the DQw6-B6 mouse. (*c*) Augmentation of DQw6 expression by a rIL-4 in the DQw6-B6 spleen cells. Thin line indicates a negative control.

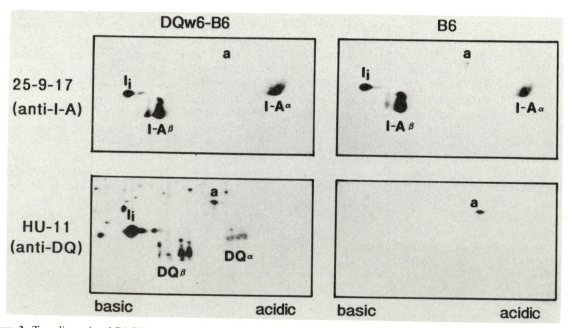

Figure 3. Two-dimensional PAGE analysis of HLA-DQw6 and I-A^b molecules expressed in the DQw6-B6 spleen cells. I_i and *a* indicate the invariant chain and actin, respectively.

and the B6 mouse. In our two-dimensional PAGE analysis, we found no evidence for xenogenic mixed class II molecules between DQw6 and I-A^b molecules.

Acquisition of Tolerance to DQw6 Molecules in the DQw6-B6 Mice

As shown in Figure 4a, lymph node cells of the B6 mice exhibited a significant MLR to DQw6-B6 spleen cells, even though the magnitude of the MLR was smaller than that of the allogeneic C3H spleen cells. On the other hand, lymph node cells from the DQw6-B6 mice did not respond to spleen cells of DQw6-positive littermates but did respond to the spleen cells of C3H mice, as did the B6 mice. With EB-TOK immunization, both DQw6-B/C F$_1$ and B/C F$_1$ strains produced an anti-DR2 antibody. The B/C F$_1$ mouse also produced an anti-DQw6 antibody, but the DQw6-B/C F$_1$ mouse did not (Fig. 4b). These observations are interpreted to mean that the DQw6-B6 mouse acquired an immunological tolerance to DQw6 molecules.

Acquisition of Immune Responsiveness to SCW in the DQw6-B6 Mice

FACS analysis of cells stained with fluorescence-conjugated antibodies showed no significant differences in the proportion of immunoglobulin-M-positive B cells, CD4$^+$CD8$^-$ T cells, CD4$^-$CD8$^+$ T cells, CD4 CD8 double-positive or CD4 CD8 double-negative T cells in thymus, lymph nodes, and spleen between DQw6-B6 and B6 mice (data not shown).

There were no differences in response to lectins such as concanavalin A, phytohemagglutinin, and pokeweed mitogen. Both B6 and DQw6-B6 mice were low responders to synthetic terpolymer L-glutamic acid:L-lysine:L-tyrosine (1:1:1), chicken egg white lysozyme, and bovine insulin; and high responders to keyhole limpet hemocyanin (KLH) or synthetic terpolymer L-glutamic acid:L-tyrosine:L-alanine (1:1:1) (GTA) (data not shown). The B6 mouse was a low responder to SCW, but the DQw6-B6 mouse acquired a high responsiveness to SCW (Fig. 5a). This difference in immune responsiveness to SCW between B6 and DQw6-B6 mice was highly reproducible in 14 mice of each strain. Dose response of the immune response to SCW (1.7–135 μg/ml) in vitro confirmed the difference in the immune response to SCW between these two strains of mice, and even in the presence of a large amount (135 μg/ml) of SCW, the B6 mouse remained a low responder (Fig. 5b). Kinetic study of the immune response to SCW (25 μg/ml) in vitro confirmed the low responsiveness of the B6 mouse during the day 2 to day 7 culture period, whereas the peak response was observed on day 4 in the DQw6-B6 mouse (Fig. 5c).

To identify the critical cell-surface molecules involved in the immune response to SCW, blocking experiments of the proliferative response of T cells with monoclonal antibodies were performed (Fig. 6a). Anti-DQ MAb, HU-11, and anti-murine CD4 MAb, GK1.5, completely inhibited the immune response of the DQw6-B6 mouse to SCW. Unexpectedly, both anti-I-A^bα MAb, 3JP, and anti-I-A^bβ MAb, 25-9-17, also completely inhibited the immune response. Inhibitory effects of the anti-class-II monoclonal antibodies were specific because HU-11 did not inhibit the proliferative response of T cells from DQw6-B6 to GTA, which was restricted by I-A^b molecules in the transgenic mouse and because both anti-I-A^b α and β MAbs, as well as HU-11, had no apparent effects on the proliferative response to KLH of T cells from the C3H mouse of the unrelated H-2^k haplotype (data not shown). Both anti-I-A^b MAbs and anti-DQ MAb, HU-11, used in this study showed no cross-reactivity to DQw6 or I-A^b molecules, respectively, in the immunofluorescence staining of B6 spleen cells or L-cell transfectants expressing DQw6 genes (data not shown). The lack of cross-reactivity of HU-11 or 25-9-17 to I-A^b or DQw6 molecules, respectively, was confirmed by two-dimensional PAGE analysis, as described above. Therefore, the inhibitory effect of anti-I-A monoclonal antibodies on the proliferative response to SCW of DQw6-B6 T cells is apparently not due to the binding of monoclonal antibodies to DQw6 molecules on the antigen-presenting cells. It was thus concluded that DQw6, I-A^b, and CD4 molecules were directly involved in the activation

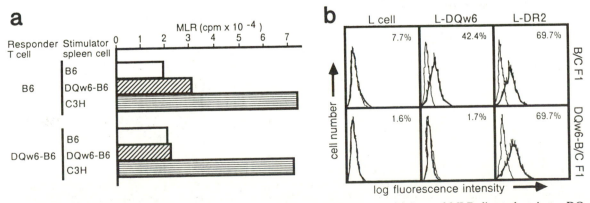

Figure 4. Acquisition of tolerance to a DQw6 molecule in the DQw6-B6 mouse. (a) Loss of MLR directed against a DQw6 molecule in the DQw6-B6 mice. (b) No production of antibodies specific to a DQw6 molecule in the HLA-DQw6 transgenic mice.

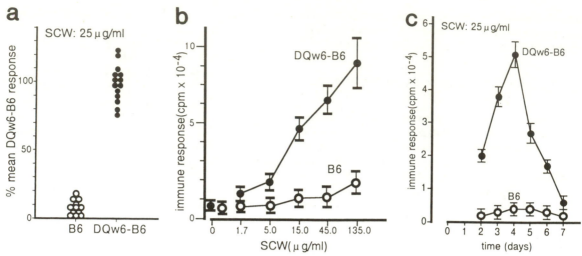

Figure 5. Acquisition of immune responsiveness to SCW in the DQw6-B6 mice. (*a*) Difference in immune responsiveness to SCW between fourteen B6 and DQw6-B6 mice. The data are a summary of five independent experiments. The immune response was expressed by percentage of the proliferative response of an individual mouse to the mean response of two or three mice, in each experiment. (*b*) Dose response of proliferative response of T cells to SCW in B6 and DQw6-B6 mice. (*c*) Kinetic study of the proliferative response of T cells to SCW in B6 and DQw6-B6 mice.

of T cells specific to SCW in DQw6-B6. A T-cell line specific to SCW and established from lymph node cells of the DQw6-B6 mice responded to SCW in the presence of murine L cells expressing DQw6A and B genes (Fig. 6b). This observation strongly suggests that the T-cell receptor of the T-cell line recognizes specifically, at least in part, SCW in the context of DQw6 molecules.

DISCUSSION

In an attempt to obtain direct evidence for the critical role of the HLA class II molecules in the regulation of the immune response, genomic genes for α and β chains of HLA-DQw6 from HLA-Dw12 haplotype were introduced into the C57BL/6(B6) strain of

mouse, and a line of HLA-DQw6 transgenic mouse was obtained. Tissue specificity of the expression of the DQw6 transgenes was exactly the same as that of I-A^b genes, and the expression of DQw6 genes was augmented by murine IL-4. Therefore, the flanking regions of the DQw6 transgenes contain promoter regions that control the tissue-specific expression and responsiveness to IL-4 of DQ genes. Murine *trans*-acting factors can interact with the promoter regions of DQw6 transgenes, thereby indicating that these factors may be highly conserved between human and mouse.

In terms of the consensus sequences in the promoter regions of human and murine class II genes, the DQA gene has a base substitution at the Y box of the 5'-flanking region, and the binding of nuclear protein to the Y box of DQA gene was markedly reduced, as

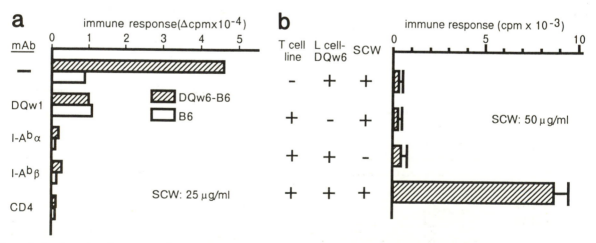

Figure 6. Involvement of DQw6, I-A^b, and CD4 molecules in the immune response to SCW of the DQw6-B6 mice. (*a*) Inhibition of the proliferative response of T cells to SCW by anti-DQ, anti-I-A^b, or anti-CD4 monoclonal antibodies in the DQw6-B6 mice. (*b*) Recognition of SCW in the context of the DQw6 molecule expressed on the murine L cell by a T-cell line established from the DQw6-B6 mice.

compared with those of other class II genes (A. Kimura et al., unpubl.). This may account for poor expression of DQ molecules in both human and DQw6-B6 non-T cells.

In humans, class II molecules, including the DQ molecule, are expressed on activated T cells (Evans et al. 1978; Charron et al. 1980), whereas the expression of class II molecules on murine activated T cells is controversial (Nagy et al. 1976; Elliott et al. 1980). FACS analysis revealed little or no expression of DQw6 molecules on the DQw6-B6 splenic T cells activated with concanavalin A. This phenomenon may be explained as follows. (1) The B6 mice do not produce, or the DQw6 transgene cannot accept, murine *trans*-acting factors inducing the expression of class II genes in the activated T cells. (2) The B6 mice produce *trans*-acting factors that inhibit the expression of class II genes in activated T cells, and the DQw6 transgenes can accept them. (3) The DQw6 transgenes have a deletion of the promoter region that controls the expression of class II genes in the activated T cells.

In recent reports (Hengartner et al. 1988; Kisielow et al. 1988; Marrack et al. 1988), it was suggested that tolerance to self major histocompatibility antigens expressed on bone-marrow-derived cells was acquired during ontogeny of the T cells in the thymus. The DQw6-B6 mice expressed DQw6 molecules in both the thymic cortex and medulla, and the transgenic mice acquired tolerance to the DQw6 molecule, at least at the T-cell level. The loss of MLR was directed against the DQw6 molecule in the DQw6-B6 mice. The DQw6-B6 mice did not produce antibodies directed against the DQw6 molecule, but it remains unclear whether the B cells also acquired tolerance to the DQ molecules.

In humans, the majority of proliferative T cells specific to SCW were restricted by HLA-DR molecules in high responders (Sone et al. 1985; Hirayama et al. 1986). We asked whether the DQ molecules were defective class II molecules that will not allow the development of DQ-restricted T cells or that cannot present SCW to T cells. Our DQw6-B6 mice contributed to the elucidation of this question. We conclude that the DQw6 molecule binds processed SCW and presents it to T cells that specifically recognize SCW in the context of the DQw6 molecules. Our interpretation for the complete blocking of the immune response to SCW by anti-I-A^b MAbs is as follows. In the DQw6-B6 strain, the majority of the SCW-specific T cells recognized SCW in the context of DQw6 molecules. On the other hand, the majority of murine CD4 (L3T4) molecules expressed on DQw6-B6 T cells may interact with I-A^b molecules on antigen-presenting cells (Fig. 7) to give a tighter interaction between SCW-specific T cells and antigen-presenting cells (Doyle and Strominger 1987; Gay et al. 1987; Sleckman et al. 1987) because of the low expression of DQw6 molecules on antigen-presenting cells or because of the low affinity to murine CD4 molecules to human DQw6 molecules, as suggested by the latter authors.

At this stage, we cannot clearly define the mecha-

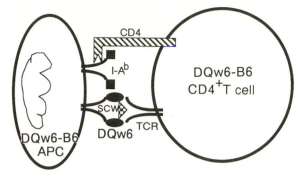

Figure 7. Scheme for the interaction of CD4$^+$ T cells and antigen-presenting cells in immune response to SCW of the DQw6-B6 mice.

nisms involved in the development of T cells specific to DQw6 plus SCW, the positive selection of thymocytes (Sha et al. 1988, Scott et al. 1989) by I-A^b molecules or DQw6 molecules in the thymic cortex. We are now generating bone marrow chimera between B6 and DQw6-B6 mice to answer this question. It will also be important to investigate the reactivity of SCW-specific T-cell hybridomas restricted by the DQw6 molecule to thymic cortical epithelium of the B6 or DQw6-B6 strains.

The HLA-DQw6 transgenic mouse can thus serve as an excellent tool for investigating the function of DQ molecules in regulation of the immune response and disease susceptibility.

ACKNOWLEDGMENTS

We thank Ronald N. Germain of the National Institutes of Health and Masao Kimoto of Saga University, Japan, for critical advice and for monoclonal antibodies; Akemi Wakisaka of Hokkaido University, Japan, for the gift of a monoclonal antibody; Kenichi Yamamura of Kumamoto University and Toshio Sone of Meiji Biomedical Research Center, Japan, for instruction on the techniques; Kazuaki Hama of Ono Pharmaceutical Co. Ltd., Japan, for murine recombinant interleukin 4; Hiroshi Egawa of Creative Research Community, Japan, for FACS analysis; and M. Ohara for helpful comments. This work was supported in part by grants 63440028 from the Ministry of Education, Science and Culture, the Science and Technology Agency, and the Ministry of Health and Welfare, Japan.

REFERENCES

Auffray, C., J.W. Lillie, D. Arnot, D. Grossberger, D. Kappes, and J.L. Strominger. 1984. Isotypic and allotypic variation of human class II histocompatibility antigen α-chain genes. *Nature* **308:** 327.

Ballet, J.J., C. Rabian-Herzog, M. Lathrop, J.F. Bourge, M. Agrapart, J. Drouet, J.M. Lalouel, and J. Dausset. 1983. Specific immune responses after booster immunization with tetanus toxoid in man. *Immunogenetics* **18:** 343.

Charron, D.J., E.G. Engleman, C.J. Benike, and H.O. McDevitt. 1980. Ia antigens on alloreactive T cells in man detected by monoclonal antibodies. *J. Exp. Med.* **152:** 127s.

Dialynas, D.P., D.B. Wilde, P. Marrack, K.A. Wall, W. Havran, G. Otten, M.R. Loken, M. Pierres, J. Kappler, and F. Fitch. 1983. Characterization of the murine antigenic determinant, designated L3T4a, recognized by monoclonal antibody GK1.5. *Immunol. Rev.* **74:** 30.

Doyle, C. and J.L. Strominger. 1987. Interaction between CD4 and class II MHC molecules mediate cell adhesion. *Nature* **330:** 256.

Elliott, B.E., Z.A. Nagy, Y. Ben-Neriah, and D. Givol. 1980. Alloactivated Lyt 1$^+$ 2$^-$ T lymphoblasts bind syngeneic Ia antigens. *Nature* **285:** 496.

Evans, R.L., T.J. Faldetta, R.E. Humphrey, D.M. Pratt, E.J. Yunis, and S.F. Schlossman. 1978. Peripheral human T cells sensitized in mixed leukocyte culture synthesize and express Ia-like antigens. *J. Exp. Med.* **148:** 1440.

Gay, D., P. Maddon, R. Sekaly, M.A. Talle, M. Godfrey, E. Long, G. Goldstein, L. Chess, R. Axel, J. Kappler, and P. Marrack. 1987. Functional interaction between human T-cell protein CD4 and the major histocompatibility complex HLA-DR antigen. *Nature* **328:** 626.

Hengartner, H., B. Odermatt, R. Schneider, M. Schreyer, G. Wälle, H.R. MacDonald, and R.M. Zinkernagel. 1988. Deletion of self-reactive T cells before entry into the thymus medulla. *Nature* **336:** 388.

Hirayama, K., Y. Nishimura, K. Tsukamoto, and T. Sasazuki. 1986. Functional and molecular analysis of three distinct HLA-DR4β-chains responsible for the MLR between HLA-Dw4,Dw15 and DKT2. *J. Immunol.* **137:** 924.

Hirayama, K., S. Matsushita, I. Kikuchi, M. Iuchi, N. Ohta, and T. Sasazuki. 1987. HLA-DQ is epistatic to HLA-DR in controlling the immune response to schistosomal antigen in humans. *Nature* **327:** 426.

Janeway, C.A., Jr., P.J. Conrad, E.A. Lerner, J. Babich, P. Wettstein, and D.B. Murphy. 1984. Monoclonal antibodies specific for Ia glycoproteins raised by immunization with activated T cells. *J. Immunol.* **132:** 662.

Kasahara, M., T. Takenouchi, H. Ikeda, K. Ogasawara, T. Okuyama, N. Ishikawa, A. Wakssaka, Y. Kikuchi, and M. Aizawa. 1983. Serologic dissection of HLA-D specificities by the use of monoclonal antibodies. *Immunogenetics* **18:** 525.

Kimoto, M. and C.G. Fathman. 1980. Antigen-reactive T cell clones I. Transcomplementing hybrid I-A-region gene products function effectively in antigen presentation. *J. Exp. Med.* **152:** 759.

Kimura, A., A. Israël, O. LeBail, and P. Kourilsky. 1986. Detailed analysis of the mouse H-2K^b promoter. *Cell* **44:** 261.

Kisielow, P., H. Blüthmann, U.D. Staerz, M. Steinmetz, and H.V. Boehmer. 1988. Tolerance in T-cell-receptor transgenic mice involves deletion of nonmature CD4$^+$8$^+$ thymocytes. *Nature* **333:** 742.

Lamb, J.R. and M. Feldmann. 1984. Essential requirement for major histocompatibility complex recognition in T-cell tolerance induction. *Nature* **308:** 72.

Long, E.O., J. Gorski, and B. Mach. 1984. Structural relationship of the SB beta-chain gene to HLA-D-region genes and murine I-region genes. *Nature* **310:** 233.

Maniatis, T., E.F. Fritsch, and J. Sambrook. 1982. *Molecular cloning: A laboratory manual,* Cold Spring Harbor Laboratory, Cold Spring Harbor, New York.

Marrack, P., D. Lo, R. Brinster, R. Palmiter, L. Burkly, R.H. Flavell, and J. Kappler. 1988. The effect of thymus environment on T cell development and tolerance. *Cell* **53:** 627.

Nagy, Z., B.E. Elliott, M. Nabholz, P.H. Krammer, and B. Pernis. 1976. Specific binding of alloantigens to T cells activated in the mixed lymphocyte reaction. *J. Exp. Med.* **143:** 648.

Nishimura, Y. and T. Sasazuki. 1983. Suppressor T cells control the HLA-linked low responsiveness to streptococcal antigen in man. *Nature* **302:** 67.

Ozato, K. and D.H. Sachs. 1981. Monoclonal antibodies to mouse MHC antigens. *J. Immunol.* **126:** 317.

Sasazuki, T., Y. Nishimura, M. Muto, and N. Ohta. 1983. HLA-linked genes controlling the immune response and disease susceptibility. *Immunol. Rev.* **70:** 51.

Sasazuki, T., N. Ohta, R. Kaneoka, and S. Kojima. 1980a. Association between HLA haplotype and low responsiveness to schistosomal worm antigen in man. *J. Exp. Med.* **152:** 314s.

Sasazuki, T., H. Kaneoka, Y. Nishimura, R. Kaneoka, M. Hayama, and H. Ohkuni. 1980b. An HLA-linked immune suppression gene in man. *J. Exp. Med.* **152:** 297s.

Sasazuki, T., Y. Kohno, I. Iwamoto, M. Tanimura, and S. Naito. 1978. Association between an HLA haplotype and low responsiveness to tetanus toxoid in man. *Nature* **272:** 359.

Schwarts, R.H. 1984. The role of gene products of the major histocompatibility complex in T cell activation and cellular interactions. In *Fundamentals of immunology* (ed. W.E. Paul), p. 379. Raven Press, New York.

Scott, B., H. Blüthmann, H.S. Teh, and H.V. Boehmer. 1989. The generation of mature T cells requires interaction of the $\alpha\beta$ T-cell receptor with major histocompatibility antigens. *Nature* **338:** 591.

Sha, W.C., C.A. Nelson, R.D. Newberry, D.M. Kranz, J.H. Russell, and D.Y. Loh. 1988. Positive and negative selection of an antigen receptor on T cells in transgenic mice. *Nature* **336:** 73.

Sleckman, B.P., A. Peterson, W.K. Jones, J.A. Foran, J.L. Greenstein, B. Seed, and S.J. Burakoff. 1987. Expression and function of CD4 in a murine T-cell hybridoma. *Nature* **328:** 351.

Sone, T., K. Tsukamoto, K. Hirayama, Y. Nishimura, T. Takenouchi, M. Aizawa, and T. Sasazuki. 1985. Two distinct class II molecules encoded by the genes within HLA-DR subregion of HLA-Dw2 and Dw12 can act as stimulating and restriction molecules. *J. Immunol.* **135:** 1288.

Todd, J.A., H. Acha-Orbea, J.I. Bell, N. Chao, Z. Fronek, C.O. Jacob, M. McDermott, A.A. Sinha, L. Timmerman, L. Steinman, and H.O. McDevitt. 1988. A molecular basis for MHC class II-associated autoimmunity. *Science* **240:** 1003.

Tsukamoto, K., M. Yasunami, A. Kimura, H. Inoko, A. Ando, T. Hirose, S. Inayama, and T. Sasazuki. 1987. DQw1 gene from HLA-DR2-Dw12 consists of six exons and expresses multiple DQw1 polypeptide through alternative splicing. *Immunogenetics* **25:** 343.

Use of Mutants to Analyze Regions on the H-2K^b Molecule for Interaction with Immune Receptors

S.G. Nathenson,* K. Kesari,* J.M. Sheil,† and P. Ajitkumar*

*Departments of Cell Biology and Microbiology and Immunology, Albert Einstein College of Medicine, Bronx, New York 10461; †Department of Microbiology, West Virginia University School of Medicine, Morgantown, West Virginia 26506

The class I genes of the murine major histocompatibility complex (MHC), H-2K, D and L, encode cell-surface-associated molecules that not only are targets in allogeneic graft rejection (Snell et al. 1976), but, current evidence suggests, also present foreign antigens processed to the form of peptides for recognition by the T-cell-antigen receptor (TCR) (Townsend et al. 1986). This latter phenomenon, called MHC restriction, is dependent on the ability of the cytotoxic T lymphocytes (CTL) to recognize a foreign antigen in the context of a self H-2 molecule (Zinkernagel and Doherty 1979).

Biochemical studies have demonstrated that the class I molecules are expressed on the surface of almost all somatic cells as heterodimers composed of a 45,000 dalton polymorphic glycoprotein (heavy chain) noncovalently associated with a 12,000 dalton invariant chain (light chain). The heavy chain, which anchors the complex in the cell membrane, consists of three amino-terminal extracellular domains approximately 90 amino acids in length (designated as α_1, α_2, and α_3), a hydrophobic transmembrane region, and a carboxy-terminal cytoplasmic portion (Nathenson et al. 1981). Essential to our understanding of the basis of MHC function is the characterization of the structural features of the highly polymorphic class I molecule that allow for interaction with antigenic peptides and with the TCR. An approach we have found useful for relating the structural features of the MHC class I molecules to their functional properties has been the characterization of MHC variants that have sustained a measurable alteration in an associated biological activity. In particular, H-2K^b mutants with limited biochemical alterations have been especially valuable for the purpose of localizing defined regions on the class I heavy chain that function as recognition sites within the immune system (Nathenson et al. 1986). In the present paper, we review some of our studies over the past few years using MHC variants obtained in different ways for probing such structure/function relationships.

MHC variants have been isolated following selection both in vivo (Bailey and Kohn 1965; Egorov 1967) and in vitro (Geier et al. 1986). The MHC mutants that were first obtained in mouse strains were selected because of their ability to promote graft rejection when tissue transplants were exchanged among otherwise syngeneic littermates (Kohn et al. 1978). These histogenic mutants ultimately were of value, not only for identifying some of the structural features of specific MHC proteins involved in transplant rejection (Nairn et al. 1980), but also for identifying an unexpected genetic mechanism responsible for diversification of class I genes (Schulze et al. 1983; Weiss et al. 1983). This process, which we have termed micro-recombination, or gene conversion, results in the transfer of short sequences of genetic information among class I genes and is thought to play a key role in the concerted evolution of H-2 products (Geliebter and Nathenson 1987). Continuous diversification in K- and D-region genes through such micro-recombinations provides an expanded repertoire of class I molecules in the population.

When correlated with protein and nucleic acid sequence information, immunological data on the MHC mutants led us to conclude that the functional regions of the H-2 molecules resided in the first two domains, and furthermore, to propose that the amino acid stretches from 70 to 90 in the α_1 domain and from 150 to 180 in the α_2 domain appeared to form recognition sites for the TCR (Nathenson et al. 1986; Zeff et al. 1988). Resolution of the three-dimensional structure of the HLA-A2 molecule by Wiley, Strominger, and their colleagues (Bjorkman et al. 1987a,b) has greatly facilitated our interpretations of the structure/function relationship of class I molecules. The salient features of this structure showed that a super domain comprising the first two domains (α_1 and α_2) formed the most membrane-distal portion of the molecule supported by the α_3 domain and β_2-microglobulin subunit. The super domain contained two α-helical regions, one formed by the α_1 domain residues 58–84 (α_1 helix) and the other by the α_2 domain residues 138–180 (α_2 helix), which formed the sides of a groove (the putative antigen-binding site) between the α helices. The residues in the eight central β strands of the antiparallel β-pleated sheet ran below the α helices and formed the floor of the groove. Thus, our hypothesis, which suggested that T-cell recognition of MHC molecules required concordant recognition of the α_1 and α_2 domains, appeared reasonable in view of the intimate proximity of these domains according to the three-dimensional structure.

Because the in-vivo-derived mutants bore clustered but multiple amino acid changes, it was not possible to experimentally determine the individual amino acid contact residues for any given CTL clone. Thus, to approach an understanding at the molecular level of the precise nature of the sites on the class I polypeptide involved in the interaction with the TCR, we embarked on a strategy to identify MHC variants with single amino acid alterations (Geier et al. 1986). Such variants were isolated in vitro following mutagenesis of established tissue culture cell lines by a procedure that selected cells expressing a specific phenotype; i.e., the loss of a particular serologic or T-cell-defined epitope (Geier et al. 1986; Sheil et al. 1986). We found that this approach yielded class I variants much more efficiently than isolation of spontaneous, histoincompatible mutant mice and allowed us to greatly expand the number of available K^b structural mutants. It also turned out that antibody selection provided a panel of K^b mutants with amino acid alterations in mostly surface residues, primarily on the α helices (Ajitkumar et al. 1988). The K^b mutants selected by allogeneic skin grafting, on the other hand, all contained at least one altered residue affecting the antigen groove, as well as surface residues on the α helices.

Selection and Sequence Determination of Somatic Cell Variants

The strategy for isolating K^b structural variants utilized an approach of negative selection against wild-type antigenic epitope(s) encoded on a particular class I molecule. Negative selection with monoclonal antibodies (MAbs) was used (Fig. 1) to isolate H-2K^b structural variants from an H-2^b × H-2^d heterozygous Abelson virus-transformed pre-B cell line, R8 (Geier et al. 1986). Mutagenized cells were treated with one of a panel of anti-K^b MAbs and complement, and the survivors of this negative selection procedure were then tested with a pool of anti-K^b MAbs by cytofluorometric analysis to distinguish putative "structural variants" from H-2K^b "loss variants." Structural variants are defined as cells expressing K^b on the cell surface as determined by positive reactivity with the anti-K^b MAb pool but lacking the antigenic site identified by the selecting monoclonal antibody. In contrast, loss variants lacked all the antigenic epitopes present on K^b as defined by the pool of monoclonal antibodies.

An additional method was employed by Sheil et al. (1986) for isolation of somatic cell K^b variants in which anti-K^b CTL clones were used for the selection rather than antibodies. For these studies, ethyl methane sulfonate (EMS)-mutagenized R8 cells were selected for the loss of an antigenic epitope defined by a single K^b-reactive CTL clone.

For determination of the site of mutation, the RNA sequencing protocol described previously was utilized (Geliebter 1987). Single nucleotide changes were documented for 16 mutants selected by antibody and 2 mutants selected by CTL (Ajitkumar et al. 1988; R. Sun et al., unpubl.). Since several mutants shared the same mutation, the final series consisted of 12 mutants with the following amino acid residue changes: 75

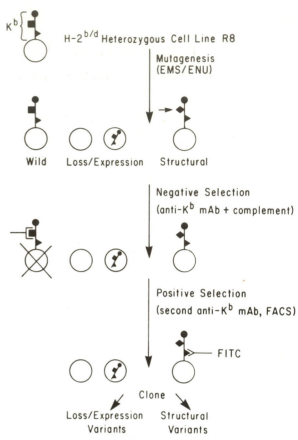

Figure 1. Isolation of H-2K^b somatic cell mutants. The heterozygous cell line R8 (H-2^b × H-2^d) was mutagenized with either EMS or ethyl nitrosourea (ENU). We postulated that at least four classes of cells would result, including (1) wild type with no changes in structure, (2) loss mutants with no detectable product, (3) expression mutants that synthesize a K^b product that is not expressed at the plasma membrane, and (4) structural mutants with an altered phenotype, as detected by a panel of monoclonal antibodies to K^b. Negative selection with a single monoclonal antibody was performed to remove wild-type K^b-expressing cells, which escaped mutagenesis. Of those that survived negative selection, positive selection was performed with a second monoclonal antibody employing FACS analysis. Cell lines were categorized as either structural variants or loss/expression variants and cloned separately for further analysis. (Reprinted, with permission, from Geier et al. 1986.)

(Arg→Gln); 80 (Thr→Ile); 82 (Leu→Pro); 82 (Leu→Phe); 90 (Gln→Asp); 138 (Met→Lys); 141 (Leu→Arg); 150 (Ala→Pro); 162 (Gly→Asp); 166 (Glu→Lys); 174 (Asn→Lys); 192 (His→Glu).

Construction of a Three-dimensional K^b Model

To locate the altered residues in a three-dimensional K^b structure, a model of the α_1 and α_2 domain portion (residues 1–182) of the molecule was constructed (Ajitkumar et al. 1988) by introducing those amino acid residues of the K^b molecule that differed from the HLA-A2 sequence into the crystallographic structure of the HLA-A2 molecule (Bjorkman et al. 1987a), using the computer graphics program FRODO (Jones 1982). The basic premise for the construction of the model was that the three-dimensional structure of the α-carbon backbone and the side-chain directions of the residues of the K^b molecule would be the same as that of the HLA-A2 molecule. This contention is supported by the following facts: (1) The K^b and the HLA-A2 molecules share the same number of residues and can be optimally aligned without any gaps or insertions; (2) the aligned sequences of the α_1 and α_2 domains of the two molecules show 73% identity, with an additional 7% conservative substitutions (Klein and Figueroa 1986); (3) the patterns of polymorphic and conserved residues present in the α helices of the α_1 and α_2 domains of the HLA-A2 molecule (Bjorkman et al. 1987b) are similar to those in the K^b molecule, giving confidence that the α helices are oriented similarly in both the molecules.

This model did not attempt to predict conformational changes of neighboring residues caused by the substitutions of the side chains of the K^b residues for those in the HLA-A2 structure. The most striking difference between the overall appearance of the K^b as compared to the A2 molecule was the much longer and deeper space in the antigen cleft produced by the loss of two bulky residues, a change at position 9 (Phe to Val) and at position 99 (Tyr to Ser). A schematic representation looking down on the top of the three-dimensional K^b model structure is given in Figure 2, showing the two α-helical regions and the groove between them, and the eight β-pleated-sheet strands forming the floor of the putative antigen peptide-binding site.

Characteristics of Altered Amino Acid Residues and Side-chain Orientation in Antibody-selected K^b Mutants, and Comparison to Changes in the In Vivo Histogenically Selected Mutants

The characteristics of the altered amino acid residue in the series of somatic K^b mutants selected by antibody are summarized in Table 1 and graphically displayed in Figure 2A. All of the altered residues were found to be located in either the α_1 or α_2 helices except for the change at position 90, which was on the loop between the α_1 and α_2 helices (Table 1, Fig. 2A). Significantly, the side chains of the variant amino acid residues pointed upward and away from the putative antigenic site except the threonine at position 80, for which the side chain projected partially upward as well as into the antigen-binding groove.

Although the in vivo mutants have also incurred changes in both the α_1 and α_2 domains, several differences from the pattern of changes of the in vitro mutants were noted (Table 2). First, several mutants had alterations in the β-sheet residues in the floor of the groove. Thus, in the mutant bm8 (amino acid residues 22, 23, 24, 30) and in the bg series bm6, 7, 9 (amino acid residues 116, 121), changes have occurred in stretches of the polypeptide chain that lined the floor of the antigen groove. Such alterations, although changing the shape and volume of the cleft, would not be expected to alter the shape of the two α helices. For the other mutants, bm3, 11, 19, and 23 (α_1 domain) and bm1, 4, and 10 (α_2 domain), the altered residues occurred in the α-helical regions of the first two domains,

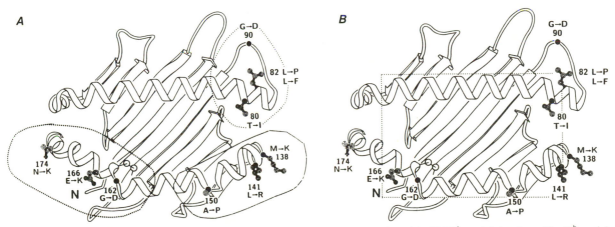

Figure 2. Location of the mutated amino acid residues on a schematic representation of the H-2K^b model structure. The K^b model depicts the α_1 and α_2 domain portion of the K^b molecule. The amino terminal is indicated by N, the β strands by flat arrow ribbons, and the α helices by coiled ribbons. Residues 1–90 form the α_1 domain, which comprises the first four β strands from the amino terminal and the α_1 helix (residues 58–84). The α_2 domain consists of residues 91–182 and is formed by the four β strands (immediately following the α_1 helix) and the α_2 helix (residues 138–180). The two α helices are separated by a groove, which is the putative antigen-binding site. Eight β strands, four from each domain, form the floor of the groove. Single amino acid substitutions are identified by one-letter codes, and their positions are indicated by numbers. The side chains shown are of the native K^b residues that underwent substitution. (A) Groups of residues contributing to the epitopes recognized by the MAbs EH-144 (Thr-80, Leu-82, Gly-90), Y-3 (Met-138, Leu-141, Ala-150), and 5F1-2-14 (Gly-162, Glu-166, Asn-174) are identified by the respective circles. (B) An area of 30 Å by 20 Å (600 Å^2), encompassing the residues Leu-82 and Glu-166, which are recognized by nearly all of the CTL clones examined in this study, is identified by the rectangle superimposed on the α helices (inclusive of the antigen-binding site in between). (Reprinted, with permission, from Ajitkumar et al. 1988.)

Table 1. Amino Acid Side-chain Orientation of Somatic K^b Mutant Altered Residues (Selected by Antibodies)

Mutant residue number	Change	Location	Orientation relative to antigen-binding site
75[a]	R → Q	α_1 helix	away from site
80	T → I	α_1 helix	into site (slightly upward)
82	L → P	α_1 helix	up and slightly into site
	L → F		
90	G → D	loop (α_1/α_2)	—
138	M → K	α_2 helix	up and away from site
141	L → R	α_2 helix	away and down from α helix
150	A → P	α_2 helix	up and away from site
162	G → D	α_2 helix	(?)
166	E → K	α_2 helix	up and away from site
174	N → K	α_2 helix	away from site

[a]Preliminary observations, J. Sheil, P. Ajitkumar, and R. Sun.

and at least one and sometimes several of the variant amino acid side chains projected into the antigen-binding groove. Thus, the major difference between the in vivo histogenically selected mutants and the antibody or CTL negatively selected mutants was the feature of orientation regarding the antigen cleft.

Binding Sites for the Monoclonal Antibodies on the H-2K^b Molecule

Earlier studies on the binding of a panel of monoclonal antibodies on cells from bm mutant mice (Hammerling et al. 1982) had indicated which domain a particular monoclonal antibody recognized on the H-

2K^b molecule. The structural variants of R8 selected by the antibodies, however, provided a more precise identification of the amino acid residues that contribute to a specific monoclonal antibody epitope. The protocol outlined in Figure 1 was aimed toward the selection of variants expressing normal amounts of structurally altered K^b molecules with only minimal conformational alterations. In such an experimental strategy, the amino acids exposed on the surface of the K^b molecule might be expected to mutate in order to disrupt the contact with the selecting antibody. The series of chemically induced K^b variants isolated as mentioned above (Geier et al. 1986) showed loss of reactivity with the selecting antibody, but retention of reactivity with

Table 2. Amino Acid Side-chain Orientation of In Vivo K^b Mutant Altered Residues (Selected by Allograft Rejection)

Mutant	Changed residue	Change	Location	Orientation relative to antigen-binding site
bm8	22	Y → F	β sheet	into site
	23	M → I	β sheet	down
	24	E → S	β sheet	into site
	30	D → N	loop	—
bm6, 7, 9	116	Y → F	β sheet	into site
	121	C → R	loop	—
bm3	77	D → S	α_1 helix	into site
	89	K → A	loop	—
bm11	77	D → S	α_1 helix	into site
	80	T → N	α_1 helix	into site
bm19	80	T → N	α_1 helix	into site
bm23	75	R → H	α_1 helix	up and out
	77	D → S	α_1 helix	into site
bm1	152	E → A	α_2 helix	into site
	155	R → Y	α_2 helix	up and into site
	156	L → Y	α_2 helix	into site
bm4	162	G → D	α_2 helix	(?)
	163	T → P	α_2 helix	into site (partial up)
	165	V → L	α_2 helix	away from site
	173	K → E	α_2 helix	away from site
	174	N → L	α_2 helix	away from site
bm10	163	T → A	α_2 helix	into site (partial up)
	165	V → M	α_2 helix	away from site
	167	W → S	α_2 helix	into site
	173	K → E	α_2 helix	away from site
	174	N → L	α_2 helix	away from site

others. About half of the independently derived mutants showed only the loss of a single epitope. These findings clearly supported the idea that antibodies bind to specific domains of the H-2 molecule (Fig. 2A), since in no case did a mutant selected with an α_1 or α_2 antibody lose an epitope for an antibody detecting a site in the other domain. The three MAbs, EH-144, 5F1-2-14, and Y-3, which were used for selection of the somatic variants, selected mutants with alterations of the amino acid residues clustered at discrete sites on the K^b molecule, as demonstrated by the three groups of residues outlined in Figure 2A.

An assessment of the most distant residues that contribute to any particular antibody-specific epitope can be used to estimate the minimum dimensions of the area of a region recognized by that monoclonal antibody. In the case of the Y-3 epitope, the distance between the α-carbon atoms of Met-138 and Ala-150 is 21 Å. This distance can be roughly accommodated by an antigen/antibody interface area of approximately 30 Å by 20 Å (600 Å^2). Such estimates for surface area of interface are also found to be well within roughly 600 Å^2 for the MAbs EH-144 and B8-24-3.

Confinement of the monoclonal antibody epitopes, for the limited number of antibodies we have examined, to the α helices is also consistent with the serological analyses of the in vivo K^{bm} mutants (Nathenson et al. 1986). The loss of K^b-specific monoclonal antibody epitopes is evident only in the mutants that have incurred mutations in the α-helical regions, e.g., bm4, 10, 3, 11, and 23; whereas bm6, 7, 8, and 9, which do not bear mutations in the exposed α-helices, have lost no known K^b-specific monoclonal antibody epitopes.

The available data suggest that the monoclonal antibodies that have been raised thus far detect spatially discrete, domain-specific sites. However, it would seem reasonable that antibodies should be able to detect a pattern of amino acid residues, including portions of the α_1 and α_2 helices and the surface residues of a peptide in the antigen cleft. That such antibodies have not yet been isolated and characterized may be due to the large number of potentially different peptides (self peptides) in the groove of a population of otherwise identical MHC molecules, thus making their detection difficult. Preliminary evidence for such an antibody for class II molecules has been reported (Janeway et al., this volume). The detailed characterization of this reagent should provide us with information on this type of recognition.

Cellular Recognition of the MHC Class I Molecule

The mouse MHC mutants have proven valuable for obtaining information on the mechanisms of both allogeneic and MHC-restricted or antigen-associated recognition. Using the cells from bm mutant mice in in vitro CTL assays, it was earlier demonstrated that the CTLs recognize conformational and not linear determinants on the MHC class I molecule (Melief et al.

1980). Thus, the observations on the cross-reactivity of mutant anti-parent primary CTLs (Melief et al. 1980; DeWaal et al. 1983) and of cloned CTL lines (Sherman 1982a,b) suggested that, irrespective of the location of mutations in the bm mutants that were used to elicit a response, the CTLs showed cross-reactivity with the targets bearing mutations in either the α_1 or α_2 domain. Therefore, each CTL clone appeared to have its own unique specificity toward the MHC molecule.

The availability of the panel of H-2K^b mutants derived in vitro from the R8 cell line offered the opportunity to refine our understanding of interaction sites on the K^b molecule at the level of single amino acid residues (Ajitkumar et al. 1988). Functional analysis of the R8 mutants was carried out using a panel of allogeneic anti-K^b CTL clones raised in bm mutant mice (Bluestone et al. 1986), as well as with several anti-K^b allogeneic CTL clones (J.M. Sheil, unpubl.). An examination of the pattern of reactivity (Table 3) of the anti-K^b CTL clones on the R8 mutants in the context of sequence information has revealed several features of T-cell recognition of the MHC molecule. As shown in the summary of the CTL results in Table 3, of the eleven substitutions tested for their effect on CTL recognition, nine were found to affect the recognition by one or more CTL clones (Arg-75, Thr-80, Leu-82, Met-138, Ala-150, Gly-162, Glu-166, Asn-174, and His-192). These residues (except His-192) are located along the α-helical regions of the two domains. Every CTL clone tested (except bm11 CTL clone 39) was found to be sensitive to the substitution of at least one residue from both the α_1 and α_2 helices. For example, recognition of the K^b molecule by bm8 CTL clone 13 was affected by changes at Thr-80, Leu-82 in the α_1 helix, as well as those at Met-138, Gly-162, and Glu-166 in the α_2 helix. That the observations are not due to artifacts of raising CTL clones in the bm mutants is suggested by the finding of a similar effect of the K^b R8 mutant changes on recognition by the two classic allogeneic anti-K^b clones raised in a K^d context (Table 3).

We interpreted the results of loss of recognition by anti-K^b CTL clones due to the alteration in K^b of a single amino acid side chain to mean that the TCR of the clone must contact the amino acid residue of K^b at that position. Thus, we concluded that the CTLs must simultaneously interact with amino acid residues in both the helical stretches of the α_1 and α_2 domains. That all of the CTL clones examined interacted with residues on the α_1 and α_2 helices is also consistent with the surface locations of the residues that we could examine. The upward orientation of the side chains from the α helices supports the idea that they interact directly with the TCR (Fig. 2A and Table 1), rather than indirectly through an alteration of a bound peptide.

It is important that two residues, whose substitutions abrogated monoclonal antibody binding but did not significantly affect the CTL recognition, were Gly-90 and Leu-141. Although Gly-90 is not located on the α helix, Leu-141 has its side chain oriented down toward

Table 3. CTL Recognition Pattern of In-vitro-selected K^b Mutants

Origin of anti-K^b CTL clones	CTL clone number	Positions of altered amino acid residues affecting CTL recognition									Positions of altered amino acid residues not affecting CTL recognition							
		α$_1$ domain			α$_2$ domain					α$_3$ domain	α$_1$ domain			α$_2$ domain				α$_3$ domain
		80	82P	82F	138	150	162	166	174	192	80	82P	90	138	141	162	166	192
bm8	4	80	82P	82F	138		162	166		192			90		141			
	6			82F	138			166			80	82P	90		141	162		192
	9	80	n.t.	82F	138*		162	n.t.		n.t.			90		n.t.			
	10		82P	n.t.	n.t.		n.t.	n.t.		n.t.	80		90		141			
	11		n.t.	82F	138		162	166*		192	80		90		141			
	12	80		82F	138			166		192	80		90		141	162		
	13		82P	82F	138		162	166		192	80		90		141	162		
	14		82P	82F	138			166		192	80				141			
	15	80*	82P	82F	n.t.		n.t.	166		192			90		141			
bm10	5	80	82P	82F*	138		162	166		192			90	138	141			192
	6	80*	82P	82F	138		n.t.	n.t.		192			90	138	141			192
	37	80	82P*	82F	138		162	166		n.t.			90	138	141			
	38	80	82P*	n.t.	n.t.		n.t.	n.t.		n.t.			n.t.	138	141			
	42	80	82P	82F	138		162	166					90	138	141			192
	47		82P	82F	138		162	166					90	138	141			192
	47		82P	82F	n.t.		n.t.	n.t.			80		90	138	n.t.			192
bm11	28			82F*				166			80	82P	90	138	141	162		192
	37		82P	82F				166*		192	80		90	138	141	162		192
	39	80	82P	82F				n.t.		192	80		90	138	141	162	166	
	41	80	82P	82F	138			n.t.		n.t.	80		90	138	n.t.	162		
clone 110 (K^d anti-K^b)	75P	80	82P	82F	138	150	162	166	174	192	80		90		141			
	75Q					150			174	75Q			90					
clone 19 (K^d and K^b)	75P	80	82P	82F	138	150		166	174	75Q 192	80		90	138	141	162	166	192

82P and 82F indicate the substitution of Pro and Phe, respectively, for Leu 82; (*) sign on the numbers indicating the positions of mutations shows partial reactivity of a particular CTL clone on the mutant having a substitution at that position; n.t. indicates not tested. 75 and 150 variants were only tested with clones 110 and 60.

the cell membrane and away from the top surface of the α_2 helix and the putative antigen-binding site and in a position consistent with noncontact to the TCR. Only one residue, His-192, which was found to affect the recognition by some CTL clones, is located in the α_3 domain, ~ 50 Å below the α helices. In the context of the three-dimensional structure, the effect of this residue on the CTL recognition most probably must be indirect, possibly due to its influence on the binding of an accessory molecule, such as CD8. Recently, the direct involvement of an amino acid residue from the α_3 domain in the CTL recognition process through CD8 binding has been shown using a mutant cell line (Potter et al. 1989).

Similar to the assessment of the approximate interface area for the antigen/antibody complex, we could estimate a potential interface area of an MHC molecule/TCR complex from the distance between two CTL-specific residues on the MHC molecule. An area of dimensions 30 Å by 20 Å (600 Å^2), which is equivalent to the interface area of an antigen/antibody complex (Amit et al. 1986), can accommodate the residues Leu-82 and Glu-166, which are recognized by nearly all of the CTL clones examined (Fig. 2B). However, our data suggest that the TCR/MHC molecule interface may even encompass a slightly larger area, since the most distantly located CTL-specific residues Leu-82 and Asn-174 reported in this paper are separated by a diagonal distance of 44 Å, which can be accommodated by an area 39 Å by 20 Å (780 Å^2). The specific physical requirement that the TCR should contact residues on both α helices necessitates such an extensive interface area.

The notion of a broad surface region of contact between the TCR and both α helices of the MHC molecule is also consistent with recent independently derived modeling studies on the TCR. These analyses postulate that the homolog of immunoglobulin CDR1, and CDR2 regions of the TCR would contact the α-helical regions of the MHC, whereas the CDR3 regions would contact the antigen peptide contained in the groove (Chothia et al. 1988; Davis and Bjorkman 1988; Claverie et al. 1989).

Does Allorecognition Involve Peptides?

At present, the question of the nature and the number of peptides involved in an allorecognition event remains unresolved. However, an indirect inference can be made from the available data on the in vivo bm mutants (Table 2). A close examination of the positions of the substituted amino acid residues and their orientations reveals that each one of them has at least one amino acid residue whose side chain points into the antigen-binding groove. This is consistent with the idea that an altered peptide may be an absolute requirement for allogenicity. In a related series of experiments on our antibody-selected K^b mutants, we have found that the entire panel of R8 mutants, except the two mutants with changes at Thr-80 (R8.24, R8.246), failed to

evoke an alloreactive response (Lewis et al. 1988). The two mutants that produced an allo response were found to have identical substitutions of Thr-80 to Ile-80. Of all the in vitro point mutations studied, only this residue (a lip residue) has its side chain pointing into the antigen-binding groove as well as slightly upward, a finding consistent with the idea that the mutation at Thr-80 is contributing to the allogenicity through a peptide. Strong support for the role of the peptide also comes from analysis of the mutants bm6, 7, and 9: 116 (Tyr → Phe), and bm8: 22 (Tyr → Phe), 23 (Met → Ile), 24 (Glu → Ser), 30 (Asp → Asn). The alterations in their K^b molecules have changes exclusively at the residues located on the β sheet or loops (Table 2). In each case, there is at least one residue with its side chain projecting into the antigen-binding groove and there are, more significantly, no changes in the residues situated along the α helices that are wild-type K^b in sequence. These observations taken together are consistent with the notion that in allogeneic recognition, the T cell recognizes a pattern formed by the residues on the α helices and on a peptide between the helices, in a manner presumed to be the basis for antigen-specific recognition as well.

SUMMARY

MHC variants isolated both in vivo (by tissue graft rejection) and in vitro (by antibody selection) were utilized to study sites on the H-2K^b molecule involved in interaction with antibodies and with the TCR. K^b mutants selected by antibodies were found to have single point mutations, which when analyzed in the context of the three-dimensional structure of a K^b molecule modeled from HLA-A2 coordinates showed that the altered residues were localized mostly to the α_1 and α_2 helices. The side chains of the variant amino acid residues pointed upward and away from the antigenic site. Analysis of the altered amino acids in the previously described tissue-graft-selected K^b mutants showed that the side chains of the variant residues occur either in the α-helical regions or in the β-pleated-sheet floor of the antigen groove, but every mutant contained at least one and sometimes several acid side chains projecting into the antigen-binding groove. Monoclonal antibody studies showed that the available monoclonal antibodies mapped to discrete domain-specific sites. Analysis of CTL recognition sites using cloned mutant anti-parent or allogeneic combinations showed that all CTL clones examined interacted with amino acid side-chain residues on both the α_1 and α_2 helices. Thus, we concluded that the CTLs must simultaneously interact with the amino acid residues in both the α-helical stretches of the α_1 and α_2 domains. Our analyses with the point mutants imply that the TCR must interact with the MHC molecule over a relatively large surface area in such an orientation that it interfaces with the two α helices, as well as with the foreign or self-peptide in the antigen-binding site between the helices. These findings, together with the observation that several of the in vivo K^b mutants induce strong alloreactions yet have changes only in the bottom of the antigen-binding groove and no alterations in the α-helical residues, are consistent with the hypothesis that in some cases alloreaction can be the result of T-cell recognition of an altered pattern on the MHC molecule due to a changed peptide in the antigen groove.

ACKNOWLEDGMENTS

We thank our collaborators and colleagues S. Geier, M. Nakagawa, J.A. Bluestone, M.A. Saper, Tom Garrett, and D.C. Wiley. The original research from the laboratory of S.G.N. was supported by U.S. Public Health Service grants AI-07289 and AI-10701, National Cancer Institute grant P30-CA-13330, and the Irvington Institute for Medical Research, and by postdoctoral fellowships to P.A. and K.K. from the Cancer Research Institute, New York. We also acknowledge the excellent secretarial assistance of Ms. Rosalie Spata.

REFERENCES

Ajitkumar, P., S.S. Geier, K.V. Kesari, F. Borriello, M. Nakagawa, J.A. Bluestone, M.A. Saper, D.C. Wiley, and S.G. Nathenson. 1988. Evidence that multiple residues on both the α-helices of the class I MHC molecule are simultaneously recognized by the T cell receptor. *Cell* 54: 47.

Amit, A.G., R.A. Mariuzza, S.E.V. Phillips, and R.J. Poljak. 1986. Three-dimensional structure of an antigen-antibody complex at 2.8 Å resolution. *Science* 233: 747.

Bailey, D.W. and H.I. Kohn. 1965. Inherited histocompatibility changes in progeny of irradiated and unirradiated mice. *Genet. Res.* 6: 330.

Bjorkman, P.J., M.A. Saper, B. Samraoui, W.S. Bennett, J.L. Strominger, and D.C. Wiley. 1987a. Structure of the human class I histocompatibility antigen, HLA-A2. *Nature* 329: 506.

———. 1987b. The foreign antigen binding site and T cell recognition regions of class I histocompatibility antigens. *Nature* 329: 512.

Bluestone, J.A., C. Langlet, S.S. Geier, S.G. Nathenson, M. Foo, and A.-M. Schmitt-Verhulst. 1986. Somatic cell variants express altered H-2K^b allodeterminants recognized by cytolytic T cell clones. *J. Immunol.* 137: 1244.

Chothia, C., D.R. Boswell, and A.M. Lesk. 1988. The outline structure of the T-cell $\alpha\beta$ receptor. *EMBO J.* 7: 3745.

Claverie, J.-M., A.P. Chalufour, and L. Bougueleret. 1989. Implications of a Fab-like structure for the T-cell receptor. *Immunol. Today* 10: 10.

Davis, M.M. and P.J. Bjorkman. 1988. T-cell antigen receptor genes and T-cell recognition. *Nature* 334: 395.

DeWaal, L.P., S.G. Nathenson, and C.J.M. Melief. 1983. Direct demonstration that cytotoxic T lymphocytes recognize conformational determinants and not primary amino acid sequences. *J. Exp. Med.* 158: 1720.

Egorov, I.K. 1967. A mutation of histocompatibility-2 locus in the mouse. *Genetika* 3: 136.

Geier, S.S., R.A. Zeff, D.M. McGovern, T.V. Rajan, and S.G. Nathenson. 1986. An approach to the study of structure-function relationships of MHC class I molecules: Isolation and serologic characterization of H-2K^b somatic cell variants. *J. Immunol.* 137: 1239.

Geliebter, J. 1987. Dideoxynucleotide sequencing of RNA and uncloned cDNA. *Focus* 9: 5.

Geliebter, J. and S.G. Nathenson. 1987. Recombination and the concerted evolution of the murine MHC. *Trends. Genetics* 3: 107.

Hammerling, G.J., E. Rusch, N. Tada, S. Kimura, and U. Hammerling. 1982. Localization of allodeterminants on H-2K^b antigens determined with monoclonal antibodies and H-2 mutant mice. *Proc. Natl. Acad. Sci.* 79: 4737.

Jones, T.A. 1982. FRODO: A graphics fitting program for macromolecules. In *Computational crystallography* (ed. D. Sayre), p. 303. Clarendon Press, Oxford.

Klein, J. and F. Figueroa. 1986. The evolution of class I MHC genes. Amino acid sequences of class I MHC molecules from mouse, rat, rabbit and man. *Immunol. Today* 7: 2.

Kohn, H.I., J. Klein, R.W. Melvold, S.G. Nathenson, D. Pious, and D.C. Shreffler. 1978. The first H-2 mutant workshop. *Immunogenetics* 7: 279.

Lewis, J., M. Foo, S.S. Geier, P. Ajitkumar, S.G. Nathenson, and J.A. Bluestone. 1988. Cytotoxic T lymphocyte recognition of novel allodeterminants expressed on in vitro selected H-2K^b mutants. *J. Immunol.* 141: 728.

Melief, C.J.M., L.P. DeWaal, M.Y. Van Der Meulen, R.W. Melvold, and H.I. Kohn. 1980. Fine specificity of alloimmune cytotoxic T lymphocytes directed against H-2K. A study with K^b mutants. *J. Exp. Med.* 151: 993.

Nairn, R., K. Yamaga, and S.G. Nathenson. 1980. Biochemistry of the gene products of murine MHC mutants. *Annu. Rev. Genet.* 14: 241.

Nathenson, S.G., J. Geliebter, G.M. Pfaffenbach, and R.A. Zeff. 1986. Murine major histocompatibility complex class I mutants: Molecular analysis and structure-function implications. *Annu. Rev. Immunol.* 4: 471.

Nathenson, S.G., H. Uehara, B.M. Ewenstein, T.J. Kindt, and J.E. Coligan. 1981. Primary structural analysis of the transplantation antigens of the murine H-2 major histocompatibility complex. *Annu. Rev. Biochem.* 50: 1025.

Potter, T.A., T.V. Rajan, R.F. Dick II, and J.A. Bluestone. 1989. Substitution at residue 227 of H-2 class I molecules abrogates recognition by CD8-dependent, but not CD8-independent, cytotoxic T lymphocytes. *Nature* 337: 73.

Schulze, D.H., L.R. Pease, S.S. Geier, A.A. Reyes, L.A. Sarmiento, R.B. Wallace, and S.G. Nathenson. 1983. Comparison of the cloned H-2K^{bm1} variant gene with the H-2K^b gene shows a cluster of seven nucleotide differences. *Proc. Natl. Acad. Sci.* 80: 2007.

Sheil, J.M., M.J. Bevan, and L.A. Sherman. 1986. Immunoselection of structural H-2K^b variants: Use of cloned cytolytic T cells to select for loss of a CTL defined allodeterminant. *Immunogenetics* 23: 52.

Sherman, L.A. 1982a. Recognition of conformational determinants on H-2 by cytolytic T lymphocytes. *Nature* 297: 511.

———. 1982b. Influence of the major histocompatibility complex on the repertoire of allospecific cytolytic T lymphocytes. *J. Exp. Med.* 155: 380.

Snell, G.D., J. Dausset, and S.G. Nathenson. 1976. *Histocompatibility*. Academic Press, New York.

Townsend, A.R.M., J. Rothbard, F.M. Gotch, G. Bahadur, D. Wraith, and A.J. McMichael. 1986. The epitopes of influenza nucleoprotein recognized by cytotoxic T lymphocytes can be defined with short synthetic peptides. *Cell* 44: 959.

Weiss, E.H., A. Mellor, L. Golden, K. Fahrner, E. Simpson, J. Hurst, and R.A. Flavell. 1983. The structure of a mutant H-2 gene suggests that the generation of polymorphism in H-2 genes may occur by gene conversion-like events. *Nature* 301: 671.

Zeff, R.A., P. Ajitkumar, J. Geliebter, and S.G. Nathenson. 1988. Localization of immune receptor recognition sites on MHC molecules through the analysis of H-2K^b mutants. In *Processing and presentation of antigens* (ed. B. Pernis and H.J. Vogel). p. 263. Academic Press, New York.

Zinkernagel, R.M. and P.C. Doherty. 1979. MHC-restricted cytotoxic T cells: Studies on the biological role of polymorphic major transplantation antigens determining T cell restriction-specificity, function, and responsiveness. *Adv. Immunol.* 27: 51.

Diversity of Class I HLA Molecules: Functional and Evolutionary Interactions with T Cells

P. Parham,* R.J. Benjamin,* B.P. Chen,* C. Clayberger,† P.D. Ennis,* A.M. Krensky,†
D.A. Lawlor,* D.R. Littman,‡§ A.M. Norment,‡ H.T. Orr,**
R.D. Salter,* and J. Zemmour*

*Department of Cell Biology and †Department of Pediatrics, Stanford University, Stanford, California 94305;
‡Department of Microbiology and Immunology and §Howard Hughes Medical Institute, University of California
at San Francisco, California 94143; **Department of Laboratory Medicine and Pathology and the
Institute of Human Genetics, University of Minnesota, Minneapolis, Minnesota 55455

In the past 5 years, the nature of major histocompatibility complex (MHC) glycoproteins, as well as the mechanism by which they restrict antigen recognition by T lymphocytes, has been clarified. These molecules bind peptides within intracellular membrane compartments, forming complexes that are then brought to the cell surface to be surveilled by antigen receptors of circulating T lymphocytes. When a threshold of molecular complementarity between T-cell receptor (TCR) and an MHC/peptide complex occurs, the T cell becomes activated, thus initiating an immune response. Through exploitation of distinct but poorly understood pathways of intracellular traffic, class I MHC molecules present peptides derived from endogenous proteins, whereas class II MHC molecules present peptides derived from exogenously synthesized proteins. It is likely that these processes of peptide presentation are central to thymic selection of the T-cell repertoire and to initiation, in the periphery, of T-cell responses to foreign antigens (for review, see Davis and Bjorkman 1988; Hedrick 1988; Marrack and Kappler 1988; Long and Jacobson 1989; Townsend and Bodmer 1989).

The essence of T-cell recognition is thus the interaction of an MHC molecule with a TCR. A consequence of this functional interdependence is that genes encoding these two diverse families of genes evolve in concert. The evolutionary origins of the interaction probably lie with a nonvariable, nonimmunological ligand-receptor system that was subsequently adapted to immunological purpose. This argues for a fundamental, intrinsic affinity between all functioning TCRs and MHC molecules of a species, a concept originally developed for immunoglobulin and MHC molecules (Jerne 1971). The similarities of class I and class II MHC molecules provide compelling evidence for their derivation from a common ancestral molecule that also interacted with TCRs. That class I and class II molecules still interact with receptors derived from a common pool confirms this supposition and reveals that genes encoding functional class I and class II genes do not evolve in an independent fashion (Rupp et al. 1985).

Although MHC molecules and TCRs both interact with a diversity of antigenic peptides, their adaptations to the challenge of antigenic diversity are quite distinct. Somatic gene rearrangements permit large numbers of different and specific TCRs, each restricted to a small number of cells, to be expressed. In contrast, the genes encoding MHC molecules are somatically stable and constitutively expressed by all cells of a given type. Diversity in antigen presentation is, in part, accomplished by codominant expression of the products of multiple class I and class II MHC genes. A second critical factor is the relative degeneracy, a lack of specificity, of the peptide-combining site of MHC molecules (Guillet et al. 1986). The kinetics of MHC peptide interactions are quite different from those observed for most antigen–antibody interactions (Buus et al. 1987) and suggest that the MHC molecule may in fact fold around the peptide in a manner that is, ironically, reminiscent of theories of antigenic instruction proposed for immunoglobulins (Pauling 1940). The unique feature of MHC genes lies not with diversity within the individual but with diversity in populations and species. Certain MHC genes are characterized by large numbers of alleles and the absence of a dominant "wild-type allele," features rarely found in eukaryotic genes. The class I MHC genes in human populations (*HLA-A,B,C*) have been particularly well characterized and provide examples par excellence of polymorphic MHC genes. Currently, some 20 alleles at the *A* locus, 40 at the *B* locus, and 11 at the *C* locus have been defined; however, this is a minimal estimate, since the number of alleles continues to increase significantly as more sensitive methods are brought to the analysis (Dupont 1989).

Structural Analysis of Class I HLA-A,B,C Polymorphism

To understand the nature of the diversity, its generation, its contribution to the functional interactions of class I HLA molecules, and its evolutionary significance for the survival of populations requires structures for many alleles and their products. This effort was initiated in the early 1970s, and the first partial amino acid sequences were presented at the previous "immunological" symposium in this series (Strominger et al. 1976). Since that time, there has been a continuing acquisition of primary structural information using first protein chemistry and then cloning of cDNA and genes (for review, see Lew et al. 1986; Strachan 1987; Parham et al. 1989b).

Patterns of HLA-A,B,C Polymorphism

Human class I molecules consist of a polymorphic MHC-encoded heavy chain, an invariant β_2-microglobulin (β_2-m), and a variable, and as yet poorly characterized, bound peptide (Bjorkman et al. 1987a). In the *HLA* gene complex there are 17–20 class I heavy-chain genes, including various pseudogenes and gene fragments. Only six genes (*HLA-A, B, C, E, F*, and *G*) are known to make β_2-m-associated products, and of these only HLA-A,B,C show the broad tissue distribution characteristic of antigen-presenting molecules (Koller et al. 1989).

Over 50 HLA-A,B,C sequences have been determined and provide the data for analysis of diversity (for review, see Parham et al. 1988, 1989a). Alleles of a locus differ by 1–100 nucleotide substitutions that, although found throughout the sequence, are concentrated in exons 2 and 3, which encode the peptide-binding domains, α_1 and α_2. Alleles of different loci are readily distinguished by 62 locus-specific substitutions, mostly in exons 4–8 encoding the α_3, transmembrane, and cytoplasmic domains. Many positions in the amino acid sequence, perhaps as many as one third of the total, exhibit polymorphism, but at most of the variable positions there are only two or three different amino acids, and one residue is usually dominant. Twenty residues show high variability, exhibiting up to eight different amino acids, and these are at positions in the three-dimensional structure where the amino acid side chain is hypothesized to contact bound peptide or TCR (Bjorkman et al. 1987b; Parham et al. 1988). However, such positions are not all variable, an effect that is more vividly illustrated by class II HLA-DR molecules in which the half of the peptide-binding groove that is contributed by the α chain is totally invariant. The helical region of the α_1 domain shows the greatest variation and, by comparison, the helix of the α_2 domain is quite conserved. In contrast, the β strands of the α_2 domain have greater variability than the corresponding strands of the α_1 domain. Alignment and comparison of allelic sequences reveal a characteristic patchwork motif, due to the sharing of small clusters of substitutions in many different combinations (Fig. 1). This is most pronounced for exons 2 and 3 encoding the α_1 and α_2 domains of HLA-B molecules (Fig. 1A).

Our general strategy has been to isolate and sequence genomic or cDNA clones encoding complete HLA-A,B heavy chains. With recent refinements in technology (Saiki et al. 1988), it has become feasible to use the polymerase chain reaction (PCR) to obtain full-length cDNA clones encoding *HLA-A, B, C* genes. The strategy taken was to design oligonucleotide primers from sequences in the 5' and 3' untranslated regions that flank the coding sequence and are relatively conserved between *HLA-A, B, C* alleles (Fig. 2A). These primers were used to amplify single-stranded cDNA, synthesized from total cellular RNA prepared from human B-cell lines of known HLA type. The amplified product, which contains a mixture of alleles, is subcloned into M13 sequencing vectors using *Sal*I and *Hin*dIII sites incorporated into the amplification primers. Analysis of over 100 randomly picked clones from such "class I libraries" has shown them all to have full-length class I HLA sequences.

Because the goal is to obtain clones faithfully encoding HLA-A,B,C molecules, which can then be expressed and used in functional studies, the errors arising from PCR amplification become of critical importance. To assess the nature and frequency of errors, an initial experiment was designed to study *HLA-A, B* genes for which considerable information was already available but for which a complete determination of their sequences would prove useful. These are the *HLA-A2* and *HLA-B7* genes of the JY cell line, the products of which may represent the most extensively studied MHC molecules. Despite the wealth of information, including the crystallographic structure of HLA-A2 (Bjorkman et al. 1987a,b), the sequences of these proteins and the genes encoding them had yet to be completed (Orr et al. 1979a,b; Sood et al. 1985).

Clones were randomly picked from a PCR-amplified JY class I library, and on the basis of preliminary sequencing, were identified as encoding either HLA-A2 or HLA-B7. Ten clones for each gene, five from each orientation, were completely sequenced using four pairs of oligonucleotide primers (Fig. 2).

Compilation of the ten *HLA-A2* sequences gave a clear consensus identical to the coding sequence of the *HLA-A2* gene obtained from the LCL-721 cell line (Koller and Orr 1985). Sequences of four of the ten cDNA clones are identical to this consensus and thus represent faithful copies of the gene. Three of the remaining clones have single nucleotide substitutions, and one clone has three substitutions; however, none of these "errors" were found in more than one clone (Table 1). Two clones have hybrid sequences with a 5' part derived from *HLA-A2* and a 3' part from *HLA-B7*. Although appearing as recombinations, these clones presumably result from premature termination of the polymerase on one cycle, with subsequent reannealing of the unfinished A2 strand to a B7 template and completion of the strand in another cycle. The "recombination" points in the two clones are different, and one clone has an additional point substitution.

The pattern to emerge from the *HLA-B7* analysis is similar to that observed for *HLA-A2*. Three clones have sequences identical to the consensus obtained from all ten, with four clones having single nonidentical substitutions, one a single base-pair deletion, and two being "recombinants" with a 5' *B7* sequence and a 3'

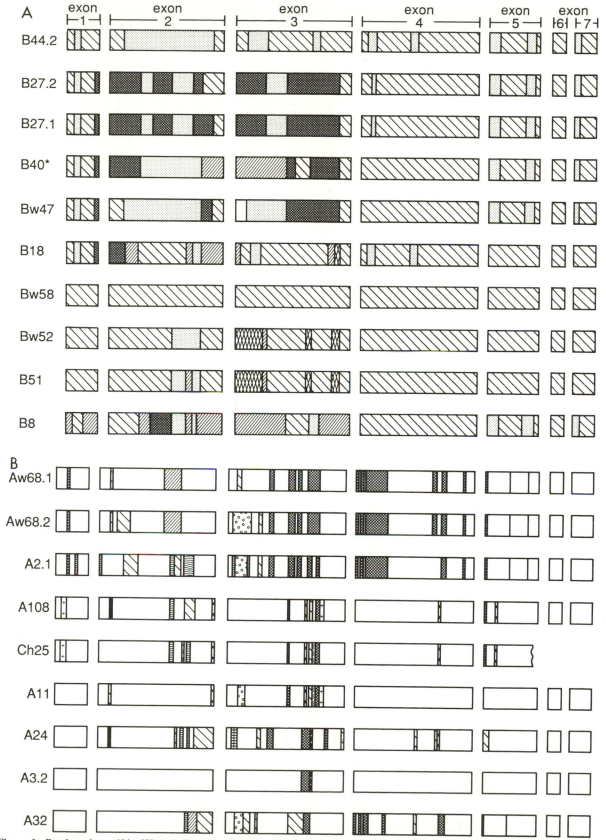

Figure 1. Patchwork motif in *HLA-A, B* sequences. The sequence relationships between representative *HLA-B* (panel *A*) and *HLA-A* (panel *B*) alleles are shown. Identical and closely related patterns of substitution are represented by similar shading. Two *ChLA-A* alleles, *A108* and *Ch25*, are included with the *HLA-A* alleles. The *Ch25* cDNA lacks exons 6 and 7 and part of exon 5.

Table 1. Analysis of PCR Errors Using B7 and A2 from the JY Cell Line

Allele	Clone	Differences from consensus
A2	1	685; G > A
	2	none
	6	none
	8	none
	9	none
	20	361; A > G, "recombination" with B7; 561–602, 652; A > G
	23	310; A > G, 538; T > C, 965; T > C
	25	recombination with B7; 917–932, 1050; T > C
	28	117; C > T
	29	293; A > G
B7	3	none
	4	none
	7	188; A > G
	10	218; C > T
	12	111; C > T, "recombination" with A2; 874–909
	21	recombination with A2; 653–734, 996; G > A
	22	914; C > T
	24	278; deletion
	26	none
	27	785; A > G

All misincorporations are transitions.

A2 sequence. One recombinant has an additional point substitution (Table 1). In contrast to the results with *HLA-A2*, the consensus sequence obtained from the *HLA-B7* clones is not identical to the cDNA sequence reported by Sood et al. (1985), since there are a total of 26 substitutions scattered throughout the coding sequence (Fig. 2B). It is likely that many, if not all, of the substitutions in the cDNA sequence are the result of sequencing errors. Comparison with over 50 *HLA-A,B,C* alleles shows that 22 of the 26 substitutions that distinguish the two B7 sequences are unique to the cDNA sequence of Sood et al. (1985), a number of unique substitutions significantly exceeding that found in any other allele. Also unusual is the fact that a majority of these substitutions (18 of 26) are silent, and only two of the seven amino acid differences are found in the extracellular domains. Comparison of other pairs of alleles always gives a predominance of replacement

over silent changes that are mostly found in exons encoding the extracellular domains (Parham et al. 1989a). Also of relevance is comparison of the B7 sequences with HLA-Bw42, a molecule found in black populations and serologically related to HLA-B7. Previous comparison of the protein sequences indicated that *HLA-Bw42* resulted from homologous recombination between *HLA-B7* and *-B8* genes (Parham et al. 1988). This was supported by nucleotide identity in exons 3–8 of the *HLA-B8* and *-Bw42* genes. It is now confirmed by the identity in exons 1 and 2 between *HLA-Bw42* and the PCR-derived sequence for *HLA-B7* (Fig. 2B). Errors have been found in another sequence by this group (Srivastava et al. 1989), and in the case of *HLA-B7*, an accumulation of erroneous silent substitutions might have resulted from reliance on the previously published protein sequence (Orr et al. 1979b) for interpretation of the sequencing gels.

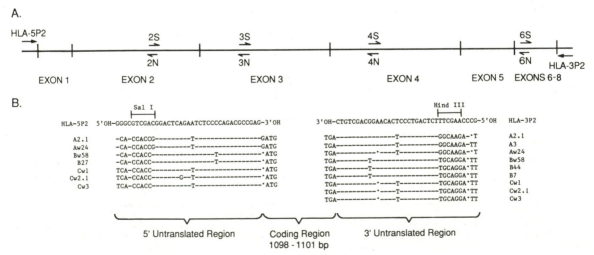

Figure 2. (*Continued on facing page.*)

C

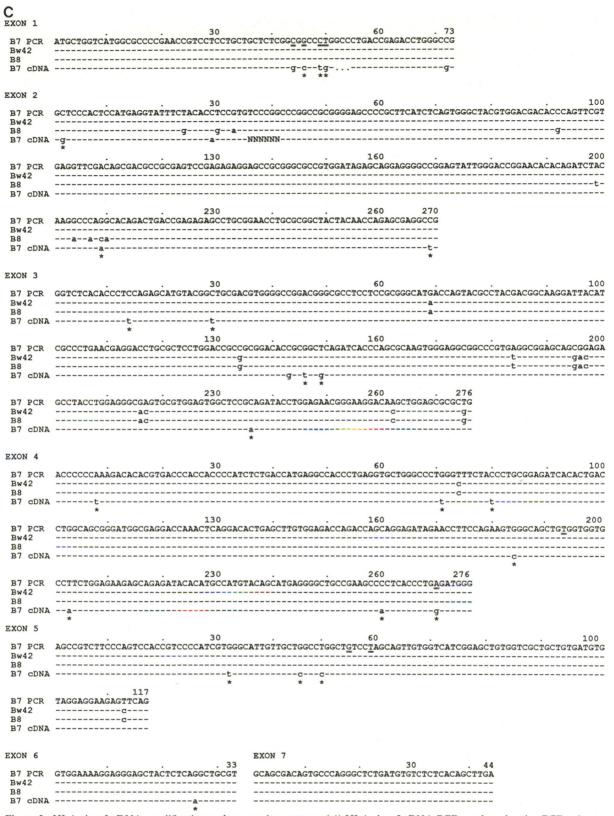

Figure 2. HLA class I cDNA amplification and sequencing strategy. (*A*) HLA class I cDNA PCR product showing PCR primers (large arrows), sequencing primers (small arrows), and exon boundaries (vertical lines). Arrowheads are at the 3′ OH end of each oligonucleotide primer and point in the direction of polymerase extension. Oligonucleotides 5P2, 2S, 3S, 4S, and 6S have sense strand sequence; 3P2, 6N, 4N, 3N, and 2N have RNA strand sequence. (*B*) Design of HLA class I cDNA PCR primers and alignment with representative *HLA-A, B,* and *C* sequences. Dashes indicate HLA-A,B,C nucleotide positions identical to HLA-5P2 and complementary to HLA-3P2. (●) Single-base gaps introduced for improved alignment. (*C*) Consensus nucleotide-coding sequence of 10 PCR clones derived from *HLA-B7* mRNA (B7-PCR) is compared to the exonic sequences of *HLA-Bw42* and *HLA-B8* genomic sequences and the *B7* cDNA sequence of Sood et al. (1985). Dashes indicate identity. (*) Substitutions found in the *B7* cDNA sequence and no other *HLA-B* locus allele. Coding substitutions are double underlined.

In conclusion, this PCR-based method gives authentic full-length class I cDNA clones with a frequency of about 30%. By comparison with conventional methods for isolation of class I cDNA, the advantages are that a full-length product is always obtained and that time is saved in the preparation and screening of libraries. One disadvantage is that multiple complete sequences must be obtained in order to determine a consensus sequence and select a faithful clone. Another is the rather high number of recombinant clones that could potentially confuse the identification of clones for previously uncharacterized alleles. Further optimization of conditions may enable the frequency of recombinant products to be reduced. Point substitutions pose less of a problem, and their frequency was low, a total of 15, all transitions being found in the 21,960 bp sequenced.

Generation of HLA-A,B,C Polymorphism

Evolutionary change results from a two-step process. First are the mutational events that create variation: in this case, new HLA-A,B,C alleles. Second are the selective events that can either eliminate new alleles or increase their frequency in the population. These include positive selection, negative or purifying selection, and neutral change through genetic drift. The conclusion to be drawn from comparison of sequences is that the extraordinary polymorphism of HLA-A,B,C genes does not stem from an unusually high rate of mutation or from specific targeting of special mutagenetic mechanisms. The difference between MHC and other genes is in selection for increased diversity that acts upon genes encoding antigen-presenting molecules (Jaulin et al. 1985; N'Guyen et al. 1985; Hughes and Nei 1988; Parham et al. 1989a). It is possible, as discussed below, that positive selection may also act to reduce polymorphism at MHC loci.

The evidence that the rate of mutation in HLA-A,B,C genes is comparable to that in other genes is as follows. No product of a new HLA-A,B,C mutation—where a child has a serological type not found in either parent—has ever been detected. If these genes were hypermutable, one would expect, in the course of the many HLA typings of families, that such novel types would have been found. *Homo sapiens* and *Pan troglodytes* (chimpanzees) are species that are estimated to have diverged between 3.7 and 7.7 million years ago (Sibley and Ahlquist 1984; Hasegawa et al. 1987). Comparison of HLA-A,B,C alleles with their chimpanzee homologs (ChLA-A,B,C) thus provides an assessment of the new mutations that have accumulated in each species during at least 3 million years of separate evolution. The result of such comparison is that (1) a majority of the polymorphisms, including silent substitutions, are common to alleles of the two species, (2) individual alleles of one species are more similar to particular alleles in the other species than to the majority of alleles from either species (Fig. 3), and (3) no species-specific features have been fixed in the alleles of

either species, although locus-specific features are shared by the corresponding alleles of both species. These observations show that much of the diversity in contemporary HLA-A,B,C genes was already present in the ancestral primate species that gave rise to humans and chimpanzees and was subsequently passed on to both species (Lawlor et al. 1988; Mayer et al. 1988). Since that time, the numbers of new polymorphisms accumulated, as most accurately assessed by silent substitutions, seem comparable to those found in other genes. These conclusions are reinforced by analysis of low-frequency subtypes of HLA-A,B molecules that are specific to particular human populations or races and represent newer alleles that originated in *Homo sapiens*. These alleles commonly differ from the more frequent subtype by a single or a small number of substitutions that can be accounted for by a single mutagenetic event. An example shown in Figure 2C is HLA-Bw42, which is specifically found in Africans and their descendants and results from an intragenic recombination between HLA-B7 and -B8 alleles.

Comparison of related alleles also permits an assessment of the nature of genetic events that produce new HLA-A,B,C alleles. The ultimate origin of all variation is, of course, in point mutations that occur in individual alleles; these are subsequently assorted into many different combinations by various recombinational mechanisms. In addition to single recombinations, as postulated in the formation of HLA-Bw42, there is considerable evidence for events that convert a short segment of sequence from one allele or gene into the homologous sequence found in another.

A common feature of eukaryotic genes is homogeneity in sequence within species but divergence between species. For example, although β_2-m is nonpolymorphic within humans, there are 96 nucleotide substitutions in the coding region between human and murine β_2-m (Suggs et al. 1981; Parnes and Seidman 1982). Although some of these species differences may be adaptive, it is also likely that others, including the 51 silent substitutions, are neutral changes resulting from genetic drift. The question then becomes why greater amounts of neutral polymorphism in protein like β_2-m are not found more frequently within species. This suggests that there are mechanisms that, in the absence of selection for diversity, will tend to homogenize alleles. The accumulating evidence indicates that nonreciprocal gene conversion events are a common, and possibly a general, feature of mammalian genes (Smithies and Powers 1986; Dover and Strachan 1987) that can act to homogenize or diversify a set of homologous sequences. In most genes, it may act as a mechanism for homogenization, as seems true for the 3′ exons (4–8) of HLA-A,B,C genes (Parham et al. 1989a). For example, within exon 4 encoding the α_3 domain, there are 13 silent (and 4 coding) substitutions that are invariant between alleles of a locus but differ between the HLA-A,B,C loci. That such presumably neutral substitutions are fixed in a family of alleles with highly divergent 5′ sequences is most readily explained in terms

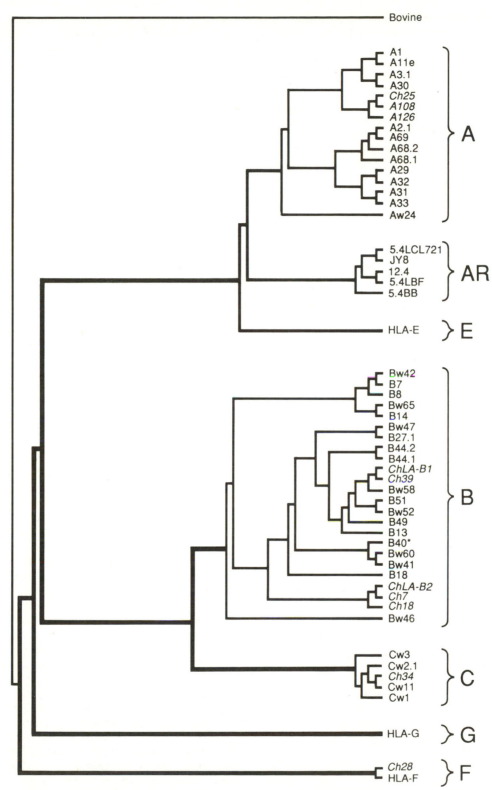

Figure 3. Tree based on parsimony depicting the relationships between human and chimpanzee class I alleles of the MHC. Analysis of the complete nucleotide sequence for the coding region of 55 alleles was initially performed by the heuristic methods of the PAUP (Swofford) program. Gaps were inserted in exon 5 as per Needleman and Wunsch (1970) to ensure optimal alignment. This inexact search produced 32 most parsimonious trees with a length of 1256. The overall consistency index was 0.536. Discrepant branching orders were resolved by using more rigorous algorithms, branch and bound and alltrees, with distinct subsets of the alleles. Data were considered unordered, and bovine sequence BL3-6 served as the outgroup to root the tree. Sequences and primary references are as in Mayer et al. (1988), Parham et al. (1989a), Trapani et al. (1989), and J. Zemmour et al. (in prep.). We thank Bo Dupont and Soo Young Yang for unpublished results.

of homogenization by localized, homologous, non-reciprocal conversions between alleles.

In contrast, the 5' exons (1, 2, and 3) exhibit a characteristic patchwork pattern of substitution that is indicative of diversification again through the agency of conversions and/or double recombinations (Fig. 1). The evidence for positive selection for diversity in the 5' exons is the relative frequency of replacement to silent substitutions, which is much greater than would be expected if the substitutions were random (Jaulin et al. 1985; N'Guyen et al. 1985; Parham et al. 1989a). This difference is particularly striking if one differentiates between functional and nonfunctional positions of diversity, as assigned from interpretation of the crystallographic structure of HLA-A2 (Bjorkman et al. 1987b; Hughes and Nei 1988). Furthermore, the frequency of the dinucleotide CpG within the 5' exons is much greater than in the 3' exons and most other eukaryotic genes. In the absence of sequence-specific selection, CpG sequences tend to mutate through specific methylation and deamination; thus, their preservation is also a marker of positive selection (Tykocinski and Max 1984).

In addition to conversion between alleles of the $HLA-A, B,$ or C loci, there is also evidence for conversions between alleles of different class I MHC loci; a particularly striking example is provided by HLA-Bw46, which has an α_1 helix donated by the linked $HLA-Cw11$ gene (Parham et al. 1989a,b). In contrast to murine class I MHC genes (Nathenson et al. 1986), where it has been a major source of diversification, this mechanism has been a minor contributor to contemporary $HLA-A, B, C$ diversity (Parham et al. 1988, 1989b). A consequence of the predominance of interallelic rather than intergenic conversion is that considerable divergence in both the conserved and polymorphic parts of the products of the $HLA-A, B,$ and C loci has occurred.

The divergence of structure in products of the $HLA-A, B, C$ loci may have functional implications. Differences in the α_1 and α_2 contribute specialization in the types of peptide bound, whereas α_3 differences affect the affinity for CD8. Extensive locus-specific differences in the transmembrane and cytoplasmic domains may determine interactions with membrane and cytoplasmic components, perhaps providing signals that distinguish the intracellular trafficking or recycling of the products of the different loci. These are critical and outstanding questions to be addressed.

Do T-cell Responses Determine the Rise and Fall of MHC Genes?

An individual's potential for T-cell responses is determined by the repertoire of peptides that can be presented and the repertoire of TCRs that can respond. The number of different MHC molecules expressed by an individual has effects on both parameters.

Greater diversity in MHC molecules, and in particular of their peptide-binding sites, enables larger num-bers of peptides to be presented; it is this effect that creates the positive evolutionary selection for MHC polymorphism and diversity. Multiple homologous, codominantly expressed loci and extensive polymorphism at these loci both contribute to increased capacity for antigen presentation.

In contrast to this simple effect upon antigen presentation, the influence of increased numbers of MHC molecules on the T-cell repertoire is complex, involving both positive and negative components (Marrack and Kappler 1988). The receptors of immature T cells are stringently selected on the basis of their interactions with MHC/peptide complexes encountered in the thymus. Although this process is poorly understood, it is thought that cells having either too weak or too strong an interaction with any self-MHC molecule are eliminated, whereas receptors of positively selected cells are of an intermediate affinity. Increasing the diversity of MHC molecules in the thymus can therefore lead to diminution of the T-cell repertoire, a thesis supported by the high frequency of alloreactive cells in mature T-cell populations and by studies with transgenic mice (Kappler et al. 1987). Each additional class I or class II molecule expressed in the thymus results in the deletion of T cells that are potentially autoreactive against that MHC molecule, but might otherwise have been positively selected for interaction with another MHC molecule. Thus, the necessity for self-tolerance means that each individual MHC molecule has the negative effect of reducing the repertoire of receptors restricted to all other MHC molecules (Matzinger et al. 1984) (Fig. 4). That class I and class II MHC-restricted T cells appear to draw their receptors from the same pool (Rupp et al. 1985) suggests there will be evolutionary interplay between the numbers of expressed class I and class II MHC products and the repertoires of class-I-restricted (mostly cytotoxic) and class-II-restricted (mostly helper) T cells. Compromise between the positive effects on antigen presentation and the negative effects on T-cell repertoire may explain why the number of class I and class II loci expressed by any individual in all species examined is limited. This burden of tolerance is not felt at the level of populations, where the advantage of increased antigen presentation can lead to greater and greater polymorphism in MHC loci.

The relationships between T cells that are positively or negatively selected by different MHC molecules suggest how evolutionary selection for advantageous immune responses, provided by particular MHC alleles or loci, could result in the reduction of polymorphism, expression, and functionality of other MHC alleles and loci. Thus, as the antigenic environment changes, there will be selection for certain MHC alleles and loci and against others. The $HLA-AR$ and $HLA-C$ loci discussed in the next section both have features suggesting that they were once selected for antigen presentation but are now in varying states of decline. The alternative to somatic deletion of the T-cell clone can thus become evolutionary deletion of the MHC molecule. An exam-

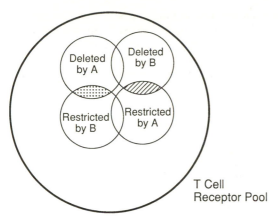

Figure 4. Cartoon showing the total TCR pool and the subsets of receptors affected by MHC molecules from two different loci, A and B. For each MHC locus there is a set of receptors that are negatively selected, and, as a consequence, the cells expressing those receptors are deleted. In addition, there is a set of receptors that are positively selected, and cells expressing those receptors enter the mature T-cell pool. Overlap between the receptors that would be positively selected by one MHC molecule and negatively selected by the other is indicated by shading. Since negative selection is dominant over positive selection, both these populations would be deleted in individuals expressing MHC A and B. If potential T-cell responses using receptors in either shaded area were particularly advantageous, there would be selection for elimination of the MHC locus responsible for the negative selection. Identical arguments can be applied to individual alleles of either the same or different loci.

ple of such a process in action is perhaps provided by the striking deletion of clones expressing $V_\beta 17$ T-cell receptors by I-E molecules in mice (Kappler et al. 1987). Elimination of I-E expression in certain H-2 haplotypes, and by a variety of different mutations (Mathis et al. 1983), releases $V_\beta 17$-containing receptors from deletion and makes them available for positive thymic selection by other MHC molecules. The differences in the numbers and polymorphism of expressed class I and class II loci in different species and in different strains of mice provide evidence for the dynamic nature of the MHC, adapting to the demands of T-cell immunity imposed by everchanging antigenic environments (Flavell et al. 1986).

Balancing of the repertoires selected by different MHC molecules means that class I molecules will influence the class-II-restricted T-cell repertoire and vice versa. Selection upon such interplay could result in linkage disequilibrium, as frequently observed between particular HLA alleles (Dupont 1989); it may also be responsible for the Syrian hamster having monomorphic class I loci and polymorphic class II loci (Streilein 1987). In an environment such as that inhabited by the Syrian hamster, in which viruses appear not to be a problem, the reduction in class I polymorphism may be in part a consequence of selection for greater diversity in class-II-restricted responses. Evidence for the changing fortunes of MHC genes can also be found in the HLA region.

HLA-AR: A Defunct Class I Antigen-presenting Gene

HLA-AR (also called 12.4 and 5.4p) is closely linked on chromosome 6 to *HLA-A* (Malissen et al. 1982; Pontarotti et al. 1988; Koller et al. 1989), and the sequences of *HLA-AR* alleles are most closely related to *HLA-A* alleles (Fig. 3). For example, *HLA-AR* alleles show identity to *HLA-A* at 47 of 62 locus-specific nucleotides that have been defined on the basis of *HLA-A,B,C* sequences. It is therefore likely that *HLA-A* and *HLA-AR* resulted from duplication of an ancestral gene, and the descendant of that duplication is now fixed in the human population. The remarkable fact is that whereas all contemporary *HLA-A* alleles are expressed and believed to function in antigen presentation, all *HLA-AR* alleles are pseudogenes. Six *HLA-AR* alleles have been sequenced, and they all have a phenylalanine encoded at position 164 instead of the cysteine that forms the essential disulfide bond of the α_2 domain (J. Zemmour et al., in prep.). In addition, five of the six alleles have a single nucleotide deletion at codon 227 in the α_3 domain. This causes a frameshift and premature termination at codon 272. If it were not for these deleterious changes, the sequences would appear to be those of functional class I HLA molecules, indicating that they were previously under selection for antigen presentation. For example, polymorphic substitutions are predominantly found in exons 2 and 3. Thus, it is likely that the duplication that led to *HLA-A* and *HLA-AR* was of a functioning allele and that in the initial period of its history, *HLA-AR* was a functioning locus. What sequence of events can have led to its downfall?

The occurrence of identical deleterious mutations in *HLA-AR* alleles by convergent evolution is improbable. It is more likely that each of the two mutations was produced once and that fixation has occurred by introduction of the mutation into other alleles through nonreciprocal conversion and by propagation of the mutant alleles. The fact that a deleterious mutation became fixed suggests that a historic change in selection took place, with the result that there was no longer any advantage to be obtained from the presentation of antigens by HLA-AR molecules, and that subsequently there may have been positive selection for their elimination. Such positive selection could derive from advantageous immune responses mediated by T cells that could only survive thymic selection in the absence of HLA-AR proteins. The causative change in selection upon the *HLA-AR* locus could have resulted from alterations in the antigenic environment, from the development of new alleles at other MHC loci that more effectively presented critical antigens, from changes in the TCR gene repertoire, or from some combination of these factors.

Once the positive functional selection on a class I locus like *HLA-AR* has been removed, it will begin to decline. Point mutations slowly accumulate; the action of conversion events, in the absence of selection for diversity, will be to homogenize and reduce poly-

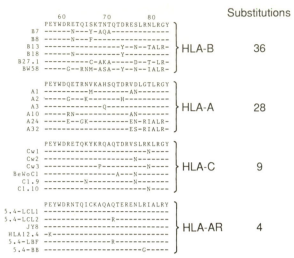

Figure 5. The amino acid sequence in the α helix of the α₁ domain for six HLA-AR, HLA-C, HLA-A, and HLA-B molecules is shown. This helix is the most variable region in class I antigen-presenting molecules. Although HLA-AR molecules are closely related to HLA-A through most of the molecule, they show greatest similarity with certain HLA-B alleles in this region.

morphism. This can be seen from comparison of the *HLA-AR* and *HLA-A* loci. For example, the α helix of the α₁ domain, which is the most variable part of HLA-A molecules, is quite homogeneous in HLA-AR (Fig. 5). The power of conversion events to homogenize alleles is suggested by the presence of both deleterious mutations in five of the six alleles. These mutations presumably had independent origins in different alleles, and it is unlikely that their combination would confer any selective advantage. Probably they have been combined through selectively neutral conversion events.

Nonclassical Class I Genes

These observations on the *HLA-AR* locus illustrate that conservation of sequence or lack of polymorphism in MHC alleles need not imply that the sequences are under positive selection for function. In this case, homogenization, or loss of diversity, may be the consequence of loss of function. What else might happen to MHC genes that are no longer useful? In a situation where selection is favoring the reduction of class I or class II diversity expressed by an individual, there are various mutational changes that could be advantageous, and not all would result in production of an obvious pseudogene like *HLA-AR*. Their critical feature would be to remove the influence of an MHC gene upon the repertoire of TCRs. One way to do this is to select for mutations that alter the patterns of tissue expression in such a way that expression on critical cells in the thymus is lost. This could result in class I genes with rather specific and different patterns of tissue expression such as *Tla*, *Qa* antigens and *HLA-F*. A second way is to prevent expression at the cell surface,

perhaps by sequestering the genes within the cell as found for *HLA-E* and *G* or by secretion as occurs for *Q10* (Chen et al. 1987; Robinson 1987; Koller et al. 1989). Thus, many nonclassical genes have properties predicted for inactivating mutations of antigen-presenting loci. These properties, combined with the lack of any known function for the products of nonclassical class I genes and the lack of correspondence between the nonclassical genes of different species (Rogers 1985), strongly suggest that these molecules are nonfunctional and are the products of genes in decline (Klein and Figueroa 1986). Of course, this does not prevent their participation in gene conversion events as observed in the mouse (Nathenson et al. 1986), but this function, as such, will be used infrequently and by a very small minority of individuals.

HLA-C: A Declining Class I Gene?

Cellular interactions are dependent on the density of the contributing cell-surface molecules, and another possible mechanism for extinguishing the role of an MHC gene in thymic selection is to reduce the level of cell-surface expression. Perhaps this is what happened to the *HLA-C* locus, the products of which are found at the cell surface at about one tenth the level of HLA-A and HLA-B molecules. Supporting the view that HLA-C molecules are in decline is the reduced diversity, especially in the α₁ helix (Fig. 5). *HLA-C* and *HLA-B* alleles have closely related sequences and are clearly the products of a gene duplication (Fig. 3). Despite this common origin, the nature of polymorphism in contemporary *HLA-B* and *C* alleles is significantly different. *HLA-B* has many more alleles with greater diversification in sequence and with substitutions concentrated at positions directly involved in contacting bound peptide and the TCR. *HLA-C* has fewer alleles differing by smaller numbers of substitutions, which are frequently at positions distant from the combining site groove. Reinforcing suspicions that HLA-C contributes little to human immunity is the absence of evidence showing antigen presentation by HLA-C to human T cells. That HLA-C molecules are still capable of antigen presentation function has been demonstrated by experiments with transgenic mice (Dill et al. 1988); whether there are sufficient HLA-C-restricted T cells for it to happen with any frequency in the human immune response is another matter.

HLA-B Polymorphism Is Bigger, but Is It Better Than That of *HLA-A*?

It is thus possible that the only human class I loci that encode functional antigen-presenting molecules are *HLA-A* and *HLA-B*. (However, even for these loci the actual number of allelic products that have been shown to present a peptide to a T cell is a minority). Major differences in the patterns of polymorphism are observed and suggest that the two loci are following distinct evolutionary paths.

There are many more *HLA-B* than *HLA-A* alleles, and they exhibit greater diversification of sequence in the peptide-binding domains and greater homogeneity of sequence in the α_3, transmembrane, and cytoplasmic domains. Comparison of human and chimpanzee sequences reveals greater similarity between *A* than *B* alleles in the two species (Parham et al. 1989a), showing that new polymorphisms have accumulated at a higher rate in *HLA-B* compared to *HLA-A*. A final difference is the existence of a high-frequency allele at the A locus, *HLA-A2*, for which there is no equivalent at the B locus. This, combined with the smaller number of *HLA-A* alleles, increases homozygosity at the *HLA-A* locus.

There are two ways of interpreting these observations. The first is to argue that decreased *HLA-A* polymorphism and diversity are the result of negative effects due to selection at another MHC locus, in a manner analogous to that hypothesized for *HLA-AR*. In this view, *HLA-A* is perceived as being in relative decline, and the high frequency of *HLA-A2* need not be associated with any particular advantage. The second view is that the relative conservation of *HLA-A* alleles is because their products are critical for immune responses against prevalent and important pathogens. In this view, *HLA-A* becomes a more optimized locus and *HLA-A2* a particularly advantageous allele. Adding to this interesting puzzle is the noticeable absence of HLA-A2 in chimpanzees (Balner et al. 1978).

Binding of CD8 to Class I MHC Antigens

Two other molecules intimately involved in the function of MHC-restricted T cells are the CD4 and CD8 glycoproteins (for review, see Littman 1987; Parnes 1989). CD4 defines T cells reactive with class II MHC molecules, and CD8 defines T cells reactive with class I MHC molecules. The derivation of both class-I- and class-II-restricted TCRs from a common pool suggests that CD8 or CD4 expression is tightly coordinated to the restriction specificity of mature T cells and that these molecules play an essential role in thymic selection (for review, see Janeway 1988). In addition, the inhibitory effects of monoclonal antibodies in in vitro assays suggested CD4 and CD8 were important for effector functions of T lymphocytes, a supposition that has subsequently been demonstrated by transfection experiments (Dembic et al. 1986). The molecular basis for these functions has been hypothesized to lie with a specific interaction between CD4 or CD8 and monomorphic sites of class I or class II MHC molecules, respectively (Swain 1981). Such interactions could contribute to adhesion between T cells and antigen-presenting cells—both in the thymus and in the periphery—and also to transmembrane signalling events that determine T-cell function following antigen recognition.

To test these ideas, an in vitro cell-binding assay to detect specific interactions between CD8 and class I MHC molecules was developed (Norment et al. 1988). Its principle is the binding of cells in suspension, which are radioactively labeled and express class I molecules, to a monolayer of attached cells expressing CD8 (Fig. 6). Class I genes are transfected into CIR, a mutant human B-cell line that expresses no endogenous HLA-A,B molecules. (It does express low levels of class I molecules, which are thought to be HLA-C; however, they have no effect on the binding assay). Transfectants of CHO cells, which have no endogenous expression of CD8, are the source of CD8. Specific binding, which is

CD8 Binding Assay

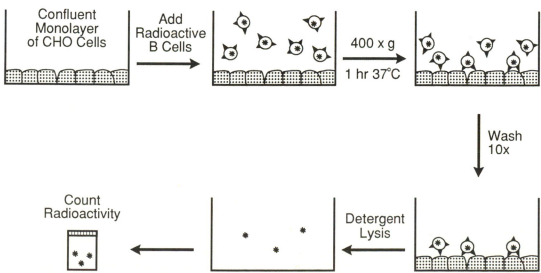

Figure 6. Cartoon of the cell–cell binding assay used to analyze the interaction between CD8 and class I MHC molecules (Norment et al. 1988).

assessed by control experiments with untransfected cells, is dependent on high levels of expression of the transfected genes. This indicates that the affinity of individual CD8 and class I MHC molecules is low and that the specific binding between cells is dependent on multipoint attachment. Background binding is relatively high and leads to signal to noise ratios of 3–10. In addition to controls with untransfected cells, the specific binding can also be assessed by using monoclonal antibodies directed against either class I MHC or CD8 as inhibitors.

Comparison of a panel of CIR transfectants, each expressing a different class I MHC molecule, produced two interesting findings (Salter et al. 1989). First, two murine class I molecules (H-2K^b and H-D^p) bound human CD8 as well as HLA-A,B molecules. Second, two closely related HLA-A molecules, HLA-Aw68.1 and HLA-Aw68.2, do not bind CD8 in this assay. This demonstration of polymorphism upsets the prevailing paradigm that classical class I molecules have a monomorphic CD8-binding site. The question of differential affinities of CD8 binding within the group of positive binding molecules is also open, since the assay is only

qualitative and the significance of the quantitative differences seen in binding is uncertain.

The discovery that HLA-Aw68.1 does not bind CD8 was extremely fortunate, since this molecule has been crystallized, and its structure has been determined. It differs at only 13 residues in the three extracellular domains from HLA-A2.1, the other MHC molecule for which an X-ray structure is available (Bjorkman et al. 1985, 1987a). These two molecules thus provide an excellent system with which to map the site of interaction between CD8 and the class I MHC molecule. Site-directed mutagenesis of *HLA-A2.1* and *HLA-Aw68.1* genes has shown that the amino acid at position 245 in the α_3 domain is solely responsible for the difference in CD8 binding between HLA-A2.1 and HLA-Aw68.1 molecules (Salter et al. 1989). This residue, which is alanine in HLA-A2.1 and all other antigen-presenting class I molecules so far sequenced, is replaced by valine in HLA-Aw68.1 and the other nonbinding molecule, HLA-Aw68.2. These results, indicating that the α_3 domain is important for CD8 interaction, are supported by observations that a mutant H-2D^d molecule, with substitution of lysine for aspartic

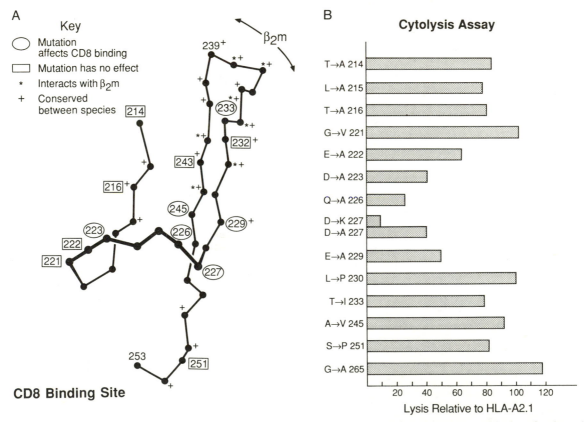

Figure 7. Mutagenesis of the α_3 domain affects CD8 binding and T-cell recognition. (*A*) Approximate positioning of amino acids 214–253 comprising β strands 3, 4, and 5 of the α_3 domain. This is viewed from the opposite side to the common representation as depicted in Fig. 2a of Bjorkman et al. (1987a) and Fig. 5B of Bjorkman et al. (1987b). Positions at which point mutations of HLA-A2.1 eliminate CD8 binding are circled and those that have no effect are in squares. Positions identified by Bjorkman et al. (1987a) as contacting β_2-m are indicated by asterisks, and the general positioning of β_2-m is shown with arrows. Residues that are conserved in class I molecules from different species are indicated by plus signs. (*B*) Lysis by a clone AMSH10 of alloreactive HLA-A2-specific cytotoxic T cells of CIR cells transfected with mutant HLA-A2 molecules having substitutions shown at the left. The lysis is given relative to target cells transfected with wild-type HLA-A2.1.

acid at position 227, cannot be recognized by CD8-dependent cytotoxic T cells (CTL) (Connolly et al. 1988; Potter et al. 1989). Residue 245, which is on the fifth strand of β sheet of the α_3 domain, is within 10.5 Å of residue 227, which is found on the loop between the third and fourth strands (Fig. 7A). This region of the α_3 domain is relatively exposed in the structure of HLA-A2 and could be accessible for binding to a protein the size of CD8.

To further investigate the class I/CD8 interaction, additional point mutations in the α_3 domain have been studied (Fig. 7A). As observed for H-2D^d, the introduction of lysine at position 227 eliminates CD8 binding, as do other mutations at positions 223, 226, 229, and 233 in this region of the α_3 domain. In contrast, more distant mutations at positions 214, 216, 221, 222, 232, 243, and 251 have no effect, as is also seen with various mutations in residues of the α_1 and α_2 domains. Clustering of mutations that eliminate CD8 binding to a region around the carboxy-terminal part of the loop, between strands 3 and 4, indicates that this part of the α_3 domain is involved in directly contacting the CD8 molecule. The sequence of the loop from residues 220 to 229—Asp.Gly.Glu.Asp.Gln.Thr.Gln.Asp.Thr.Glu.—is noticeably acidic, and mutations that remove acidic residues generally lead to loss of CD8 binding. The importance of acidic residues is also suggested by a mutant in which an additional acidic residue was introduced at position 221 and gave increased CD8 binding.

The effects observed in the CD8-binding assay can be correlated with recognition and cytolysis by T cells. Molecules that have lost CD8 binding are less efficiently recognized by CTL (Fig. 7B).

These results focus attention on the subtypes of HLA-Aw68 and the function of these molecules in antigen presentation. Experiments to prime alloreactive and antigen-specific CTL with HLA-Aw68 have been negative. However, and as found for the H-2D^d mutant, CTL that are primed with a cross-reactive molecule, such as HLA-A2 or HLA-Aw69, can in a secondary response react with HLA-Aw68 (Gaston et al. 1985). These results suggest that the loss in CD8 binding reduces the capacity of HLA-Aw68 to select for T cells in the thymus. As such, HLA-Aw68 appears to be a molecule that has lost, or is losing, function and may provide another example of a mechanism that is being used to reduce the polymorphism and functional effect of an MHC locus, in this case HLA-A. Alternatively, the loss of CD8 binding may lead to a functional advantage, perhaps the selection of higher-affinity T cells, which have so far eluded detection. Answers to these questions will come from further study of the capacity of HLA-Aw68 to bind peptides and interact with T cells.

The location of the CD8-binding site of class I MHC molecules has been a topic for speculation. On the basis of similarities between the immunoglobulin-like domains of CD8 and the variable regions of TCR, Davis and Bjorkman (1988) proposed that CD8 interacts with class I molecules in a manner analogous to the TCR

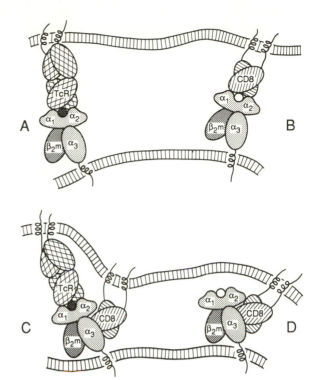

Figure 8. Cartoon of hypothesized interactions between class I MHC molecules, CD8 and the TCR. *A* and *B* are as depicted by Davis and Bjorkman (1988). *(A)* Interaction between TCR, a specific peptide (●), and the α_1 and α_2 domains of class I MHC molecules. *(B)* The analogous interaction of the V-like domains of CD8 with the α_1 and β_2 domains of class I MHC, which has nonspecific peptide bound (○). *C* and *D* give possible interactions if the α_3 domain of class I MHC molecules provides the binding site of CD8. *(C)* TCR and CD8 both binding to the complex of class I MHC and specific peptide; *(D)* CD8 interacting with the complex of class I MHC and nonspecific peptide.

(Fig. 8A,B). If this is true, then CD8 and a TCR could not simultaneously interact with the same class I MHC molecule (Fig. 8C). Our results with the CD8/class I MHC cell-binding assay implicate a localized region of the α_3 domain in the binding site of CD8 (Fig. 8D) and argue against a direct involvement of the helices of the α_1 and α_2 domains as hypothesized previously (Davis and Bjorkman 1988). This leaves open the possibility of simultaneous interaction of CD8 and TCR, with the identical class I MHC molecule being the critical interaction that initiates T-cell responses (Fig. 8C).

CONCLUDING REMARKS

A characteristic of class I MHC molecules is their diversity and polymorphism. Comparison of allelic sequences in humans and chimpanzees shows that diversity is accumulated gradually over the lifetimes of many species and does not involve any unusual mechanisms or rates of mutation that are specific to these genes. Rather, it is the unique nature of the evolutionary selection for advantageous T-cell immunity that is responsible for the diversity. Variation is found through-out the molecule and affects the interactions of class I MHC molecules with antigenic peptides, TCRs, the CD8 proteins, and possibly other cellular components. Combined analysis of natural variants and site-directed mutants is enabling the functional sites of class I molecules involved in these interactions to be mapped.

Within the individual, MHC diversity probably has two opposing effects on T-cell immunity, which serve to limit the numbers and polymorphism of MHC loci expressed. These are increased antigen presentation due to diversity in peptide-binding domains (α_1 and α_2) and decreased TCR repertoire due to the establishment of self-tolerance. The limiting effect of self-tolerance is not imposed on populations, and diversity for antigen presentation becomes the dominant effect and can lead to extraordinary polymorphism. That MHC molecules can both present antigens and delete T cells means that, depending on the antigenic environment, there can be evolutionary selection for the presence or elimination of particular MHC alleles or loci. This can result in the advantageous diversification, homogenization, or extinction of particular loci. Examples of different patterns of polymorphism at four human class I MHC loci support this thesis. Since receptors restricted by all MHC loci—class I and class II—are derived from the same pool, polymorphisms at any one locus will affect the functional potential at other loci. In essence, the different MHC molecules are in competition with each other. Thus, positive selection for responses that are restricted by one MHC molecule, or set of molecules, can result in the elimination of others. Such a dynamic functional interplay between the products of different MHC loci should result in the continuing, but gradual, rise and fall of polymorphism and functionality at different MHC loci in response to changing antigenic conditions. This can explain the remarkable diversity in the numbers of MHC loci and their expression between species and populations.

REFERENCES

Balner, H., W. van Vreeswijk, J.H. Roger, and J. D'Amaro. 1978. The major histocompatibility complex of chimpanzees: Identification of several new antigens controlled by the A and B loci of ChLA. *Tissue Antigens* 12: 1.

Bjorkman, P.J., J.L. Strominger, and D.C. Wiley. 1985. Crystallization and X-ray diffraction studies on the histocompatibility antigens HLA-A2 and HLA-A28 from human cell membranes. *J. Mol. Biol.* 186: 205.

Bjorkman, P.J., M.A. Saper, B. Samraoui, W.S. Bennett, J.L. Strominger, and D.C. Wiley. 1987a. Structure of the human class I histocompatibility antigen, HLA-A2. *Nature* 329: 506.

———. 1987b. The foreign antigen binding site and T cell recognition regions of class I histocompatibility antigens. *Nature* 329: 512.

Buus, S., A. Sette, S.M. Colon, C. Miles, and H.M. Grey. 1987. The relation between major histocompatibility complex (MHC) and the capacity of Ia to bind immunogenic peptides. *Science* 235: 1353.

Chen, Y.-T., Y. Obata, E. Stockert, T. Takahashi, and L.J.

Old. 1987. Tla-region genes and their products. *Immunol. Res.* 6: 30.

Connolly, J.M., T.A. Potter, E.-M. Wormstall, and T.H. Hansen. 1988. The Lyt-2 molecule recognizes residues in the class I α_3 domain in allogeneic cytotoxic T cell responses. *J. Exp. Med.* 168: 325.

Davis, M.M. and P.J. Bjorkman. 1988. T-cell antigen receptor genes and T-cell recognition. *Nature* 334: 395.

Dembic, Z., W. Haas, S. Weiss, J. McCubrey, H. Kiefer, H. von Boehmer, and M. Steinmetz. 1986. Transfer of specificity by murine α and β T-cell receptor genes. *Nature* 320: 232.

Dill, O., F. Kievits, S. Koch, P. Ivanyi, and G.J. Hammerling. 1988. Immunological function of HLA-C antigens in HLA-Cw3 transgenic mice. *Proc. Natl. Acad. Sci.* 85: 5664.

Dover, G.A. and T. Strachan. 1987. Molecular drive in the evolution of the immune superfamily of genes: The initiation and spread of novelty. In *Evolution and vertebrate immunity* (ed. G. Kelsoe and D.H. Schulze), p. 15. University of Texas Press, Austin.

Dupont, B., ed. 1989. *Immunobiology of HLA*, vol. 1: *Histocompatibility testing 1987*. Springer-Verlag, New York.

Flavell, R.A., H. Allen, C.C. Burkly, D.H. Sherman, G.L. Waneck, and G. Widera. 1986. Molecular biology of the H-2 histocompatibility complex. *Science* 233: 437.

Gaston, J.S.H., A.B. Rickinson, and M.A. Epstein. 1985. The role of HLA antigens in the control of the cytotoxic T-cell response to Epstein-Barr virus: A family study. *Cell. Immunol.* 94: 231.

Guillet, J.-G., M.-Z. Lai, T.J. Briner, J.A. Smith, and M.L. Gefter. 1986. Interaction of peptide antigens and class II major histocompatibility complex antigens. *Nature* 324: 260.

Hasegawa, M., H. Kishino, and T. Yano. 1987. Man's place in Hominoidea as inferred from molecular clocks of DNA. *J. Mol. Evol.* 26: 132.

Hedrick, S.M. 1988. Specificity of the T cell receptor for antigen. *Adv. Immunol.* 43: 193.

Hughes, A.L. and M. Nei. 1988. Patterns of nucleotide substitution at major histocompatibility complex class I loci reveals overdominant selection. *Nature* 335: 167.

Janeway, C.A. 1988. Accessories or coreceptors? *Nature* 335: 208.

Jaulin, C., A. Perrin, J.P. Abastado, B. Duman, J. Papamatheakis, and P. Kourilsky. 1985. Polymorphism in mouse and human class I H-2 and HLA genes is not the result of random independent point mutations. *Immunogenetics* 22: 453.

Jerne, N.K. 1971. The somatic generation of immune recognition. *Eur. J. Immunol.* 1: 1.

Kappler, J.W., N. Roehm, and P. Marrack. 1987. T cell tolerance by clonal elimination in the thymus. *Cell* 49: 273.

Klein, J. and F. Figueroa. 1986. Evolution of the major histocompatibility complex. *CRC Crit. Rev. Immunol.* 6: 295.

Koller, B.H. and H.T. Orr. 1985. Cloning and complete sequence of an HLA-A2 gene: Analysis of two HLA-A alleles at the nucleotide level. *J. Immunol.* 134: 2727.

Koller, B.H., D.E. Geraghty, R. DeMars, L. Duvick, S.S. Rich, and H.T. Orr. 1989. Chromosomal organization of the human major histocompatibility complex class I gene family. *J. Exp. Med.* 169: 469.

Lawlor, D.A., F.E. Ward, P.D. Ennis, A.P. Jackson, and P. Parham. 1988. HLA-A and B polymorphisms predate the divergence of humans and chimpanzees. *Nature* 335: 268.

Lew, A.M., E.P. Lillehoj, E.P. Cowan, W.L. Maloy, M.R. van Schravendijk, and J.E. Coligan. 1986. Class I genes and molecules: An update. *Immunology* 57: 3.

Littman, D.R. 1987. The structure of the CD4 and CD8 genes. *Annu. Rev. Immunol.* 5: 561.

Long, E.O. and S. Jacobson. 1989. Pathways of viral antigen processing and presentation to CTL: Defined by the mode of virus entry. *Immunol. Today* 10: 45.

Malissen, M., B. Malissen, and B.R. Jordan. 1982. Exon/

intron organization and complete nucleotide sequence of an HLA gene. *Proc. Natl. Acad. Sci.* **79**: 893.

Marrack, P. and J. Kappler. 1988. The T-cell repertoire for antigen and MHC. *Immunol. Today* **9**: 308.

Mathis, D.J., C. Benoist, V.E. Williams, M. Kanter, and H.O. McDevitt. 1983. Several mechanisms can account for defective Eα gene expression in different mouse haplotypes. *Proc. Natl. Acad. Sci.* **80**: 273.

Matzinger, P., R. Zamoyska, and H. Waldmann. 1984. Self-tolerance is H-2-restricted. *Nature* **308**: 738.

Mayer, W.E., M. Jonker, D. Klein, P. Ivanyi, G. van Seventer, and J. Klein. 1988. Nucleotide sequences of chimpanzee MHC class I alleles: Evidence for trans-species mode of evolution. *EMBO J.* **7**: 2765.

Nathenson, S.G., J. Geliebter, G.M. Pfaffenbach, and R.A. Zeff. 1986. Murine major histocompatibility complex class-I mutants: Molecular analysis and structure-function implications. *Annu. Rev. Immunol.* **4**: 471.

Needleman, S.B. and C.D. Wunsch. 1970. A general method applicable to the search for similarities in the amino acid sequence of two proteins. *J. Mol. Biol.* **48**: 443.

N'Guyen, C., R. Sodoyer, J. Trucy, T. Strachan, and B.R. Jordan. 1985. The HLA-AW24 gene: Sequence, surroundings and comparison with the HLA-A2 and HLA-A3 genes. *Immunogenetics* **21**: 479.

Norment, A.M., R.D. Salter, P. Parham, V.H. Engelhard, and D.R. Littman. 1988. Cell-cell adhesion mediated by CD8 and MHC class I molecules. *Nature* **336**: 79.

Orr, H.T., J.A. Lopez de Castro, D. Lancet, and J.L. Strominger. 1979a. Complete amino acid sequence of a papain-solubilized human histocompatibility antigen, HLA-B7. 2. Sequence determination and search for homologies. *Biochemistry* **18**: 5711.

Orr, H.T., J.A. Lopez de Castro, P. Parham, H.L. Ploegh, and J.L. Strominger. 1979b. Comparison of amino acid sequences of two human histocompatibility antigens, HLA-A2 and HLA-B7: Location of putative alloantigenic sites. *Proc. Natl. Acad. Sci.* **76**: 4395.

Parham, P., D.A. Lawlor, C.E. Lomen, and P.D. Ennis. 1989a. Diversity and diversification of HLA-A,B,C alleles. *J. Immunol.* **142**: 3937.

Parham, P., D.A. Lawlor, R.D. Salter, C.E. Lomen, P.J. Bjorkman, and P.D. Ennis. 1989b. HLA-A,B,C: Patterns of polymorphism in peptide binding proteins. In *Immunobiology of HLA*, vol. 2: *Immunogenetics and histocompatibility* (ed. B. Dupont), p. 10. Springer-Verlag, New York.

Parham, P., C.E. Lomen, D.A. Lawlor, J.P. Ways, N. Holmes, H.L. Coppin, R.D. Salter, A.M. Wan, and P.D. Ennis. 1988. The nature of polymorphism in HLA-A, -B, -C molecules. *Proc. Natl. Acad. Sci.* **85**: 4005.

Parnes, J.R. 1989. Molecular biology and function of CD4 and CD8. *Adv. Immunol.* **44**: 265.

Parnes, J.R. and J.G. Seidman. 1982. Structure of wild-type and mutant mouse β_2-microglobulin genes. *Cell* **29**: 661.

Pauling, L. 1940. A theory of the structure and process of formation of antibodies. *J. Am. Chem. Soc.* **62**: 2643.

Pontarotti, P., G. Chimini, C. Nguyen, J. Boretto, and B.R. Jordan. 1988. CpG islands and HTF islands in the HLA class I region: Investigation of the methylation status of class I genes leads to precise physical mapping of the HLA-B and -C genes. *Nucleic Acids Res.* **16**: 6767.

Potter, T.A., T.V. Rajan, R.F. Dick II, and J.A. Bluestone. 1989. Substitution at residue 227 of H-2 class I molecules abrogates recognition by CD8-dependent, but not CD8-independent, cytotoxic T lymphocytes. *Nature* **337**: 73.

Robinson, P.J. 1987. Structure and expression of polypeptides encoded in the mouse Qa region. *Immunol. Res.* **6**: 46.

Rogers, J.H. 1985. Family organization of mouse H-2 class I genes. *Immunogenetics* **21**: 343.

Rupp, F., H. Acha-Orbea, H. Hengartner, R. Zinkernagel, and R. Joho. 1985. Identical V_β T-cell receptor genes used in alloreactive cytotoxic and antigen plus I-A specific helper T cells. *Nature* **315**: 425.

Saiki, R.K., D.H. Gelfand, S. Stoffel, S.J. Scharf, R. Higuchi, G.T. Horn, K.B. Mullis, and H.A. Erlich. 1988. Primer-directed enzymatic amplification of DNA with a thermostable DNA polymerase. *Science* **239**: 487.

Salter, R.D., A.M. Norment, B.P. Chen, C. Clayberger, A.M. Krensky, D.R. Littman, and P. Parham. 1989. Polymorphism in the α_3 domain of HLA-A molecules affects binding to CD8. *Nature* **338**: 345.

Sibley, C.G. and J.E. Ahlquist. 1984. The phylogeny of the hominoid primates, as indicated by DNA-DNA hybridization. *J. Mol. Evol.* **20**: 2.

Smithies, O. and P.A. Powers. 1986. Gene conversions and their relation to homologous chromosome pairing. *Philos. Trans. R. Soc. Lond. B* **312**: 291.

Sood, A.K., J. Pan, P.A. Biro, D. Pereira, R. Srivastava, V.B. Reddy, B.W. Duceman, and S.M. Weissman. 1985. Structure and polymorphism of class I MHC antigen mRNA. *Immunogenetics* **22**: 101.

Srivastava, R., M.J. Chorney, S.K. Lawrance, J. Pan, Z. Smith, C.L. Smith, and S.M. Weissman. 1989. Correction. *Proc. Natl. Acad. Sci.* **86**: 650.

Strachan, T. 1987. Molecular genetics and polymorphism of class I HLA antigens. *Brit. Med. Bull.* **43**: 1.

Streilein, J.W. 1987. Studies on an MHC exhibiting limited polymorphism. In *Evolution and vertebrate immunity* (ed. G. Kelsoe and D.H. Schulze), p. 379. University of Texas Press, Austin.

Strominger, J.L., D.L. Mann, P. Parham, R. Robb, T. Springer, and C. Terhorst. 1976. Structure of HL-A A and B antigens isolated from cultured human lymphocytes. *Cold Spring Harbor Symp. Quant. Biol.* **41**: 323.

Suggs, S.V., R.B. Wallace, T. Hirose, E.H. Kawashima, and K. Itakura. 1981. Use of synthetic oligonucleotides as hybridization probes: Isolation of cloned cDNA sequences for human β_2-microglobulin. *Proc. Natl. Acad. Sci.* **78**: 6613.

Swain, S.L. 1981. Significance of Lyt phenotypes: Lyt2 antibodies block activities of T cells that recognized class-1 major histocompatibility complex antigens regardless of their function. *Proc. Natl. Acad. Sci.* **78**: 7101.

Swofford, D.L. *Phylogenetic analysis using parsimony, version 2.4* (computer program). Illinois Natural History Survey, Champaign, Illinois.

Townsend, A. and H. Bodmer. 1989. Antigen recognition by class I-restricted T lymphocytes. *Annu. Rev. Immunol.* **7**: 601.

Trapani, J.A., S. Mizuno, S.H. Kang, S.Y. Yang, and B. Dupont. 1989. Molecular mapping of a new public HLA class I epitope shared by all HLA-B and HLA-C antigens and defined by a monoclonal antibody. *Immunogenetics* **29**: 25.

Tykocinski, M.L. and E.E. Max. 1984. CG dinucleotide clusters in MHC genes and in 5' demethylated genes. *Nucleic Acids Res.* **12**: 4385.

Structural Features of Peptides Recognized by H-2K^d-restricted T Cells

J.L. MARYANSKI,* J.-P. ABASTADO,†§ G. CORRADIN,‡ AND J.-C. CEROTTINI*

*Ludwig Institute for Cancer Research, Lausanne Branch, 1066 Epalinges, Switzerland;
†Unité de Biologie Moléculaire, Institut Pasteur, Paris, France; ‡Institute of Biochemistry,
University of Lausanne, 1066 Epalinges, Switzerland

We have recently developed a model system to study the recognition of antigens by major histocompatibility complex (MHC) class-I-restricted T cells (Maryanski et al. 1986a,b, 1988; Pala et al. 1988b). Cytotoxic T lymphocyte (CTL) clones were derived from DBA/2 (H-2^d) mice immunized with syngeneic P815 cells transfected with HLA-CW3 or HLA-A24 genes. The H-2K^d-restricted CTL clones obtained in this manner lysed not only P815-HLA transfectant target cells, but also untransfected (HLA$^-$) P815 cells incubated with synthetic peptides corresponding to region 170-182 of the CW3 or A24 molecules. The two HLA alleles differ only at residue 173 (Lys for CW3 and Glu for A24) within that region.

To analyze in more detail the presumed interaction of the HLA peptides with the K^d restriction element, we performed functional competition assays. For CTL that recognize CW3 or A24 mutually exclusively, we demonstrated (Maryanski et al. 1988) that the peptide corresponding to the nonrecognized allele could compete with the antigenic HLA peptide for recognition on P815 target cells. Moreover, the HLA peptides and another K^d-restricted peptide from influenza nucleoprotein (NP 147-158) could compete with each other for recognition by the appropriate CTL (Pala et al. 1988a). A modified NP peptide, NP 147-158 (R$^-_{156}$) containing a deletion of Arg-156, that was found to be 1000 times more active as an antigen than the natural sequence (Bodmer et al. 1988) was likewise at least 30-fold more potent as a competitor for the HLA peptides (Pala et al. 1988a). Other peptides from NP that are recognized by T cells in the context of other MHC class I molecules either failed to compete with the HLA peptides or were only marginally active. These results support the hypothesis that both the CW3 and A24 peptides and peptide NP 147-158 bind to the same site or to overlapping sites on the K^d restriction molecule.

For peptides recognized in the context of MHC class II molecules, the analysis of substituted peptides has allowed the identification of residues that are critical for peptide-MHC interaction (Allen et al. 1987; Sette et al. 1987). In a recent study (J. Maryanski et al., in prep.), we found that HLA residues Tyr-171, Thr-178, and Leu-179 appear to be critical for the function of the

peptides as efficient competitors. In the present paper, we expand that analysis by comparing truncated and substituted HLA peptides in terms of their relative efficiency as competitors and as antigens.

As an approach for the identification of critical residues on the K^d restriction element, we analyzed peptide recognition on L cells (H-2^k) transfected with intradomain K^d/D^d hybrid recombinant molecules (Maryanski et al. 1987, 1989). Replacement of K^d residues 152, 155, and 156 with those of D^d appeared to alter the specificity of peptide recognition. In the present paper, we have examined the relative efficiency of different peptides to compete with the CW3 peptide on L cells that express either the normal K^d molecule or K^d/D^d hybrids. We find that the NP peptides that are very efficient competitors on K^d targets are relatively inefficient on K^d/D^d recombinants that show altered patterns of peptide recognition by HLA-specific CTL. The HLA peptides and peptide NP 147-158 (R$^-_{156}$) that compete with each other for recognition on K^d targets both contain a tyrosine residue that appears to be crucial for competitor function (J. Maryanski et al., in prep.). The results of this competition study on recombinant K^d/D^d targets, however, suggest that these peptides may nevertheless interact somewhat differently with the MHC molecules.

EXPERIMENTAL PROCEDURES

Cells. The isolation of K^d-restricted, HLA-specific CTL clones from DBA/2 (H-2^d) mice immunized with syngeneic P815 cells transfected with HLA-CW3 or HLA-A24 genes is presented elsewhere (Maryanski et al. 1986a, 1988). CTL clones are designated by the HLA gene expressed by the P815 transfectant used for immunization. The derivation of L cells expressing either K^d or the K^d/D^d recombinant complementary DNA clones R8, R9, and R9.5 is described in detail elsewhere (Abastado et al. 1987; Maryanski et al. 1989).

Peptides. Peptide synthesis and purification were carried out as described previously (Maryanski et al. 1986b).

Cytolytic assay. Target cells (10^6) were labeled with 150 μCi sodium [^{51}Cr] chromate as described previously (Cerottini et al. 1974) for 1 hour at 37°C and washed

§Present address: National Institutes of Health, Building 6, Room 311, Bethesda, Maryland 20892.

three times. Labeled targets (2×10^3 in 50-μl volumes) were added to wells of V-bottom microtiter plates containing 100-μl volumes of the appropriate peptide diluted in DME supplemented with 5% FCS and HEPES. CTL (6×10^3 cells) were added in 50-μl volumes. Assays with P815 or L-cell targets were incubated for 4 or 5 hours, respectively, after which time the supernatants (100 μl) were harvested for counting. For competition experiments, the target cells were incubated for 15 minutes with the competitor peptide (100-μl volume) before addition of a suboptimal concentration of the antigenic peptide (50-μl volume). CTL (50-μl volume) were added after a further 15-minute incubation at room temperature. The percentage of lysis was calculated as $100 \times$ ([experimental – spontaneous release]/[total – spontaneous release]). The percentage of control lysis was calculated as $100 \times$ ([% lysis with competitor-background lysis]/[% lysis without competitor-background lysis]). Background lysis represents the percentage of lysis of the target cells in the absence of peptides. The relative competitor efficiency of the peptides was calculated for the peptide concentration required to obtain 50% or 70% control lysis.

RESULTS

Truncated or Substituted HLA Peptides Define Critical Residues

A series of CTL clones specific for HLA-CW3 or HLA-A24 were isolated from DBA/2 (H-2^d) mice immunized with syngeneic P815 cells transfected with the corresponding HLA genes (Maryanski et al. 1986a, 1988). The clones recognize synthetic peptides corresponding to region 170-182 of the HLA molecules (Fig. 1) in association with K^d as a restriction element (Maryanski et al. 1987). Within this region, A24 and CW3 differ only at position 173, which corresponds to glutamic acid for A24 and lysine for CW3. Some CTL clones (CW3/10.1 and A24/10.1) recognize either the CW3 or the A24 peptide, whereas others (CW3/1.1 and A24/12.2) recognize both (Fig. 1). The same pattern of reactivity was found on P815 HLA transfectant target cells (Maryanski et al. 1988).

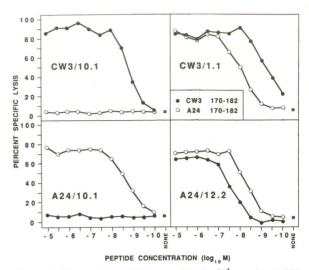

Figure 1. Recognition of HLA peptides by K^d-restricted CTL clones. The lysis of P815 target cells in the presence of the indicated concentrations of peptides CW3 170-182 (●) or A24 170-182 (○) by CTL clones CW3/10.1, A24/10.1, CW3/1.1, and A24/12.2 is shown.

In an analysis of different length peptides, we found that truncated CW3 and A24 peptides corresponding to residues 172-182 or 173-182 were not recognized by any of the HLA-specific CTL clones tested (Maryanski et al. 1988). HLA peptides having a common carboxyl terminus at position 182 but varying in length from 13 to 15 residues were recognized by CTL but with different efficiencies. Such differences might be due, at least in part, to differences in the affinity of the peptides for K^d. In the absence of an in vitro binding assay, we developed a functional competition assay to compare the relative peptide affinities indirectly (Maryanski et al. 1988).

In the present study, different length synthetic peptides corresponding to sequences within region 169–182 of the HLA-CW3 molecule were assayed both as antigens for recognition on P815 target cells by three different CW3-specific CTL clones and as competitors for the homologous A24 170-182 peptide recognized by a CTL clone specific for A24. The efficiency of the different peptides relative to peptide CW3 170-182 was calculated, and the data are summarized in Table 1. For

Table 1. Comparison of the Efficiency of Truncated CW3 Peptides as Competitors and as Antigens

Peptide	Sequence	Relative peptide efficiency as[a]			
			antigen for CTL clone		
		competitor[b]	CW3/10.1	CW3/1.1	CW3/701.1
CW3 170-182	– R Y L K N G K E T L Q R A	1.0	1.0	1.0	1.0
CW3 172-182	– – – L K N G K E T L Q R A	<0.04	<0.0003	<0.0001	<0.0003
CW3 171-182	– – Y L K N G K E T L Q R A	0.22	0.12	0.16	0.014
CW3 169-182	R R Y L K N G K E T L Q R A	0.10	0.06	0.07	0.05
CW3 169-182 (R169L)	L R Y L K N G K E T L Q R A	0.67	0.62	0.60	0.50
CW3 170-180	– R Y L K N G K E T L Q – –	0.87	<0.01	<0.02	<0.01
CW3 169-180	R R Y L K N G K E T L Q – –	~0.04	<0.0003	<0.0001	<0.0003

[a]Relative to peptide CW3 170–182.
[b]Peptides were compared as competitors for recognition of peptide A24 170–182 by CTL clone A24/10.1.

several peptides, the relative efficiency of the peptide as a competitor clearly correlated with its relative efficiency as an antigen. For example, the efficiency of peptide CW3 169-182 as a competitor was 0.1 compared to peptide 170-182, and its relative efficiency as an antigen ranged from 0.07 to 0.05 for the three CTL clones. The decreased efficiency of the longer peptide was not due solely to the presence of an additional amino acid (residue 169) at the amino terminus, but depended on the nature of that residue. Thus, replacement of Arg-169 with leucine (peptide CW3 169-182 [R169L]) resulted in a nearly complete recovery of the activity of the peptide in terms of both competition and antigenic recognition.

The removal of residue 170 (peptide CW3 171-182) decreased the efficiency of the peptide as a competitor by approximately 5-fold. A similar decrease in the potency of the peptide as an antigen was observed for two of the CTL clones (CW3/10.1 and CW3/1.1). However, in confirmation of our previous results (Maryanski et al. 1988), peptide CW3 171-182 was approximately 100-fold less efficient as an antigen than peptide CW3 170-182 for CTL clone CW3/701.1. No competition could be demonstrated in this system for truncated peptide CW3 172-182, and this peptide was not recognized by any of the three CTL clones. In contrast, another 11-residue peptide (CW3 170-180) was nearly as efficient as the full-length peptide (CW3 170-182) as a competitor, but was not recognized.

Similar results were obtained with truncated peptides from within the same region (170-182) of the HLA-A24 molecule. As shown in Figure 2, the truncated peptide A24 170-180 was as efficient as the full-length peptide A24 170-182 as a competitor for antigenic peptide CW3

170-182, whereas a peptide truncated at the amino-terminal end (A24 172-182) was more than 10-fold reduced. Neither of the truncated peptides was recognized by A24-specific CTL clones (Maryanski et al. 1988 and data not shown). From these results, it appears that residues crucial for the interaction of HLA peptides with the K^d restriction element are contained within region 170-180 of the HLA molecules.

In another study (J.L. Maryanski et al., in prep.), we identified three HLA residues (Tyr-171, Thr-178, and Leu-179) that appear to be important for competition in terms of their sensitivity to amino acid substitution (summarized in Table 2). The most critical residue appeared to be Tyr-171, in that its replacement with alanine reduced the efficiency of the A24 peptide as a competitor by more than 100-fold. The substituted A24 peptides that were poor competitors were likewise not recognized as antigen by the A24-specific CTL clone A24/10.1 and the cross-reactive clone CW3/1.1 (Table 2). The patterns of recognition of substituted A24 peptides that still functioned as competitors differed for the two CTL clones. For CTL clone CW3/1.1, substitutions at positions 174 (Asn to Leu), 175 (Gly to Thr), 176 (Lys to Arg or Asn), or 177 (Glu to Asp) of the A24 peptide resulted in a loss of recognition. CTL clone A24/10.1 failed to recognize A24 peptides with replacements at position 173 (Glu to Lys), 175 (Gly to Thr), or 177 (Glu to Asp).

Comparison of K^d-restricted Peptides as Competitors on Modified K^d Molecules

The cross-competition observed between HLA and NP peptides that are recognized in the context of K^d was interpreted as an indication that these peptides bind to the same site or to overlapping sites on the MHC molecule (Pala et al. 1988a). In a recent study (J. Maryanski et al., in prep.), we found that the Tyr-148 residue in peptide NP 147-158 (R$^-_{156}$) was critical for its activity as a competitor. Thus, for both HLA and NP peptides, tyrosine residues may form part of the K^d-binding motif. The activity of the peptides as competitors on modified K^d molecules might provide clues as to whether the HLA and NP peptides interact with identical residues on the MHC molecule. We showed previously (Maryanski et al. 1987, 1989) that the HLA peptides can be recognized on a limited series of hybrid K^d/D^d molecules, but that the fine specificity of peptide recognition was altered for some CTL clones on the recombinants compared to K^d. The hybrid K^d/D^d molecules R9 and R9.5 provided an informative pair of recombinants in that analysis. The R9.5 molecule contains the K^d sequence from the amino terminus (residue 1) up to residue 172 followed by the D^d sequence. L cells transfected with R9.5 were recognized as well as the K^d controls (in the presence of HLA peptides) by all of the K^d-restricted CTL clones tested. In contrast, the pattern of peptide recognition was altered for recombinants R8 and R9. R9 differs from R9.5 only at residues 152, 155, and 156, whereas R8 contains two

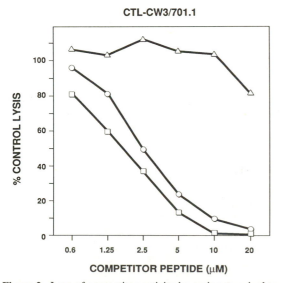

Figure 2. Loss of competitor activity by amino-terminal truncation of peptide A24 170-182. The competition experiment was performed with CTL-CW3/701.1, antigenic peptide CW3 170-182 (0.05 μM), and competitor peptides A24 170-182 (○), 170-180 (□), and 172-182 (△). Control lysis in the absence of competitors was 51%.

Table 2. Substituted A24 Peptides Define Residues Critical for Recognition by K^d-restricted CTL

Peptide	Sequence	competitor[a]	A24/10.1	CW3/1.1
			antigen for CTL clone[b]	
A24	R Y L E N G K E T L Q R A	++++[c]	++++	+++
CW3	- - - K - - - - - - - - -	++++	-	++++
186C1	- A - - - - - - - - - - -	-	-	-
100	- - - - - - - K - - - -	+	-	-
132B	- - - - - - - D - - - -	+	-	-
136	- - - - - - - - - A - - -	+	-	-
137	- - - - - - - - - K - - -	+	-	-
B7	- - - - - - D K - E - -	+	-	-
99	- - - - - - - D - - - -	+++	-	-
AV	- - - - - - - - - E - -	+++	++++	+++
135A	- - A - - - - - - - - -	+++	+++++	+++
145A	- - - - - T - - - - - -	+++	-	-
145C	- - - - - - R - - - - -	+++++	++++	-
D^d/L^d	- - - K - - N A - - L - T	+++++	-	-
K^d	- - - - L - N - - - L - T	+++++	-	-
87	- - - - L - N - - - - - T	++++	-	-
88	- - - - L - - - - - - T	++++	+++	+/-
AIII	- - - - L - - - - - - -	+++++	+++	+/-
AVIII	- - - - - - - - - - - T	n.t.[d]	+++	+++
AII	- - - - - - N - - - - -	++++	+++	-

[a]Competition experiments were performed with CTL clone CW3/701.1 and antigenic peptide CW3 170–182, as in Fig. 2, except for peptide CW3 170–182, which was assayed as a competitior for peptide A24 170–182 recognized by CTL A24/10.1. Data from J. Maryanski et al. (in prep.).

[b]Peptides were titrated as in Fig. 1 for recognition by CTL clones A24/10.1 and CW3/1.1.

[c]Activity relative to peptide A24 170–182: (++++) 100%; (−) <1%; (+) 10–20%; (+++) 50–100%; (+++++) >100%.

[d]Not tested.

further D^d substitutions at positions 138 and 148 (Abastado et al. 1987; Maryanski et al. 1989). As illustrated in Table 3, CTL clones CW3/10.1 and A24/10.1 recognize CW3 and A24 peptides, respectively, on R9.5 and on K^d targets but not on R8 or R9 target cells. In contrast, CTL clone CW3/701.1 recognizes peptide CW3 170-182 not only on R9.5 and K^d, but also on R8 and R9. In addition, the latter clone recognizes the A24 peptide on R8 and R9 target cells, but not on R9.5 or on K^d target cells.

With CTL clone CW3/701.1, it was thus possible to compare the efficiency of different peptides as competitors for the CW3 peptide on targets that express modified H-2 molecules. The most striking difference observed was the low level of competition obtained with NP peptides on the R8 and R9 targets compared to

that on the R9.5 and K^d targets (Fig. 3). This was the case both for the natural NP 147-158 sequence and for the variant peptide, NP 147-158 (R^-_{156}). In contrast, for peptides corresponding to region 170-182 of the K^d and D^d molecules, the relative efficiency of the peptides was similar on all four recombinant targets (Fig. 4). Peptide B7 170-182 was likewise a poor competitor on the four targets.

DISCUSSION

For several CW3 peptides of different lengths, we found a quantitative correlation between the relative activity of the peptides as competitors and as antigens (Table 1). These results would be expected in cases where the modification of the peptide affected the af-

Table 3. Recognition of HLA Peptides on Hybrid K^d/D^d Molecules

CTL clone	Peptide	H-2 residue	L-cell transfectant				
			D^d	R8	R9	R9.5	K^d
		152	A	A	A	D	D
		155	R	R	R	Y	Y
		156	D	D	D	Y	Y
CW3/701.1	CW3		−	+	+	+	+
	A24		−	+	+	−	−
CW3/10.1	CW3		−	−	−	+	+
	A24		−	−	−	−	−
A24/10.1	CW3		−	−	−	−	−
	A24		−	−	−	+	+

Compiled from Maryanski et al. (1987, 1989).

CTL - CW3/701.1

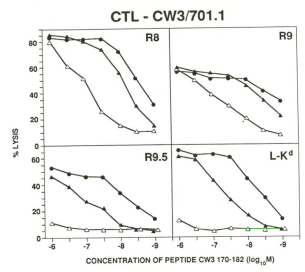

Figure 3. Reduced efficiency of NP peptides as competitors on hybrid K^d/D^d targets R8 and R9. The competition experiment was performed with CTL clone CW3/701.1 and antigenic peptide CW3 170-182 at the indicated concentrations. L-cell targets transfected with K^d or with R8, R9, or R9.5 hybrid cDNA (see Table 3) were incubated with medium (●) as a control or with competitor peptides NP 147-158 (▲) or NP 147-158 (R$^-_{156}$) (△) at 2×10^{-5} M.

CTL - CW3 / 701.1

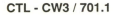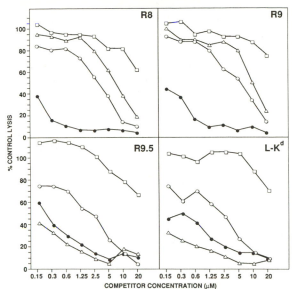

Figure 4. Competition on target cells that express different hybrid K^d/D^d molecules discriminates peptide NP 147-158 (R$^-_{156}$) from other competitors. The competition experiment was performed with CTL clone CW3/701.1 and antigenic peptide CW3 170-182 (0.1 μM) in the presence of the indicated concentrations of competitor peptides K^d 170-182 (●), D^d 170-182 (○), B7 170-182 (□), or NP 147-158 (R$^-_{156}$) (△). The control lysis for R8, R9, R9.5, and L-K^d target cells was 73%, 41%, 48%, and 66%, respectively.

finity of the peptide for K^d without altering significantly the presentation of the peptide as antigen to the T-cell receptor. This was the case for peptides CW3 169-182 and CW3 169-182 (R169L) that were less active than peptide CW3 170-182 by approximately tenfold and twofold, respectively, both as competitors and as antigens for three different CTL clones. For peptide CW3 171-182, a similar correlation was found for CTL clones CW3/10.1 and CW3/1.1, but for another CTL clone, CW3/701.1, the relative efficiency of the peptide as an antigen was tenfold lower than its relative efficiency as a competitor (Table 1). The latter CTL clone could also be distinguished from the former two clones in that it was more sensitive to iodination of peptide CW3 170-182 on the Tyr-171 residue (J. Maryanski and G. Corradin, unpubl.).

Substituted A24 peptides containing replacements at positions 171 (Tyr to Ala), 178 (Thr to Lys or Asp), or 179 (Leu to Ala or Lys) that correspond to the putative K^d-binding motif were not recognized by CTL clones A24/10.1 and CW3/1.1 that recognize the A24 peptide (Table 2). The reduction in the efficiency of these substituted peptides as antigen compared to peptide A24 170-182 exceeded by more than tenfold the reduction in their relative efficiency as competitors (Table 2 and J. Maryanski, unpubl.). By this analysis, it appears that the effects of these substitutions are not limited to reductions in the affinity of the peptides for K^d. Several alternative consequences might include alterations in (1) peptide conformation, (2) the site of interaction on the K^d molecule, and (3) peptide sensitivity to hydrolysis.

For substituted A24 peptides that functioned at least as well as the original A24 peptide as competitors, recognition patterns varied with the CTL clone analyzed (Table 2). Amino acid substitutions that result in loss of recognition by a particular CTL clone, but that fail to affect competitor activity, may identify residues that interact directly with the T-cell receptor. Alternatively, the loss of antigenic activity could be due to a more indirect effect, for instance, a change in peptide conformation. In our view, the present information is insufficient for constructing a model of the HLA peptides as they bind to K^d.

Our results suggest that the tyrosine residue shared by the HLA peptides and peptide NP 147-158 (R$^-_{156}$) has a critical role in the interaction of the peptides with the K^d molecule (Table 2 and J. Maryanski et al., in prep.). We are currently analyzing other peptides recognized in the context of K^d to determine whether the finding might be more general. It is noteworthy that a peptide corresponding to the influenza hemagglutinin transmembrane region that is recognized by K^d-restricted CTL contains two tyrosine residues (Braciale et al. 1987) of as yet undetermined function. A tyrosine residue in the peptide might be expected to interact with another hydrophobic residue in the MHC molecule. Within the region defined as the presumed antigen-binding site for MHC class I molecules (Bjorkman et al. 1987a,b), the K^d molecule contains numerous candidates including tyrosine, phenylalanine, and tryptophan residues (Kvist et al. 1983).

Although the HLA and NP peptides appear to share a critical tyrosine residue for interaction with K^d, the competition experiments presented herein suggest that they may not interact identically with K^d or hybrid K^d/D^d molecules. The NP peptides NP 147-158 and NP 147-158 (R^-_{156}) were found to be poor competitors on the R8 and R9 recombinant target cells compared to their activity on R9.5 and K^d targets (Figs. 3 and 4). One interpretation for these results is that the NP peptides have a lower affinity for R8 and R9 than for R9.5 and K^d, whereas the affinity of the HLA peptides and the K^d and D^d peptides is similar for all four MHC molecules. Alternatively, the NP peptides might have the same affinity for K^d and the K^d/D^d recombinant molecules, and the peptides corresponding to region 170-182 of HLA and H-2 might have a higher affinity for R8 and R9 than for R9.5 or the original K^d molecule. Without a direct binding assay, we cannot distinguish between these possibilities. The differential relative activity of the NP and K^d or D^d peptides on target cells that differ only in the expression of altered MHC molecules also provides strong evidence that the inhibition between peptides is due to a direct interaction of the peptides with the MHC molecules. A nonspecific, noncompetitive inhibition by the NP peptides, for example, would be expected to be the same relative to the other peptides on target cells that express different MHC molecules.

The analysis of truncated and substituted HLA peptides as competitors provides preliminary clues for understanding the basis of the interaction of the peptides with the K^d restriction molecule. The simplest interpretation of our results would be that peptide residues Tyr-171, Thr-178, and Leu-179 interact directly with the K^d molecule. On the basis of this model, we have recently designed functional competitor analogs by expressing the Tyr...Thr-Leu motif in different molecular contexts (J. Maryanski et al., in prep.). We synthesized peptide analogs in which the tyrosine residue was separated from the Thr-Leu pair by a short stretch of oligoproline or oligo-glycine spacers. These analogs were functional competitors for HLA and NP peptides recognized in the context of K^d. The reduced structural complexity of poly-proline analogs may be advantageous for molecular modeling studies.

ACKNOWLEDGMENTS

We thank K. Muhlethaler and F. Penea for excellent technical assistance and A. Zoppi for help in the preparation of the manuscript.

REFERENCES

Abastado, J.-P., C. Jaulin, M.-P. Schutze, P. Langlade-Demoyen, F. Plata, K. Ozato, and P. Kourilsky. 1987. Fine mapping of epitopes by intradomain K^d/D^d recombinants. *J. Exp. Med.* **166**: 327.

Allen, P.M., G.R. Matsueda, R.J. Evans, J.B. Dunbar, G.R. Marshall, and E.R. Unanue. 1987. Identification of the T-cell and Ia contact residues of a T-cell antigenic epitope. *Nature* **327**: 713.

Bjorkman, P.J., M.A. Saper, B. Samraoui, W.S. Bennett, J.L. Strominger, and D.C. Wiley. 1987a. Structure of the human class I histocompatibility antigen, HLA-A2. *Nature* **329**: 506.

———. 1987b. The foreign antigen binding site and T cell recognition regions of class I histocompatibility antigens. *Nature* **329**: 512.

Bodmer, H.C., R.M. Pemberton, J.B. Rothbard, and B.A. Askonas. 1988. Enhanced recognition of a modified peptide antigen by cytotoxic T cells specific for influenza nucleoprotein. *Cell* **52**: 253.

Braciale, T.J., V.L. Braciale, M. Winkler, I. Stroynowski, L. Hood, J. Sambrook, and M.-J. Gething. 1987. On the role of the transmembrane anchor sequence of influenza hemagglutinin in target cell recognition by class I MHC-restricted, hemagglutinin-specific cytolytic T lymphocytes. *J. Exp. Med.* **166**: 678.

Cerottini, J.-C., H.D. Engers, H.R. MacDonald, and K.T. Brunner. 1974. Generation of cytotoxic T lymphocytes in vitro. I. Response of normal and immune mouse spleen cells in mixed lymphocyte cultures. *J. Exp. Med.* **140**: 703.

Kvist, S., L. Roberts, and B. Dobberstein. 1983. Mouse histocompatibility genes: Structure and organization of a K^d gene. *EMBO J.* **2**: 245.

Maryanski, J.L., J.-P. Abastado, and P. Kourilsky. 1987. Specificity of peptide presentation by a set of hybrid mouse class I MHC molecules. *Nature* **330**: 660.

Maryanski, J.L., R.S. Accolla, and B.R. Jordan. 1986a. H-2 restricted recognition of cloned HLA class I gene products expressed in mouse cells. *J. Immunol.* **136**: 4340.

Maryanski, J.L., J.-P. Abastado, H.R. MacDonald, and P. Kourilsky. 1989. Intradomain H-2K^d/D^d recombinants define the same regions as crucial for recognition by alloreactive or major histocompatibility complex-restricted cytolytic T cells. *Eur. J. Immunol.* **19**: 193.

Maryanski, J.L., P. Pala, J.-C. Cerottini, and G. Corradin. 1988. Synthetic peptides as antigens and competitors in recognition by H-2-restricted cytolytic T cells specific for HLA. *J. Exp. Med.* **167**: 1391.

Maryanski, J.L., P. Pala, G. Corradin, B.R. Jordan, and J.-C. Cerottini. 1986b. H-2 restricted cytolytic T cells specific for HLA can recognize a synthetic HLA peptide. *Nature* **324**: 578.

Pala, P., H.C. Bodmer, R.M. Pemberton, J.-C. Cerottini, J.L. Maryanski, and B.A. Askonas. 1988a. Competition between unrelated peptides recognized by H-2K^d restricted T cells. *J. Immunol.* **141**: 2298.

Pala, P., G. Corradin, T. Strachan, R. Sodoyer, B.R. Jordan, J.-C. Cerottini, and J.L. Maryanski. 1988b. Mapping of HLA epitopes recognized by H-2 restricted CTL specific for HLA using recombinant genes and synthetic peptides. *J. Immunol.* **140**: 871.

Sette, A., S. Buus, S. Colon, J.A. Smith, C. Miles, and H.M. Grey. 1987. Structural characteristics of an antigen required for its interaction with Ia and recognition by T cells. *Nature* **328**: 395.

Class I MHC-restricted Cytotoxic Responses to Soluble Protein Antigen

F.R. Carbone, N.A. Hosken, M.W. Moore, and M.J. Bevan

Department of Immunology, Research Institute of Scripps Clinic, La Jolla, California 92037

Peripheral T lymphocytes that use the α and β receptor chains to recognize foreign antigen can be classified on the basis of the type of major histocompatibility complex (MHC) molecule with which they interact. Thus, T cells recognize antigen in association with the class I glycoproteins of the MHC (H-2K, D, or L in mice), or their recognition of foreign antigen may be restricted by the MHC class II molecules (I-A and I-E in mice). This subdivision correlates perfectly with the expression by the T cell of the accessory molecules CD8 (for class I) and CD4 (for class II). There is recent, direct evidence to explain this perfect correlation, namely, that these accessory molecules on the T cell interact with the relatively conserved regions of the MHC glycoproteins on the antigen-presenting cell (Potter et al. 1989; Salter et al. 1989). It is fair to say that most class-I-restricted, CD8[+] T cells are cytotoxic T lymphocytes (CTL), whereas most class-II-restricted, CD4[+] T cells are helper T cells. This classification is not perfect, however. There are many examples of class-II-restricted, CD4[+] T cells that behave (at least in vitro) as very effective killer cells (Braciale et al. 1987; Jacobson et al. 1989).

CD4[+] T-cell responses are readily induced in mice by immunization with almost any foreign protein. The most studied antigens are the readily available, inexpensive proteins such as hen egg ovalbumin, lysozyme, myoglobin, etc. Antigen-presenting cells that express class II "process" such endocytosed foreign antigens and present denatured or degraded fragments of the antigen in association with class II molecules on their surface for T-helper-cell recognition. Since the early 1980s, a large number of linear peptides, 10–20 residues long, have been identified that associate with class II molecules and mimic the form of antigen recognized by CD4[+] helper T cells.

Class-I-restricted T-cell responses are not readily induced by the intravenous, subcutaneous, or intraperitoneal injection of any of the common protein antigens that induce CD4[+] T cells. Rather, class-I-restricted CD8[+] cytolytic responses are induced by replicating antigens, most notably infectious viruses. The same virus that has been inactivated, say by UV light irradiation, will be unable to induce class-I-restricted responses, while remaining an effective inducer of helper T-cell and antibody responses (Braciale and Yap 1978; Morrison et al. 1986). Class-I-restricted T-cell responses are also induced against some intracellular

bacteria, tumor antigens, minor histocompatibility antigens expressed on MHC-matched cells, or antigens expressed by cells as a result of gene transfection. Like class-II-restricted responses, however, all of these class-I-associated epitopes seem to be peptide degradation products of the nominal antigen (Townsend and Bodmer 1989). The rule that splits the world of T-cell antigens seems to be that class-II-restricted responses are induced by soluble proteins that come from outside the antigen-presenting cell and can be endocytosed—exogenous antigens; whereas class-I-restricted responses are mounted to antigens synthesized within the presenting cell as a result of infection or anomalous gene expression—endogenous antigens.

Most of the classic class-I-restricted antigens are either not defined biochemically, e.g., tumor antigens or minor H antigens, or if they are defined, they are not readily available in large quantity, e.g., viral glycoproteins, viral polymerases, or viral nucleoproteins. To study the proposed endogenous or cytosolic pathway of class-I-restricted processing and presentation, we wished to convert some of the readily available antigens, such as ovalbumin (OVA) or β-galactosidase (β-Gal), to class-I-restricted immunogens. If we can learn how to get nonreplicating antigens to serve as class-I-restricted antigens, this may have significance in designing more effective viral or bacterial vaccines *without* using the agent in infectious form.

RESULTS AND DISCUSSION

Induction of Class I MHC-restricted CTL Using OVA-expressing Transfectants

At the initiation of our studies, it had already been shown that gene transfection served to generate cell lines expressing appropriate class I MHC-associated determinants from foreign proteins (Townsend et al. 1985; Maryanski et al. 1986). Such transfectants could, in turn, elicit CTL of the desired specificity after in vivo immunization (Maryanski et al. 1986). OVA was chosen as our initial antigen, since it has been studied extensively as a T-helper antigen, the soluble protein is readily available, and the OVA gene and cDNA are already available. OVA cDNA inserted into an appropriate expression vector was transfected into EL4 cells (a C57BL/6 thymoma) to generate an OVA-producing EL4 subline designated as E.G7-OVA. Immunization

CARBONE ET AL.

of C57BL/6 mice with this transfectant, followed by secondary in vitro stimulation of spleen cells, generated E.G7-OVA-specific CTL. These CTL were of the CD8$^+$4$^-$ phenotype and specific for a determinant mapped by the peptide OVA(258-276) in association with H-2K^b (Moore et al. 1988).

Introduction of Soluble OVA into the Class I Antigen-presentation Pathway

Coincubation of native OVA and EL4 failed to sensitize these cells for lysis by the class-I-restricted CTL, consistent with the notion that class-I-associated antigenic processing usually requires some form of endogenous expression (Germain 1986). To ascertain whether this reflected an absolute requirement for de novo protein synthesis or perhaps some form of specialized antigen localization not usually accessible to exogenous proteins, we introduced soluble OVA directly into the cell cytoplasm via the osmotic lysis of pinosomes (Okada and Rechsteiner 1982). In this technique, cells are incubated at 37°C in hypertonic medium containing the macromolecule of interest and then rapidly diluted to hypotonicity. Under such conditions, pinosomes containing the protein of interest swell and burst, releasing their contents into the cytoplasm. Significantly, this approach resulted in successful sensitization of target cells using the native protein (Moore et al. 1988). Results from a typical experiment are shown in Table 1. Only target cells that were allowed to take up OVA during the first incubation, in hypertonic media, proved to be effective targets for the transfectant-specific CTL. This observation was subsequently extended to a second protein antigen, β-Gal, using a H-2L^d-restricted β-Gal-specific CTL line kindly provided by H.G. Rammensee of the Max-Planck Institute in Tübingen. Thus, cytoplasmic localization of proteins may be a general requirement for class-I-associated antigen processing.

Table 1. Introduction of OVA into the Class I Pathway of Antigen Presentation

Treatment of EL4 target cells		% Lysis by CTL
first incubation	second incubation	
Hypertonic, +OVA	hypotonic	65
Hypertonic, −OVA	hypotonic	0
Hypertonic, −OVA	hypotonic, +OVA	2
Isotonic, +OVA	hypotonic	6
Isotonic, +OVA	isotonic	7

EL4 cells were incubated with or without 20 mg/ml native OVA for a first incubation of 10 min and then diluted 30-fold for a second incubation of 2 min. Cells were rested for 6 hr and then used as targets in a ^{51}Cr-release assay with a C57BL/6 anti-E.G7-OVA CTL line at an effector:target ratio of 6:1.

Processing of Soluble Protein Introduced into the Cell Cytoplasm

The processing and class-I-restricted presentation of OVA introduced directly into the cell cytoplasm takes approximately 45–60 minutes (Hosken et al. 1989). This was estimated by glutaraldehyde treatment of cells at successive times after cytoplasmic loading and assessment of their susceptibility toward CTL lysis. These kinetics are comparable to those measured for the transport of the newly synthesized H-2K molecule itself to the cell surface (Williams et al. 1985). Since this result could suggest that peptide may only associate with nascent class I molecules, we ascertained whether inhibition of protein synthesis affected class-I-restricted presentation of OVA introduced into the cell cytoplasm.

When EL4 target cells were treated with cyclohexamide (10–100 μg/ml), protein synthesis (as measured by [^{3}H]leucine incorporation) was inhibited to greater than 99%. However, cells treated with cyclohexamide for up to 6 hours prior to OVA loading were still able to process and present the protein to OVA-specific CTL. Moreover, as shown in Table 2, the kinetics and extent

Table 2. Effect of Cyclohexamide on the Kinetics of Class-I-restricted OVA Presentation

Time of glutaraldehyde fixation (min)	OVA loaded	CTL-mediated lysis of targets			
		no cyclohexamide pretreatment		cyclohexamide pretreated targets	
		−OVA$_{242-276}$	+OVA$_{242-276}$	−OVA$_{242-276}$	+OVA$_{242-276}$
0	−	−	++	−	++
15	+	−	++	−	++
30	+	−	++	−	++
45	+	+	++	+	++
60	+	++	++	++	++
90	+	++	++	++	++
Unfixed	+	++	++	++	++

Target cells were pretreated with cyclohexamide for 2 hr, loaded with OVA in the presence of cyclohexamide, fixed with glutaraldehyde at the times indicated or left unfixed, and incubated in a 3-hr ^{51}Cr-release assay with H-2K^b-restricted, OVA-specific CTL. Cyclohexamide was present at 100 μg/ml throughout. (−) No lysis, (+) partial sensitization, (++) maximal sensitization for lysis.

of sensitization for lysis of cyclohexamide-treated target cells were identical to those of control cells. Therefore, association of peptides derived from intracellularly degraded antigen does not require the ongoing synthesis of the class I MHC molecules to which they ultimately bind.

How and where antigens are fragmented within target cells for presentation to class-I-restricted T cells remains unknown. Intracellular proteins are known to be degraded by a number of ATP-dependent pathways that are either lysosomal or nonlysosomal (Ciechanover 1987). Since it has been shown that lysosomotropic agents have no effect on class-I-antigen presentation (Morrison et al. 1986), it is likely that nonlysosomal processing is required for class-I-antigen presentation. In particular, Bigelow et al. (1981) have shown that proteins artificially delivered into cells are degraded predominantly within the cytosol rather than the lysosomes.

The best-characterized mechanism involved in cytosolic protein degradation is the ubiquitin-dependent pathway. Ubiquitin-mediated proteolysis is initiated by the covalent linkage of ubiquitin to ϵ-NH$_2$ groups of lysine residues within the protein substrate. Reductive methylation of the ϵ-NH$_2$ of the lysines completely inhibits ubiquitin-mediated protein degradation in reticulocyte lysates without affecting ubiquitin-independent pathways (Katznelson and Kulke 1983; Tanaka et al. 1983). Therefore, if ubiquitin linkage to ϵ-NH$_2$ groups is a requirement for class-I-restricted antigen degradation, then methylation of all ϵ-NH$_2$ groups should inhibit processing of any protein introduced directly into the cell cytoplasm. However, as shown in Table 3, this was found not to be the case for OVA. Both the naive OVA and the completely methylated protein effectively sensitized EL4 for lysis by the E.G7-OVA-specific CTL line after they were directly introduced into the cell cytoplasm. Both the native and methylated forms of the protein were ineffective at CTL targeting after exogenous addition. CNBr treat-

ment that generates the CN-OVA and CN-methyl-OVA digest releases the active fragments and consequently permits CTL recognition. These results suggest that, at least for OVA, the ubiquitin-mediated degradation mechanism may play no role in the processing events required for class I MHC antigen presentation.

Primary In Vitro Stimulation of Peptide-specific CTL

The studies described above served to show that exogenous, native protein could not be processed for class I MHC presentation. In contrast, appropriate peptides could successfully sensitize targets for CTL recognition. This sensitization presumably results from direct association of the peptide determinant to cell-surface MHC, since glutaraldehyde-fixed cells served as effective CTL targets (Hosken et al. 1989). Given these observations, we reasoned that if a protein such as OVA were "processed" before in vivo immunization to release class-I-binding fragments, then the peptides may elicit a class-I-restricted CTL response. However, in experiments using OVA peptides, we found that, in fact, these fragments could induce measurable in vitro primary CTL responses from *normal*, unimmunized H-2^b splenocytes (Carbone et al. 1988). This is exemplified by the results shown in Figure 1. When the synthetic fragment OVA(258-276), which is efficiently recognized by H-2K^b, E.G7-OVA-specific CTL, was

Table 3. Effect of Reductive Methylation of OVA on Class-I-restricted Presentation

Target cell	Treatment of targets	Lysis of CTL
EL4	—	−
E.G7-OVA	—	+++
EL4	OVA load	+++
EL4	CN-OVA	+++
EL4	native OVA	−
EL4	methyl-OVA load	+++
EL4	CN-methyl-OVA	+++
EL4	methyl OVA	−

Ovalbumin was denatured, alkylated, and reductively methylated to completion (Jentoft and Dearborn 1979). Native and methylated OVA were also fragmented with CNBr to release the target determinant required for CTL recognition. Target cells were loaded via the osmotic lysis of pinosomes with either native or methylated OVA before addition to a CTL assay. Alternatively, exogenous CN-OVA, CN-methyl-OVA, native OVA, or methyl-OVA was added directly to the CTL assay. E.G7-OVA-specific CTL were derived by the method of Carbone and Bevan (1989).

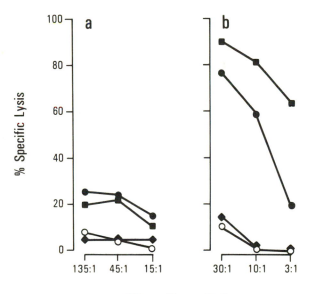

Effector/Target Ratio

Figure 1. Induction of CTL by primary peptide immunization. (*a*) Spleen cells from C57BL/6 mice were cultured for 5 days with 10 μg/ml H-2K^b-restricted peptide, OVA(258−276), and then assayed for CTL activity. (*b*) Effectors derived from the primary cultures were restimulated twice with peptide and then assayed for CTL activity 5 days after the last stimulation. Specific lysis in a 4-hr ^{51}Cr-release assay is shown for EL4 cells alone (○) or in the presence of 10 μg/ml OVA(258-276) (■) or 100 μg/ml CNBr-cleaved OVA (●) and for the OVA-producing transfectant E.G7-OVA (◆).

incubated with naive C57BL/6 splenocytes, peptide-specific effectors were readily detected after 5 days in culture (Fig. 1a). This activity is extremely weak when compared to the primary response to cells expressing allogeneic class I MHC antigens, but it can be effectively expanded by repetitive in vitro peptide stimulation (Fig. 1b). However, as is also shown in Figure 1, in no instance were these effectors capable of lysing E.G7-OVA, which expresses the target antigen as a result of endogenous presentation. This failure could not be attributed to an inadvertent priming against peptide contaminants associated with the synthesis, since the effectors clearly cross-reacted with the natural OVA fragments generated after CNBr cleavage. Moreover, peptide recognition was H-2K^b-restricted (not shown), consistent with the presentation of this determinant to E.G7-OVA-specific CTL derived from in vivo transfectant priming. These and related results (Carbone et al. 1988) suggest that the class-I-restricted T cells generated by direct in vitro peptide priming reflect a population of effectors that differ from the physiologically relevant CTL that are likely to be active in vivo.

Although the exact nature of this difference remains uncertain, we have speculated that the peptide-induced CTL are in fact low-affinity T cells that result as a consequence of an artificially high density of peptide/MHC complexes on the antigen-presenting cell (Carbone et al. 1988). Thus, the important distinction between these peptide-induced T cells and the more physiologically relevant class-I-restricted cells that arise as a consequence of virus or transfectant immunization is not that the former are derived by in vitro compared to in vivo priming, but that the *direct* binding of peptide to MHC elicits T cells of presumably lower affinity compared to antigen presentation via the appropriate intracellular pathway.

Use of Proteins or Peptide to Immunize Class-I-restricted T Cells In Vivo

We have shown that soluble proteins can be introduced into the intracellular pathway of class-I-restricted presentation by direct injection into the cell cytoplasm. Clearly, this approach lends itself to the priming of a physiologically relevant CTL response in vivo. This was confirmed in the results shown in Table 4. In this experiment, both the CTL targeting epitope of OVA(258-276) and intact, soluble OVA injected intravenously failed to prime a class-I-restricted response. In contrast, when animals were primed by injecting syngeneic spleen cells that had been loaded with antigen via the osmotic lysis of pinosomes, physiologically relevant CTL specific for E.G7-OVA were induced. These T cells were specific for the H-2K^b-restricted peptide OVA(258-276), which clearly was not immunogenic on its own. Despite these results, it would be inaccurate to generalize that *all* exogenous proteins fail to elicit appropriate CTL responses in vivo. There have been several reports of the use of purified viral proteins to elicit virus-specific, class-I-restricted T-cell responses (Tevethia et al. 1980; Wraith and Askonas 1985). Furthermore, we have found that at least one relatively large fragment from OVA can elicit physiologically relevant CTL (Carbone and Bevan 1989). As shown in Table 5, E.G7-OVA-specific priming was observed in C57BL/6 mice that are primed with either soluble OVA(229-276) peptide or syngeneic spleen cells pulsed with this peptide. In contrast, spleen cells pulsed with the OVA(258-276) determinant failed to generate a response, confirming that this peptide is not immunogenic (Table 4). It should be added that in vivo immunization using certain OVA digests occasionally gave an enhanced *peptide*-specific CTL response that did not cross-react on the OVA-expressing transfectant, E.G7-OVA. This activity probably resulted from a direct peptide/MHC interaction comparable to that associated with the primary CTL response shown in Figure 1. The above results demonstrate that some, but not all, forms of exogenous antigens can elicit a class-I-restricted response after in vivo immunization. Consequently, this would necessitate a specialized cell or mechanism operating in vivo that allows these antigens to enter the appropriate class I processing and presentation pathway.

In conclusion, we have shown that exogenous, soluble proteins can enter the class-I-restricted antigen-processing pathway if they are introduced directly into the cell cytoplasm. This can be achieved in vitro by the technique of osmotic lysis of pinosomes and can be exploited to generate class-I-restricted T cells specific for defined antigens. Further studies, using CTL directed against soluble proteins, should provide us with

Table 4. OVA-loaded Splenocytes Prime a Class-I-restricted CTL Response In Vivo

	% Lysis of ^{51}Cr targets[b]	
In vivo immunization[a]	E.G7-OVA	EL4
Saline	0	8
OVA (300 μg)	0	5
OVA(258-276) (30 μg)	7	10
OVA-loaded spleen cells	54	10

[a]C57BL/6 mice were immunized i.v. Splenocytes from these mice were stimulated for 5 days in vitro with irradiated E.G7-OVA cells. Syngeneic spleen cells (10^7) were loaded with OVA at 10 mg/ml.
[b]Lysis was measured at an effector:target rato of 30:1.

Table 5. The Synthetic Peptide OVA229–276 Primes for Transfectant-specific CTL

	% Lysis of ^{51}Cr targets[b]	
In vivo immunization[a]	E.G7-OVA	EL4
Saline	4	3
OVA(258-276)-pulsed splenocytes	4	1
OVA(229-276)-pulsed splenocytes	35	4
OVA(229-276) (500 μg)	32	4

[a]C57BL/6 mice were immunized i.v. as indicated. Syngeneic spleen cells (10^8) were pulsed with 0.2 mM peptide, and then 2×10^7 cells were injected per animal.
[b]Lysis at effector:target ratio of 20:1.

insights into the mechanisms associated with class-I-restricted antigen presentation.

ACKNOWLEDGMENTS

This work was supported in part by grants AI-19499 and AI-19335 from the National Institutes of Health. F.R.C. is the recipient of an Arthritis Foundation Fellowship. N.A.H. is a graduate student in the Department of Biology at the University of California, San Diego, and is the recipient of a National Science Foundation Graduate Fellowship.

REFERENCES

Bigelow, S., R. Hough, and M. Rechsteiner. 1981. The selective degradation of injected proteins occurs principally in the cytosol rather than in lysosomes. *Cell* **25**: 83.

Braciale, T.J. and K.L. Yap. 1978. Role of viral infectivity in the induction of influenza virus-specific cytotoxic T cells. *J. Exp. Med.* **147**: 1236.

Braciale, T.J., L.A. Morrison, M.T. Sweetser, J. Sambrook, M.J. Gething, and V.L. Braciale. 1987. Antigen presentation pathways to class I and class II MHC-restricted T lymphocytes. *Immunol. Rev.* **98**: 95.

Carbone, F.R. and M.J. Bevan. 1989. Induction of ovalbumin cytotoxic T cells by *in vivo* peptide immunization. *J. Exp. Med.* **169**: 603.

Carbone, F.R., M.W. Moore, J.M. Shiel, and M.J. Bevan. 1988. Induction of cytotoxic T lymphocytes by primary *in vitro* stimulation with peptides. *J. Exp. Med.* **167**: 1767.

Ciechanover, A. 1987. Mechanism of energy-dependent intracellular protein breakdown: The ubiquitin-mediated proteolytic pathway. In *Lysosomes: Their role in protein breakdown* (ed. H. Glaumann and F.J. Ballard), p. 561. Academic Press, London.

Germain, R.N. 1986. The ins and outs of antigen processing and presentation. *Nature* **322**: 687.

Hosken, N.A., M.J. Bevan, and F.R. Carbone. 1989. Class I restricted presentation occurs without internalization or processing of antigenic peptides. *J. Immunol.* **142**: 1079.

Jacobson, S., R.P. Sekaly, C.L. Jacobson, H.F. McFarland, and E.O. Long. 1989. HLA Class II-restricted presentation of cytoplasmic measles virus antigens to cytotoxic T cells. *J. Virol.* **63**: 1756.

Jentoft, N. and D.G. Dearborn. 1979. Labeling of proteins by reductive methylation using sodium cyanoborohydride. *J. Biol. Chem.* **254**: 4359.

Katznelson, R. and R.G. Kulka. 1983. Degradation of microinjected methylated and unmethylated proteins in hepatoma tissue culture cells. *J. Biol. Chem.* **258**: 9597.

Maryanski, J.L., P. Pala, G. Corradin, B.R. Jordan, and J.C. Cerrottini. 1986. H-2 restricted cytotoxic T cells specific for HLA can recognize a synthetic HLA peptide. *Nature* **324**: 578.

Moore, M.W., F.R. Carbone, and M.J. Bevan. 1988. Introduction of soluble protein into the class I pathway of antigen processing and presentation. *Cell* **54**: 777.

Morrison, L.A., A.E. Lukacher, V.L. Braciale, D. Fan, and T.J. Braciale. 1986. Differences in antigen presentation to MHC class I- and class II-restricted influenza virus-specific cytolytic T lymphocyte clones. *J. Exp. Med.* **163**: 903.

Okada, C.Y. and M. Rechsteiner. 1982. Introduction of macromolecules into cultured mammalian cells by the osmotic lysis of pinocytic vesicles. *Cell* **29**: 33.

Potter, T.A., T.V. Rajan, F.R. Dick II, and J.A. Bluestone. 1989. Substitution at residue 227 of H-2 class I molecules abrogates recognition by CD8-dependent, but not CD8-independent, cytotoxic T lymphocytes. *Nature* **337**: 73.

Salter, R.D., A.M. Normant, B.P. Chen, C. Clayberger, A.M. Krensky, D.R. Littman, and P. Parham. 1989. Polymorphism in the α_3 domain of HLA-A molecules affects binding to CD8. *Nature* **338**: 345.

Tanaka, K., L. Waxman, and A. Goldberg. 1983. ATP serves two distinct roles in protein degradation, one requiring and one independent of ubiquitin. *J. Cell. Biol.* **96**: 1580.

Tevethia, S.S., D.C. Flyer, and R. Tjian. 1980. Biology of simian virus 40 (SV40) transplantation antigen (TrAg). VI. Mechanism of induction of SV40 transplantation immunity in mice by purified SV40 T antigen (D2 protein). *Virology* **107**: 13.

Townsend, A.R.M. and H. Bodmer. 1989. Antigen presentation by class I-restricted T lymphocytes. *Annu. Rev. Immunol.* **7**: 601.

Townsend, A.R.M., F.M. Gotch, and J. Davey. 1985. Cytotoxic T cells recognize fragments of influenza nucleoprotein. *Cell* **42**: 457.

Williams, D.B., S.J. Swiedler, and G.W. Hart. 1985. Intracellular transport of membrane glycoproteins: Two closely related histocompatibility antigens differ in their rates of transit to the cell surface. *J. Cell. Biol.* **101**: 725.

Wraith, D.C. and B.A. Askonas. 1985. Induction of influenza A virus cross-reactive cytotoxic T cells by a nucleoprotein/haemagglutinin preparation. *J. Gen. Virol.* **66**: 1327.

A Peptide Derived from the α-Helical Region of Class I MHC Blocks CTL Engagement of the Class I MHC Molecule

T.I. Munitz,[*] J. Schneck,[†] J.E. Coligan,[‡] W.L. Maloy,[‡] J.P. Henrich,[*]
S.O. Sharrow,[*] D.H. Margulies,[†] and A. Singer[*]

[*]Experimental Immunology Branch, National Cancer Institute, [†]Molecular Biology Section, Laboratory of Immunology
and [‡]Biological Resources Branch, National Institute of Allergy and Infectious Diseases,
National Institutes of Health, Bethesda, Maryland 20892

Murine class I major histocompatibility complex (MHC) antigens are polymorphic cell-surface glycoproteins originally described as transplantation antigens responsible for mediating allogenic skin graft rejections (Snell et al. 1976). These complex molecules have also been shown to play an important role in immune responses by presenting antigen to cytolytic T cells, allowing them to recognize foreign antigens in an MHC-restricted fashion (Zinkernagel and Doherty 1979). More current studies propose that foreign antigens in the form of peptidic fragments are presented to cytotoxic T lymphocytes (CTL) in association with the class I molecule (Maryanski et al. 1986; Townsend et al. 1986; Braciale et al. 1987; Staertz et al. 1987; Takahashi et al. 1988). Although recognition and processing of nominal antigens is well documented (Schwartz et al. 1978; Corradin and Chiller 1979; Maryanski et al. 1986; Townsend et al. 1986; Braciale et al. 1987; Schwartz 1987), questions concerned with the nature of T-cell recognition sites on MHC molecules remain. The three-dimensional structure of the class I molecule has recently been described (Bjorkman et al. 1987a,b). The model shows two upwardly extended α-helical domains separated by a β-stranded groove that forms the floor of the molecule. The floor of the molecule is the putative antigen-binding site, whereas the exposed surfaces of the α-helical regions are thought to be potential binding sites for T-cell receptors. In our study, we wanted to investigate further the importance of the α-helical region in the interaction of the T-cell receptor with the H-2K^b molecule.

To investigate one potential T-cell recognition site from an exposed α-helical region of the class I molecule, a peptide whose sequence is identical to H-2K^b in the region of the H-2K^{bm10} mutation (peptide Kb163-174) was synthesized and analyzed for its ability to influence T-cell recognition (Bjorkman et al. 1987a,b; Maloy et al. 1987; Schneck et al. 1989). As a negative control peptide for our experiments, a peptide from a nonexposed portion of the H-2K^b molecule (Kb37-50) was also synthesized. We found that Kb163-174 was able to inhibit lysis of an H-2K^b target cell when cocultured with an H-2K^{bm10} anti-H-2K^b CTL clone or line. In addition, inhibition of lysis of H-2K^b target cells was

observed by CTL directed toward other regions of the K^b molecule as well as bulk third-party anti-H-2K^b CTL. Surprisingly, pretreatment experiments showed that inhibition by the peptide was at the level of the effector T cell and not at the level of the target cell. Furthermore, Kb163-174 was able to block conjugate formation between anti-K^b CTL effectors and K^b-bearing target cells, providing direct physical evidence that the peptide interferes with the physical association of the effector T cell with the target H-2K^b molecule. Thus, as suggested by these results, amino acid residues 163–174 define a site used by alloreactive T cells to engage the H-2K^b molecule.

MATERIALS AND METHODS

Mice. Mice used in this study were purchased from The Jackson Laboratory (Bar Harbor, Maine) or were bred in our animal colony. The genotypes of mouse strains used in this study at the H-2 K, IA, D loci are C57BL/10SnJ (B10), b,b,b; B10.BR, k,k,k; B10.YBR, b,b,d; B6.C-H-2^{bm1} (bm1), bm1,b,b; B6.C-H-2^{bm3} (bm3), bm3,b,b; B6.C-H-2^{bm6} (bm6), bm6,b,b; B6.C-H-2^{bm8} (bm8), bm8,b,b; B6.C-H-2^{bm10} (bm10), bm10,b,b; BALB/cJ, d,d,d; (BALB/cJ × C57BL/6J)F$_1$(CB6F$_1$), d,d,d, x b,b,b.

Concanavalin-A-induced supernatant (Con-A SN). Con-A SN was the supernatant from Con-A-stimulated BALB/c spleen cells prepared as described previously (Kruisbeek et al. 1980). The residual Con A was neutralized by the addition of 0.2 M α-methy-D-mannoside and was used in mixed lymphocyte cultures at a final concentration of 12.5%.

Peptides Kb163-174 and Kb37-50. All peptides were synthesized by solid-phase methodology using an automated peptide synthesizer. The peptides were then purified by gel filtration chromatography on a P-2 column (Bio-Rad Labs) and subsequently analyzed by amino acid composition and reversed-phase high-performance liquid chromatography (HPLC). Inhibitory effects of K^b peptide were maintained even when using different lots of purified peptide as well as HPLC-purified peptide. A peptide concentration of 100 μg/ml equals a final concentration of 63 μM for Kb163-174 and 56 μM for Kb37-50. All peptides were maintained as stock solutions of 10 mg/ml in phosphate-buffered saline (PBS) and stored at $-20°C$.

In vitro generation of CTL. Primary CTL were generated by mixed lymphocyte cultures of 5×10^6 spleen cells from normal unprimed responder mice and 5×10^6 (2000 R) stimulator spleen cells established in 2-ml cultures of complete RPMI medium supplemented with 10% FCS. All cultures were incubated at 37°C in 7.5% CO_2-humidified air. Cells were harvested, washed, counted, and assayed for their ability to lyse ^{51}Cr-labeled blasted spleen-cell, L-cell, or tumor-cell targets in a 4-hour ^{51}Cr-release assay. Cell lines were maintained by weekly restimulation with 2×10^6 to 5×10^6 (2000 R) stimulator spleen cells. In addition, 12.5% Con-A SN and 15–20 units of human recombinant interleukin-2 were added to each well. Cloned CTL were generated by expanding serially diluted cultures from cell lines and were maintained as individual cell lines as described above. An H-2K^{bm10} anti-H-2K^b CTL clone, clone 37, was originally described by Bluestone et al. (1986) and was maintained in our laboratory.

Peptide inhibition assay. Cells from primary cultures were harvested on day 5 (no sooner than day 3 poststimulation for clones and lines), washed, counted, and diluted out according to desired effector to target (E/T) ratio. Then either media alone or K^b peptides were added just prior to the addition of ^{51}Cr-labeled target cells. Cells were cocultured 4 hours for splenic or tumor cell targets and 6 hours for L-cell target cells. CTL were assayed in triplicate at each of four E/T ratios. Percent specific lysis = 100 × (experimental release − spontaneous release)/(maximum release − spontaneous release). Standard errors were routinely less than 5% specific lysis.

Peptide pretreatment assay. In these assays, either the bm10 anti-B10 CTL line or the ^{51}Cr-labeled EL4 target cells were cultured for 1 hour at 4°C with 200 μg/ml of peptide Kb163-174, Kb37-50, or medium alone. Cells were washed once in serum containing medium, resuspended in fresh medium, counted, diluted to an appropriate concentration, and assayed for lysis of the labeled EL4 target cells in a 4-hour ^{51}Cr-release assay. There was no significant change in cell viability at the end of the pretreatment, as determined by trypan blue exclusion. One lytic unit was defined as the number of effector cells required to lyse 30% of 10^5 target cells.

Conjugate formation assay. Conjugate formation assays were performed using modified methods described previously (Perez et al. 1985). Effector CTL lines were harvested on day 4 or 5 poststimulation. Fresh spleen cells used as targets were processed into a single cell suspension, and the red blood cells were lysed. Both cell populations were then washed once in phosphate-buffered saline (PBS) (pH 7.2). CTL were resuspend-ed to 2×10^6 cells/ml in PBS (pH 7.2), and spleen cells were resuspended to 20×10^6 cells/ml. The appropriate volume of 1 mM fluorescein isothiocyanate (FITC) (Sigma) in ethanol was added to the CTL line, and 1 mM rhodamine isothiocyanate (Research Organics, Inc., Cleveland, Ohio) in ethanol was added to the spleen cells to yield a final concentration of 10 μM. After a 10-minute incubation at 37°C, the cells were washed once with complete medium. They were then subjected to density gradient sedimentation on lympho-lyte M (Cedar Lane, Hornby, Ontario) to remove dead cells, washed once, and resuspended in complete medium to a concentration of 1×10^7 cells/ml. CTL were transferred to 200-μl microfuge tubes and pre-incubated at room temperature for 10 minutes with either media alone, 20 μg Kb163-174, or 20 μg Kb37-50. Next, spleen cell targets were added to each tube, centrifuged for 1 second in a Beckman microfuge, and incubated for 10 minutes at room temperature. Cells were gently resuspended with a Pasteur pipet and immediately diluted into 1 ml staining medium (Hanks balanced salt solution + 0.1% sodium azide + 0.1% bovine serum albumin) at 0°C.

These conjugate mixtures were maintained on ice for no more than 2 hours until analyzed using a modified BD FACS II Dual Laser System flow cytometer employing the manufacturer's filters and photomultipliers (Becton-Dickinson Immunocytochemistry Systems). FITC was excited using 488 nm (argon ion laser), and XRITC was excited using 590 nm (Rhodamine 6G pumped dye laser). Data collection was triggered using forward light scatter, gated to exclude most of unconjugated target spleen cells (which were significantly smaller than effector cells. Fluorescence data were collected, using 3-decade logarithmic amplification, on 50K forward light scatter events. Data were collected, stored, and analyzed using NIH-designed hardware interface and PDP11/84 computer system (Digital Equipment Corporation, Maynard, Maryland). The percentage of effectors in conjugates was calculated using the following equation: (total no. of effector cells in conjugates/total no. of effector cells) × 100.

Anti-H-2K^b CTL Are Specifically Blocked by Kb163-174

We began our investigation by examining the effect of a peptide derived from the α-helical region between amino acid residues 163 and 174 of H-2K^b on an al-loreactive CTL clone whose specificity was directed toward this region of the H-2K^b molecule. Lysis of H-2K^b target cells by an allospecific H-2K^{bm10} anti-H-2K^b CTL clone (clone 37) was blocked by peptide Kb163-174 (Table 1). The inability of Kb163-174 to block lysis of an H-2L^d target cell by an allospecific anti-H-2L^d clone (clone DF$_1$) demonstrates the specificity of inhibition by this peptide (Table 1). A control peptide from a different region of the H-2K^b molecule, between amino acids 37 and 50, was unable to block target cell lysis by either of the CTL clones

Table 1. Inhibition of CTL Recognition of Target Cells by K^b-derived Peptides

Responder cell		Stimulator cell		Target	% Target cell lysis in presence of		
			MHC antigen		media	Kb peptide	
type	strain	strain	disparity (a.a.)			163–174	37–50
Clone	Clone 37 (bm10 anti-B10)	B10	K^b (163–174)	EL4[a]	52	2	41
Clone	DF1 (B6 anti-B10.YBR)	B10.YBR	L^d	T1.1.1[b]	44	76	47
Cell line	bm10	B10	K^b (163–174)	EL4	58	31	54
Primary	bm10	B10	K^b (163–174)	EL4	32	8	36
Primary	bm1	B10	K^b (152, 155, 156)	EL4	48	10	48
Primary	bm3	B10	K^b (77, 89)	EL4	25	6	23
Primary	bm6	B10	K^b(116, 121)	EL4	42	17	n.d.
Primary	bm8	B10	K^b (22, 23, 24, 30)	EL4	36	17	n.d.
Primary	B10.BR	B10	H-2^b	I-3[c]	29	18	30
Primary	B10	B10.BR	H-2^k	I-3	28	35	27

n.d., not determined; a.a., amino acid.
[a]EL4 is an H-2^b murine tumor cell line.
[b]T1.1.1 is a C3H-derived murine L-cell line transfected with H-$2L^d$.
[c]I-3 is a C3H-derived murine L-cell line transfected with H-$2K^b$.

(Table 1). To assess if blockade of clone 37 by Kb163-174 was unique to the clone or a general characteristic of H-$2K^{bm10}$ anti-H-$2K^b$ CTL effectors, we examined a heterogeneous H-$2K^{bm10}$ anti-H-$2K^b$ CTL line. We found that Kb163-174 was able to block lysis of H-$2K^b$ target cells by a heterogeneous H-$2K^{bm10}$ anti-H-$2K^b$ CTL line (Table 1). Furthermore, this peptide was found to block heterogeneous primary H-$2K^{bm10}$ anti-H-$2K^b$ response cultures (Table 1). These experiments demonstrate that H-$2K^{bm10}$ anti-H-$2K^b$ CTL clone, line, or primary cultures can be blocked by a peptide whose sequence is identical to H-$2K^b$ between amino acids 163 and 174 corresponding to the region of the H-$2K^{bm10}$ mutation.

To assess whether the inhibition by peptide Kb163-174 was limited to H-$2K^{bm10}$ anti-H-$2K^b$ CTL specific for the region between amino acids 163 and 174 or whether this was a much broader anti-H-$2K^b$ effect, we tested the ability of this peptide to block anti-H-$2K^b$

CTL derived from primary response cultures whose allospecificity was directed toward regions of the H-$2K^b$ molecule distinct from amino acids 163 and 174. Surprisingly, peptide Kb163-174 was able to inhibit lysis of H-$2K^b$ target cells by primary H-$2K^{bm10}$ anti-H-$2K^b$ CTL cultures as well as by H-$2K^{bm1}$, H-$2K^{bm3}$, H-$2K^{bm6}$, and H-$2K^{bm8}$ anti-H-$2K^b$ CTL cultures in which peptide Kb163-174 represents a self-sequence rather than a foreign sequence (Table 1). Finally, lysis of an H-$2K^b$-positive transfected L-cell line, I-3, by primary B10.BR anti-B10 (H-2^k anti-H-2^b) CTL effectors was also inhibited by peptide Kb163-174 (Table 1). In contrast, lysis of the same transfected L-cell line I-3 by primary B10 anti-B10.BR (H-2^b anti-H-2^k) CTL effectors was not inhibited by peptide Kb163-174 (Table 1). Therefore, peptide Kb163-174 was able to specifically inhibit anti-K^b CTL effectors whether the region of the H-$2K^b$ molecule between amino acids 163 and 174 served as a foreign site or as a self site.

Table 2. Prepulsing of Effectors and Targets with K^b Peptides

Expt.	Effector	Prepulsing peptide[a]		Target[b]	Prepulsing Peptide		% Specific lysis			Lytic units
		163–174	37–50		163–174	37–50				
						E/T:	10	3	1	
1	bm10 anti-B10 (CTL line)	−	−	EL4	−	−	40	33	23	45
		+	−	EL4	−	−	30	22	8	8
		−	+	EL4	−	−	40	31	22	37
2	bm10 anti-B10 (CTL line)	−	−	EL4	−	−	60	48	28	141
		−	−	EL4	+	−	54	43	28	100
		−	−	EL4	−	+	60	55	33	174
3	bm10 anti-B10 (CTL line)	−	−	EL4	−	−	62	56	51	2249
		+	−	EL4	−	−	48	43	32	285
		−	+	EL4	−	−	64	58	45	1822

[a]Peptide concentration used was 100 μg/tube.
[b]EL4 is an H-2^b thymoma.

Table 3. Specificity of Peptide Blockade of CTL Generated from Dual Reactive Response Cultures

Responder	K^b peptide (16 μg)	E:T	Target cell[a] % specific lysis	
			T1.1.1 (L^d)	I-3 (K^b)
B10.BR anti-CB6F$_1$ (k anti-dxb)	media	30	22.5	19.8
	163–174	30	17.2	9.6
	37–50	30	23.0	21.2

[a]L-cell transfectants.

Peptide Kb163-174 Blocks at the Level of the Effector T Cell

To determine whether Kb163-174 was blocking at the level of the effector cell or the target cell, we performed pretreatment experiments in which either anti-K^b CTL effector cells or K^b-expressing target cells were preincubated with the peptides. These experiments showed that preincubation of effector T cells from an H-2K^{bm10} anti-H-2K^b CTL line with peptide Kb163-174 specifically inhibited their ability to lyse K^b target cells (Table 2). This is emphasized by a decrease in lytic activity of greater than 80%. In contrast, preincubation of target cells with Kb163-174 had no specific effect on their ability to be lysed by the anti-K^b CTL line.

To further investigate the site of action of the effector T cell, we looked at the effect of Kb163-174 to inhibit lysis of a single effector cell population with two distinct receptor-mediated allospecificities. To accomplish this, we harvested CTL from a single B10.BR anti-CB6F$_1$ response culture that contained both anti-K^b and anti-L^d effector cells. As can be seen in Table 3, inhibition of lysis by Kb163-174 was observed when B10.BR anti-CB6F$_1$ (H-2^k anti-H-2^{dxb}) CTL cultures were tested on target cells expressing H-2K^b, but no inhibition of lysis was observed when the same effector cell population was tested on target cells expressing H-2L$^{d \cdot}$. Thus, peptide Kb163-174 inhibits lysis of anti-H-2K^b CTL but not anti-L^d CTL, even when both CTL populations are genetically identical and are generated simultaneously in a single response culture.

Peptide Kb163-174 Specifically Blocks H-2K^{bm10} Anti-H-2K^b Conjugate Formation

From our previous studies, it was evident that peptide Kb163-174 was able to specifically block allorecognition of H-2K^b-bearing target cells by anti-H-2K^b CTL effectors. Therefore, we wanted to investigate the pos-

sible effect this peptide might have on the physical interaction between the CTL effector cell and its target cell. Peptide Kb163-174 was tested for its ability to block conjugate formation between Tim-411, an H-2K^{bm10} anti-H-2K^b CTL line, and its specific H-2K^b target, B10. Table 4 illustrates the ability of Kb163-174 to significantly block the vast majority of conjugates formed between Tim-411 and an H-2K^b target cell. Conversely, there was no inhibitory effect observed with the addition of the control peptide, Kb37-50.

DISCUSSION

In the present paper, we have demonstrated that a soluble peptide with a sequence identical to H-2K^b between amino acids 163 and 174, the region of the H-2K^{bm10} mutation, was able to block allorecognition of H-2K^b target cells by H-2K^{bm10} anti-H-2K^b CTL clone, line, or bulk cultures. These results show that blockade was a general characteristic of H-2K^{bm10} anti-H-2K^b CTL effectors and was not unique to a selected clonal population. In addition, Kb163-174 was able to inhibit the formation of allospecific conjugates, which provides physical evidence that this peptide interferes with the engagement of the K^b molecule by anti-H-2K^b CTL effectors. Surprisingly, this peptide was able to block primary CTL effectors whose allospecificity was directed toward various regions of the H-2K^b molecule and for whom peptide Kb163-174 represented a self site. Thus, blockade appears to be independent of the region between amino acids 163 and 174 being recognized as a foreign site but dependent on the anti-H-2K^b specificity of the effector T cell. Therefore, our experiments provide evidence that the α-helical region of K^b between amino acids 163 and 174 is a necessary binding site for many anti-H-2K^b T cell effectors.

Surprisingly, blocking of anti-K^b CTL by Kb163-174 appears to be at the level of the effector T cell, as

Table 4. Specific Blockade of Conjugate Formation by Kb163-174 Peptide

Effector cells	Kb peptide[a]	% Effector cells in conjugates with		Net K^b-specific conjugates
		B10	bm10	
Tim-411[b]	None	23.8	8.8	15.0
	163–174	12.9	9.0	3.9
	37–50	24.5	10.0	14.5

[a]20 μg/tube of peptide was used in this assay.
[b]Tim-411 is an H-2K^{bm10} anti-H-2K^b CTL line.

shown by preincubation experiments. One possible explanation for this finding that we considered was that the peptide bound to MHC molecules on the anti-H-2K^b CTL effectors, turning them into targets for other CTL effectors present in the CTL population. However, contrary to this possibility, peptide Kb163-174 never sensitized targets for killing by anti-H-2K^b CTL. Furthermore, ^{51}Cr-labeling of the CTL effectors themselves revealed that they neither lysed themselves nor each other upon addition of peptide Kb163-174 (data not shown). Another possible explanation for the direct effect of peptide Kb163-174 on anti-K^b CTL was that it bound to an adhesion molecule, possibly CD8, on the surface of anti-K^b effector CTL. However, anti-L^d CTL responses were equally dependent on CD8 as were anti-K^b CTL, yet the peptide only blocked anti-K^b lysis. Consequently, we think the most straightforward interpretation of these data is that Kb163-174 interferes with CTL lysis of K^b target cells by binding directly to the clonotypic receptor on anti-K^b CTL. The high concentrations required for this blocking imply that the affinity of this interaction is low.

In conclusion, we think the present results demonstrate the importance of an exposed region of the α-helical domain for T-cell recognition by identifying the area between amino acids 163 and 174 as a necessary binding site on the H-2K^b molecule required for contact by the clonotypic T-cell receptor.

REFERENCES

Bjorkman, P.J., M.A. Saper, B. Samraoui, W.S. Bennett, J.L. Strominger, and D.C. Wiley. 1987a. Structure of the human class I histocompatibility antigen, HLA-A2. *Nature* **329:** 506.

———. 1987b. The foreign antigen binding site and T cell recognition regions of class I histocompatibility antigens. *Nature* **329:** 512.

Bluestone, J.A., C. Langlet, S.S. Geier, S.G. Nathenson, M. Foo, and A.-M. Schmitt-Verhulst. 1986. Somatic cell variants express altered H-2K^b allodeterminants recognized by cytolytic T cell clones. *J. Immunol.* **137:** 1244.

Braciale, T.J., V.L. Braciale, M. Winkler, I. Stroynowski, L. Hood, J. Sambrook, and M.J. Gething. 1987. On the role of the transmembrane anchor sequence of influenza hemagglutinin in target cell recognition by class I MHC-restricted, hemagglutinin-specific cytolytic T lymphocytes. *J. Exp. Med.* **166:** 678.

Corradin, G. and J.M. Chiller. 1979. Lymphocyte-specificity to protein antigen. II. Fine specificity of T-cell activation with cytochrome C and derived peptides as antigenic probes. *J. Exp. Med.* **149:** 436.

Kruisbeek, A.M., J.M. Zijlstra, and T.J. Krose. 1980. Distinct effects of T cell growth factors and thymic epithelial factors on the generation of cytotoxic T lymphocyte subpopulations. *J. Immunol.* **125:** 995.

Maloy, W.L. 1987. Comparison of the primary structure of class I molecules. *Immunol. Rev.* **6:** 11.

Maryanski, J.L., P. Pala, G. Corridan, B.R. Jordan, and J.C. Cerottini. 1986. H-2 restricted cytolytic T cells specific for HLA can recognize a synthetic HLA peptide. *Nature* **324:** 578.

Perez, P., J.A. Bluestone, D.A. Stephany, and D.M. Segel. 1985. Quantitative measurements of the specificity and kinetics of conjugate formation between cloned cytotoxic T lymphocytes and splenic target cells by dual parameter flow cytometry. *J. Immunol.* **134:** 478.

Schneck, J., W.L. Maloy, J.E. Coligan, and D.H. Margulies. 1989. Inhibition of an allospecific T cell hybridoma by soluble class I proteins and peptides: Estimation of the affinity of a T cell receptor for MHC. *Cell* **55:** 47.

Schwartz, R.H. 1987. Immune response (Ir) genes of the murine major histocompatibility complex. *Adv. Immunol.* **38:** 31.

Schwartz, R.H., J.A. Berzofsky, C.L. Horton, A.N. Schechter, and D.H. Sachs. 1978. Genetic control of the T lymphocyte proliferative response to staphylococcal nuclease: Evidence for multiple MHC-linked Ir gene control. *J. Immunol.* **120:** 1741.

Snell, G.D., J. Dauwwet, and S.G. Nathenson. 1976. *Histocompatibility*. Academic Press, New York.

Staertz, U.D., H. Korasyama, and A.M. Garner. 1987. Cytotoxic T lymphocytes against a soluble protein. *Nature* **329:** 449.

Takahashi, H., J. Cohen, C. DeLisi, B. Moss, R.N. Germain, and J.A. Berzofsky. 1988. An immunodominant epitope of the human immunodeficiency virus envelope glycoprotein gp160 recognized by class I major histocompatibility complex molecule-restricted murine cytotoxic T lymphocytes. *Proc. Natl. Acad. Sci.* **85:** 3105.

Townsend, A.R.M., J. Rothbard, F.M. Gotch, G. Bahadur, D. Wraith, and A.J. McMichael. 1986. The epitopes of influenza nucleoprotein by cytotoxic T lymphocytes can be defined with short synthetic peptides. *Cell* **44:** 959.

Zinkernagel, R.M. and P.C. Doherty. 1979. MHC-restricted cytotoxic T cells: Studies on the biological role of polymorphic major transplantation antigens determining T cell restriction-specificity, function and responsiveness. *Adv. Immunol.* **27:** 51.

Molecular Definition of a Mitochondrially Encoded Mouse Minor Histocompatibility Antigen

K. FISCHER LINDAHL,* E. HERMEL,† B.E. LOVELAND,‡ S. RICHARDS,§
C.-R. WANG, AND H. YONEKAWA**

*Howard Hughes Medical Institute and the *Departments of Microbiology and Biochemistry
and the †Graduate Immunology Program,
University of Texas Southwestern Medical Center, Dallas, Texas 75235-9050*

Mta, the maternally transmitted antigen of the mouse, is an exceptional minor histocompatibility (H) antigen. Like other minor H antigens, it causes slow skin-graft rejection (Chan and Fischer Lindahl 1985) and is readily detected by cytotoxic T lymphocytes (CTLs) (Fischer Lindahl et al. 1980) but does not induce an alloantibody response. Unlike other minor H antigens, Mta shows extrachromosomal, matroclinous inheritance (Fischer Lindahl et al. 1980; Fischer Lindahl and Bürki 1982; Fischer Lindahl and Hausmann 1983), and the CTLs specific for Mta do not exhibit standard H-2 restriction (Fischer Lindahl et al. 1980). We undertook the study of Mta in the hope that this exception would illuminate the rules for what CTLs can recognize.

Genetic analysis of wild mice with variant Mta phenotypes led to the identification of two genes that jointly determine the epitopes of Mta: *Mtf* and *Hmt* (Fischer Lindahl et al. 1983, 1986). Four allelic forms of *Mtf*, the maternally transmitted factor, have been identified to date (Hirama and Fischer Lindahl 1985), and they each determine immunologically distinct forms of Mta (Fischer Lindahl et al. 1989). *Hmt* is closely linked to the major histocompatibility complex (MHC) of the mouse, 1–2 cM distal of *H-2D* (Fischer Lindahl et al. 1983).

The proximity of *Hmt* to large clusters of MHC class I genes, the H-2 unrestricted recognition of Mta, and the requirement for β_2-microglobulin for Mta expression led us to propose that *Hmt* encodes an MHC class I gene, which acts as a restriction element for the CTL recognition of a ligand encoded by *Mtf* (Fischer Lindahl et al. 1983, 1987; Fischer Lindahl 1985). To prove this hypothesis, we had only to identify and isolate the genes involved and examine how their products interact.

Present addresses: ‡Centre for Molecular Biology and Medicine, Monash University, Clayton, Victoria 3168, Australia; §GeneScreen, Dallas, Texas 75207; **Tokyo Metropolitan Institute of Medical Science, Bunkyo-ku, Tokyo 113, Japan.

RESULTS

MTF Peptide

The only genes in mice known to be strictly maternally transmitted are the mitochondrial genes (Fischer Lindahl 1985). The rare alleles of *Mtf* (β, γ, and δ) are associated with unique mitochondrial genomes (Ferris et al. 1983; C.-R. Wang et al., in prep.; U. Gyllensten and E.M. Prager, pers. comm.), and in somatic cell hybrids, the MTF phenotypes segregate with mitochondrial DNA (mtDNA) (Smith et al. 1983; Huston et al. 1985; B.E. Loveland et al., in prep.). However, the assumption that *Mtf* is encoded by the mitochondrial genome entailed no obvious mechanism for how it could affect a cell-surface character, although a multitude of models were proposed (Hirama and Fischer Lindahl 1985; Rodgers et al. 1986; Han et al. 1987, 1989). Mitochondria import proteins from the cytoplasm on a large scale, but no mitochondrial protein is known to be exported.

Whereas other minor H genes have been defined by genetic recombination to chromosomal intervals spanning millions of base pairs at the least, *Mtf* offered the advantage that the mitochondrial genome is small (16,300 bp), and the sequence of one, from L cells derived from C3H mice of *Mtf*$^\alpha$ type, was already known (Bibb et al. 1981). We therefore decided to sequence the mtDNA from mice of β, γ, and δ types to discover exactly where the mitochondrial genomes for the four *Mtf* types differ. The mtDNAs of α, β (from strain NZB/BlNJ), and γ mice (from the MilP line, derived from a wild mouse caught near Pavia, Italy) differ from each other by 0.6% in their nucleotide sequence and that of δ mice (the SUB-SHH stock from Shanghai) differs from these by 3%. The complete sequences will be published elsewhere (H. Yonekawa et al.; C.-R. Wang et al.; both in prep.).

Table 1 lists the number of amino acid substitutions among the four types in the 13 known mitochondrially encoded proteins. The substitutions are all single and generally conservative, scattered over the genomes. Only four proteins, ND1, ND2, ND5, and ND6, differ

Table 1. Amino Acid Substitutions between the 13 Proteins Encoded by Mitochondrial Genomes of Different *Mtf* Types

	α	β	γ
δ	36	40	39
γ	16	17	
β	15		

among all four types. Given current insights into antigen recognition by T cells, it was reasonable to assume that *Mtf* encodes peptides that escape the mitochondria and are presented on the cell surface by an MHC class I molecule encoded by *Hmt*. The simplest model stated that MTF is a single peptide.

There is one and only one position where all four types differ from each other: at the amino terminus of the ND1 protein, a 30-kD hydrophobic subunit of NADH dehydrogenase, or complex I (Fig. 1). If this is *Mtf*, we reasoned that we should be able to confer a new Mta phenotype on a target cell by the addition of a synthetic peptide of the corresponding sequence (Townsend et al. 1986). Unfortunately, it was not known whether translation of mouse ND1 starts at GUG, aligning it with cow and human counterparts (Anderson et al. 1982), or three codons later at AUU, as proposed by Bibb et al. (1981). We therefore tested three peptides with the α sequence: the 26-amino-acid-long ND1α1-26 and the 17-amino-acid-long ND1α1-17, both with formylmethionine in position 1 and isoleucine in positions 4 and 6, and the 23-amino-acid-long ND1α4-26, starting with formylmethionine in position 4. In addition, we tested ND1β1-17, which differs from ND1α1-17 only by an alanine in position 6. The results of these assays will appear in detail elsewhere (B.E. Loveland et al., in prep.), and they can be summarized as follows:

1. If added overnight to cells with β or δ *Mtf*, the ND1α1-26 peptide, but not ND1α4-26, transformed these cells into targets for CTLs that were specific for the α form of Mta. The activity of ND1α1-17 is indistinguishable from that of ND1α1-26. The cells treated with the peptide were at least as susceptible

to lysis as cells with the proper mitochondrial genome. Thus, it can be concluded that the amino terminus of ND1 is indeed a minor H antigen and that translation of ND1 starts at position 1 from a GUG codon.

2. ND1β1-17 confers susceptibility to β-specific CTLs if added to *Mtf*^α target cells. ND1α1-17 and ND1β1-17 show specificity in their ability to confer susceptibility to α- and β-specific CTLs, respectively. Thus, the allelic forms of *Mtf* can be accounted for by a single, conservative amino acid substitution.

3. Target cells carrying the standard *Hmt*^a allele can be transformed but not target cells with the *Hmt*^b null allele, further confirming that the synthetic peptides mimic the endogenous *Mtf* product.

4. Full sensitivity to killing is achieved with a peptide concentration of 100 nM; thus, the MTF peptide is active within the same range as has been described for viral peptides presented by standard H-2 class I molecules (Townsend et al. 1986).

5. The target cells generated by addition of synthetic peptide compete fully with the natural target cells of appropriate mitochondrial genotype for the recognition by CTLs, thus showing that the ND1 peptide alone generates all the epitopes of Mta.

Perhaps the most surprising of our findings is the fact that only one of the many differences in the mitochondrial proteins of mice with different *Mtf* types gives rise to a CTL response. This point is illustrated further in Figure 2. Even though there are 36 potentially antigenic differences between δ and α mitochondria, the killing of target cells with *Mtf*^α mitochondria can be fully inhibited by competitors treated with an ND1α peptide; untreated competitors with rat or *Mtf*^β mitochondria do not inhibit.

Although Bastin et al. (1987) had shown that CTLs are able to discriminate between a glutamic and an aspartic residue in a viral peptide, we were still impressed by how small the difference is between the allelic forms of MTF (Fig. 3). The absence or presence of a single methyl group is sufficient to induce a CTL response, given proper help (K. Fischer Lindahl et al., in prep.).

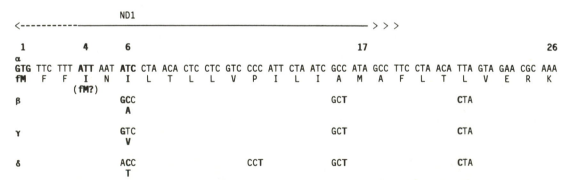

Figure 1. Sequence of the 5′ end of the mitochondrial ND1 gene in *Mtf*^α mice, starting from the first base after the tRNA^Leu gene. The translation into the ND1α1-26 peptide is given in one-letter code, and position 4, the alternative start codon, is indicated. For the β, γ, and δ mice, only those codons with a change (boldface type) are shown; only the change in the sixth codon caused an amino acid replacement.

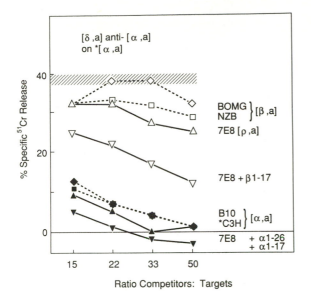

Figure 2. The amino terminus of ND1 is the only mitochondrial peptide recognized by CTLs specific for Mta. The killer cells were from (SHB × BALB.B)F₁ mice (*Mtf^δ*) immunized with BALB.B (*Mtf^α*) cells, and they were stimulated and assayed as described previously (B.E. Loveland et al., in prep.) at a ratio of 27:1 on ⁵¹Cr-labeled concanavalin A lymphoblast target cells from C3H/HeJ mice (*Mtf^α*). Cold target competitors, used in the indicated ratios, were lymphoblasts from *Mtf^α* or *Mtf^β* mice on the 7E8 hybridoma, which has rat mitochondria (ρ) and carries the mouse *Hmt^α* gene. The hybridoma cells were cultured with the ND1 peptides indicated at a concentration of 400 nM for 46 hr before the assay. We explain the partial inhibition by 7E8 + ND1β1-17 as the combined effect of two weakly cross-reacting determinants (ρ and β).

MHC Class I Genes in the *Hmt* Region

The demonstration that MTF is a peptide and that the allelic forms are due to single amino acid differences is very strong support for our model of Hmt as a restriction element. We started our search for the gene with the genetic definition of the *Hmt* region on chromosome 17, which we can now limit by two recombinational breakpoints, R4-e and R4-l, thought to be less than 0.7 cM apart. Two further breakpoints have been useful in the subdivision of the *Hmt* region: the end of the distal *t* inversion and the *t^w18* duplication (Richards et al. 1989). We are in the process of mapping *Hmt* relative to the distal *t* inversion, using two *t* haplotypes that differ for *H-2*, *Hmt*, and *Tpx-1*. In

α Ile β Ala
γ Val δ Thr

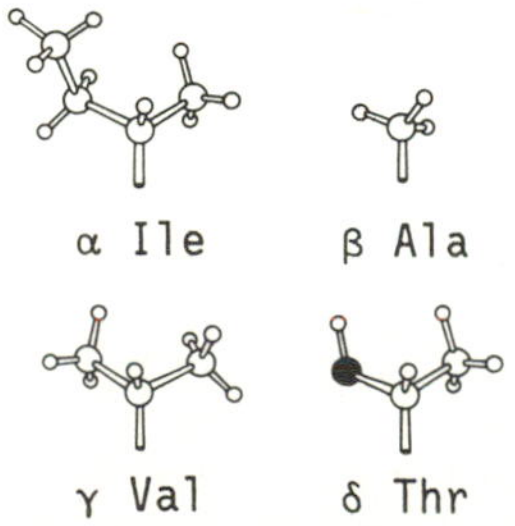

Figure 3. Histoincompatibility reduced ad absurdum: The allelic forms of the MTF minor H antigen. Oxygen is black.

recombinants between these haplotypes, *Hmt* segregates with *H-2*, showing that it is included in the *t* inversion, rather than with *Tpx-1*, as it would if it were outside (Z. Zhu et al., unpubl.).

Our R4-l haplotype carries the *Hmt* region from *Mus musculus castaneus (Hmt^b)* on a chromosome 17 otherwise derived from the laboratory mice C3H and C3H.SW (*Hmt^a*). Because of the genetic divergence of the strains involved, this haplotype is well suited for analysis of restriction-fragment-length polymorphisms (RFLPs). On the assumption that *Hmt* belongs to the family of MHC class I genes, we have screened digests of genomic DNA from the recombinant and parental strains with a probe for the conserved exon 4. We found several fragments that must map to the *Hmt* region (Fischer Lindahl et al. 1987), and we have cloned two of these from band libraries (S. Richards et al. 1989; C.-R. Wang, in prep.). The same panel of strains has also been used to map two previously cloned MHC class I genes, *Thy19.4* (Brorson et al. 1989) and *Mb1* (Singer et al. 1988), to the *Hmt* region. The currently known MHC class I genes of the *Hmt* region are listed in Table 2. Because they all have characteristic conserved RFLPs in *t* haplotypes, they must lie within the *t* inversion and therefore belong to the proximal end of the *Hmt* region, closest to *Tla*.

The extremely low level of expression of *Thy19.4*, except in the thymus, and negative results from transfection experiments suggest that it is not *Hmt*. Similarly, the lack of evidence for expression of the endogenous *Mb1* gene rules out that it is *Hmt*. The *Mb1* probe cross-hybridizes with a second fragment that also was mapped to the *Hmt* region; this could represent a sixth class I gene in that region.

C3R1 was cloned as a 5-kb *Eco*RI fragment, containing the 3′ end of the class I gene. With a probe derived from this clone, two cosmids with the complete gene have been isolated, one of which contains an additional, intact class I gene, *CRW2*. Because *C3R1* has a stop codon in the third exon, and no mRNA was found with an exon 3 probe, it is a poor candidate for *Hmt*. *CRW2* is interesting in that exons 2 and 3 differ strikingly from all other class I genes (although the glycosylation site in the α₁ and the two cysteines in the α₂ domain are conserved), whereas exon 4 shows a normal level of similarity and the gene encodes a proper transmembrane region and a short cytoplasmic tail. *CRW2* appears to be an intact class I gene, but we do not yet know whether it is expressed.

R4B2 was cloned from *Hmt^b* DNA as a 17-kb *Bgl*II fragment. We have since isolated the homolog from *Hmt^a* mice in the form of one cosmid and several cDNA clones. The amino acid sequence of *R4B2* shows about 15%, 65%, 55%, 80%, and 30% similarity to known class I genes for exons 1, 2, 3, 4, and 5, respectively. It has a single glycosylation site at residue 86 in the α₁ domain, a hydrophobic transmembrane domain, and a cytoplasmic tail of 8 amino acids. *R4B2* mRNA is easily detectable in thymus, spleen, lymph nodes, liver, and kidney (C.-R. Wang, in prep.).

Table 2. MHC Class I Genes in the *Hmt* Region

Gene[1]	Clones	Similarity to L[d] (%)			Intron 3 length (kb)	Deduced protein exons	Glycosylation sites		Expression
		α_1	α_2	α_3					
Thy19.4	genomic	59	61	77[2]	0.7	346 amino acids	α_1:	86, 90	thymus (scarce) >
	cDNA[3]	68	68	88[4]		5 exons	α_2:	176	other tissues and
							α_3:	256	cell lines
Mb1[5]	genomic	38	39	59[2]	0.6	320 amino acids	α_1:	85	none detected in
		55	54	75[4]		5 exons	α_3:	222	tissues and cell lines
C3R1	genomic[6]	not done		62[2]	>1.1	stop codon in exon 3	not done		none detected (exon 3 probe) in tissues and transfectants
CRW2	genomic[6]	34	48	77[2]	0.5	>5 exons	α_1:	86	not done
R4B2	genomic	65	60	82[2]	1.0	325 amino acids	α_1:	86	thymus > spleen,
	cDNA	69	70	86[4]		5 exons + 3′UT			liver, and kidney > testis ≫ brain

[1]Sources: Singer et al. (1988); Brorson et al. (1989); S. Richards et al.; C.-R. Wang (both in prep.).
[2]Amino acids.
[3]The cDNA clone was neither full length nor completely spliced.
[4]Nucleotides.
[5]The *Hmt* region contains an additional gene, about which nothing is known, that cross-hybridizes with the *Mb1* probe.
[6]*C3R1* and *CRW2* are present on the same cosmid.

We have transfected a cosmid with the *R4B2* gene from an *Hmt*[a] mouse into a fibroblast line from an *Hmt*[b] mouse, which does not express Mta. The preliminary results showed that some of the transfectants could be lysed by CTLs specific for Mta and that they could present the ND1β1-17 peptide, suggesting that we may have found *Hmt* (B.E. Loveland, unpubl.).

The properties of *R4B2* are consistent with what we know about *Hmt*. Both have a wide tissue distribution (Fischer Lindahl et al. 1980; Rodgers et al. 1986). Unlike Qa2, the Mta target antigen is not sensitive to phospholipase C, suggesting that Hmt has a proper transmembrane anchor rather than a phosphatidylinositol linkage (B.E. Loveland and D. Mann, unpubl.). Upon tunicamycin treatment, *Mtf*[a]:*Hmt*[a] target cells become sensitive to lysis by CTLs specific for MTF[β], suggesting that *Hmt* has N-linked carbohydrate(s) (Han et al. 1987). *R4B2* shares a number of conserved, structurally important residues (Brown et al. 1988) and has sufficient sequence similarity to other MHC class I genes to suggest that it would fold in the same manner. It is worth noting that no charged residues point directly into the groove or peptide-binding site (C.-R. Wang, in prep.).

T-cell Receptor for Mta

Several clones with γ/δ T-cell receptors (TCRs) have been found to recognize antigens encoded in the distal end of the MHC, possibly in the *Hmt* region (Tonegawa et al.; Houlden et al.; both this volume), suggesting that the MHC class Ib molecules may be the restriction elements for γ/δ TCRs (Raulet 1989; Strominger 1989). It was therefore of considerable interest to determine what type of TCR is used by CTLs specific for Hmt or Mta.

We tested four lines of T cells from C3H.R4-1 mice (*Hmt*[b]) that had been immunized in vivo with C3H/HeJ cells, which differ only by the *Hmt*[a] region and prime CTLs specific for either Hmt[a] alone or the Mta complex of Hmt[a] + MTF[α]. The lines had been cultured for over 100 days in vitro with *Hmt*[a] cells, either exclusively from C3H/HeJ (124.1) or later from BOM (*Mtf*[β], 124.2), C57BL/10 (*Mtf*[α], 124.3), or SHG5F1 (*Mtf*[δ], 131) to select the CTLs that recognize Hmt[a], irrespective of the MTF ligand. In all cases, we could

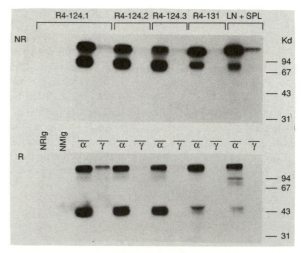

Figure 4. Immunoprecipitation of TCRs from CTLs specific for Hmt or Mta. Cells ($1–5 \times 10^7$), either from long-term cultures of *Hmt*[b] cells (R4) stimulated with *Hmt*[a] cells (for details, see text) or fresh lymph node and spleen cells, were labeled with ^{125}I by the lactoperoxidase method. The washed cells were lysed, the precleared lysates were immunoprecipitated with rabbit anti-TCRα or anti-TCRγ serum and protein A–Sepharose, and the samples were electrophoresed under nonreducing (NR) or reducing (R) conditions. The anti-TCR sera were a gift from Drs. K. Maeda and S. Tonegawa.

immunoprecipitate a labeled TCR complex with an antiserum specific for TCRα, but not with one specific for TCRγ (Fig. 4). Thus, we conclude that these CTLs use the α/β and not the γ/δ TCR.

DISCUSSION

A Model Minor H Antigen

Mta is the first minor H antigen to be defined in molecular terms, and the exception has revealed itself as the prototype of the rule: All H antigens are complexes of an MHC molecule and a peptide ligand. The ND1 protein that MTF is derived from is one of many subunits of NADH dehydrogenase, an enzyme complex located in the mitochondrial inner membrane. There is no obvious reason why this peptide, which is usually buried deep inside the cell, should be a transplantation antigen.

Boon and his co-workers have recently succeeded in cloning and identifying a number of tumor-specific transplantation antigens (De Plaen et al. 1988; Boon et al., this volume). Like MTF, they are short peptides derived from intracellular proteins common to many cells, and the antigenic form of the peptide differs from that of normal cells by a conservative amino acid substitution such as arginine to histidine. Whereas the mutation in the case of the tumor antigen P91A is thought to create an agretope, we know that all four alleles of MTF are presented, and the polymorphic residue is therefore more likely to interact directly with the TCR.

Generalizing from these two systems, it is to be expected that minor H antigens will all prove to be short peptides that differ within a species by single conservative amino acid substitutions. Although derived from cellular proteins, the peptides no longer bear any relation to the function of those proteins, most of which will be located inside the cell. The cloning of more minor H antigens is not a direct way to the discovery of interesting genes, with the possible exception of H-Y, the male-specific antigen (Simpson 1986).

It is likely that any protein can become a minor H antigen if a mutation occurs to create a variant of a component peptide suitable for presentation by an MHC molecule. It will therefore never be feasible to define all the minor H antigens of an individual as the MHC can be described. To prevent the complications that minor H antigens cause in bone marrow transplantation, one might aim for an understanding of the rules that determine which peptide a given MHC molecule can present (Grey et al., this volume). It may be possible to construct nonantigenic peptides that compete with all antigenic peptides for presentation and thus prevent their recognition (Maryanski et al.; Madden et al., both this volume).

Nonpolymorphic H Molecules

The tools of classic immunogenetics detect and consider only those H molecules that show allelic variation. A difference in the MHC molecule affects a large number of complexes and gives rise to a strong T-cell response, whereas a change in a peptide ligand affects only a few complexes and causes a correspondingly weaker reaction (Matzinger and Bevan 1977). Our earlier failure to obtain experimental evidence for this model is quite likely explained by the majority of these ligands being nonpolymorphic (Langhorne and Fischer Lindahl 1982). Such ligands can be detected if they have a unique tissue distribution (Marrack and Kappler 1988).

Although the nature of our analysis has emphasized the different forms of Mta, the antigen is actually almost nonpolymorphic. A stroke of luck originally led us to immunize the only laboratory mice that are not Mtf^α, and hundreds of wild mice were screened to find Mtf^γ and Mtf^δ mice (Ferris et al. 1983; Fischer Lindahl and Hausmann 1983). Similarly, variants of Hmt are limited to t haplotypes or (sub)species like $M.\ m.\ castaneus$, $M.\ m.\ bactrianus$, or $M.\ m.\ spretus$ (Fischer Lindahl 1986).

Our results with Hmt prove that MHC class I molecules other than the classic ones, such as H-2K, H-2D, and H-2L, can present antigens to T cells. It is worth noting that if the presenting molecule is not polymorphic, the T-cell recognition will appear to be nonrestricted. In view of the evidence that it may be a requirement for folding and export (Townsend et al., this volume), we believe that all MHC class I molecules carry a peptide ligand. Just as the approach of molecular biology uncovered the existence of the majority of the MHC class I genes (Steinmetz et al. 1982), the detection of the molecules they encode and the ligands these molecules bind will require new techniques if they are not polymorphic.

Origin of MTF

Knowing what Mtf is raises a number of questions that could not be asked before. Of these, the most pressing is the origin of the peptide. The position of the peptide at the amino terminus of ND1 and the conservation of 23 hydrophobic amino acids followed by Glu-Arg-Lys (K. Fischer Lindahl et al., in prep.) suggested that it might be a cleavable signal sequence for insertion of ND1 in the inner mitochondrial membrane. However, the very similar ND1 proteins from cows and the *Neurospora* homolog are not cleaved (Zauner et al. 1985; Yagi and Hatefi 1988).

Han et al. (1989) have reported experiments to suggest that MTF disappears from cells with a half-life on the order of 6 hours in the presence of chloramphenicol, an inhibitor of mitochondrial protein synthesis. This would suggest that the peptide is generated as an immediate result of mitochondrial protein synthesis, perhaps by degradation of malfolded or excess unassembled ND1 subunits. Complex I has more than 25 subunits, of which only 7 are synthesized in the mitochondria, and it would be surprising if they were all produced in stoichiometric amounts. The alternative model—that MTF is liberated during the normal turn-over of mitochondrial proteins—would predict the existence of a large pool of precursors and relative insensitivity to chloramphenicol (Hirama and Fischer Lindahl 1985).

It is also possible that MTF is synthesized as a pep-tide, perhaps from a short mRNA. We do not know the size of the natural MTF peptide. The smallest ND1 peptide we tested is 17 amino acids long, and it is likely that the carboxy-terminal residues are superfluous. The critical polymorphic residue is in position 6, and it is possible that when ND1α4-26 was inactive, it was be-cause the wrong residue was in position 4 or it was too short at the amino terminus, or both. The ND1 pep-tides were all virtually insoluble (B.E. Loveland et al., in prep.), and one would predict that MTF would al-ways be inserted in a membrane. We have no notion of how it escapes the mitochondria.

Understanding the origin of MTF might answer the riddle of why no other mitochondrial peptide acts as a minor H antigen (Fischer Lindahl et al. 1986; B.E. Loveland et al., in prep.). One may speculate that MTF has a unique function, perhaps related to its position as the first translation product from the L-strand tran-script, which encodes 12 of the 13 mitochondrial pro-teins. Alternatively, one may postulate that only MTF survives proteolytic degradation, that only MTF can be bound by Hmt, that only MTF is immunogenic, or that MTF is immunodominant (Ametani et al.; Scherer et al.; both this volume). Some of these possibilities can be tested by direct immunization with other mitochon-drial peptides.

The Privileged Interaction of Hmt and MTF

Hmt is not yet known to present any other peptide ligand, nor does MTF appear to be presented in im-munogenic form by any other MHC class I molecule (K. Fischer Lindahl, unpubl.). We do not know why Hmt and MTF specifically associate with each other to form Mta. The hydrophobic nature of the binding site encoded by the *R4B2* gene may be part of the answer, but there were no other features in the sequence to suggest a unique function. We must discover where the components of Mta are synthesized, where they first interact, and how they are transported to the cell mem-brane.

We frequently observe that addition of a self-peptide, e.g., ND1α peptide to *Mtf*$^\alpha$ cells, leads to increased susceptibility to lysis, suggesting that the MTF peptide is limiting in cells that are not growing vigorously (B.E. Loveland et al., in prep.). The added peptide might exchange with other kinds of peptides bound by Hmt, it might assist in the folding of more Hmt molecules (Townsend et al., this volume), or, perhaps least likely, it might bind to unoccupied grooves. Although we see plateau activity with 100 nM peptide concentration, this is a maximum estimate of the affinity of the interaction, because the peptide is added to the cells as a particulate suspension and the local concentration may be much higher.

It will be critical for our evaluation of the biological role of Hmt to understand the nature of the null allele *Hmt*^{b}. Our failure to raise a CTL response against an Hmt^b:MTF$^\alpha$ complex could mean either that no Hmt^b is expressed, that it does not bind MTF$^\alpha$, or that the complex is not immunogenic (K. Fischer Lindahl, unpubl.).

There is little evidence, other than its origin (Fischer Lindahl 1985), to support the notion that MTF plays a role in mitochondrial function or regulation (Han et al. 1989). Instead, one may consider the possibility that Hmt represents a third mode of antigen presentation, devoted to antigens synthesized by intracellular para-sites, such as *Rickettsia*, *Chlamydia*, and *Listeria*, which, like mitochondria, are isolated from the cell cytoplasm by their membranes. Reports of nonrestrict-ed CTL responses to such antigens may reflect restric-tion by a nonpolymorphic MHC molecule like Hmt (Kaufman et al. 1988). This is compatible with the notion that MHC class I molecules present special an-tigens to cells with γ/δ TCRs (Strominger 1989). As the presentation of nuclearly encoded minor H antigens may be a by-product of the mechanism for presentation of viral antigens by standard MHC class I molecules, so the presentation of a mitochondrial H antigen may be a by-product of the ability of Hmt to present parasite antigens.

ACKNOWLEDGMENTS

We thank Lynn DeOgny and Dr. Clive Slaughter for advice and synthesis of peptides, Drs. Keiji Maeda and Susumu Tonegawa for antisera, Irene Carlo, Annie Eubanks, Jannett Marshall-Holmes, Margaretan Stol-fo, and Danny Clark for technical assistance, and Julie McCorkle for preparation of the manuscript. E.H. was supported by the Texas Ladies Auxiliary of Veterans of Foreign Wars.

REFERENCES

Anderson, S., A.T. Bankier, B.G. Barrell, M.H.L. deBruijn, A.R. Coulson, J. Drouin, I.C. Eperon, D.P. Nierlich, B.A. Roe, F. Sanger, P.H. Schreier, A.J.H. Smith, R. Staden, and I.G. Young. 1982. Comparison of the human and bovine mitochondrial genomes. In *Mitochondrial genes* (ed. P. Slonimski et al.), p. 5. Cold Spring Harbor Laboratory, Cold Spring Harbor, New York.

Bastin, J., J. Rothbard, J. Davey, I. Jones, and A. Townsend. 1987. Use of synthetic peptides of influenza nucleoprotein to define epitopes recognized by class I-restricted cytotoxic T lymphocytes. *J. Exp. Med.* **165:** 1508.

Bibb, M.J., R.A. Van Etten, C.T. Wright, M.W. Walberg, and D.A. Clayton. 1981. Sequence and gene organization of mouse mitochondrial DNA. *Cell* **26:** 167.

Brorson, K.A., S. Richards, S.W. Hunt III, H. Cheroutre, K. Fischer Lindahl, and L. Hood. 1989. Analysis of a new class I gene mapping to the *Hmt* region of the mouse. *Immunogenetics* **30:** 273.

Brown, J.H., T. Jardetzky, M.A. Saper, B. Samraoui, P.J.

Bjorkman, and D.C. Wiley. 1988. A hypothetical model of the foreign antigen binding site of Class II histocompatibility molecules. *Nature* 332: 845.

Chan, T. and K. Fischer Lindahl. 1985. Skin graft rejection due to a maternally transmitted antigen, Mta. *Transplantation* 39: 477.

De Plaen, E., C. Lurquin, A. Van Pel, B. Mariamé, J.-P. Szikora, T. Wölfel, C. Sibille, P. Chomex, and T. Boon. 1988. Immunogenic (tum⁻) variants of mouse tumor P815: Cloning of the gene of tum⁻ antigen P91A and identification of the tum⁻ mutation. *Proc. Natl. Acad. Sci.* 85: 2274.

Ferris, S.D., U. Ritte, K. Fischer Lindahl, E.M. Prager, and A.C. Wilson. 1983. Unusual type of mitochondrial DNA in mice lacking a maternally transmitted antigen. *Nucleic Acids Res.* 11: 2917.

Fischer Lindahl, K. 1985. Mitochondrial inheritance in mice. *Trends Genet.* 1: 135.

———. 1986. Genetic variants of histocompatibility antigens from wild mice. *Curr. Top. Microbiol. Immunol.* 127: 272.

Fischer Lindahl, K. and K. Bürki. 1982. Mta, a maternally inherited cell surface antigen of the mouse, is transmitted in the egg. *Proc. Natl. Acad. Sci.* 79: 5362.

Fischer Lindahl, K. and B. Hausmann. 1983. Cytoplasmic inheritance of a cell surface antigen in the mouse. *Genetics* 103: 483.

Fischer Lindahl, K., M. Bocchieri, and R. Riblet. 1980. Maternally transmitted target antigen for unrestricted killing by NZB T lymphocytes. *J. Exp. Med.* 152: 1583.

Fischer Lindahl, K., B. Hausmann, and V.M. Chapman. 1983. A new *H-2*-linked class I gene whose expression depends on a maternally inherited factor. *Nature* 306: 383.

Fischer Lindahl, K., B. Hausmann, and J.-L. Guénet. 1989. Distinct epitopes of the maternally transmitted antigen, Mta, determined by three allelic forms of the cytoplasmic gene *Mtf. J. Immunogenet.* (in press).

Fischer Lindahl, K., B.E. Loveland, and C.S. Richards. 1987. The end of *H-2*. In *H-2 antigens: Genes, molecules, function* (ed. C.S. David), p. 327. Plenum Press, New York.

Fischer Lindahl, K., B. Hausmann, P.J. Robinson, J.-L. Guénet, D.C. Wharton, and H. Winking. 1986. Mta, the maternally transmitted antigen, is determined jointly by the chromosomal *Hmt* and the extrachromosomal *Mtf* genes. *J. Exp. Med.* 163: 334.

Han, A.C., J.R. Rodgers, and R.R. Rich. 1987. Unglycosylated Mtaᵃ expresses an Mtaᵇ-like determinant. *Immunogenetics* 25: 234.

———. 1989. An unexpectedly labile mitochondrially encoded protein is required for Mta expression. *Immunogenetics* 29: 258.

Hirama, M. and K. Fischer Lindahl. 1985. Mouse mitochondria and the cell surface. In *Achievements and perspectives of mitochondrial research: Biogenesis* (ed. E. Quagliariello et al.), vol. II, p. 445. Elsevier, Amsterdam.

Huston, M.M., R. Smith III, R. Hull, D.P. Huston, and R.R. Rich. 1985. Mitochondrial modulation of maternally transmitted antigen: Analysis of cell hybrids. *Proc. Natl. Acad. Sci.* 82: 3286.

Kaufmann, S.H.E., H.-R. Rodewald, E. Hug, and G. De Libero. 1988. Cloned *Listeria monocytogenes* specific non-MHC-restricted Lyt-2⁺ T cells with cytolytic and protective activity. *J. Immunol.* 140: 3173.

Langhorne, J. and K. Fischer Lindahl. 1982. Role of non-H-2 antigens in the cytotoxic T cell response to allogeneic H-2. *Eur. J. Immunol.* 12: 101.

Marrack, P. and J. Kappler. 1988. T cells can distinguish between allogeneic major histocompatibility complex products on different cell types. *Nature* 332: 840.

Matzinger, P. and M.J. Bevan. 1977. Hypothesis: Why do so many lymphocytes respond to major histocompatibility antigens? *Cell. Immunol.* 29: 1.

Raulet, D.H. 1989. Antigens for γ/δ T cells. *Nature* 339: 342.

Richards, S., M. Bucan, K. Brorson, M.C. Kiefer, S.W. Hunt III, H. Lehrach, and K. Fischer Lindahl. 1989. Genetic and molecular mapping of the *Hmt* region of the mouse. *EMBO J.* 8: (in press).

Rodgers, J.R., R. Smith, III, M.M. Huston, and R.R. Rich. 1986. Maternally transmitted antigen. *Adv. Immunol.* 38: 313.

Simpson, E. 1986. The H-Y antigen and sex reversal. *Cell* 44: 813.

Singer, D.S., J. Hare, H. Golding, L. Flaherty, and S. Rudikoff. 1988. Characterization of a new subfamily of class I genes in the H-2 complex of the mouse. *Immunogenetics* 28: 13.

Smith, R., III, M.M. Huston, R.N. Jenkins, D.P. Huston, and R.R. Rich. 1983. Mitochondria control expression of a murine cell surface antigen. *Nature* 306: 599.

Steinmetz, M., A. Winoto, K. Minard, and L. Hood. 1982. Clusters of genes encoding mouse transplantation antigens. *Cell* 28: 489.

Strominger, J.L. 1989. The γδ T cell receptor and class Ib MHC-related proteins: Enigmatic molecules of immune recognition. *Cell* 57: 895.

Townsend, A.R.M., J. Rothbard, F.M. Gotch, G. Bahadur, D. Wraith, and A.J. McMichael. 1986. The epitopes of influenza nucleoprotein recognized by cytotoxic T lymphocytes can be defined with short synthetic peptides. *Cell* 44: 959.

Yagi, T. and Y. Hatefi. 1988. Identification of the dicyclohexylcarbodiimide-binding subunit of NADH-ubiquinone oxidoreductase (Complex I). *J. Biol. Chem.* 263: 16150.

Zauner, R., J. Christner, G. Jung, U. Borchart, W. Machleidt, A. Videira, and S. Werner. 1985. Identification of the polypeptide encoded by the *URF-1* gene of *Neurospora crassa* mtDNA. *Eur. J. Biochem.* 150: 447.

Cloning and Expression of the Neonatal Rat Intestinal Fc Receptor, a Major Histocompatibility Complex Class I Antigen Homolog

N.E. SIMISTER* and K.E. MOSTOV†

*Whitehead Institute for Biomedical Research, Cambridge, Massachusetts 02142; †Department of Anatomy, University of California at San Francisco, California 94143

Although the immune system of the late fetus is capable of antibody synthesis, it is normally sheltered from foreign antigens. Because a pregnant or nursing mammal is exposed to roughly the same antigenic environment as the newborn, a mother's immunological experience is directly relevant to the needs of her offspring. Maternal IgG is transmitted to fetal or neonatal mammals and provides humoral immunity during the first weeks of independent life. Humans are born with IgG that was transported across the placenta. In contrast, cattle are agammaglobulinemic at birth and receive IgG from colostrum. There is some prenatal transfer in mice and rats, by way of the uterine lumen and fetal yolk sac, but most IgG is obtained from colostrum and milk. Receptors for the Fc region of IgG (FcRn, *neonatal*) mediate its internalization at the apical surface of intestinal epithelial cells of the suckling rat. The pH in the gut lumen is 6.0–6.5 (Rodewald 1976), which is optimal for binding of IgG to the FcR (Jones and Waldman 1972). IgG does not bind its receptor at the serosal fluid pH of 7.4 (Jones and Waldman 1972) and therefore dissociates when undergoing transcytosis to the basolateral membrane (Fig. 1). Transmission of ingested IgG to the circulation can be detected shortly after birth in the rat and peaks 10–14 days later, coincidentally with IgG binding by intestinal brush borders. Transport stops naturally at 3 weeks of age, when the rats are weaned, but it can be terminated prematurely by administration of cortisone acetate (Halliday 1959; Morris and Morris 1974) or thyroxine (Israel et al. 1987).

FcRs have been purified from intestinal epithelial cells of suckling rats in several laboratories (Rodewald and Kraehenbuhl 1984; Jakoi et al. 1985; Simister and Rees 1985). Detergent-solubilized intestinal FcRs isolated by affinity chromatography on immobilized rat or human IgG are resolved by SDS-PAGE under reducing conditions into components with relative molecular masses of 45–53 kD (p51) and approximately 14 kD (p14). We identified the smaller component as β_2-microglobulin (β_2m) serologically and by partial amino acid sequence (Simister and Mostov 1989). Association of β_2m with p51 was confirmed by cross-linking in intestinal epithelial cell brush borders by dithiobis(succinimidyl propionate) (DSP). Complementary DNAs were cloned that encode the Fc-binding subunit p51

(Simister and Mostov 1989). Its predicted primary structure has three extracellular domains and a transmembrane region all homologous to the corresponding domains of major histocompatibility complex (MHC) class I antigens. Expression of the p51 cDNA in rat and mouse fibroblast lines confers IgG binding, with the pH dependence observed in vivo. This is the first time that a function has been assigned to an MHC antigen-related molecule.

METHODS

Protein sequencing. We isolated brush borders from epithelial cells of the proximal third of the small intestine of 11-day-old Wistar rats (Charles River). Membrane proteins were solubilized in 3-([3-cholamidopropyl] dimethylammonio)-1-propane sulfonate (CHAPS) in 50 mM sodium phosphate (pH 6.5) and cycled over an affinity matrix of human or rat IgG coupled to agarose. The physiological pH dependence of IgG binding (Jones and Waldman 1972) allowed us to elute FcRs by shifting the pH from 6.5 to 8.0 (Simister and Rees 1985). The receptor was denatured in 6 M urea/ 20 mM Tris-HCl (pH 7.2), diluted with five parts 0.1% trifluoroacetic acid (TFA), and loaded onto an RP300 high-performance liquid chromatography (HPLC) column (Brownlee). Fractions eluted in an acetonitrile gradient in 0.1% TFA were analyzed by SDS-PAGE. p14 was eluted at approximately 32% and p51 at approximately 70% acetonitrile. p14 and p51 were electroblotted onto Immobilon polyvinylidene difluoride (PVDF, Millipore) and sequenced directly from membrane strips (Matsudaira 1987). Additionally, p51 was digested with staphylococcal V8 protease in ammonium phosphate buffer (pH 7.8). Cleavage peptides were separated by SDS-PAGE and blotted onto PVDF for sequencing.

Antisera. We raised antisera in New Zealand white rabbits against the putative receptor subunits, using gel slices containing p51 or p14 cut out after SDS-PAGE as immunogen.

Cross-linking. Brush borders were incubated in suspension with the thiol-cleavable cross-linking reagent DSP (1 mM from a 100× stock in dimethylformamide [DMF]) for 4 hours at 4°C. Ethanolamine (50 mM, pH

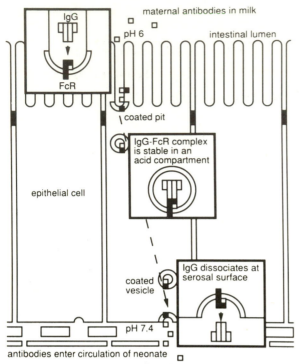

Figure 1. Schematic diagram of IgG transport across the intestinal epithelium of the neonatal rat.

8.0) was added to quench the reaction. Control samples were prepared by adding DMF alone. The brush borders were collected by centrifugation. Membrane proteins were extracted, and affinity chromatography was done as described previously. Cross-linked and control samples were electrophoresed under reducing and nonreducing conditions. We electroblotted the separated proteins onto nitrocellulose and probed the filters with anti-p51 or anti-human β_2m. Alkaline phosphatase-conjugated goat anti-rabbit IgG was used as a second layer and developed with 5-bromo-4-chloro-3-indolyl phosphate/nitro blue tetrazolium.

Cloning.   A cDNA library was made in λgt11 from RNA of epithelial cells of the proximal small intestine of 11-day-old rats. Two clones were selected using anti-p51. Restriction fragments of both cDNAs were subcloned into m13, mp18, and mp19 vectors and sequenced by the dideoxy method (Sanger et al. 1977). The smaller clone was identical to the 5' 925 bp of the larger 1038-bp clone. An *Eco*RI/*Sac*I fragment comprising the 5' 350 bp was used as a probe to screen a neonatal rat intestinal library with inserts greater than 1.5 kb. Filters were hybridized at 42°C in 5× SSC (standard sodium citrate, 150 mM NaCl, 15 mM Na citrate), 50% formamide, 5× Denhardt's solution (1× Denhardt's = 0.02% each of Ficoll, bovine serum albumin [BSA], and polyvinylpyrrolidione), 0.1% SDS, and 100 mg/ml sheared salmon sperm DNA and washed in 0.1× SSC at 60°C. Two cDNAs were obtained (1570 and 1540 bp), which had nucleotide sequences identical with one another at their 5' and 3'

ends and included the sequences of the smaller clones at their 3' ends (except for a G substituted in the poly[A] tail of the smaller). Both strands of these clones were sequenced with at least twofold redundancy.

Sequence alignment.   MHC class I sequences of each species (and subclass) that had the most identity with p51 were selected from the NBRF Protein and New data bases, using FASTA (Pearson and Lipman 1988). A multiple alignment was generated, using ALNED (Protein Information Resource Staff, unpubl.), and was regapped manually in the transmembrane and cytoplasmic domains to align stop-transfer sequences.

Northern blots.   RNAs (25 μg total RNA, except adult small intestine: 1 μg poly[A]$^+$ RNA) were fractionated by electrophoresis in 1.5% agarose/formaldehyde gels and transferred to nylon membranes (GeneScreen Plus, New England Nuclear) by passive diffusion in 20× SSC. Hybridization was in 5× SSC, 50% formamide, 5× Denhardt's solution, 0.1% SDS, and 100 mg/ml sheared salmon sperm DNA at 42°C with a ^{32}P-labeled DNA probe primed with random hexanucleotides from the 925-bp cDNA. The membrane was washed in 0.1× SSC at 50°C. Probes encoding the exoplasmic (plus signal) and cytoplasmic domains were made, using as templates *Mae*III/*Bgl*II (nucleotides 170–1090) and *Sfa*NI (nucleotides 1170–1300) restriction fragments, respectively. These were hybridized with blots under the conditions described above. The filters were washed in 0.1× SSC at 65°C. Washed filters were air-dried and exposed at −70°C to pre-flashed Kodak XAR-5 film with an intensifying screen for the times indicated.

Expression.   Most of the 5'- and 3'-untranslated sequences were removed from the 1570-bp FcRn cDNA by digestion with *Mae*III, and the 5' overhangs were filled in using Klenow fragment. *Bam*HI linkers were added. The resulting 1.2-kb construct was subcloned into the *Bam*HI site of the retroviral expression vector pWE (R.C. Mulligan et al., unpubl.; Fig. 2) and transfected into Ψ2 or ΨAM packaging cells (Cone and Mulligan 1984). Retroviral supernatants were used to infect murine 3T3 fibroblasts and Rat-1 fibroblasts. Clones resistant to G418 were selected and expanded (Korman et al. 1987; Breitfeld et al. 1989).

Metabolic labeling and immunoprecipitation.   The cell lines 3T3 and Rat-1 and their retrovirus-infected derivatives were maintained in Dulbecco's modified Eagle's medium (DME) with 10% fetal bovine serum (FBS), 100 units/ml penicillin, and 100 μg/ml streptomycin in 5% CO$_2$. For pulse-chase experiments, confluent or nearly confluent cell monolayers on 35-mm dishes were depleted of cysteine for 30 minutes in cysteine-free DME, supplemented with 5% FBS previously dialyzed against 150 mM NaCl, and with 20 mM Na HEPES (pH 7.3). Cells were pulse-labeled for 30 minutes with 100 μCi/ml [^{35}S]cysteine (Amersham; ~700–1100 Ci/mmole) in the same medium. Labeled

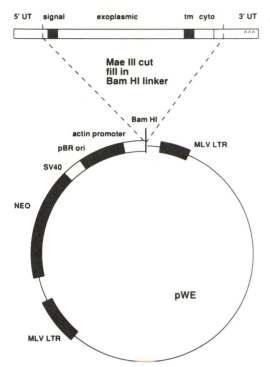

Figure 2. Strategy of subcloning FcRn p51 cDNA for retro-virus-mediated expression.

cells were harvested immediately (time zero) or after chasing the proteins labeled during synthesis through their maturation pathways for 1–4 hours in complete DME (which contains unlabeled cysteine).

To harvest the cells, we removed the labeling or chase medium and rinsed the dish with phosphate-buffered saline (PBS). The cells were then scraped into 0.5 ml of SDS lysis buffer (0.5% SDS, 150 mM NaCl, 5 mM EDTA, 100 units/ml trasylol, 20 mM ethanol-amine-HCl at pH 8.1), transferred to 1.5-ml microcentrifuge tubes and boiled for 5 minutes, cooled on ice, and sonicated for 2×30 seconds (Branson sonicator with cup horn). To each lysate, 0.5 ml of 2.5% Triton dilution buffer (2.5% Triton X-100, 100 mM NaCl, 5 mM EDTA, 100 units/ml trasylol, 0.1% NaN$_3$, 50 mM ethanolamine-HCl at pH 8.6) was added. Before immunoprecipitation, samples were precleared with 2 μl of normal rabbit serum (1 hr at room temperature) and 100 μl of a 20% (v/v) slurry of protein A–Sepharose (Sigma; 30 min at room temperature). The beads were spun down. The supernatants were transferred to new tubes and incubated with 2 μl of anti-p51 (overnight at 4°C). Immune complexes were precipitated with protein A–Sepharose, as described above. Beads were washed by brief centrifugation (10 sec) and resuspension in 1 ml of wash buffer. Five washes in mixed micelle buffer (1% Triton X-100, 0.2% SDS, 150 mM NaCl, 5% w/v sucrose, 5 mM EDTA, 100 units/ml trasylol, 0.1% NaN$_3$, 20 mM ethanolamine-HCl at pH 8.6) and two in final wash buffer (15 mM NaCl, 5 mM EDTA, 100 units/ml trasylol, 0.1% NaN$_3$, 20 mM ethanolamine-HCl at pH 8.6) were done. Finally, the beads were boiled in SDS-gel sample buffer. Eluted proteins were analyzed on 10% polyacrylamide gels, which were then dehydrated in glacial acetic acid and fluorographed using 22% (w/v) 2,5-diphenyloxazole (PPO) in acetic acid.

IgG binding and internalization. Human IgG (ICN Immunochemicals) was labeled with ^{125}I-labeled iodide to a specific activity of 0.5–1 mCi/nmole, using Iodogen (Pierce), according to the manufacturers' instructions.

Murine 3T3 and Rat-1 fibroblasts and clones expressing FcRn were grown to confluence or near confluence on 35-mm dishes. The cells were first washed with PBS and 1 mM KI (pH 6.0 or 7.4) at 4°C. Then ^{125}I-labeled IgG (10^7 cpm/ml, $\sim 10^{-8}$ M) in PBS, 1 mM KI, 1% ovalbumin (pH 6.0 or 7.4), with or without 0.5 mg/ml unlabeled IgG (3.3×10^{-6} M), was added to the dish. The cells were allowed to bind and internalize IgG at 37°C for 1 hour. Unbound ligand was removed with three washes of PBS and 1 mM KI (pH 6.0 or 7.4) at 4°C. Cells were dissolved in 2×0.5 ml of 0.1 M NaOH and transferred to vials. The bound radioligand was measured in a gamma counter.

To correct the results for variations in the number of cells on dishes of different cell lines, binding data were normalized to total protein per dish. Protein in the cell solubilisates was determined by the bicinchoninic acid method (Smith et al. 1985) (BCA, Pierce). Standards were prepared using BSA.

RESULTS

Light Chain of FcRn Is β_2m

The amino-terminal 19 amino acids of p14 were found to be IQKTPQIQVYSRHPPENGK and are identical to those of rat β_2m (Poulik and Smithies 1979). To look for a cell-surface association between p51 and β_2m, we affinity-purified FcRn after cross-linking brush border proteins in situ with DSP. FcRn from DSP-treated brush borders contained a species of approximately 62 kD that was lost on reduction of DSP disulfide bonds (Fig. 3). This band was detected by both anti-p51 and anti-β_2m sera on Western blots and therefore represents a p51/β_2m heterodimer. β_2m has been shown previously to form a noncovalent heterodimer with products of the MHC class I genes (Nathenson et al. 1981; Ploegh et al. 1981) and with CD1 (T6) antigens (Kahn-Perles et al. 1985; Boumsell et al. 1986). The identification of p14 as β_2m suggested that the larger subunit of FcRn resembled an MHC class I heavy chain.

Cloning the FcRn Heavy Chain

We investigated the possibility of the larger subunit of FcRn resembling an MHC class I heavy chain by molecular cloning. Using the anti-p51 serum, we selected clones from a λgt11 library of duodenum and jejunum of 11-day-old rats. These were used as probes to

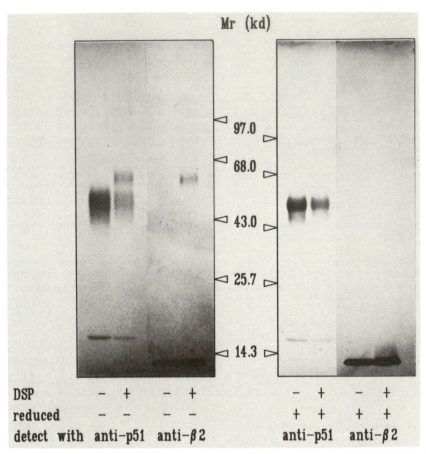

Figure 3. Immunoblot analysis of FcRn prepared with or without cross-linking of brush border proteins with DSP. The blots were probed using antisera to the FcRn heavy chain p51 or to β_2m.

obtain full-length clones. Two positive clones (1570 and 1540 bp) were sequenced completely (Fig. 4). An initiation AUG codon flanked by ribosome-binding site consensus nucleotides (Kozak 1986) followed approximately 200 bp of 5'-untranslated sequence. Translation of the nucleotide sequence revealed a probable amino-terminal signal sequence, a putative extracellular region with four sites of potential N glycosylation, a single membrane-spanning domain, and a 40-amino-acid cytoplasmic tail. The amino-terminal sequence predicted, using the von Heijne algorithm (von Heijne 1986), was confirmed by the sequence AEPXL-PLMYXLAAVXDL from the amino terminus of HPLC-purified p51. Furthermore, predicted internal sequences matched the sequences (E153↑)XEFLLTS-XPE and (E259↑)XLAQPLTVDL from V8 proteinase fragments (where ↑ shows the site of cleavage, which is on the carboxy-terminal side of glutamic acid residues under the conditions used).

FcRn Heavy-chain mRNA Transcribed in Intestine and Other Tissues

Probes made from the 925-bp cDNA (which encodes the cytoplasmic, transmembrane, and α_2 and α_3 ex-

oplasmic domains) hybridized on Northern blots with 1.7- and 3.1-kb messages in RNA from the proximal half of the small intestine of suckling rats (Fig. 5a). These mRNAs are less abundant in the distal half of the small intestine. Trace hybridization with an mRNA of approximately 1.7 kb from the small intestine, brain, heart, kidney, liver, pancreas, and spleen of adult rats was detected. The approximately 1.7-kb mRNA was detected by probes made from restriction fragments encoding either the exoplasmic and signal sequences or the cytoplasmic tail of p51 in RNA from neonatal rat proximal small intestine and from adult rat spleen (Fig. 5b).

Expression of FcRn in Fibroblast Cell Lines

Biosynthetic incorporation of [35S]cysteine into the products of retrovirus-infected 3T3 and Rat-1 cells shows that the immunoprecipitable FcRn heavy chain is made during a 30-minute labeling period as a 47-kD precursor that is converted during a 4-hour chase to a 52- to 60-kD protein (Fig. 6), presumably by the maturation in the Golgi of high mannose N-linked oligosaccharide chains to complex type.

```
   1  TCAGTTCTGTAATTAATTAACTAACGTGATCAAATGAAGGTCACACAGGAGCACTCCTGTCGTCTTGGACTGCGTTCTCCATCCCACCATCCAGTGCCCTGGTCTACGAAG  120

 121  AGTCCACAGGGACCTTGTGAAGAATCAACAAGGCGGGTCCAGAGAGTCACGTGTGCCTTCCACTCCGGTCGCCCCTGTCGCCCCTGTCGGTCTCCTCAGCCTC         240
                                                                      MetGlyMetSerGlnProGlyValLeuLeuSerLeu         -11
      -22

 241  TTATTGGTCCTCGCCTCAGACCTGGGAGCGGAGCCCCGTCTCCCACTGATGTATCATCTTCGACGTGTCTGACTTATCAACGGGGCCTTCCCTTTCTGGCCACGGGCTGGCTG  360
 -10  LeuLeuValLeuLeuProGlnThrTrpGlyAlaGluProArgLeuProLeuMetTyrHisLeuAlaAlaValSerAspLeuSerThrGlyProSerPheProAlaThrGlyTrpLeu  30
                                             -1 +1

 361  GGTGCTCAGCAATATCTGACCTACAACAACCTGCGCAGGAGGTGACCCCTGTGGGCCTGGATATGGAAAACCAGGTGTCTTGGTATTGGGAGAAGGAGACCACGATCTGAAAAGC  480
  31  GlyAlaGlnGlnTyrLeuThrTyrAsnAsnLeuArgGlnGluAlaAspProCysGlyAlaTrpIleTrpGluAsnGlnValSerTrpTyrTrpGluLysGluThrThrAspLeuLysSer  70

 481  AAAGAACAGCTCTTCTTGGAGGCCATCAGGACCCTGGAGAACCAAATAAATGGGACCTTCACACTGCAGGGCCTGCTGAACTGGCCCTGATAATTCTTCATTGCCCACGGCT    600
  71  LysGluGlnLeuPheLeuGluAlaIleArgThrLeuGluAsnGlnIleAsnGlyThrPheThrLeuGlnGlyLeuLeuAsnSerGluLeuAlaProAspAsnSerLeuProThrAla  110
                                                                                              ---CHO----

 601  GTGTTTGCCCTCAATGTGAGGAGTTCAACCCAAGAGTTCAACCCAGAGCAACTGATATCGTTGGTAATCTGTGATGAAGCAACCTGAGGCGGGC           720
 111  ValPheAlaLeuAsnGlyGlyGluPheMetArgPheAsnProArgThrGlyAsnTrpSerGlyTrpProGluThrAspIleValGlyAsnLeuTrpMetLysGlnProGluAlaAlaLeu  150
                                                ---CHO----

 721  AGGAAGGAGAGCGAGTTCCGTAACTTCTTGTCCTGAGAGGCCGCCACCTGAGGAGGAGCCGCCATCTATGGCGCCGAAGGCCCGTCCT   840
 151  ArgLysGluSerGluPheLeuSerCysProGluArgLeuLeuGluThrSerCysProGluValGluArgGlyHisLeuLeuGlnGlyAsnLeuGluTrpLysGluProProSerMetArgLeuLysAlaArgPro  190

 841  GGCAACTCTCGCCTCCAGTACTGACCTGTGCTGTTTCTCCTTCTACCCGCGAGCTCAAGTTTCGATTCTGCCAATGGCTAGCCTCAGGCTCTGGGAATTGCAGCACTGTCCC  960
 191  GlyAsnSerGlySerSerValLeuThrCysAlaAlaPheSerPheTyrProGluLeuLysPheArgPheTyrProGluLeuLysPheArgPheLeuGlnAlaSerGlyLeuAlaSerGlyLeuAsnCysSerThrGlyPro  230
                                                                                              ---CHO----

 961  AATGGTGATGATCTTTCCATGCATGGTCATTGCTAGAGGTCAAAGTGGAGATGAACACCATTACCAATGTCAAGTGGAGCATGAGGGGCTGGCCCAGCCTCCACTGTGGACCTAGAT  1080
 231  AsnGlyAspAspSerPheHisAlaTrpSerLeuLeuGluValLysArgGlyAspGluHisHisTyrGlnCysGlnValAlaGlyGlnGlyLeuAlaGlnProLeuThrValAspLeuAsp  270

1081  TCGCCCCGCAGATCTTCTGCTCCGGAATCATTCTTGGTTTATTGCTGGTAGTGGCAGTCCCATCCAGAGGGTGTGCTGCTATGGAACAGGATGCGAAGTGGGCTGCAGCCCCA  1200
 271  SerProAlaArgSerSerValProValAlaGlyIleIleLeuGlyLeuLeuLeuValValValAlaIleAlaGlyGlyValAlaAlaMetArgSerGlyLeuProAlaPro  310
      ================================================================

1201  TGGCTTTCTCTCAGTGGTGATGACTCTGGCGACCTATTGCCTGGTGGAACTTGCCCCCGAGGCTGAACCTCAAGGTGTAAATGCCTTCCGGCCACTTCCTGATGCCAACCCAGGCCC  1320
 311  TrpLeuSerLeuSerGlyAspAspSerGlyAspLeuLeuProGlyGlyAsnLeuProGlyGlnGlyValAsnAlaPheProAlaThrSer  344

1321  CATACCCATTGCAGCCTGTGGGGCTGTGTGACCTCCTGAACTGTCTCTGAGCCTCCGTGGCTGCTTCAGTTTC  1440

1441  CCCTCTTAATGTCAATGGCTATTCCATCTCCACATAAATTGGGCCCAAATCTGTGTGCATCGTTATTCCAGTTTCAGGCAGCCGAATAAATTGAACAAGTTTGAGAAAAAAAA  1560

1561  AAAAAAAAAAAAA  1573
```

Figure 4. Complete nucleotide sequence and deduced amino acid sequence of the FcRn large subunit p51. The potential ATG start is indicated by asterisks (*) over the initiation site consensus nucleotides. The predicted amino terminus after signal cleavage is indicated by +1 under Ala. Four potential sites for N-linked glycosylation (Asn-X-Ser or Asn-X-Thr), the hydrophobic membrane-spanning segment, and the polyadenylation signal AATAAA in the 3'-untranslated sequence are underlined.

575

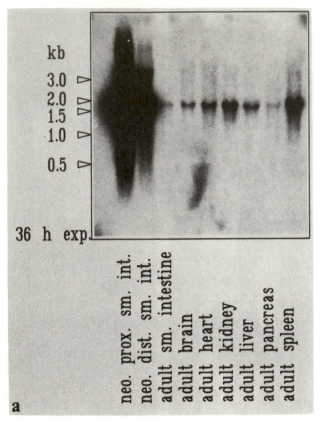

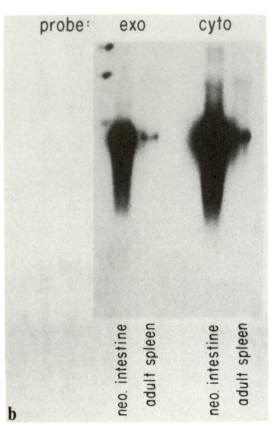

Figure 5. (*a*) Northern blot of RNA from neonatal (neo) and adult rat tissues, probed with a 925-bp cDNA from a clone immunoselected with antiserum to the FcRn large subunit p51. (*b*) Northern blot of RNA from neonatal rat small intestine and adult rat spleen, probed with cDNAs encoding either the signal and exoplasmic (exo) or cytoplasmic (cyto) domains of p51.

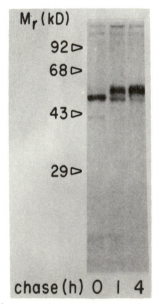

Figure 6. FcRn heavy chain immunoprecipitated from lysates of murine 3T3 fibroblasts infected with a retroviral vector that contains the FcRn heavy-chain cDNA. Cells were pulse-labeled with [^{35}S]cysteine and chased with unlabeled cysteine for the times indicated.

Clones expressing the most FcRn heavy chains were selected on the basis of metabolic labeling and immunoprecipitation, normalized for protein as a measure of cell number. These were designated rfcr4 (Rat-1) and mfcr5 (3T3). Clones rfcr4 and mfcr5 specifically bound 20-fold and 7-fold more IgG (in a 1-hr experiment) than their respective parental lines at pH 6.0 (Fig. 7). No specific binding was detected at pH 7.4. The greater binding and uptake by rfcr4 compared with mfcr5 reflects a higher level ($\sim 3\times$) of FcRn expression by the rat clone (data not shown).

DISCUSSION

Homology with MHC Class I Antigens

Computed alignments of p51 with MHC class I heavy-chain sequences show significant identity (ALIGN [Dayhoff et al. 1983] scores of 6–15 s.d.) in all three extracellular domains (Fig. 8). In the X-ray crystallographic structure of HLA-A2 (Bjorkman et al. 1988), domains α_1 and α_2 each comprise four β-strands, followed by two or four α-helices, and pair so that the helices are the walls and the strands are the floor of a groove, proposed as the site of antigen presentation. In

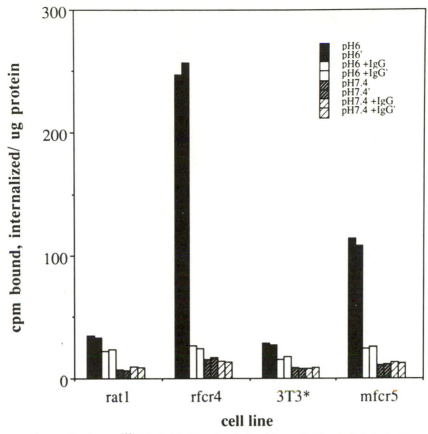

Figure 7. Binding and internalization of ^{125}I-labeled IgG by Rat-1 fibroblasts, Rat-1 cells infected with a retroviral vector that contains the FcRn heavy-chain cDNA (rfcr4), murine 3T3 fibroblasts infected with vector alone (3T3*), and 3T3 cells infected with a retroviral vector that contains the FcRn heavy-chain cDNA (mfcr5). Duplicate assays were done at pH 6.0 or pH 7.4, with or without competing unlabeled IgG. Counts were normalized for total protein to allow for variation in the number of cells on a plate.

the α_1 and α_2 sequences of p51, helix residues that point toward the β-strands in the HLA-A2 model are notably conserved, including a region of every-fourth-residue identity in the carboxy-terminal part of each domain (residues marked s in Fig. 8), corresponding to one face of each long α-helix. Few residues on the other faces of the HLA-A2 helices, which contain presumed recognition sites for the T-cell receptor (TCR) and for antigen, are conserved in p51. Some β_2m contacts are conserved, as expected (marked β in Fig. 8).

The homology between p51 and the MHC class I antigens is greatest in the immunoglobulin-like domain, α_3 (35–37% identity, compared with 27–30% in α_1 and 22–29% in α_2). An unpaired cysteine in α_3 might participate in the formation of disulfide-linked dimers between p51 molecules, which have been observed previously (Simister and Rees 1985). The functional size of FcRn in situ in enterocyte brush borders, determined by radiation inactivation, is consistent with the molecular weight of a p51 dimer (Simister and Rees 1985). This model is attractive because the ligand is a dimer of IgG heavy chains.

FcRn is much more divergent from classic class I

transplantation antigens than are Qa and Tla antigens, which are encoded in the MHC. The persistent integrity of the MHC throughout evolution is striking, yet the human CD1 antigens (whose heavy chains show significant class I homology and bind both β_2m and CD8) map outside it (Calabi and Milstein 1986). FcRn heavy chain is as divergent from the CD1s as are classic and nonclassic class I sequences but has amino acid identities with CD1a,b, and c that are not shared by MHC class I molecules. This may be because FcRn and CD1 had a common ancestor after diverging from the MHC lineage, or it may represent the survival of residues lost to the rapidly diverging MHC. The binding of IgG (through immunoglobulin C domains) is a simpler function than the concomitant recognition by HLA-A2, for example, of processed antigen, TCR (immunoglobulin V domains), and CD8 (immunoglobulin V domains). FcRn may therefore resemble an ancestral receptor for an immunoglobulin domain more closely than MHC class I antigens do. No functions of Qa, Tla, and CD1 have been identified, but the very different biological roles of FcRn and classic MHC class I antigens illustrate that the uses of these homologs may be diverse.

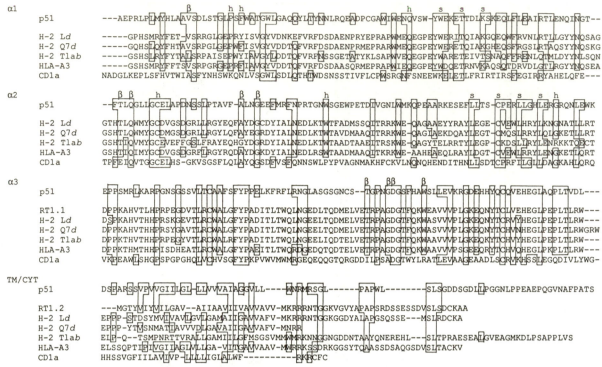

Figure 8. Domain-by-domain comparison of the primary structures of p51, rat (RT1.1, RT1.2 [Kastern 1985]), mouse (H-2L^d [Evans et al. 1982; Moore et al. 1982], H-2Q7^d [Steinmetz et al. 1981], H-2Tla^b [Obata et al. 1985]), and human (HLA-A3 [Strachan et al. 1984]) MHC class I heavy-chain sequences and the thymocyte differentiation antigen CD1a (Martin et al. 1987). Identities with the p51 sequence are boxed. Symbols above p51 residues refer to the crystallographic structure of HLA-A2 (Bjorkman et al. 1988): (h) Conserved residues (mostly in β-strands), whose side chains point toward helices; (s) conserved residues (in α-helices) that face β-strands; (β) conserved residues that contact β_2m. HLA-A2 and HLA-A3 are 95% identical in their extracellular domains; all of the marked residues are common to both.

Predicting the IgG-binding Site

Comparison with MHC class I antigens suggests three candidate regions for the IgG-binding site: the binding sites for the T cell receptor and processed antigen and for CD8. Amino acids involved in TCR and antigen recognition in HLA-A2 are found on the upper and inner faces of the α-helices of the α_1 and α_2 domains. CD8 binds close to residues 227 and 245 in α_3 (Connolly et al., 1988). The pH dependence of IgG binding (binding at pH 6.5; none at 7.5) suggests the involvement of a charged group on the receptor or in Fc with a pK_a between 6.5 and 7.5. Histidine residues ionize in this range, as may lysine and arginine if in a hydrophobic environment. Histidines 250 and 251 in α_3 of FcRn lie close to the site of CD8 binding of classic class I molecules (Parham 1989), and the predicted α-helices of α_1 and α_2 are rich in basic amino acids. Ultimately, localization of the binding site must await mutagenesis studies.

Cytoplasmic Tail

The predicted membrane-spanning domain of p51 is related to human and (weakly) to rodent class I transmembrane regions. The cytoplasmic tails show little identity, perhaps because MHC class I molecules and p51 need different cytoplasmic sorting signals. Tyrosine residues in the cytoplasmic tail of some receptors—LDL receptor (Davis et al., 1987), cation-independent mannose 6-phosphate receptor (P. Lobel and S. Kornfeld, pers. comm.), and polymeric immunoglobulin receptor (P. Breitfeld and K. Mostov, unpubl.)—are required for internalization through coated pits. Phenylalanine and tryptophan can substitute for tyrosine in the LDL receptor tail. We hypothesize that either the cytoplasmic tryptophan or phenylalanine of p51 (there is no tyrosine) allows its coated-pit-mediated endocytosis. The cytoplasmic tail contains five serines (S305 has a basic amino acid to its carboxy-terminal side, as do many protein kinase C substrates [Edelman et al. 1987]) and one threonine residue. We do not know whether FcRn is phosphorylated in vivo.

Functional Expression of FcRn

Cloned p51, expressed in rat and mouse fibroblasts (Rat-1 and 3T3), is first detected in pulse-chase experiments as a 47-kD putative rough endoplasmic reticulum (RER) form. This molecular weight is consistent with the presence of high mannose oligosaccharide chains at the four potential sites of N-linked glycosylation of the 38.5-kD polypeptide predicted by the cDNA sequence.

Association of β_2m with the heavy chains of class I transplantation antigens is, with few exceptions (Allen et al. 1986), obligatory for their export to the cell surface (Arce-Gomez et al. 1982). The precursor form of p51 undergoes oligosaccharide processing in the Golgi of both cell lines. These results show that murine β_2m is sufficiently homologous to that of rat to associate with FcRn heavy chain and allow its export from the endoplasmic reticulum.

The expression of p51 in fibroblast lines of rodent origin dramatically increased their specific binding and uptake of IgG at pH 6.0, but no specific binding could be measured at pH 7.4. This requirement for a slightly acidic pH for binding is characteristic of FcRn in situ in neonatal rat intestinal segments (Jones and Waldman 1972) and enterocyte brush borders (Wallace and Rees 1980) and was used to purify solubilized p51 by affinity chromatography on immobilized IgG.

Is FcRn Unique?

mRNAs from cells of the small intestine of suckling rats hybridize with a probe encoding exoplasmic, trans-membrane, and cytoplasmic sequences of p51. The two mRNAs, 1.7 and 3.1 kb, are more abundant in the proximal half of the small intestine, which is the site of IgG transport (Rodewald 1970), than in the distal half, where there are fewer transporting cells (Rodewald 1970). The longest cDNA clone is presumably a full-length or nearly full-length transcript of the 1.7-kb mRNA. The larger message might represent a nuclear RNA or derive from the use of an alternate polyadenylation signal. The same probe hybridized at trace levels with an mRNA of approximately 1.7 kb from the intestine and other tissues of adult rats. As the DNA encoding the exoplasmic and membrane-spanning domains of FcRn has up to 55% identity with murine MHC class I genes, it seemed possible that the signal in other tissues might represent rat MHC class I mRNA. The high-stringency blot, using probes specific for the signal/exoplasmic and cytoplasmic domains, tests this, because the cytoplasmic sequence has no MHC homology. The 1.7- and 3.1-kb messages were detected by both probes in rat spleen RNA, although at a much lower abundance than intestinal RNA from the neonate. This shows that an mRNA homologous or identical to that of FcRn is transcribed in tissues other than the intestine. The data do not show whether this message is present in tissue-specific cell types or in leukocytes isolated together with the tissues.

FcRn is unrelated to $Fc_\gamma RI$, the macrophage receptor with high affinity for monomeric IgG (Allen and Seed 1989), or to macrophage or lymphocyte $Fc_\gamma RII$ isoforms or neutrophil $Fc_\gamma RIII$, which bind immune complexes (Lewis et al. 1986; Ravetch et al. 1986; Stuart et al. 1987; Hibbs et al. 1988; Simmons and Seed 1988; Stengelin et al. 1988). However, earlier observations suggest that a subset of leukocyte $Fc_\gamma Rs$ are associated with β_2m: Antisera to β_2m inhibit FcR-mediated killing of opsonized cells (Solheim et al. 1976) and induce cell-surface rearrangement of $Fc_\gamma Rs$ on human peripheral lymphocytes (Sarmay and Gergely 1983). Cells of the Burkitt's lymphoma-derived line Daudi do not make β_2m and fail to express class I human leukemic A (HLA) antigens at their surface (Arce-Gomez et al. 1982); their capacity to bind irrelevant IgG1 monoclonal antibodies is enhanced by transfection with a cDNA encoding β_2m (Seong et al. 1988). This may indicate that some Daudi $Fc_\gamma Rs$ must associate with β_2m to reach the cell surface. We therefore speculate that FcRs related to MHC class I antigens are not unique to the intestinal epithelium of suckling rodents.

ACKNOWLEDGMENTS

We thank P. Matsudaira and S. Blackmon for protein sequencing; J. Brown, M. Saper, and D. Wiley for discussing HLA-A2 structure; P. Parham for suggesting possible IgG-binding sites; B. Thorens for adult rat RNAs; S. Ross and J. Harris for preparing intestinal epithelial cells; and H. Lodish for reading the manuscript. N.E.S. is supported by the Cancer Research Institute/F.M. Kirby Foundation. The study was funded by the Hood Foundation and the National Institutes of Health.

REFERENCES

Allen, H., J. Fraser, D. Flyer, S. Calvin, and R. Flavell. 1986. Beta 2-microglobulin is not required for cell surface expression of the murine class I histocompatibility antigen H-2D^b or of a truncated H-2D^b. *Proc. Natl. Acad. Sci.* **83:** 7447.

Allen, J.M. and B. Seed. 1989. Isolation and expression of functional high-affinity Fc receptor complementary DNAs. *Science* **243:** 378.

Arce-Gomez, B., E.A. Jones, C.J. Barnstable, E. Solomon, and W. Bodmer. 1982. The genetic control of HLA-A and B antigens in somatic cell hybrids: Requirement for beta 2-microglobulin. *Tissue Antigens* **11:** 96.

Bjorkman, P.J., M.A. Saper, B. Samraoui, W.S. Bennet, J.L. Strominger, and D.C. Wiley. 1988. Structure of the human class I histocompatibility antigen, HLA-A2. *Nature* **239:** 506.

Boumsell, L., M. Amniot, B. Raynal, V. Gay-Bellile, B. Caillou, and A. Bernard. 1986. Epitopic groups of CD1 molecules. In *Leukocyte typing II* (ed. E.L. Reinherz et al.), p. 289. Springer-Verlag, New York.

Breitfeld, P., J.E. Casanova, J.M. Harris, N.E. Simister, and K.E. Mostov. 1989. Expression and analysis of the polymeric immunoglobulin receptor in Madin-Darby canine kidney cells using retroviral vectors. *Methods Cell Biol.* **32:** 329.

Calabi, F. and C. Milstein. 1986. A novel family of human major histocompatibility complex-related genes not mapping to chromosome 6. *Nature* **323:** 540.

Cone, R.D. and R.C. Mulligan. 1984. High efficiency gene transfer into mammalian cells: Generation of helper-free recombinant virus with broad mammalian host range. *Proc. Natl. Acad. Sci.* **81:** 6349.

Connolly, J.M., T.A. Potter, E.M. Wormstall, and T.H. Hansen. 1988. The Lyt2 molecule recognizes residues in the class I alpha 3 domain in allogeneic cytotoxic T cell responses. *J. Exp. Med.* **168:** 325.

Davis, C.G., I.R. van Driel, D.W.Russel, M.S. Brown, and J.L. Goldstein. 1987. The low density lipoprotein receptor: Identification of amino acids in the cytoplasmic domain required for rapid endocytosis. *J. Biol. Chem.* **262:** 4075.

Dayhoff, M.O., W.C. Barker, and L.T. Hunt. 1983. Establishing homologies in protein sequences. *Methods Enzymol.* **91:** 524.

Edelman, A.M., D.K. Blumenthal, and E.G. Krebs. 1987. Protein serine/threonine kinases. *Annu. Rev. Biochem.* **56:** 567.

Evans, G.A., D.H. Margulies, R.D. Camerini-Otero, K. Ozato, and J.G. Seidman. 1982. Structure and expression of a mouse major histocompatibility antigen gene, H-2Ld. *Proc. Natl. Acad. Sci.* **79:** 1994.

Halliday, R. 1959. The effect of steroid hormones on the absorption of antibodies by the young rat. *J. Endocrinol.* **18:** 56.

Hibbs, M.L., L. Bonadonna, B.M. Scott, I.F.C. McEnzie, and P.M. Hogarth. 1988. Molecular cloning of a human immunoglobulin G Fc receptor. *Proc. Natl. Acad. Sci.* **85:** 2240.

Israel, E.J., K.Y. Pang, P.R. Harmatz, and W.A. Walker. 1987. Structural and functional maturation of rat gastrointestinal barrier with thyroxine. *Am. J. Physiol.* **252:** G762.

Jakoi, E.R., J. Cambier, and S. Saslow. 1985. Transepithelial transport of maternal antibody: Purification of IgG receptor from newborn rat intestine. *J. Immunol.* **135:** 3360.

Jones, E.A. and T.A. Waldman. 1972. The mechanism of intestinal uptake and transcellular transport of IgG in the neonatal rat. *J. Clin. Invest.* **51:** 2916.

Kahn-Perles, B., J. Wietzerbin, D.H. Caillol, and F. Lemonnier. 1985. Delineation of three subsets of class I human T antigens (HTA) on MOLT-4 cells: Serologic and regulatory relationship to HLA class I antigens. *J. Immunol.* **134:** 1759.

Kastern, W. 1985. Characterization of two class I major histocompatibility rat cDNA clones, one of which contains a premature termination codon. *Gene* **34:** 227.

Korman, A.J., J.D. Frantz, J.L. Strominger, and R.C. Mulligan. 1987. Expression of human class II major histocompatibility complex antigens using retroviral vectors. *Proc. Natl. Acad. Sci.* **84:** 2150.

Kozak, M. 1986. Point mutations define a sequence flanking the AUG initiator codon that modulates translation by eukaryotic ribosomes. *Cell* **44:** 283.

Lewis, V.A., T. Koch, H. Plutner, and I. Mellman. 1986. Characterization of a cDNA clone for a mouse macrophage-lymphocyte Fc receptor. *Nature* **324:** 372.

Martin, L.H., F. Calabi, F.-A. Lefebvre, C.A.G. Bilsland, and C. Milstein. 1987. Structure and expression of the human thymocyte antigens CD1a, CD1b and CD1c. *Proc. Natl. Acad. Sci.* **84:** 9189.

Matsudaira, P. 1987. Sequence from picomole quantities of proteins electroblotted onto polyvinylidene difluoride membranes. *J. Biol. Chem.* **262:** 10035.

Moore, K.H., B.T. Sher, Y. Sun H., K.A. Eakle, and L. Hood. 1982. DNA sequence of a gene encoding a BALB/c mouse Ld transplantation antigen. *Science* **215:** 679.

Morris, B. and R. Morris. 1974. The effects of cortisone acetate on stomach evacuation and the absorption of ^{125}I-labelled globulins in young rats, *J. Physiol.* **240:** 79.

Nathenson, S.G., H. Uehara, and B.M. Ewenstein. 1981. Primary structural analysis of the transplantation antigens of the murine H-2 major histocompatibility complex. *Annu. Rev. Biochem.* **50:** 1025.

Obata, Y., Y.-T. Chen, E. Stockert, and L.J. Old. 1985. Structural analysis of TL genes of the mouse. *Proc. Natl. Acad. Sci.* **82:** 5475.

Parham, P. 1989. MHC meets mother's milk. *Nature* **337:** 118.

Pearson, W.R. and D.J. Lipman. 1988. Improved tools for biological sequence comparison. *Proc. Natl. Acad. Sci.* **85:** 2444.

Ploegh, H.L., H.T. Orr, and J.L. Strominger. 1981. Major histocompatibility antigens: The human (HLA-A, -B, -C) and murine (H-2K, H-2D) class I molecules. *Cell* **24:** 287.

Poulik, M.D. and O. Smithies. 1979. Partial amino acid sequences of rabbit and rat beta 2-microglobulins. *Mol. Immunol.* **16:** 731.

Ravetch, J.V., A.D. Luster, R. Weinshank, J. Kochan, A. Pavlovec, D.A. Portnoy, J. Humes, Y.C.E. Pan, and J. Unkeless. 1986. Structural heterogeneity and functional domains of murine immunoglobulin G Fc receptors. *Science* **234:** 718.

Rodewald, R. 1970. Selective antibody transport in the proximal small intestine of the neonatal rat. *J. Cell. Biol.* **45:** 635.

———. 1976. pH-dependent binding of immunoglobulins to intestinal cells of the neonatal rat. *J. Cell Biol.* **71:** 666.

Rodewald, R. and J.-P. Kraehenbuhl. 1984. Receptor-mediated transport of IgG. *J. Cell. Biol.* **99:** 159s.

Sanger, F., S. Nicklen, and R. Coulson. 1977. DNA sequencing with chain-terminating inhibitors. *Proc. Natl. Acad. Sci.* **74:** 5463.

Sarmay, G. and J. Gergely. 1983. Activation of lymphocytes alters Fc receptor and beta2-microglobulin relationship on the lymphocyte surface. *Cell. Immunol.* **78:** 73.

Seong, R.H., C.A. Clayberger, A.M. Krensky, and J.R. Parnes. 1988. Rescue of Daudi cell HLA expression by transfection of the mouse beta 2-microglobulin gene. *J. Exp. Med.* **167:** 288.

Simister, N.E. and K.E. Mostov. 1989. An Fc receptor structurally related to MHC class I antigens. *Nature* **337:** 184.

Simister, N.E., and A.R. Rees. 1985. Isolation and characterization of an Fc receptor from neonatal rat small intestine. *Eur. J. Immunol.* **15:** 733.

Simmons, D. and B. Seed. 1988. The Fcg receptor of natural killer cells is a phospholipid-linked membrane protein. *Nature* **333:** 568.

Smith, P.K., R.I. Krohn, G.T. Hermanson, A.K. Mallia, F.H. Gartner, M.D. Provenzano, E.K. Fujimoto, N.M. Goeke, B.J. Olson, and D.C. Klenk. 1985. Measurement of protein using bicinchoninic acid. *Anal. Biochem.* **150:** 76.

Solheim, B.G., E. Thorsby, and E. Moller. 1976. Inhibition of the Fc receptor of human lymphoid cells by antisera recognizing determinants of the HLA system. *J. Exp. Med.* **143:** 1568.

Steinmetz, M., K.W. Moore, J.G. Frelinger, B.T. Sher, F.-W. Shen, E.A. Boyse, and L. Hood. 1981. A pseudogene homologous to mouse transplantation antigens: Transplantation antigens are encoded by eight exons that correlate with protein domains. *Cell* **25:** 683.

Stengelin, S., I. Stamenkovic, and B. Seed. 1988. Isolation of cDNAs for two distinct human Fc receptors by ligand affinity cloning. *EMBO J.* **7:** 1053.

Strachan, T., R. Sodoyer, M. Damotte, and B.R. Jordan. 1984. Complete nucleotide sequence of a functional class I HLA gene, HLA-A3: Implications for the evolution of HLA genes. *EMBO J.* **3:** 887.

Stuart, S.G., M.L. Troustine, D.J.T. Vaux, T. Koch, C.L. Martens, I. Mellman, and K.W. Moore. 1987. Isolation and expression of cDNA clones encoding a human receptor for IgG (FcgRII). *J. Exp. Med.* **166:** 1668.

von Heijne, G. 1986. A new method for predicting signal sequence cleavage sites. *Nucleic Acids Res.* **14:** 4683.

Wallace, K.H. and A.R. Rees. 1980. Studies on the immunoglobulin-G Fc-fragment receptor from neonatal rat small intestine. *Biochem. J.* **188:** 9.

Variation in HLA Expression on Tumors: An Escape from Immune Response

M.E.F. Smith, J.G. Bodmer, A.P. Kelly, J. Trowsdale, S.C. Kirkland, and W.F. Bodmer
Imperial Cancer Research Fund, Lincoln's Inn Fields, London, WC2A 3PX United Kingdom

HLA-A, B, C, and HLA-D antigens are polymorphic heterodimeric surface-membrane glycoproteins. HLA-A, B, C heavy chains are encoded at three highly polymorphic loci (A, B, and C) in the major histocompatibility (HLA) region of chromosome 6, whereas the light-chain β_2-microglobulin is encoded on chromosome 15. β_2-Microglobulin is required for the surface expression of the mature HLA-A, B, C molecule. Both α and β chains of HLA-D molecules map to loci in the DR, DQ, and DP subregions of the HLA region, most of which are polymorphic. HLA-A, B, C, and HLA-D molecules control the recognition of antigen by T lymphocytes. Cytotoxic T lymphocytes usually recognize antigen in the context of HLA-A, B, C molecules, whereas helper T lymphocytes recognize antigen in the context of HLA-D. Different HLA allele products mapping to the same locus vary in their ability to present alternative antigen epitopes (McMichael et al. 1986; Gotch et al. 1987; Möller 1987).

The lack of surface-membrane HLA-A, B, C expression in some tumor-derived cell lines led to the suggestion that tumors expressing novel antigenic determinants could escape cytotoxic T lymphocyte attack through the selective outgrowth of HLA-A, B, C loss variants (Brodsky et al. 1979b; Travers et al. 1982). Immunohistochemical techniques have shown that a proportion of many tumors lack HLA-A, B, C expression in vivo. For example, although normal colorectal epithelium consistently strongly expresses HLA-A, B, C antigens, these molecules are undetectable on approximately 10% of colorectal adenocarcinomas (Momburg et al. 1986; Richman 1987). Selective losses of individual HLA-A, B, C allele products from colorectal adenomas and adenocarcinomas have been described recently (Rees et al. 1988; Smith et al. 1988), and they also are likely to be of functional importance in tumor escape from immune attack.

HLA-D antigens are not constitutively expressed by normal colorectal epithelium, but their expression can be induced by cytokines such as γ-interferon (IFN-γ) (Pallone et al. 1988; for review, see Bodmer 1987). The expression of HLA-D antigens on many colorectal adenocarcinomas (Moore et al. 1986) could therefore be a normal response to cytokines (Lampert et al. 1985). The abnormal situation is seen in colorectal carcinomas and carcinoma-derived cell lines that fail to express HLA-D antigens in response to IFN-γ and other similar stimuli (Pfizenmaier et al. 1985; Moore et

al. 1986; Richman 1987). Failure of tumors to express HLA-D antigens in response to cytokines could be selected for either through a decreased presentation of novel tumor antigens to the immune system or through tumor escape from HLA-D-restricted cytotoxic T lymphocyte killing.

In this paper, we update and review data published previously on HLA-A, B, C expression in colorectal adenocarcinomas (Smith et al. 1988, 1989) and present further data on the expression of HLA antigens in colorectal carcinoma cell lines.

MATERIALS AND METHODS

Tissues and immunohistochemistry. Samples from 10 colorectal adenomas (9 from familial adenomatous polyposis patients) and 31 colorectal adenocarcinomas from a total of 41 patients were studied. Histologically normal colonic mucosa was separately sampled from 7 of the adenoma patients and 16 of the adenocarcinoma patients. Tissues were snap frozen in liquid-nitrogen-cooled isopentane and subsequently stored under liquid nitrogen before cryostat sectioning at 7 μm thickness. The sections were immunohistochemically stained by a peroxidase–anti-peroxidase technique (Smith et al. 1989), using monoclonal antibodies (MAbs) recognizing monomorphic and polymorphic determinants on HLA-A, B, C antigens.

Cell lines. The following colorectal carcinoma cell lines were studied: SW620, SW837, and SW1222 (Leibovitz et al. 1976); HT29 (Fogh and Trempe 1975); LS174T (Tom et al. 1976); LoVo (Drewinko et al. 1976); HCA-7 and HCA-46 (Kirkland and Bailey 1986); and CC20 and CC22 (Greenhalgh and Kinsella 1985). CC20 and CC22 are separate cell lines grown from the same primary colonic adenocarcinoma. All cell lines were grown as monolayers on tissue culture plastic (Nunc) and on glass slides, with or without 1000 IU/ml of human recombinant IFN-γ for 24 hours. Molt 4, an acute lymphocytic-leukemia-derived cell line (Minowada et al. 1972) and Raji, a Burkitt-lymphoma-derived B-lymphocytic cell line (Epstein and Barr 1965), were used as controls in the mRNA analysis.

ELISA. A galactosidase-antigalactosidase enzyme-linked immunosorbent assay (ELISA) (Durbin and Bodmer 1987) was performed on the colorectal carcinoma cell lines. Following trypsinization, the cells were pipetted to form a single-cell suspension, washed, and plated at a density of 5×10^4 cells/well in 96-well microtiter plates (Dynatek).

Monoclonal antibodies. The following monoclonal antibodies were used at dilutions determined by preliminary titration experiments: BBM.1 detects β_2-microglobulin (Brodsky et al. 1979a); HC-10 detects HLA-A, B, C free heavy chain, with a preference for HLA-B products (Stam et al. 1986); PA2.6 detects a monomorphic determinant on β_2-microglobulin-associated HLA-A, B, C antigens (Brodsky et al. 1979b); 142.2 detects HLA-A1 and HLA-Aw36 (J. Bodmer, unpubl.); MA2.1 detects HLA-A2 and HLA-B17 (McMichael et al. 1980); BB7.2 detects HLA-A2 and HLA-Aw69 (Brodsky et al. 1979b); GAP A3 detects HLA-A3 (Berger et al. 1982); 116.5.28 detects HLA-Bw4 (K. Gelsthorpe, pers. comm.); 126.39 detects HLA-Bw6 (K. Gelsthorpe, pers. comm.); L243 detects HLA-DR (Lampson and Levy 1980); and RR1/1 detects intercellular adhesion molecule 1 (ICAM-1) (Rothlein et al. 1986).

mRNA and Northern blotting. mRNA was prepared from cell lines using standard guanidinium isothiocyanate methods. Northern blotting procedures were also standard, and both techniques were described by Maniatis et al. (1982). The following probes were used: DRα cDNA (Lee et al. 1982); TGFβ (Derynck et al. 1985); ICAM-1 (Simmons et al. 1988); invariant chain (Ii) (Claesson et al. 1983).

RESULTS

HLA-A, B, C Expression in Colorectal Tumors

The tumor cells of 27 of 31 colorectal adenocarcinomas expressed HLA-A, B, C antigens strongly and fairly uniformly, as detected by MAb PA2.6, which is directed against a monomorphic determinant. One tumor showed very heterogeneous HLA-A, B, C expression, two showed uniformly weak expression, and a single case showed no detectable expression. In this last case, the reactivity of tumor cells with MAb HC-10 (recognizing free HLA-A, B, C heavy chains), but not with MAb BBM.1 (recognizing β_2-microglobulin), indicates that a loss of β_2-microglobulin underlies the absence of mature HLA-A, B, C molecules. Selective

losses of individual HLA-A, B, C allele products were studied using monoclonal antibodies to polymorphic determinants in the 28 adenocarcinomas that strongly expressed (focally in one case) HLA-A, B, C antigens. Complete selective losses recognized by strong staining of tumor stroma and, when available, normal colorectal mucosa, but no staining of tumor cells was common, being present in 8 of 28 cases. Complete loss of HLA-A2 and HLA-Bw4 was seen in 7 of 14 and 4 of 14 cases, respectively (Fig. 1; Table 1). Interestingly, the four cases that lost HLA-Bw4 also lost HLA-A2. Complete losses of HLA-A1, HLA-A3 and HLA-Bw6 were seen infrequently or not at all (Table 1). All normal colorectal epithelium strongly expressed HLA-A, B, C antigens, and, furthermore, no example of selective loss of an HLA-A, B, C allele product was seen in the normal epithelium.

All ten adenomas expressed HLA-A, B, C antigens strongly and uniformly, as detected by MAb PA2.6. Two adenomas, however, showed focal loss of an HLA-B product.

HLA-A, B, C Expression in Colorectal Carcinoma Cell Lines

ELISA detected strong although variable HLA-A, B, C expression using MAb PA2.6 in nine of the ten colorectal carcinoma cell lines (Fig. 2A). Some of these lines, such as LS174T, have been described previously as having significantly reduced HLA-A, B, C expression (Travers et al. 1982). HLA-A, B, C expression was virtually absent in the cell line LoVo, as also described previously (Brodsky et al. 1979b) (Fig. 2A). The induction of increased HLA-A, B, C antigen expression by IFN-γ was very variable. For example, there was no induction in LoVo, very minor induction in LS174T (from an initially low level) and in HCA-7, but much more pronounced induction especially in CC20 as well as in SW620, SW1222, and SW837, all from initially low levels (Fig. 2A).

Peripheral blood lymphocytes were available from the patient from whose colorectal carcinoma the cell line HCA-7 had been grown. The lymphocyte HLA-A, B, C typing by a standard microlymphocytotoxicity assay (Bodmer and Bodmer 1979) was A1,2; B37,51(Bw4). In contrast, an immunohistochemical HLA-A, B, C typing of HCA-7 cells grown on glass slides was A2;Bw4, suggesting tumor loss of HLA-A1

Table 1. Complete Losses of HLA-A, B, C Allele Products in 28 Colorectal Adenocarcinomas

	HLA					
	A1	A2	A3	B17	Bw4	Bw6
			(no. of cases)			
Stroma +ve[a]	7	14	6	1	14	22
Tumor −ve[b]	0	7	1	0	4	0

[a]Tumor stroma positive for HLA-A, B, C allele products.
[b]Tumor cells completely negative and tumor stroma positive for HLA-A, B, C allele products.

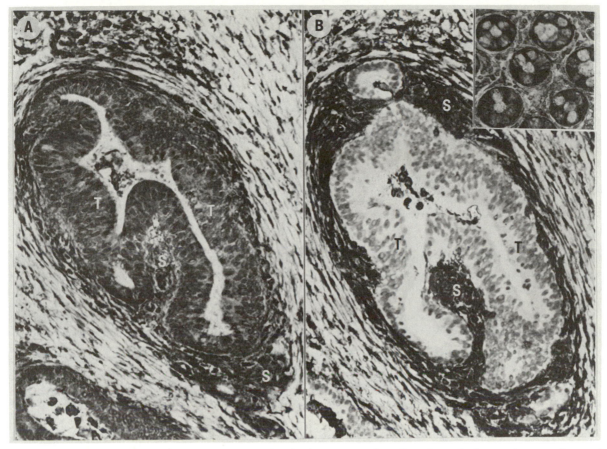

Figure 1. Immunoperoxidase-stained hematoxylin-counterstained cryostat sections of a colorectal adenocarcinoma and normal colonic epithelium from the same patient. There is strong expression of HLA-Bw4 antigen (using MAb 116.5.28) on both stroma (S) and tumor (T) cells (*A*). HLA-A2 antigen (using MAb MA2.1) is present on stromal cells but has been lost from tumor cells (*B*). (*Inset*) HLA-A2 antigen (using MAb MA2.1) is present on normal colonic epithelium. Magnifications: (*A, B*) 200 × ; (*inset*) 150 × .

antigen. MAb 142.2 failed to detect the HLA-A1 antigen immunohistochemically on HCA-7 cells, even following IFN-γ treatment.

HLA-DR and ICAM-1 Expression in Colorectal Carcinoma Cell Lines

Induction of HLA-DR (as recognized by MAb L243) with IFN-γ was very variable among the ten cell lines studied (Fig. 2B). For example, IFN-γ caused substantial HLA-DR induction in HCA-7, HCA-46, and SW1222 but induced no, or very little, HLA-DR expression in SW620, CC20, CC22, and LoVo. LS174T, SW837, and HT29 showed intermediate levels of HLA-DR induction. In contrast, IFN-γ induced very substantial increases in ICAM-1 expression in all ten cell lines studied (Fig. 2C), showing that none of the lines lacked a general ability to respond to IFN-γ, such as might be due, for example, to absence of an IFN-γ receptor.

Analysis of mRNA after IFN Induction in Colorectal Carcinoma Cell Lines

To establish the molecular basis of the results of the experiments with monoclonal antibodies, various cell lines were treated with IFN-γ, and RNA was extracted to run on Northern blots as shown in Figure 3. Figure 3, A and B, shows that class II (DRα) and Ii mRNAs were induced in SW1222 cells, as expected, but that the SW620 extracts showed very low, if any, expression after induction. As shown in Figure 3C, the lack of expression in SW620 was not due to a general failure of IFN-γ to affect gene expression after its interaction with the cells, because ICAM-1 transcripts were equally inducible in all the cells. The results with Raji and Molt 4 served as positive and negative controls, respectively. These results were extended at the mRNA level to LoVo and CC20. In these two cell lines, the Ii mRNA was induced similarly to SW1222, and there was very slight induction of DR mRNA (data not shown). These data confirm and extend the results from the antibody-

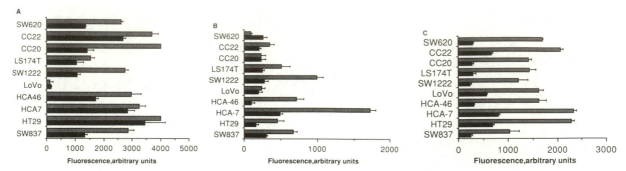

Figure 2. ELISA on colorectal carcinoma cell lines comparing inducibility of HLA-A,B,C antigens (*A*) using MAb PA2.6, HLA-DR antigens (*B*) using MAb L243, and ICAM-1 (*C*) using MAb RR1/1, by IFN-γ. Solid columns represent expression with no IFN-γ; hatched columns, with IFN-γ. Data shown represents the mean ± standard deviation of three determinations. Maximum readout equals 4000 arbitrary fluorescence units.

binding studies described earlier. There have been reports that TGFβ can down-regulate class II expression (Czarniecki et al. 1988). To test this, Northern blots were probed with a TGFβ cDNA. The levels of this transcript were low in all the cells examined, and IFN-γ did not appear to affect the level.

DISCUSSION

Normal colorectal epithelium strongly expresses HLA-A, B, C molecules and does not show selective expression of individual HLA-A, B, C allele products. Therefore, in colorectal adenocarcinoma, the absence or weak expression of all HLA-A, B, C molecules (seen in 10% of cases in our series) (Momburg et al. 1986; Richman 1987) or the selective loss of individual allele products (seen in 50% of cases for HLA-A2 in our series) (Rees et al. 1988) are abnormal phenotypes that must have been selected for in tumor progression. HLA-A, B, C molecules control the recognition of antigen by cytotoxic T lymphocytes. This suggests that the outgrowth of HLA-A, B, C lacking tumor mutants could occur through their ability to escape destruction

by cytotoxic T lymphocytes. Because different HLA-A, B, C allele products vary in their ability to present the same antigen epitope to cytotoxic T lymphocytes, the loss of some tumor HLA-A, B, C allele products with the retention of others, as described in this paper, could also confer on tumor cells substantial resistance to cytotoxic T lymphocyte attack.

The focal selective losses of HLA-B products seen in two of ten adenomas may represent precursors to the more extensive selective losses seen in adenocarcinomas.

In the ten colorectal carcinoma cell lines studied for in vitro models of HLA-A, B, C loss, only LoVo showed complete or almost complete absence of HLA-A, B, C antigens, which was, moreover, not affected by IFN-γ. This loss has been shown previously to be secondary to the loss of β_2-microglobulin (Travers et al. 1982). HCA-7 may be an in vitro model for the selective loss of an individual HLA-A, B, C allele product with probable HLA-A1 antigen loss. Other variations in HLA-A, B, C expression, namely, relatively low levels, even after IFN-γ, as in LS174T, and low basal levels, as in SW620 and SW837, may also reflect some lesser effects of immune selection. The molecular bases for these HLA-A, B, C losses and variations in expression are currently under investigation.

A normal counterpart to the loss of HLA-A, B, C expression from tumors is their absence from the majority of trophoblasts. This protects the trophoblast from maternal cellular immune attack and therefore provides the simplest explanation for why the fetus survives as an allograft. This also explains why choriocarcinomas, which are trophoblast-derived tumors, also lack HLA-A, B, C, and are therefore not influenced by HLA incompatibility (for review, see Bodmer 1987). However, a normal cell type that never expressed HLA-A, B, C could be a considerable disadvantage as it could harbor viruses in a protected environment, because virus-infected cells would not be susceptible to normal T-cell immune attack. It is therefore of considerable interest that preliminary experiments in our laboratory (A. Thomas, pers. comm.) suggest that HLA-A, B, C expression can, under ap-

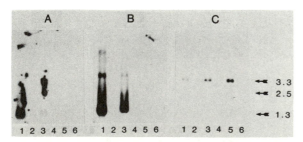

Figure 3. Northern blots comparing inducibility of DRα (*A*), Ii (*B*), and ICAM-1 (*C*). Total RNA (8 μg) was run in each lane, and the gels were blotted as described in Materials and Methods. The filter was then hybridized and exposed to film under standard conditions, as described in literature from Amersham, using the multiprime system for probe labeling (membrane transfer and detection methods, Amersham). (Lane *1*) Raji; (lane *2*) Molt 4; (lane *3*) SW1222 with IFN-γ induction; (lane *4*) SW1222 without IFN-γ; (lanes *5* and *6*) SW620 with and without IFN-γ induction, respectively.

propriate circumstances, readily be induced in trophoblasts. This emphasizes the significance of the usual lack of HLA-A, B, C expression in trophoblasts as seen by immunohistochemistry in placental histological sections. The molecular basis for the lack of HLA-A, B, C expression in tumors may sometimes involve mutations affecting the processes that normally control expression in the trophoblast, perhaps by *trans*-acting DNA-binding proteins.

HLA-D antigen expression does not occur constitutively in colorectal epithelium but can be induced by IFN-γ (Pallone et al. 1988). Sometimes, the invasion of colorectal mucosa by adenocarcinoma cells induces HLA-D antigen expression in nonneoplastic crypts (Richman 1987). However, in a microenvironment inducive to HLA-D antigen expression, the adenocarcinoma cells, themselves, sometimes fail to express HLA-D antigens (Moore et al. 1986; Richman 1987). This, too, is an abnormal tumor phenotype that must have been selected for, perhaps through an advantage of a decreased ability to present novel tumor antigens to the immune system or through escape from HLA-D antigen-restricted cytotoxic T lymphocyte attack.

The in vitro counterpart of this phenomenon probably occurs in the colorectal carcinoma cell lines SW620, CC20, CC22, and LoVo in which IFN-γ fails to induce HLA-DR antigens. The increase in ICAM-1 expression induced by IFN-γ in these cell lines demonstrates a striking specificity for HLA-D in the resistance to interferon, making it most probable that the lack of induction of HLA-D antigens is specifically selected for in tumor progression. In these colorectal carcinoma cell lines, the failure of IFN-γ to induce HLA-DR expression, in combination with its ability to induce molecules such as ICAM-1, is reminiscent of the B lymphocytes of HLA-D-deficient severe combined immunodeficiency (SCID) syndrome patients (Lisowska-Grospierre et al. 1985). This SCID syndrome is inherited as an autosomal recessive condition and is associated with the absence of a DNA-binding protein (RF-X) that normally binds to the X box of the HLA-DRα promoter (Reith et al. 1988). This raises the possibility that a mutation causing a similar defect, but occurring at the somatic level during tumor progression, is responsible for the failure of IFN-γ to induce HLA-D expression in some colorectal carcinoma cell lines.

We have described several abnormal phenotypes with regard to the expression of immunoregulatory molecules in colorectal neoplasia. These include loss of all HLA-A, B, C molecules, selective loss of individual HLA-A, B, C allele products, reduced expression and inducibility of HLA-A, B, C molecules, the lack of inducibility of HLA-D antigens by IFN-γ, and the loss of lymphocyte-function-associated antigen 3, described elsewhere (Smith et al. 1989). All of these tumor phenotypes are likely to be selected for in tumor progression by conferring a growth advantage through resistance to immune destruction. They thus constitute indirect evidence for the frequent existence of novel tumor antigens, initially detectable by the host immune system, in colorectal adenocarcinoma. The colorectal carcinoma cell lines with abnormal expression of major histocompatibility antigens described in this paper will probably be the best cell types in which, initially, to detect and characterize such tumor-specific antigens. The recently described ability of T lymphocytes to recognize proteins that have an intracellular location and are not expressed in their native state on the cell-surface membrane (Townsend et al. 1985, 1986) extends the range of candidate tumor-specific antigens to intracellular mutant oncogene products. In this context, mutant *ras* and p53 genes, whose protein products occur in subsurface membrane and nuclear locations, respectively, have been identified in colorectal adenocarcinomas (Vogelstein et al. 1988; Baker et al. 1989). Their protein products could therefore be the target of a T-cell immune response. The identification of tumor-specific antigens early in tumor progression, before the outgrowth of mutant tumor cells resistant to immune attack, is an important goal because tumor cells at this early stage may be susceptible to immunotherapy.

ACKNOWLEDGMENTS

We are grateful to the Imperial Cancer Research Fund Colorectal Unit and Pathology Department, St Mark's Hospital, London, for providing tumor tissue, to Boehringer Ingelheim for recombinant human IFN-γ, and to K. Gelsthorpe (116.5.28 and 126.39), H. Ploegh (HC-10), T.A. Springer (RR1/1 and TS2/9), and Genetic Systems (142.2) for monoclonal antibodies.

REFERENCES

Baker, S.J., E.R Fearon, J.M. Nigro, S.R. Hamilton, A.C. Preisinger, J.M. Jessup, P. van Tuinen, D.H. Ledbetter, D.F. Barker, Y. Nakamura, R. White, and B. Vogelstein. 1989. Chromosome 17 deletions and p53 gene mutations in colorectal carcinomas. *Science* **244:** 217.

Berger, A.E., J.E. Davis, and P. Cresswell. 1982. Monoclonal antibody to HLA-A3. *Hybridoma* **1:** 87.

Bodmer, W.F. 1987. The HLA system: Structure and function. *J. Clin. Pathol.* **40:** 948.

Bodmer, W.F. and J.G. Bodmer. 1979. Cytofluorochromasia for HLA-A, -B, -C and DR typing. In *NIAID manual of tissue typing techniques* (ed. J.G. Ray), p. 46. National Institutes of Health Publication No. 80-545.

Brodsky, F.M., W.F. Bodmer, and P. Parham. 1979a. Characterization of a monoclonal anti-β₂-microglobulin antibody and its use in the genetic and biochemical analysis of major histocompatibility antigens. *Eur. J. Immunol.* **9:** 536.

Brodsky, F.M., P. Parham, C.J. Barnstable, M.J. Crumpton, and W.F. Bodmer. 1979b. Monoclonal antibodies for analysis of the HLA system. *Immunol. Rev.* **47:** 3.

Claesson, L., D. Larhammar, L. Rask, and P.A. Peterson. 1983. cDNA clone for the human invariant γ chain of class II histocompatibility antigens and its implications for the protein structure. *Proc. Natl. Acad. Sci.* **80:** 7395.

Czarniecki, C.W., H.H. Chiu, G.H.W. Wong, S.M. McCabe and M.A. Palladino. 1988. Transforming growth factor-β1 modulates the expression of class II histocompatibility antigens on human cells. *J. Immunol.* **140:** 4217.

Derynck, R., J.A. Jarrett, E.Y. Chen, D.H. Eaton, J.R. Bell, R.K. Assoian, A.B. Roberts, M.B. Sporn, and D.V. Goeddel. 1985. Human transforming growth factor-β complementary DNA sequence and expression in normal and transformed cells. *Nature* **316**: 701.

Drewinko, B., M.M. Romsdahl, L.Y. Yang, M.J. Ahearn, and J.M. Trujillo. 1976. Establishment of a human carcinoembryonic antigen-producing colon adenocarcinoma cell line. *Cancer Res.* **36**: 467.

Durbin, H. and W.F. Bodmer. 1987. A sensitive microimmunoassay using β-galactosidase/anti-β-galactosidase complexes. *J. Immunol. Methods* **97**: 19.

Epstein, M.A. and Y.M. Barr. 1965. Characteristics and mode of growth of a tissue culture strain (EB1) of human lymphoblasts from Burkitt's Lymphoma. *J. Natl. Cancer Inst.* **34**: 231.

Fogh, J. and G. Trempe. 1975. New human tumor cell lines. In *Human tumor cells in vitro* (ed. J. Fogh), p. 115. Plenum Press, New York.

Gotch, F., J. Rothbard, K. Howland, A. Townsend, and A. McMichael. 1987. Cytotoxic T lymphocytes recognise a fragment of influenza virus matrix protein in association with HLA-A2. *Nature* **326**: 881.

Greenhalgh, D.A. and A.R. Kinsella. 1985. c-Ha-*ras* not c-Ki-*ras* activation in three colon tumour cell lines. *Carcinogenesis* **6**: 1533.

Kirkland, S.C. and I.G. Bailey. 1986. Establishment and characterisation of six human colorectal adenocarcinoma cell lines. *Br. J. Cancer* **53**: 779.

Lampert, I.A., S. Kirkland, S. Farrell, and L.K. Borysiewicz. 1985. HLA-DR expression in a human colonic carcinoma cell line. *J. Pathol.* **146**: 337.

Lampson, L.A. and R. Levy. 1980. Two populations of Ia-like molecules on a human B cell line. *J. Immunol.* **125**: 293.

Lee, J.S., J. Trowsdale, and W.F. Bodmer. 1982. cDNA clones coding for the heavy chain of human HLA-DR antigen. *Proc. Natl. Acad. Sci.* **79**: 545.

Leibovitz, A., J.C. Stinson, W.B. McCombs, C.E. McCoy, K.C. Mazur, and N.D. Mabry. 1976. Classification of human colorectal adenocarcinoma cell lines. *Cancer Res.* **36**: 4562.

Lisowska-Grospierre, B., D.J. Charron, C. de Préval, A. Durandy, C. Griscelli, and B. Mach. 1985. Defect in the regulation of major histocompatibility complex class II gene expression in human HLA-DR negative lymphocytes from patients with combined immunodeficiency syndrome. *J. Clin. Invest.* **76**: 381.

McMichael, A.J., F.M. Gotch, and J. Rothbard. 1986. HLA B37 determines an influenza A virus nucleoprotein epitope recognised by cytotoxic T lymphocytes. *J. Exp. Med.* **164**: 1397.

McMichael, A.J., P. Parham, N. Rust, and F.M. Brodsky. 1980. A monoclonal antibody that recognizes an antigenic determinant shared by HLA A2 and B17. *Hum. Immunol.* **1**: 121.

Maniatis, T., E.F. Fritsch, and J. Sambrook. 1982. *Molecular cloning: A laboratory manual.* Cold Spring Harbor Laboratory, Cold Spring Harbor, New York.

Minowada, J., T. Ohnuma, and G.E. Moore. 1972. Rosette-forming human lymphoid cell lines. 1. Establishment and evidence for origin of thymus-derived lymphocytes. *J. Natl. Cancer Inst.* **49**: 891.

Möller, G. 1987. Antigen requirements for activation of MHC restricted responses. *Immunol. Rev.* **98**: 1.

Momburg, F., T. Degener, E. Bacchus, G. Moldenhauer, G.J. Hämmerling, and P. Möller. 1986. Loss of HLA-A,

B,C and *de novo* expression of HLA-D in colorectal cancer. *Int. J. Cancer* **37**: 179.

Moore, M., A.K. Ghosh, D. Johnston, and A.J. Street. 1986. Expression of MHC class II products on human colorectal cancer. *J. Immunogenet.* **13**: 201.

Pallone, F., S. Fais, and M.R. Capobianchi. 1988. HLA-D region antigens on isolated human colonic epithelial cells: Enhanced expression in inflammatory bowel disease and *in vitro* induction by different stimuli. *Clin. Exp. Immunol.* **74**: 75.

Pfizenmaier, K., H. Bartsch, P. Scheurich, B. Seliger, U. Ucer, K. Vehmeyer, and G.A. Nagel. 1985. Differential γ-interferon response of human colon carcinoma cells: Inhibition of proliferation and modulation of immunogenicity as independent effects of γ-interferon on tumor cell growth. *Cancer Res.* **45**: 3503.

Rees, R.C., A.-M. Buckle, K. Gelsthorpe, V. James, C.W. Potter, K. Rogers, and G. Jacob. 1988. Loss of polymorphic A and B locus HLA antigens in colon carcinoma. *Br. J. Cancer* **57**: 374.

Reith, W., S. Satola, C. Herrero Sanchez, I. Amaldi, B. Lisowska-Grospierre, C. Griscelli, M.R. Hadam, and B. Mach. 1988. Congenital immunodeficiency with a regulatory defect in MHC class II gene expression lacks a specific HLA-DR promoter binding protein, RF-X. *Cell* **53**: 897.

Richman, P.I. 1987. "Monoclonal antibodies for the study of differentiation in normal and neoplastic human colorectal epithelium." Ph.D. thesis. London University.

Rothlein, R., M.L. Dustin, S.D. Marlin, and T.A. Springer. 1986. A human intercellular adhesion molecule (ICAM-1) distinct from LFA-1. *J. Immunol.* **137**: 1270.

Simmons, D., M.W. Makgoba, and B. Seed. 1988. ICAM, an adhesion ligand of LFA-1, is homologous to the neural cell adhesion molecule NCAM. *Nature* **331**: 624.

Smith, M.E.F., W.F. Bodmer, and J.G. Bodmer. 1988. Selective loss of HLA-A,B,C locus products in colorectal adenocarcinoma. *Lancet* **I**: 823.

Smith, M.E.F., S.G.E. Marsh, J.G. Bodmer, K. Gelsthorpe, and W.F. Bodmer. 1989. Loss of HLA-A,B,C allele products and lymphocyte function-associated antigen 3 in colorectal neoplasia. *Proc. Natl. Acad. Sci.* **86**: 5557.

Stam, N.J., H. Spits, and H.L. Ploegh. 1986. Monoclonal antibodies raised against denatured HLA-B locus heavy chains permit biochemical characterization of certain HLA-C locus products. *J. Immunol.* **137**: 2299.

Tom, B.H., L.P. Rutzky, M.M. Jakstys, R. Oyashu, C.I. Kaye, and B.D. Kahan. 1976. Human colonic adenocarcinoma cells. I. Establishment and description of a new line. *In Vitro* **12**: 180.

Townsend, A.R.M., F.M. Gotch, and J. Davey. 1985. Cytotoxic T cells recognize fragments of the influenza nucleoprotein. *Cell* **42**: 457.

Townsend, A.R.M., J. Rothbard, F.M. Gotch, G. Bahadur, D. Wraith, and A.J. McMichael. 1986. The epitopes of influenza nucleoprotein recognized by cytotoxic T lymphocytes can be defined by short synthetic peptides. *Cell* **44**: 959.

Travers, P.J., J.L. Arklie, J. Trowsdale, R.A. Patillo, and W.F. Bodmer. 1982. Lack of expression of HLA-ABC antigens in choriocarcinoma and other human tumor cell lines. *Nat. Cancer Inst. Monogr.* **60**: 175.

Vogelstein, B., E.R. Fearon, S.R. Hamilton, S.E. Kern, A.C. Preisinger, M. Leppert, Y. Nakamura, R. White, A.M.M. Smits, and J.L. Bos. 1988. Genetic alterations during colorectal-tumor development. *N. Engl. J. Med.* **319**: 525.

Genes Coding for T-cell-defined Tum⁻ Transplantation Antigens: Point Mutations, Antigenic Peptides, and Subgenic Expression

T. BOON, A. VAN PEL, E. DE PLAEN, P. CHOMEZ, C. LURQUIN, J.-P. SZIKORA, C. SIBILLE, B. MARIAMÉ, B. VAN DEN EYNDE, B. LETHÉ, AND V. BRICHART
Ludwig Institute for Cancer Research, Brussels Branch, Brussels 1200, Belgium;
Cellular Genetics Unit, University of Louvain, Brussels, Belgium

The antigens encoded by class I and class II genes of the major histocompatibility complex (MHC) are an exception among transplantation antigens in that they elicit not only T-cell-mediated rejection responses, but also antibody responses. Immunoprecipitation could therefore be used to isolate and characterize these antigenic proteins. From there, it was possible to clone and sequence the MHC genes (Ploegh et al. 1980). For the other transplantation antigens, notably, mouse minor histocompatibility antigens, tumor-specific transplantation antigens (TSTAs), and male-specific antigen H-Y, repeated attempts have failed consistently to produce specific antibodies. As a result, the structure of these antigenic molecules and the identity of the encoding genes have remained completely unknown. We have developed a gene transfection approach aimed at identifying directly the genes that code for this type of antigen. It was applied to transplantation antigens that arise on mouse tumor cells when they are treated with mutagenic agents; however, this approach should be applicable to all of the transplantation antigens that can be identified with cytolytic T lymphocytes (CTLs).

Tum⁻ Antigens

In vitro mutagen treatment of mouse tumor cells generates at high frequency stable immunogenic variants that are rejected by syngeneic mice (Boon and Kellermann 1977; Boon 1983). Because of their failure to form tumors, these variants were named tum⁻, as opposed to the original tum⁺ cell, which produces progressive tumors. With a dose of N-methyl-N'-nitro-N-nitrosoguanidine resulting in survival of about 0.1% of the treated tumor cells, the frequency of tum⁻ variants usually ranges between 1% and 20% of the survivors. This phenomenon has been observed on a large number of mouse tumor cell lines of various types and also with a guinea pig fibrosarcoma (Contessa et al. 1981; Frost et al. 1983; Zbar et al. 1984). Most tum⁻ variants express new transplantation antigens not found on the original tum⁺ cell. The existence of these tum⁻ antigens was first demonstrated in vivo by cross-immunization experiments (Boon and Van Pel 1978).

We have studied a series of tum⁻ variants derived from mastocytoma P815, a tumor induced in a DBA/2 mouse with methylcholanthrene (Uyttenhove et al. 1980). From clonal tum⁺ line P1, we obtained more than 30 different tum⁻ variants, which rarely produce progressive tumors, even when they were injected at doses exceeding 1000 times a tumorigenic dose of P1. When we restimulated in vitro spleen cells of syngeneic mice that had rejected these variants, we obtained CTLs that lysed preferentially the immunizing tum⁻ variant (Boon et al. 1980). From these lymphocytes, we were able to isolate stable CTL clones (Maryanski et al. 1982), some of which appeared to be directed against a TSTA of P815: They lysed P1 and all P815-derived cells but not syngeneic control tumors. Others recognized the immunizing tum⁻ variant, but neither the original tum⁺ cell nor the other tum⁻ variants derived from P815. They therefore defined new tum⁻ antigens specific for each variant. A systematic study of the tum⁻ antigens found on P815 variants revealed their considerable diversity: No antigen was found twice among the 15 tum⁻ variants that were analyzed.

By in vitro immunoselection with anti-tum⁻ CTL clones, it was also possible to demonstrate that some tum⁻ variants carry several tum⁻ antigens: Cells were isolated that were resistant to the selecting CTLs but still sensitive to other anti-tum⁻ CTL clones directed against the same variant (Maryanski and Boon 1982). Similar results were obtained after in vivo escape of some variants. For example, tum⁻ variant P91 occasionally produces progressive tumors in DBA/2 mice. These "escaping" tumors usually appear after a much longer delay than those produced by tum⁺ cells. When cells were collected from these tumors and cultured in vitro, they were found to be resistant against the majority of anti-P91 CTL clones but not against all of them. This defined at least two tum⁻ antigens present on variant P91:P91A (lost in vivo) and P91B (Fig. 1) (Maryanski et al. 1983a). In addition, these experiments clearly demonstrated that the tum⁻ antigens defined in vitro with CTLs play an important role in the rejection of tum⁻ variants. Likewise, we found that antigen-loss variants identified in vitro by immuno-

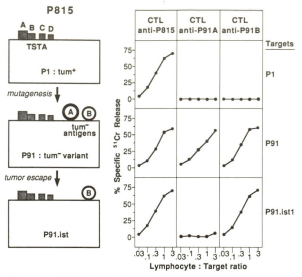

Figure 1. TSTA and tum⁻ antigens present on the original P815 line P1, on tum⁻ variant P91, and on the rare tumors (P91.ist) that arise after injection of P91 cells into DBA/2 mice. The CTL clones were derived from spleen cells obtained from mice that had rejected variant P91. They were incubated with their target for 4 hr.

selection with CTLs had regained the capacity to produce progressive tumors in syngeneic mice. Similar experiments performed with anti-tum⁺ CTL clones identified four different TSTAs on P815 (Uyttenhove et al. 1983).

To find an explanation that could reconcile the remarkably high frequency of tum⁻ variants with their stability and also to understand the source of their diversity, it appeared essential to identify the antigenic molecules: Would these molecules belong to a family encoded by related genes or would they represent an array of completely unrelated structures? We failed to obtain antibodies directed against tum⁻ antigens in all of our attempts. Therefore, we undertook to clone directly the relevant genes on the basis of their ability to produce the antigens recognized by the anti-tum⁻ CTLs.

Transfection of Tum⁻ Genes

Somatic cell hybrids obtained by fusion of P1 with P815 tum⁻ variants were found to express the tum⁻ antigens of the parental variant (Maryanski et al. 1983b). This dominant expression of the tum⁻ antigen opened the possibility of using gene transfection to clone the gene.

Whereas the transfection of genes coding for surface antigens recognized by antibodies had been demonstrated earlier (Kavathas and Herzenberg 1983), we faced the obligation of detecting our transfectants with CTLs. This implied that the recipient cell must be a good target for CTLs and must express the same H-2 haplotype as P815 (Zinkernagel and Doherty 1974). The fibroblast lines commonly used for DNA transfection by the calcium phosphate precipitation technique

are not very good targets for CTLs, but the tum⁺ cell P1 was ideal in this respect. Unfortunately, like most cell growing in suspension, it proved to be a very poor DNA recipient. However, we were able to select a highly transfectable variant, P1.HTR, by submitting P1 to repeated cycles of transfections with a selectable marker (Van Pel et al. 1985). P1.HTR has an efficiency of transfection of approximately 10^{-4} compared with 10^{-6} for P1. Endocytosis of calcium-precipitated DNA occurs at least tenfold more efficiently in P1.HTR than in P1 (Goethals et al. 1987).

It was reasonable to expect that the antigen would be expressed by only one allele of the relevant gene. Taking into account the size of the mammalian genome (6.10^6 kb) and the observation that recipients of calcium-phosphate-precipitated DNA integrate on the average approximately 1000 kb (Perucho et al. 1980), it appeared that a minimum of 6000 transfectants would have to be screened, a number in good agreement with the results obtained with surface antigens (Kavathas and Herzenberg 1983). Testing all of these transfectants individually for CTL lysis appeared impractical. We therefore explored the possibility of detecting transfectants by their ability to stimulate the proliferation of CTL clones directed against the relevant antigen. Anti-tum⁻ CTL clones were identified that showed a considerable increase in proliferation when the proper target was present. Most importantly, we found that mixtures of cells expressing tum⁻ antigens (e.g., P91) and cells that did not (e.g., P1.HTR) at a 1:30 ratio could provide a clearly recognizable stimulation of these CTL clones (Fig. 2). On the basis of this test, we set out to cotransfect P1.HTR cells with plasmid pSVtk-neoβ carrying the selectable *neo* gene and with DNA of variant P91, as outlined in Figure 2. Transfectants expressing tum⁻ antigen P91A were obtained at a frequency of 1/13,000 (Wölfel et al. 1987). These transfectants were not lysed by CTL directed against tum⁻ antigen P91B, confirming that P91A and P91B were independent antigens encoded by different genes.

Isolation of Cosmids Expressing Tum⁻ Antigens

We failed in our attempts to retrieve gene P91A from the transfectants on the basis of its linkage with the cotransfected *neo* gene. However, transfections performed with size-selected DNA indicated that genomic fragments smaller than 30 kb were capable of transfecting the expression of the antigen. We therefore decided to build and transfect a cosmid library because cosmids accept inserts up to 45 kb. We counted on identifying the P91A gene either by retrieving the transfected gene through the cosmidic sequences or by applying sibling selection to a positive subgroup of the cosmid library. The major problem associated with the transfection of a cosmid library is that it requires an enormous amplification: Each cosmid must be amplified 10^8 times to provide enough DNA for transfection. There is therefore a high risk of losing the representativity of the

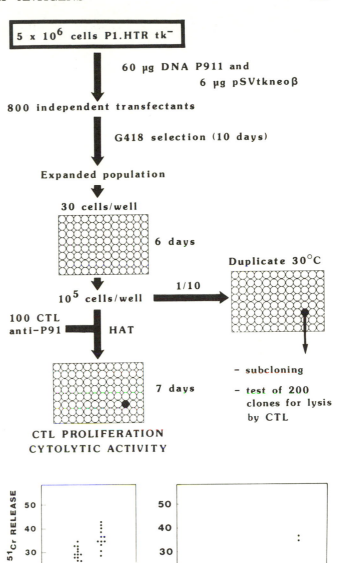

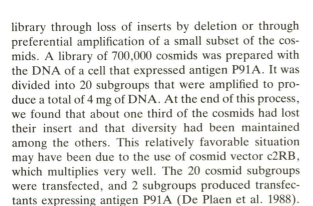

Figure 2. (*Top*) Outline of the transfection and detection procedures. (*Bottom left*) Control stimulation of an anti-P91A CTL clone with a population containing a minority of P91 cells. Microcultures contained 100 anti-P91A CTLs and no stimulating cells (*A*), 2000 P91 cells (*B*), 2000 P91 and 60,000 P1.HTR cells (*C*), or 60,000 P1.HTR cells (*D*). After 7 days, the lytic activity of the microcultures was tested against the appropriate tum⁻ variant. Each point represents the lytic activity of a single microculture. (*Bottom right*) Identification of microcultures containing antigen-expressing transfectants. For each of the three transfection groups shown here, 96 microcultures, each containing 30 geneticin-resistant transfectants, were allowed to multiply so as to reach 60,000 cells. One hundred anti-P91A CTLs were then added. One week later, the cytolytic activity of half the content of each microculture was assayed on 2000 chromium-labeled P91 cells for 4 hr. Each point represents the lytic activity of a single microculture. In group *3*, the two microcultures with a lytic activity exceeding 25% were subcloned and found to contain cells that were lysed by anti-P91A CTL.

library through loss of inserts by deletion or through preferential amplification of a small subset of the cosmids. A library of 700,000 cosmids was prepared with the DNA of a cell that expressed antigen P91A. It was divided into 20 subgroups that were amplified to produce a total of 4 mg of DNA. At the end of this process, we found that about one third of the cosmids had lost their insert and that diversity had been maintained among the others. This relatively favorable situation may have been due to the use of cosmid vector c2RB, which multiplies very well. The 20 cosmid subgroups were transfected, and 2 subgroups produced transfectants expressing antigen P91A (De Plaen et al. 1988).

For the isolation of the sequences expressing antigen P91A, we benefited from an observation of Lau and

Kan (1983), who demonstrated that a gene transfected in a cosmid can often be retrieved by simply packaging the DNA of the transfectant into bacteriophage λ components. This may be due to tandem integration of cosmids resulting in the positioning of the gene between two *cos* sites with proper orientation and distance. When we applied this to the DNA of our first cosmid transfectant, we obtained two different cosmid species. One of them proved capable of transferring at high frequency the expression of the antigen (De Plaen et al. 1988). Various restriction fragments of this cosmid were subcloned and transfected. We identified a 3.9-kb fragment that transferred the expression of the antigen. Surprisingly, when this fragment was subdivided further, we found that an 800-bp fragment was

Table 1. Frequencies of Transfection and Cosmid Rescue Obtained with Various Antigens

Antigen	Transfection with genomic DNA[a] (No. of transfectants expressing antigen/no. of drug-resistant transfectants)	Transfection with cosmid library (No. of independent cosmids transferring antigen/no. of independent cosmids in library)	Success rate for cosmid recovery by direct DNA packaging of transfectant DNA[b] (No. of independent transfectants from which a cosmid transferring expression of antigen was recovered/total no. of independent cosmid transfectants)
tum⁻			
P91A	7/90,000	2/700,000	1/3
P91B	1/26,000	0/1,200,000	
P35B	3/35,000	5/700,000	1/9
P35A	0/35,000	0/700,000	
P198	2/9,000	3/400,000	1/8
TSTA			
P1.A	3/30,000	1/2,100,000	2/2

[a]Genomic DNA was cotransfected with a plasmid conferring resistance to geneticin or hygromycin, as shown in Fig. 2.
[b]DNA of all the independent cosmid transfectants expressing the tum⁻ antigen was packaged in phage λ components. The number of these transfectants was often higher than that of the positive cosmids because several independent transfectants were obtained with the same group of cosmids. The cosmids resulting from direct packaging were tested by transfection.

still capable of transferring expression at high efficiency, even though it was suspected and later confirmed to contain only a small part of the gene. With this 800-bp fragment, which was devoid of repetitive sequences, it was possible to identify cosmids containing both alleles of the entire P91A gene, as well as cDNA clones of the homologous mRNA.

The procedure that led to the isolation of tum⁻ gene P91A was applied with success to the cloning of tum⁻ genes P35B and P198, which encode antigens expressed by other tum⁻ variants derived from P815 (J.-P. Szikora et al., unpubl.). Recently, we have been able to obtain cosmid transfectants for TSTA P1A present on

P815. This was achieved by using as transfection recipient a P1A⁻ antigen-loss variant selected from the P1.HTR line with an anti-P1A CTL clone (B. Van den Eynde and B. Lethé, unpubl.). Table 1 provides a survey of the frequencies of transfection and cosmid rescue obtained for the various antigens. As expected, the retrieval of the tum⁻ genes by direct packaging was not successful with every cosmid transfectant.

Tum⁻ Genes and Tum⁻ Mutations

Northern blots probed with the 800-bp fragment of gene P91A revealed a single mRNA species of 2.2 kb.

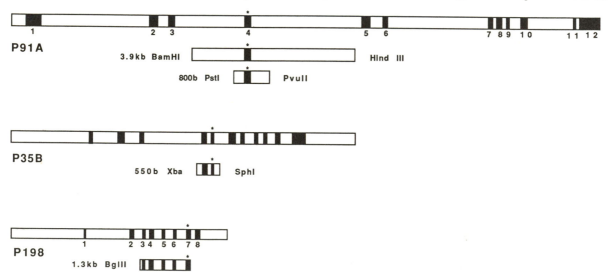

Figure 3. General structure of genes P91A, P35B, and P198 and subgenic fragments that transfer the expression of tum⁻ antigens. Solid regions represent exons. Those of gene P35B are not numbered because they may be additional 5′ exons that are not yet identified. (∗) The exon containing the tum⁻ mutation.

The band was of equal intensity for tum⁻ variant P91 and for P1, which does not express the antigen. The expression of antigen P91A is therefore not due to the activation of a silent gene.

The structure of gene P91A is shown in Figure 3. It comprises 12 exons spread over 14 kb (Lurquin et al. 1989). It does not show any similarity with immunoglobulin, T-cell receptor, or MHC genes. The complete sequence was obtained; it is unrelated to any sequence presently recorded in the main data banks.

Additional evidence for the role of this gene was provided by the study of three "escaping" tumors obtained with variant P91. These variants, which had lost the expression of gene P91A, all showed deletions in one allele of the gene (Lurquin et al. 1989).

A sequence comparison of the normal and tum⁻ alleles of gene P91A indicated that they differ by a point mutation in the exon, which is present in the transfecting 800-bp fragment (Fig. 4). This tum⁻ mutation is a G → A transition that changes an arginine into a histidine in the main open reading frame of the gene.

By site-directed mutagenesis performed on the 800-bp fragment derived from the normal allele, we confirmed that this mutation is indeed responsible for the expression of the antigen (De Plaen et al. 1988).

Southern blots of P1 and P91 DNAs were hybridized with probes corresponding to various regions of the genes. They always gave identical bands for both cells. Therefore, it appears that no gene rearrangement occurred in the transition between the normal and the tum⁻ allele (Lurquin et al. 1989).

The study of the tum⁻ alleles of genes P35B and P198 also revealed that they differ from the normal alleles by a point mutation in an exon (Fig. 4). The general structures and the sequences of the three tum⁻ genes isolated so far are completely unrelated (Fig. 3).

Antigenic Peptides

The main open reading frame of gene P91A encodes a protein of 60 kD, which does not have a typical amino-terminal signal sequence (Lurquin et al. 1989).

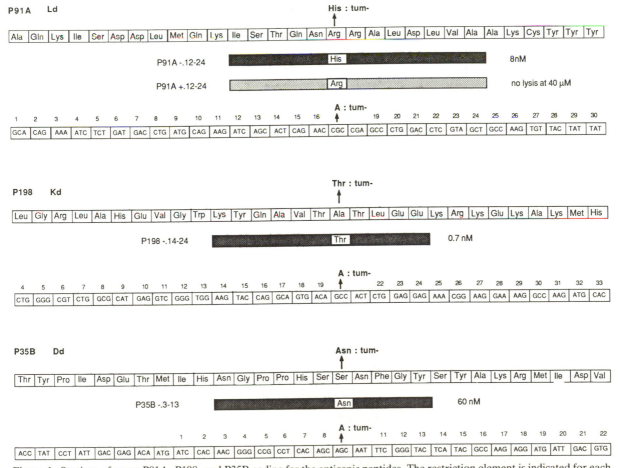

Figure 4. Sections of genes P91A, P198, and P35B coding for the antigenic peptides. The restriction element is indicated for each gene. Numbering of codons starts at the first codon of the relevant exon. The tum⁻ mutation and resulting amino acid change are indicated. Synthetic peptides corresponding to the mutant (P91A−.12-24) and normal (P91A + .12-24, etc.) sequences of the genes are indicated by boxes. They were tested for their ability to render P1.HTR cells susceptible to lysis by anti-tum⁻ CTLs. The concentration indicated to the right of each peptide provided 50% of the lysis obtained at saturating concentration of peptide.

In vitro translation was performed by incubating a rabbit reticulocyte extract with an mRNA produced by transcribing a quasi-full-length cDNA cloned in pSP65. A product of the expected size was produced. The addition of dog pancreas microsomes did not change the molecular weight, even though the sequence of P91A contains two potential N-glycosylation sites (D. Godelaine et al., unpubl.). Antigen P91A is therefore very unlikely to be borne by a membrane protein. However, this is hardly surprising, considering the recent demonstration that CTLs can recognize influenza antigens corresponding to endogenous proteins remaining inside the cell, because CTLs recognize small peptides that bind to surface class I MHC molecules (Townsend et al. 1985, 1986a,b). On the basis of this evidence, we examined whether we could also identify a small peptide that would trigger the lysis of P815 cells by anti-P91A CTLs. In our search for this peptide, we were guided by the location of the tum⁻ mutation. A short peptide (Fig. 4) corresponding to the mutant sequence induced the lysis of P1 by anti-P91A CTLs. Transfection and peptide studies with H-2^k fibroblasts, which also expressed K^d, D^d, or L^d, demonstrated that antigen P91A is associative with L^d. Antigenic peptides corresponding to the sequence surrounding the tum⁻ mutation were also obtained for genes P35B and P198 (Fig. 4). They associate with D^d and K^d, respectively.

Studies with P91A peptides enabled us to define the role of the tum⁻ mutation precisely. A priori, the mutation could influence either the production of the antigenic peptide or its ability to associate with the L^d molecule (i.e., the *antigen restriction tope*, or *agretope*) or the epitope presented to T cells by the peptide-MHC complex. Having the antigenic P91A peptide, we prepared the homologous peptide corresponding to the normal allele of the gene. This peptide did not induce lysis by anti-P91A CTLs nor did it compete with the tum⁻ peptide. Moreover, we found that the tum⁻ peptide competed effectively to prevent a cytomegalovirus-derived peptide from inducing lysis by CTLs directed against an L^d-associative cytomegalovirus antigen. The tum⁺ P91A peptide did not compete (Lurquin et al. 1989). This indicates that the P91A tum⁻ mutation generates the agretope of the antigen but does not exclude that it also influences the epitope of the peptide.

Expression of Tum⁻ Antigens by Promoterless Subgenic Fragments

In the course of cloning gene P91A, we made the surprising observation that expression of the tum⁻ antigen was obtained by transfecting an 800-bp restriction fragment, which comprised only the mutated exon 4 and parts of the surrounding introns (Fig. 3). Similar results were obtained with other restriction fragments ranging from 3.9 kb to 175 bp, which contained the whole or part of exon 4. Subgenic fragments of the P198 and the P35B genes also transfected the expression of the tum⁻ antigens (Fig. 3). In all of these experiments, we transfected these fragments cloned in M13 or pUC vectors, which are not expression vectors. This DNA was cotransfected with selective plasmid pSVtk-neoβ, and the neo^r transfectant population was either tested directly for chromium lysis with anti-tum⁻ CTL or it was subcloned and the clones tested individually for sensitivity to the CTL. When both tests were performed on the same population, they showed good agreement.

We were able to rule out that expression by promoterless subgenic fragments required homologous recombination of the transfected exon with the resident genes. First, we identified a transfectant that had integrated a single copy of the transfected P91A exon in a location that was clearly outside the resident gene, as indicated by a supplementary band on the Southern blot. We then submitted this transfectant to CTL selection and obtained an antigen-loss variant. It had lost the extra band. This demonstrated that the antigen was produced by the exon integrated outside the homologous resident genes in the original transfectant.

Next, we determined that transfected subgenic fragments express the antigen with good efficiency. By transfecting a low amount of the P91A 800-bp fragment, we obtained seven transfectants that had integrated one copy and one that had integrated two copies. For three of these transfectants, we could detect a significant amount of lysis by anti-P91A CTL. The same conclusion was reached by a different approach. We cloned the entire P91A gene, as well as the gene amputated from the promoter and the three first exons in a λ vector. When the neo^r populations transfected with these two constructs were analyzed in a chromium release assay, they showed almost equal sensitivity to anti-P91A CTL (Table 2). We conclude that each transfected subgenic fragment has at least a 25% chance to produce a measurable amount of antigen.

How can transfected subgenic fragments express tum⁻ antigens efficiently? One explanation could be that these fragments often integrate in the middle of an active gene, leading to the synthesis of a composite mRNA, followed by the splicing of exon 4 to a preceding exon and the production of a chimeric protein. The degradation of this protein would produce the appropriate peptide. However, it is difficult to conceive how

Table 2. Transfection of Entire or Truncated P91A Gene

Effector to target ratio	Specific lysis with anti P91A CTL (%)		
	no insert	gene P91A	gene P91A − exons 1,2,3
3:1	3	49	33
1:1	0	28	24
0.3:1	0	12	15
0.1:1	0	3	5
0.03:1	0	1	2

P1.HTR cells were cotransfected with DNA of pSVtk-neoβ and λ EMBL3A containing either no insert, the entire P91A gene, or the gene from which the promoter region and the first three exons had been removed. The population of neo^r transfectants was tested for lysis by an anti-P91A CTL clone in a chromium release assay.

this could ensure the expression of the antigen by more than a very small proportion of the fragments, considering the relatively small part (~1%) of the genome thought to be occupied by active genes, unless transfected DNA integrates preferentially in active regions of the genome or unless one considers that the promoter of the cotransfected *neo* gene can direct the synthesis of a composite mRNA that includes the transfected exon. It is well known that cotransfected genes are usually strongly linked (Perucho et al. 1980); however, in the case of the *neo* gene, this would involve an abnormal splicing event bypassing an exon present on the plasmid. In addition, the ribosome would encounter a stop signal near the end of the *neo* exon and would have to reinitiate at a downstream start codon, a process that does not occur efficiently in eukaryotes (Kozak 1989). Another possible explanation is that a transcript covering the mutated exon initiates at a "cryptic promoter" site in the prokaryotic DNA of the vector that carries the fragment. However, there are difficulties here, too, because for long fragments such as the 3.9-kb P91A fragment (Fig. 3), the ribosome would have to go through an intronic region replete with stop and start codons, before it could reach a start codon leading to the synthesis of the region covering the antigenic peptide.

Because of the difficulty of explaining our phenomenon with the mechanisms just described, we ex-

plored an alternative hypothesis, namely, that the transcription and translation that produce the antigenic peptide are both initiated in the region covered by the subgenic fragment. As a first step, we examined whether translational starts located in the 800-bp P91A fragment were used to produce the antigen. The results of a number of site-directed mutagenesis experiments carried out on this fragment are summarized in Figure 5. As expected, the expression of the antigen was abolished by the transformation into a stop codon (TAG) of codon 10 of exon 4 (Fig. 4), a codon located immediately before the sequence encoding the antigenic peptide (Fig. 5). However, the transformation of codon 2 of exon 4 into a stop (TAG) codon preserved most of the expression. When the ATG in position 9 was transformed into an ATC in addition to this stop, expression was completely suppressed. This suggested that the ATG in position 9 serves as start codon for a significant fraction of the antigen. However, it is not the only start codon used to produce the antigen, because when no stop codon was introduced upstream, its transformation into an ATC did not abolish antigenicity. Another important start codon appears to be located at the end of intron 3, because antigenicity was completely suppressed when we introduced a stop codon 20 nucleotides before the beginning of exon 4 (Fig. 5), in addition to inactivating the ATG in position 9. These experiments, however, must be interpreted

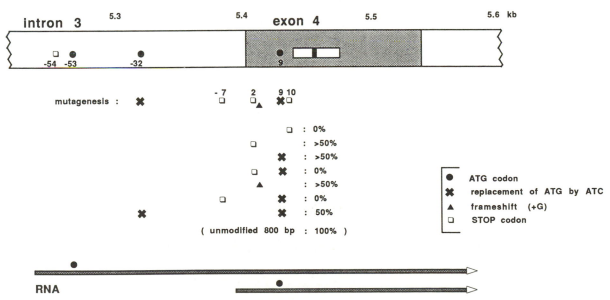

Figure 5. (*Top*) Exon 4 of gene P91A and part of the preceding intron. The start codon in position 9 of exon 4 is indicated, as well as two start codons in the same reading frame at the end of intron 3 (the numbering indicates the distance in codons moving back from the first position of exon 4). The stop codon in location −54 is the last stop codon of intron 3 in that reading frame. The white box in exon 4 indicates the location of the antigenic peptide. (*Center*) Changes introduced in the 800-bp fragment of gene P91A by site-directed mutagenesis are indicated, with their effect on the antigenicity of the transfectants. The values are rough approximations drawn from several experiments. They represent the lysis of the transfectants by anti-P91A CTLs as a percentage of that observed after transfection of the intact 800-bp fragment. The frameshift involved the addition of a G between codons 3 and 4 of exon 4. (*Bottom*) Two hypothetical RNA species compatible with the results.

with some caution because we do not know the exact relation between the amount of synthesis of the protein comprising the antigenic peptide region and the amount of lysis by CTLs observed on the transfectants. Nevertheless, these results strongly suggest that in the 800-bp fragment, there are two start codons involved in the protein synthesis that eventually leads to the antigenic peptide: one at the end of intron 3 and one at the beginning of exon 4. The use of a start codon in intron 3 is incompatible with an exclusive role for the hypothesis described previously that involves the splicing of exon 4 to a preceding exon, but a combination of the splicing and cryptic promoter hypotheses cannot be completely excluded. On the other hand, the use of these two start codons could be explained easily if two species of local messenger, such as those shown in Figure 5, were used for the production of antigenic peptide.

If transfected subgenic fragments are expressed through a local transcription process, it is conceivable that this may reflect a process that also occurs in intact genes for the production of antigenic peptides (Boon and Van Pel 1989). Subgenic regions, which we named "peptons," because they eventually produce peptides, could be transcribed into local messengers (Fig. 6). These "p-RNAs" would be initiated a short distance upstream of the region coding for the antigenic peptides. How long they should extend downstream from this region is not clear.

As a first test of this pepton hypothesis, we inactivated some start codons and introduced various stop codons or frameshifts on the entire P91A gene cloned in a λ vector. The antigenicity of cells transfected with these constructs was examined. We found that the ATG located at the beginning of exon 4 functions as a start codon for the production of a minor, but significant, fraction of the antigen in cells transfected with the entire P91A gene. Moreover, the introduction of a frameshift very near the 3' end of exon 3, combined with the inactivation of the ATG of exon 4, preserved a significant amount of antigenicity on the transfectants. This strongly suggests that similar to the 800-bp fragment, a start codon located at the end of intron 3 plays a significant role in the production of antigenic peptide by the intact gene. Finally, the transformation of the first ATG codon of the long open reading frame of gene P91A into ATC had no significant effect on the antigenicity of the transfectants.

CONCLUSIONS

The demonstration of the recognition of MHC-bound peptides by T-cell receptors clearly constitutes a major breakthrough in our understanding of T-cell immunology (Shimonkevitz et al. 1983, 1984; Allen et al. 1984; Babbitt et al. 1985; Buus et al. 1986, 1987). The extension of these results to the recognition of antigens by CTLs, first achieved for influenza antigens and later

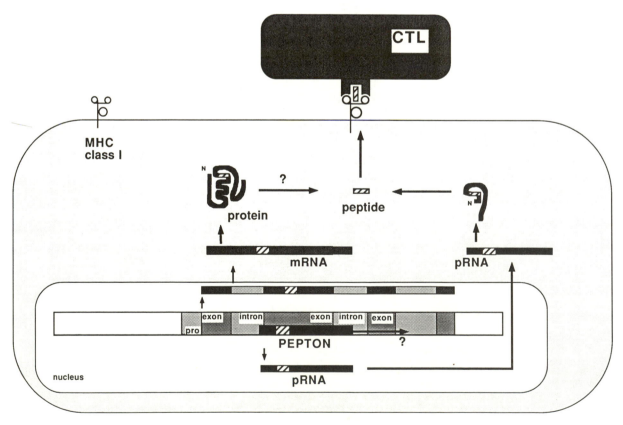

Figure 6. Pepton hypothesis.

confirmed in other systems (Townsend et al. 1986a; Maryanski et al. 1988), proved of considerable help in our understanding of tum⁻ antigens.

Our data provide an explanation for the high frequency, stability, and diversity of tum⁻ variants. They result from mutations in unrelated genes, and it is likely that such mutations can occur in most, if not all, genes to produce new antigenic peptides and thereby new transplantation antigens. It therefore appears that T-cell receptors, MHC molecules, and peptide-producing processes constitute a rather elaborate immunosurveillance mechanism capable of monitoring the integrity of our genome.

The ability of promoterless subgenic fragments to express tum⁻ antigens in transfectants proved of great use in locating rapidly the region of the gene that codes for the antigenic peptide. It remains a puzzling observation that we find difficult to explain in classic terms; hence, the pepton hypothesis. More pertinent data are clearly needed before we can assess the value of this hypothesis, and many aspects remain undefined, but its essential feature clearly resides in the possibility of producing antigenic peptides independently of the expression of the normal products of the genes. It is worth noting that this offers two interesting possibilities regarding immunosurveillance. A problem with immunosurveillance is how to avoid having the MHC molecules occupied predominantly by a few peptide species derived from a few proteins that are synthesized by the cell in very large amounts. Peptons might provide a solution by ensuring a basal level of peptide production that would be roughly equal for all genes because it would not depend on the activity of the classic promoter of the genes. Another possibility regards tolerance. The expression of peptons in thymic cells could enable these cells to present to the T lymphocytes the whole self repertoire of antigenic peptide without the need—and the consequence—of expressing all of the genes that are active in the various types of differentiated cells.

The method that ensured the cloning of the genes coding for tum⁻ antigens should, in principle, be applicable to other transplantation antigens, notably, TSTAs and minor histocompatibility antigens. On the basis of our results, it is tempting to believe that like tum⁻ antigens, TSTAs arise by a mutational mechanism acting throughout the whole genome. This would explain their high diversity (Prehn 1975). For tumors induced with chemical carcinogens, it was proposed that concomitantly to the mutation that affects an oncogene, another mutation occurring in a completely unrelated gene creates a TSTA (Boon 1983). It is also conceivable that as cells age, they undergo a number of mutations that generate new antigenic peptides. As long as the clonal progeny of each cell remains small, as would be expected for normal tissues, the chance of an encounter with the relevant T cell could remain extremely low. If one of these cells becomes malignant, these antigens could become targets for the immune system.

REFERENCES

Allen, P.M., D. Strydom, and E.R. Unanue. 1984. Processing of lysozyme by macrophage: Identification of the determinant recognized by two T cell hybridomas. *Proc. Natl. Acad. Sci.* **81:** 2489.

Babbitt, B., P. Allen, G. Matsueda, E. Haber, and E.R. Unanue. 1985. Binding of immunogenic peptides to Ia histocompatibility molecules. *Nature* **317:** 359.

Boon, T. 1983. Antigenic tumor cell variants obtained with mutagens. *Adv. Cancer Res.* **39:** 121.

Boon, T. and O. Kellermann. 1977. Rejection by syngeneic mice of cell variants obtained by mutagenesis of a malignant teratocarcinoma cell line. *Proc. Natl. Acad. Sci.* **74:** 272.

Boon, T. and A. Van Pel. 1978. Teratocarcinoma cell variants rejected by syngeneic mice: Production of mice immunized with these variants against other variants and against the original malignant cell line. *Proc. Natl. Acad. Sci.* **75:** 1519.

———. 1989. T cell-recognized antigenic peptides derived from the cellular genome are not protein degradation products but can be generated directly by transcription and translation of short subgenic regions. A hypothesis. *Immunogenetics* **29:** 75.

Boon, T., J. Van Snick, A. Van Pel, C. Uyttenhove, and M. Marchand. 1980. Immunogenic variants obtained by mutagenesis of mouse mastocytoma P815. II. T Lymphocyte-mediated cytolysis. *J. Exp. Med.* **152:** 1184.

Buus, S., A. Sette, S. Colon, D. Jenis, and H. Grey. 1986. Isolation and characterization of antigen-Ia complexes involved in T cell recognition. *Cell* **47:** 1071.

Buus, S., A. Sette, S. Colon, C. Miles, and H.M. Grey. 1987. The relation between major histocompatibility complex (MHC) restriction and the capacity of Ia to bind immunogenic peptides. *Science* **235:** 1353.

Contessa, A., A. Bonmassar, A. Giampietri, A. Circolo, A. Goldin, and M. Fioretti. 1981. In vitro generation of a highly immunogenic subline of L1210 leukemia following exposure to 5-(3,3′-dimethyl-1-triazeno) imidazole-4-carboxamide. *Cancer Res.* **41:** 2476.

De Plaen, E., C. Lurquin, A. Van Pel, B. Mariamé, J.-P. Szikora, T. Wölfel, C. Sibille, P. Chomez, and T. Boon. 1988. Immunogenic (tum⁻) variants of mouse tumor P815: Cloning of the gene of tum⁻ antigen P91A and identification of the tum⁻ mutation. *Proc. Natl. Acad. Sci.* **85:** 2274.

Frost, P., R. Kerbel, E. Bauer, R. Tartamella-Biondo, and W. Cefalu. 1983. Mutagen treatments as a means for selecting immunogenic variants from otherwise poorly immunogenic malignant murine tumors. *Cancer Res.* **43:** 125.

Goethals, A., P. Courtoy, C. Lurquin, A. Van Pel, E. De Plaen, T. Boon, and P. Baudhuin. 1987. The efficiency of transfection of mammalian cells is directly related to endocytosis of DNA. *Arch. Int. Physiol. Biochim.* **95:** B202.

Kavathas, P. and L.A. Herzenberg. 1983. Stable transformation of mouse L cells for human membrane T-cell differentiation antigens, HLA and β-microglobulin: Selection by fluorescence-activated cell sorting. *Proc. Natl. Acad. Sci.* **80:** 524.

Kozak, M. 1989. The scanning model for translation: An update. *J. Cell Biol.* **108:** 229.

Lau, Y.-F. and Y.W. Kan. 1983. Versatile cosmid vectors for the isolation, expression and rescue of gene sequences: Studies with the human alpha-globin gene cluster. *Proc. Natl. Acad. Sci.* **80:** 5225.

Lurquin, C., A. Van Pel, B. Mariamé, E. De Plaen, J.P. Szikora, C. Janssens, J. Lejeune, M.J. Reddehase, and T. Boon. 1989. Structure of the gene coding for tum⁻ antigen P91A. A peptide encoded by the mutated exon is recognized with Lᵈ by cytolytic T cells. *Cell* **58:** 293.

Maryanski, J.L. and T. Boon. 1982. Immunogenic variants obtained by mutagenesis of mouse mastocytoma P815. IV. Analysis of variant-specific antigens by selection of antigen-loss variants with cytolytic T cell clones. *Eur. J. Immunol.* **12:** 406.

Maryanski, J.L., M. Marchand, C. Uyttenhove, and T. Boon. 1983a. Immunogenic variants obtained by mutagenesis of mouse mastocytoma P815. VI. Occasional escape from host rejection due to antigen-loss secondary variants. *Int. J. Cancer* **31:** 119.

Maryanski, J.L., P. Pala, J.-C. Cerottini, and G. Corradin. 1988. Synthetic peptides as antigens and competitors in recognition by H-2-restricted cytolytic T cells specific for HLA. *J. Exp. Med.* **167:** 1391.

Maryanski, J.L., J. Szpirer, C. Szpirer, and T. Boon. 1983b. Immunogenic variants obtained by mutagenesis of mouse mastocytoma P815. Dominant expression of variant antigens in somatic cell hybrids. *Somatic Cell Genet.* **9:** 345.

Maryanski, J.L., J. Van Snick, J.-C. Cerottini, and T. Boon. 1982. Immunogenic variants obtained by mutagenesis of mouse mastocytoma P815. III. Clonal analysis of the syngeneic cytolytic T lymphocyte response. *Eur. J. Immunol.* **12:** 401.

Perucho, M., D. Hanahan, and M. Wigler. 1980. Genetic and physical linkage of exogenous sequences in transformed cells. *Cell* **22:** 309.

Ploegh, H., H. Orr, and J. Strominger. 1980. Molecular cloning of a human histocompatibility antigen cDNA fragment. *Proc. Natl. Acad. Sci.* **77:** 6081.

Prehn, R.T. 1975. Relationship of tumor immunogenicity to concentration of the oncogene. *J. Nat. Cancer Inst.* **55:** 189.

Shimonkevitz, R., J. Kappler, P. Marrack, and H.M. Grey. 1983. Antigen recognition by H-2 restricted T cells. I. Cell-free antigen processing. *J. Exp. Med.* **158:** 303.

Shimonkevitz, R., S. Colon, J. Kappler, P. Marrack, and H.M. Grey. 1984. Antigen recognition by H-2 restricted T cells. A tryptic ovalbumin peptide that substitute for processed antigen. *J. Immunol.* **133:** 2067.

Townsend, A.R.M., F.M. Gotch, and J. Davey. 1985. Cytotoxic T cells recognize fragments of the influenza nucleoprotein. *Cell* **42:** 457.

Townsend, A.R.M., J. Bastin, K. Gould, and G.G. Brownlee. 1986a. Cytotoxic T lymphocytes recognize influenza haemagglutinin that lacks a signal sequence. *Nature* **324:** 575.

Townsend, A.R.M., J. Rothbard, F.M. Gotch, G. Bahadur, D. Wraith, and A.J. McMichael. 1986b. The epitopes of influenza nucleoprotein recognized by cytotoxic T lymphocytes can be defined with short synthetic peptides. *Cell* **44:** 959.

Uyttenhove, C., J. Maryanski, and T. Boon. 1983. Escape of mouse mastocytoma P815 after nearly complete rejection is due to antigen-loss variants rather than immunosuppression. *J. Exp. Med.* **157:** 1040.

Uyttenhove, C., J. Van Snick, and T. Boon. 1980. Immunogenic variants obtained by mutagenesis of mouse mastocytoma P815. I. Rejection by syngeneic mice. *J. Exp. Med.* **152:** 1175.

Van Pel, A., E. De Plaen, and T. Boon. 1985. Selection of highly transfectable variant from mouse mastocytoma P815. *Somat. Cell Mol. Genet.* **11:** 467.

Wölfel, T., A. Van Pel, E. De Plaen, C. Lurquin, J.L. Maryanski, and T. Boon. 1987. Immunogenic (tum⁻) variants obtained by mutagenesis of mouse mastocytoma P815. VIII. Detection of stable transfectants expressing a tum⁻ antigen with a cytolytic T cell stimulation assay. *Immunogenetics* **26:** 178.

Zbar, B., S. Sukumar, Y. Tanio, N. Terata, and J. Hovis. 1984. Antigenic variants isolated from a mutagen-treated guinea pig fibrosarcoma. *Cancer Res.* **44:** 5079.

Zinkernagel, R.M. and P.C. Doherty. 1974. Restriction of in vitro T cell mediated cytotoxicity in lymphocytic choriomeningitis within a syngeneic or semiallogeneic system. *Nature* **248:** 701.

Immunosurveillance of Virus-induced Tumors

C.J.M. Melief,* W.L.E. Vasmel,* R. Offringa,† E.J.A.M. Sijts,* E.A. Matthews,*
P.J. Peters,‡ R.H. Meloen,§ A.J. van der Eb,† and W.M. Kast*
*Division of Immunology, The Netherlands Cancer Institute, Antoni van Leeuwenhoek Huis, 1066 CX Amsterdam;
†Sylvius Laboratory, University of Leiden, Leiden; ‡Laboratory of Cell Biology, Center for Electron Microscopy,
University of Utrecht, Utrecht; §Central Veterinary Institute, Lelystad, The Netherlands

T-cell immunity is of paramount importance in the defense against viruses and virus-induced tumors (Klein 1973; Zinkernagel and Doherty 1979; Doherty 1985; Kast et al. 1986; Zijlstra and Melief 1986). Virus-induced tumors can evade T-cell immunity by down-regulation of class I major histocompatibility complex (MHC) expression (Bernards et al. 1983; Schrier et al. 1983; Hui et al. 1984) or by failure to express viral antigens (Green 1983; van der Hoorn et al. 1985; Vasmel et al. 1989). The relevance of class I MHC down-regulation in evasion of T-cell immunity by adenovirus type 12 (Ad12) early region 1 (E1)-induced tumors (Bernards et al. 1983; Schrier et al. 1983) is supported by our recent demonstration of eradication of large Ad5 E1-induced tumors, without down-regulated class I MHC expression, by cloned E1-specific cytotoxic T lymphocytes (CTL) (Kast et al. 1989). In this paper, we review the evidence from our laboratory for the remarkable efficiency of tumor eradication by CTL and the importance of class I down-regulation in evasion of this form of immunity. This work deals with human adenovirus-induced tumors in mice. As a second major mechanism of evasion of T-cell immunity by virus-induced tumors, we have observed failure to express viral antigens despite presence of viral genomes in murine leukemia virus (MLV)-induced primary lymphomas. If evasion of T-cell immunity by virus-induced tumors by these mechanisms is bad news, this is counterbalanced by the rarity of such escapes and by the fact that relatively small numbers of T cells can eradicate very large established tumors when given in combination with recombinant interleukin-2 (rIL-2).

METHODS AND EXPERIMENTAL PROCEDURES

All methods and procedures are described by Kast et al. (1989) and Vasmel et al. (1989).

Oncogenicity of Rodent Cells Transformed by E1 of Human Adenoviruses

Human adenoviruses use at least two genes to achieve the fully transformed state in infected rodent cells or in cells transfected with the crucial left 10% of the viral genome, representing the E1 region (Bernards and van der Eb 1984; Branton et al. 1985; van der Eb and Oostra 1985). This situation resembles the coope-ration between the cellular oncogenes myc and ras in cell transformation (Land et al. 1983; Murray et al. 1983; Ruley 1983). Moreover, one of the crucial E1 genes of adenoviruses, the E1A gene, shows functional similarity to the c-myc gene (Bernards and van der Eb 1984; Kingston et al. 1984). Recently, it was shown that the adenovirus E1A proteins bind to the retinoblastoma (Rb) gene product, providing evidence for a physical link between an oncogene (E1A) and an anti-oncogene (Rb gene). Possibly the E1A products inactivate the Rb protein (Whyte et al. 1988). SV40 large T antigen contains a region with structural similarity to conserved domain 2 of adenovirus E1A. This region likewise interacts with the Rb gene product (DeCaprio et al. 1988) and can substitute for the transforming domain of the Ad E1A product (Moran 1988). Furthermore, the human papillomavirus (HPV) type 16 E7 gene encodes regions homologous to the conserved regions 1 and 2 of Ad E1A, which have been shown to be essential for transformation (Phelps et al. 1988). Several HPV types, including type 16, have been implicated in precancerous cervical lesions as well as in carcinoma in situ and invasive cervical carcinoma in women (zur Hausen and Schneider 1987). Human adenoviruses, in contrast, have so far not been implicated in the causation of cancer in human beings. Nonetheless, their structural and functional similarity with other human DNA viruses, some of which are implicated in human cancer, as well as their transforming ability in rodents and the availability of oncogenic and nononcogenic serotypes, makes adenovirus-induced oncogenesis in rodents an attractive cancer research model.

Oncogenesis by E1 and Tumor Immunity

The availability of oncogenic (Ad12) and nononcogenic (Ad2, Ad5) serotypes of adenoviruses and the involvement of both E1A and E1B genes in cell immortalization, transformation, and oncogenesis has allowed the use of genetic recombinants between oncogenic and nononcogenic viral genomes to identify regions crucial for these functions (for review, see Bernards and van der Eb 1984; van der Eb et al. 1984; Branton et la. 1985; van der Eb and Oostra 1985). Although the E1B region of Ad12 contributes more strongly to the oncogenic state in nude mice than the

E1B region of Ad5 (Schrier et al. 1983), the E1A region of Ad12, as opposed to the E1A region of Ad5, probably also contributes strongly to the oncogenic potential in immunocompetent animals by suppressing class I MHC gene expression. The mechanism of this is probably evasion of class I MHC-restricted T-cell immunity, notably evasion of destruction by tumor-directed CTL. This is supported by the fact that cells expressing Ad12 E1A are less susceptible to allospecific CTL than those expressing Ad5 E1A (Bernards et al. 1983; van der Eb et al. 1984; Sawada et al. 1985); by the fact that transfection of an H-2 class I gene into Ad12-transformed cells, associated with high expression of the newly introduced gene, led to loss of oncogenicity (Tanaka et al. 1985); and by our observation that Ad5 E1A-specific CTL are extremely efficient in the eradication of Ad5 E1-induced tumors in T-cell deficient nude mice (see below). Admittedly, all of these arguments are indirect or, especially in the case of the class I MHC gene transfection experiment, can also be explained in terms of different sensitivity to natural killer (NK) cells based on the difference in MHC expression. The literature on the relationship of NK sensitivity and MHC expression shows contrasting effects. With various tumor lines unrelated to adenovirus transformation, an inverse relationship between class I MHC expression and NK susceptibility was observed (Ljunggren and Kärre 1985; Piontek et al. 1985; Harel-Bellan et al. 1986; Kärre et al. 1986; Storkus et al. 1987; Ljunggren et al. 1988). In contrast, however, in adenovirus-transformed cells, low MHC expression was associated with low NK susceptibility (Sawada et al. 1985; Kenyon and Raska 1986; Cook and Lewis 1987; Cook et al. 1987; Kast et al. 1989). These findings can be reconciled by assuming that the relationship between NK susceptibility and class I MHC expression is indirect. Whereas gamma interferon (IFN-γ) is known to up-regulate class I MHC expression and simultaneously to down-regulate NK susceptibility, Ad12 E1A down-regulates class I MHC expression but does not alter the low NK susceptibility of control normal mouse embryo cells (Kast et al. 1989). Neither IFN-γ and Ad E1A, nor the mutagenesis and selection used in the tumor systems in which the relationship NK susceptibility/class I MHC expression was first observed, are limited in their effects to class I MHC expression only. An argument in favor of a direct relationship is the reduced NK sensitivity of Daudi cells following transfection with the β2M gene, restoring HLA class I expression in these cells (Quillet et al. 1988). To further investigate this issue, small cell lung carcinoma (SCLC) cells lacking class I MHC expression and showing marked susceptibility to NK lysis were rendered positive for HLA class I antigens by two methods: treatment with IFN-γ or transfection with HLA class I genes. Although both methods resulted in increased levels of class I antigens, only the interferon-treated cells showed reduced susceptibility to NK lysis. NK lysis of cells positive for class I MHC as a result of transfection remained unaffected (Stam et al. 1989). In

another recent report, susceptibility to NK lysis was also independent of target cell HLA class I expression (Leiden et al. 1989). These contrasting findings can only be understood by assuming that the relationship between NK susceptibility and class I MHC expression is indirect or, alternatively, only holds for certain tumor systems and/or certain class I MHC alleles.

The evidence generated so far in our own studies (see below) favors the idea that different susceptibility to CTL lysis of Ad5 and Ad12 E1-transformed cells on the basis of down-regulated class I MHC expression on Ad12-transformed cells is a more likely explanation for the difference in oncogenicity between these cells than differential susceptibility to NK lysis. Although Ad5 E1A-transformed cells show much higher susceptibility to NK lysis than Ad12 E1A-transformed cells, they showed comparable tumorigenicity in T-cell-deficient nude mice that have high levels of NK activity (Clark et al. 1981; Kast et al. 1986; and see below). This confirms observations made in rats (Bernards et al. 1983; Schrier et al. 1983).

The down-regulation of class I MHC expression by Ad12 E1 is relative rather than absolute (Bernards et al. 1983; van der Eb et al. 1984; Sawada et al. 1985), is a function of the first exon of Ad12 E1A, and can be reversed by Ad5 E1A (van der Eb et al. 1984) or treatment with IFN-γ (Eager et al. 1985; 1989; Hayashi et al. 1985). Recent evidence suggests that the reduction in MHC expression is at least in part due to a decreased rate of initiation of transcription of class I MHC genes (Ackrill and Blair 1988; Friedman and Ricciardi 1988; A.J. van der Eb et al., unpubl.).

Generation and Specificity of Ad E1-specific CTL in H-2^b Mice

We explored the hypothesis that down-regulation of class I MHC expression is an important mechanism whereby Ad E1-transformed cells can evade destruction by class I MHC-restricted CTL. To this end, we first investigated the importance of Ad E1-specific CTL in a situation in which such a CTL response is most likely to occur, namely, following immunization with Ad5 E1-transformed cells in immunocompetent mice. C57BL/6 (B6, H-2K^{b}D^b) mice were immunized with syngeneic embryo cells, transformed by transfection with the Ad5 E1 region. After repeated stimulation of T cells from the spleen of immunized mice in bulk culture, several lines of Ad5 E1-specific CD8$^+$ CTL clones were expanded in the presence of Ad5-specific stimulator cells and rIL-2. These CTL clones were obtained by limiting dilution in the presence of irradiated specific stimulator cells, rIL-2, and irradiated syngeneic spleen cells as "feeder cells." All clones, like secondary Ad5-specific bulk CTL, were specific for the Ad5 E1A region, because Ad5 E1A/Ad12 E1B, but not Ad12 E1A/Ad5 E1B-transfected target cells, both of B6 origin, were specifically lysed. (In the case of Ad12 E1A/Ad5 E1B targets, IFN-γ treated targets were used to up-regulate class I MHC expression

[Table 1] [Kast et al. 1989].) All clones, like secondary Ad5-specific bulk CTL, were restricted by the H-2D^b molecule as established by cytotoxicity against B10.A(5R) (K^{b}D^d) and B10.A(4R) (K^{k}D^b) target cells transfected with Ad5 E1A/Ad5 E1B. Of these cells, only the B10.A(4R) H-2 recombinant cells were specifically lysed (Table 1) (Kast et al. 1989). That D^b is the restriction element was confirmed by the observation that Ad5 E1-transformed cells of the bm13 and bm14 D^b mutants were lysed poorly or not at all, respectively, by B6 Ad5-specific CTL. These findings suggested that Ad5-specific CTL raised in H-2^b mice recognize one or a limited number of immunodominant E1A epitopes in the context of the D^b class I MHC molecule. This was proven by peptide analysis (see below).

Eradication of Ad E1-induced Tumors by E1A-specific CTL

CTL clone 5 (CTL 5) grew particularly well, showed monoclonal T-cell receptor β rearrangement, and was used for immunotherapy to establish the in vivo potency of these CTL cells. After i.v. injection into B6 nude mice, Ad5-specific CTL 5 (10^7 cells) caused complete regression within 12 days of s.c. Ad5 tumor masses up to 10 cm^3 of B6 origin, provided 10^5 units of rIL-2 were given simultaneously as a depot in incomplete Freund's adjuvant at a s.c. site distant from the tumor (Kast et al. 1989). Treatment with rIL-2 alone had no effect on these tumors. Ad12 E1A/12 E1B tumors, the recombi-

nant 12 E1A/5 1B tumors, and Ad5 tumors of BALB/c origin did not go into regression after treatment with Ad5-specific CTL plus rIL-2, but the recombinant tumor 5 E1A/12 E1B of B6 origin completely disappeared after treatment, showing that the in vivo specificity of tumor rejection was the same as that of the in vitro CTL activity (Ad5 E1A-specific, H-2D^b-restricted) (Table 1).

Next, we evaluated the possibility of bystander killing of an MHC disparate tumor by CTL activated in the same animal by the specifically recognized tumor. Conceivably, the specific CTL, once activated, might nonspecifically kill MHC (or antigen) disparate tumors. However, injection of the appropriate tumor (B6, H-2^b, Ad5 E1A/Ad5 E1B) recognized by CTL 5 and of a second tumor (BALB/c, H-2^d, Ad5 E1A/Ad5 E1B) not recognized by these CTL at two different sites in the same animal, followed by therapy with CTL 5 and rIL-2, led to regression of only the tumor recognized by CTL 5, excluding nonspecific bystander killing of tumor cells by in vivo activated CTL (Kast et al. 1989).

Specific Immunologic "Memory"

After complete cure of nude mice carrying B6 Ad5 tumors with CTL 5, the animals were given a second Ad5 tumor s.c. Such an Ad5 tumor grew exponentially as in previously untreated mice, unless rIL-2 was given simultaneously, in which case tumor outgrowth was completely and permanently prevented. In control previously untreated mice, rIL-2 had no effect, and all

Table 1. Lytic Activity In Vitro and Tumor Eradication In Vivo Mediated by Ad5 E1-specific CTL Clone 5

Target/tumor cells[a]	Activity of CTL clone 5	
	lysis in vitro[b]	tumor eradication in vivo[c]
B6 (5 E1A/5 E1B) (K^b, D^b)	+	+
B6 (12 E1A/12 E1B) (K^b, D^b)	−	−
B6 (12 E1A/5 E1B) (K^b, D^b)	−	−
B6 (5 E1A/12 E1B) (K^b, D^b)	+	+
B6 (−/−) (K^b, D^b)	−	nontumorigenic
4R (5 E1A/5 E1B) (K^k, D^b)	+	+
5R (5 E1A/5 E1B) (K^b, D^d)	−	−
BALB/c (5 E1A/5 E1B) (K^d, D^d)	−	−

Summarized from Kast et al. (1989).
[a] Mouse embryo cells of H-2 haplotypes as indicated transfected with Ad5 E1A/Ad5 E1B, Ad12 E1A/Ad12 E1B, or recombinant E1 regions as indicated and control nontransfected (−/−) cells.
[b] Measured by ^{51}Cr release at effector/target ratios of 20:1 to 1.25:1.
[c] Measured by rejection of established tumors in B6 (nu/nu) mice after i.v. injection of 1×10^7 to 2×10^7 to cloned CTL and s.c. implantation of 5×10^5 units of rIL-2 in incomplete Freund's adjuvant plus 0.5% BSA.

animals eventually died with progressive tumors (Kast et al. 1989). This finding suggested the existence of CTL clone "memory" up to 3 months after the first tumor was successfully treated. Further experiments showed that in the treated mice at this time, following stimulation of spleen cells by specific stimulator cells and rIL-2, CTL are demonstrable with the same clonal T-cell receptor β rearrangement as in the originally injected CTL 5 (Kast et al. 1989).

We confirmed that Ad5 E1-transformed cells, in contrast to Ad12 E1-transformed cells, are markedly susceptible to lysis by NK cells in vitro, in agreement with the literature (Kast et al. 1989). The nude mice in which the in vivo experiments were carried out have high levels of NK activity. It is therefore unlikely that NK cells are highly effective in coping with these tumors, and an apparent discrepancy exists between in vitro and in vivo sensitivity to NK lysis. These data correspond to the finding that rIL-2 alone somewhat delayed tumor outgrowth, if given simultaneously with s.c. tumor cell inoculation, and had no effect at all on established tumors.

The combined data indicate that it would be very advantageous for Ad5 tumors to down-regulate class I MHC expression to evade the highly effective CTL response. Indeed, the lack of class I MHC down-regulation by Ad5 E1A might be one of the main reasons why Ad5 E1-transformed cells fail to grow out in immunocompetent animals. Compared to the CTL, NK cells appear to have little therapeutic activity against Ad5-transformed cells. Experiments with ^{35}S-labeled CTL 5 cells showed that the CTL specifically home to the tumor site later than about 24 hours following i.v. infusion. Before that time, only nonspecific localization in liver is seen. Ultrastructural studies carried out by P. Peters and H.J. Geuze (University of Utrecht) have indicated that Ad5-specific CTL actually pass the endothelium within the tumor and are found within areas of necrosis from day 2 of therapy onward. Ad5-specific CTL 5 have the ultrastructural appearance of large activated cells with many perforin containing lytic granules within the cytoplasm.

Identification of Ad E1A Peptide Recognized by D[b]-restricted CTL Clones

The results obtained so far show a remarkably efficient therapeutic effect obtained with a single dose of CTL and rIL-2 and associated with the existence of long-term CTL memory. To address the question whether an E1A peptide sequence itself was recognized in the context of H-2D[b] or a sequence of an unknown cellular protein induced by E1A, we tried to identify whether any of the E1A peptides synthesized by PEPSCAN was recognized. The E1A gene encodes three proteins of 6 kD, 27 kD, and 32 kD synthesized from 9S, 12S, and 13S mRNA species, respectively. The 27-kD and 32-kD proteins are the major proteins found in transformed cells, are identical except for an extra 46-amino-acid sequence present in the 32-kD protein,

and consist of 243 and 289 residues, respectively (van Ormondt and Galibert 1984). The 6-kD protein consists of 55 residues, 26 of which are shared with the 27-kD and 32-kD proteins (van Ormondt and Galibert 1984). The PEPSCAN analysis, originally developed to probe viral epitopes defined by antibodies (Geysen et al. 1984) and later used for the mapping of a T-cell epitope defined by a T-helper clone in proliferation assay (van der Zee et al. 1989), was adapted by us to map and characterize epitopes defined by CTL in collaboration with R.H. Meloen and co-workers at the Central Veterinary Institute in Lelystad. In this analysis, all possible 316 peptides of 12 residues with overlaps of 11 residues of the 3 Ad5 E1A proteins referred to were synthesized on solid supports as described previously (van der Zee et al. 1989). The peptides were detached with formic acid (van der Zee et al. 1989), and after desiccation, the resolubilized peptides were incubated with the target cells during the ^{51}Cr-release assay. The peptide recognized by D[b]-restricted Ad5 E1A-specific CTL 5 runs from position 232 to 247 of the E1A amino acid sequence and has the sequence CDSGPSNTPPEIHPVV (Kast et al. 1989). This sequence is not present in Ad12 E1A proteins. This explains the failure of Ad5 E1A-specific CTL to lyse Ad12 E1-transformed tumor cells, even if class I MHC expression on the latter cells is restored by IFN-γ. Further analysis showed that the 8-mer PSNTPPEI, constituting the core of the original 16-amino-acid sequence, is the smallest peptide optimally recognized by CTL clone 5 (Kast et al. 1989). All of 10 independently derived Ad5 E1A-specific CTL clones recognize the same peptide.

Primary Virus-induced Lymphomas Evade T-cell Immunity by Failure to Express Viral Antigens

Lymphoma induction by MLV results from a complex series of oncogenic events in virus-infected cells (Melief et al. 1986; Zijlstra and Melief 1986; Bishop 1987). The development of lymphomas is strongly influenced by the H-2 complex. This probably reflects the fact that virus-infected and virus-transformed cells do not grow out to overt lymphomas in the presence of H-2-restricted MLV-specific T-helper and CTL responses (for review, see Zijlstra and Melief 1986). T-cell immunosurveillance will fail, however, if tumor cells do not express the appropriate MHC molecule and/or viral peptide at the cell surface. Indeed, various so-called "virus-negative" variant murine lymphoma lines have been reported that are resistant against T-cell-mediated destruction. However, these lines arose under forced circumstances, such as long-term culture of tumor cells (Green 1983) or in vivo selection under exogenous CTL therapy (van der Hoorn et al. 1985). Class I MHC gene expression was found to exert an important influence on tumorigenesis and metastasis in studies with established cell lines (Eisenbach et al. 1984; Hui et al. 1984; Wallich et al. 1985).

Table 2. Viral Antigen and MHC Expression in Primary MCF 1233 MLV-induced T-cell Lymphomas of H-2 Nonresponder-type Mice: Nonresponder Lymphomas

Number of lymphomas per number tested	Viral antigen expression	MHC expression	
		class I	class II
15/17	+	+	−
2/17	+	−	−

Data summarized from Vasmel et al. (1989)

We therefore decided to conduct a systematic investigation of tumor selection mechanisms, involving viral antigen and MHC cell-surface expression, during primary lymphomagenesis by a mink cell focus-inducing isolate of MLV. We had shown previously that the H-2 complex strongly influences lymphoma incidence of neonatal infection of H-2 congenic C57BL mice with this virus (Vasmel et al. 1988). Resistance against early T lymphoma in this study is dominant, maps to the H-2 I-A region, and is associated with high levels of anti-MLV envelope antibodies. A high percentage (64%) of animals of susceptible (nonresponder) strains (H-2 I-$A^{k,d}$) developed T-cell lymphomas with a mean latency of 37 weeks. In responder strains (H-2 I-$A^{b,bm12,b/k}$), only 14% of the mice developed T lymphomas with a longer latency of 57 weeks (Vasmel et al. 1988).

We then asked ourselves how the latter lymphomas had escaped from the apparently strong I-A-mediated antiviral immune response. To this end, viral antigen and class I and II MHC expression were measured by cytofluorimetry with a panel of monoclonal and polyclonal antibodies on the cell surface of 11 rare T lymphomas from responder-type strains. As a control, cell-surface expression of viral antigens and MHC molecules was also measured on the surface of 17 randomly chosen T lymphomas from nonresponder strains. The anti-MLV antibodies included anti-*env* monoclonal antibodies reactive with the highly conserved $gp70^F$ epitope, the $p15E^c$ epitope, and the gp70/p15E complex, a polyclonal anti-p30 serum. This analysis showed that all 17 nonresponder tumors expressed high levels of both *env* and *gag* viral proteins, whereas 15 of these 17 tumors expressed high levels of H-2 class I, K, and D antigens (Table 2).

In contrast, 10 of 11 responder lymphomas lacked *env* and/or *gag* determinants (Table 3). The only responder lymphoma with both strong *env* and *gag* expression did not express H-2K and D antigens (Table

3). Multiple reintegrated proviruses were found in the DNA of both responder and nonresponder lymphomas (Vasmel et al. 1989). Low or absent viral antigen expression was confirmed at the cytoplasmic and RNA levels. Various molecular mechanisms appear to cause the reduced or absent viral antigen expression. Upon passage in nude mice, the viral antigen "low" phenotype was stable in some tumors, whereas other tumors showed reexpression of viral antigens (Vasmel et al. 1989).

In this latter category of tumors, the antiviral T-cell response appears to actively suppress viral antigen expression or select a minor component within the tumor cells lacking viral antigen expression. In this model, failure to express viral antigen is a more frequent cause of escape from surveillance than down-regulation of MHC expression.

In conclusion, the strong antiviral immune response in responder-type mice strongly reduces T-lymphoma incidence (Vasmel et al. 1988). The few T lymphomas that escape from this response have achieved this only by virtue of poor or absent viral antigen expression, or more rarely, down-regulation of class I MHC expression.

DISCUSSION AND GENERAL CONCLUSIONS

Class I MHC-restricted CTL are remarkably potent in eradication of murine tumors transformed by the E1 region of human Ad5. In H-2^b mice, these CTL are directed against a peptide encoded by the viral nuclear oncogene E1A. By serology, E1A proteins are not demonstrable at the cell surface. Thus, these results strengthen the notion that effective antitumor CTL responses can be directed against internal viral or cellular proteins (see also Boon et al., this volume). During primary lymphomagenesis by MLV, numerous escapes from immunosurveillance, largely due to failure

Table 3. Decreased Viral Antigen or MHC Expression in Primary MCF 1233 MLV-induced T-cell Lymphomas of H-2 Responder-type Mice: Responder T Lymphomas

Number of lymphomas per number tested	Viral antigen expression	MHC expression	
		class I	class II
9/11	± or −	+	−
1/11	+	−	−
1/11	(+)[a]	(+)[b]	−

Data summarized from Vasmel et al. (1989).
[a] Absence of p30 but not $gp70^F$ expression.
[b] Absence of K^b but not D^b expression.

of viral antigen expression, were noted. However, no escapes from treatment with cloned CTL were observed. Presumably, the time span available for escapes is too short under these conditions. Within 2 weeks, all Ad E1-induced tumors had completely regressed following CTL infusion combined with IL-2 administration.

These findings argue in favor of the hypothesis that viral oncogene-induced tumors can evade CTL-mediated destruction by decreasing their class I expression, as observed in Ad12 E1-transformed cells. On the other hand, in lymphomagenesis by MLV, failure to express viral antigens, rather than down-regulation of MHC expression, is the most frequent mechanism of escape from T-cell surveillance. Thus, depending on the system studied, either failure to express viral antigens or down-regulation of class I MHC expression allows evasion of T-cell surveillance.

Future efforts should nevertheless be directed at exploiting the remarkable potency of CTL in the therapy of human tumors, since under therapy with established cloned CTL, the possibility of escape from immune destruction may be remote because the cancer cells are taken by surprise in a massive and deadly assault.

ACKNOWLEDGMENTS

We thank A.C. Voordouw and C.J.M. Leupers for contributions to these studies. We also express our gratitude to Eurocetus B.V. for a generous gift of rIL-2.

REFERENCES

Ackrill, A.M. and G.E. Blair. 1988. Regulation of major histocompatibility class I gene expression at the level of transcription in highly oncogenic adenovirus transformed rat cells. *Oncogene* 3: 483.

Bernards, R. and A.J. van der Eb. 1984. Adenoviruses: Transformation and oncogenicity. *Biochim. Biophys. Acta* 783: 187.

Bernards, R., P.I. Schrier, A. Houweling, J.L. Bos, A.J. van der Eb, M. Zijlstra, and C.J.M. Melief. 1983. Tumorigenicity of cells transformed by adenovirus type 12 by evasion of T-cell immunity. *Nature* 305: 776.

Bishop, M. 1987. The molecular genetics of cancer. *Science* 235: 305.

Branton, P.E., S.T. Bayley, and F.N. Graham. 1985. Transformation by human adenoviruses. *Biochim. Biophys. Acta* 780: 67.

Clark, E.A., L.D. Shultz, and S.B. Pollack. 1981. Mutations in mice that influence NK activity. *Immunogenetics* 12: 601.

Cook, J.L. and A.M. Lewis. 1987. Immunological surveillance against DNA virus-transformed cells: Correlations between NK cytolytic competence and tumor susceptibility of athymic rodents. *J. Virol.* 61: 2155.

Cook, J.L., D.L. May, A.M. Lewis, and T.A. Walker. 1987. Transformation by human adenoviruses. *J. Virol.* 61: 3510.

DeCaprio, J.A., J.W. Ludlow, J. Figge, J.Y. Shew, C.-M. Huang, W.-H. Lee, E. Marsilio, E. Paucha, and D.M. Livingston. 1988. SV40 large tumor antigen forms a specific complex with the product of the retinoblastoma susceptibility gene. *Cell* 54: 275.

Doherty, P.C. 1985. T cells and viral infections. *Br. Med. Bull.* 41: 7.

Eager, K.B., K. Pfizenmaier, and R.P. Ricciardi. 1989. Modulation of major histocompatibility complex (MHC) class I genes in adenovirus 12 transformed cells: Interferon-γ increases class I expression by a mechanism that circumvents E1A induced-repression and tumor necrosis factor enhances the effect of interferon-γ. *Oncogene* 4: 39.

Eager, K.B., J. Williams, D. Breiding, S. Pan, B. Knowles, E. Appella, and R.P. Ricciardi. 1985. Expression of histocompatibility antigens H-2K, -D, and -L is reduced in adenovirus-12-transformed mouse cells and is restored by interferon-γ. *Proc. Natl. Acad. Sci.* 82: 5525.

Eisenbach, L., N. Hollander, L. Greenfeld, H. Yakor, S. Segal, and M. Feldman. 1984. The differential expression of H-2K versus H-2D antigens, distinguishing high-metastatic from low-metastatic clones, is correlated with the immunogenic properties of the tumor cells. *Int. J. Cancer* 34: 567.

Friedman, D.J. and R.P. Ricciardi. 1988. Adenovirus type 12 E1A gene represses accumulation of MHC class I mRNAs at the level of transcription. *Virology* 165: 303.

Geysen, M.H., R.H. Meloen, and S.J. Barteling. 1984. Use of peptide synthesis to prove viral antigens for epitopes to a resolution of a single amino acid. *Proc. Natl. Acad. Sci.* 81: 3998.

Green, W.R. 1983. The specificity of H-2 restricted cytotoxic T lymphocytes directed to AKR/Gross leukemia virus-induced tumors. I. Isolation of a selectively resistant variant tumor subclone. *Eur. J. Immunol.* 13: 863.

Harel-Bellan, A., A. Quillet, C. Marchiol, R. De Mars, T. Tursz, and D. Fraddizi. 1986. Natural killer susceptibility of human cells may be regulated by genes in the HLA region on chromosome 6. *Proc. Natl. Acad. Sci.* 83: 5688.

Hayashi, H., K. Tanaka, F. Jay, G. Khoury, and G. Jay. 1985. Modulation of the tumorigenicity of human adenovirus-12-transformed cells by interferon. *Cell* 43: 263.

Hui, K.H., F. Grosveld, and H. Festenstein. 1984. Rejection of transplantable AKR-leukemia cells following MHC DNA-mediated cell transformation. *Nature* 311: 750.

Kast, W.M., A.M. Bronkhorst, L.P. De Waal, and C.J.M. Melief. 1986. Cooperation between cytotoxic and helper T lymphocytes in protection against lethal Sendai virus infection. Protection by T cells is MHC-restricted and MHC-regulated: A model for MHC-disease associations. *J. Exp. Med.* 164: 723.

Kast, W.M., R. Offringa, P.J. Peters, A.C. Voordouw, R.H. Meloen, A.J. van der Eb, and C.J.M. Melief. 1989. Eradication of adenovirus E1-induced tumors by E1A specific cytotoxic T lymphocytes. *Cell* (in press).

Kärre, K., H.G. Ljunggren, G. Piontek, and R. Kiessling. 1986. Selective rejection of H-2 deficient lymphoma variants suggests alternative immune defence strategy. *Nature* 319: 675.

Kenyon, D.J. and K. Raska. 1986. Region E1A of highly oncogenic adenovirus 12 in transformed cells protects against NK but not LAk cytolysis. *Virology* 155: 644.

Klein, G. 1973. Tumor immunology. *Transplant. Proc.* 5: 31.

Kingston, R.E., A.S. Baldwin, and P.S. Sharp. 1984. Regulation of heat shock protein 70 expression by c-*myc*. *Nature* 312: 280.

Land, H., L.F. Parada, and R.A. Weinberg. 1983. Tumorigenic conversion of primary embryo cells requires at least two cooperating oncogenes. *Nature* 304: 596.

Leiden, J.M., B.A. Karpinski, L. Gottschalk, and J. Kornbluth. 1989. Susceptibility to NK cell-mediated cytolysis is independent of target cell class I HLA expression. *J. Immunol.* 142: 2140.

Ljunggren, H.G. and K. Kärre. 1985. Host resistance directed selectively against H-2-deficient lymphoma variants. *J. Exp. Med.* 162: 1745.

Ljunggren, H.G., C. Öhler, P. Höglund, T. Yamasaki, G. Klein, and K. Kärre. 1988. Afferent and efferent cellular interactions in natural resistance directed against MHC class I deficient tumor grafts. *J. Immunol.* 140: 671.

Melief, C.J.M., M. Zijlstra, W.L.E. Vasmel, E.A. Matthews, R.M. Slater, and A. Berns. 1986. Mechanisms of lymphoma induction by retroviruses. *Prog. Immunol.* **6**: 664.

Moran, E. 1988. A region of SV40 large T antigen can substitute for a transforming domain of the adenovirus E1A products. *Nature* **334**: 168.

Murray, M.J., J.M. Cunningham, L.F. Parada, F. Dautry, P. Lebowitz, and R.A. Weinberg. 1983. The HL-60 transforming sequence: A *ras* oncogene coexisting with altered *myc* genes in hematopoietic tumors. *Cell* **33**: 749.

Phelps, W.C., C.L. Yee, K. Münger, and P.M. Howley. 1988. The human papillomavirus type 16 E7 gene encodes transactivation and transformation and transformation functions similar to those of adenovirus E1A. *Cell* **53**: 539.

Piontek, G.E., K. Taniguchi, H.G. Ljunggren, A. Grönberg, R. Kiessling, G. Klein, and K. Kärre. 1985. YAC-1 MHC class I variants reveal an association between decreased NK sensitivity and increased H-2 expression after interferon treatment of in vivo passage. *J. Immunol.* **135**: 4281.

Quillet, A., F. Presse, C. Marchiol-Fournigault, A. Harel-Bellan, M. Benbijnan, H. Ploegh, and D. Fradelize. 1988. Increased resistance to non-MHC-restricted cytotoxicity related to HLA A, B expression: Direct demonstration using β2-microglobulin-transfected Daudi cells. *J. Immunol.* **141**: 17.

Ruley, H.E. 1983. Adenovirus early region 1A enables viral and cellular transforming genes to transform primary cells in culture. *Nature* **304**: 602.

Sawada, Y., B. Föhring, T.E. Shenk, and K. Raska. 1985. Tumorigenicity of adenovirus-transformed cells: Region E1A of adenovirus 12 confers resistance to natural killer cells. *Virology* **147**: 413.

Schrier, P.I., R. Bernards, R.T.M.J. Vaessen, A. Houweling, and A.J. van der Eb. 1983. Expression of class I major histocompatibility antigens switched off by highly oncogenic adenovirus 12 in transformed rat cells. *Nature* **305**: 771.

Stam, N.J., W.M. Kast, A.C. Voordouw, E.B. Pastoors, F.A. van der Hoeven, C.J.M. Melief, and H.L. Ploegh. 1989. Lack of correlation between levels of MHC class I antigen and susceptibility to lysis of small cellular lung carcinoma (SCLC) by natural killer cells. *J. Immunol.* **142**: 4113.

Storkus, W.J., D.N. Howell, R.D. Salter, J.R. Dawson, and P. Cresswell. 1987. NK susceptibility varies inversely with target cell class I HLA antigen expression. *J. Immunol.* **138**: 1657.

Tanaka, K., K.J. Isselbacher, G. Khoury, and G. Jay. 1985. Oncogenesis by the expression of a major histocompatibility complex class I gene. *Science* **228**: 26.

van der Eb, A.J. and B.A. Oostra. 1985. Expression of class I major histocompatibility antigens in adenovirus transformed cells. In *Adenoviruses* (ed. W. Doerfler), vol. 10, p. 343. Martinus Nijhoff, Boston.

van der Eb, A.J., R. Bernards, P.I. Schrier, J.L. Bos, R.T. Vaessen, A.G. Jochemsen, C.J.M. Melief. 1984. Altered expression of cellular genes in adenovirus transformed cells. *Cancer Cells* **2**: 501.

van der Hoorn, F., T. Lahaye, V. Müller, M.A. Ogle, and H.D. Engers. 1985. Characterization of gP85^gag as an antigen recognized by Moloney leukemia virus-specific cytolytic T cell clones that function in vivo. *J. Exp. Med.* **162**: 128.

van der Zee, R., W. Van Eden, R.H. Meloen, A. Noordzij, and J.D.A. Van Embden. 1989. Efficient mapping and characterization of a T cell epitope by the simultaneous synthesis of multiple peptides. *Eur. J. Immunol.* **19**: 43.

Van Ormondt, H. and F. Galibert. 1984. Nucleotide sequences of adenovirus DNAs. *Curr. Top. Microbiol. Immunol.* **110**: 75.

Vasmel, W.L.E., E.J.A.M. Sijts, C.J.M. Leupers, E.A. Matthews, and C.J.M. Melief. 1989. Primary virus-induced lymphomas evade T cell immunity by failure to express viral antigens. *J. Exp. Med.* **169**: 1233.

Vasmel, W.L.E., M. Zijlstra, T. Radaszkiewicz, C.J.M. Leupers, R.E.Y. De Goede, and C.J.M. Melief. 1988. Major histocompatibility complex class II-regulated immunity to murine leukemia virus protects against early T- but not late B-cell lymphomas. *J. Virol.* **62**: 3156.

Wallich, R., N. Bulbue, G.J. Hämmerling, S. Katzav, S. Segal, and M. Feldman. 1985. Abrogation of metastatic properties of tumour cells by de novo expression of H-2K antigens following H-2 gene transfection. *Nature* **315**: 301.

Whyte, P., K.J. Buchkovich, J.M. Horowitz, S.H. Friend, M. Raybuck, R.A. Weinberg, and E. Harlow. 1988. Association between an oncogene and an anti-oncogene: The adenovirus E1A proteins bind to the retinoblastoma gene product. *Nature* **334**: 124.

Zijlstra, M. and C.J.M. Melief. 1986. Virology, genetics and immunology of murine lymphomagenesis. *Biochim. Biophys. Acta* **865**: 197.

Zinkernagel, R.M. and P.C. Doherty. 1979. MHC restricted cytotoxic T-cells, studies on the biological role of polymorphic major transplantation antigens determining T-cell restriction-specificity, function and responsiveness. *Adv. Immunol.* **27**: 51.

zur Hausen, H. and A. Schneider. 1987. The role of papillomaviruses in human anogenital cancer. In *The papovaviridae: The papillomaviruses* (ed. P.M. Howley and N. Salzman), p. 245. Plenum Press, New York.